Biomaterials and Regenerative Medicine

Written by world-leading experts, this book focuses on the role of biomaterials in stem cell research and regenerative medicine. Emphasizing basic principles and methodology, it covers stem cell interactions, fabrication technologies, design principles, physical characterization, and biological evaluation, across a broad variety of systems and biomaterials. Topics include:

- Stem cell biology, including embryonic stem cells, iPS cells, HSCs, and progenitor cells
- Modern scaffold structures, including biopolymer, bioceramic, micro- and nanofiber, ECM and biohydrogel
- Advanced fabrication technologies, including computer-aided tissue engineering and organ printing
- Cutting-edge drug delivery systems and gene therapy techniques
- Medical applications spanning hard and soft tissues, the cardiovascular system, and organ regeneration

With a contribution by Nobel laureate Shinya Yamanaka, this is a must-have reference for anyone in the field of biomaterials, stem cell biology and engineering, tissue engineering and regenerative medicine.

Peter X. Ma is the Richard H. Kingery Endowed Collegiate Professor at the University of Michigan. A recent winner of the Clemson Award (2013) from the Society of Biomaterials and a Distinguished Scientist Award (Isaac Schour Memorial Award 2013) from the International Association for Dental Research, he is a Fellow of the American Institute for Medical and Biological Engineering (AIMBE), a Fellow of the International Union of Societies for Biomaterials Science and Engineering (IUSBSE), and a Fellow of the American Association for the Advancement of Science.

"The field of regenerative medicine is changing medical practice, and the opportunities for the future are immense. This text describes the many ways that biomaterials are critically important in the field: biomaterials can serve as scaffolds to guide tissue remodeling, as matrices that signal cells to grow or differentiate, and as reservoirs for the slow release of paracrine signals.

"Professor Ma, an internationally known materials scientist, leads an impressive collection of experts in documenting the state of the art in biomaterials design and synthesis for regenerative medicine."

W. Mark Saltzman
Yale University

Biomaterials and Regenerative Medicine

Edited by

Peter X. Ma

University of Michigan

CAMBRIDGE
UNIVERSITY PRESS

CAMBRIDGE
UNIVERSITY PRESS

University Printing House, Cambridge CB2 8BS, United Kingdom

Cambridge University Press is part of the University of Cambridge.

It furthers the University's mission by disseminating knowledge in the pursuit of education, learning and research at the highest international levels of excellence.

www.cambridge.org
Information on this title: www.cambridge.org/9781107012097

First published 2014

Printed in the United Kingdom by Clays, St Ives plc

A catalog record for this publication is available from the British Library

Library of Congress Cataloging in Publication data
Biomaterials and regenerative medicine / [edited by] Peter X. Ma.
p. ; cm.
Includes bibliographical references.
ISBN 978-1-107-01209-7 (Hardback)
I. Ma, Peter X., editor of compilation.
[DNLM: 1. Biocompatible Materials. 2. Tissue Engineering–methods. 3. Regenerative Medicine–methods. 4. Stem Cells–cytology. 5. Tissue Scaffolds. QT 37]
R857.M3
610.28–dc23 2013038000

ISBN 978-1-107-01209-7 Hardback

Contents

Contributors

Vineet Agrawal
University of Pittsburgh

Pedro Alvarez
Carnegie Mellon University

Anthony Atala
The Wake Forest Institute for Regenerative Medicine

Stephen F. Badylak
University of Pittsburgh

Hojae Bae
Harvard Medical School

Vince Beachley
Johns Hopkins University

Mohammod Bhuyan
University of Texas at El Paso

Thomas Boland
University of Texas at El Paso

Gulden Camci-Unal
Harvard Medical School

Yilin Cao
Shanghai Jiao Tong University School of Medicine

Xanthippi Chatzistavrou
University of Michigan

Mo Chen
Columbia University Medical Center

Y. Eugene Chen
University of Michigan

Loraine L. Y. Chiu
University of Toronto

Shoko Cho
Columbia University Medical Center

Fu-zhai Cui
Tsinghua University

Sashka Dimitrievska
Yale University

Ziming Dong
Zhengzhou University

Amy Donovan
Carnegie Mellon University

Jennifer H. Elisseeff
The Johns Hopkins University

Mildred Embree
Columbia University Medical Center

Megan J. Farrell
University of Pennsylvania

Kai Feng
University of Michigan

William V. Giannobile
University of Michigan

Erin D. Grassl
Medtronic Inc.

Robert E. Guldberg
Georgia Institute of Technology

Melanie J. Gupte
University of Michigan

Jeffrey Mark Halpern
Case Western Reserve University

Qudus Hamid
Drexel University

Jesper Hjortnaes
Harvard Medical School

Kelan Hlavaty
Northwestern University

Jeffrey O. Hollinger
Carnegie Mellon University

Jeremy M. Holzwarth
University of Michigan

Akitsu Hotta
Kyoto University

Eric W. Hsu
Carnegie Mellon University

Jiang Hu
University of Michigan

Chang Hun Lee
Columbia University Medical Center

Mayumi Ito
New York University

Nan Jiang
Columbia University Medical Center

Xiaobing Jin
University of Michigan

F. Kurtis Kasper
Rice University

Ali Khademhosseini
Harvard Medical School

Nora T. Khanarian
Columbia University

Kyobum Kim
Rice University

Kimi Kong
Columbia University Medical Center

Johnny Lam
Rice University

Nancy M. Lee
Columbia University

Xiaoming Li
Beihang University

Linheng Li
Stowers Institute for Medical Research

Mon-Tzu A. Li
Georgia Institute of Technology

Chien-Chi Lin
Indiana University-Purdue University Indianapolis

Wei Liu
Shanghai Jiao Tong University School of Medicine

Shiguang Liu
Carnegie Mellon University

Steven Lu
Rice University

Helen H. Lu
Columbia University

Peter X. Ma
University of Michigan

David Mack
University of Washington

Jeremy J. Mao
Columbia University Medical Center

Robert L. Mauck
University of Pennsylvania

Geeta Mehta
University of Michigan

Avital Mendelson
Columbia University Medical Center

Antonios G. Mikos
Rice University

Zubad Newaz
University of Michigan

Hemin Nie
Columbia University Medical Center

Laura E. Niklason
Yale University

Petros Papagerakis
University of Michigan

Milica Radisic
University of Toronto

Horst A. von Recum
Case Western Reserve University

Mehmet Remzi Dokmeci
Harvard Medical School

Daniel Reyna-Soriano
University of Texas at El Paso

Pamela Gehron Robey
National Institutes of Health

Jorge I. Rodríguez-Dévora
University of Texas at El Paso

Edward A. Sander
University of Iowa

Stephanie K. Seidlits
Northwestern University

Bhranti Shah
Columbia University Medical Center

Lonnie D. Shea
Northwestern University

Yusuke Shiozawa
University of Michigan

Arun R. Shivats
Carnegie Mellon University

Lyndsey Shutte
Carnegie Mellon University

Jacob A. Simson
The Johns Hopkins University

Aleksander Skardal
The Wake Forest Institute for Regenerative Medicine

Nicole Slawny
University of Michigan

Gary D. Smith
University of Michigan

Ian O. Smith
University of Michigan

Jessica Snyder
Drexel University

Shay Soker
The Wake Forest Institute for Regenerative Medicine

Marissa R. Solomon
Columbia University

Wei Sun
Drexel University & Tsinghua University

Takahiro Suzuki
Columbia University Medical Center

Russell Taichman
University of Michigan

Makoto Takeo
New York University

Andrei D. Taut
University of Michigan

Robert T. Tranquillo
University of Minnesota

Brent A. Uhrig
Georgia Institute of Technology

Aparna Venkatraman
Stowers Institute for Medical Research

Chengyang Wang
Drexel University

Jing Wang
University of Michigan

Zhe Wang
Sichuan University

Xuejun Wen
Virginia Commonwealth University

Nick J. Willett
Georgia Institute of Technology

Zhanwen Xiao
Sichuan University

Yun Xiao
University of Toronto

Changqing Xie
University of Michigan

Tao Xu
University of Texas at El Paso

Shinya Yamanaka
Kyoto University

Bangcheng Yang
Sichuan University

Rujing Yang
Columbia University Medical Center

Bo Yang
University of Michigan

Pamela C. Yelick
Tufts University

Zhanpeng Zhang
University of Michigan

Xingdong Zhang
Sichuan University

Yuanyuan Zhang
The Wake Forest Institute for Regenerative Medicine

Weibo Zhang
Tufts University

Boyang Zhang
University of Toronto

Meng Zhao
Stowers Institute for Medical Research

Preface

Regenerative medicine aims to regenerate tissues and organs for medical therapies by harnessing the regenerative potentials of various stem cells. Stem cells include embryonic stem cells, multipotent adult stem cells, tissue specific stem cells, and induced pluripotent stem cells. These stem cells are the driving force for regeneration. There is a growing recognition of the effect of the three-dimensional (3D) matrix microenvironment on the fate and function of stem cells. A key challenge facing regenerative medicine is to generate 3D microenvironments (matrix, signals, supporting cells etc.) that can recapitulate those in development or healing to maintain stemness, to accelerate proliferation, or to direct the stem cells to differentiate toward a specific therapeutic lineage. Biomaterials can serve as 3D matrices; they can play critical roles in creating the 3D microenvironments for stem cells to facilitate regeneration. As the interactions and the overlap of the fields of biomaterials, stem cells, and regenerative medicine are rapidly growing, there is an urgent need for understanding of, and technologies to utilize, the interactions between biomaterials and stem cells for regenerative medicine.

This book, *Biomaterials and Regenerative Medicine*, overviews the state-of-the-art knowledge on stem cells, interactions of biomaterials with stem cells, biomaterials design for regenerative medicine, and the animal models and clinical applications of biomaterials for regeneration. While providing a comprehensive overview of the field, the emphasis is on the design principles, fabrication technologies, physical characterization, and biological evaluation of the biomaterials for stem cell research and regenerative medicine.

The book aims to serve as a textbook for senior undergraduate students and graduate students in the fields of biomaterials, stem cell biology, regenerative medicine, tissue engineering, controlled release, biomedical engineering, biomedical sciences, life sciences, and surgery. This book is also intended to serve as a reference book for researchers, scientists, engineers, and medical doctors who are involved in biomaterials, stem cells, and regenerative medicine.

Considering the strong interdisciplinary and multidisciplinary nature of the topics covered in this book, I had to invite experts from various disciplines to participate in this project. I am extremely grateful to all the contributors, who are the authorities of their disciplines, including a Nobel laureate in Physiology or Medicine (Dr. Shinya Yamanaka), for their time and efforts in making this a high-quality book.

I would like to express my appreciation of two extremely capable assistants for me on this project, Mss. Deborah Keedy and Elizabeth Rodriguez, for tracking the progress of each chapter, and communicating with the authors, reviewers, and publisher on a daily basis. I also enjoyed the professional interactions with the editorial staff at Cambridge University Press during the entire process. Finally, I would like to express my gratitude to my family (Chaoying, Judy, Jane, and Leon) for their understanding and support for this very exciting and laborious project.

Peter X. Ma, PhD
Richard H. Kingery Endowed Collegiate Professor
Department of Biologic and Materials Sciences
Department of Biomedical Engineering
Macromolecular Science and Engineering Center
Department of Materials Science and Engineering
The University of Michigan
Ann Arbor, MI, USA

PART I

Introduction to stem cells and regenerative medicine

1

Embryonic stem cells

Nicole Slawny and Gary D. Smith

1.1 Preimplantation embryo development sets the stage for pluripotency

Regenerative medicine has the potential to revolutionize health care by offering the promise of replacement cells, tissues, and organs to combat injury, disease, and aging. In an ideal setting, stem cell therapies would begin with a pluripotent cell that by definition is able to give rise to any cell formed in the embryo. Additionally this would most likely require that the stem cells could self-renew or were able to divide and give rise to either more pluripotent stem cells or progressively more differentiated cells under the control of extrinsic cues. Stem cells are biological cells found in multicellular organisms, that can mitotically divide and differentiate into specialized cell types and can self-renew to produce more stem cells. There are two broad types of stem cells: embryonic stem cells and adult stem cells. Embryonic stem cells originate from the inner cell mass of the preimplantation embryo and are considered pluripotent whereas *in situ* adult stem cells are considered multipotent. Embryonic stem cells (ESCs) possess characteristics that make them a potentially outstanding starting material for use in regenerative medicine. They are unique among cultured cells because they have an apparently limitless capacity to self-renew in vitro, as well as being pluripotent. Because of these extraordinary properties, ESCs have been an intense focus of research for more than 30 years.

In order to fully understand the basic properties of ESCs and how they are generated, it is important to consider the events of embryonic development that surround the timing of their formation. The events and molecular signaling required for embryonic development have been explored to a large extent using the laboratory mouse as a model system due to there being very limited material for experimentation and the inherent moral complexities of studies utilizing human embryos (Vassena *et al.*, 2011; Cockburn and Rossant, 2010). Therefore early mouse development will be used to illustrate the events critical to generating pluripotency in ESCs and other cells. While some developmental events are certainly conserved among all mammalian species, other aspects of rodent embryologic development beyond the scope of this chapter have made their ESCs unique and more amenable for use as a model system (Brons *et al.*, 2007; Tesar *et al.*, 2007; Nichols and Smith, 2009; Rossant, 2008). A more complete understanding of these species-specific differences may be important if hESCs are to be utilized to their fullest potential to improve human health.

Following fertilization of the egg by sperm the preimplantation embryo undergoes a series of cell divisions that generate smaller cells known as blastomeres (Figure 1.1).

Early cleavage divisions result in an eight-cell embryo when compaction or an increase in intracellular adhesion is initiated, an event believed to create the first molecular differences in polarity between blastomeres. Continued cell divisions give rise to a 32-cell morula where the first cell-fate choice occurs in the embryo. Cells on the outside differentiate into trophectoderm that gives rise to part of the placenta, while cells on the inside become the inner cell mass. The specification of trophectoderm versus inner cell mass occurs

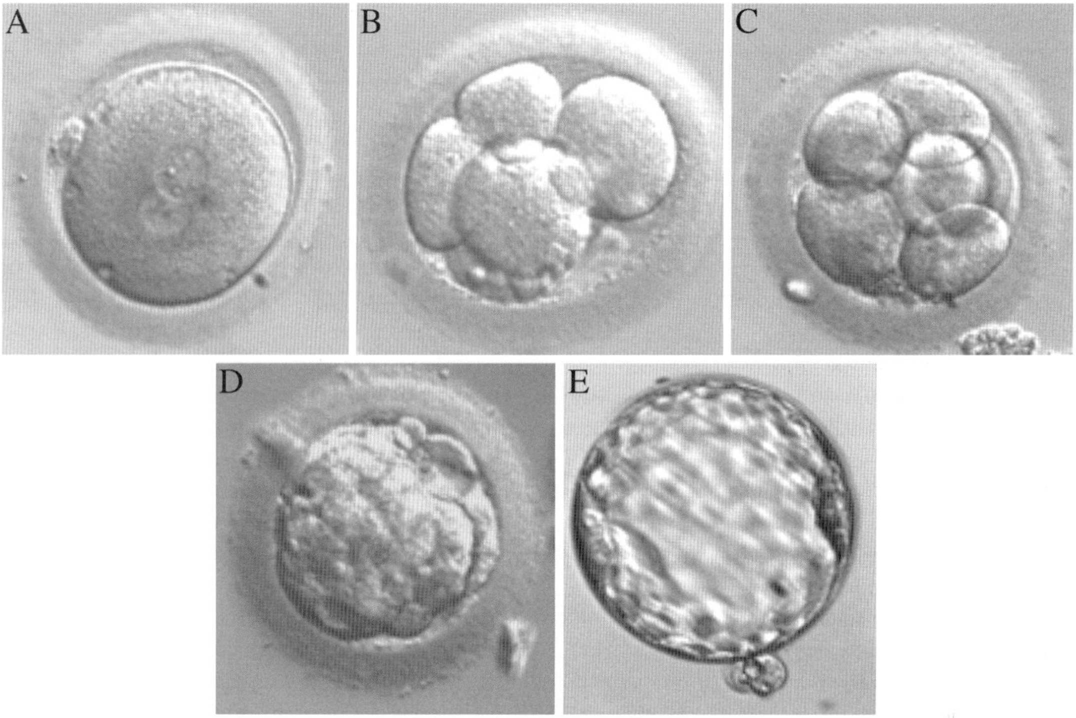

Figure 1.1 Cleavage- and blastocyst-stage human embryos. It is important to note that preimplantation mouse and human embryo development are extremely similar in morphological characteristics. A. Pronuclear stage embryo immediately following fertilization. The haploid nuclei of both the sperm and the egg are clearly visible. B. Four-cell embryo cultured for two days. C. Eight-cell embryo cultured for three days. D. Morula-stage embryo illustrating compaction of blastomeres cultured for four days. E. Human blastocyst, the stage at which the inner cell mass is removed to culture human embryonic stem cells (culture day six). All images kindly provided by Sandra Mojica, Gary Smith, and the University of Michigan Taubman Consortium for Stem Cell Therapies.

via a combination of asymmetrical/symmetrical cell divisions, cell polarity, and differential gene expression, the control of which is still debated (Arnold and Robertson, 2009; Rossant and Tam, 2009; Zernicka-Goetz *et al.*, 2009). The maintenance of the inner cell mass requires the formation of a blastocoel, a fluid-filled cavity in the center of the embryo now called a blastocyst: the stage from which ESCs are frequently derived.

Lineage allocation in the preimplantation mouse embryo continues with the segregation of blastocyst inner cell mass into the epiblast, which differentiates into the embryo proper, and subjacent primitive endoderm, which gives rise to extra-embryonic tissues that play key roles in further directing embryo development. It was initially supposed that inner-cell-mass cells were uniform and assumed different cell fates based on undefined positional cues (Dziadek, 1979). More recently it was demonstrated that, prior to differentiation, cells of the inner cell mass express either Nanog (epiblast marker) or Gata6 (primitive endoderm marker) in a "salt and pepper" pattern, indicating that the inner cell mass is not a homogeneous population (Chazaud *et al.*, 2006). The model proposed on the basis of this work suggested that expression of Nanog versus Gata6 controlled the expression of different cell-surface adhesion molecules, allowing the cells to physically sort into two distinct populations. Recently, it has been shown that up-regulation of fibroblast growth factor (FGF)/mitogen-activated protein kinase (MAPK) signaling in the inner cell mass converts the entire population to primitive endoderm cells, whereas blocking FGF/MAPK converts the entire population to epiblast cells (Yamanaka *et al.*, 2010). Cells within the inner cell mass express FGF4 (Nichols *et al.*, 1998; Yuan *et al.*, 1995) and the FGF4-null mouse completely lacks primitive endoderm development (Feldman *et al.*, 1995), suggesting that signaling within the inner cell mass promotes primitive endoderm fate (Yamanaka *et al.*, 2010). While a type of pluripotent stem cell can still be generated from the epithelized epiblast even after embryo implantation, differentiation of Gata6-expressing primitive endoderm has been shown to be inhibitory to the derivation of ESCs from the blastocyst (Brook and Gardner, 1997).

While they are not fully specified until after embryo implantation, primordial germ cells are embryonic precursors that differentiate into sex-specific gametes that come together to generate the pluripotent embryo of the next generation. Extra-embryonic tissues secrete bone morphogenic proteins that signal to roughly six cells in the adjacent epiblast to differentiate into primordial germ cells (Tam and Snow, 1981, Ohinata *et al.*, 2005; Ying *et al.*, 2001; Ying and Zhao, 2001). Thus, primordial germ cells begin to express germ-line-specific transcription factors, undergo rapid mitotic cell division, and migrate into the genital ridges between 10 and 13 days *post coitum* (dpc) (Godin *et al.*, 1990; Gomperts *et al.*, 1994; Molyneaux *et al.*, 2001). Once in the genital ridges, inherited epigenetic imprinting marks, for example X chromosome inactivation, are erased and sex-specific differentiation of gametes determines the timing and specificity of remethylation (Lucifero *et al.*, 2002, 2004; Davis *et al.*, 1999, 2000). These two embryonic populations of cells, inner cell mass and primordial germ cells, were the starting material from which the entire scientific investigation of pluripotent stem cells began.

1.2 A brief history of pluripotent cells

Pioneering work analyzing teratocarcinomas, malignant tumors now known to be initiated by embryonic germ cells, demonstrated that these tumors contained poorly organized somatic cells derived from all three embryonic germ layers, namely ectoderm, endoderm, and mesoderm, in addition to harboring a stem cell component (Kleinsmith and Pierce, 1964). Embryonic carcinoma stem cells (Figure 1.2) provided the first tissue culture system of pluripotency and differentiation used to model embryologic development (Kahan and Ephrussi, 1970; Rosenthal *et al.*, 1970). Defining requirements for culturing embryonic carcinoma stem cells (Martin and Evans, 1974, 1975) and maintaining their pluripotency paved the way for the first derivations of mouse (mESCs) and later human (hESCs) embryonic stem cells (Figure 1.2) from the inner cell mass of preimplantation blastocysts (Evans and Kaufman, 1981; Martin, 1981; Thomson *et al.*, 1998; Reubinoff *et al.*, 2000). Even more striking experiments demonstrated that embryonic carcinoma stem cells injected into mouse blastocysts could form not only tumors (Rossant and McBurney, 1982) but also normal cells in chimeric mice derived from both the recipient blastocyst and the injected embryonic carcinoma stem cells (Mintz and Illmensee, 1975; Papaioannou *et al.*, 1975; Illmensee and Mintz, 1976). The ability of cells injected into the blastocyst to contribute to all tissues of the resulting mouse embryo is currently one of the more stringent tests used to demonstrate pluripotency (Jaenisch and Young, 2008; Kuijk *et al.*, 2011). While embryonic carcinoma cells have historical importance, it is relevant to note that they likely have little relevance for regenerative medicine.

Teratocarcinomas arise at high frequency in the 129 mouse strain (Stevens and Little, 1954), but also can be induced to form in other mouse strains by transplanting either 7-dpc mouse embryos (Solter *et al.*, 1970) or genital ridges from 12.5-dpc embryos (Stevens, 1967) into ectopic sites such as under the kidney capsule or into the testis. Recall that at 12.5 dpc the genital ridges contain primordial germ cells (Ewen and Koopman, 2010; Saga, 2008). Given that they can drive teratocarcinoma formation, it is not surprising that pluripotent embryonic germ cell lines have been derived from mouse and human primordial germ cells that closely resemble ESCs (Resnick *et al.*, 1992; Matsui *et al.*, 1992; Durcova-Hills *et al.*, 2001; Shamblott *et al.*, 1998).

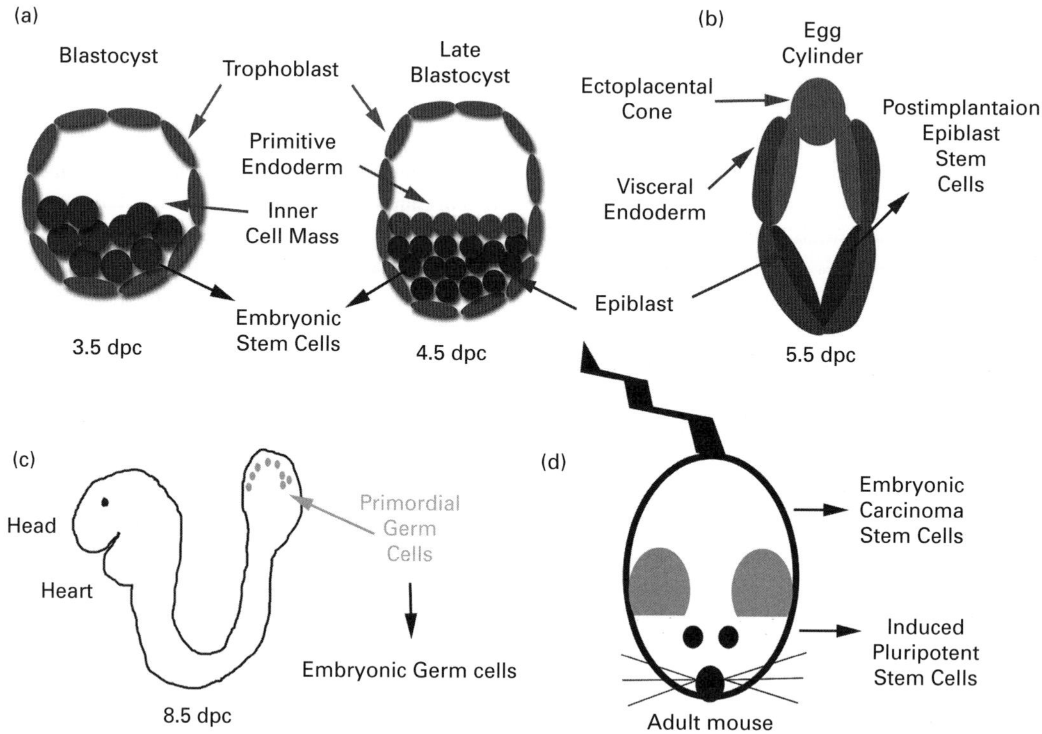

Figure 1.2 Embryonic stages of mouse stem cell derivation. (a) Embryonic stem cells can be derived from the inner cell mass of the blastocyst or from the preimplantation epiblast in the late blastocyst. (b) Postimplantation epiblast stem cells are derived from the epiblast of the egg cylinder stage. The ectoplacental cone is an extra-embryonic structure that forms a portion of the placenta. (c) Embryonic germ cell lines are derived from primordial germ cells harvested from the 8.5 dpc mouse embryo. (d) Embryonic carcinoma stem cell lines are derived from teratocarcinomas in adult mice. Induced pluripotency cells can be derived from nearly any somatic cell in the adult mouse.

More recently, pluripotent stem cells have been derived from perhaps unforeseen sources (Figure 1.2), for instance from the postimplantation mouse epiblast (Tesar *et al.*, 2007; Brons *et al.*, 2007). While postimplantation epiblast stem cells can differentiate into cells of all three germ layers in vitro and generate teratomas (benign tumors derived from embryonic germ cells or injected pluripotent stem cells containing all three germ layers when injected into immunocompromised mice) they are unable to contribute to chimeras, suggesting that there are some important functional differences from mESCs (Tesar *et al.*, 2007; Brons *et al.*, 2007). Even more unexpected was the demonstration that terminally differentiated cells such as fibroblasts could be induced to form pluripotent stem cells by the expression of only four factors, namely Oct3/4, Sox2, c-Myc, and Klf4 (Takahashi and Yamanaka, 2006; Okita *et al.*, 2007). Induced pluripotent stem cells (Figure 1.2) are morphologically and functionally similar to mESCs and can generate teratomas as well as contribute cells to chimeras when injected into the blastocyst. By comparing the properties and developmental potential of all of these pluripotent stem cells one can begin to draw conclusions about the origin of ESCs and how to improve their production and control their differentiation for use in regenerative medicine. It is also important to recognize that ESCs are pluripotent (can give rise to all endoderm, mesoderm, and ectoderm cells) as well as being able to colonize the germline and contribute to germ cells.

1.3 Properties and origins of pluripotent stem cells

The pluripotency of ESCs is controlled at multiple levels, including a poised chromatin state with a large transcriptome, a core set of transcription factors that inhibit differentiation, a unique cell cycle that promotes proliferation and inhibits differentiation and extracellular signaling molecules that stimulate or inhibit key signal transduction pathways. The chromatin in ESC DNA tends to have an abundance of trimethylation of Lysine 4 of histone H3 (H3K4) and acetylation of histone 4 (H4Ac) that generally marks areas of open chromatin with concomitant gene activity (Azuara *et al.*, 2006). The large regions of open chromatin result in widespread gene expression, but expression is at low levels, leading to the suggestion that ESC are "primed" to differentiate (Efroni *et al.*, 2008). While histone marks associated gene inactivation, such as trimethylation of Lysine 27 of histone H3 (H3K27) are more rare, they are concentrated on promoters of lineage specific genes (Azuara *et al.*, 2006; Bernstein *et al.*, 2006). These promoter regions are also the targets of repression by the core transcription factors Oct3/4, Sox2, and Nanog discussed in detail below (Boyer *et al.*, 2005). Regions of DNA marked with both closed (H3K27) and open (H3K4) chromatin histone marks are considered bivalent and thought to represent the pluripotent state, creating the unique situation in which ESCs are poised for differentiation yet held in an undifferentiated state (Azuara *et al.*, 2006; Bernstein *et al.*, 2006).

Three core transcription factors maintain the undifferentiated state of ESCs: Oct3/4 (Nichols *et al.*, 1998), Sox2 (Nichols *et al.*, 1998; Avilion *et al.*, 2003), and Nanog (Mitsui *et al.*, 2003; Chambers *et al.*, 2003). Oct3/4 is a POU domain transcription factor that represses the trophectoderm lineage and promotes the inner cell mass lineage by forming a repressive complex with the cdx2 transcription factor (Niwa *et al.*, 2005; Ralston and Rossant, 2008). Sox2 is a member of the SRY-related HMG box gene family that, like Oct3/4, is required for survival of epiblast cells (Avilion *et al.*, 2003). Oct3/4 and Sox2 frequently co-regulate gene expression by binding adjacent sites (POU/HMG sites) within gene promoters, and can reciprocally regulate their own promoters (Chew *et al.*, 2005). Nanog is a homeobox protein, with no known homology to other proteins, that occupies many of the same gene promoters as Oct3/4 and Sox2 (Boyer *et al.*, 2005; Chambers *et al.*, 2003; Mitsui *et al.*, 2003), indicating that these three transcription factors work in concert to maintain the balance of pluripotency versus differentiation of mESCs. While these factors form the core of the pluripotency regulation machinery, there are many other factors that regulate the expression of the core factors, such as Tcf3 (Cole *et al.*, 2008; Pereira *et al.*, 2006; Tam *et al.*, 2008), Stat3 (Wu *et al.*, 2009), and Klf4 (Chen *et al.*, 2008).

The ESCs and the epiblast spend the majority of the cell cycle in S phase with a very short G1 phase (Burdon *et al.*, 2002; White *et al.*, 2005), unlike somatic cells, where G1 predominates. These differences not only produce the rapid cycling of the epiblast and ESCs, but also may play an important role in inhibiting differentiation and maintaining pluripotency. The most crucial decision point in the cell cycle, i.e. to proliferate, differentiate, quiesce, senesce, or apoptose, occurs at the G1 checkpoint (Blomen and Boonstra, 2007). Spending minimal amounts of time in the G1 phase had also been suggested to prevent differentiation by insulating cells from growth factor signaling (Orford and Scadden, 2008; Burdon *et al.*, 1999). In fact, many of the mechanisms that maintain ESC pluripotency are directed at keeping the cells rapidly dividing. Moreover, exit from the cell cycle is considered a prerequisite for differentiation due to differential requirements for organization of the cytoskeleton in both processes (Grosshans and Wieschaus, 2000).

Initially culture of mESCs relied on co-culture with a layer of mitotically inactivated fibroblast feeder cells (Evans and Kaufman, 1981; Martin, 1981) until it was discovered that they were providing the cytokine leukemia inhibitory factor (LIF) to activate Stat3 (Niwa *et al.*, 1998; Matsuda *et al.*, 1999), after which it became possible to simply supplement media with LIF (Smith *et al.*, 1988). While LIF was critical for mESC pluripotency, it required cooperation of proteins found in fetal calf serum including BMP4, a member of the TGF-β signaling family (Ying *et al.*, 2001), to induce the expression of inhibitor of differentiation (Id) genes. Subsequent investigations have demonstrated that inhibition of FGF/MAPK with and without inhibition of glycogen synthase kinase-3 (GKS-3) using small-molecule inhibitors can maintain pluripotency in serum-free conditions without LIF (Ying *et al.*, 2008). Alternatively, hESCs are routinely maintained on a fibroblast feeder layer because LIF is unable to prevent their differentiation (Thomson *et al.*, 1998; Reubinoff *et al.*, 2000; Humphrey *et al.*, 2004). Addition of BMP-4 to hESC cultures induces their differentiation into trophectoderm (Xu *et al.*, 2002), which is striking because mESCs are unable to form trophectoderm unless there is a reduction in expression of Oct3/4 (Niwa *et al.*, 2000). Because exposure to BMP promotes differentiation, hESCs are cultured in knock-out serum replacement (KOSR; Invitrogen) with the addition of high levels of basic fibroblast growth factor (bFGF) (Xu *et al.*, 2005a, 2005b) to inhibit signaling by any BMP present in KOSR and maintain their pluripotency (Amit *et al.*, 2000). The striking differences in culture requirements for mESCs versus hESCs likely reflect differences in the developmental timing between mouse and human embryos that may enable mouse epiblast cells to linger in the pluripotent state longer than human epiblast cells (Nichols and Smith, 2009).

Growth factor requirements for hESCs more closely resemble those required for postimplantation epiblast stem cells: absence of LIF, but inclusion of FGF and activin (Brons *et al.*, 2007; Tesar *et al.*, 2007). In addition, both cell types have a relatively flattened morphology, can differentiate into trophectoderm when exposed to BMP-4, and cannot be maintained at single-cell densities (Nichols and Smith, 2011). These observations have led to the hypothesis that mESCs represent an earlier state of pluripotency with greater developmental potential than hESCs, which may be more representative of the postimplantation epiblast and therefore have a more restricted developmental potential (Rossant, 2008; Nichols and Smith, 2009). In fact, postimplantation epiblast stem cells cannot contribute to chimeras when injected into the blastocyst even though they can form all three germ layers in vitro (Brons *et al.*, 2007; Tesar *et al.*, 2007). Experiments involving injection of hESCs into human blastocysts cannot be performed due to obvious moral issues; however, they have been injected into mouse blastocysts (James *et al.*, 2006). Despite some rare but promising integration of hESCs into very early mouse embryos, there can be no conclusions about the ability of hESCs to colonize recipient blastocysts. Recent experiments have demonstrated that both hESCs and postimplantation epiblast stem cells can be converted to cells much more similar to mESCs by expression of Oct3/4, Klf4, and Klf2 in hESCs and by Klf4 alone in postimplantation epiblast stem cells (Hanna *et al.*, 2010; Guo *et al.*, 2009).

The observed similarities among mESCs, embryonic carcinoma stem cells, and embryonic germ cells, as well as experimental results suggesting that, while pre-implantation epiblast (i.e. inner cell mass that is not primitive endoderm) cells were the definitive source of mESCs, only three cell lines could be derived from an entire epiblast (recall that just six epiblast cells give rise to primordial germ cells), led to a hypothesis that the embryologic origin of ESCs was germ cells (Gardner and Brook, 1997; Zwaka and Thomson, 2005). Indeed, mESCs and embryonic carcinoma stem cells express genes considered to be markers of primordial germ cells, and during induced pluripotent stem cell formation expression of primordial germ cell markers precedes expression of pluripotency genes (Xu *et al.*, 2011; Tang *et al.*, 2010). In turn, primordial germ cells and germ cells express the core pluripotency transcription factors: Oct3/4, Sox2, and Nanog (Yabuta *et al.*, 2006; Ohinata *et al.*, 2005; Avilion *et al.*, 2003; Chambers *et al.*, 2003; Yamaguchi *et al.*, 2005). However, refinement of mESC derivation conditions by including inhibitors of FGF/MAPK and GSK-3 signaling, likely driving more of the inner cell mass to adopt an epiblast fate instead of a primitive endoderm fate, illustrated that the number of mESC cell lines derived per embryo could be increased far above the number of primordial germ cells found in the epiblast (Nichols and Smith,

2011). Therefore there appear to be two distinct times during embryologic development when pluripotent cells are created, corresponding to the preimplantation inner cell mass and primordial germ cells which carry pluripotency to the next generation (Nichols and Smith, 2011). While a great deal has been learned about the pluripotent state, many questions still remain. In order to safely and effectively utilize ESCs for cell replacement therapies and regenerative medicine we will need to know exactly how a true pluripotent state is created as well as how to end that state and begin controlled differentiation. Only by studying all pluripotent cells, namely ESCs, embryonic germ cells, embryonic carcinoma stem cells, induced pluripotent stem cells, and postimplantation epiblast stem cells, will we be able to completely understand the pluripotent state and how to utilize this state for regenerative medicine.

1.4 Derivation of human embryonic stem cells

The first step in derivation of hESC lines is the ethical acquisition of appropriate starting material, which is most commonly supernumerary embryos from assisted reproductive technology (ART). These are either cryopreserved embryos donated by couples that are no longer pursuing family building or, alternatively, non-cryopreserved or frozen embryos that have been judged to be genetically abnormal by preimplantation genetic screening (Harper and Sengupta, 2012) for aneuploidy or preimplantation genetic diagnosis (Kuliev and Rechitsky, 2011) for single-gene disorders. Those embryos which are tested and found to be genetically abnormal can be considered unsuitable for transfer to a patient's uterus. To maintain the highest ethical standards regarding informed consent, the information given to donors should include that their embryos will be used for hESC derivation, that there are alternatives to donation for hESC derivation, that they might not receive direct medical benefit, that resulting hESC lines may result in a commercial product for which they will receive no payment, and, finally, that they may withdraw consent until the embryos are used. There should be no monetary or medical compensation for embryo donation (Fraga *et al.*, 2011; Murdoch *et al.*, 2012; Hasegawa *et al.*, 2010). Also the embryo donor's personal information must be carefully protected to ensure confidentiality. Because there is significant debate about the morality of destroying embryos to derive hESC lines, it is of utmost importance that all embryo research is carried out observing the highest ethical standards.

Supernumerary embryos from ART are frequently frozen at the two pronuclear stages, namely early cleavage stage or blastocyst stage (Figures 1.1 and 1.3) and therefore need to be thawed and cultured until the inner cell mass appears within the blastocyst on day 5 or 6 in order to derive hESC lines. Appropriate culture conditions are critical for successful embryo maturation and have been extensively refined by clinics performing in-vitro fertilization (IVF) to ensure the highest possible rates of successful embryo maturation (Hasegawa *et al.*, 2010; Stojkovic *et al.*, 2004). There are several commercially available media and protocols used to culture human embryos using two sequential media (Ilic *et al.*, 2009; Bongso and Tan, 2005), a single medium (Biggers and Summers, 2008), or even co-culture with various types of supporting cells (Kattal *et al.*, 2008) all in an attempt to closely model the in-vivo niche of the fallopian tube. Once the embryos have reached the blastocyst stage they are graded on the basis of morphology (Bongso and Tan, 2005). The blastocysts with the best morphology routinely give rise to hESC lines at the highest frequency; however, several groups have been successful at deriving lines from clinically inferior embryos (Mitalipova *et al.*, 2003; Lerou *et al.*, 2008; Gavrilov *et al.*, 2011).

The next step in hESC derivation is to isolate the inner cell mass from the surrounding trophoblast cells (Figure 1.3). In many cases trophoblast cells are killed by immunosurgery utilizing antibodies and complement (Solter and Knowles, 1975). However, this procedure exposes xenomaterials to the hESC culture, which could introduce either disease causing agents or foreign proteins into the cells, potentially increasing the likelihood of rejection if they are used for regenerative therapies in the future (Fraga *et al.*, 2011; Hasegawa *et al.*, 2010; Vazin and Freed, 2010).

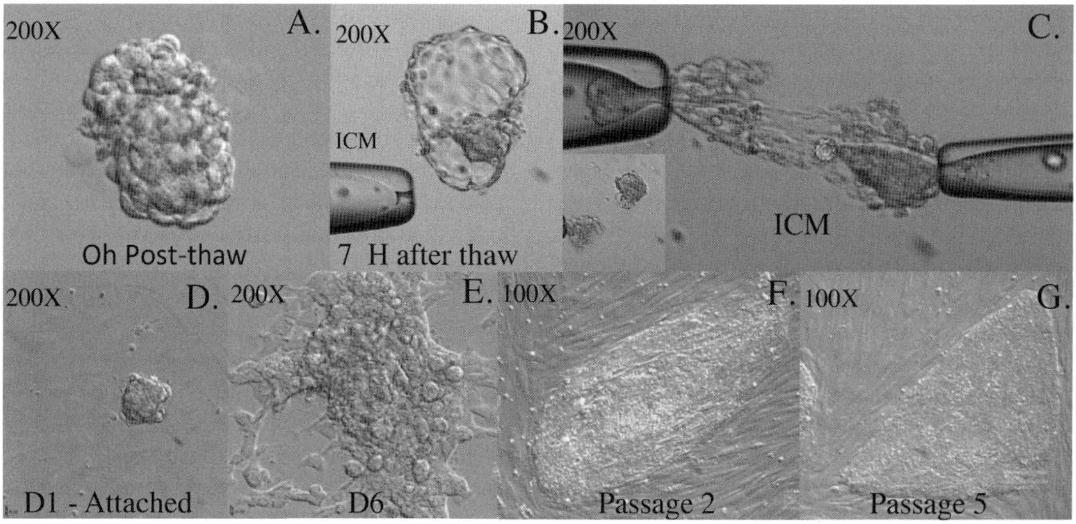

Figure 1.3 Derivation of human embryonic stem cells. A. Cryopreserved blastocyst-stage embryo immediately after thawing. B. Seven hours after thawing the inner cell mass (ICM) is clearly visible. C. Laser-assisted separation of the ICM from the trophoblast. The laser target used for aiming is visible in the center of the frame. Isolated ICM pictured in insert. D. After one day in culture, the ICM has attached to a layer of mitotically inactive mouse or human fibroblast feeder cells. E. Following 6 days of ICM expansion, the center of the explant is removed and plated onto a new layer of fibroblast feeder cells. F. Newly derived hESC line after two passages on inactivated fibroblasts. G. Newly derived hESC line after five passages on inactivated fibroblasts. All images kindly provide by Sandra Mojica, Gary Smith, and the University of Michigan Taubman Consortium for Stem Cell Therapies.

Alternatively, trophoblast cells can be removed by microdissection using fine needles (Strom *et al.*, 2007; Amit and Itskovitz-Eldor, 2002) or with lasers (Figure 1.3) originally used to remove single or multiple blastomeres for preimplantation genetic diagnosis/screening (Turetsky *et al.*, 2008). Because destruction of embryos to generate hESC is so controversial, techniques to generate cell lines from single blastomeres of human embryos that in theory would allow for continued development to term on the basis of results from embryos subjected to preimplantation genetic diagnosis/screening have been proposed (Klimanskaya *et al.*, 2006; Chung *et al.*, 2008). While this is not yet commonplace, one could imagine an opportunity for hESC banking for children conceived by IVF much as umbilical cord blood cells are currently banked.

Once the inner cell mass has been isolated it is typically plated on a layer of feeder cells to enable primary expansion. Since the original protocols (Reubinoff *et al.*, 2000; Thomson *et al.*, 1998) were based on mESC derivation protocols, these were often mouse embryonic fibroblasts. Owing to the discovery that mouse feeder cells and fetal calf serum resulted in the expression of non-human surface antigens on hESCs that could precipitate immune rejection in humans (Martin *et al.*, 2005), current protocols now commonly use human embryonic fibroblasts or other human cell feeder layers (Amit *et al.*, 2003; Choo *et al.*, 2004; Lee *et al.*, 2004). As discussed earlier, hESC are characteristically maintained in Dulbecco's Modified Eagle's Medium-based medium with KOSR and bFGF. A great deal of investigation has centered on developing feeder-free, xeno-free, completely defined conditions in which to derive, expand, and maintain pluripotent hESCs, enabling adoption of good manufacturing practice standards (Ahrlund-Richter *et al.*, 2009; Unger *et al.*, 2008; Rajala *et al.*, 2010). Currently there are several commercially available defined xeno-free media that can maintain hESC pluripotency in the absence of feeder layers (Hasegawa *et al.*, 2010). It should be noted that there is some evidence that the absence of feeder layers causes increased chromosomal instability, thereby necessitating increased karyotypic vigilance (Catalina *et al.*, 2008). However, recently numerous investigative groups have demonstrated long-term expansion of karyotypically normal, undifferentiated hESCs on fully defined and xeno-free substrates such as hydrogels (Villa-Diaz *et al.*, 2010; Melkoumian *et al.*, 2010) and recombinant laminin (Rodin *et al.*, 2010).

Expanded hESCs are passaged mechanically by cutting larger colonies into smaller clumps and replating them. Differentiated cells can also be eliminated from cultures during passage. Manually dissecting colonies is labor-intensive and inhibitory to rapid expansion. However, use of enzymatic or chemical agents to passage hESCs has been shown to increase the risk of chromosomal instability (Catalina *et al.*, 2008; Mitalipova *et al.*, 2005). Therefore, currently mechanical dissection is the best way to maintain the bulk of a hESC line, with enzymatic and chemical passage methods being used only sparingly (Hasegawa *et al.*, 2010). Once established, hESC lines need to be characterized to determine whether they are pluripotent (Englund *et al.*, 2010). Immunohistochemistry or fluorescence-activated cell sorting (FACS) can be used to look for surface antigens found on pluripotent cells, such as SSEA-3, SSEA-4, and/or TRA-1-60, TRA-1-81 as well as expression of pluripotency markers such as Oct3/4 and Nanog. Karyotyping should be done on early, middle, and late passages to demonstrate chromosomal stability. The cells should be subjected to the in-vitro differentiation assay of embryoid body formation. When ESC are grown in suspension culture as embryoid bodies, floating aggregates of cells, they spontaneously differentiate into all three germ layers: ectoderm, mesoderm, and endoderm. The presence of ectoderm, mesoderm, and endoderm contributions in the embryoid body can be confirmed with immunocytochemistry with linage-specific antibodies or with PCR and linage-specific mRNA/cDNA primers. However, there are significant differences in the organization of the embryo and an embryoid body. Lineage allocation in an embryoid body is far more chaotic; there is no organized geometry, formation of an anterior visceral endoderm (AVE) (an embryonic organizing center), node, or primitive streak. Finally, the ESCs should be used to generate teratomas in immunocompromised mice, considered the gold standard of pluripotency with hESCs.

1.5 Pluripotent stem cells in regenerative medicine

Currently a major disadvantage of using ESCs in cell replacement therapies is their potential to generate teratocarcinomas or teratomas, or simply undergo uncontrolled levels of proliferation that result in graft overgrowth. One of the most scientifically sound ways to approach this problem is to gain sufficient understanding of the embryonic development necessary to differentiate ESCs to the level of the resident tissue stem cell or even fully differentiated cell, then transplant those cells with a "suicide" transgene (e.g. thymidine kinase driven by a cyclin gene promoter) that could be used to kill cells if they re-enter cell cycle (Fareed and Moolten, 2002; Schuldiner *et al.*, 2003). Alternatively, several cell surface antigens have been identified that can be used in conjunction with FACS to remove tumor-initiating cells from a population of differentiated ESCs prior to implantation (Tang *et al.*, 2011).

Another major obstacle in the use of ESCs in regenerative medicine is immunogenicity of implanted cells. While elimination of foreign proteins and disease-causing agents from ESC culture conditions is important, major histocompatibility (MHC), minor histocompatibility (mHC), and blood group antigen (ABO) differences between donor ESC and graft recipients can all precipitate rejection of ESC transplants (Drukker and Benvenisty, 2004; Lui *et al.*, 2009). There are several methods that may be employed to avoid rejection. Seemingly the most simple would be to match MHC, mHC, and ABO antigens between hESC lines and recipients, as is done for organ transplantation. Unfortunately, this would require an enormous bank of hESC lines because of the massive number of haplotype combinations. In fact, hESC line ethnic diversity appears to be poor, likely due to the fact that most donor embryos are leftovers from ART (Mosher *et al.*, 2010; Laurent *et al.*, 2010). Alternatively, somatic cell nuclear transfer could be used to place the nucleus of a somatic cell from the patient into a donor oocyte that could be parthenogenetically activated and used to generate patient-specific hESC lines (Drukker and Benvenisty, 2004; Mai *et al.*, 2007; Kim *et al.*, 2007). Unfortunately, this technology is dependent on obtaining donor oocytes, which is currently problematic. More importantly, despite numerous attempts, human SCNT has resulted in few, if any, successful derivations of blastocysts (Li *et al.*, 2009) and only one hESC line (Trivedi *et al.*, 2006). Finally, there is a possibility of hematopoetic stem cells derived from hESCs being used to induce immune tolerance prior to transplantation of hESC-derived cells or tissues (Lui *et al.*, 2009; Drukker and Benvenisty, 2004; Trivedi *et al.*, 2006). Therefore, while rejection by the immune system is still a difficult impediment for regenerative medicine, scientific progress may present reasonable solutions in the not too distant future.

Another caveat in cell replacement therapy is that placing new cells into a diseased environment might yield nothing but dead cells because the diseased tissue/organ is producing a deficient microenvironment. Careful studies with ESCs may enable co-transplantation of stem cells with supporting cells that promote survival and colonization and thereby improve patient outcomes. Currently we lack a sufficiently complete understanding of embryologic development to allow for the differentiation of every cell type needed in the body. In addition, most ESC differentiation protocols are plagued by relatively low yields and contamination with undesired cell types and undifferentiated cells. However, our knowledge base is constantly expanding and in the future we will be able to use lessons learned from development to hypothetically generate each cell type needed for transplantation (Cohen and Melton, 2011; Murry and Keller, 2008). Finally, other practical shortcomings of using ESCs for regenerative medicine such as problems in scale-up, defined and predictable protocols for directed differentiation, and methods of cell delivery must be explored

Induced pluripotent stem cells are a tremendously exciting discovery that initially had the potential to eliminate the immunogenicity issues currently faced by ESC therapies, because they can be derived directly from the somatic cells of the recipient patient. However, a recent report suggests that aberrant gene expression in induced pluripotent stem cells may generate an immune response even in syngeneic hosts (Zhao *et al.*, 2011). Current induced pluripotent stem cell derivation protocols require the use of potent oncogenes to induce pluripotency with a high efficiency, which increases their potential to generate tumors (Lee *et al.*, 2009). There are also some questions of variability in the pluripotency of induced pluripotent stem cells derived from different cell types and regarding whether they retain a "cellular memory" that could restrict their developmental potential (Hu *et al.*, 2010; Kim *et al.*, 2010; Kulkeaw *et al.*, 2010). Despite these issues, induced pluripotent stem cells make an excellent tool to further our understanding of pluripotency and differentiation as well as potentially improving understanding of somatic nuclear cell transfer. Preimplantation genetic diagnosis of embryos created by ART has generated an opportunity of using genetically abnormal embryos to produce disease-specific hESC lines that have the potential to dramatically increase our understanding of human genetic diseases. In the same way, induced pluripotent stem cells can be derived from people with genetic diseases, again providing a model system to investigate human disease at the cellular level. The discovery of induced pluripotent stem cells was heralded as justification for the elimination of funding and research with hESCs due to the controversy surrounding destruction of human embryos. Given the current problems with immunogenicity, use of oncogenes for derivation, and variability in induced pluripotent stem cells, the most prudent course of action is to continue to explore ESCs and induced pluripotent stem cell models together in order to develop the best possible system for regenerative medicine (Lee *et al.*, 2009).

The ultimate translational goal for stem cell research is to generate large quantities of cells that can be used safely to derive cells, tissues, and organs for transplantation. ESCs and potentially induced pluripotent stem cells will make excellent starting materials for regenerative therapy. Currently both cell types have limitations that make their clinical use difficult, but science is overcoming those barriers. In October of 2010 the Geron corporation received FDA approval for the first Phase I clinical trial of a hESC-derived product. They injected oligodendrocyte progenitor cells, GRNOPC1, into patients with fresh severe spinal cord injuries in order to assess safety and tolerability of the cells. While this clinical trial is an exciting step forward, there is still much to be learned about pluripotent cells and their end products before they can be routinely used for therapies. In November of 2011, Geron discontinued the study to focus on cancer research. Geron's chief executive officer commented that "in the current environment of capital scarcity and uncertain economic conditions, we intend to focus our resources on advancing our two novel and promising oncology drug candidates" (Stein, 2011). In 2010 Advanced Cell Technology began studies aimed at improving the vision of patients with Stargardt's macular dystrophy and dry age-related macular degeneration. In this trial patients' eyes are injected with retinal pigmented epithelial cells derived from hESCs. At present no definitive findings from this study have been produced, yet an article published in the *Lancet* in January 2012 stated that preliminary findings appear to be promising (Schwartz *et al.*, 2012).

REFERENCES

Ahrlund-Richter, L., De Luca, M., Marshak, D. R. *et al.* 2009. Isolation and production of cells suitable for human therapy: challenges ahead. *Cell Stem Cell*, **4**, 20–6.

Amit, M., Carpenter, M. K., Inokuma, M. S. *et al.* 2000. Clonally derived human embryonic stem cell lines maintain pluripotency and proliferative potential for prolonged periods of culture. *Developmental Biol.*, **227**, 271–8.

Amit, M. and Itskovitz-Eldor, J. 2002. Derivation and spontaneous differentiation of human embryonic stem cells. *J. Anatomy*, **200**, 225–32.

Amit, M., Margulets, V., Segev, H. *et al.* 2003. Human feeder layers for human embryonic stem cells. *Biol. Reproduction*, **68**, 2150–6.

Arnold, S. J. and Robertson, E. J. 2009. Making a commitment: cell lineage allocation and axis patterning in the early mouse embryo. *Nature Rev. Molec. Cell Biol.*, **10**, 91–103.

Avilion, A. A., Nicolis, S. K., Pevny, L. H. *et al.* 2003. Multipotent cell lineages in early mouse development depend on SOX2 function. *Genes Development*, **17**, 126–40.

Azuara, V., Perry, P., Sauer, S. *et al.* 2006. Chromatin signatures of pluripotent cell lines. *Nature Cell Biol.*, **8**, 532–8.

Bernstein, B. E., Mikkelsen, T. S., Xie, X. *et al.* 2006. A bivalent chromatin structure marks key developmental genes in embryonic stem cells. *Cell*, **125**, 315–26.

Biggers, J. D. and Summers, M. C. 2008. Choosing a culture medium: making informed choices. *Fertility Sterility*, **90**, 473–83.

Blomen, V. A. and Boonstra, J. 2007. Cell fate determination during G1 phase progression. *Cellular Molec. Life Sci.: CMLS*, **64**, 3084–104.

Bongso, A. and Tan, S. 2005. Human blastocyst culture and derivation of embryonic stem cell lines. *Stem Cell Rev.*, **1**, 87–98.

Boyer, L. A., Lee, T. I., Cole, M. F. *et al.* 2005. Core transcriptional regulatory circuitry in human embryonic stem cells. *Cell*, **122**, 947–56.

Brons, I. G., Smithers, L. E., Trotter, M. W. *et al.* 2007. Derivation of pluripotent epiblast stem cells from mammalian embryos. *Nature*, **448**, 191–5.

Brook, F. A. and Gardner, R. L. 1997. The origin and efficient derivation of embryonic stem cells in the mouse. *Proc. Nat. Acad. Sci. USA*, **94**, 5709–12.

Burdon, T., Smith, A. and Savatier, P. 2002. Signalling, cell cycle and pluripotency in embryonic stem cells. *Trends Cell Biol.*, **12**, 432–8.

Burdon, T., Stracey, C., Chambers, I., Nichols, J. and Smith, A. 1999. Suppression of SHP-2 and ERK signalling promotes self-renewal of mouse embryonic stem cells. *Developmental Biol.*, **210**, 30–43.

Catalina, P., Montes, R., Ligero, G. *et al.* 2008. Human ESCs predisposition to karyotypic instability: is a matter of culture adaptation or differential vulnerability among hESC lines due to inherent properties? *Molec. Cancer*, **7**, 76.

Chambers, I., Colby, D., Robertson, M. *et al.* 2003. Functional expression cloning of Nanog, a pluripotency sustaining factor in embryonic stem cells. *Cell*, **113**, 643–55.

Chazaud, C., Yamanaka, Y., Pawson, T. and Rossant, J. 2006. Early lineage segregation between epiblast and primitive endoderm in mouse blastocysts through the Grb2-MAPK pathway. *Developmental Cell*, **10**, 615–24.

Chen, X., Xu, H., Yuan, P. *et al.* 2008. Integration of external signaling pathways with the core transcriptional network in embryonic stem cells. *Cell*, **133**, 1106–17.

Chew, J. L., Loh, Y. H., Zhang, W. *et al.* 2005. Reciprocal transcriptional regulation of Pou5f1 and Sox2 via the Oct4/Sox2 complex in embryonic stem cells. *Molec. Cellular Biol.*, **25**, 6031–46.

Choo, A. B., Padmanabhan, J., Chin, A. C. and Oh, S. K. 2004. Expansion of pluripotent human embryonic stem cells on human feeders. *Biotechnol. Bioeng.*, **88**, 321–31.

Chung, Y., Klimanskaya, I., Becker, S. *et al.* 2008. Human embryonic stem cell lines generated without embryo destruction. *Cell Stem Cell*, **2**, 113–7.

Cockburn, K. and Rossant, J. 2010. Making the blastocyst: lessons from the mouse. *J. Clinical Investigation*, **120**, 995–1003.

Cohen, D. E. and Melton, D. 2011. Turning straw into gold: directing cell fate for regenerative medicine. *Nature Rev. Genetics*, **12**, 243–52.

Cole, M. F., Johnstone, S. E., Newman, J. J., Kagey, M. H. and Young, R. A. 2008. Tcf3 is an integral component of the core regulatory circuitry of embryonic stem cells. *Genes Development*, **22**, 746–55.

Davis, T. L., Trasler, J. M., Moss, S. B., Yang, G. J. and Bartolomei, M. S. 1999. Acquisition of the H19 methylation imprint occurs differentially on the parental alleles during spermatogenesis. *Genomics*, **58**, 18–28.

Davis, T. L., Yang, G. J., McCarrey, J. R. and Bartolomei, M. S. 2000. The H19 methylation imprint is erased and re-established differentially on the parental alleles during male germ cell development. *Human Molec. Genetics*, **9**, 2885–94.

Drukker, M. and Benvenisty, N. 2004. The immunogenicity of human embryonic stem-derived cells. *Trends Biotechnol.*, **22**, 136–41.

Durcova-Hills, G., Ainscough, J. and McLaren, A. 2001. Pluripotential stem cells derived from migrating primordial germ cells. *Differentiation; Res. Biol. Diversity*, **68**, 220–6.

Dziadek, M. 1979. Cell differentiation in isolated inner cell masses of mouse blastocysts in vitro: onset of specific gene expression. *J. Embryol. Exp. Morphol.*, **53**, 367–79.

Efroni, S., Duttagupta, R., Cheng, J. *et al.* 2008. Global transcription in pluripotent embryonic stem cells. *Cell Stem Cell*, **2**, 437–47.

Englund, M. C., Caisander, G., Noaksson, K. *et al.* 2010. The establishment of 20 different human embryonic stem cell lines and subclones; a report on derivation, culture, characterisation and banking. *In vitro Cellular Developmental Biol. Animal*, **46**, 217–30.

Evans, M. J. and Kaufman, M. H. 1981. Establishment in culture of pluripotential cells from mouse embryos. *Nature*, **292**, 154–6.

Ewen, K. A. and Koopman, P. 2010. Mouse germ cell development: from specification to sex determination. *Molec. Cellular Endocrinol.*, **323**, 76–93.

Fareed, M. U. and Moolten, F. L. 2002. Suicide gene transduction sensitizes murine embryonic and human mesenchymal stem cells to ablation on demand – a fail-safe protection against cellular misbehavior. *Gene Therapy*, **9**, 955–62.

Feldman, B., Poueymirou, W., Papaioannou, V. E., Dechiara, T. M. and Goldfarb, M. 1995. Requirement of FGF-4 for postimplantation mouse development. *Science*, **267**, 246–9.

Fraga, A. M., Souza de Araújo, É. S., Stabellini, R., Vergani, N. and Pereira, L. V. 2011. A survey of parameters involved in the establishment of new lines of human embryonic stem cells. *Stem Cell Rev.*, **7**(4), 775–81.

Gardner, R. L. and Brook, F. A. 1997. Reflections on the biology of embryonic stem (ES) cells. *Int. J. Developmental Biol.*, **41**, 235–43.

Gavrilov, S., Marolt, D., Douglas, N. C. *et al.* 2011. Derivation of two new human embryonic stem cell lines from nonviable human embryos. *Stem Cells Int.*, **2011**, 765378.

Godin, I., Wylie, C. and Heasman, J. 1990. Genital ridges exert long-range effects on mouse primordial germ cell numbers and direction of migration in culture. *Development*, **108**, 357–63.

Gomperts, M., Garcia-Castro, M., Wylie, C. and Heasman, J. 1994. Interactions between primordial germ cells play a role in their migration in mouse embryos. *Development*, **120**, 135–41.

Grosshans, J. and Wieschaus, E. 2000. A genetic link between morphogenesis and cell division during formation of the ventral furrow in Drosophila. *Cell*, **101**, 523–31.

Guo, G., Yang, J., Nichols, J. *et al.* 2009. Klf4 reverts developmentally programmed restriction of ground state pluripotency. *Development*, **136**, 1063–9.

Hanna, J., Cheng, A. W., Saha, K. *et al.* 2010. Human embryonic stem cells with biological and epigenetic characteristics similar to those of mouse ESCs. *Proc. Nat. Acad. Sci. USA*, **107**, 9222–7.

Harper, J. C. and Sengupta, S. B. 2012. Preimplantation genetic diagnosis: state of the ART 2011. *Human Genetics*, **131**, 175–86.

Hasegawa, K., Pomeroy, J. E. and Pera, M. F. 2010. Current technology for the derivation of pluripotent stem cell lines from human embryos. *Cell Stem Cell*, **6**, 521–31.

Hu, B. Y., Weick, J. P., Yu, J. *et al.* 2010. Neural differentiation of human induced pluripotent stem cells follows developmental principles but with variable potency. *Proc. Nat. Acad. Sci. USA*, **107**, 4335–40.

Humphrey, R. K., Beattie, G. M., Lopez, A. D. *et al.* 2004. Maintenance of pluripotency in human embryonic stem cells is STAT3 independent. *Stem Cells*, **22**, 522–30.

Ilic, D., Giritharan, G., Zdravkovic, T. *et al.* 2009. Derivation of human embryonic stem cell lines from biopsied blastomeres on human feeders with minimal exposure to xenomaterials. *Stem Cells Development*, **18**, 1343–50.

Illmensee, K. and Mintz, B. 1976. Totipotency and normal differentiation of single teratocarcinoma cells cloned by injection into blastocysts. *Proc. Nat. Acad. Sci. USA*, **73**, 549–53.

Jaenisch, R. and Young, R. 2008. Stem cells, the molecular circuitry of pluripotency and nuclear reprogramming. *Cell*, **132**, 567–82.

James, D., Noggle, S. A., Swigut, T. and Brivanlou, A. H. 2006. Contribution of human embryonic stem cells to mouse blastocysts. *Developmental Biol.*, **295**, 90–102.

Kahan, B. W. and Ephrussi, B. 1970. Developmental potentialities of clonal in vitro cultures of mouse testicular teratoma. *J. Nat. Cancer Inst.*, **44**, 1015–36.

Kattal, N., Cohen, J. and Barmat, L. I. 2008. Role of coculture in human in vitro fertilization: a meta-analysis. *Fertility Sterility*, **90**, 1069–76.

Kim, D. S., Lee, J. S., Leem, J. W. *et al.* 2010. Robust enhancement of neural differentiation from human ES and iPS cells regardless of their innate difference in differentiation propensity. *Stem Cell Rev.*, **6**, 270–81.

Kim, K., Lerou, P., Yabuuchi, A. *et al.* 2007. Histocompatible embryonic stem cells by parthenogenesis. *Science*, **315**, 482–6.

Kleinsmith, L. J. and Pierce, G. B., Jr. 1964. Multipotentiality of single embryonal carcinoma cells. *Cancer Res.*, **24**, 1544–51.

Klimanskaya, I., Chung Y., Becker S., Lu S. J. and Lanza R. 2006. Human embryonic stem cell lines derived from single blastomeres. *Nature*, **444**, 481–485.

Kuijk, E. W., Chuva De Sousa Lopes, S. M., Geijsen, N., Macklon, N. and Roelen, B. A. 2011. The different shades of mammalian pluripotent stem cells. *Human Reproduction Update*, **17**, 254–71.

Kuliev, A. and Rechitsky, S. 2011. Polar body based preimplantation genetic diagnosis for Mendelian disorders. *Molec. Human Reproduction*, **17**, 275–85.

Kulkeaw, K., Horio, Y., Mizuochi, C., Ogawa, M. and Sugiyama, D. 2010. Variation in hematopoietic potential of induced pluripotent stem cell lines. *Stem Cell Rev.*, **6**, 381–9.

Laurent, L. C., Nievergelt, C. M., Lynch, C. *et al.* 2010. Restrictemphasised ethnic diversity in human embryonic stem cell lines. *Nature Methods*, **7**, 6–7.

Lee, H., Park, J., Forget, B. G. and Gaines, P. 2009. Induced pluripotent stem cells in regenerative medicine: an argument for continued research on human embryonic stem cells. *Regen. Med.*, **4**, 759–69.

Lee, J. B., Song, J. M., Lee, J. E. *et al.* 2004. Available human feeder cells for the maintenance of human embryonic stem cells. *Reproduction*, **128**, 727–35.

Lerou, P. H., Yabuuchi, A., Huo, H. *et al.* 2008. Human embryonic stem cell derivation from poor-quality embryos. *Nature Biotechnol.*, **26**, 212–14.

Li, J., Liu, X., Wang, H. *et al.* 2009. Human embryos derived by somatic cell nuclear transfer using an alternative enucleation approach. *Cloning Stem Cells*, **11**, 39–50.

Lucifero, D., Mann, M. R., Bartolomei, M. S. and Trasler, J. M. 2004. Gene-specific timing and epigenetic memory in oocyte imprinting. *Human Molec. Genetics*, **13**, 839–49.

Lucifero, D., Mertineit, C., Clarke, H. J., Bestor, T. H. and Trasler, J. M. 2002. Methylation dynamics of imprinted genes in mouse germ cells. *Genomics*, **79**, 530–8.

Lui, K. O., Waldmann, H. and Fairchild, P. J. 2009. Embryonic stem cells: overcoming the immunological barriers to cell replacement therapy. *Current Stem Cell Res. Therapy*, **4**, 70–80.

Mai, Q., Yu, Y., Li, T. *et al.* 2007. Derivation of human embryonic stem cell lines from parthenogenetic blastocysts. *Cell Res.*, **17**, 1008–19.

Martin, G. R. 1981. Isolation of a pluripotent cell line from early mouse embryos cultured in medium conditioned by teratocarcinoma stem cells. *Proc. Nat. Acad. Sci. USA*, **78**, 7634–8.

Martin, G. R. and Evans, M. J. 1974. The morphology and growth of a pluripotent teratocarcinoma cell line and its derivatives in tissue culture. *Cell*, **2**, 163–72.

Martin, G. R. and Evans, M. J. 1975. Differentiation of clonal lines of teratocarcinoma cells: formation of embryoid bodies in vitro. *Proc. Nat. Acad. Sci. USA*, **72**, 1441–5.

Martin, M. J., Muotri, A., Gage, F. and Varki, A. 2005. Human embryonic stem cells express an immunogenic nonhuman sialic acid. *Nature Med.*, **11**, 228–32.

Matsuda, T., Nakamura, T., Nakao, K. *et al.* 1999. STAT3 activation is sufficient to maintain an undifferentiated state of mouse embryonic stem cells. *EMBO J.*, **18**, 4261–9.

Matsui, Y., Zsebo, K. and Hogan, B. L. 1992. Derivation of pluripotential embryonic stem cells from murine primordial germ cells in culture. *Cell*, **70**, 841–7.

Melkoumian, Z., Weber, J. L., Weber, D. M. *et al.* 2010. Synthetic peptide-acrylate surfaces for long-term self-renewal and cardiomyocyte differentiation of human embryonic stem cells. *Nature Biotechnol.*, **28**, 606–10.

Mintz, B. and Illmensee, K. 1975. Normal genetically mosaic mice produced from malignant teratocarcinoma cells. *Proc. Nat. Acad. Sci. USA*, **72**, 3585–9.

Mitalipova, M., Calhoun, J., Shin, S. *et al.* 2003. Human embryonic stem cell lines derived from discarded embryos. *Stem Cells*, **21**, 521–6.

Mitalipova, M. M., Rao, R. R., Hoyer, D. M. *et al.* 2005. Preserving the genetic integrity of human embryonic stem cells. *Nature Biotechnol.*, **23**, 19–20.

Mitsui, K., Tokuzawa, Y., Itoh, H. *et al.* 2003. The homeoprotein Nanog is required for maintenance of pluripotency in mouse epiblast and ES cells. *Cell*, **113**, 631–42.

Molyneaux, K. A., Stallock, J., Schaible, K. and Wylie, C. 2001. Time-lapse analysis of living mouse germ cell migration. *Developmental Biol.*, **240**, 488–98.

Mosher, J. T., Pemberton, T. J., Harter, K. *et al.* 2010. Lack of population diversity in commonly used human embryonic stem-cell lines. *New England J. Med.*, **362**, 183–5.

Murdoch, A., Braude, P., Courtney, A. *et al.* 2012. The procurement of cells for the derivation of human embryonic stem cell lines for therapeutic use: recommendations for good practice. *Stem Cell Rev.*, **8**, 91–9.

Murry, C. E. and Keller, G. 2008. Differentiation of embryonic stem cells to clinically relevant populations: lessons from embryonic development. *Cell*, **132**, 661–80.

Nichols, J. and Smith, A. 2009. Naive and primed pluripotent states. *Cell Stem Cell*, **4**, 487–92.

Nichols, J. and Smith, A. 2011. The origin and identity of embryonic stem cells. *Development*, **138**, 3–8.

Nichols, J., Zevnik, B., Anastassiadis, K. *et al.* 1998. Formation of pluripotent stem cells in the mammalian embryo depends on the POU transcription factor Oct4. *Cell*, **95**, 379–91.

Niwa, H., Burdon, T., Chambers, I. and Smith, A. 1998. Self-renewal of pluripotent embryonic stem cells is mediated via activation of STAT3. *Genes Development*, **12**, 2048–60.

Niwa, H., Miyazaki, J. and Smith, A. G. 2000. Quantitative expression of Oct-3/4 defines differentiation, dedifferentiation or self-renewal of ES cells. *Nature Genetics*, **24**, 372–6.

Niwa, H., Toyooka, Y., Shimosato, D. *et al.* 2005. Interaction between Oct3/4 and Cdx2 determines trophectoderm differentiation. *Cell*, **123**, 917–29.

Ohinata, Y., Payer, B., O'Carroll, D. *et al.* 2005. Blimp1 is a critical determinant of the germ cell lineage in mice. *Nature*, **436**, 207–13.

Okita K., Ichisaka T. and Yamanaka S. 2007. Generation of germline-competent induced pluripotent stem cells. *Nature*, **448**, 313–17.

Orford, K. W. and Scadden, D. T. 2008. Deconstructing stem cell self-renewal: genetic insights into cell-cycle regulation. *Nature Rev. Genetics*, **9**, 115–28.

Papaioannou, V. E., McBurney, M. W., Gardner, R. L. and Evans, M. J. 1975. Fate of teratocarcinoma cells injected into early mouse embryos. *Nature*, **258**, 70–3.

Pereira, L., Yi, F. and Merrill, B. J. 2006. Repression of Nanog gene transcription by Tcf3 limits embryonic stem cell self-renewal. *Molec. Cellular Biol.*, **26**, 7479–91.

Rajala, K., Lindroos, B., Hussein, S. M. *et al.* 2010. A defined and xeno-free culture method enabling the establishment of clinical-grade human embryonic, induced pluripotent and adipose stem cells. *PloS One*, **5**, e10246.

Ralston, A. and Rossant, J. 2008. Cdx2 acts downstream of cell polarization to cell-autonomously promote trophectoderm fate in the early mouse embryo. *Developmental Biol.*, **313**, 614–29.

Resnick, J. L., Bixler, L. S., Cheng, L. and Donovan, P. J. 1992. Long-term proliferation of mouse primordial germ cells in culture. *Nature*, **359**, 550–1.

Reubinoff, B. E., Pera, M. F., Fong, C. Y., Trounson, A. and Bongso, A. 2000. Embryonic stem cell lines from human blastocysts: somatic differentiation in vitro. *Nature Biotechnol.*, **18**, 399–404.

Rodin, S., Domogatskaya, A., Strom, S. *et al.* 2010. Long-term self-renewal of human pluripotent stem cells on human recombinant laminin-511. *Nature Biotechnol.*, **28**, 611–15.

Rosenthal, M. D., Wishnow, R. M. and Sato, G. H. 1970. In vitro growth and differetiation of clonal populations of multipotential mouse cells derived from a transplantable testicular teratocarcinoma. *J. Nat. Cancer Inst.*, **44**, 1001–14.

Rossant, J. 2008. Stem cells and early lineage development. *Cell*, **132**, 527–31.

Rossant, J. and McBurney, M. W. 1982. The developmental potential of a euploid male teratocarcinoma cell line after blastocyst injection. *J. Embryol. Exp. Morphol.*, **70**, 99–112.

Rossant, J. and Tam, P. P. 2009. Blastocyst lineage formation, early embryonic asymmetries and axis patterning in the mouse. *Development*, **136**, 701–13.

Saga, Y. 2008. Mouse germ cell development during embryogenesis. *Current Opinion Genetics Development*, **18**, 337–41.

Schuldiner, M., Itskovitz-Eldor, J. and Benvenisty, N. 2003. Selective ablation of human embryonic stem cells expressing a "suicide" gene. *Stem Cells*, **21**, 257–65.

Schwartz S. D., Hubschman J. P., Heilwell G. *et al.* 2012. Embryonic stem cell trials for macular degeneration: a preliminary report. *Lancet*, **379**, 713–20.

Shamblott, M. J., Axelman, J., Wang, S. *et al.* 1998. Derivation of pluripotent stem cells from cultured human primordial germ cells. *Proc. Nat. Acad. Sci. USA*, **95**, 13726–31.

Smith, A. G., Heath, J. K., Donaldson, D. D. *et al.* 1988. Inhibition of pluripotential embryonic stem cell differentiation by purified polypeptides. *Nature*, **336**, 688–90.

Solter, D. and Knowles, B. B. 1975. Immunosurgery of mouse blastocyst. *Proc. Nat. Acad. Sci. USA*, **72**, 5099–102.

Solter, D., Skreb, N. and Damjanov, I. 1970. Extrauterine growth of mouse egg-cylinders results in malignant teratoma. *Nature*, **227**, 503–4.

Stein, R. 2011. *First Human Embryonic Stem Cell Therapy in People Discontinued.* Washington Post, November 14.

Stevens, L. C. 1967. Origin of testicular teratomas from primordial germ cells in mice. *J. Nat. Cancer Inst.*, **38**, 549–52.

Stevens, L. C. and Little, C. C. 1954. Spontaneous testicular teratomas in an inbred strain of mice. *Proc. Nat. Acad. Sci. USA*, **40**, 1080–7.

Stojkovic, M., Lako, M., Strachan, T. and Murdoch, A. 2004. Derivation, growth and applications of human embryonic stem cells. *Reproduction*, **128**, 259–67.

Strom, S., Inzunza, J., Grinnemo, K. H. *et al.* 2007. Mechanical isolation of the inner cell mass is effective in derivation of new human embryonic stem cell lines. *Human Reproduction*, **22**, 3051–8.

Takahashi, K. and Yamanaka, S. 2006. Induction of pluripotent stem cells from mouse embryonic and adult fibroblast cultures by defined factors. *Cell*, **126**, 663–76.

Tam, P. P. and Snow, M. H. 1981. Proliferation and migration of primordial germ cells during compensatory growth in mouse embryos. *J. Embryol. Exp. Morphol.*, **64**, 133–47.

Tam, W. L., Lim, C. Y., Han, J. *et al.* 2008. T-cell factor 3 regulates embryonic stem cell pluripotency and self-renewal by the transcriptional control of multiple lineage pathways. *Stem Cells*, **26**, 2019–31.

Tang, C., Lee, A. S., Volkmer, J. P. *et al.* 2011. An antibody against SSEA-5 glycan on human pluripotent stem cells enables removal of teratoma-forming cells. *Nature Biotechnol.*, **29**, 829–34.

Tang, F., Barbacioru, C., Bao, S. *et al.* 2010. Tracing the derivation of embryonic stem cells from the inner cell mass by single-cell RNA-Seq analysis. *Cell Stem Cell*, **6**, 468–78.

Tesar, P. J., Chenoweth, J. G., Brook, F. A. *et al.* 2007. New cell lines from mouse epiblast share defining features with human embryonic stem cells. *Nature*, **448**, 196–9.

Thomson, J. A., Itskovitz-Eldor, J., Shapiro, S. S. *et al.* 1998. Embryonic stem cell lines derived from human blastocysts. *Science*, **282**, 1145–7.

Trivedi, H. L., Mishra, V. V., Vanikar, A. V. *et al.* 2006. Embryonic stem cell derived and adult hematopoietic stem cell transplantation for tolerance induction in a renal allograft recipient: a case report. *Transplantation Proc.*, **38**, 3103–8.

Turetsky, T., Aizenman, E., Gil, Y. *et al.* 2008. Laser-assisted derivation of human embryonic stem cell lines from IVF embryos after preimplantation genetic diagnosis. *Human Reproduction*, **23**, 46–53.

Unger, C., Skottman, H., Blomberg, P., Dilber, M. S. and Hovatta, O. 2008. Good manufacturing practice and clinical-grade human embryonic stem cell lines. *Human Molec. Genetics*, **17**, R48–53.

Vassena, R., Boue, S., Gonzalez-Roca, E. *et al.* 2011. Waves of early transcriptional activation and pluripotency program initiation during human preimplantation development. *Development*, **138**, 3699–709.

Vazin, T. and Freed, W. J. 2010. Human embryonic stem cells: derivation, culture, and differentiation: a review. *Restorative Neurol. Neurosci.*, **28**, 589–603.

Villa-Diaz, L. G., Nandivada, H., Ding, J. *et al.* 2010. Synthetic polymer coatings for long-term growth of human embryonic stem cells. *Nature Biotechnol.*, **28**, 581–3.

White, J., Stead, E., Faast, R. *et al.* 2005. Developmental activation of the Rb-E2F pathway and establishment of cell cycle-regulated cyclin-dependent kinase activity during embryonic stem cell differentiation. *Molec. Biol. Cell*, **16**, 2018–27.

Wu, D., Pang, Y., Ke, Y. *et al.* 2009. A conserved mechanism for control of human and mouse embryonic stem cell pluripotency and differentiation by shp2 tyrosine phosphatase. *PloS One*, **4**, e4914.

Xu, C., Rosler, E., Jiang, J. *et al.* 2005a. Basic fibroblast growth factor supports undifferentiated human embryonic stem cell growth without conditioned medium. *Stem Cells*, **23**, 315–23.

Xu, R. H., Chen, X., Li, D. S. *et al.* 2002. BMP4 initiates human embryonic stem cell differentiation to trophoblast. *Nature Biotechnol.*, **20**, 1261–4.

Xu, R. H., Peck, R. M., Li, D. S. *et al.* 2005b. Basic FGF and suppression of BMP signaling sustain undifferentiated proliferation of human ES cells. *Nature Methods*, **2**, 185–90.

Xu, X., Pantakani, D. V., Luhrig, S. *et al.* 2011. Stage-specific germ-cell marker genes are expressed in all mouse pluripotent cell types and emerge early during induced pluripotency. *PloS One*, **6**, e22413.

Yabuta, Y., Kurimoto, K., Ohinata, Y., Seki, Y. and Saitou, M. 2006. Gene expression dynamics during germline specification in mice identified by quantitative single-cell gene expression profiling. *Biol. Reproduction*, **75**, 705–16.

Yamaguchi, S., Kimura, H., Tada, M., Nakatsuji, N. and Tada, T. 2005. Nanog expression in mouse germ cell development. *Gene Expression Patterns: GEP*, **5**, 639–46.

Yamanaka, Y., Lanner, F. and Rossant, J. 2010. FGF signal-dependent segregation of primitive endoderm and epiblast in the mouse blastocyst. *Development*, **137**, 715–24.

Ying, Q. L., Wray, J., Nichols, J. *et al.* 2008. The ground state of embryonic stem cell self-renewal. *Nature*, **453**, 519–23.

Ying, Y., Qi, X. and Zhao, G. Q. 2001. Induction of primordial germ cells from murine epiblasts by synergistic action of BMP4 and BMP8B signaling pathways. *Proc. Nat. Acad. Sci. USA*, **98**, 7858–62.

Ying, Y. and Zhao, G. Q. 2001. Cooperation of endoderm-derived BMP2 and extraembryonic ectoderm-derived BMP4 in primordial germ cell generation in the mouse. *Developmental Biol.*, **232**, 484–92.

Yuan, H., Corbi, N., Basilico, C. and Dailey, L. 1995. Developmental-specific activity of the FGF-4 enhancer requires the synergistic action of Sox2 and Oct-3. *Genes Development*, **9**, 2635–45.

Zernicka-Goetz, M., Morris, S. A. and Bruce, A. W. 2009. Making a firm decision: multifaceted regulation of cell fate in the early mouse embryo. *Nature Rev. Genetics*, **10**, 467–77.

Zhao, T., Zhang, Z. N., Rong, Z. and Xu, Y. 2011. Immunogenicity of induced pluripotent stem cells. *Nature*, **474**, 212–15.

Zwaka, T. P. and Thomson, J. A. 2005. A germ cell origin of embryonic stem cells? *Development*, **132**, 227–33.

2

Induced pluripotent stem cells

Akitsu Hotta and Shinya Yamanaka

2.1 Introduction to iPS cells

Induced pluripotent stem cells, or iPS cells, have quite similar characteristics to embryonic stem (ES) cells, such as pluripotency and unlimited self-renewal, yet can be derived from somatic cells without using embryos [1]. "Pluripotency" is defined as the ability to differentiate in response to extrinsic cues into all somatic lineages that comprise the entire body, including the germ line. An unlimited self-renewal capacity allows a large amount of stem cells to be cultured and grown in the laboratory. Such unique cell identities are programmed in the gene-expression patterns and epigenetic modification patterns of ES cells, and are quite different from other somatic cells. However, the somatic cells can be "reprogrammed" to confer ES cell-like pluripotency by introducing a cocktail of genes (so-called reprogramming factors) - typically Oct4, Sox2, Klf4, and c-Myc. Therefore, iPS cells hold great promise not only for basic biological studies of cell-fate decisions, but also for medical applications. In this chapter, we first summarize a number of methodologies developed to derive iPS cells, and later discuss the recent progress and challenges in the clinical application of iPS cells.

2.2 Cells of origin

Many different types of somatic cells have been reprogrammed to pluripotency to generate iPS cells (Table 2.1). Fibroblasts were the first cell type to be reprogrammed [2, 3], and are one of the most widely used cell types so far, because of the well-established culture conditions, distinct morphology from ES cells, high susceptibility to retroviral vector transduction, and their innate ability to serve as feeder cells. Some particular cell types, especially somatic stem cells or progenitor cells, express a number of reprogramming factors endogenously, which presumably allows low-level transduction of some exogenous reprogramming factor(s). For example, adult neural stem cells [4] and dermal papilla cells [5] endogenously express Sox2 and c-Myc, which allows iPS cells to be derived using only two reprogramming factors (i.e. Oct4 and Klf4), although the resulting reprogramming efficiency is lower than that obtained for cells reprogrammed using the four factors. Keratinocytes are an attractive cell source because of their higher reprogramming efficiency [6]. However, the cultivation and expansion of keratinocytes is challenging [7]. In the hematopoietic lineage, the differentiation stage of the cells influences the efficiency of their reprogramming. Hematopoietic stem/progenitor cells generate iPS cells better than do terminally differentiated B and T cells [8].

There are many choices available regarding the origin of cells to generate iPS cells, but there has been debate about which cell type would be the best for generating clinically relevant iPS cells. There is no simple answer to this question, but the following aspects have to be taken into consideration: the accessibility of the cells, burden on the patient during acquisition, robustness of culture, genetic stability, and ease of reprogramming. For example, some somatic stem cells, such as neural stem cells in the brain, reprogram efficiently, but are rarely accessible during normal

Table 2.1 Cell of origin for iPS cell derivation

Type	Cell name	Original tissue	Remarks	Reference
Amniotic fluid (AF)	AF/CVS cells	Amniotic fluid/chorionic villus sampling		[9]
	AFDCs (AF-derived cells)	Amniotic fluid		[10]
	AF skin cells	Amniotic fluid		[11]
Blood	Mobilized $CD34^+$ hematopoietic stem/ progenitor cells	Human peripheral blood		[12]
	T lymphocytes	Heparinized human peripheral blood, Ficoll-Hypaque density gradient and $CD3^+$ isolation, IL-2 and anti-CD3 antibody activation		[13]
	T lymphocytes	Human peripheral blood, $CD34^+$, mononuclear cells (PBMCs), Ficoll-Hypaque density gradient		[14]
	T lymphocytes	Heparinized human peripheral blood, Ficoll-Hypaque density gradient and $CD3^+$ isolation, IL-2 and anti-CD3 antibody activation		[15]
	Mononuclear (MNC) blood cells (mature peripheral blood T and myeloid cells)	Human peripheral blood, Ficoll-Hypaque density gradient, IL-7/G-CSF, GM-CSF, IL-3, IL-6	Lower efficiency than fibroblasts	[16]
Bone marrow	B lymphocyte	Mouse bone marrow/spleen	OSKM + C/EBPα or OSKM + shPax5	[17]
	Adult bone marrow mononuclear cells (BM MNCs)	Mouse bone marrow		[18]
Brain	Adult neural stem cells	Mouse	Oct4 + Klf4 or Oct4 + c-Myc is sufficient to reprogram	[19]
	Adult neural stem cells	Mouse	Oct4 alone is sufficient (but results in low chimerism)	[20]
	Astrocytes	Human cerebral tissue	Higher efficiency than fibroblasts	[21]
	Meningiocytes	Newborn mouse meningeal membrane in skull		[22]
Embryo	Mouse embryonic fibroblasts (MEF)	E12.5–14.5 embryo		[2]
Fat	Adult human adipose stem cells	Lipo-aspiration	Feeder-free	[23]
	Adipose-derived mesenchymal stem cells	Mouse stromal vascular fraction (SVF) from white adipose tissue/ human white preadipocytes (hWP) and adipose-derived mesenchymal stem (hADS) cells	ADSCs can serve as feeders	[24]

Table 2.1 (cont.)

Type	Cell name	Original tissue	Remarks	Reference
Liver	Primary hepatocytes	Mouse liver	Albumin-expressing hepatocytes, low mortality of chimeric mice	[25]
Pancreas	Pancreatic beta cells	Mouse pancreatic islet	Insulin-positive beta cells	[26]
Skin	Tail-tip fibroblasts	Mouse tail		[2]
	Human dermal fibroblasts (HDFs)	Foreskin, skin biopsy		[3]
	Keratinocytes	Foreskin epidermis/plucked human hair	Higher efficiency than fibroblasts	[6]
	Dermal papilla cells	Mouse	Oct4 + Klf4 is sufficient to reprogram	[5]
	Melanocytes	Mouse epidermis/R545 mouse melanoma cells, human foreskin	Higher efficiency than fibroblasts, Sox2 dispensable	[27]
Stomach	Gastric epithelial cells	Mouse stomach	Low mortality of chimeric mice	[25]
Tooth	Mesenchymal-like stem/progenitor cells of dental tissue	Stem cells from exfoliated deciduous teeth (SHED), stem cells from apical papilla (SCAP), and dental pulp stem cells (DPSCs).		[28]
	Dental pulp cells	Extracted teeth		[29]
Umbilical cord	Cord blood	$CD133^+$ mononuclear cells from human umbilical cord blood	Oct4 + Sox2 is sufficient to reprogram	[30]
	Human cord blood (CB)-derived endothelial cells (ECs)	High expression of endothelial markers (CD31, CD146) and no expression of monocyte markers (CD45, CD14)		[31]

circumstances. Other tissue samples may be available in the case of surgery or samples from clinical testing. Cord blood and peripheral blood have been collected and stored in established cell banks. Such existing banks should be useful for initiating iPS cell banks.

2.3 Factor delivery

In the first iPS cell derivation experiment, a retroviral vector was used to introduce the reprogramming factors, because of its high co-transduction efficiency and nature of self-inactivation in stem cells due to transcriptional silencing [2]. Since this first demonstration, many different methods have been developed to introduce the reprogramming factors, such as lentiviral vectors, adenoviral vectors, *piggyBac* transposon vectors, Sendai viral vectors, plasmid (minicircle) vectors, and episomal vectors, as well as non-DNA-based methods such as protein transduction or RNA transduction (Table 2.2). There are advantages and disadvantages for each of these methods.

For in-vitro use, such as disease modeling and drug screening, practically any method can be used, so long as full pluripotency is demonstrated by the stringent tests available [32]. Retroviral vectors are still the primary method used to derive iPS cells for in-vitro use, since their high transduction efficiency allows

Table 2.2 The delivery methods used to generate human iPS cells

Type	Vector	Form in target cells	Reprogrammed cell types	Reference
Virus	Retroviral vector	Integration into chromosomes	Many cell types	[3]
	Lentiviral vector	Integration into chromosomes	Many cell types	[33]
	Adenoviral vector	Viral linear dsDNA in the nucleus	Human embryonic fibroblasts	[34]
	Sendai virus vector	Viral ssRNA in the cytoplasm	Human dermal fibroblasts, human activated T cells	[35]
DNA	Episomal plasmid	Episomal circular dsDNA	Newborn foreskin fibroblasts, human dermal fibroblasts, dental pulp cells	[36, 37]
	piggyBac transposon vector	Integration into chromosomes, removable by expression of transposase	Mouse embryonic fibroblasts, human embryonic fibroblasts	[38–40]
	Minicircle vector	Supercoiled circular dsDNA	Human adipose stem cells	[41]
Protein	Protein	Tagged protein transported into the nucleus	Human newborn fibroblasts	[42]
RNA	mRNA	Messenger RNA	hESC-derived fibroblasts, human fetal fibroblasts, neonatal foreskin fibroblasts, skin fibroblasts	[43]
	miRNA	Micro RNA	Mouse and human adipose stromal cells, human dermal fibroblasts	[44]

reproducible generation of many clones, retroviral silencing serves as a marker of full reprogramming, and random integrations into chromosomes allow one to distinguish individual iPS cell clones, and thus avoid cross-contamination.

When considering the medical applications of stem cells, safety is the first and foremost issue. The risk of each method needs to be evaluated, ensuring the patient's safety. First, permanent integration of reprogramming factors, especially by retroviral and lentiviral vectors, carries the risk of insertional mutagenesis, potentially leading to the reactivation of inactive oncogenes or the disruption of tumor-suppressor genes. Reactivation of the reprogramming factors themselves could also lead to an increased risk of tumorigenesis, since reprogramming factor combinations often contain well-known oncogenes (such as c-Myc). Re-reprogramming after differentiation or resistance to differentiation is also a possibility, which may lead to teratoma formation. In this regard, non-integrating methods would be preferable to generate iPS cells intended for transplantation. At the same time, proper induction of full reprogramming is of foremost importance, because partially or inadequately reprogrammed cells have a much higher tumorigenic propensity. To avoid improper reprogramming, it is important to maintain high-level expression of the reprogramming factors for a sufficient duration (i.e. 1–2 weeks or longer). Possible cell damage and genomic instability due to repeated transfection should also be taken into account. To consolidate the reprogramming method for clinical use, further optimization of the transduction methods, or refinement of the factor combinations, will be necessary.

2.4 Reprogramming factors

Regarding the reprogramming factors, a cocktail of Oct4 (also known as Pou5f1), Sox2, Klf4, and c-Myc was initially used for iPS cell generation, but subsequent studies have identified dozens of factors that can replace one of these four, or can be used in combination to enhance the reprogramming efficiency (Table 2.3). For instance, other Sox family members (Sox1, 3, 15, 17, or 18) can replace Sox2, Klf family

Table 2.3 Additional reprogramming factors that have been reported

Introduced gene	Gene name	Remarks	Species	Reference
p53 (Trp53) deficiency	(i.e. p53 shRNA, dominant negative form, or genetic knockout)	Increased efficiency	Mouse and human	[49–53]
Mdm2	Transformed mouse 3T3 cell double minute 2	Increased efficiency	Human	[49]
p21 shRNA, p19 Arf shRNA, or 16 Ink4a shRNA		Increased efficiency	Mouse	[50]
Bcl2	B-cell leukemia/lymphoma 2	Increased efficiency	Mouse	[50]
Sall4	Sal-like 4 (Drosophila)	Increased efficiency	Mouse and human	[54]
Cdh1 (E-cadherin)	Cadherin 1, type 1, E-cadherin (epithelial)	Increased efficiency	Mouse	[55]
PRC2 complex	Jarid2, Mtf2, and esPRC2p48 (E130012A19Rik)	Increased efficiency	Mouse	[56]
lincRNA-RoR	Large intergenic non-coding RNA	Increased efficiency	Human	[57]
miR-93, miR-106b, miR-17, or miR-106a	Micro RNA	Increased efficiency	Mouse	[58]
miR-302b and miR-372	Micro RNA	Increased efficiency	Human	[59]
n-Myc	Myelocytomatosis oncogene	Replaced c-Myc	Mouse	[45, 47]
L-Myc	Myelocytomatosis oncogene	Replaced c-Myc	Mouse and human	[45, 48]
Tbx3	T-box 3	Replaced c-Myc	Mouse	[60]
Utf1 and p53 shRNA	Undifferentiated embryonic cell transcription factor 1	Replaced c-Myc	Mouse	[61]
Rem2	RAS (RAD and GEM) like GTP binding 2	Replaced c-Myc	Human	[62]
Yap1	Yes-associated protein	Replaced c-Myc	Mouse	[63]
miR-291–3p, miR-294, miR-295, or miR-302d	Micro RNA	Replaced c-Myc	Mouse	[64]
Klf2 or Klf5	Kruppel-like factor family	Replaced Klf4	Mouse	[45, 46]
Esrrb, or Esrrg	Estrogen-related receptor, beta/ estrogen-related receptor, gamma	Replaced Klf4 or c-Myc	Mouse	[46]
Glis1	GLIS family zinc finger 1	Replaced Klf4 or c-Myc	Mouse and human	[65]
Nanog and Lin28	Nanog homeobox/lin-28 homolog (*C. elegans*)	Replaced Klf4 and c-Myc	Human	[33]
SV40 large T antigen		Replaced Klf4 and c-Myc	Human	[66]
Sox1, Sox3, Sox15, Sox17, or Sox18	SRY-box containing gene family	Replaced Sox2	Mouse	[48]
Prmt5	Protein arginine methyltransferase 5	Replaced Sox2 and c-Myc	Mouse	[67]
Nr5a2, Nr1i2, or Nr5a1	Nuclear receptor subfamily	Replaced Oct4	Mouse	[68]
Tcl1a	T-cell leukemia/lymphoma protein 1A	Replaced Oct4	Human	[69]
miR-302/367 cluster	miR-302a, miR-302b, miR-302c, miR-302d, and miR-367	Replaced Oct4, Sox2, Klf4, and c-Myc	Mouse and human	[70]
miR-200c, miR-302s, and miR-369s	Micro RNA	Replaced Oct4, Sox2, Klf4, and c-Myc	Mouse and human	[44]

members (Klf2 or Klf5) can replace Klf4 [45, 46], and Myc family members (n-Myc or L-Myc) can replace c-Myc [47, 48]. The question comes down to which combination of genes is the best for iPS cell generation, since the choice of factor combinations can alter the characteristics of the resultant iPS cells. For instance, simply omitting c-Myc from the four-factor combination not only reduces the efficiency of iPS cell induction, but also alters the iPS cell characteristics, and, in mice, significantly reduces their capacity for germline transmission [45, 48]. A comprehensive and combinatorial evaluation would be required in order to better understand the effects of factor combinations.

It is of note that two independent groups recently reported the generation of iPS cells by the introduction of ES cell-specific microRNAs (miRNAs), without the use of gene transduction [44, 70]. These miRNAs are members of an endogenous small RNA family, generally associated with translational inhibition and/or degradation of protein-coding mRNAs. Successful induction of iPS cells with miRNAs suggests that either suppression of key gene networks is sufficient for inducing pluripotency (i.e. suppression of suppressors can indirectly activate genes) or some miRNAs may function to activate genes. Further studies will be required in order to elucidate the mechanisms of miRNA-mediated reprogramming.

2.5 Selection of good-quality iPS cells

Because of the heterogeneous and stochastic process of iPS cell induction, some selection process is essential in order to establish high-quality iPS cells. In mouse iPS cell induction experiments, transgenic mice with a reporter gene (i.e. fluorescent protein or antibiotic resistance gene) are used to identify and enrich for cells that have activated pluripotency-associated genes. In the derivation of first-generation iPS cells, the expression of Fbx15 was used as a reporter. However, many of these cells were found to be incompletely reprogrammed. Subsequent studies showed that Oct4 and Nanog are more determinate markers to identify iPS cells [71–73]. For human experiments, cell morphology [3], live-cell staining with cell surface markers such as TRA-1-81 [74], live imaging techniques [75], and transgenic reporter systems [76] have all been used to establish iPS cell clones. To assess the successful reprogramming of somatic cells to a pluripotent state, it is essential to analyze multiple markers in comparison with their expression in native ES cells. The expression of late-onset markers activated during the end stages of reprogramming (i.e. Nanog, Oct4, or Rex1) serves as a more stringent criterion than that of early-onset markers (i.e. alkaline phosphatase or Fbx15).

Retroviral silencing may be used to assess the full reprogramming of both mouse and human iPS cells, although this requires the use of retroviral transduction for factor delivery, or of integrated reporters. The phenomenon of transcriptional suppression of Moloney-murine leukemia virus (MoMLV) in pluripotent stem cells and early embryos has been known for 30 years, yet it seems that additional unidentified silencing mechanisms exist, since lentiviral vectors are also silenced after iPS cell induction [77]. One must analyze dozens of clones in order to identify an iPS cell clone in which all the retroviral transgenes are completely silenced, but such a clone tends to be of better quality than the other clones expressing reprogramming transgenes even at a low level. Removal of transgenes by recombination technology (such as Cre-loxP or *piggyBac* transposase) is an elegant system to excise transgenes and prevent long-term factor expression, although additional cloning steps are required [38, 40, 78]. It remains unknown whether artificially removed clones are equivalent to naturally silenced clones.

2.6 Issues and challenges for future applications

2.6.1 Tumorigenicity

Differentiated cells from pluripotent stem (ES/iPS) cells have potential therapeutic value; however, residual undifferentiated cells are oncogenic and problematic for cell transplantation therapy. If undifferentiated pluripotent stem cells are injected into immunodeficient animals, the cells may grow into a cell mass with randomly differentiated tissue structures, forming an encapsulated tumor, or teratoma. Teratoma formation is often used as an assay to test the pluripotency of iPS cells in vivo; however, measures must be taken to avoid this happening in a patient. From animal experiments, we know that, even if only a small percentage of contaminating undifferentiated cells persists, there is a substantial risk of teratoma formation [79, 80]. Importantly, the level of residual undifferentiated cells tends to correlate with the initial quality of iPS cells. Therefore, it is critical to develop a solid and secure method to derive high-quality iPS cells [79]. Complementary to this, it is necessary to establish efficient and robust differentiation protocols to reduce the propensity for undifferentiated cell contamination, or to provide reliable and reproducible cell purification methods to isolate differentiated cells prior to transplantation.

2.6.2 Heterogeneity: culture artifact or characteristic in nature?

In general, iPS cells can be derived from somatic cells by introducing a cocktail of reprogramming factors. The establishment of iPS cell lines itself is technically simple and highly reproducible by laboratories around the world. However, there are considerable quality variations among the established iPS cell lines depending on the derivation method and the culture conditions. Introduction of a set of reprogramming factors does not necessarily guarantee the acquisition of full pluripotency, since the transition from a somatic cell to a pluripotent state involves several hurdles that are associated with dynamic cellular and epigenetic changes. It is important to study the partially reprogrammed cells that fail to pass these hurdles in order to better understand the reprogramming process, since there may be opportunities to use these metastable cells to direct them toward particular cell lineages. However, from the perspective of clinical application, it is important to establish iPS cells that closely resemble ES cells; in this way we can easily adapt iPS cells to the culture conditions, assay methods, and differentiation protocols established for ES cells.

We still do not fully understand the heterogeneity of iPS cells, since ES cell culture itself is known to be heterogeneous [81], even though the cell sources (early embryo) and derivation methods (outgrowth) between ES cell lines are less variable than those of iPS cells. It could simply be that the heterogeneity of pluripotent stem cells is a reverse side of cell plasticity, but further studies are needed in order to elucidate the differences between ES and iPS cells for practical use.

2.6.3 Immunogenicity

As long as the cells are derived from the patient him/herself, it is reasonable to assume that autologously transplanted cells would not encounter serious immune rejection, compared with allogeneic transplantation. However, the reality might not be so simple. The cultivation of iPS cells or ES cells generally requires animal products (i.e. serum or serum replacement) in media to support cell growth. To provide proper cell surface matrix and growth factors, mouse embryonic fibroblasts (MEFs) are often used as feeder cells. However, co-culture of human cells with mouse cells or animal products may transfer unknown pathogens or endogenous antigens to the cells. In fact, Martin *et al.* showed that human ES cells maintained on MEF feeders with regular ESC media incorporate non-human-type sialic acid Neu5Gc [82].

To ensure that they are non-immunogenic and to improve their safety for personalized medicine, iPS cells have to be cultured without animal products. Lamin-rich soluble basement membrane extracted from EHS sarcoma (termed "Matrigel™") is a well-established material for feeder-free culture, but it has a poorly defined composition and is non-human in origin. For human iPS cell derivation, the use of autologous feeder cells [83] and xeno-free conditions (recombinant proteins and human materials) [84] should be considered in order to avoid contamination with animal products. In fact, human iPS cells derived under animal-product-free conditions showed no detectable level of non-human sialic acid Neu5Gc [85]. Recent reports have demonstrated more defined culture surfaces for human ES cell culture, including recombinant human laminin-511 protein [86], synthetic acrylate surfaces conjugated with peptides from vitronectin or bone sialoprotein [87], the synthetic polymer PMEDSAH [88], and combinatorial polymers [89]. Such defined surfaces are an attractive solution for culture prior to clinical applications, but new technology will need to be tested on several iPS cell lines to ensure that these technologies provide reproducible results.

2.6.4 Genetic stability

Cultivating cells in a dish is an artificial environment, and is different from the in-vivo situation. It has long been known that routine cell culture can induce genetic mutations. Exploring this possibility, recent reports have demonstrated that some human iPS cells acquire de-novo mutations in exons [90], copy-number variations (CNVs) [91–93], or chromosomal abnormalities [94]. The aberration of chromosomes is an ultimate case of genomic instability, and such cells should not be used for clinical applications. Single-nucleotide polymorphisms (SNPs) and gain or loss of small genomic locus (CNVs) are the major genetic variations present among individuals, and even healthy individuals have some level of genetic mutation. The risk of such genetic mutations associated with cellular reprogramming or long-term culture remains to be determined, especially if the safety and functionality of the end products is to be maintained. Keeping the passage number low to minimize the cultivation time is a basic and fundamental technique for any cell culture, however, in the case of iPS cell derivation, early-passage iPS cells might not yet be fully reprogrammed [95]. Faster reprogramming kinetics might be better in this context; however, rapid changes in cell state may enhance genetic instability. Further studies are needed in order to evaluate this point.

2.7 Disease modeling and drug screening

The ability to generate an unlimited supply of patient-derived, disease-relevant cell types is the most important aspect of iPS cell technology. To study disease mechanisms and drug efficacy, in-vitro cell models are of the utmost importance for many researchers. Since iPS cells can be derived from easily accessible somatic cells (such as skin or peripheral blood cells), there are tremendous ongoing efforts to establish iPS cell lines from patients who suffer from severe genetic diseases. Such iPS cell lines, so-called "disease iPS cells" or "patient-specific iPS cells," can be cultured and maintained in a dish indefinitely, and, furthermore, they may also be differentiated into the affected cell type for a given disease.

As listed in Table 2.4, over two dozen papers have reported in-vitro disease modeling using iPS cells within the past few years. So far, these disease-modeling studies have shown the proof of principle that iPS technology can recapitulate disease genotypes and many phenotypes that are mainly known from previous studies. Disease modeling is not trivial, in so far as there are many challenges regarding recapitulation of disease phenotypes in vitro, such as the differentiation of iPS cells into the desired cell type, the maturation and aging of differentiated cells to recapitulate late-onset diseases, and the development of appropriate control cells for comparison [96]. Monogenic and cell-autonomous effects are relatively easy to recapitulate in a culture dish; however, there are numerous diseases that are caused by complex and multiple genetic factors, non-cell-autonomous effects, and/or environmental factors. As cell differentiation protocols and genetic manipulation tools improve, we should eventually be able to overcome these issues.

Once disease-associated phenotypes have been recapitulated using patient-derived cells, it will be possible to begin testing the efficacy of potentially therapeutic drugs in vitro. Not only does this entail screening newly synthesized drugs, but also we can use such cells for toxicology tests in order to minimize the unexpected side effects of therapeutic drugs. The impact on drug development and human health will be enormous. It is our hope that disease-associated iPS cells will lead us to find new treatments that can improve patients' lives in the near future.

2.8 Clinical applications for cell therapy

The clinical application of iPS cells for cell-replacement therapy would be one of the most exciting

Table 2.4 A list of disease models using human iPS cells

Disease	Mutated gene region	Symptoms	Reference
Amyotrophic lateral sclerosis (ALS)	SOD1 heterozygous L144F	Degeneration of motor neurons	[97]
Spinal muscular atrophy (SMA)	Mutation in SMN1 gene	Degeneration of lower α-motor neurons	[98]
Familial dysautonomia	IKBKAP (IkB kinase complex-associated protein)	Disorder of the autonomic nervous system	[99]
Parkinson's disease	Genetic cause unidentified	Degeneration of the central nervous system	[78]
Parkinson's disease	LRRK2 (leucine-rich repeat kinase 2)	Degeneration of the central nervous system	[100]
Rett syndrome	MECP2 (methyl CpG binding protein)	Neurodevelopmental disorder	[101, 102]
Angelman syndrome	Maternal 15q11–13 imprinting, UBE3A	Neurodevelopmental disorder	[103]
Prader–Willi syndrome	Paternal 15q11–13 imprinting, snoRNAs HBII-85	Neurodevelopmental disorder	[103, 104]
Fragile X syndrome	FMR1 (fragile X mental retardation 1)	Neurodevelopmental disorder	[105]
Huntington's disease	Huntingtin (HTT)	Neurodegenerative disorder	[106]
Friedreich ataxia	Extension of a GAA repeat of the FXN gene	Degeneration of sensory neurons in the spinal cord	[107]
Schizophrenia	Genetic cause unidentified	Neurodevelopmental disorder	[108]
Gyrate atrophy	Ornithine-δ-aminotransferase (OAT)	Degeneration of the retinal pigmented epithelium	[109]
Duchenne muscular dystrophy (DMD)	Deletion of exon 4–43 of the DMD (dystrophin) gene	Degeneration of skeletal muscle	[110]
Timothy syndrome (Long-QT syndrome)	CACNA1C (Ca^{2+}-channel, voltage-dependent, L-type, alpha 1C subunit)	Cardiac disorder	[111]
Long QT Syndrome Type 2	KCNH2 (K^{+} voltage-gated channel, subfamily H, member 2)	Cardiac disorder	[112]
Type-I diabetes	Autoimmunity	Degeneration of insulin-producing beta cells of the pancreas	[113]
Hutchinson–Gilford progeria	LMNA (lamin A)	Accelerated aging	[114, 115]
LEOPARD syndrome	PTPN11 heterozygous T468M	Disorders of the skin, skeletal and cardiovascular system	[116]
β-Thalassemia	HBB (β-hemoglobin) misregulation	Anemia due to misregulation of HBB	[9, 117]
Sickle-cell anemia	HBB (β-hemoglobin) mutation	Abnormal red blood cells	[9]
Fanconi anemia	FANCA (Fanconi anemia, complementation group A)	Bone-marrow failure due to DNA instability	[118]
Chronic myeloid leukemia (CML)	Chromosomal translocations	Leukemia	[119]
Down syndrome	Trisomy 21	Defects in cognitive activity and physical growth	[120]

applications of the technology, since it may overcome the issues of donor shortage and immune-system rejection. However, in general, there will be a long and winding road ahead before the clinical application of such cells can be realized. Currently, two clinical trials in the USA have received clearance from the US Food and Drug Administration (FDA) to use derivatives from human ES cells. One trial will use the retinal pigment epithelium derived from human ES cells to treat macular degeneration. A biotechnology company (Advanced Cell Technology Inc.) received FDA clearance for Phase I/II clinical trials for Stargardt's macular degeneration and dry age-related macular degeneration in November 2010 and January 2011, respectively.

In another trial initiated in October 2010, a patient with spinal cord injury was enrolled in the first clinical trial which involved the transplantation of oligodendrocyte progenitor cells derived from human ES cells. The original research paper upon which this trial was based was published in 2005 [121], and the first approval from the FDA was given in January 2009. This Phase I clinical trial, which was initially led by Geron Corporation, is intended to evaluate the safety and tolerability of such cells. Therefore, we should not necessarily expect therapeutic outcomes, but the results of this trial would have a massive impact on any subsequent pluripotent stem-cell-based therapies. If these trials can demonstrate a clinical benefit without severe side effects associated with the use of pluripotent stem cells, it would encourage researchers, patients, and law-makers to move forward with clinical application of iPS cells.

2.9 Direct conversion to bypass the reprogramming process

Successful reprogramming of somatic cells by using only a handful of genes has changed our view of cell plasticity in mammals. The concept of cell reprogramming by a combination of transcriptional factors has been applied to direct cell conversion, such as converting fibroblasts into neurons [122–124], neural progenitors [125], hematopoietic progenitors [126], cardiomyocytes [127], cartilage [128], and hepatocytes [129, 130]. For in-vitro applications, quickly proliferating iPS cells might be more advantageous than somatic cell-based direct conversions, since somatic cells in general have very limited proliferation potential. At this point, it is too early to say whether these technologies are feasible for in-vivo clinical applications, because we still have little information about the nature of these cells.

2.10 Conclusion

iPS cells hold promise as a cell source for regenerative medicine; they can be derived from easily accessible somatic cells, yet can regain the unlimited proliferation and enormous differentiation potential associated with ES cells. Still, we do not fully understand the characteristics and limitations of iPS cells, since it has still only been a few years since the iPS cell technology was first developed. There are many issues that need to be resolved before direct clinical applications can be realized. These issues include artifacts of transgene over-expression, partial reprogramming (including epigenetic memory of the original somatic cells), the heterogeneity of culture, genetic stability over time, and immunogenicity after transplantation. To evaluate these issues, animal models and other cell types, such as embryonic stem cells, remain useful and important. We are still in the process of characterizing and optimizing the methods for inducing iPS cells. It may take several years to see the first results of iPS-cell-based therapy, but we need to continue improving the reprogramming technology in preparation for future clinical applications.

ACKNOWLEDGEMENTS

We thank Drs. Kazutoshi Takahashi and Knut Woltjen for their critical reading of the manuscript, and our lab members for their comments.

REFERENCES

[1] Yamanaka, S. and Blau, H. M. 2010. Nuclear reprogramming to a pluripotent state by three approaches. *Nature*, **465**(7299), 704–12.

[2] Takahashi, K. and Yamanaka, S. 2006. Induction of pluripotent stem cells from mouse embryonic and adult fibroblast cultures by defined factors. *Cell*, **126**(4), 663–76.

[3] Takahashi, K., Tanabe, K., Ohnuki, M. *et al.* 2007. Induction of pluripotent stem cells from adult human fibroblasts by defined factors. *Cell*, **131**(5), 861–72.

[4] Kim, J. B., Zaehres, H., Wu, G. *et al.* 2008. Pluripotent stem cells induced from adult neural stem cells by reprogramming with two factors. *Nature*, **454**(7204), 646–50.

[5] Tsai, S.-Y., Clavel, C., Kim, S. *et al.* 2010. Oct4 and Klf4 reprogram dermal papilla cells into induced pluripotent stem cells. *Stem Cells*, **28**(2), 221–8.

[6] Aasen, T., Raya, A., Barrero, M. J. *et al.* 2008. Efficient and rapid generation of induced pluripotent stem cells from human keratinocytes. *Nature Biotechnol.*, **26**(11), 1276–84.

[7] Aasen, T. and Belmonte, J. 2010. Isolation and cultivation of human keratinocytes from skin or plucked hair for the generation of induced pluripotent stem cells. *Nature Protoc.*, **5**, 371–82.

[8] Eminli, S., Foudi, A., Stadtfeld, M. *et al.* 2009. Differentiation stage determines potential of hematopoietic cells for reprogramming into induced pluripotent stem cells. *Nature Genetics*, **41**(9), 968–76.

[9] Ye, L., Chang, J. C., Lin, C. *et al.* 2009. Induced pluripotent stem cells offer new approach to therapy in thalassemia and sickle cell anemia and option in prenatal diagnosis in genetic diseases. *Proc. Nat. Acad. Sci. USA*, **106**(24), 9826–30.

[10] Li, C., Zhou, J., Shi, G. *et al.* 2009. Pluripotency can be rapidly and efficiently induced in human amniotic fluid-derived cells. *Hum. Mol. Genet.*, **18**(22), 4340–9.

[11] Galende, E., Karakikes, I., Edelmann, L. *et al.* 2010. Amniotic fluid cells are more efficiently reprogrammed to pluripotency than adult cells. *Cell Reprogram.*, **12**(2), 117–25.

[12] Loh, Y. H., Agarwal, S., Park, I. H. *et al.* 2009. Generation of induced pluripotent stem cells from human blood. *Blood*, **113**(22), 5476–9.

[13] Seki, T., Yuasa, S., Oda, M. *et al.* 2010. Generation of induced pluripotent stem cells from human terminally differentiated circulating T cells. *Cell Stem Cell*, **7**(1), 11–14.

[14] Loh, Y. H., Hartung, O., Li, H. *et al.* 2010. Reprogramming of T cells from human peripheral blood. *Cell Stem Cell*, **7**(1), 15–19.

[15] Brown, M. E., Rondon, E., Rajesh, D. *et al.* 2010. Derivation of induced pluripotent stem cells from human peripheral blood T lymphocytes. *PLoS One*, **5**(6), e11373.

[16] Staerk, J., Dawlaty, M. M., Gao, Q. *et al.* 2010. Reprogramming of human peripheral blood cells to induced pluripotent stem cells. *Cell Stem Cell*, **7**(1), 20–4.

[17] Hanna, J., Markoulaki, S., Schorderet, P. *et al.* 2008. Direct reprogramming of terminally differentiated mature B lymphocytes to pluripotency. *Cell*, **133**(2), 250–64.

[18] Kunisato, A., Wakatsuki, M., Kodama, Y. *et al.* 2010. Generation of induced pluripotent stem (iPS) cells by efficient reprogramming of adult bone marrow cells. *Stem Cells Dev.*, **19**(2), 229–38.

[19] Kim, J. B., Zaehres, H., Wu, G. *et al.* 2008. Pluripotent stem cells induced from adult neural stem cells by reprogramming with two factors. *Nature*, **454**, 646–50.

[20] Kim, J. B., Sebastiano, V., Wu, G. *et al.* 2009. Oct4-induced pluripotency in adult neural stem cells. *Cell*, **136**(3), 411–19.

[21] Ruiz, S., Brennand, K., Panopoulos, A. D. *et al.* 2010. High-efficient generation of induced pluripotent stem cells from human astrocytes. *PLoS One*, **5**, e15526.

[22] Qin, D., Gan, Y., Shao, K. *et al.* 2008. Mouse meningiocytes express Sox2 and yield high efficiency of chimeras after nuclear reprogramming with exogenous factors. *J. Biol. Chem.*, **283**(48), 33730–5.

[23] Sun, N., Panetta, N. J., Gupta, D. M. *et al.* 2009. Feeder-free derivation of induced pluripotent stem cells from adult human adipose stem cells. *Proc. Nat. Acad. Sci. USA*, **106**(37), 15720–5.

[24] Sugii, S., Kida, Y., Kawamura, T. *et al.* 2010. Human and mouse adipose-derived cells support feeder-independent induction of pluripotent stem cells. *Proc. Nat. Acad. Sci. USA*, **107**(8), 3558–63.

[25] Aoi, T., Yae, K., Nakagaura, M. *et al.* 2008. Generation of pluripotent stem cells from adult mouse liver and stomach cells. *Science*, **321**, 699–702.

[26] Stadtfeld, M., Brennand, K. and Hochedlinger, K. 2008. Reprogramming of pancreatic Beta cells into induced pluripotent stem cells. *Curr. Biol.*, **18**(12), 890–4.

[27] Utikal, J., Maherali, N., Kulalert, W. and Hochedlinger, K. 2009. Sox2 is dispensable for the reprogramming of melanocytes and melanoma cells into induced pluripotent stem cells. *J. Cell Sci.*, **122**(19), 3502–10.

[28] Yan, X., Qin, H., Qu, C. *et al.* 2010. iPS cells reprogrammed from mesenchymal-like stem/progenitor cells of dental tissue origin. *Stem Cells Dev.*, **19**(4), 469–80.

[29] Tamaoki, N., Takahashi, K., Tanaka, T. *et al.* 2010. Dental pulp cells for induced pluripotent stem cell banking. *J. Dent. Res.*, **89**(8), 773–8.

[30] Giorgetti, A., Montserrat, N., Aasen, T. *et al.* 2009. Generation of induced pluripotent stem cells from human cord blood using OCT4 and SOX2. *Cell Stem Cell*, **5**(4), 353–7.

[31] Haase, A., Olmer, R., Schwanke, K. *et al.* 2009. Generation of induced pluripotent stem cells from human cord blood. *Cell Stem Cell*, **5**(4), 434–41.

[32] Daley, G. Q., Lensch, M. W., Jaenisch, R. *et al.* 2009. Broader implications of defining standards for the pluripotency of iPSCs. *Cell Stem Cell*, **4**, 200–1; author reply 202.

[33] Yu, J., Vodyanik, M. A., Smuga-Otto, K. *et al.* 2007. Induced pluripotent stem cell lines derived from human somatic cells. *Science*, **318**(5858), 1917–20.

[34] Zhou, W. and Freed, C. R. 2009. Adenoviral gene delivery can reprogram human fibroblasts to induced pluripotent stem cells. *Stem Cells*, **27**(11), 2667–74.

[35] Fusaki, N., Ban, H., Nishiyama, A. *et al.* 2009. Efficient induction of transgene-free human pluripotent stem cells using a vector based on Sendai virus, an RNA virus that does not integrate into the host genome. *Proc. Jap. Acad. Ser. B Phys. Biol. Sci.*, **85**(8), 348–62.

[36] Yu, J., Hu, K., Smuga-Otto, K. *et al.* 2009. Human induced pluripotent stem cells free of vector and transgene sequences. *Science*, **324**(5928), 797–801.

[37] Okita, K., Matsumura, Y., Sato, Y. *et al.* 2011. A more efficient method to generate integration-free human iPS cells. *Nature Methods*, **8**(5), 409–12.

[38] Woltjen, K., Michael, I. P., Mohseni, P. *et al.* 2009. piggyBac transposition reprograms fibroblasts to induced pluripotent stem cells. *Nature*, **458**(7239), 766–70.

[39] Kaji, K., Norrby, K., Paca, A. *et al.* 2009. Virus-free induction of pluripotency and subsequent excision of reprogramming factors. *Nature*, **458**(7239), 771–5.

[40] Yusa, K., Rad, R., Takeda, J. *et al.* 2009. Generation of transgene-free induced pluripotent mouse stem cells by the piggyBac transposon. *Nature Methods*, **6**(5), 363–9.

[41] Jia, F., Wilson, K. D., Sun, N. *et al.* 2010. A nonviral minicircle vector for deriving human iPS cells. *Nature Methods*, **7**(3), 197–9.

[42] Kim, D., Kim, C. H., Moon, J. I. *et al.* 2009. Generation of human induced pluripotent stem cells by direct delivery of reprogramming proteins. *Cell Stem Cell*, **4**, 472–6.

[43] Warren, L., Manos, P. D., Ahfeldt, T. *et al.* 2010. Highly efficient reprogramming to pluripotency and directed differentiation of human cells with synthetic modified mRNA. *Cell Stem Cell*, **7**(5), 618–30.

[44] Miyoshi, N., Ishii, H., Nagano, H. *et al.* 2011. Reprogramming of mouse and human cells to pluripotency using mature microRNAs. *Cell Stem Cell*, **8**, 633–8.

[45] Nakagawa, M., Koyanagi, M., Tanabe, K. *et al.* 2008. Generation of induced pluripotent stem cells without Myc from mouse and human fibroblasts. *Nature Biotechnol.*, **26**(1), 101–6.

[46] Feng, B., Jiang, J., Kraus, P. *et al.* 2009. Reprogramming of fibroblasts into induced pluripotent stem cells with orphan nuclear receptor Esrrb. *Nature Cell Biol.*, **11**(2), 197–203.

[47] Blelloch, R., Venere, M., Yen, J. and Ramalho-Santos, M. 2007. Generation of induced pluripotent stem cells in the absence of drug selection. *Cell Stem Cell*, **1**, 245–247.

[48] Nakagawa, M., Takizawa, N., Narita, M., Ichisaka, T. and Yamanaka, S. 2010. Promotion of direct reprogramming by transformation-deficient Myc. *Proc. Nat. Acad. Sci. USA*, **107**(32), 14152–7.

[49] Hong, H., Takahashi, K., Ichisaka, T. *et al.* 2009. Suppression of induced pluripotent stem cell generation by the p53–p21 pathway. *Nature*, **460**(7259), 1132–5.

[50] Kawamura, T., Suzuki, J., Wang, Y. V. *et al.* 2009. Linking the p53 tumour suppressor pathway to somatic cell reprogramming. *Nature*, **460**(7259), 1140–4.

[51] Li, H., Collado, M., Villasante, A. *et al.* 2009. The Ink4/Arf locus is a barrier for iPS cell reprogramming. *Nature*, **460**(7259), 1136–9.

[52] Marion, R. M., Strati, K., Li, H. *et al.* 2009. A p53-mediated DNA damage response limits reprogramming to ensure iPS cell genomic integrity. *Nature*, **460**(7259), 1149–53.

[53] Utikal, J., Polo, J. M., Stadtfeld, M. *et al.* 2009. Immortalization eliminates a roadblock during cellular reprogramming into iPS cells. *Nature*, **460**(7259), 1145–8.

[54] Tsubooka, N., Ichisaka, T., Okita, K. *et al.* 2009. Roles of Sall4 in the generation of pluripotent stem cells from blastocysts and fibroblasts. *Genes Cells*, **14**(6), 683–94.

[55] Chen, T., Yuan, D., Wei, B. *et al.* 2010. E-cadherin-mediated cell–cell contact is critical for induced pluripotent stem cell generation. *Stem Cells*, **28**(8), 1315–25.

[56] Zhang, Z., Jones, A., Sun, C. W. *et al.* 2011. PRC2 complexes with JARID2, MTF2, and esPRC2p48 in ES cells to modulate ES cell pluripotency and somatic cell reprogramming. *Stem Cells*, **29**(2), 229–40.

[57] Loewer, S., Cabili, M. N., Guttman, M. *et al.* 2010. Large intergenic non-coding RNA-RoR modulates reprogramming of human induced pluripotent stem cells. *Nature Genet.*, **42**(12), 1113–7.

[58] Li, Z., Yang, C. S., Nakashima, K. and Rana, T. M. 2011. Small RNA-mediated regulation of iPS cell generation. *EMBO J*, **30**, 823–34.

[59] Subramanyam, D., Lamouille, S., Judson, R. L. *et al.* 2011. Multiple targets of miR-302 and miR-372 promote reprogramming of human fibroblasts to induced pluripotent stem cells. *Nature Biotechnol.*, **29**, 443–8.

[60] Han, J., Yang, H., Zhang, J. *et al.* 2010. Tbx3 improves the germ-line competency of induced pluripotent stem cells. *Nature*, **463**(7284), 1096–100.

[61] Zhao, Y., Yin, X., Qin, H. *et al.* 2008. Two supporting factors greatly improve the efficiency of human iPSC generation. *Cell Stem Cell*, **3**(5), 475–9.

[62] Edel, M. J., Menchon, C., Menendez, S. *et al.* 2010. Rem2 GTPase maintains survival of human embryonic stem cells as well as enhancing reprogramming by regulating p53 and cyclin D1. *Genes Development*, **24** (6), 561–73.

[63] Lian, I., Kim, J., Okazaura, H. *et al.* 2010. The role of YAP transcription coactivator in regulating stem cell self-renewal and differentiation. *Genes Development*, **24** (11), 1106–18.

[64] Judson, R. L., Babiarz, J. E., Venere, M. and Blelloch, R. 2009. Embryonic stem cell-specific microRNAs promote induced pluripotency. *Nature Biotechnol.*, **27**(5), 459–61.

[65] Maekawa, M., Yamaguchi, K., Nakamura, T. *et al.* 2011. Direct reprogramming of somatic cells is promoted by maternal transcription factor Glis1. *Nature*, **474**, 225–9.

[66] Mali, P., Ye, Z., Hommond, H. H. *et al.* 2008. Improved efficiency and pace of generating induced pluripotent stem cells from human adult and fetal fibroblasts. *Stem Cells*, **26**, 1998–2005.

[67] Nagamatsu, G., Kosaka, T., Kawasumi, M. *et al.* 2011. A germ cell-specific gene, Prmt5, works in somatic cell reprogramming. *J. Biol. Chem.*, **286**(12), 10641–8.

[68] Heng, J. C., Feng, B., Han, J. *et al.* 2010. The nuclear receptor Nr5a2 can replace Oct4 in the reprogramming of murine somatic cells to pluripotent cells. *Cell Stem Cell*, **6**(2), 167–74.

[69] Picanço-Castro, V., Russo-Carbolante, E., Reis, L. C. J. *et al.* 2011. Pluripotent reprogramming of fibroblasts by lentiviral-mediated insertion of SOX2, C-MYC and TCL-1A. *Stem Cells Dev.*, **20**(1), 169–80.

[70] Anokye-Danso, F., Trivedi, C. M., Juhr, D. *et al.* 2011. Highly efficient miRNA-mediated reprogramming of mouse and human somatic cells to pluripotency. *Cell Stem Cell*, **8**, 376–88.

[71] Okita, K., Ichisaka, T. and Yamanaka, S. 2007. Generation of germline-competent induced pluripotent stem cells. *Nature*, **448**, 313–317.

[72] Maherall, N., Sridharan, R., Xie, W. *et al.* 2007. Directly reprogrammed fibroblasts show global epigenetic remodeling and widespread tissue contribution. *Cell Stem Cell*, **1**, 55–70.

[73] Wernig, M., Meissner, A., Foreman, R. *et al.* 2007. In vitro reprogramming of fibroblasts into a pluripotent ES-cell-like state. *Nature*, **448**, 318–324.

[74] Lowry, W. E., Richter, L., Yachechko, R. *et al.* 2008. Generation of human induced pluripotent stem cells from dermal fibroblasts. *Proc. Nat. Acad. Sci. USA*, **105**(8), 2883–8.

[75] Chan, E. M., Ratansirintrawoot, S., Park, I. H. *et al.* 2009. Live cell imaging distinguishes bona fide human iPS cells from partially reprogrammed cells. *Nature Biotechnol.*, **27**(11), 1033–7.

[76] Hotta, A., Cheung, A. Y. L., Farra, N. *et al.* 2009. Isolation of human iPS cells using EOS lentiviral vectors to select for pluripotency. *Nature Methods*, **6**(5), 370–6.

[77] Hotta, A. and Ellis, J. 2008. Retroviral vector silencing during iPS cell induction: an epigenetic beacon that signals distinct pluripotent states. *J. Cell Biochem.*, **105**, 940–8.

[78] Soldner, F., Hockemeyer, D., Beard, C. *et al.* 2009. Parkinson's disease patient-derived induced pluripotent stem cells free of viral reprogramming factors. *Cell*, **136**(5), 964–977.

[79] Miura, K., Okada, Y., Aoi, T. *et al.* 2009. Variation in the safety of induced pluripotent stem cell lines. *Nature Biotechnol.*, **27**(8), 743–5.

[80] Wernig, M., Zhao, J. P., Pruszak, J. *et al.* 2008. Neurons derived from reprogrammed fibroblasts functionally integrate into the fetal brain and improve symptoms of rats with Parkinson's disease. *Proc. Nat. Acad. Sci. USA*, **105**(15), 5856–61.

[81] Osafune, K., Caron, L., Borowiak, M. *et al.* 2008. Marked differences in differentiation propensity among human embryonic stem cell lines. *Nature Biotechnol*, **26**(3), 313–15.

[82] Martin, M. J., Muotri, A., Gage, F. and Varki, A. 2005. Human embryonic stem cells express an immunogenic nonhuman sialic acid. *Nature Med.*, **11**(2), 228–32.

[83] Takahashi, K., Narita, M., Yokura, M., Ichisaka, T. and Yamanaka, S. 2009. Human induced pluripotent stem cells on autologous feeders. *PLoS One*, **4**(12), e8067.

[84] Rodriguez-Piza, I., Richaud-Patin, Y., Vassena, R. *et al.* 2009. Reprogramming of human fibroblasts to induced pluripotent stem cells under xeno-free conditions. *Stem Cells*, **28**(1), 36–44.

[85] Hayashi, Y., Chan, T., Warashina, M. *et al.* 2010. Reduction of N glycolylneuraminic acid in human induced pluripotent stem cells generated or cultured under feeder- and serum-free defined conditions. *PLoS One*, **5**(11), e14099.

[86] Rodin, S., Domogatskaya, A., Ström, S. *et al.* 2010. Long-term self-renewal of human pluripotent stem cells on human recombinant laminin-511. *Nature Biotechnol.*, **28**(6), 611–15.

[87] Melkoumian, Z., Weber, J. L., Weber, D. M. *et al.* 2010. Synthetic peptide-acrylate surfaces for long-term self-renewal and cardiomyocyte differentiation of human embryonic stem cells. *Nature Biotechnol.*, **28**, 606–10.

[88] Villa-Diaz, L. G., Nandivada, H., Ding, J. *et al.* 2010. Synthetic polymer coatings for long-term growth of human embryonic stem cells. *Nature Biotechnol.*, **28**, 581–3.

[89] Mei, Y., Saha, K., Bogatyrev, S. R. *et al.* 2010. Combinatorial development of biomaterials for clonal growth of human pluripotent stem cells. *Nature Mater.*, **9**(9), 768–78.

[90] Gore, A., Li, Z., Fung, H. L. *et al.* 2011. Somatic coding mutations in human induced pluripotent stem cells. *Nature*, **471**, 63–7.

[91] Laurent, L. C., Ulitsky, I., Slavin, I. *et al.* 2011. Dynamic changes in the copy number of pluripotency and cell proliferation genes in human ESCs and iPSCs during reprogramming and time in culture. *Cell Stem Cell*, **8**, 106–18.

[92] Hussein, S. M., Batada, N. N., Vuoristo, S. *et al.* 2011. Copy number variation and selection during reprogramming to pluripotency. *Nature*, **471**, 58–62.

[93] Martins-Taylor, K., Nisler, B. S., Taapken, S. M. *et al.*, 2011. Recurrent copy number variations in human induced pluripotent stem cells. *Nature Biotechnol.*, **29**, 488–91.

[94] Mayshar, Y., Ben-David, U., Neta, L. *et al.* 2010. Identification and classification of chromosomal aberrations in human induced pluripotent stem cells. *Cell Stem Cell*, **7**(4), 521–31.

[95] Chin, M. H., Mason, M. J., Xie, W. *et al.* 2009. Induced pluripotent stem cells and embryonic stem cells are distinguished by gene expression signatures. *Cell Stem Cell*, **5**(1), 111–23.

[96] Saha, K. and Jaenisch, R. 2009. Technical challenges in using human induced pluripotent stem cells to model disease. *Cell Stem Cell*, **5**, 584–95.

[97] Dimos, J. T., Rodolfa, K. T., Niakan, K. K. *et al.* 2008. Induced pluripotent stem cells generated from patients with ALS can be differentiated into motor neurons. *Science*, **321**, 1218–21.

[98] Ebert, A. D., Yu, J., Rose, F. F., Jr. *et al.* 2009. Induced pluripotent stem cells from a spinal muscular atrophy patient. *Nature*, **457**(7227), 277–80.

[99] Lee, G., Papapetrou, E. P., Kim, H. *et al.* 2009. Modeling pathogenesis and treatment of familial dysautonomia using patient-specific iPSCs. *Nature*, **461**(7262), 402–6.

[100] Nguyen, H. N., Byers, B., Cord, B. *et al.* 2011. LRRK2 mutant iPSC-derived DA neurons demonstrate increased susceptibility to oxidative stress. *Cell Stem Cell*, **8**(3), 267–80.

[101] Marchetto, M. C. N., Carromeu, C., Acab, A. *et al.* 2010. A model for neural development and treatment of rett syndrome using human induced pluripotent stem cells. *Cell*, **143**(4), 527–39.

[102] Cheung, A. Y., Horvath, L. M., Grafodatskaya, D. *et al.* 2011. Isolation of MECP2-null Rett Syndrome patient hiPS cells and isogenic controls through X-chromosome inactivation. *Human Molec. Genetics*, **20**(11), 2103–15.

[103] Chamberlain, S. J., Chen, P.-F., Ng, K. Y. *et al.* 2010. Induced pluripotent stem cell models of the genomic imprinting disorders Angelman and Prader–Willi syndromes. *Proc. Nat. Acad. Sci. USA*, **107**(41), 17668–73.

[104] Yang, J., Cai, J., Zhang, Y. *et al.* 2010. Induced pluripotent stem cells can be used to model the genomic imprinting disorder Prader–Willi syndrome. *J. Biol. Chem.*, **285**(51), 40303–11.

[105] Urbach, A., Bar-Nur, O., Daley, G. Q. *et al.* 2010. Differential modeling of fragile X syndrome by human embryonic stem cells and induced pluripotent stem cells. *Cell Stem Cell*, **6**(5), 407–11.

[106] Zhang, N., An, M. C., Montoro, D. and Ellerby, L. M. 2010. Characterization of human Huntington's disease cell model from induced pluripotent stem cells. *PLoS Curr.*, **2**, RRN1193.

[107] Liu, J., Verma, P. J., Evans-Galea, M. V. *et al.* 2011. Generation of induced pluripotent stem cell lines from Friedreich ataxia patients. *Stem Cell Rev.*, **7**(3), 703–13.

[108] Brennand, K. J., Simone, A., Jou, J. *et al.* 2011. Modelling schizophrenia using human induced pluripotent stem cells. *Nature*, **473**(7346), 221–5.

[109] Howden, S., Gore, A., Li, Z. *et al.* 2011. Genetic correction and analysis of induced pluripotent stem cells from a patient with gyrate atrophy. *Proc. Nat. Acad. Sci. USA*, **108**, 6537–42.

[110] Kazuki, Y., Hiratsuka, M., Takiguchi, M. *et al.* 2010. Complete genetic correction of iPS cells from Duchenne muscular dystrophy. *Molec. Ther.*, **18**, 386–93.

[111] Yazawa, M., Hsueh, B., Jia, X. *et al.* 2011. Using induced pluripotent stem cells to investigate cardiac phenotypes in Timothy syndrome. *Nature*, **471**(7337), 230–4.

[112] Itzhaki, I., Maizels, L., Huber, I. *et al.* 2011. Modelling the long QT syndrome with induced pluripotent stem cells. *Nature*, **471**(7337), 225–9.

[113] Maehr, R., Chen, S., Snitow, M. *et al.* 2009. Generation of pluripotent stem cells from patients with type 1 diabetes. *Proc. Nat. Acad. Sci. USA*, **106**(37), 15768–73.

[114] Liu, G. H., Barkho, B. Z., Ruiz, S. *et al.* 2011. Recapitulation of premature ageing with iPSCs from Hutchinson–Gilford progeria syndrome. *Nature*, **472** (7342), 221–5.

[115] Zhang, J., Lian, Q., Zhu, G. *et al.* 2011. A human iPSC model of Hutchinson Gilford progeria reveals vascular smooth muscle and mesenchymal stem cell defects. *Cell Stem Cell*, **8**(1), 31–45.

[116] Carvajal-Vergara, X., Sevilla, A., D'Souza, S. L. *et al.* 2010. Patient-specific induced pluripotent stem-cell-derived models of LEOPARD syndrome. *Nature*, **465** (7299), 808–12.

[117] Papapetrou, E. P., Lee, G., Malani, N. *et al.* 2011. Genomic safe harbors permit high beta-globin transgene expression in thalassemia induced pluripotent stem cells. *Nature Biotechnol.*, **29**, 73–8.

[118] Raya, Á., Rodríguez-Pizà, I., Guenechea, G. *et al.* 2009. Disease-corrected haematopoietic progenitors from Fanconi anaemia induced pluripotent stem cells. *Nature*, **460**(7251), 53–9.

[119] Hu, K., Yu, J., Suknuntha, K. *et al.* 2011. Efficient generation of transgene-free induced pluripotent stem cells from normal and neoplastic bone marrow and cord blood mononuclear cells. *Blood*, **117**(14), e109–19.

[120] Park, I.-H., Arora, N., Huo, H. *et al.* 2008. Disease-specific induced pluripotent stem cells. *Cell*, **134**, 877–886.

[121] Keirstead, H. S., Nistor, G., Bernal, G. *et al.* 2005. Human embryonic stem cell-derived oligodendrocyte progenitor cell transplants remyelinate and restore locomotion after spinal cord injury. *J. Neurosci.*, **25** (19), 4694–705.

[122] Vierbuchen, T., Ostermeier, A., Zhiping, P. *et al.* 2010. Direct conversion of fibroblasts to functional neurons by defined factors. *Nature*, **463**(7284), 1035–41.

[123] Caiazzo, M., Dell'Anno, M. T., Dvoretskova, E. *et al.* 2011. Direct generation of functional dopaminergic neurons from mouse and human fibroblasts. *Nature*, **476**, 224–232.

[124] Pfisterer, U., Kirkeby, A., Torper, O. *et al.* 2011. Direct conversion of human fibroblasts to dopaminergic neurons. *Proc. Nat. Acad. Sci. USA*, **108**(25), 10343–8.

[125] Kim, J., Su, S. C., Wang, H. *et al.* 2011. Direct reprogramming of mouse fibroblasts to neural progenitors. *Proc. Nat. Acad. Sci. USA*, **108**(19), 7838–43.

[126] Szabo, E., Rampalli, S., Risueno, R. M. *et al.* 2010. Direct conversion of human fibroblasts to multilineage blood progenitors. *Nature*, **468**(7323), 521–6.

[127] Ieda, M., Fu, J. D., Delgado-Olguin, P. *et al.* 2010. Direct reprogramming of fibroblasts into functional cardiomyocytes by defined factors. *Cell*, **142**(3), 375–86.

[128] Hiramatsu, K., Sasagawa, S., Outani, H. *et al.* 2011. Generation of hyaline cartilaginous tissue from mouse adult dermal fibroblast culture by defined factors. *J. Clin. Investigation*, **121**(2), 640–57.

[129] Huang, P., He, Z., Ji, S. *et al.* 2011. Induction of functional hepatocyte-like cells from mouse fibroblasts by defined factors. *Nature*, **475**(7356), 386–9.

[130] Sekiya, S. and Suzuki, A. 2011. Direct conversion of mouse fibroblasts to hepatocyte-like cells by defined factors. *Nature*, **475**(7356), 390–3.

3

Connective tissue stem and progenitor cells

Pamela Gehron Robey

3.1 History

The concept that post-natal tissues self-renew, and do so by means of a stem/progenitor cell, is not a new one, being based on observations made around 1900, primarily in the field of hematology. While this concept was originally thought to apply to tissues with a high rate of turnover (blood, the gastrointestinal tract, epidermis), studies over the past few decades have demonstrated that virtually all tissues, including connective tissues, have the ability to self-renew, albeit at different rates, depending on the demands imposed upon them [1]. Methods to establish cell cultures in vitro were first attempted in the late 1800s and early 1900s by a number of investigators, namely Bernard, Roux, Harrison, and others [2], but it is Alexis Carrel who is credited with the methodology employed to establish and maintain connective tissue cells in vitro [3]. With subsequent refinements in the following years, connective tissue cell cultures rapidly became an essential tool in cell physiology and molecular biology. Perhaps the first real evidence of stem/progenitor cells within a population of connective tissue cells emerged in the late 1960s, when Alexander Friedenstein and coworkers isolated clones of rapidly adherent bone marrow stromal cells (BMSCs), derived from a single cell, a colony-forming unit-fibroblast (CFU-F). Approximately 10%–20% of single CFU-F-derived strains had the ability to form bone, hematopoiesis-supportive stroma, and marrow adipocytes upon in-vivo transplantation in open systems, and cartilage as well in closed systems. Friedenstein and his collaborator, Maureen Owen, later called these cells "multipotent bone marrow stromal stem cells" [4, 5]; more recently, the term "skeletal stem cell" has been coined [6].

3.2 Connective tissue stem/progenitor cells in tissue engineering and regenerative medicine

Over the last several decades, putative stem/progenitor cells have been isolated from a long list of connective tissues. These cells have been collectively termed "mesenchymal stem cells" or more recently "mesenchymal stromal cells" ("MSCs"), because of their adherence to tissue culture plastic, fibroblastic morphology, and expression of cell surface markers [7]. How similar or dissimilar "MSCs" are from different connective tissues, and whether they are true stem/progenitor cells, is not well known [8]. Nonetheless, these populations may be useful in the reconstruction of connective tissues.

3.2.1 Reconstruction of connective tissues

So, one may ask, are stem/progenitor cells really essential for reconstruction of a given connective tissue? The answer most likely is that sometimes they are and sometimes they are not, and that it depends on the rate of tissue turnover. In tissues that undergo turnover very slowly, if at all (such as cartilage), the use of more mature populations of cells will undoubtedly fit the bill. But, in cases where tissue turnover is required, stem/progenitor cells are a necessary ingredient in any type of construct for long-term efficacy.

While the dynamics of tissue turnover and the need for stem/progenitor cells have been well established for rapidly self-renewing tissues such as blood, skin, and intestine, and for bone, the same is not the case for many connective tissues. In adipose tissue, there are scenarios where the size of adipocytes waxes and wanes without the formation of new adipocytes from stem/progenitor cells, and others where the birth of new adipocytes does occur, depending on the metabolic status of the host [9]. In caries formation in the tooth, when there is a breach in the protective enamel and dentin coating, dental pulp stem cells form reparative dentin [10], but it is not clear to what extent dental pulp and its stem cell undergo turnover with time. The same question of rate of tissue turnover applies to the dermis. While the epidermis undergoes very rapid turnover, it is not clear what the rate is for the more stable dermal layer of skin.

3.2.2 Connective tissue cells in another form of regenerative medicine

While not a topic of this book, strictly speaking, it cannot be ignored that different populations of "MSCs" are currently being tested in another form of regenerative medicine. In this case, cells are being either directly injected into injured tissues or systemically infused. Given the seemingly encouraging results in pre-clinical models, there are numerous Phase I/II clinical trials ongoing around the world with different types of "MSCs" for the treatment of acute GVHD, inflammatory bowel disease, and cardiovascular disease, as a few examples. However, efficacy has been variable. This variability may be due to the source of the "MSCs," how they are expanded in vitro, the route of administration, clinical trial designs, and differences in outcome measures. It remains to be seen whether this type of cell-based therapy will withstand the test of time and critical analyses, and lead to evidence-based changes in current clinical practice. Furthermore, it will be extremely important to determine the timing and mode of delivery, and the mechanism of action (the nature of the cytokines and growth factors needed for a particular indication, whether cell-cell contact is required, etc.).

3.3 Methods of isolation and expansion of connective tissue stem/progenitor cells

Numerous methods have been published for the isolation of cells from virtually every connective tissue in the body, but the methods generally fall into three techniques: (1) aspiration and lavage (bone marrow and bone), (2) explantation, and (3) enzymatic release (Figure 3.1 – A).

While on the surface it would seem that explantation and enzymatic release would result in similar populations of cells, this need not necessarily be the case. Cells that emerge from explant cultures may have different properties (the ability to disassemble surrounding matrix and to migrate) from those that are liberated from matrix enzymatically, and this method may isolate only a subpopulation of cells within the tissue. On the other hand, enzymatic digestion undoubtedly results in a more efficient release of all of the cells present in the tissue, but enzyme preparations may be toxic to certain types of cells. Comparison of the two methods is not often performed, but it has been reported that explants are preferable to enzymatic release in the derivation of adipose-derived stromal cells [11].

For bone, marrow aspiration or extensive lavage of trabecular surfaces is commonly used for isolation of BMSCs [12]. Isolation of BMSCs generally does not require the use of enzymatic digestion of marrow, although enzymatic release has been found to be necessary for optimal isolation of murine BMSCs [13]. While aspirates are less invasive than core biopsies, aspirates are often contaminated with peripheral blood when large volumes are obtained, even with frequent repositioning of the aspiration needle, and excess peripheral blood can have a negative impact on growth of BMSCs [14]. More mature osteogenic cells can be generated by a number of methods, including using a series of enzymatic treatments, or obtained from explant cultures of bone fragments without or with collagenase pre-treatment [12]. While

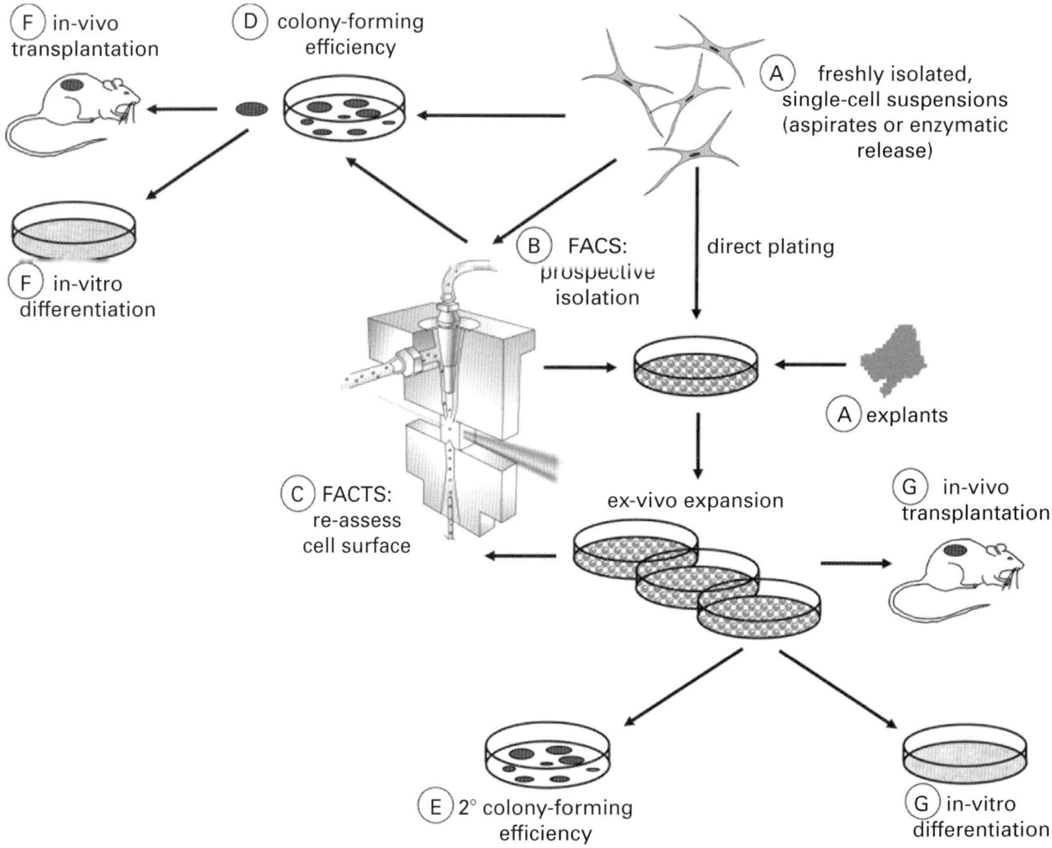

Figure 3.1 Isolation and characterization of connective tissue cell populations.

relatively acellular, explant cultures of cementum have been used to culture cementoblast-like cells [15]. Because dentin is acellular (contains only odontoblastic processes), neither explantation nor enzymatic release can be used. Both explant and enzymatic treatments have been utilized to obtain dental pulp cells and periodontal ligament cells (which form cementum as well as a PDL-like structure). With respect to cartilage, enzymatic digestion is required, however, cells that are released very rapidly undergo dedifferentiation in monolayer culture, and micromass [16], or pellet cultures [17] are required in order for them to maintain their phenotype. Soft tissues, obtained by fine-needle aspiration or by biopsy, are typically cultivated by either explantation or enzymatic release of cells. Numerous variations (too lengthy to list here) on these two types of method have been published for specific tissues.

The efficacy of ex-vivo expansion of connective tissue cells with high quality is highly dependent on the culture conditions. Each particular cell type has its own needs that must be adequately tested, even when growing cells from one animal species to another. Media compositions and supplements can have a profound effect on cell growth. In particular, fetal bovine serum (FBS) often needs to be lot-selected, and, in some cases, it has been shown that heat-inactivation can have a negative effect on cell growth [18]. It would be preferable to be able to substitute FBS with a totally defined cocktail of growth factors and cytokines that will maintain normal cell growth, and some types of supplements are currently available. However, those that adequately support growth are prohibitively expensive, and it is not likely that they could be used in scale-up procedures. Of note, current FDA regulations do not prohibit the use of FBS, but do require that FBS components be eliminated as much as possible during the final stages of clinical-grade cell preparation.

In addition to the media used, the nature of tissue culture plastic varies from one company to another, and can have a dramatic influence on cell growth. One plastic can be better than another, depending on what type of connective tissue cell is being expanded. Atmospheric conditions also cannot be ignored. Depending on the composition and buffering of the medium used, CO_2 levels need to be adjusted to maintain a physiological pH. More recently, it has been determined that O_2 levels also influence cell growth, and it has been suggested that hypoxic conditions (2%) are more amenable to maintaining stem cells within different populations of connective tissue cells than normoxic conditions (20%) [19]. However, more work is needed in this area, and it is likely that different connective stem/progenitor populations have different requirements. With regard to culture conditions, it is apparent that one size does not fit all. While this type of testing would appear to be elementary, it is often not performed. For example, the ex-vivo cultivation of murine BMSCs has very different requirements from that of human BMSCs [20], a fact that is often not recognized. This most likely applies to cells from other tissues as well.

3.4 Characterization

Having established cells in culture, characterization of the cell population and the subset of stem/progenitor cells within it is a critical step in devising procedures for use of the cell populations in tissue engineering. How cells grow in a laboratory setting is not necessarily recapitulated upon scale-up using large numbers of large flasks, cell factories, or bioreactors. Characterization of the efficacy of cell populations generated by large-scale production depends on in-depth analyses, using a variety of assays based on clonal and nonclonal populations of cells.

3.4.1 Cell-surface markers

Cell sorting is essential to define the character of freshly isolated cells (Figure 3.1 – B), but it is not practical to achieve sufficient numbers of cells for connective tissue regeneration by FACS without ex-vivo expansion. Nonetheless, assessment of the cell surface profile after cell expansion does provide key information on the nature of the cell population (Figure 3.1 – C). Owing to the fact that cell surface markers can change in vitro, loss of a marker can be indicative of over-expansion and senescence. A long list of markers has been associated with connective tissue cells ("MSCs") [7, 21]. In addition to being negative for hematopoietic markers, they are also negative for endothelial markers such as CD31 (PECAM-1) and CD62E (E-Selectin). In humans, connective tissue stem/progenitor cells are usually positive (but sometimes inconsistently so) for CD13 (aminopeptidase N), CD29 (β_1 integrin subunit), CD44 (hyaluronan receptor), CD49α (α_1 integrin subunit, VLA), CD63 (lysosomal membrane-associated glycoprotein 3, LAMP3), CD 73 (ecto-5′-nucleotidase), CD90 (Thy-1), CD105 (endoglin), and CD106 (VCAM-1, $\alpha_4\beta_1$ integrin ligand) [21]. Many of these markers are involved in important biological processes, such as cell–matrix interactions (CD29, CD44, CD49a). Some of these markers may be critically important in the biological function of connective tissue stem/progenitors, such as CD105/endoglin, which is the regulatory subunit of the TGF-β receptor that modulates responses to TGF-β. Recent studies have also indicated that it is important to assess expression of CD146 (Muc18, MCAM) [22] and CD106 (VCAM-1) [23], both of which have been suggested to regulate interactions with endothelial cells.

3.4.2 Colony-forming efficiency

It is unlikely that clinical protocols for regeneration of connective tissues would rely on the use of clonal strains due to the number of population doublings that would be required in order to achieve a sufficient number of cells. However, interrogation of a primary population for the presence of potential stem/progenitor cells by performing clonogenic assays is necessary in order to ensure that stem/progenitor cells are present (Figure 3.1 – D). Because of the lack of specific markers to isolate a stem/progenitor cell from more mature cells, an estimate of the number of stem/progenitor cells can be determined by employing the colony-forming efficiency assay. In this assay, single-cell suspensions are plated at low density ($(0.14–14.0) \times 10^3$ nucleated cells/cm^2 for bone marrow aspirates, $(0.007–3.5) \times 10^3$ nucleated cells/cm^2 for bone core biopsies) [21]. When this assay is performed on phenotype-purified BMSCs, or non-bone-marrow cells released from tissues by enzymatic digestion, or initially grown from explants, the clonal density is 1.63 cells/cm^2 due to the fact that hematopoietic cells, which are non-adherent in human samples, are under-represented in soft connective tissues compared with bone marrow. Within 2–3 hours of plating, a single CFU-F adheres, and within 24–48 hours proliferates to form a colony, demonstrating density-independent growth [24]. The colony-forming efficiency for BMSCs ranges from 10–50 per 10^5 nucleated cells, and substantial deviations signify either inadequate culture conditions, or a potential skeletal pathology [25]. For other connective tissues, the colony-forming efficiency is reported to be much higher than for BMSCs and the range is very broad (due to the different culture conditions and plating densities that have been used). However, within a given laboratory, a normal range should be established for connective tissues from normal donors. As in bone marrow, deviations from this normal range would be indicative of either inadequate culture conditions or a pathological condition, and consequently that particular population of cells would not necessarily be appropriate for tissue regeneration. After ex-vivo expansion, colony-forming efficiency can be re-interrogated (second-degree colony-forming efficiency) (Figure 3.1 – E). However, it must be noted that, in the secondary assay, transiently amplifying cells (cells that are more differentiated than stem/progenitor cells, but still proliferative) are also enumerated, and the colony-forming efficiency may appear to increase, but that does not signify an increase in the number of stem/progenitor cells. However, a dramatic decrease or loss of colonies would again signify an undesirable outcome of ex-vivo expansion.

3.4.3 Potency and self-renewal

In characterizing populations of connective tissue cells that may be contemplated for tissue regeneration, it is essential to have an in-depth understanding of the differentiation capacities of the stem/progenitor cell within the population. Differentiation assays performed on the population as a whole (Figure 3.1 – G) are useful in making sure that the stem/progenitor cell within the population has not been lost during ex-vivo expansion. However, clonal analysis and subsequent assays that rigorously demonstrate differentiation potential and self-renewal (the two defining features of a stem cell), are absolutely essential to support the claims that stem/progenitor cells reside within the population (Figure 3.1 – F). Furthermore, as will be presented elsewhere in this book, the scaffold that maybe used in tissue regeneration must be supportive both of the differentiation potential and of self-renewal in order for reconstruction to be successful [12].

3.4.3.1 Differentiation potential

As an example of the required documentation of the existence of a multipotent cell in a connective tissue cell population, evidence has been provided for the existence of multipotent cells in bone marrow stroma [5]. When a series of clonal strains (i.e. the clonal strain arises from a single CFU-F) was transplanted in vivo, only ~10%–20% of the single-cell-derived strains were found to recreate a bone/marrow organ [26]. This points to the fact that multipotent cells are a fraction of the population, and that not all BMSCs, not even all CFU-Fs, are multipotent. That is not to say that the BMSC population, or any other connective cell population, as a whole, with its subset of multipotent cells, is inferior in any way, it is only to say that it is necessary to document the existence of multipotent (or unipotent) stem cells within the population via clonal

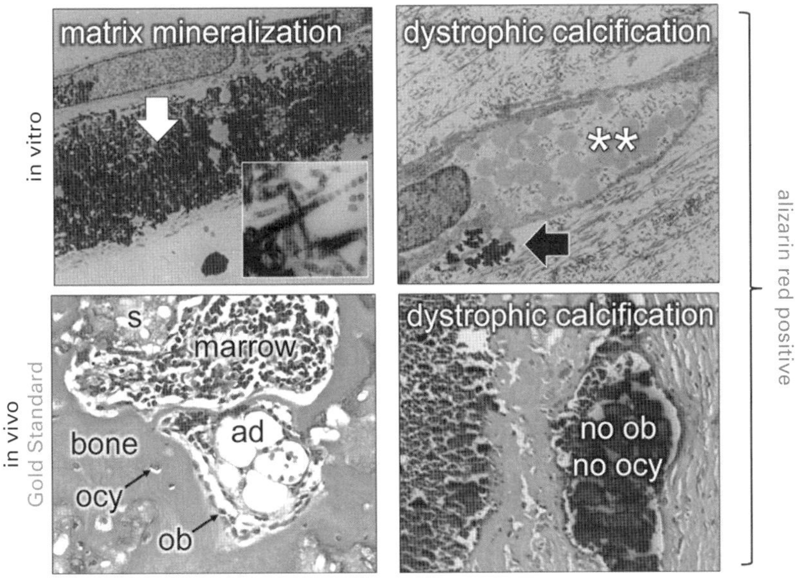

Figure 3.2 Distinguishing features of matrix mineralization and bone formation versus dystrophic calcification, in vitro and in vivo.

analysis (Figure 3.1 – D) and appropriate differentiation assays, which primarily rely on in-vivo transplantation, although, in some cases, in-vitro assays are required (Figure 3.1 – F). These principles can and should be applied to all connective tissue cell populations.

Unfortunately, in-vitro assays that supposedly depict osteogenic and adipogenic differentiation potential have, in most instances, become poor substitutes for in-vivo transplantation. The prolonged treatment of cells at high density with high levels of β-glycerolphosphate can induce dystrophic calcification rather than matrix mineralization [27]. Alizarin red S or von Kossa staining cannot distinguish between dystrophic calcification (induced by dead and dying cells) and matrix mineralization [27]. See Figure 3.2.

The situation is even more complicated when using in-vitro assays to characterize cells that form bone (BMSCs, trabecular bone cells, periosteal cells), in comparison with cells that form dentin (dental pulp cells) or cementum (cementum explants, periodontal ligament cells). In this scenario, true matrix mineralization can be detected in vitro. However, the nature of the mineralized matrix can be assessed only by electron microscopic techniques, not at the light microscope level. The size and shape of apatite crystals and their organization in the organic matrix are quite different in bone, dentin, and cementum, and these differences have an effect on the mechanical properties displayed by each tissue [12].

For adipogenic assays, cells sometimes accumulate lipid from serum components rather than synthesizing them de novo [28], and sometimes this assay can be misleading. For example, dental pulp cells can be induced to form adipocyte-like cells in culture; however, upon in-vivo transplantation, dental pulp cells form dentin and a pulp-like complex, devoid of adipocytes (and, of note, adipocytes in dental pulp have never been documented, even in pathological conditions).

For chondrogenesis, the best assays utilize micromass or pellet cultures, but the results are often reported in terms of alcian blue (which will also stain osteoid) positivity, or safranin O (which is also a nuclear stain in addition to being a cartilage matrix stain). Reliable results for cartilage require histological evidence of chondrocytes lying in lacunae, surrounded

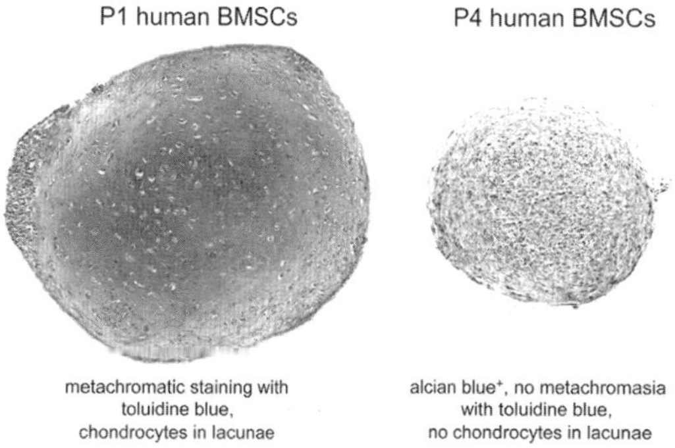

Figure 3.3 Histological determination of cartilage formation by pellet cultures.

by matrix that stains metachromatically (purple) with toluidine blue. See Figure 3.3.

It is due to the over-utilization of these in-vitro assays that one would conclude from the current literature that virtually any connective cell population (clonal or non-clonal) has the ability to form bone, fat, or cartilage. Few researchers have performed in-vivo transplantation assays on cells derived from non-skeletal connective tissues (not treated with BMPs) to show that mineralized matrix (rather than dystrophic calcification) is formed, with osteocytes and osteoblasts of donor origin. Lastly, mRNA expression of some markers indicative of a differentiated cell phenotype is often used as evidence for osteogenic, adipogenic, and chondrogenic phenotype; however, it is often the case that their level of expression is marginal compared with that of BMSCs, and that the pattern of expression does not match the pattern exhibited by BMSCs with time during differentiation. Thus, expression of markers is not sufficient to establish the differentiation potential of the cell population.

It is also difficult to determine what the appropriate differentiation assay would be for other types of adherent, clonogenic fibroblastic cells that are derived from umbilical cord blood or Wharton's jelly, or from different portions of the placenta, or the uterine wall, for example. What would their inherent differentiation capacity be? Without knowing what these cells do in vivo, design of appropriate differentiation assays remains a difficult task.

3.4.3.2 Self-renewal

Evidence of self-renewal of connective tissue stem/progenitors remains to be documented in most instances. It is often stated that extensive ex-vivo proliferation demonstrates self-renewal. However, extensive proliferation does not indicate that the ex-vivo expanded cells have maintained their differentiation capacity, or that they have self-renewed, in the absence of appropriate defining assays. Owing to the solid, rather than fluid, nature of connective tissues, assays of self-renewal are challenging. The most rigorous assay of self-renewal is based on the serial repopulation assay of the hematopoietic system, which serves as a model upon which to base the necessary proof of self-renewal of connective tissue/stem progenitor cells. In this assay, hematopoiesis is ablated either chemically or by irradiation of a recipient mouse, and a purified population of donor hematopoietic stem cells is introduced in order to re-establish hematopoiesis in that mouse. Subsequently, donor hematopoietic stem cells are re-isolated and introduced into a second marrow-ablated recipient, hematopoiesis is re-established, and, again, donor hematopoietic cells are re-isolated [29]. Using this model, a serial transplantation assay has recently been reported to demonstrate the self-renewal of skeletal stem cells [22].

3.5 Sources of connective tissue stem/progenitor cells

There has been great progress in generating connective tissue cell populations for tissue engineering. However, there are two factors, in addition to the tissue source, that must be taken into consideration in protocols for connective tissue regeneration: (1) autologous (self) vs. allogeneic (non-self); and (2) embryonic origin.

3.5.1 Autologous versus allogeneic cell sources

It has been reported that BMSCs (and other "MSCs") are immune-privileged; that is, that BMSCs (and maybe other "MSCs") can escape rejection when used in an allogeneic setting [30]. While this may be true when allogeneic or xenogeneic BMSCs are introduced into developing embryos prior to establishment of the immune system, there are results that indicate that allogeneic and xenogeneic BMSCs are indeed rejected when infused systemically into immune competent recipients [31]. They are even more likely to be rejected when they are induced to differentiate into any differentiated cell type, owing to their expression of histocompatibility antigens. Thus, for regeneration of a differentiated connective tissue, cells will most likely have to be autologous in order to avoid the need for immunosuppression of the recipient.

3.5.2 Embryonic origin of cell sources

With respect to the embryonic origin, as an example, bones in the facial region of the skull derive from neuroectoderm, while those in the axial and appendicular skeleton derive from mesoderm [32], and recent results indicate that cells from these two different embryonic sources are not identical [33]. Oral surgeons have long noted that transplantation of iliac crest (mesodermally derived) into the jawbones (neuroectodermally derived) does not last long-term [34], suggesting some sort of incompatibility. These findings may very well apply to the use of any type of connective stem/progenitor cell population for tissue regeneration. It appears that embryonic origin may matter!

3.5.3 Post-natal sources of connective tissue/stem progenitor cells

As is described elsewhere in this book, there are multiple applications of cells for regeneration of bone (see Chapter 26), dental and periodontal tissues (see Chapters 31–33), cartilage (see Chapter 28), skin (Chapter 34), and tendon and ligament (see Chapter 29).

What has not been covered in this book, but deserves mention, is the case of stem/progenitor cells derived from adipose tissue [35], muscle [36], umbilical cord [37], and stromal-like cells [38, 39] and fibrocytes [40] found in the circulation. However, issues described in this chapter with regard to isolation, characterization, and demonstration of differentiation potential and self-renewal also pertain to these other cell types. In particular, it has been highly touted that adipose-derived stromal cells are a suitable source of cells for bone regeneration. However, the vast majority of the results in support of this claim have come from studies performed in vitro, and, interestingly, it has been reported recently that, in a calvarial critically sized defect, adipose-derived stromal cells did not form bone, but apparently induced cells in the dura mater to do so, and did not persist beyond two weeks [41].

3.6 Summary and conclusions

Great strides have been made in the establishment of cells from different connective tissues, their characterization, and their potential usage in tissue engineering. Rapid progress is being made in moving these studies from the bench to clinical reality. Nonetheless, future studies are needed in order to better understand the biological nature and differentiation capacities of connective tissue stem/progenitor cells. In particular, the field would be better served if one were to focus on the inherent character of local connective tissue stem/progenitor cells, due to the fact that they will most likely be the most reliable source of cells for reconstruction of specific connective tissues. While induced pluripotent cells are on the horizon, it is likely that it will take some time to establish methods for their consistent differentiation into specific cell types. What better cell to teach them how than a tissue-specific post-natal stem/progenitor cell? The more that we know about them, the better we will be able to utilize them.

ACKNOWLEDGEMENTS

This work was supported, in part, by the Division of Intramural Research of the National Institute of Dental and Craniofacial Research, a part of the Intramural Research Program, the National Institutes of Health, Department of Health and Human Services, USA.

REFERENCES

[1] Robey, P. G. 2000. Stem cells near the century mark. *J. Clin. Invest.*, **105**(11), 1489–91.

[2] Witkowski, J. A. 1979. Alexis Carrel and the mysticism of tissue culture. *Med. Hist.*, **23**(3), 279–96.

[3] Carrel, A. 1913. Contributions to the study of the mechanism of the growth of connective tissue. *J. Exp. Med.*, **18**(3), 287–98.

[4] Friedenstein, A. J., Chailakhyan, R. K. and Gerasimov, U. V. 1987. Bone marrow osteogenic stem cells: in vitro cultivation and transplantation in diffusion chambers. *Cell Tissue Kinet.*, **20**(3), 263–72.

[5] Owen, M. and Friedenstein, A. J. 1988. Stromal stem cells: marrow-derived osteogenic precursors. *Ciba Found. Symp.*, **136**, 42–60.

[6] Bianco, P. and Robey, P. G. 2004. Skeletal stem cells. In Lanza, R. P., editor. *Handbook of Adult and Fetal Stem Cells.* San Diego, CA: Academic Press; pp. 415–24.

[7] Dominici, M., Le Blanc, K., Mueller, I. *et al.* 2006. Minimal criteria for defining multipotent mesenchymal stromal cells. The International Society for Cellular Therapy position statement. *Cytotherapy*, **8**(4), 315–17.

[8] Bianco, P., Robey, P. G. and Simmons, P. J. 2008. Mesenchymal stem cells: revisiting history, concepts, and assays. *Cell Stem Cell*, **2**(4), 313–19.

[9] Spalding, K. L, Arner, E., Westermark, P. O. *et al.* 2008. Dynamics of fat cell turnover in humans. *Nature*, **453**(7196), 783–7.

[10] Gronthos, S., Brahim, J., Li, W. *et al.* 2002. Stem cell properties of human dental pulp stem cells. *J. Dent. Res.*, **81**(8), 531–5.

[11] Priya, N., Sarcar, S., Majumdar, A. S. and Sundarraj, S. 2012. Explant culture: a simple, reproducible, efficient and economic technique for isolation of mesenchymal stromal cells from human adipose tissue and lipoaspirate. *J. Tissue Eng. Regen. Med.*, **27**, 1–9.

[12] Robey, P. G. 2011. Cell sources for bone regeneration: the good, the bad, and the ugly (but promising). *Tissue Eng. Part B Rev.*, **17**(6), 423–30.

[13] Suire, C., Brouard, N., Hirschi, K. and Simmons, P. J. 2012. Isolation of the stromal-vascular fraction of mouse bone marrow markedly enhances the yield of clonogenic stromal progenitors. *Blood*, **119**(11), e86–95.

[14] Kharlamova, L. A. 1975. Colony formation inhibition in human bone marrow stromal cells exposed to a factor formed in vitro by peripheral blood leukocytes [in Russian]. *Biull. Éksp. Biol. Med.*, **80**(7), 89–91.

[15] Grzesik, W. J., Cheng, H., Oh, J. S. *et al.* 2000. Cementum-forming cells are phenotypically distinct from bone-forming cells. *J. Bone Miner. Res.*, **15**(1), 52–9.

[16] Langille, R. M. and Solursh, M. 1990. Formation of chondrous and osseous tissues in micromass cultures of rat frontonasal and mandibular ectomesenchyme. *Differentiation*, **44**(3), 197–206.

[17] Angele, P., Kujat, R., Nerlich, M. *et al.* 1999. Engineering of osteochondral tissue with bone marrow mesenchymal progenitor cells in a derivatized hyaluronan–gelatin composite sponge. *Tissue Eng.*, **5**(6), 545–54.

[18] Kuznetsov, S. A., Mankani, M. H. and Robey, P. G. 2000. Effect of serum on human bone marrow stromal cells: ex vivo expansion and in vivo bone formation. *Transplantation*, **70**(12), 1780–7.

[19] Ivanovic, Z. 2009. Hypoxia or in situ normoxia: the stem cell paradigm. *J. Cell Physiol.*, **219**(2), 271–5.

[20] Kuznetsov, S. and Robey, P. G. 1996. Species differences in growth requirements for bone marrow stromal fibroblast colony formation in vitro. *Calcified Tissue Int.*, **59** (4), 265–70.

[21] Bianco, P., Kuznetsov, S., Riminucci, M. and Robey, P. G. 2006. Postnatal skeletal stem cells. *Meth. Enzymol.*, **419**, 117–48.

[22] Sacchetti, B., Funari, A., Michienzi, S. *et al.* 2007. Self-renewing osteoprogenitors in bone marrow sinusoids can organize a hematopoietic microenvironment. *Cell*, **131**, 324–36.

[23] Chou, D. B., Sworder, B., Bouladoux, N. *et al.* 2012. Stromal-derived IL-6 alters the balance of myeloerythroid progenitors during *Toxoplasma gondii* infection. *J. Leukoc. Biol.*, **92**(1), 123–31.

[24] Friedenstein, A. J. 1976. Precursor cells of mechanocytes. *Int. Rev. Cytol.*, **47**, 327–59.

[25] Kuznetsov, S. A., Mankani M. H., Bianco, P. and Robey, P. G. 2009. Enumeration of the colony-forming units–fibroblast from mouse and human bone marrow in normal and pathological conditions. *Stem Cell Res.*, **2** (1), 83–94.

[26] Kuznetsov, S. A., Krebsbach, P. H., Satomura, K. *et al.* 1997. Single-colony derived strains of human marrow stromal fibroblasts form bone after transplantation in vivo. *J. Bone Miner. Res.*, **12**(9), 1335–47.

[27] Bonewald, L. F., Harris, S. E., Rosser, J. *et al.* 2003. Von Kossa staining alone is not sufficient to confirm that

mineralization in vitro represents bone formation. *Calcif. Tissue Int.*, **72**(5), 537–47.

[28] Diascro, D. D, Jr., Vogel, R. L., Johnson, T. E. *et al.* 1998. High fatty acid content in rabbit serum is responsible for the differentiation of osteoblasts into adipocyte-like cells. *J. Bone Miner. Res.*, **13**(1), 96–106.

[29] Szilvassy, S. J., Humphries, R. K., Lansdorp, P. M., Eaves, A. C. and Eaves, C. J. 1990. Quantitative assay for totipotent reconstituting hematopoietic stem cells by a competitive repopulation strategy. *Proc. Nat. Acad. Sci. USA*, **87**(22), 8736–40.

[30] Liechty, K. W., MacKenzie, T. C., Shaaban, A. F. *et al.* 2000. Human mesenchymal stem cells engraft and demonstrate site-specific differentiation after in utero transplantation in sheep. *Nature Med.*, **6**(11), 1282–6.

[31] Eliopoulos, N., Stagg, J., Lejeune, L., Pommey, S. and Galipeau, J. 2005. Allogeneic marrow stromal cells are immune rejected by MHC class I- and class II-mismatched recipient mice. *Blood*, **106**(13), 4057–65.

[32] Olsen, B. R., Reginato, A. M. and Wang, W. 2000. Bone development. *Annu. Rev. Cell Dev. Biol.*, **16**, 191–220.

[33] Akintoye, S. O., Lam, T., Shi, S. *et al.* 2006. Skeletal site-specific characterization of orofacial and iliac crest human bone marrow stromal cells in same individuals. *Bone*, **38**(6), 758–68.

[34] Burnette, E. W., Jr. 1972. Fate of an iliac crest graft. *J. Periodontol.*, **43**(2), 88–90.

[35] Minteer, D., Marra, K. G. and Rubin, J. P. 2013. Adipose-derived mesenchymal stem cells: biology and potential applications. *Adv. Biochem. Eng. Biotechnol.*, **129**, 59–71.

[36] Shadrach, J. L. and Wagers, A. J. 2011. Stem cells for skeletal muscle repair. *Philos. Trans. R. Soc. Lond. B Biol. Sci.*, **366**(1575), 2297–306.

[37] Fan, C. G., Zhang, Q. J. and Zhou, J. R. 2011. Therapeutic potentials of mesenchymal stem cells derived from human umbilical cord. *Stem Cell Rev.*, **7**(1), 195–207.

[38] Kuznetsov, S. A., Mankani, M. H., Gronthos, S. *et al.* 2001. Circulating skeletal stem cells. *J. Cell Biol.*, **153**(5), 1133–40.

[39] Hong, H. S., Lee, J., Lee, E. *et al.* 2009. A new role of substance P as an injury-inducible messenger for mobilization of D29(+) stromal-like cells. *Nature Med.*, **15**(4), 425–35.

[40] Grieb, G., Steffens, G., Pallua, N., Bernhagen, J. and Bucala, R. 2011. Circulating fibrocytes – biology and mechanisms in wound healing and scar formation. *Int. Rev. Cell Mol. Biol.*, **291**, 1–19.

[41] Levi, B., James, A. W., Nelson, E. R. *et al.* 2010. Human adipose derived stromal cells heal critical size mouse calvarial defects. *PLoS One*, **5**(6), e11177.

4

Hematopoietic stem cells and their niches

Geeta Mehta, Yusuke Shiozawa and Russell Taichman

4.1 Introduction

Hematopoietic stem cells (HSCs) are a type of adult stem cell that give rise to all cells in the blood lineage. In adult mammals, they reside in the spongy bone marrow of the long bones. HSCs are not only the most widely studied stem cells, but also the most common cells used in transplantation in the clinic. Since blood is the most commonly transplanted tissue in clinical settings, this makes HSCs an important candidate in establishing better treatments for hematological malignancies.

They have been widely studied for the last 40 years, and the literature on HSCs covers a diverse range of topics. Since it is impossible to cover all aspects of HSC biology in one chapter, here we will focus briefly on the origins of HSCs and their microenvironments, or niches, the isolation methods of HSCs, the standard assays for detection of HSC activity, in-vitro expansion of HSCs, their clinical relevance, and the potential role of the HSC niches in cancer metastases.

4.2 Definition of HSCs

HSCs can self-renew themselves, differentiate into all types of blood cells, mobilize out of bone marrow, and undergo apoptosis. The bone marrow is the classic source of HSCs, along with fetal liver, umbilical cord, aorta-gonad-mesonephros (AGM) region and peripheral blood. About 1 in every 100,000 cells in the marrow is a long-term, blood-forming stem cell; other cells present include stromal cells, stem cells of mesenchymal origin (MSCs), blood progenitor cells, and mature and maturing lymphoid and myeloid cells. Hematopoiesis is the process by which HSCs develop into mature blood cells. According to the monophyletic theory, a single type of stem cell gives rise to all mature blood cells in the body. HSCs divide by all three possible modes of division: asymmetric divisions (one identical stem cell and one daughter), symmetric renewal (two identical stem cells) or symmetric commitment (two daughter cells) [1–4]. The hematopoietic organ includes a range of maturing hematopoietic cells originating from the proliferation, commitment, and differentiation of blood-born HSCs and progenitors, which seed the marrow [5]. Enucleated erythrocytes are one of the progenies of HSCs formed by differentiation of erythroid progenitors, and are turned over every 21 days over the entire lifetime of humans.

Long-term reconstituting HSCs (LT-HSCs), the most primitive HSCs, can both self-renew and differentiate into daughter progenies in the long term, and are thought to be quiescent or slow-cycling cells. These cells self-renew themselves throughout the lifespan of the organism; therefore, they are very important for developing HSC-based cell therapies. They also provide the constant supply of myeloid and lymphoid cells in the marrow, as well as in the circulatory system. Short-term reconstituting HSCs (ST-HSCs), are believed to be actively cycling cells and can sustain hematopoiesis for only a few weeks. LT-HSCs and ST-HSCs create daughter progenies that are multipotent progenitors (MPPs, which can differentiate into multiple lineages), oligopotent progenitors (which can differentiate into more than one lineage), and unipotent progenitors (which can differentiate into only one lineage). HSCs are rather heterogeneous cells, and have complex kinetics of repopulation, with significantly varying ability to create daughter cells of different lineages [6–9]. They can be categorized by the ratio of lymphoid to myeloid progenies that they produce, and classified as myeloid-biased, lymphoid-biased, or balanced. Moreover, each of these specific classes of HSCs creates progenies in which lineage commitment and proliferation rates are driven by epigenetically predetermined factors rather than being stochastic or dependent on the microenvironment [7, 8, 10]. However, the microenvironment around the HSCs is extremely important in their self-renewal and the maintenance of their epigenetic programs, and can also influence the fate choices of myeloid and lymphoid progenies (even though they may be interpreted differently by each of these lineage progenies). Thus, the relationship and balance between cell-intrinsic and cell-extrinsic regulation of HSCs and their progenies will continue to fascinate researchers and clinicians interested in controlling HSC phenotypes.

4.3 HSCs during development

Although the site of the initial emergence of hematopoiesis is highly debated, during ontogeny the mammalian hematopoiesis is accepted to occur in three distinct waves: (1) primitive hematopoiesis, (2) definitive but transient hematopoiesis, and (3) definitive and persistent hematopoiesis established by HSCs. In each of these waves, increasingly mature hematopoietic cells engraft in emerging niches [11, 12]. The first and second hematopoietic waves originate from the yolk sac where common precursors of the hematopoietic and endothelial lineages, called "hemangioblasts," play a crucial role [13–16]. The developing organs that serve as niches for embryonic hematopoiesis and HSCs are shown in Figure 4.1.

The early erythroid and some committed lymphoid precursors appear at the yolk sac and paraaortic splanchnopleura (P-Sp)/AGM region around embryonic day 7 (E7) in mice [17]. By E10.5, the AGM-derived cells have relocated to the fetal liver, which becomes the predominant hematopoietic organ supporting HSCs' expansion. The liver sustains hematopoietic activity throughout the remainder of in-utero development, and serves as a hematopoietic niche all the way up to a few weeks post-natally [18–20]. Spleen and bone marrow also become supportive niches for HSCs apart from the fetal liver, and hematopoiesis fully develops at these sites by E18 [21]. Circulating HSCs from the fetal liver finally make the bone marrow their permanent niche that sustains hematopoiesis throughout adult life [15, 22, 23]. Along with HSCs, other defined stem-cell populations concurrently emerge at the hematopoietic niches.

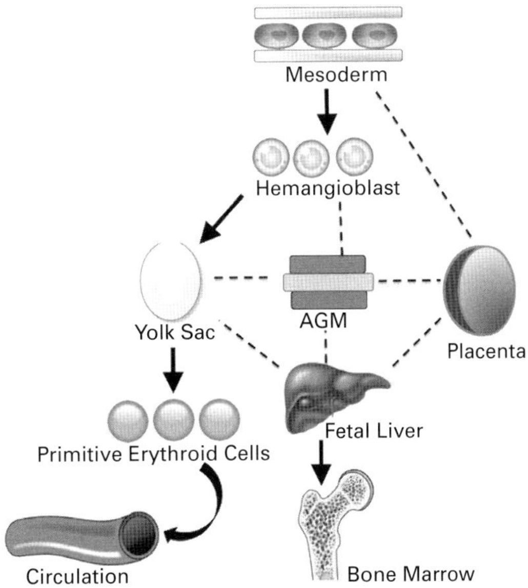

Figure 4.1 HSC Ontogeny: Development of hematopoiesis and HSCs at different anatomic sites (and interactions between these sites) in a fetus. Bipotent hemangioblast progenitors (of hematopoietic and endothelial lineages) arise from mesodermal cells in the embryo. These progenitors migrate into the yolk sac, aorta-gonad-mesonephros (AGM) region, spleen (mice), thymus (humans), and placental regions to give rise to primitive and definitive hematopoiesis. Hematopoietic stem cells are generated in these sites before migrating to fetal liver for expansion, from where they migrate to bone marrow at around the time of birth. Reproduced from [178] with permission of the Nature Publishing Group.

In humans, hematopoiesis is initiated in the yolk sac during the third week of fetal development [24]. Blood starts to circulate in the fetus around day 21 of gestation, followed by emergence of hematopoietic cells in the aorta and viteline artery in the P-Sp and the AGM between 4–6 weeks of gestation. Hematopoiesis appears in the fetal liver by 5 weeks of gestation. The liver sustains hematopoiesis until mid-gestation, when the bone marrow becomes the primary site of hematopoiesis. In humans the spleen is never considered a major hematopoietic organ (unlike in mice). The thymus also develops as a hematopoietic organ in humans and becomes anatomically mature by 15 weeks of gestation [25]. Moreover, the circulating fetal peripheral blood is a source of progenitors and hematopoietic progenitors are observed in circulation by 7 weeks of gestation. Bone marrow hematopoiesis begins by 11 weeks of gestation, and, by 10 weeks after birth, it remains the major HSC niche and hematopoiesis organ [26, 27].

When the adult bone marrow hematopoiesis is compromised due to bone marrow infiltration, hemoglobinopathies, and myeloproliferative disorders, in adult mammals, extramedullary hematopoiesis is established in spleen, liver, muscle, thymus, and adipose tissue [28–34].

4.4 HSC niches

Bone marrow is the primary site of HSCs in adult mammals. Within the marrow discrete areas of residence have been noted for HSCs, areas that have been termed "niches." In vivo the HSC niche is composed of an intricate blend of extracellular matrix (ECM) proteins, soluble protein factors, immobilized protein factors, proteoglycans, small-molecule signals, mineralized tissue, and numerous adjacent cell types, which vary in space and time. These components present the HSCs with biochemical signals, and the HSCs are continually sensing these inputs, processing the signals through signal transduction and gene regulation networks, and executing cell behavioral or fate choices [35–42]. In the secure confines of the bone marrow, HSCs can produce an estimated 500 billion cells per day [43].

The features of an in-vivo HSC niche include a small number of HSCs surrounded by supporting cells, low oxygen tension [44–47], close proximity of HSCs to sinusoidal endothelial cells as well as to osteoblasts on the endosteum, and pericytes and megakaryocytes near the sinusoids, and adhesive and soluble signals between HSCs and surrounding cells [48, 49]. Osteoblasts and other stromal supporting cells (including endothelial cells, pericytes, MSCs, macrophages, megakaryocytes, adipocytes, and fibroblasts) play a central role in hematopoiesis, and produce many factors essential for the survival, self-renewal, and maturation of HSCs [29, 48–53]. Endosteal and perivascular in-vivo bone marrow niches of HSCs are represented in Figure 4.2.

An important feature of the HSC niche is that the cells are arranged in a three-dimensional (3D) structure. In fact, 3D cultures of HSCs have been reported to increase the expansion of HSCs in vitro [54–63]. Some of these studies have included culturing of HSCs on collagen beads, with capillaries of endothelial cells, in porous hydroxyapatite disks, on silk fiber matrices, in porous biomatrix Cellfoam, on collagen-coated porous polyvinyl formal resin, on tantalum-coated porous biomaterial, on porous bovine collagen microspheres, and on 3D bone marrow spheroids [55, 57, 59, 64–69].

The bone marrow ECM is composed of collagen (types I, III, and IV), adhesive proteins (e.g. fibronectin and laminin), and structural macromolecules (e.g. proteoglycans and glycosaminoglycans) [70]. MSCs and fibroblasts make type I and III collagen fibers to create a 3D architecture, on which hematopoietic cells are supported by the matrix proteins (laminin and fibronectin) and proteoglycan-bound growth factors. Many hematopoietic microenvironments exist within the marrow, created by varied interactions of binding proteins, cytokines, and cells, and are conducive to the differentiation of specific lineages and maturational stages of cells [71–74]. HSCs live in intimate connection with the cells and ECM in the bone marrow. Adhesion molecules play a role in mobilization, attachment to the ECM, and in transmitting signals that regulate HSC self-renewal and progenitor differentiation.

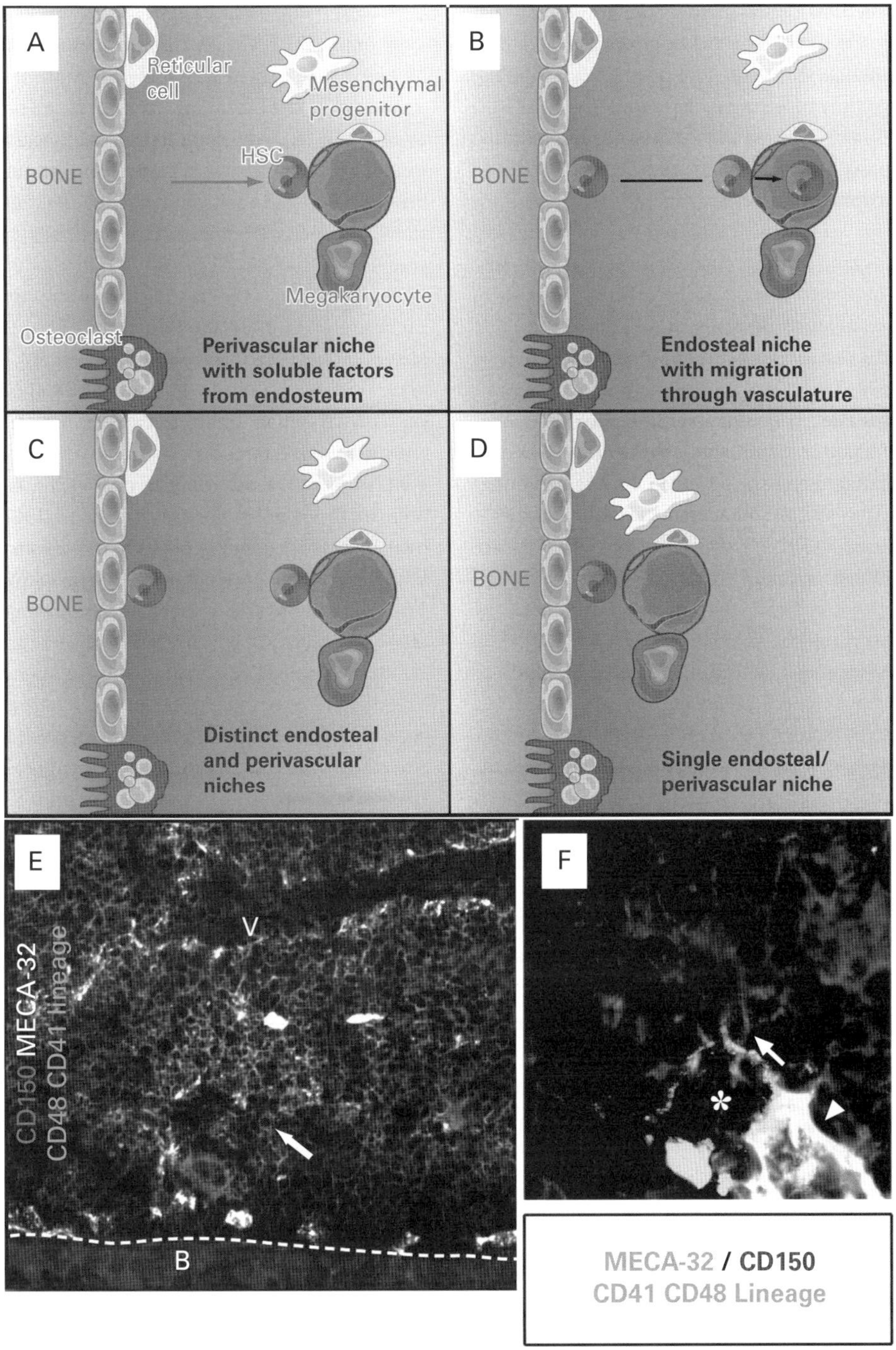

Figure 4.2 HSC niches in the bone marrow. HSCs have been proposed to be close to the endosteal and the perivascular cells in the bone marrow. A, B, C, and D represent different configurations of the HSC niches. (A) HSCs either reside near sinusoids,

In their niches, the rare HSCs are surrounded by a heterogeneous population of supporting cells, which provides them with soluble and adhesive signals. For example, in the mouse bone marrow there is one HSC per 30,000 bone marrow cells. HSCs need supporting cells to provide adhesive and soluble signals and to mediate cellular processes such as self-renewal, proliferation, differentiation, mobilization, homing, and apoptosis. The literature also supports the idea that primitive quiescent HSCs are located in the regions of very low oxygen tension (close to 1%) while the more differentiated progenitors are found at higher oxygen levels [44, 75, 76].

Osteoblasts have been known to regulate HSC activities for a long time [77–79]. Increase in the bone-lining spindle-shaped osteoblasts enhances the HSC number in the marrow, and their depletion mobilized the HSCs to the spleen [80–82]. MSCs, identified using nestin expression, are spatially associated with HSCs, and constitute an essential HSC niche component by highly expressing HSC maintenance genes (SCF, IL-7, OPN, VCAM1, Ang-1, and CXCL12) [40]. Similarly to nestin$^+$ MSCs, adipo-osteogenic progenitors called CXCL12-abundant reticular (CAR) cells support putative HSCs and are found in endosteal and perivascular niches [83, 84]. Moreover, self-renewing CD45$^-$, CD146$^+$ perivascular MSC-like progenitors in the human marrow can generate bone as well as functional marrow when transplanted under the skin of immunodeficient mice [85]. Likewise, CD45$^-$, CD105$^+$ osteoprogenitors can support formation of an HSC niche in a kidney capsule. Calcium-ion receptors on the surfaces of HSCs allow them to follow the Ca^{2+} gradient in response to bone remodeling and navigate their homing to the endosteum [86]. In-vitro studies have demonstrated that the survival of HSCs in co-culture with osteoblasts requires intimate cell-to-cell contact. This suggests that the osteoblast-derived factors that support HSC maintenance are membrane-anchored and/or require the engagement of cell-to-cell adhesion molecules, produced in very small quantities, and are rapidly turned over [87]. As an example, survival of HPCs on osteoblasts is dependent upon the engagement of VLA-4 ($\alpha_4\beta_1$) and VLA-5 ($\alpha_5\beta_1$) receptors [87].

Regulation of HSC fate involves multiple highly orchestrated pathways that determine the cell cycle status, mobilization, and gene expression profile. The genes involved in HSC self-renewal are HOXB4, WNT proteins, Notch-1, Sonic hedgehog, GATA2, AML1, p18, MPL, STAT5, and p21 [88]. For example, overexpression of Hoxb4 strongly enhances HSC regeneration, and mice deficient in both Hoxb3 and Hoxb4 have defects in endogenous hematopoiesis and diminished number of hematopoietic progenitors due to insufficient expansion of HSCs. It has been shown that elevated reactive oxygen species causes progressive bone marrow failure resulting from a defect in HSC function in mice [89]. Further, Notch-1 and Tie-2 receptors are believed to be instrumental in the homing to endosteal HSC niche and quiescence of the HSCs, respectively [80, 90].

HSCs do not grow as independent autonomous units; instead, they are completely surrounded by the marrow microenvironment, which is defined by cell-to-cell interactions, cell-to-ECM interactions, and exposure to variable concentrations and combinations of soluble factors including cytokines. The HSC supporting cells not only provide a scaffold to the developing stem cells and progenitor cells, but also produce transmembrane ligands, extracellular matrix components, and soluble proteins. HSCs are exposed *in situ* to

Caption for Figure 4.2 (*cont.*) adhering to the perivascular cells while being influenced by endosteal cells' secreted factors, or (B) may be close to endosteal surface and frequently migrate through perivascular niches under the control of perivascular cells. (C) HSCs might reside in functionally unequivalent spatially distinct endosteal or perivascular niches at different stages in their life cycle, or (D) HSCs might reside in a single niche created by endosteal and perivascular cells [91]. (E) Mouse bone marrow section showing an HSC (CD150$^+$CD48$^-$CD41$^-$Lin$^-$, white arrow) close to the endosteum (white line) and a sinusoid (white, B, bone; V, blood vessel). (F) An optical section of the bone marrow showing an HSC (CD150$^+$CD48$^-$CD41$^-$Lin$^-$, white arrow) close to a sinusoid (* indicates lumen of sinusoid) and megakaryocyte (arrowhead) and surrounded by hematopoietic progenitor cells [107]. Reprinted from [91, 107] with kind permission from Cell Press.

many different growth factors, some soluble, some bound to ECM, and some bound to adjacent cells. Frequent cell-to-cell signaling occurs when HSCs are in cell-to-cell contact with stromal cells, committed hematopoietic progenitor cells (HPCs), and other HSCs. ECM of bone marrow acts in concert with cell-to-cell interactions and soluble factors to regulate the HSC. Adhesion of HSCs and HPCs to the marrow ECM inhibits cellular proliferation and prevents apoptosis, both of which lead to long-term survival of quiescent HSCs. Numerous molecules within the HSC membranes mediate signals from the ECM, including integrins, immunoglobulin-like molecules, cadherins, selectins, and mucins [29, 79, 91–93].

4.5 Sources of HSCs

HSCs can be isolated from various tissues in mammals. Some of the prominent sources of HSCs are the bone marrow, cord blood, and peripheral blood.

4.5.1 Bone marrow

During homeostasis, most adult HSCs reside in the bone marrow, making it a primary source of these cells. In rodents, the HSCs are isolated from the femurs, tibias, humeri, and iliac crest. In humans, HSCs are predominantly isolated from the iliac crest.

4.5.2 Cord blood

Umbilical cord blood (UCB) is a rich source of HSCs, and is readily available through cord blood banks. Since 1989, umbilical cord blood banks have been established in six continents and over one million cord blood collections have been performed. Although cord blood transplantation has a low risk of graft versus host disease (GVHD), the limited number of cells collected from single donors poses a challenge for clinical use of UCB [94]. For this reason, expansion of UCB HSCs is an active field of research [95]. Apart from UCB, amniotic fluid is also a source of HSCs.

4.5.3 Peripheral blood

At any given time, a small fraction of HSCs will be circulating in the peripheral blood (PB). HSCs can also be mobilized out of the bone marrow to the peripheral blood by treatment with granulocyte colony-stimulating factor (G-CSF) or granulocyte-macrophage colony-stimulating factor (GM-CSF) (which is ineffective in 15%–20% of patients) [96]. Combination of G-CSF with plerixafor (1,1′-[1,4-phenylenebis (methylene)]bis [1,4,8,11-tetraazacyclotetradecane] or AMD3100), which is an antagonist for CXCR4 and an allosteric agonist of CXCR7, increases the frequency of HSC mobilization out of the marrow [97]. In peripheral blood HSC isolation, leukapheresis is used to return the red blood cells to the donor, isolating only the HSCs and hematopoietic progenitor cells [98].

4.6 Isolation of HSCs

HSC identification and isolation is performed by analysis of the expression, or lack of expression, of specific cell surface markers via fluorescence-activated cell sorting (FACS). Since no single specific marker that can positively identify HSCs has yet been discovered, a combination of surface markers is used for HSC isolation.

Isolation of murine HSCs relies on the positive expression of the tyrosine kinase receptor c-Kit (CD117) and the membrane glycoprotein Sca-1, in parallel with the lack of markers of terminal differentiation (Ter119, Gr-1, Mac-1, B220, CD4, and CD8), collectively known as lineage markers. The resulting c-Kit$^+$, Sca-1$^+$, Lineage$^-$ population, commonly referred to as LSK cells, as seen in Figure 4.3, contains cells capable of hematopoietic reconstitution (the LT-HSC, ST-HSC, and MPPs) [99, 100]. The LSK population is further enriched to obtain HSCs with long-term reconstitution ability by combination with other surface markers. Some such combinations for murine HSCs are LSK Thy^{Low} [101], LSK CD34$^-$ (0.004% of bone marrow cells) [102] and LSK CD34$^{-/Low}$ Flk2$^-$ [103]. HSCs can also be enriched by their ability to efflux Hoechst dye and identified as side population

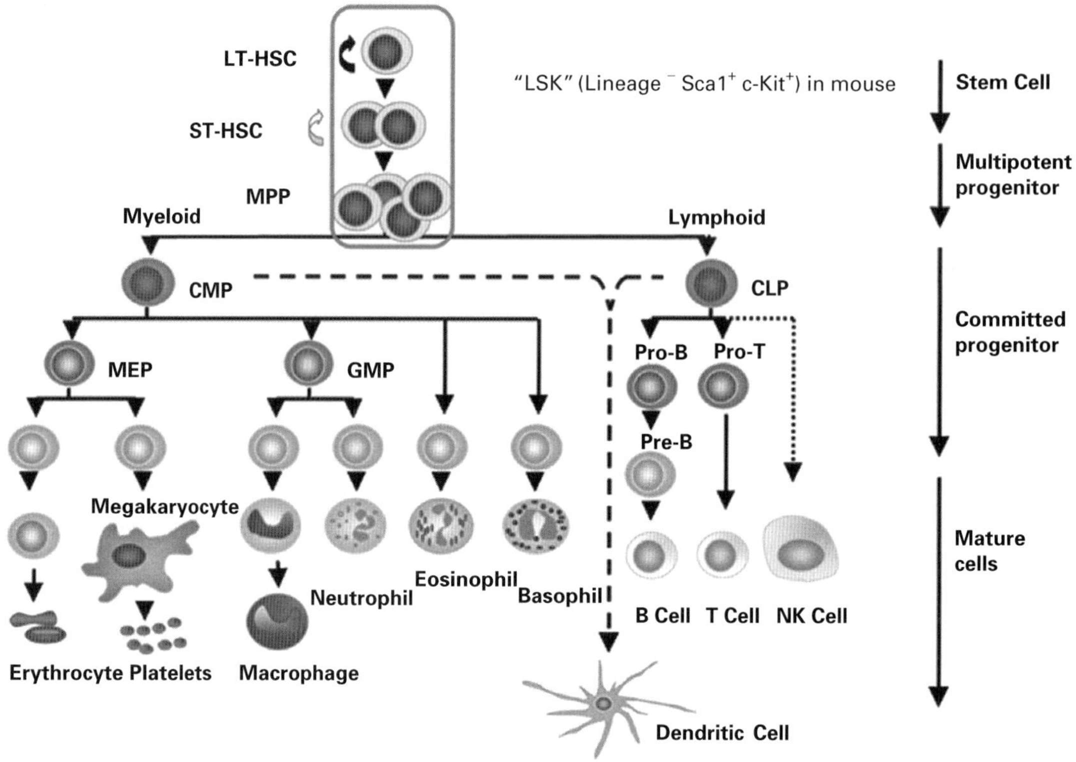

Figure 4.3 Differentiation and the hierarchy of hematopoietic cells. Legend: LT-HSC, long-term repopulating HSC; ST-HSC, short-term repopulating HSC; MPP, multipotent progenitor; CMP, common myeloid progenitor; CLP, common lymphoid progenitor; MEP, megakaryocyte/erythroid progenitor; GMP, granulocyte-macrophage progenitor. The highlighted pluripotent population, LT-HSC, ST-HSC, and MPP are Lin^-, $Sca\text{-}1^+$, and $c\text{-}kit^+$ as shown [179]. Reproduced by permission of the Nature Publishing Group.

(SP); such cells are identified as low-fluorescence-emitting cells when Hoechst 33342 red and blue fluorescence signals are plotted against each other [99, 104]. The SP cells are highly enriched in HSCs and are capable of sustaining multilineage and long-term engraftment in mice.

Other methods to isolate murine HSCs include the use of markers such as endothelial protein C receptor (EPCR) [105], Tie-2 [90], and endoglin [106]. Others have identified the signaling lymphocytic activation molecule (SLAM) family markers to identify LT-HSC ($CD150^+$, $CD41^-$, $CD48^-$, 0.0067% of the bone marrow cells), MPP ($CD150^-$, $CD41^+$, $CD48^-$), and restricted progenitors ($CD150^-$, $CD41^+$, $CD48^+$) [107]. Many laboratories use a combination of the LSK and $CD150^+$, $CD41^-$, $CD48^-$ markers to isolate enriched HSCs from murine bone marrow [108, 109].

Isolation strategies for human HSCs are not as well developed as those for murine HSCs due to a lack of methods to separate enriched HSCs from MPPs and lineage-restricted progenitors. $CD34^+$ cells are routinely used in transplantation in the clinic as well as in xenografts, making them among the positive identifiers of human HSCs. HSCs can be enriched further on the basis of CD38 [110], CD45RA [111], Thy1 (CD90) [112–114], and CD49f [115] expression. Within the Lin^-, $CD34^+$, $CD38^-$ fraction, HSCs can be further enriched by high efflux of the mitochondrial dye rhodamine-123 (Rho^{Low}) [116]. To date, Lin^-, $CD34^+$, $CD38^-$, $CD45RA^-$, $Thy1^+$, Rho^{Low}, $CD49f^+$ are the most enriched human HSCs [115].

4.7 Assays for HSCs activity

The stem cell activity of HSCs and HPCs is detected by a variety of in-vitro and in-vivo assays that measure proliferation of cells (quantified by the number of cells produced) and their differentiation potential (assessed by the number of different lineages represented in daughter cells). The assays fall under two categories: (1) long-term assays, where the HSCs and progenies go through high number of divisions (>15) in more than 5 weeks; and (2) short-term assays, where progenitors divide 5–10 times in less than 3 weeks. Some of the gold-standard assays for determining HSC functional activity are listed below.

4.7.1 Colony-formation unit (CFU) assay

CFU is an established and popular in-vitro short-term semi-solid assay in which the test cells are placed in a viscous medium (methylcellulose or agar) with defined cytokine concentrations and composition. Over a period of 2 weeks, each HPC undergoes clonal expansion and differentiation into daughter colonies. At the end of 12–14 days, the colonies are quantified and categorized according to size, color, composition, and disposition into colony-forming unit lymphocyte (CFU-L), colony-forming unit granulocyte erythroid monocyte megakaryocyte (CFU-GEMM, the most primitive myeloid), colony-forming unit granulocyte monocyte (CFU-GM), colony-forming unit granulocyte (CFU-G), colony-forming unit monocyte (CFU-M), colony-forming unit megakaryocyte (CFU-Meg) colony-forming unit erythroid (CFU-E), and immature burst-forming unit erythroid (BFU-E). The numbers and types of colonies formed in the CFU assay indicate the stage of differentiation of the HPCs in culture. The proliferative potential of the progenitors is easy to ascertain in clonal assays such as CFU or single-cell cultures, where the progeny of each progenitor remains well separated and its size is roughly proportional to the proliferative potential. However, CFU by itself is not considered a functional assay for HSCs.

4.7.2 Long-term culture initiation assay (LT-IC)

LTC-IC is an in-vitro long-term assay that detects test cells capable of continuously forming myeloid cells for 4 weeks in culture, when co-cultured on mitotically inactivated feeder layer cells [117, 118]. The colonies produced by the test cells are assessed by CFU assay. Poisson statistics and the method of maximum likelihood are then utilized to calculate the frequency of LTC-IC in the test cell sample. This is another retrospective assay in which the LTC-IC cells in the initial test cells are identified 5–8 weeks after being placed in culture. LTC-ICs are upstream of the CFUs.

4.7.3 Cobblestone area formation assay (CAFC)

CAFC is an in-vitro long-term assay that quantifies the frequencies of different hematopoietic cells forming a cobblestone area (defined as a group of flattened and optically dense cells) underneath and in close contact with the feeder layer cells after co-culture for 6–12 weeks [119, 120].

4.7.4 Competitive repopulating unit (CRU) assay

CRU is a long-term in-vivo assay that quantifies the ability of test cells to rescue the hematopoietic organ in a lethally (or partially) myeloablated host. In a CRU assay, limiting doses of donor test cells are transplanted into groups of myeloablated, congenic recipient mice (for mouse-to-mouse transplantation) or severe combined immune-deficient (SCID) mice (for human-to-mouse xenografts), along with helper cells (to ensure the survival of the host when the test cells contain low or non-detectable CRU) [121–123]. Four months after transplantation hematopoietic myeloid and lymphoid chimerism is measured in the peripheral blood samples of hosts via flow cytometry and antibody combinations that determine donor-derived cells and lineage-specificity. Poisson statistics and the method of maximum likelihood are utilized to calculate the CRU frequency in the test cells on the basis of the proportion of negative recipients at each cell dose. The CRU assay identifies the LT-HSCs that have the capacity to home into the bone marrow of the host and produce MPPs in the long-term (>4 months), and is the most widely used in-vivo assay for studies involving HSCs.

4.8 In-vitro HSC expansion

HSCs, when isolated and then cultured in vitro, quickly lose the expression of key antigens on their cell surface [124]. They undergo differentiation as the time in culture increases. Many research groups have developed innovative solutions to prolong the self-renewal capacity or "stemness" of HSCs in in-vitro cultures, such as co-culturing with different support cells, exposure to media rich in cytokines found in the bone marrow, growing HSCs in different extracellular substrates, using serum-free media, changing metabolic parameters, using non-contact co-cultures, and changing gene expression (over-expression, deletion of a certain gene) either in HSCs or in support cells [56, 125–133]. Even with all these ways to elongate the self-renewal capacity of HSCs in vitro, current state-of-the-art expansion is dramatically lower than the in-vivo capacity of expansion of HSCs, which is 8400-fold [131, 134, 135]. Some of the techniques for in-vitro HSC expansion are discussed below:

4.8.1 Cytokine cocktails

Cytokines have been used extensively in in-vitro expansion of HSCs and HPCs, either alone or in combination cocktails. More than 30 hematopoietic factors that contribute to proliferation and differentiation of HSCs or HPCs have been cloned and identified. Examples of some of these factors are erythropoietin (EPO), thrombopoietin (TPO), G-CSF, GM-SCF, interleukin (IL)-1, IL-3, IL-6, soluble IL-6 receptor (sIL-6R), IL-11, stem cell factor (SCF), Flt-3/Flt-2 ligand (FL), bone morphogenic factor 4 (BMP 4), BMP 7, Notch ligand, Wnt 3a, and, fibroblast growth factor-1 (FGF-1), all of which have demonstrated significant expansion of HSCs and HPCs [134, 136–139]. Expansion of hematopoietic cells is assessed by measuring CFCs, CAFCs, and LTC-ICs in a variety of culture conditions across different labs, which makes it difficult to make comparisons and sometimes leads to conflicting data.

4.8.2 Co-cultures

Given that in vivo the hematopoietic supporting cells regulate and maintain HSCs and HPCs, these cells have been co-cultured with a variety of supporting cells from different sources since 1974 [117]. Feeder layers or non-contact co-cultures with bone marrow stromal cells, osteoblasts, endothelial cells, MSCs, and fibroblasts (both primary cells and cell lines such as MS-5, ST-2, PA-6, and OP-9) have supported in-vitro expansion of HSCs and HPCs. In feeder-layer co-cultures, direct cell-to-cell contact between HSCs/HPCs and supporting cells provides physical adhesion as well as regulatory signal information crosstalk between the cells involved, while in non-contact cultures, soluble regulatory cytokines, chemokines, and growth factors secreted by supporting cells regulate the self-renewal, amplification, proliferation, and differentiation of HSCs and HPCs.

4.8.3 Bioreactors

Dynamic bioreactor systems where nutrient levels, oxygen tension, pH, and soluble signals can be carefully monitored and controlled have been developed to expand HSCs and HPCs and FDA approved for clinical use [140]. Ideally, under optimized conditions these systems can mass produce expanded hematopoietic cells for clinical uses. With online monitoring, automated feeding strategies, and frequent sampling, bioreactors provide a better control of culture parameters, with lower contamination risk, while supporting high cell densities and supporting (feeder-layer) cells. The following are some examples of the most popular hematopoietic bioreactors.

Perfusion bioreactor. In continuous-perfusion bioreactors, cell culture medium is continuously exchanged over the culture time. These bioreactors support expansion of HSCs with cytokine supplementation with or without the feeder layer by optimizing growth factor levels, oxygen tension, and the size of the cell growth area [141, 142].

Microfluidic bioreactors, in which a few HSCs and primary bone marrow cells (hundreds of cells) can be cultured in nanoliter volumes of fluids under defined microenvironments, have an advantage over conventional bioreactors or other macroscopic culture systems in that the small volume allows even one or a few HSCs to condition the culture environment significantly. Such microbioreactors have been successfully utilized to expand HSCs and HPCs in 3D co-cultures with supporting cells, and to differentiate them toward myeloid and erythroid lineages [143, 144]. Microfluidic devices enable greater control of the in-vitro cell microenvironment than do conventional culture systems, and active convective fluid flow in the devices can regulate the chemical as well as the mechanical environment. Microbioreactors allow additional functionality to control autocrine/paracrine factors, local nutrient/mitogenic gradients, continuous perfusion, micrometer control of topology and composition of substrate, and easy integration with sensing and analysis tools [145–147].

Fixed-bed or packed-bed bioreactors. These comprise a scaffold for HSC attachment and culture to recreate elements of the bone marrow ECM. In these bioreactors, HSCs are co-cultured on scaffolds (beds) on which the supporting cells have been attached [148].

Stirred bioreactors. These provide homogeneous concentrations of nutrients in a batch, fed-batch, and perfusion mode [149, 150].

Although bioreactors have the promise of clinic-ready HSCs, the optimization of culture conditions and the cues required to approximate the in-vivo expansion rates is an ongoing challenge.

4.8.4 Metabolic cues

Apart from the cytokines, soluble, secreted and matrix factors that drive HSC and HPC phenotypes via interconnected signaling pathways, the metabolic environment around them can also influence their self-renewal and proliferation. Cross *et al.* postulated that the amplification of hematopoietic cells is dependent on a defined and limiting nutrient (which includes pH and oxygen tension) environment presented by their niches [151]. In vivo, HSCs reside in low-oxygen-tension endosteal and perivascular niches [44–47]. Human UCB CD133$^+$ hematopoietic cells have higher survival and CFU frequency when cultured at 1% oxygen and low glucose (<1 mM). These metabolic cues coordinate with signaling pathways to tightly control the HSC expansion in specialized niches where it is rate-limited by the metabolite availability, thereby supporting a supply of LT-HSCs, reducing DNA damage, and avoiding the long-term selection of activating mutations in signaling pathways.

4.9 Clinical relevance of HSCs

Bone marrow transplantation, which was pioneered more than 40 years ago, is now being successfully used for treatment of about 40 different diseases. Transplantation of HSCs and HPCs from bone marrow, UCB, and peripheral blood, has radically changed the treatment and cure of multiple myeloma, aplastic anemia, and other hematopoietic malignancies [152].

Bone marrow transplantation is clinically useful for leukemia and lymphoma (such as acute lymphoblastic leukemia (ALL), acute myeloblastic leukemia (AML), chronic myelogenous leukemia (CML), multiple myeloma, Hodgkin's disease, and non-Hodgkin's lymphoma), as well as inherited blood disorders (such as β-thalassemia, aplastic anemia, globoid cell leukodystrophy, Blackfan–Diamond syndrome, sickle-cell anemia, severe combined immunodeficiency, and X-linked lymphoproliferative syndrome) [153, 154]. Some inborn errors of metabolism may also be treated with bone marrow transplants, including Hunter's syndrome, Hurler's syndrome, Lesch–Nyhan syndrome, and osteopetrosis [155]. Transplants are also applicable to bone marrow rescue following high-dose chemotherapy for the treatment of solid tumors [156]. Additionally, cord blood transplants may also be applied in the future toward other autoimmune diseases, such as diabetes, rheumatoid arthritis, and system lupus erythematosis, in an effort to reconstitute or reprogram the immune system [157].

Given that the true expansion of human HSCs from UCB, bone marrow, or peripheral blood is not currently possible without losing their self-renewal properties, there remains an unmet need for the generation and expansion of HSCs from embryonic stem cells (ESCs) and from reprogramming of adult cell-derived induced pluripotent cells (iPSCs), both of which routes are currently being actively investigated [158–160]. ESCs and iPSCs are differentiated into HSCs and HPCs by stimulation with cytokine and growth factor cocktails as well as co-culture with supporting feeder-layer cells. Some of the signaling pathways that have been identified as important for development of HSCs include Wnt, Notch, BMPs, and the transcription factors Runx1, SIL/TAL, and GATA [161], and might be useful for driving the pluripotent cells into hematopoietic lineage. These approaches can be applied toward obtaining autologous inherited-diseases gene-corrected HSCs from patient-derived iPSCs after homologous recombination, thereby avoiding the use of semi-randomly integrating vectors with potential genotoxicity. Studies on how to improve the yield of HSCs and HPCs from iPSCs and ESCs are under way.

4.10 HSC niches in cancer metastasis

The bone and bone marrow become unwitting hosts to cancer cells when tumors metastasize to their niches. In fact, the malignancy of cancers is determined by their metastases (or dissemination) to distant organs, with nearly 80% of patients with advanced breast or prostrate cancer suffering from bone and bone marrow metastasis, leading to over 90% fatality in cancer patients [162]. To date, no cure for this chronic malignancy has been found [163, 164]. Moreover, in spite of clinical importance, the underlying cellular and molecular mechanisms driving bone marrow metastasis of solid cancers remain elusive, and are the topic of intensive research.

Primary tumors from organs such as breast, prostrate, lung, and thyroid become malignant and start distributing tumor cells through the blood circulation to various organs. Circulating tumor cells invade through the endothelial layer and basement membrane and reach the secondary site, such as bone and bone marrow. In order to home to the bone marrow, the tumor cells use similar molecular pathways that the HSCs typically use, such as the CXCR4/CXCL12 axis [165, 166]. Moreover, tumor cells overexpress certain receptors (such as CXCR4/CXCR7, CXCR6, CD44, VLA-4, Axl/Mer, and Anxa2-R), which are activated by the ligands secreted or expressed by the bone marrow cells (such as SDF-1, CXCL16, hyaluron, fibronectin (FN), GAS-6, and Anxa2) [167–169]. Once localized to the bone and bone marrow, these disseminated tumor cells (DTCs) may engage the microenvironment, or niche, through specific cell-to-cell adhesive interactions. These stimuli are believed to cause DTCs to resist chemotherapy, maintain a quiescent state, or self-renew and spread to secondary sites [170–172]. On the other hand, the niche constituent cells are also activated by the DTCs to secrete factors that drive DTCs' proliferation and survival, thereby creating a more metastatic and aggressive tumor. Some of the growth factors and molecules that might have play a role in this crosstalk are transforming growth factor-β (TGF-β), platelet-derived growth factor (PDGF), insulin growth factors 1 and 2 (IGF-1,2), RANKL/Osteoprotegrin (RANKL/OPG), FGF, BMP, Runx2, VEGF, IL-6, endothelins, and Wnt [168, 173–175].

Importantly, our group has recently found that prostate cancer (PCa) cells directly compete with HSCs for occupancy of the bone marrow niche [176]. On increasing the niche constituent osteoblasts in vivo (via PTH injections) metastasis of PCa was enhanced, whereas on decreasing the number of osteoblasts, PCa metastasis was reduced. Moreover, disseminated PCa can be mobilized out of the niche by using CXCR4 inhibitor (AMD3100) that typically mobilizes HSCs out of the marrow. Although further study will clearly be needed, these data suggest that bone marrow niche is a potential therapeutic target for bone metastatic disease.

4.11 Future directions

Although we have made substantial progress toward understanding the biology of HSCs, we are still far away from recreating bone marrow microenvironments, expanding HSCs ex vivo at high efficiencies, understanding niche homeostatic and metastatic interactions, and uncovering the complexities of the kinetics of self-renewal and differentiation. The following are some of the issues to keep in mind as research on these topics continues.

4.11.1 Biological questions

The bone marrow niche is one of the most well-known microenvironments for adult HSCs. Although it has been established that osteoblasts and other supporting cells (including MSCs, endothelial cells, adipocytes, and fibroblasts) play central roles in hematopoiesis, and produce many factors essential for the survival, self-renewal, and maturation of HSCs, it still needs to be determined whether HSCs play a role in establishing an inductive microenvironment. Most reports on the topic are from the perspective of how the object under evaluation impacts HSC proliferation, differentiation, homing, quiescence, and migration, but not the other way around. Thus, it is important to identify the roles HSCs play in the niche and how they influence marrow cells (MSCs, osteoblasts, and endothelial cells) to create an inductive microenvironment, and to study how their function is altered in hematopathologies and marrow metastasis. Recent work by our group has demonstrated that HSCs are able to induce the differentiation of osteoblasts from immature MSCs [177]. Yet it is very difficult and resource-straining to perform this type of study in animal models. Therefore, in-vitro studies can be formulated to find out the influence HSCs can have on MSCs and stromal cells of the marrow niche, including endothelial cells and osteoblasts. In such studies, different variations of abnormal HSCs in cultures can be configured where small populations of HSCs and stromal cells can be easily studied in simulated microenvironments.

Other biological issues that remain to be understood in the context of the HSC bone marrow niche are the following.

- The role of supporting cells (osteoblasts, MSCs, perivascular cells, etc.) in getting pre-HSCs and HSCs to differentiate.
- The role of supporting cells in hematopoietic malignancies and bone marrow metastasis.
- The operational structure of the bone marrow microenvironment (and how it is different in leukemia and bone marrow metastasis).
- Interactions between cell-associated growth factors (provided by supporting cells) and growth factor receptors (on HSCs) that are important for
  - proliferation of HSCs (e.g. G-CSF, GM-CSF, etc.),
  - niche localization or homing of HSCs (e.g. ICAMs, Jagged1, CD 164, etc.), and
  - survival and quiescence of HSCs (e.g. VCAM-1, N-Cadherin, Ang-1, etc.).

Understanding the molecular mechanisms underlying these cell-to-cell interactions (mediated by cell-surface or secreted molecules) holds the key to HSC biology and is of biological and clinical interest.

4.11.2 High-throughput screening

In the bone marrow HSC niches, a heterogeneous population of cells (support cells and HSCs) co-habitates in a hierarchical and structurally functional manner to maintain bone marrow as a complex organ. The definition of microenvironment and mimicking the in-vivo marrow processes are not straightforward tasks due to the highly transient processes and the largely undefined heterogeneous environment. Therefore, high-throughput screening technologies are needed in order to test various parameters that capture the networks of communication in the bone marrow, and can influence HSC fate choices.

4.11.3 Design of experiments (DOE)

The process control of hematopoiesis has been difficult to achieve due to the complexity and interactions of the cells, cues, and signals involved. The variability of cell type, transient kinetics, high sensitivity, and specificity to extrinsic factors, and interaction of a multitude of these factors affecting cellular behavior pose significant challenges to process characterization. Considering the example of HSC expansion in vitro, this lack of characterization and control is highly undesirable and can result in low quality, yield, and purity of the final LT-HSC produced in expansion cultures. Full factorial designs will be essential in future studies in order to screen out a large number of parameters and experimental conditions that do not allow a drastic increase in LT-HSC expansion. In order for such a design of experiments to be successful and insightful, the interactions among all variables must also be accounted for. Kinetic models of LT-HSC expansion might also be necessary in conjunction with DOE for predictive analysis.

4.11.4 Real-time process monitoring for iPSC and ESC hematopoietic differentiation

Real-time and on line monitoring of key process parameters will provide vital information for making decisions about the optimized culture conditions for generating a high yield of HSCs from pluripotent stem cells. The current monitoring techniques for cell bioprocesses will have to be applied to the simultaneous monitoring of the key process variables: (a) pH, dissolved oxygen tension, carbon dioxide tension, and temperature; (b) nutrients and metabolites; (c) growth factors; and (d) cell viability and density.

4.12 Conclusions

HSCs are the most widely studied adult stem cells, which can self-renew and form hematopoietic cells of all lineages. They have had an eventfull history, which is rich in the discovery of regulatory networks that control them as well as the niche constituent cells. Although many important components of the HSC niche and the key players responsible for HSC phenotypes have been discovered, the picture of HSCs and their niches is yet not complete. HSCs are distributed among different niches within the marrow on the basis of their lineage hierarchy and functional requirements provided by molecular signals and from the niche in which they reside. Further, the role of HSCs and their niches in cancer metastasis is being elucidated by new studies. In the next few years, we will also witness the development of robust methods to generate and expand HSCs both from embryonic and from adult-derived iPSCs. As the picture of HSCs and their niches begins to unfold, and we gain a better understanding of the way niches maintain HSC in vivo, this knowledge will be crucial to design novel HSC culture strategies to propagate them ex vivo for clinical applications.

ACKNOWLEDGEMENTS

We apologize to those authors whose work has not been included in this review due to space limitations. This work is directly supported by the National Cancer Institute (CA163124, CA093900, DK082481, DE020721), the Fund for Cancer Research, the Department of Defense (W81XWH-11-1-0636), the Prostate Cancer Foundation, NIH SPORE in prostate cancer grant P50 CA69568, and the Cancer Center support grant P30 CA46592.

REFERENCES

[1] Giebel, B., Zhang, T., Beckmann, J. *et al.* 2006. Primitive human hematopoietic cells give rise to differentially specified daughter cells upon their initial cell division. *Blood*, **107**(5), 2146–52.

[2] Kiel, M. J., He, S., Ashkenazi, R. *et al.* 2007. Haematopoietic stem cells do not asymmetrically segregate chromosomes or retain BrdU. *Nature*, **449**(7159), 238–42.

[3] Punzel, M., Liu, D., Zhang, T. *et al.* 2003. The symmetry of initial divisions of human hematopoietic progenitors is altered only by the cellular microenvironment. *Exp. Hematol.*, **31**(4), 339–47.

[4] Ema, H., Takano, H., Sudo, K. and Nakauchi, H. 2000. In vitro self-renewal division of hematopoietic stem cells. *J. Exp. Med.*, **192**(9), 1281–8.

[5] Morrison, S. J. and Weissman, I. L. 1995. Heterogeneity of hematopoietic stem cells: implications for clinical

applications. *Proc. Assoc. Am. Physicians,* **107**(2), 187–94.

[6] Sieburg, H. B., Cho, R. H., Dykstra, B. *et al.* 2006. The hematopoietic stem compartment consists of a limited number of discrete stem cell subsets. *Blood,* **107**(6), 2311–16.

[7] Muller-Sieburg, C. E., Cho, R. H., Karlsson, L., Huang, J. F. and Sieburg, H. B. 2004. Myeloid-biased hematopoietic stem cells have extensive self-renewal capacity but generate diminished lymphoid progeny with impaired IL-7 responsiveness. *Blood,* **103**(11), 4111–18.

[8] Muller-Sieburg, C. E., Cho, R. H., Thoman, M., Adkins, B. and Sieburg, H. B. 2002. Deterministic regulation of hematopoietic stem cell self-renewal and differentiation. *Blood,* **100**(4), 1302–9.

[9] Dykstra, B., Kent, D., Bowie, M. *et al.* 2007. Long-term propagation of distinct hematopoietic differentiation programs in vivo. *Cell Stem Cell,* **1**(2), 218–29.

[10] Challen, G. A., Boles, N. C., Chambers, S. M. and Goodell, M. A. 2010. Distinct hematopoietic stem cell subtypes are differentially regulated by TGF-β_1. *Cell Stem Cell,* **6**(3), 265–78.

[11] Moore, M. A. S. 2004. Ontogeny of the hematopoietic system. In Lanza, R. P., Weissman, I., Thomas, J. *et al.*, editors. *Handbook of Stem Cells.* Boston, MA: Elsevier Academic.

[12] Jaffredo, T., Nottingham, W., Liddiard, K. *et al.* 2005. From hemangioblast to hematopoietic stem cell: an endothelial connection? *Exp. Hematol.,* **33**(9), 1029–40.

[13] Kennedy, M., Firpo, M., Choi, K. *et al.* 1997. A common precursor for primitive erythropoiesis and definitive haematopoiesis. *Nature,* **386**(6624), 488–93.

[14] Muller, A. M., Medvinsky, A., Strouboulis, J., Grosveld, F. and Dzierzak, E. 1994. Development of hematopoietic stem cell activity in the mouse embryo. *Immunity,* **1**(4), 291–301.

[15] Cumano, A., Ferraz, J. C., Klaine, M., Di Santo, J. P. and Godin, I. 2001. Intraembryonic, but not yolk sac hematopoietic precursors, isolated before circulation, provide long-term multilineage reconstitution. *Immunity,* **15**(3), 477–85.

[16] Yoder, M. C., Hiatt, K., Dutt, P. *et al.* 1997. Characterization of definitive lymphohematopoietic stem cells in the day 9 murine yolk sac. *Immunity,* **7**(3), 335–44.

[17] Palis, J., Robertson, S., Kennedy, M., Wall, C. and Keller, G. 1999. Development of erythroid and myeloid progenitors in the yolk sac and embryo proper of the mouse. *Development,* **126**(22), 5073–84.

[18] Wolf, N. S., Bertoncello, I., Jiang, D. and Priestley, G. 1995. Developmental hematopoiesis from prenatal to young-adult life in the mouse model. *Exp. Hematol.,* **23**(2), 142–6.

[19] Harrison, D. E., Zhong, R. K., Jordan, C. T., Lemischka, I. R. and Astle, C. M. 1997. Relative to adult marrow, fetal liver repopulates nearly five times more effectively long-term than short-term. *Exp. Hematol.,* **25**(4), 293–7.

[20] Kurata, H., Mancini, G. C., Alespeiti, G., Migliaccio, A. R. and Migliaccio, G. 1998. Stem cell factor induces proliferation and differentiation of fetal progenitor cells in the mouse. *Br. J. Haematol.,* **101**(4), 676–87.

[21] Grossi, C. E., Velardi, A. and Cooper, M. D. 1985. Postnatal liver hemopoiesis in mice: generation of pre-B cells, granulocytes, and erythrocytes in discrete colonies. *J. Immunol.,* **135**(4), 2303–11.

[22] de Bruijn, M. F., Speck, N. A., Peeters, M. C. and Dzierzak, E. 2000. Definitive hematopoietic stem cells first develop within the major arterial regions of the mouse embryo. *EMBO J.,* **19**(11), 2465–74.

[23] Medvinsky, A. L. and Dzierzak, E. A. 1998. Development of the definitive hematopoietic hierarchy in the mouse. *Dev. Comp. Immunol.,* **22**(3), 289–301.

[24] Tavian, M. and Peault, B. 2005. Embryonic development of the human hematopoietic system. *Int. J. Dev. Biol.,* **49** (2–3), 243–50.

[25] Marshall, C. 2006. Intraembryonic development of hematopoietic stem cells during human ontogeny: expression analysis. In Godin, I. and Cumano, A., editors. *Hematopoietic Stem Cell Development.* Georgetown, TX; New York: Landes Bioscience/Eurekah.com; Kluwer Academic/Plenum Publishers, pp. 142–53.

[26] Tavian, M., Biasch, K., Sinka, L., Vallet, J. and Peault, B. 2010. Embryonic origin of human hematopoiesis. *Int. J. Dev. Biol.,* **54**(6–7), 1061–5.

[27] Robin, C., Ottersbach, K., de Bruijn, M. *et al.* 2003. Developmental origins of hematopoietic stem cells. *Oncol. Res.* **13**(6–10), 315–21.

[28] Morrison, S. J., Wright, D. E. and Weissman, I. L. 1997. Cyclophosphamide/granulocyte colony-stimulating factor induces hematopoietic stem cells to proliferate prior to mobilization. *Proc. Nat. Acad. Sci. USA,* **94**(5), 1908–13.

[29] Taichman, R. S. 2005. Blood and bone: two tissues whose fates are intertwined to create the hematopoietic stem-cell niche. *Blood,* **105**(7), 2631–9.

[30] Han, J., Koh, Y. J., Moon, H. R. *et al.* 2010. Adipose tissue is an extramedullary reservoir for functional hematopoietic stem and progenitor cells. *Blood,* **115**(5), 957–64.

[31] Cardier, J. E. and Barbera-Guillem, E. 1997. Extramedullary hematopoiesis in the adult mouse liver is associated with specific hepatic sinusoidal endothelial cells. *Hepatology*, **26**(1), 165–75.

[32] McKinney-Freeman, S. L., Jackson, K. A., Camargo, F. D. *et al.* 2002. Muscle-derived hematopoietic stem cells are hematopoietic in origin. *Proc. Nat. Acad. Sci. USA*, **99**(3), 1341–6.

[33] Kawada, H. and Ogawa, M. 2001. Bone marrow origin of hematopoietic progenitors and stem cells in murine muscle. *Blood*, **98**(7), 2008–13.

[34] Massberg, S., Schaerli, P., Knezevic-Maramica, I. *et al.* 2007. Immunosurveillance by hematopoietic progenitor cells trafficking through blood, lymph, and peripheral tissues. *Cell*, **131**(5), 994–1008.

[35] Adams, G. B. and Scadden, D. T. 2006. The hematopoietic stem cell in its place. *Nature Immunol.*, **7**(4), 333–7.

[36] Jang, J. H. and Schaffer, D. V. 2006. Microarraying the cellular microenvironment. *Molec. Syst. Biol.*, **2**, 39.

[37] Yin, T. and Li, L. 2006. The stem cell niches in bone. *J. Clin. Invest.*, **116**(5), 1195–201.

[38] Song, J., Kiel, M. J., Wang, Z. *et al.* 2010. An in vivo model to study and manipulate the hematopoietic stem cell niche. *Blood*, **115**(13), 2592–600.

[39] Purton, L. E. and Scadden, D. T. 2008. *The Hematopoietic Stem Cell Niche.* Cambridge, MA: StemBook.

[40] Mendez-Ferrer, S., Michurina, T. V., Ferraro, F. *et al.* 2010. Mesenchymal and haematopoietic stem cells form a unique bone marrow niche. *Nature*, **466**(7308), 829–34.

[41] Li, Z. and Li, L. 2006. Understanding hematopoietic stem-cell microenvironments. *Trends Biochem. Sci.*, **31**(10), 589–95.

[42] Kirouac, D. C. and Zandstra, P. W. 2006. Understanding cellular networks to improve hematopoietic stem cell expansion cultures. *Curr. Opin. Biotechnol.*, **17**(5), 538–47.

[43] Fliedner, T. M., Graessle, D., Paulsen, C. and Reimers, K. 2002. Structure and function of bone marrow hemopoiesis: mechanisms of response to ionizing radiation exposure. *Cancer Biother. Radiopharm.*, **17**(4), 405–26.

[44] Levesque, J. P., Winkler, I. G., Hendy, J. *et al.* 2007. Hematopoietic progenitor cell mobilization results in hypoxia with increased hypoxia-inducible transcription factor-1 alpha and vascular endothelial growth factor A in bone marrow. *Stem Cells*, **25**(8), 1954–65.

[45] Eliasson, P. and Jonsson, J. I. 2010. The hematopoietic stem cell niche: low in oxygen but a nice place to be. *J. Cell Physiol.*, **222**(1), 17–22.

[46] Parmar, K., Mauch, P., Vergilio, J. A., Sackstein, R. and Down, J. D. 2007. Distribution of hematopoietic stem cells in the bone marrow according to regional hypoxia. *Proc. Nat. Acad. Sci. USA*, **104**(13), 5431–6.

[47] Winkler, I. G., Barbier, V., Wadley, R. *et al.* 2010. Positioning of bone marrow hematopoietic and stromal cells relative to blood flow in vivo: serially reconstituting hematopoietic stem cells reside in distinct nonperfused niches. *Blood*, **116**(3), 375–85.

[48] Ehninger, A. and Trumpp, A. 2011. The bone marrow stem cell niche grows up: mesenchymal stem cells and macrophages move in. *J. Exp. Med.*, **208**(3), 421–8.

[49] Wilson, A. and Trumpp, A. 2006. Bone-marrow haematopoietic-stem-cell niches. *Nature Rev. Immunol.*, **6**(2), 93–106.

[50] Scadden, D. T. 2006. The stem-cell niche as an entity of action. *Nature*, **441**(7097), 1075–9.

[51] Kopp, H. G., Avecilla, S. T., Hooper, A. T. and Rafii, S. 2005. The bone marrow vascular niche: home of HSC differentiation and mobilization. *Physiology (Bethesda)*, **20**, 349–56.

[52] Rafii, S., Mohle, R., Shapiro, F., Frey, B. M. and Moore, M. A. 1997. Regulation of hematopoiesis by microvascular endothelium. *Leuk. Lymphoma*, **27**(5–6), 375–86.

[53] Feugier, P., Jo, D. Y., Shieh, J. H. *et al.* 2002. Ex vivo expansion of stem and progenitor cells in co-culture of mobilized peripheral blood CD34+ cells on human endothelium transfected with adenovectors expressing thrombopoietin, c-kit ligand, and Flt-3 ligand. *J. Hematother. Stem Cell Res.*, **11**(1), 127–38.

[54] Rookmaaker, M. B., Verhaar, M. C., Loomans, C. J. *et al.* 2005. CD34+ cells home, proliferate, and participate in capillary formation, and in combination with CD34− cells enhance tube formation in a 3-dimensional matrix. *Arterioscler. Thromb. Vasc. Biol.*, **25**(9), 1843–50.

[55] Braccini, A., Wendt, D., Jaquiery, C. *et al.* 2005. Three-dimensional perfusion culture of human bone marrow cells and generation of osteoinductive grafts. *Stem Cells*, **23**(8), 1066–72.

[56] Takagi, M. 2005. Cell processing engineering for ex-vivo expansion of hematopoietic cells. *J. Biosci. Bioeng.*, **99**(3), 189–96.

[57] Kim, H. S., Lim, J. B., Min, Y. H. *et al.* 2003. Ex vivo expansion of human umbilical cord blood CD34+ cells in a collagen bead-containing 3-dimensional culture system. *Int. J. Hematol.*, **78**(2), 126–32.

[58] Li, Y., Ma, T., Kniss, D. A., Yang, S. T. and Lasky, L. C. 2001. Human cord cell hematopoiesis in three-dimensional nonwoven fibrous matrices: in vitro

simulation of the marrow microenvironment. *J. Hematother. Stem Cell Res.*, **10**(3), 355–68.

[59] Banu, N., Rosenzweig, M., Kim, H., Bagley, J. and Pykett, M. 2001. Cytokine-augmented culture of haematopoietic progenitor cells in a novel three-dimensional cell growth matrix. *Cytokine*, **13**(6), 349–58.

[60] Tun, T., Miyoshi, H., Ema, H., Nakauchi, H. and Ohshima, N. 2000. New type of matrix support for bone marrow cell cultures: in vitro culture and in vivo transplantation experiments. *Asaio J.*, **46**(5), 522–6.

[61] Bagley, J., Rosenzweig, M., Marks, D. F. and Pykett, M. J. 1999. Extended culture of multipotent hematopoietic progenitors without cytokine augmentation in a novel three-dimensional device. *Exp. Hematol.*, **27**(3), 496–504.

[62] Rosenzweig, M., Pykett, M., Marks, D. F. and Johnson, R. P. 1997. Enhanced maintenance and retroviral transduction of primitive hematopoietic progenitor cells using a novel three-dimensional culture system. *Gene Ther.*, **4**(9), 928–36.

[63] Wang, T. Y., Brennan, J. K. and Wu, J. H. 1995. Multilineal hematopoiesis in a three-dimensional murine long-term bone marrow culture. *Exp. Hematol.*, **23**(1), 26–32.

[64] Bagley, J., Rosenzweig, M., Marks, D. F. and Pykett, M. J. 1999. Extended culture of multipotent hematopoietic progenitors without cytokine augmentation in a novel three-dimensional device. *Exp. Hematol.*, **27**(3), 496–504.

[65] de Barros, A. P., Takiya, C. M., Garzoni, L. R. *et al.* 2010. Osteoblasts and bone marrow mesenchymal stromal cells control hematopoietic stem cell migration and proliferation in 3D in vitro model. *PLoS One*, **5**(2), e9093.

[66] Konstantinov, S. M., Mindova, M. M., Gospodinov, P. T. and Genova, P. I. 2004. Three-dimensional bioreactor cultures: a useful dynamic model for the study of cellular interactions. *Ann. NY Acad. Sci.*, **1030**, 103–15.

[67] Rossi, M. I., Barros, A. P., Baptista, L. S. *et al.* 2005. Multicellular spheroids of bone marrow stromal cells: a three-dimensional in vitro culture system for the study of hematopoietic cell migration. *Braz. J. Med. Biol. Res.*, **38**(10), 1455–62.

[68] Tun, T., Miyoshi, H., Ema, H., Nakauchi, H. and Ohshima, N. 2000. New type of matrix support for bone marrow cell cultures: in vitro culture and in vivo transplantation experiments. *Asaio J.*, **46**(5), 522–6.

[69] Wang, T. Y., Brennan, J. K. and Wu, J. H. 1995. Multilineal hematopoiesis in a three-dimensional murine long-term bone marrow culture. *Exp. Hematol.*, **23**(1), 26–32.

[70] Campbell, A. D. and Wicha, M. S. 1988. Extracellular matrix and the hematopoietic microenvironment. *J. Lab. Clin. Med.*, **112**(2), 140–6.

[71] Dao, M. A., Hashino, K., Kato, I. and Nolta, J. A. 1998. Adhesion to fibronectin maintains regenerative capacity during ex vivo culture and transduction of human hematopoietic stem and progenitor cells. *Blood*, **92**(12), 4612–21.

[72] Campbell, A. D., Long, M. W. and Wicha, M. S. 1987. Haemonectin, a bone marrow adhesion protein specific for cells of granulocyte lineage. *Nature*, **329**(6141), 744–6.

[73] Weinstein, R., Riordan, M. A., Wenc, K. *et al.* 1989. Dual role of fibronectin in hematopoietic differentiation. *Blood*, **73**(1), 111–16.

[74] Greenberger, J. S. 1991. The hematopoietic microenvironment. *Crit. Rev. Oncol. Hematol.*, **11**(1), 65–84.

[75] Parmar, K., Mauch, P., Vergilio, J. A., Sackstein, R. and Down, J. D. 2007. Distribution of hematopoietic stem cells in the bone marrow according to regional hypoxia. *Proc. Nat. Acad. Sci. USA*, **104**(13), 5431–6.

[76] Sipkins, D. A., Wei, X., Wu, J. W. *et al.* 2005. In vivo imaging of specialized bone marrow endothelial microdomains for tumour engraftment. *Nature*, **435**(7044), 969–73.

[77] Taichman, R. S. and Emerson, S. G. 1994. Human osteoblasts support hematopoiesis through the production of granulocyte colony-stimulating factor. *J. Exp. Med.*, **179** (5), 1677–82.

[78] Taichman, R. S., Reilly, M. J., Emerson, S. G. 1996. Human osteoblasts support human hematopoietic progenitor cells in vitro bone marrow cultures. *Blood*, **87** (2), 518–24.

[79] Taichman, R. S. and Emerson, S. G. 1998. The role of osteoblasts in the hematopoietic microenvironment. *Stem Cells*, **16**(1), 7–15.

[80] Calvi, L. M., Adams, G. B., Weibrecht, K. W. *et al.* 2003. Osteoblastic cells regulate the haematopoietic stem cell niche. *Nature*, **425**(6960), 841–6.

[81] Zhang, J., Niu, C., Ye, L. *et al.* 2003. Identification of the haematopoietic stem cell niche and control of the niche size. *Nature*, **425**(6960), 836–41.

[82] Visnjic, D., Kalajzic, Z., Rowe, D. W. *et al.* 2004. Hematopoiesis is severely altered in mice with an induced osteoblast deficiency. *Blood*, **103**(9), 3258–64.

[83] Omatsu, Y., Sugiyama, T., Kohara, H. *et al.* 2010. The essential functions of adipo-osteogenic progenitors as

the hematopoietic stem and progenitor cell niche. *Immunity*, **33**(3), 387–99.

[84] Sugiyama, T., Kohara, H., Noda, M. and Nagasawa, T. 2006. Maintenance of the hematopoietic stem cell pool by CXCL12–CXCR4 chemokine signaling in bone marrow stromal cell niches. *Immunity*, **25**(6), 977–88.

[85] Sacchetti, B., Funari, A., Michienzi, S. *et al.* 2007. Self-renewing osteoprogenitors in bone marrow sinusoids can organize a hematopoietic microenvironment. *Cell*, **131**(2), 324–36.

[86] Adams, G. B., Chabner, K. T., Alley, I. R. *et al.* 2006. Stem cell engraftment at the endosteal niche is specified by the calcium-sensing receptor. *Nature*, **439**(7076), 599–603.

[87] Jung, Y., Wang, J., Havens, A. *et al.* 2005. Cell-to-cell contact is critical for the survival of hematopoietic progenitor cells on osteoblasts. *Cytokine*, **32**(3–4), 155–62.

[88] Seita, J. and Weissman, I. L. 2010. Hematopoietic stem cell: self-renewal versus differentiation. *Wiley Interdiscip. Rev. Syst. Biol. Med.*, **2**(6), 640–53.

[89] Ito, K., Hirao, A., Arai, F. *et al.* 2004. Regulation of oxidative stress by ATM is required for self-renewal of haematopoietic stem cells. *Nature*, **431**(7011), 997–1002.

[90] Arai, F., Hirao, A., Ohmura, M. *et al.* 2004. Tie2/angiopoietin-1 signaling regulates hematopoietic stem cell quiescence in the bone marrow niche. *Cell*, **118**(2), 149–61.

[91] Morrison, S. J. and Spradling, A. C. 2008. Stem cells and niches: mechanisms that promote stem cell maintenance throughout life. *Cell*, **132**(4), 598–611.

[92] Wilson, A. and Trumpp, A. 2006. Bone-marrow haematopoietic-stem-cell niches. *Nature Rev. Immunol.*, **6**(2), 93–106.

[93] Yin, T. and Li, L. 2006. The stem cell niches in bone. *J. Clin. Invest.*, **116**(5), 1195–201.

[94] Broxmeyer, H. E. 2008. *Cord Blood Hematopoietic Stem Cell Transplantation*. Cambridge, MA: StemBook.

[95] Hofmeister, C. C., Zhang, J., Knight, K. L., Le, P. and Stiff, P. J. 2007. Ex vivo expansion of umbilical cord blood stem cells for transplantation: growing knowledge from the hematopoietic niche. *Bone Marrow Transplant.* **39**(1), 11–23.

[96] Hoggatt, J. and Pelus, L. M. 2011. Mobilization of hematopoietic stem cells from the bone marrow niche to the blood compartment. *Stem Cell Res. Ther.*, **2**(2), 13.

[97] Kessans, M. R., Gatesman, M. L. and Kockler, D. R. 2010. Plerixafor: a peripheral blood stem cell mobilizer. *Pharmacotherapy*, **30**(5), 485–92.

[98] Devine, H., Tierney, D. K., Schmit-Pokorny, K. and McDermott, K. 2010. Mobilization of hematopoietic stem cells for use in autologous transplantation. *Clin. J. Oncol. Nurs.*, **14**(2), 212–22.

[99] Okada, S., Nakauchi, H., Nagayoshi, K. *et al.* 1992. In vivo and in vitro stem cell function of c-kit- and Sca-1-positive murine hematopoietic cells. *Blood*, **80**(12), 3044–50.

[100] Osawa, M., Nakamura, K., Nishi, N. *et al.* 1996. In vivo self-renewal of c-Kit+ Sca-1+ Lin(low/−) hemopoietic stem cells. *J. Immunol.*, **156**(9), 3207–14.

[101] Morrison, S. J., Lagasse, E. and Weissman, I. L. 1994. Demonstration that Thy(lo) subsets of mouse bone marrow that express high levels of lineage markers are not significant hematopoietic progenitors. *Blood*, **83**(12), 3480–90.

[102] Osawa, M., Hanada, K., Hamada, H. and Nakauchi, H. 1996. Long-term lymphohematopoietic reconstitution by a single CD34-low/negative hematopoietic stem cell. *Science*, **273**(5272), 242–5.

[103] Christensen, J. L. and Weissman, I. L. 2001. Flk-2 is a marker in hematopoietic stem cell differentiation: a simple method to isolate long-term stem cells. *Proc. Nat. Acad. Sci. USA*, **98**(25), 14541–6.

[104] Goodell, M. A., Rosenzweig, M., Kim, H. *et al.* 1997. Dye efflux studies suggest that hematopoietic stem cells expressing low or undetectable levels of CD34 antigen exist in multiple species. *Nature Med.*, **3**(12), 1337–45.

[105] Balazs, A. B., Fabian, A. J., Esmon, C. T. and Mulligan, R. C. 2006. Endothelial protein C receptor (CD201) explicitly identifies hematopoietic stem cells in murine bone marrow. *Blood*, **107**(6), 2317–21.

[106] Chen, C. Z., Li, M., de Graaf, D. *et al.* 2002. Identification of endoglin as a functional marker that defines long-term repopulating hematopoietic stem cells. *Proc. Nat. Acad. Sci. USA*, **99**(24), 15468–73.

[107] Kiel, M. J., Yilmaz, O. H., Iwashita, T., Terhorst, C. and Morrison, S. J. 2005. SLAM family receptors distinguish hematopoietic stem and progenitor cells and reveal endothelial niches for stem cells. *Cell*, **121**(7), 1109–21.

[108] Chen, J., Ellison, F. M., Keyvanfar, K. *et al.* 2008. Enrichment of hematopoietic stem cells with SLAM and LSK markers for the detection of hematopoietic stem cell function in normal and Trp53 null mice. *Exp. Hematol.*, **36**(10), 1236–43.

[109] Jung, Y., Wang, J., Song, J. *et al.* 2007. Annexin II expressed by osteoblasts and endothelial cells regulates stem cell adhesion, homing, and engraftment following transplantation. *Blood*, **110**(1), 82–90.

[110] Hao, Q. L., Shah, A. J., Thiemann, F. T., Smogorzewska, E. M. and Crooks, G. M. 1995. A functional comparison of CD34+CD38− cells in cord blood and bone marrow. *Blood*, **86**(10), 3745–53.

[111] Mayani, H., Dragowska, W. and Lansdorp, P. M. 1993. Characterization of functionally distinct subpopulations of CD34+ cord blood cells in serum-free long-term cultures supplemented with hematopoietic cytokines. *Blood*, **82**(9), 2664–72.

[112] Baum, C. M., Weissman, I. L., Tsukamoto, A. S., Buckle, A. M. and Peault, B. 1992. Isolation of a candidate human hematopoietic stem-cell population. *Proc. Nat. Acad. Sci. USA*, **89**(7), 2804–8.

[113] Craig, W., Kay, R., Cutler, R. L. and Lansdorp, P. M. 1993. Expression of Thy-1 on human hematopoietic progenitor cells. *J. Exp. Med.*, **177**(5), 1331–42.

[114] Majeti, R., Park, C. Y. and Weissman, I. L. 2007. Identification of a hierarchy of multipotent hematopoietic progenitors in human cord blood. *Cell Stem Cell*, **1**(6), 635–45.

[115] Notta, F., Doulatov, S., Laurenti, E. *et al.* 2011. Isolation of single human hematopoietic stem cells capable of long-term multilineage engraftment. *Science*, **333** (6039), 218–21.

[116] McKenzie, J. L., Takenaka, K., Gan, O. I., Doedens, M. and Dick, J. E. 2007. Low rhodamine 123 retention identifies long-term human hematopoietic stem cells within the Lin-CD34+CD38− population. *Blood*, **109** (2), 543–5.

[117] Dexter, T. M., Allen, T. D., and Lajtha, L. G. 1977. Conditions controlling the proliferation of haemopoietic stem cells in vitro. *J. Cell Physiol.*, **91**(3), 335–44.

[118] Coulombel, L., Eaves, A. C. and Eaves, C. J. 1983. Enzymatic treatment of long-term human marrow cultures reveals the preferential location of primitive hemopoietic progenitors in the adherent layer. *Blood*, **62**(2), 291–7.

[119] Ploemacher, R. E., van der Sluijs, J. P., Voerman, J. S. and Brons, N. H. 1989. An in vitro limiting-dilution assay of long-term repopulating hematopoietic stem cells in the mouse. *Blood*, **74**(8), 2755–63.

[120] Breems, D. A., Blokland, E. A., Neben, S. and Ploemacher, R. E. 1994. Frequency analysis of human primitive haematopoietic stem cell subsets using a cobblestone area forming cell assay. *Leukemia*, **8**(7), 1095–104.

[121] Purton, L. E. and Scadden, D. T. 2007. Limiting factors in murine hematopoietic stem cell assays. *Cell Stem Cell*, **1**(3), 263–70.

[122] Matsuzaki, Y., Kinjo, K., Mulligan, R. C. and Okano, H. 2004. Unexpectedly efficient homing capacity of purified murine hematopoietic stem cells. *Immunity*, **20**(1), 87–93.

[123] Benveniste, P., Cantin, C., Hyam, D. and Iscove, N. N. 2003. Hematopoietic stem cells engraft in mice with absolute efficiency. *Nature Immunol.*, **4**(7), 708–13.

[124] Zhang, C. C. and Lodish, H. F. 2005. Murine hematopoietic stem cells change their surface phenotype during ex vivo expansion. *Blood*, **105**(11), 4314–20.

[125] Sharma, S., Gurudutta, G. U., Satija, N. K. *et al.* 2006. Stem cell c-KIT and HOXB4 genes: critical roles and mechanisms in self-renewal, proliferation, and differentiation. *Stem Cells Dev.*, **15**(6), 755–78.

[126] Mikkola, H. K. and Orkin, S. H. 2006. The journey of developing hematopoietic stem cells. *Development*, **133** (19), 3733–44.

[127] Kirouac, D. C. and Zandstra, P. W. 2006. Understanding cellular networks to improve hematopoietic stem cell expansion cultures. *Curr. Opin. Biotechnol.*, **17**(5), 538–47.

[128] Cheung, A. M., Kwong, Y. L., Liang, R. and Leung, A. Y. 2006. Stem cell model of hematopoiesis. *Curr. Stem Cell Res. Ther.*, **1**(3), 305–15.

[129] Sorrentino, B. P. 2004. Clinical strategies for expansion of haematopoietic stem cells. *Nature Rev. Immunol.*, **4** (11), 878–88.

[130] Bellantuono, I. 2004. Haemopoietic stem cells. *Int. J. Biochem. Cell. Biol.*, **36**(4), 607–20.

[131] Sauvageau, G. and Iscove, N. N. and Humphries, R. K. 2004. In vitro and in vivo expansion of hematopoietic stem cells. *Oncogene*, **23**(43), 7223–32.

[132] Uher, F., Hajdu, M. and Vas, V. 2003. Self-renewal and differentiation of hematopoietic stem cells: a molecular approach. *Acta Microbiol. Immunol. Hung.*, **50**(1), 3–21.

[133] Madlambayan, G. J., Rogers, I., Casper, R. F. and Zandstra, P. W. 2001. Controlling culture dynamics for the expansion of hematopoietic stem cells. *J. Hematother. Stem Cell Res.*, **10**(4), 481–92.

[134] Dahlberg, A., Delaney, C. and Bernstein, I. D. 2011. Ex vivo expansion of human hematopoietic stem and progenitor cells. *Blood*, **117**(23), 6083–90.

[135] Huang, G. P., Pan, Z. J., Jia, B. B. *et al.* 2007. Ex vivo expansion and transplantation of hematopoietic stem/progenitor cells supported by mesenchymal stem cells from human umbilical cord blood. *Cell Transplant.*, **16**(6), 579–85.

[136] Rose-John, S. 2006. Designer cytokines for human haematopoietic progenitor cell expansion: impact for tissue regeneration. *Handb. Exp. Pharmacol.* **174**, 229–47.

[137] Dolznig, H., Kolbus, A., Leberbauer, C. *et al.* 2005. Expansion and differentiation of immature mouse and human hematopoietic progenitors. *Methods Molec. Med.*, **105**, 323–44.

[138] Kelly, S. S., Sola, C. B., de Lima, M. and Shpall, E. 2009. Ex vivo expansion of cord blood. *Bone Marrow Transplant.*, **44**(10), 673–81.

[139] Robb, L. 2007. Cytokine receptors and hematopoietic differentiation. *Oncogene*, **26**(47), 6715–23.

[140] Cabrita, G. J., Ferreira, B. S., da Silva, C. L. *et al.* 2003. Hematopoietic stem cells: from the bone to the bioreactor. *Trends Biotechnol.*, **21**(5), 233–40.

[141] Koller, M. R., Emerson, S. G. and Palsson, B. O. 1993. Large-scale expansion of human stem and progenitor cells from bone marrow mononuclear cells in continuous perfusion cultures. *Blood*, **82**(2), 378–84.

[142] Palsson, B. O., Paek, S. H., Schwartz, R. M. *et al.* 1993. Expansion of human bone marrow progenitor cells in a high cell density continuous perfusion system. *Biotechnology (NY)*, **11**(3), 368–72.

[143] Didwania, M., Didwania, A., Mehta, G. *et al.* 2011. Artificial hematopoietic stem cell niche: bioscaffolds to microfluidics to mathematical simulations. *Curr. Top. Med. Chem.*, **11**(13), 1599–605.

[144] Mehta, G. 2008. *Microenvironmental Control in Microfluidic Bioreactors for Long Term Culture of Bone Marrow Cells.* Ann Arbor, MI: University of Michigan.

[145] Mehta, G., Torisawa, Y. and Takayama, S. 2008. Engineering cellular microenvironments with microfluidics. In Gomez, F. A., editor. *Biological Applications of Microfluidics.* Hoboken, NJ: John Wiley and Sons, pp. 87–114.

[146] Shim, J., Bersano-Begey, T. F., Zhu, X. *et al.* 2003. Micro- and nanotechnologies for studying cellular function. *Curr. Top. Med. Chem.*, **3**(6), 687–703.

[147] Walker, G. M., Zeringue, H. C. and Beebe, D. J. 2004. Microenvironment design considerations for cellular scale studies. *Lab. Chip*, **4**(2), 91–7.

[148] Meissner, P., Schroder, B., Herfurth, C. and Biselli, M. 1999. Development of a fixed bed bioreactor for the expansion of human hematopoietic progenitor cells. *Cytotechnology*, **30**(1–3), 227–34.

[149] Sandstrom, C. E., Bender, J. G., Miller, W. M. and Papoutsakis, E. T. 1996. Development of novel perfusion chamber to retain nonadherent cells and its use for comparison of human "mobilized" peripheral blood mononuclear cell cultures with and without irradiated bone marrow stroma. *Biotechnol Bioeng.*, **50**(5), 493–504.

[150] Zandstra, P. W., Eaves, C. J. and Piret, J. M. 1994. Expansion of hematopoietic progenitor cell populations in stirred suspension bioreactors of normal human bone marrow cells. *Biotechnology (NY)*, **12**(9), 909–14.

[151] Cross, M., Alt, R. and Niederwieser, D. 2008. The case for a metabolic stem cell niche. *Cells Tissues Organs*, **188**(1–2), 150–9.

[152] de la Morena, M. T. and Gatti, R. A. 2010. A history of bone marrow transplantation. *Immunol. Allergy Clin. North Am.*, **30**(1), 1–15.

[153] Pulsipher, M. A. and Woolfrey, A. 2001. Nonmyeloablative transplantation in children. Current status and future prospects. *Hematol. Oncol. Clin. North Am.*, **15**(5), 809–34 and vii–viii.

[154] Mehta, P., Locatelli, F., Stary, J. and Smith, F. O. 2010. Bone marrow transplantation for inherited bone marrow failure syndromes. *Pediatr. Clin. North Am.*, **57**(1), 147–70.

[155] Boelens, J. J., Prasad, V. K., Tolar, J., Wynn, R. F. and Peters, C. 2010. Current international perspectives on hematopoietic stem cell transplantation for inherited metabolic disorders. *Pediatr. Clin. North Am.*, **57**(1), 123–45.

[156] Eide, M. B., Lauritzsen, G. F., Kvalheim, G. *et al.* 2011. High dose chemotherapy with autologous stem cell support for patients with histologically transformed B-cell non-Hodgkin lymphomas. A Norwegian multicentre phase II study. *Br. J. Haematol.*, **152**(5), 600–10.

[157] Weissman, I. L. and Shizuru, J. A. 2008. The origins of the identification and isolation of hematopoietic stem cells, and their capability to induce donor-specific transplantation tolerance and treat autoimmune diseases. *Blood*, **112**(9), 3543–53.

[158] Orlovskaya, I., Schraufstatter, I., Loring, J. and Khaldoyanidi, S. 2008. Hematopoietic differentiation of embryonic stem cells. *Methods*, **45**(2), 159–67.

[159] Sakamoto, H., Tsuji-Tamura, K. and Ogawa, M. 2010. Hematopoiesis from pluripotent stem cell lines. *Int. J. Hematol.*, **91**(3), 384–91.

[160] Huber, T. L. 2010. Dissecting hematopoietic differentiation using the embryonic stem cell differentiation model. *Int. J. Dev. Biol.*, **54**(6–7), 991–1002.

[161] Chen, M. J., Yokomizo, T., Zeigler, B. M., Dzierzak, E. and Speck, N. A. 2009. Runx1 is required for the endothelial to haematopoietic cell transition but not thereafter. *Nature*, **457**(7231), 887–91.

[162] Bendre, M., Gaddy, D., Nicholas, R. W. and Suva, L. J. 2003. Breast cancer metastasis to bone: it is not all about PTHrP. *Clin. Orthop. Relat. Res.*, **415**(Suppl.), S39–S45.

[163] Sweeney, K. J., Boland, P. J. and King, T. 2007. The management of asymptomatic skeletal breast cancer: a paradigm shift. *Ann. Surg. Oncol.*, **14**(9), 2430–1.

[164] Coleman, R. E. 2006. Clinical features of metastatic bone disease and risk of skeletal morbidity. *Clin. Cancer Res.*, **12**(20, Part 2), 6243s–9s.

[165] Sun, Y. X., Wang, J., Shelburne, C. E. *et al.* 2003. Expression of CXCR4 and CXCL12 (SDF-1) in human prostate cancers (PCa) in vivo. *J. Cell Biochem.*, **89**(3), 462–73.

[166] Sun, Y. X., Schneider, A., Jung, Y. *et al.* 2005. Skeletal localization and neutralization of the SDF-1(CXCL12)/CXCR4 axis blocks prostate cancer metastasis and growth in osseous sites in vivo. *J. Bone Miner. Res.*, **20**(2), 318–29.

[167] Shiozawa, Y., Havens, A. M., Pienta, K. J. and Taichman, R. S. 2008. The bone marrow niche: habitat to hematopoietic and mesenchymal stem cells, and unwitting host to molecular parasites. *Leukemia*, **22**(5), 941–50.

[168] Mishra, A., Shiozawa, Y., Pienta, K. J. and Taichman, R. S. 2011. Homing of cancer cells to the bone. *Cancer Microenviron.*, **4**(3), 221–235.

[169] Shiozawa, Y., Pienta, K. J. and Taichman, R. S. 2011. Hematopoietic stem cell niche is a potential therapeutic target for bone metastatic tumors. *Clin. Cancer Res.*, **17**(17), 5553–8.

[170] Alix-Panabieres, C., Riethdorf, S. and Pantel, K. 2008. Circulating tumor cells and bone marrow micrometastasis. *Clin. Cancer Res.*, **14**(16), 5013–21.

[171] Morrissey, C. and Vessella, R. L. 2007. The role of tumor microenvironment in prostate cancer bone metastasis. *J. Cell Biochem.*, **101**(4), 873–86.

[172] Wikman, H., Vessella, R. and Pantel, K. 2008. Cancer micrometastasis and tumour dormancy. *Apmis*, **116**(7–8), 754–70.

[173] Reddi, A. H., Roodman, D., Freeman, C. and Mohla, S. 2003. Mechanisms of tumor metastasis to the bone: challenges and opportunities. *J. Bone Miner. Res.*, **18**(2), 190–4.

[174] Psaila, B., Kaplan, R. N., Port, E. R. and Lyden, D. 2006. Priming the "soil" for breast cancer metastasis: the pre-metastatic niche. *Breast Dis.*, **26**, 65–74.

[175] Keller, E. T., Zhang, J., Cooper, C. R. *et al.* 2001. Prostate carcinoma skeletal metastases: cross-talk between tumor and bone. *Cancer Metastasis Rev.*, **20**(3–4), 333–49.

[176] Shiozawa, Y., Pedersen, E. A., Havens, A. M. *et al.* 2011. Human prostate cancer metastases target the hematopoietic stem cell niche to establish footholds in mouse bone marrow. *J. Clin. Invest.*, **121**(4), 1298–312.

[177] Jung, Y., Song, J., Shiozawa, Y. *et al.* 2008. Hematopoietic stem cells regulate mesenchymal stromal cell induction into osteoblasts thereby participating in the formation of the stem cell niche. *Stem Cells*, **26**(8), 2042–51.

[178] Huang, X., Cho, S. and Spangrude, G. J. 2007. Hematopoietic stem cells: generation and self-renewal. *Cell Death Differ.*, **14**(11), 1851–9.

[179] Larsson, J. and Karlsson, S. 2005. The role of Smad signaling in hematopoiesis. *Oncogene*, **24**(37), 5676–92.

5

Using biomaterials for fetal stem cell isolation, expansion and directed-differentiation

David Mack, Aleksander Skardal, Shay Soker and Anthony Atala

5.1 Introduction

Stem cells are defined by their unique ability to self-renew and produce progeny that differentiate into specialized cells. Naturally occurring stem cells are usually broken down into three principal categories. Embryonic stem cells (ESCs) are derived from the inner cell mass of a preimplantation embryo and are considered pluripotent, meaning able to produce cell types of all three germ layers. Second, adult somatic stem cells exist at a very low frequency in almost all tissues and organs of the body and are usually considered lineage-restricted to the subset of cell types that make up their tissue of origin. Lastly, fetal stem cells can be obtained from various fetal tissues, including primordial germ cells, blood, liver, bone marrow and amniotic fluid, as well as extra-embryonic tissues such as the placenta and umbilical cord. In terms of multipotentiality these fetal stem cells lie somewhere between ESCs and more committed adult somatic stem cells. A new fourth, artificially generated type of stem cell now exists, namely the so-called induced pluripotent stem (iPS) cell, which results from the transcriptional reprogramming of a terminally differentiated somatic cell. Each one of these stem cell types has advantages and disadvantages in cell-based therapies and undoubtedly no one cell type will fit all applications. For example, ES cells are attractive because of their inherent plasticity, but their derivation elicits ethical concerns and the likelihood of forming teratomas after transplantation makes them, for now, a therapeutic dead end. Adult somatic stem cells, like bone marrow mesenchymal stromal cells (BM-MSCs) are being used clinically [45, 62], but their applications are restricted by limited proliferative capacity in culture and a predisposition to differentiate down primarily mesenchymal lineages. iPS cells have been shown to be genetically unstable and also have the potential to form teratomas after transplantation [33], especially if the efficiency of the differentiation protocols is not optimized. Fetal stem cells can be isolated from two distinct sources, the fetus proper and the extra-embryonic support tissues such as the amniotic fluid, placenta, and umbilical cord (especially Wharton's jelly) [1]. Isolating stem cells from the fetus is replete with moral, ethical, and legal concerns and will therefore not be discussed further here. The use of fetal stem cells from extra-embryonic tissues, on the other hand, elicits no ethical or moral concerns because their isolation does not put a developing fetus at risk. The fact that cells forming the extra-embryonic tissues arise early in gestation and are subsequently separated from the developing fetus may endow the resident stem cells with a higher degree of plasticity than that of adult somatic stem cells. This has been shown in various cases where stem cells from these tissues have been differentiated toward adipogenic, osteogenic, myogenic, endothelial, neuronal, and hepatic lineages [25]. Important for their clinical utility, however, is that this more primitive character is not accompanied by teratoma formation after transplantation. Equally important to their broad-range therapeutic potential is the complementary immunomodulatory activity and immunoprivileged status. For example, just like MSCs, amniotic-fluid-derived stem (AFS) cells secrete a wide range of cytokines and chemokines that suppress innate and adaptive immune systems [16, 61]. Lastly, but not insignificantly for their application to cellular therapies, fetal stem cells can be isolated in large numbers simply because extra-embryonic tissues are relatively large and discarded en masse after birth [59].

Even with a highly plastic, plentiful and immunologically advantageous fetal stem cell population, our inability to guide the differentiation and behavior of these cells in vitro and in vivo has limited their therapeutic application. One of the principal deficiencies hindering our ability to manipulate stem cells is our lack of understanding of the native microenvironment of the tissue of origin. Stem cell homeostasis and activation is controlled by the bidirectional communication with the surrounding support cells of the niche. How biophysical and biochemical signals are sensed and integrated into the three-dimensional (3D) regulatory network of the stem cell is poorly understood. At the heart of this inadequate understanding is our knowledge of the niche composition. What is needed is a systematic inquiry into the biomaterials that comprise the niche and the role each material plays in determining the fate of the resident stem cells. This chapter will explore how biomaterials can be used in two-dimensional (2D) and 3D applications to support fetal stem cells in their undifferentiated state as well as participate in the directed differentiation down various lineages. In particular, this review will focus on those soft hydrogel biomaterials that currently have the most potential to make significant impact in stem cell applications and niche design. The fetal stem cell niche, especially in extra-embryonic tissues, does not have the same direct impact on stem cell differentiation as does the adult somatic stem cell niche, as illustrated in the colon crypt or hair bulge, for example. However, it is likely that the same universal principles governing cell-matrix interactions and signal transduction apply to all stem cell microenvironments and can be exploited for the purpose of directed differentiation in the laboratory for regenerative medicine applications.

Cell-based therapies have the potential to revolutionize the treatment of injuries, degenerative diseases, and the general effects of aging. However, several major limitations must be overcome to enable the wide utilization of this approach. Probably the biggest deficiency is the lack of suitable strategies to reproducibly isolate and expand, and then robustly differentiate, stem cell populations into useful lineages. The systematic integration of biomaterials into the isolation and expansion phases, regardless of the originating stem cell source, will almost certainly increase survivability, promote culture uniformity, and provide context for inductive signals during differentiation. Therefore, it is plausible that in the near future we will develop simple strategies that will allow the economical translation of this approach into the clinic.

5.2 A brief introduction to the stem cell niche

The stem cell niche is the in-vivo biophysical, biochemical, and cellular microenvironment responsible for the temporal and spatial regulation of stem cell survival, self-renewal, and differentiation [27]. A niche must have anatomical and functional dimensions (range of signaling) that protect the stem cells from depletion but also protect the "host" from over-exuberant proliferation (cancer). Elements of the niche can be broken down into extracellular matrix components, cell-cell contact, paracrine and humoral factors and metabolism as an indicator of tissue state. The integration between these elements ensures coordinated interpretation of complex external signals, which in turn drives proper tissue function, homeostasis and regeneration of aged, injured, or diseased tissues and organs. As an indication of the power of the niche, studies have shown that simply providing an instructive cell-free scaffold to a native, defective niche can direct the resident stem cells toward normal differentiation and function [5, 22, 24]. Here we explore the physical properties of the niche microenvironment that are likely key aspects of stem cell regulation – the specific polymer and protein makeup, the dimensionality (2D versus 3D), and mechanical properties such as stiffness and shear stresses.

5.2.1 Properties of the stem cell niche

In terms of composition, precise knowledge is somewhat lacking, and thus one must extrapolate from other work exploring how stem cells interact with the ECM. The authors of a number of studies have shown that MSC survival and self-renewal is highly dependent on successful integrin binding [30, 96]. It has also been suggested that N-cadherins are important, but somewhat less so, for hematopoietic stem cell (HSC) propagation and differentiation [48]. This seems to hold true for other stem cell types, insofar as ES cells are consistently differentiated into neural progenitors by culturing them on integrin-binding, laminin-containing substrates. Blocking the integrin subunits decreased the ability of ES cells to differentiate down the neural lineage [58].

The exact makeup of stem cell niches is also not well understood, and therefore much of our knowledge is based on well-known developmental environments. Developing tissues are generally low in ECM components such as collagen type I, but high in components such as collagen type IV and hyaluronic acid (HA). It has been shown that some stem cells, specifically HSCs, can synthesize HA in the niche, which in turn binds to cells, causing them to slow their proliferation and preventing differentiation into granulocytes [69]. As an example of the ultimate developmental environment, the amniotic fluid contains high levels of HA early in gestation, but those levels decrease as the pregnancy progresses, with a concomitant increase in the level of collagen type I [23]. Amniotic fluid, along with the amniotic membrane, has been known for a long time to promote scar-free healing and regeneration. Later in gestation and in adults the healing processes are dominated by the presence of collagen type I, resulting in fibrotic healing. Other ECM proteins and polymers, such as fibronectin, laminin, heparan sulfate, and elastin, can also have a pronounced effect on stem cells.

It is also important to consider the mechanical nature of the niche. Characteristics such as dimensionality, fluid shear stress, and elastic moduli can greatly impact stem cells, such as by preferentially maintaining stemness versus differentiating. Higher fluid stresses similar to that of blood flow can initiate endothelial differentiation in ESCs [103], and mechanical deformations or strains like those in mechanically active tissues such as a beating heart or dilating arteries can induce MSC differentiation toward smooth muscle [52]. Two-dimensional cell culture has long been a well-established method for the study of cell physiology and behavior. Expanding cells on plastic is still the preferred method for rapid propagation of large numbers of cells for use in other applications. However, this requires cells to adhere to abnormally stiff substrates. Moreover, since every tissue has a unique 3D architecture, a 2D cell culture cannot accurately model the in-vivo physiology and near microgravity of stem cell environments [66]. Even tissues that exist as monolayers, such as epithelial or endothelial cell sheets residing on semi-permeable basal membranes, allow 3D signaling and soluble molecule diffusion from both sides of the membranes and from adjacent cells. On plastic, cells do not have this capability. Thus, it is important that 3D environments are used for long-term in-vitro cell expansion and for creating tissues [6]. The application of biomaterials for the artificial construction of 3D microenvironments will continue to be an important tool for niche mimicry as researchers attempt to control expansion and directed differentiation of various stem cell populations.

In general, it is believed that stem cell niches are low-fluid-shear-stress environments (LFSSs) that do not mechanically induce differentiation, thus allowing stem cell self-renewal and expansion. The LFSSs experienced by cells immobilized in the body can be modeled using culture methods involving soft 3D hydrogels or rotating-wall-vessel (RWV) bioreactor cultures, in which cells tumble in suspension or adhere to suspended biomaterial microcarriers [9, 36]. The LFSS conditions experienced in an RWV bioreactor can be used to establish 3D organotypic cell aggregates on microcarriers that model the structure and function of in-vivo human tissues [68, 98]. Human primary breast carcinoma cells, that are normally limited to one or two passages in monolayer culture, had increased proliferative activity as aggregates in RWV bioreactors, staying viable for over 56 days [8]. HepG2 hepatic carcinoma spheroids expressed phenotypes similar to those seen in normal hepatocytes in vivo, such as increased cell–cell adhesion and G1 cell cycle arrest levels, reduced apoptosis, and increased ability for angiogenesis [56].

It has also been shown that the mechanical properties of a substrate directly influence stem cell behavior, particularly differentiation. Various stem cell types show a specific preference to differentiate toward a given tissue type when cultured in or on a substrate that mimics the elastic modulus of that tissue. In a seminal example explored by Engler *et al.*, when MSCs were cultured on polyacrylimide substrates at 0.1–1, 8–17, and 25–40 kPa, coated with collagen type I, the cells were directed toward neural, muscle, and osteogenic lineages, respectively [31]. Such stiffness-directed behavior has also been shown by using softer alginate hydrogels to increase neural stem cell differentiation shown by increased levels of neural markers [4]. Likewise, muscle stem cells were shown to self-renew on lower-stiffness polyethylene glycol (PEG)–laminin hydrogels at 12 kPa, but not on stiff plastic surfaces [38]. The fact that stiffness plays an important role in stem cell lineage specification highlights the importance of measuring the mechanical properties of actual stem cell niches.

5.2.2 Designing and mimicking the stem cell niche

Our limited understanding of stem cell microenvironments has recently been put to effective use with the advent of synthetic niches for in-vitro expansion of stem cells that is physiologically superior to 2D culture on plastic. The important attributes for generating engineered stem cell niches include the biochemical signals, extracellular matrix molecules, biomechanical cues, and architecture and geometry of the microenvironment [46]. Cell–cell contacts and growth factor presentation are important, but, because the ECM is what physically retains stem cells in their niche [26], this section focusses primarily on design concepts and application of synthetic ECM hydrogels to mimic stem cell niches. Balancing cellular proliferation and attachment is important, given that a substrate with too many strong adherent sites could negatively affect the cells' ability to move. It has been postulated that stem cells, once they have left their native niche, can migrate through tissues to sites of injury and secrete trophic factors and/or differentiate into specialized cells. If an engineered stem cell niche contains too high a concentration of cell attachment sites, such as strongly cell-adherent collagen type I, the attached cells might maintain viability and even proliferate, but may suffer stunted migratory abilities. In a study that explored this issue, it was shown that both proliferation and migration increased in HA hydrogels containing cell-adherent arginine-glycine-aspartic acid peptide (RGD) and matrix metalloproteinase (MMP) degradable crosslinkers allowing cell-induced matrix degradation and remodeling [54]. In an AFS cell therapy application for wound healing, we observed that cells delivered in strongly adherent collagen–fibrin gels were unable to migrate out of the gel and into the underlying tissue. We are now investigating other hydrogels that may be more permissive in order to support increased stem cell motility.

Mechanical properties also play a role in the decision of a stem cell to remain undifferentiated and divide symmetrically or to divide asymmetrically and allow one daughter cell to differentiate [31]. For example, increasing the stiffness of an RGD-containing alginate gel from 3.3 kPa to 12.4 kPa increased adipose progenitor cell self-renewal and angiogenic capacity, while inhibiting adipogenic differentiation [17]. When hematopoietic stem cells and progenitor cells were cultured on softer tropoelastin substrates instead of plastic, expansion of undifferentiated cells increased more than two-fold [42]. Furthermore, a photopolymerizable methacrylamide material was developed in which neural stem/progenitor cells showed preferential differentiation towards neurons at $E' < 1$ kPa, oligodendocytes at $E' > 7$ kPa, or astrocytes on substrates at $E' < 3.5$ kPa [55]. The potential impact of mechanical properties is not limited to applications in which differentiation is the primary objective. For example, we demonstrated that a decreased level of substrate stiffness induced a more mobile phenotype in amniotic-fluid-derived stem cells. In this state, AFS cells secrete migratory factors that recruit other AFS cells or attract endothelial cells and stimulate their angiogenic phenotype [90].

Bidirectional communication between the resident stem cell and the surrounding "support cells" allows integration and interpretation of complex external signals that need to directly impact what type of cell division a stem cell undergoes. Therefore, the marriage of stem cell biology and biomaterials will not only contribute to our basic understanding of how the niche regulates stem cell behavior but also help us identify new approaches for the propagation and forced differentiation of stem cells for regenerative medicine applications.

5.3 Practical applications of biomaterials for the manipulation of stem cells

Most applications in regenerative medicine require large numbers of cells. Cellular therapies need to deliver a sufficient number of cells to ensure engraftment and functionality at the target site. Should the delivery be systemic, the cell number has to be even higher, since it is assumed that only a small percentage of the injected cells will reach the target site. Another example requiring high cell numbers is the building of functional organs from the ground up. Whatever the method is, be it rapid prototyping, organ printing, or repopulation of decellularized tissue, the number of cells required is on the order of 1×10^9 per cm^3, making the total number of cells needed for almost any organ truly massive.

Unfortunately, it is difficult to supply large numbers of clinical-grade stem cells. Harvesting primary cells from tissues usually results in many cells dying ex vivo, and often only a subpopulation of these cells consists of "true" stem cells. Furthermore, if the cells are for autologous treatment there is a limit on the total number of cells that can be harvested because of the risk to the patient. With lower starting numbers of cells, they must be expanded in the laboratory, but standard expansion in regular tissue culture plastic dishes has practical limitations as well as the mismatch between the mechanical properties of the authentic niche and those of the tissue culture dish, as mentioned above. Conventional plasticware has limited surface area, requiring multiple passaging, splitting, and seeding steps that become time-consuming and expensive, given the amount of materials and culture media required. One advantage of 3D platforms is the ability to culture at least one order of magnitude more cells per unit volume than is possible with 2D approaches.

5.3.1 Hydrogel biomaterials as tools for stem cell applications

Because materials have a direct effect on the lineage determination and function of cells, it is important to choose the correct material for the specific application. In general, the primary purpose of hydrogel biomaterials is to mimic natural cell microenvironments in a way that is more simple and deconstructed, in order to enable a particular cell or tissue behavior. Here we explore a variety of biomaterial advances that have been implemented with stem cell technologies or that have the potential to be useful in such applications, with specific attention to hydrogels since discussion of them constitutes the bulk of the stem-cell-relevant biomaterial literature. Hydrogel biomaterials are particularly relevant to stem cell research since, being gels, they are soft materials, and the stem cell niche is often regarded as being soft as well. Tissues in the body have a wide range of stiffnesses (Figure 5.1). That of brain tissue is usually only 0.5–2 kPa and that of bone is over 50 kPa, yet standard procedures culture cells from these tissues on the same plastic surfaces that are at over 100,000 kPa [99].

Experiments currently under way in our laboratory are focussed on determining the optimal substrate stiffness for the propagation and differentiation of fetal stem cells from amniotic fluid and placenta. Immunohistochemistry revealed increased expression of genes associated with mesenchymal stem cells (CD44, CD90, CD105, and N-cadherin) in cells cultured on softer substrates, confirming that substrate stiffness alone can have profound effects on gene expression and thus alter the potential uses of these fetal stem cells [90]. In fact, growing these cells routinely on plastic in 2D culture could irreversibly alter their therapeutic potential. Hydrogels can support a range of elastic moduli, matching the mechanical properties of most tissues, with the exception of tooth and bone. In most cases, hydrogels are formed by crosslinks between polymer chains, although some are formed between proteins or

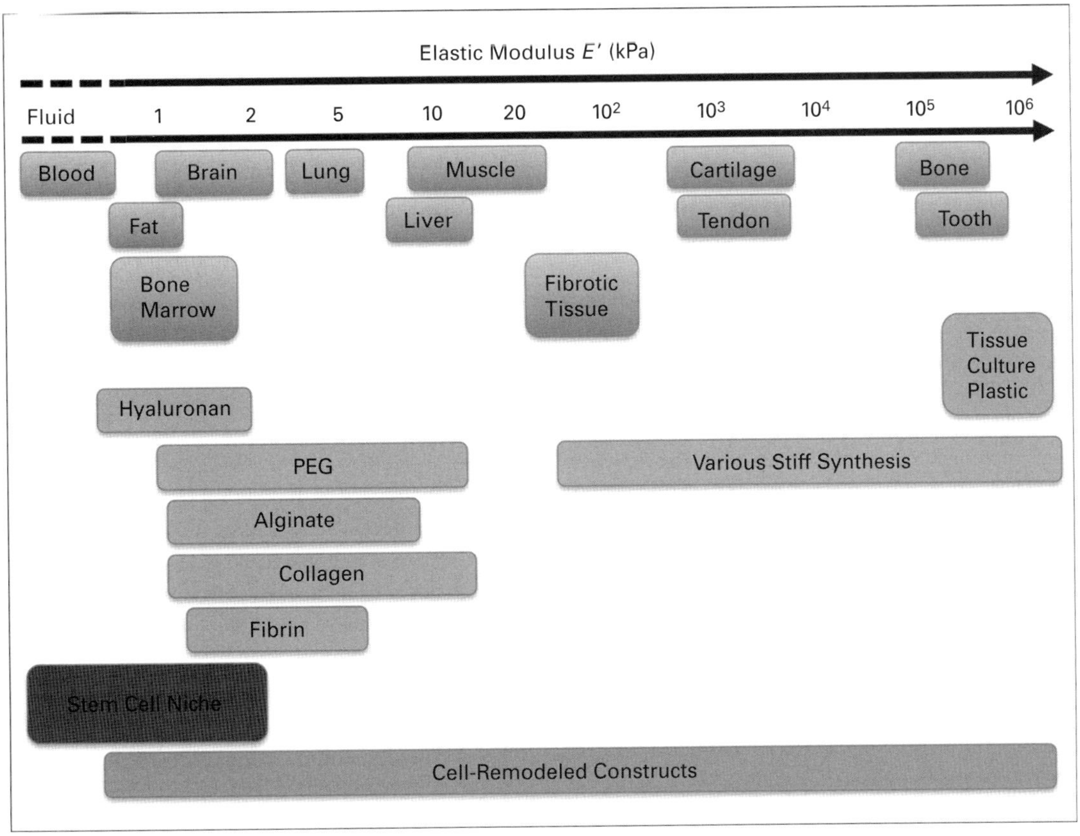

Figure 5.1 Tissues and organs in the body span a range of elastic moduli, or stiffnesses. However, tissue culture plastic, which traditionally has been used for the majority of in-vitro cell cultures, is several orders of magnitude stiffer than most tissue types, and falls short of being an optimal substrate in biomedical applications. The stem cell niche is also often described as being of low stiffness. Since hydrogels can mimic the elastic modulus of soft tissue and the potentially soft environment of a niche, they are more suitable to be used for stem cell and tissue engineering applications than classical plastic culture environments.

peptides. These crosslinks can be covalent, ionic, or physical interactions. Hydrogels can be comprised of synthetic materials, natural materials, or both. However, since natural sources contribute bioactivity to the hydrogels, they will receive most of our attention here, although synthetic hydrogels are discussed to some extent as well. Synthesis of biologically useful hydrogels may provide cell niches that are tailorable microenvironments allowing scientists to move away from 2D settings to more favorable 3D environments that increase the potential for physiological and clinical applications [72]. The materials described below were implemented in a variety of stem-cell-based applications and were able to control cell differentiation, expansion, and migration. Additionally, some biomaterials can help to maintain stemness or secretion of therapeutic factors over time in culture. Some hydrogels are formed in such ways that they can easily encapsulate stem cells for cell therapy delivery or in-vitro engineering of tissues and organs.

5.3.1.1 Synthetic polymer hydrogels

A range of synthetic materials have been used as hydrogels for applications in regenerative medicine. Synthetic polymers have one primary advantage – precise control over their chemical and physical properties can be achieved. Scientists can maintain precise chemical control over molecular weight, functional groups, and hydrophobicity/hydrophilicity at a monomer level. As a result, crosslinking rates and mechanical properties can be precisely controlled. Polyethylene glycol (PEG) and polyacrylamide are examples of synthetic polymers that are commonly used in biomedical applications. PEG has long been used as medical device coatings to control host immune responses or appended to drug constructs to reduce degradation in vivo. It can also be manipulated to form a variety of hydrogels for stem cell culture and differentiation. PEG is often modified with acrylate groups to create a photopolymerizable polyethylene glycol diacrylate (PEGDA) in which cells can quickly be encapsulated.

The same features that allow such precise control over the properties of synthetic biomaterials also translate into an inherent drawback. All biological interfacing or function has to be artificially preprogrammed into the material, since these materials typically have no active natural attachment sites that interact with cells. For example, PEG requires covalent attachment of cell-adhesion peptides such as RGD peptides or other natural proteins in order to allow cell adherence. Alternatively, many hydrogels have been synthesized from natural polymers and peptides or synthetically modified natural polymers or peptides. Examples include collagen, hyaluronic acid, alginate, fibrin, and silk.

5.3.1.2 Collagen

Collagen is one of the natural materials most commonly used as a cell substrate, since it is the most abundant component of the ECM in most tissues. Isolation and purification procedures are well established, particularly for collagen type I, and supplying collagens for surface coatings and gels for cell culture. Inherent in the collagen structure are important amino acid sequences that allow cells to adhere and proliferate via integrin binding. However, in normal tissue and extracellular matrix, collagen is only one of many components. Collagen biomaterial matrices are indeed useful and have yielded many important biological advances, but ~100% collagen matrices may limit cell migration and locomotion due to strong cell attachment. Furthermore, collagen primarily contains hydrophobic peptide motifs. Hence, when used as an implant, collagen gels often exclude water and contract, potentially resulting in decreased function, decreased diffusion of nutrients and gases, and cell death. Collagen has been used extensively in tissue culture, but its implementation for stem cell work may now be limited due to the recent development of other biomaterials with superior properties.

5.3.1.3 Hyaluronic acid

Hyaluronic acid (HA), or hyaluronan, is a unique and versatile macromolecule with great promise for tissue engineering [3]. It is a non-sulfated glycosaminoglycan (GAG) consisting of repeating disaccharide units and is present in connective tissues as a major constituent of the ECM [50]. Unmodified HA has been used clinically for over three decades [51] in applications such as treatment of damaged joints [35, 84]. It is commonly modified to be a useful and robust biomaterial that can be crosslinked or loaded with other functional molecules [80]. Physical forms include electrospun fibers, sponges, films, and hydrogels – all of which can be used in regenerative medicine applications [13]. For use with stem cells, hydrogels are most common.

Hydrogels derived from HA are often implemented by photocrosslinking methacrylate groups appended to the HA chains that can undergo radical polymerization by photocrosslinking to form soft hydrogels, referred to here as MA-HA hydrogels. Photocrosslinkable HA hydrogels have been used in many settings, from cutaneous and corneal wound healing [60] to prototype vessel structure bioprinting [93]. Thiol-modification of HA also yields a material via which hydrogels can be formed through Michael-type addition crosslinking. Akin to MA-HA, thiol-modified HA, particularly a thiolated carboxymethyl HA (CMHA-S), has been implemented in many tissue engineering applications such as wound healing [49], tumor modeling [57], and bioprinting of cellularized structures [92].

5.3.1.4 Alginate

Alginate is a popular choice for regenerative medicine applications because it is easy to form into a hydrogel in the presence of calcium ions. This has made alginate the material of choice for microencapsulation of cells. Easily available alginic sodium salt, or sodium alginate, which is unmodified, is easily crosslinked into calcium alginate hydrogel microspheres [83]. These constructs have been extensively used for creating hydrogels containing immobilized liver cells or pancreatic islets [74]. Without chemical modification, alginate is a rather simplistic material, and its use for stem cell culture is limited unless one incorporates cell-adherent motifs. Alginate materials suffer one other drawback. The reagents commonly used for creating cell-laden hydrogel microspheres, such as $CaCl_2$, the crosslinking reagent, as well as sodium citrate and ethylenediaminetetraacetic acid (EDTA), commonly used chelators, have been shown to have a detrimental effect on MSC survival during the encapsulation process [21]. However, due to the ease with which alginate gels can be formed, it remains a common choice as a material for cell encapsulation.

5.3.1.5 Fibrin and silk

Other natural-sourced hydrogels, such as those based on fibrin and silk, have been developed and implemented for culture of various tissues types, but have not been subjected to use with stem cells to the same extent as have the biomaterials discussed above. However, these materials have been used for differentiation of stem cells into skin, cartilage, bone or dental tissue, and adipose. Fibrin is comprised of fibrinogen monomers that are joined by thrombin-mediated crosslinking. It has an important role in blood clotting, wound healing, and tumor growth. It has been used clinically as a hemostatic agent and sealant in surgery. More recently, fibrin gels have been used as a scaffold for regenerative medicine due to their quick crosslinking rates and mechanical properties [2]. Silk is a different protein biomaterial that has been implemented for tissue engineering applications. It has low immunogenicity, slow degradation rates, and strong mechanical properties. These properties make silk appropriate as a stable supportive material for long-term cell culture or in-vivo implantations [18].

5.3.2 Biomaterial stem cell utilities

5.3.2.1 Differentiation

The most comprehensively researched application of hydrogel biomaterials with respect to stem cells is induction of directed differentiation. Much work has focussed on osteogenic and chrondrogenic environments, although other tissue types have been investigated. MSCs were induced to undergo chondrogenesis in PEGDA gels in vitro [102] and in vivo in mice with a hyaluronic acid supplement [87]. In many applications, additional materials must be added to support cell attachment. PEG gels with RGD peptide sequences or phosphate groups promoted human MSC viability by enhancing cell–matrix interactions [73]. Similarly, PEG–RGDS gels increased survival and chondrogenesis of MSCs, resulting in more collagen, aggrecan, and GAG production [82]. On varying the composition of PEG hydrogels and by adding chondroitin sulfate, matrix metalloproteinase-sensitive peptides, or HA, encapsulated MSCs could make zone-specific cartilage-like tissue of varying compressive modulus [67]. On adding phospho-ester to PEG, hydrogels induced MSCs to express bone-related markers and secrete osteocalcin, osteonectin, and alkaline phosphatase, resulting in increased mineralization and bone-like tissue [101]. In a thermoreversible and biodegradable Pluronic F127 hydrogel also containing HA, potential for adipose-derived stem cells (ADSCs) to undergo chondrogenesis was shown [44]. The F127 hydrogels have also been used for adipogenic differentiation of MSCs in the presence of adipogenic factors [100]. Dextran–PEG hydrogels in which both chondrocytes and ESCs could be maintained in culture for 3 weeks, after which both cell types produced cartilaginous tissue, have been created [43].

Other work has focussed on the impact of physical and spatial cues from the substrates on stem cells. In the subsequent examples the substantial control over synthetic polymer materials allowed targeted manipulation of the substrate morphologies that the cells would experience. Polyacrylimide gels with topographical patterns comprised of square and hexagonal posts of varying sizes and gap distances were formed. After coating with collagen, seeded MSCs displayed substantial morphological differences depending on the surface patterns [79]. By using a photomasking technique, surface wrinkles were patterned in poly(2-hydroxyethyl methacrylate) surfaces in lamellar or hexagonal patterns on which human MSCs were seeded. On lamellar patterned surfaces, MSCs differentiated into an osteogenic lineage, while, on hexagonally patterned surfaces, MSCs differentiated into an adipogenic lineage [39].

Photocrosslinkable MA–HA hydrogels substrates were recently used for manipulation of stem cell culture, particularly controlled differentiation [14]. Human embryonic stem cells cultured in 3D in MA–HA hydrogels were able to maintain their undifferentiated state for cell expansion, while differentiation could be selectively induced within the same hydrogel by exposure to soluble factors [37]. In the same MA–HA hydrogels MSCs could successfully undergo chondrogenesis, and increased their collagen secretion rates in comparison with that in PEG hydrogels [20]. Furthermore, co-cultures of MSCs with articular chondrocytes in MA–HA hydrogels resulted in increased mechanical properties and improved ECM production of tissue-engineered cartilage constructs [10]. MA–HA hydrogels have also been implemented with a double-crosslinking method to create internally 3D patterned hydrogels to spatially control encapsulated MSC spreading, which in turn could control adipogenic or osteogenic differentiation [47]. Undifferentiated human adipose-derived stem cells encapsulated in CMHA-S hydrogels underwent angiogenesis and adipogenesis, showing the feasibility of engineering adipose tissue [32]. CMHA-S hydrogels have also been used to support liver stem cell expansion and differentiation into hepatocytes [85].

Endothelial progenitor cells (EPCs) seeded on fibrin gels showed increased cell viability as well as increased Oct 3/4 and Nanog expression compared with cultures on fibronectin-coated plastic. Additionally, when transitioned onto Matrigel for angiogenesis studies, the EPCs cultured on fibrin secreted higher levels of cell-recruitment cytokines [7]. A PEGylated version of a fibrin gel induced differentiation of ADSCs into endothelial and pericyte-like cells expressing CD31 and von Willebrand Factor (vWF), and formed a vascularized dermal-like matrix [65]. Fibrin gels supported differentiation of bone marrow stromal cells into chondrocytes with higher levels of aggrecan and collagen II, and increased GAG deposition [41]. PEGylated fibrin was demonstrated to successfully support the formation of dental tissue. Cells derived from dental pulp and periodontal ligaments were combined with fibrin to create constructs that were implanted in mice that had increased alkaline phosphatase levels, osteoblast gene expression, and dentin markers, that had a collagenous matrix with mineral deposition [34].

Although not so commonly used, silk biomaterials have recently been combined with stem cells. ADSCs were co-cultured with endothelial cells in silk hydrogels to produce adipose-like tissue [18]. Silk has also been shown to be useful for chondrogenesis. In a silk–elastin protein polymer material, MSCs cultured with transforming growth factor β_3 (TGF-β_3) resulted in round cells embedded in a chondrogenic matrix with increased aggregan, collagen type II, and collagen type X expression [40]. Likewise, in a silk–fibroin gel, ESC-derived MSCs increased secretion of GAGs, and expressed cartilage-related genes [97].

5.3.2.2 Expansion and migration

Hydrogels may also be useful for 3D stem cell expansion and recovery. Generally, recovery of cells, once they have been encapsulated within a substrate, is difficult and requires harsh enzymatic or chemical treatment that can potentially impact cell viability and function. By combining CMHA-S materials with a cleavable PEGDA-like crosslinker, MSCs could be expanded with the benefits of 3D culture, and then recovered for future implantation or therapies using a mild enzyme-free treatment [104]. In other examples of expansion, spermatogonial stem cells showed increased cell attachment, viability, and proliferation in RGD-conjugated alginate hydrogels [19]. Collagen has been used for several tissue-specific applications.

For example, in an effort to improve engraftment of stem cells for treatment of Parkinson's disease, epidermal growth factor (EGF) was bound to a collagen hydrogel, leading to increased expansion rates of NSCs [28]. Thiol-crosslinkable CMHA-S HA hydrogels have also been used for work with stem cell culture. When loaded with hepatocyte growth factor (HGF), these gels can be used for long-term recruitment of endogenous stem cells to injury or implant sites [105]. Conjugation of RGD peptides to alginate improved MSC mobilization, which in turn, enhanced endothelial cell tube formation [11].

5.3.2.3 Delivery and cell therapy

Hydrogels are also implemented with stem and progenitor cells as delivery vehicles for cell therapy. Cells are resuspended in hydrogel precursor solution, after which the solutions polymerize and are implanted into animals. Alternatively, hydrogel precursor solutions containing cells can be injected into animals and undergo *in situ* polymerization at the target site. Various hydrogels, including alginate, chitosan, fibrin, collagen, and HA, have been explored for this purpose. A cell–hydrogel drug delivery model was demonstrated in which erythropoietin (EPO)-secreting C2C12 myoblasts were encapsulated in RGD-conjugated alginate hydrogels, which increased cell viability and prolonged function. After implantation in mice, the cell-adherent alginate hydrogels supported cell viability and EPO secretion for 300 days [75]. Similarly, chitosan microspheres in which ADSCs could be delivered were developed. When collagen gels were used in vitro to simulate the in-vivo implantation site, the chitosan microspheres supported ADSC viability and then allowed cells to migrate out into the surrounding collagen [64].

Biomaterials have also been used as repositories for GFs that can then slowly release those GFs over time after implantation or in in-vitro cultures to recruit cells or induce biological function. This technology has been widely explored. Examples include heparin-conjugated HA hydrogels for extended release of growth factors such as vascular endothelial growth factor (VEGF), fibroblast growth factor (FGF), and platelet-derived growth factor (PDGF) to induce angiogenesis [29, 76–78, 81]. Fibrin gels have also been used for releasing GFs. For example, fibrin gels containing VEGF were printed adjacent to collagen gels containing NSCs. Release of VEGF from the fibrin resulted in increased viability of the NSCs as well as morphological changes and migration toward the fibrin gels [53].

In unpublished work from our laboratory, we bioprinted AFS cells in a fibrin–collagen hybrid gel to treat full thickness wounds in mice. This treatment resulted in wound healing rates that were significantly better than those obtainable with gel-alone treatments, and resulted in increased angiogenesis and vessel maturity in the regenerated skin due to higher levels of trophic factors being secreted from the AFS cells [89]. Currently we are transitioning to a photocrosslinkable version of the thiolated HA discussed above for a similar application due to its fast gelling times that are beneficial for bioprinting, cell permissiveness, and the natural anti-inflammatory properties of HA.

5.3.2.4 Maintenance of stemness and therapeutic potential

Until recently, much work regarding mechanical properties of hydrogels and their impacts on stem cells has focussed on how modulation of the elastic modulus of a substrate or microenvironment affects differentiation [31]. However, pluripotency and the ability to differentiate into target cell types is not the only important use for stem cells. As with MSCs, we have observed that fetal stem cells, when in the right environment, are effective at releasing trophic factors that can induce angiogenesis and regeneration. Our group has recently been investigating the effects of elastic modulus on expression of several common stem cell markers in AFS cells and its impact on potential therapeutic effectiveness [90]. We found that, by transitioning AFS cells from hard plastic surfaces to polymer substrates with elastic modulus near 2 kPa, we were able to induce increased surface marker expression of CD44, CD90, CD105, and N-cadherin. AFS cells cultured on softer surfaces secreted factors that induced increased recruitment of other AFS cells and endothelial cells. Additionally, conditioned media produced from AFS cells on soft substrates were more effective at inducing endothelial tube formation in vitro than were conditioned media from AFS cells cultured on substrates with high elastic moduli, including plastic dishes used for tissue culture.

A similar phenomenon was noted when ESCs were cultured on poly-L-lysine–HA nanofilm of varying stiffness and chemistry. More highly crosslinked, and thus stiffer, films supported increased cell attachment and proliferation. However, on these stiffer films, expression of genes commonly expressed in the inner cell mass from where the ESCs were derived decreased. Only on softer, less-crosslinked films did the ESCs remain in colonies that maintained pluripotency [12].

5.3.2.5 Organ and tissue engineering

Use of hydrogels has also been combined with other techniques to generate viable prototype tissues. Small-scale tissues and organoids may be useful for increased effectiveness for drug and toxicology screening. Larger tissues and organs may, one day, be used for implantation in to patients with diseased, damaged, or missing tissues in place of current treatments such as organ transplants from donors. Examples include artificial tracheas that were fabricated by creating fibroblast and collagen hydrogel tubes, supported by collagen rings containing osteogenically induced MSCs. These constructs were implanted into rats with tracheal defects, allowing the treated rats to breathe successfully [63]. Composite hydrogels were generated by crosslinking collagen type II and HA and seeding with rat MSCs to give tissue constructs with similarities to the nucleus pulposus. Since these materials also had the appropriate swelling and stability characteristics, this approach might be useful for intervertebral disk repair, regeneration, or replacement [15].

A commonly investigated area in tissue engineering is development of functional arterial grafts and vasculature. Tubular tissue constructs have been created by mixing fibrinogen, thrombin, calcium chloride, and fibroblasts and injecting the mixture into cylindrical molds with internal mandrels to create lumens. Afterwards, the grafts were conditioned in a perfusion bioreactor, resulting in a tissue-engineered vascular graft that could withstand the burst pressures after implantation in rat and ovine models [95]. We recently explored the platform technology of bioprinting as a method to create cellularized hydrogel constructs in order to generate vessel-like tube tissue construct prototypes. We used thiol-modified HA and gelatin as the basis of the hydrogel in combination with one of three crosslinking modalities to support extrusion and deposition to build 3D tube structures. In one method we used a four-arm PEG-based tetra-acrylate crosslinker to make high-aspect-ratio cell-containing hydrogel cylinders that were stacked by a bioprinting device to form constructs that fused over time in culture to form cellularized tubes [94]. Additionally, we combined MA–HA with a novel methacrylated gelatin component for two-step photopolymerization bioprinting to create cellularized tube constructs. Lastly, we implemented thiophilic gold nanoparticles to act as nanoscale crosslinkers between thiolated HA and gelatin. These dynamically crosslinkable hydrogels allowed extrusion of the cell-loaded gels into tube structures that continued to stiffen over time in culture. Cells remained viable for 4 weeks, remodeling the matrix and secreting collagen.

5.4 Future implementation

Combinations of novel hydrogel biomaterials with stem cells hold extensive potential for implementation both in research and in the clinic. Biomaterials can be used as tools and platform technologies in vitro such as stem cell expansion and differentiation prior to implantation or generation of tissues and organs for implantation and for drug testing. Likewise, biomaterials can be used in vivo for therapeutic applications as cell delivery vehicles.

We discussed several approaches in which biomaterials were used to modulate differentiation, expansion, and maintenance of stemness during in-vitro expansion. This will likely be a growing area of interest as the potential for cell therapies to treat disease is increasing. We are exploring this area by taking advantage of the properties of hydrogels. The low elastic modulus, or stiffness, of most hydrogels is believed to be similar to that of some stem cell niches. As a result, we believe that we may be able to isolate and expand stem cells on such materials, and maintain the properties that make stem cells so interesting during expansion. The HA hydrogels may have great potential due to their mechanical properties, as described above, and the fact that HA is present at high levels in developing tissues at the time when stem cells are actively proliferating and differentiating. Interestingly, the cell-surface HA receptor, CD44, is commonly expressed on many types of stem cells.

An additional application of stem cells and biomaterials is the production of small drug testing constructs by culturing stem cells with terminally differentiated functional cells on hydrogel microcarriers in simulated microgravity with rotating-wall vessel bioreactors. This is an economical and simple method for creating large numbers of customized tissue organoids that can be transitioned to high-throughput drug and toxicology screening for development of therapeutic agents. We have demonstrated the feasibility of this approach by producing several proof-of-concept models using tumor cell lines of the intestinal epithelium [91], breast, and lung [88].

As we have noted in recent in-vitro and in-vivo experiments, AFS cells, and likely other FSCs, are effective at inducing angiogenesis. As more research focusses on engineering whole tissues or organs, induction of angiogenesis will become increasingly important. One of the main limitations to generating human-scale organs is the difficulty of supplying sufficient oxygen and nutrients to the entire engineered construct. As a construct grows in size, the efficiency of diffusion of oxygen and nutrients – which is the method by which most small-scale constructs receive support – decreases. However, to generate viable large-scale organs, the constructs must contain internal vascular networks to supply oxygen and nutrients to areas that bulk diffusion cannot effectively address. Three main approaches have been explored to this end. First, incorporation of growth factors such as VEGF, bFGF, and HGF has been used to induce vascularization of ischemic tissues. These soluble signals recruit and induce endothelial cells to form vascular structures in tissue-engineered constructs. Second, inclusion of endothelial cells within scaffolds and tissue constructs can provide vascularization. Generally, endothelial cells self-organize within their environment to form vessels. Coupling this approach with GF loading further improves formation of stable vasculature. Lastly, an additional approach to this problem is to pre-pattern or prevascularize networks of voids inside the constructs to act as artificial vasculature [70, 71]. Again, coupling this approach with GF and endothelial cell loading can further increase its effectiveness. Incorporating populations of stem cells that support angiogenesis, such as AFS cells, together with the endothelial cells or endothelial precursor cells into the constructs may also prove successful. Under the correct conditions, these approaches have the potential to form functional vascular networks that may support tissue viability.

5.5 Conclusions

How materials are designed has the potential to determine the commercial or clinical success of stem cell therapy. Beyond scientific excellence, one must consider the end user. To become a paradigm-shifting discovery or a financial success, a material needs to be easily usable both by clinicians and by researchers. Modular systems, containing finite components that can each be easily prepared and tailored toward multiple clinical and research objectives, will be more likely to succeed [86].

REFERENCES

[1] Abdulrazzak, H., Moschidou, D., Jones, G. and Guillot, P. V. 2010. Biological characteristics of stem cells from foetal, cord blood and extraembryonic tissues. *J. R. Soc. Interface*, **7**(Suppl. 6), S689–706.

[2] Ahmed, T. A., Dare, E. V. and Hincke, M. 2008. Fibrin: a versatile scaffold for tissue engineering applications. *Tissue Eng. Part B Rev.*, **14**(2), 199–215.

[3] Allison, D. D. and Grande-Allen, K. J. 2006. Hyaluronan: a powerful tissue engineering tool. *Tissue Eng.*, **12**(8), 2131–40.

[4] Banerjee, A., Arha, M., Choudhary, S. *et al.* 2009. The influence of hydrogel modulus on the proliferation and differentiation of encapsulated neural stem cells. *Biomaterials*, **30**(27), 4695–9.

[5] Barakat, O., Abbasi, S., Rodriguez, G. *et al.* 2012. Use of decellularized porcine liver for engineering humanized liver organ. *J. Surg. Res.*, **173**(1), e11–25.

[6] Barrila, J., Radtke, A. L., Crabbe, A. *et al.* 2010. Organotypic 3D cell culture models: using the rotating wall vessel to study host-pathogen interactions. *Nature Rev. Microbiol.*, **8**(11), 791–801.

[7] Barsotti, M. C., Magera, A., Armani, C. *et al.* 2011. Fibrin acts as biomimetic niche inducing both differentiation and stem cell marker expression of early human endothelial progenitor cells. *Cell Prolif.*, **44**(1), 33–48.

[8] Becker, J. L. and Blanchard, D. K. 2007. Characterization of primary breast carcinomas grown in three-dimensional cultures. *J. Surg. Res.*, **142**(2), 256–62.

[9] Begley, C. M. and Kleis, S. J. 2000. The fluid dynamic and shear environment in the NASA/JSC rotating-wall perfused-vessel bioreactor. *Biotechnol. Bioeng.*, **70**(1), 32–40.

[10] Bian, L., Zhai, D. Y., Mauck, R. L. and Burdick, J. A. 2011. Coculture of human mesenchymal stem cells and articular chondrocytes reduces hypertrophy and enhances functional properties of engineered cartilage. *Tissue Eng. Part A*, **17**(7–8), 1137–45.

[11] Bidarra, S. J., Barrias, C. C., Barbosa, M. A., Soares, R. and Granja, P. L. 2010. Immobilization of human mesenchymal stem cells within RGD-grafted alginate microspheres and assessment of their angiogenic potential. *Biomacromolecules*, **11**(8), 1956–64.

[12] Blin, G., Lablack, N., Louis-Tisserand, M. *et al.* 2010. Nano-scale control of cellular environment to drive embryonic stem cells selfrenewal and fate. *Biomaterials*, **31**(7), 1742–50.

[13] Burdick, J. A. and Prestwich, G. D. 2011. Hyaluronic acid hydrogels for biomedical applications. *Adv Mater.*, **23** (12), H41–H56.

[14] Burdick, J. A. and Vunjak-Novakovic, G. 2009. Engineered microenvironments for controlled stem cell differentiation. *Tissue Eng. Part A*, **15**(2), 205–19.

[15] Calderon, L., Collin, E., Velasco-Bayon, D. *et al.* 2010. Type II collagen-hyaluronan hydrogel – a step towards a scaffold for intervertebral disc tissue engineering. *Eur. Cell Mater.*, **20**, 134–48.

[16] Caplan, A. I. 2007. Adult mesenchymal stem cells for tissue engineering versus regenerative medicine. *J. Cell Physiol.*, **213**(2), 341–7.

[17] Chandler, E. M., Berglund, C. M., Lee, J. S. *et al.* 2011. Stiffness of photocrosslinked RGD-alginate gels regulates adipose progenitor cell behavior. *Biotechnol. Bioeng.*, **108**(7), 1683–92.

[18] Choi, J. H., Bellas, E., Vunjak-Novakovic, G. and Kaplan, D. L. 2011. Adipogenic differentiation of human adipose-derived stem cells on 3D silk scaffolds. *Methods Mol. Biol.*, **702**, 319–30.

[19] Chu, C., Schmidt, J. J., Carnes, K. *et al.* 2009. Three-dimensional synthetic niche components to control germ cell proliferation. *Tissue Eng. Part A*, **15**(2), 255–62.

[20] Chung, C. and Burdick, J. 2009. Influence of three-dimensional hyaluronic acid microenvironment on mesechymal stem cell chondrogenesis. *Tissue Eng. Part A*, **15**, 243–54.

[21] Cohen, J., Zaleski, K. L., Nourissat, G. *et al.* 2011. Survival of porcine mesenchymal stem cells over the alginate recovered cellular method. *J. Biomed. Mater. Res. A*, **96**(1), 93–9.

[22] Crapo, P. M., Medberry, C. J., Reing, J. E. *et al.* 2012. Biologic scaffolds composed of central nervous system extracellular matrix. *Biomaterials*, **33**(13), 3539–47.

[23] Dahl, L. B., Kimpton, W. G., Cahill, R. N., Brown, T. J. and Fraser, R. E. 1989. The origin and fate of hyaluronan in amniotic fluid. *J. Dev. Physiol.*, **12**(4), 209–18.

[24] Dainese, L., Guarino, A., Burba, I. *et al.* 2012. Heart valve engineering: decellularized aortic homograft seeded with human cardiac stromal cells. *J. Heart Valve Dis.*, **21**(1), 125–34.

[25] De Coppi, P., Bartsch, G., Jr., Siddiqui, M. M. *et al.* 2007. Isolation of amniotic stem cell lines with potential for therapy. *Nature Biotechnol.*, **25**(1), 100–6.

[26] Dellatore, S. M., Garcia, A. S. and Miller, W. M. 2008. Mimicking stem cell niches to increase stem cell expansion. *Curr. Opin. Biotechnol.*, **19**(5), 534–40.

[27] Discher, D. E., Mooney, D. J. and Zandstra, P. W. 2009. Growth factors, matrices, and forces combine and control stem cells. *Science*, **324**(5935), 1673–77.

[28] Egawa, E. Y., Kato, K., Hiraoka, M., Nakaji-Hirabayashi, T. and Iwata, H. 2011. Enhanced proliferation of neural stem cells in a collagen hydrogel incorporating engineered epidermal growth factor. *Biomaterials*, **32**(21), 4737–43.

[29] Elia, R., Fuegy, P. W., VanDelden, A. *et al.* 2010. Stimulation of in vivo angiogenesis by *in situ* crosslinked, dual growth factor-loaded, glycosaminoglycan hydrogels. *Biomaterials*, **31**(17), 4630–8.

[30] Ellis, S. J. and Tanentzapf, G. 2010. Integrin-mediated adhesion and stem-cell-niche interactions. *Cell Tissue Res.*, **339**(1), 121–30.

[31] Engler, A. J., Sen, S., Sweeney, H. L. and Discher, D. E. 2006. Matrix elasticity directs stem cell lineage specification. *Cell*, **126**(4), 677–89.

[32] Flynn, L., Prestwich, G. D., Semple, J. L. and Woodhouse, K. A. 2009. Adipose tissue engineering in vivo with adipose-derived stem cells on naturally derived scaffolds. *J. Biomed. Mater. Res. A*, **89**(4), 929–41.

[33] Fu, X. and Xu, Y. 2012. Challenges to the clinical application of pluripotent stem cells: towards genomic and functional stability. *Genome Med.*, **4**(6), 55.

[34] Galler, K. M., Cavender, A. C., Koeklue, U. *et al.* 2011. Bioengineering of dental stem cells in a PEGylated fibrin gel. *Regen Med.*, **6**(2), 191–200.

[35] Galus, R., Antiszko, M. and Włodarski, P. 2006. Clinical applications of hyaluronic acid. *Pol. Merkur Lek.*, **20**(119), 606–8.

[36] Gao, H., Ayyaswamy, P. S. and Ducheyne, P. 1997. Dynamics of a microcarrier particle in the simulated microgravity environment of a rotating-wall vessel. *Microgravity Sci. Technol.*, **10**(3), 154–65.

[37] Gerecht, S., Burdick, J. A., Ferreira, L. S. *et al.* 2007. Hyaluronic acid hydrogel for controlled self-renewal and differentiation of human embryonic stem cells. *Proc. Nat. Acad. Sci. USA*, **104**(27), 11298–303.

[38] Gilbert, P. M., Havenstrite, K. L., Magnusson, K. E. *et al.* 2010. Substrate elasticity regulates skeletal muscle stem cell self-renewal in culture. *Science*, **329**(5995), 1078–81.

[39] Guvendiren, M. and Burdick, J. A. 2010. The control of stem cell morphology and differentiation by hydrogel surface wrinkles. *Biomaterials*, **31**(25), 6511–18.

[40] Haider, M., Cappello, J., Ghandehari, H. and Leong, K. W. 2007. In vitro chondrogenesis of mesenchymal stem cells in recombinant silk-elastinlike hydrogels. *Pharm. Res.*, **25**(3), 692–9.

[41] Ho, S. T., Cool, S. M., Hui, J. H. and Hutmacher, D. W. 2010. The influence of fibrin based hydrogels on the chondrogenic differentiation of human bone marrow stromal cells. *Biomaterials*, **31**(1), 38–47.

[42] Holst, J., Watson, S., Lord, M. S. *et al.* 2010. Substrate elasticity provides mechanical signals for the expansion of hemopoietic stem and progenitor cells. *Nature Biotechnol.*, **28**(10), 1123–8.

[43] Jukes, J. M., van der Aa, L. J., Hiemstra, C. *et al.* 2010. A newly developed chemically crosslinked dextran poly(ethylene glycol) hydrogel for cartilage tissue engineering. *Tissue Eng. Part A*, **16**(2), 565–73.

[44] Jung, H. H., Park, K. and Han, D. K. 2010. Preparation of TGF-β_1-conjugated biodegradable pluronic F127 hydrogel and its application with adipose-derived stem cells. *J. Controll. Release*, **147**(1), 84–91.

[45] Keating, A. 2012. Mesenchymal stromal cells: new directions. *Cell Stem Cell*, **10**(6), 709–16.

[46] Keung, A. J., Healy, K. E., Kumar, S. and Schaffer, D. V. 2010. Biophysics and dynamics of natural and engineered stem cell microenvironments. *Wiley Interdiscip. Rev. Syst. Biol. Med.*, **2**(1), 49–64.

[47] Khetan, S. and Burdick, J. A. 2010. Patterning network structure to spatially control cellular remodeling and stem cell fate within 3-dimensional hydrogels. *Biomaterials*, **31**(32), 8228–34.

[48] Kiel, M. J., Acar, M., Radice, G. L. and Morrison, S. J. 2009. Hematopoietic stem cells do not depend on N-cadherin to regulate their maintenance. *Cell Stem Cell*, **4**(2), 170–9.

[49] Kirker, K. R., Luo, Y., Morris, S. E., Shelby, J. and Prestwich, G. D. 2004. Glycosaminoglycan hydrogels as supplemental wound dressings for donor sites. *J. Burn Care Rehabil.*, **25**(3), 276–86.

[50] Knudson, C. B. and Knudson, W. 2001. Cartilage proteoglycans. *Semin. Cell. Dev. Biol.*, **12**(2), 69–78.

[51] Kuo, J. W. 2006. *Practical Aspects of Hyaluronan Based Medical Products*. Boca Raton, FL: CRC/Taylor & Francis.

[52] Kurpinski, K., Chu, J., Hashi, C. and Li, S. 2006. Anisotropic mechanosensing by mesenchymal stem cells. *Proc. Nat. Acad. Sci. USA*, **103**(44), 16095–100.

[53] Lee, Y. B., Polio, S., Lee, W. *et al.* 2010. Bio-printing of collagen and VEGF-releasing fibrin gel scaffolds for neural stem cell culture. *Exp. Neurol.*, **223**(2), 645–52.

[54] Lei, Y., Gojgini, S., Lam, J. and Segura, T. 2011. The spreading, migration and proliferation of mouse mesenchymal stem cells cultured inside hyaluronic acid hydrogels. *Biomaterials*, **32**(1), 39–47.

[55] Leipzig, N. D. and Shoichet, M. S. 2009. The effect of substrate stiffness on adult neural stem cell behavior. *Biomaterials*, **30**(36), 6867–78.

[56] Li, C. L., Tian, T., Nan, K. J. *et al.* 2008. Survival advantages of multicellular spheroids vs. monolayers of HepG2 cells in vitro. *Oncol. Rep.*, **20**(6), 1465–71.

[57] Liu, Y., Shu, X. Z. and Prestwich, G. D. 2007. Tumor engineering: orthotopic cancer models in mice using cell-loaded, injectable, cross-linked hyaluronan-derived hydrogels. *Tissue Eng.*, **13**(5), 1091–101.

[58] Ma, W., Tavakoli, T., Derby, E. *et al.* 2008. Cell–extracellular matrix interactions regulate neural differentiation of human embryonic stem cells. *BMC Dev. Biol.*, **8**, 90.

[59] Marcus, A. J. and Woodbury, D. 2008. Fetal stem cells from extra-embryonic tissues: do not discard. *J. Cell Mol. Med.*, **12**(3), 730–42.

[60] Miki, D., Dastgheib, K., Kim, T. *et al.* 2002. A photopolymerized sealant for corneal lacerations. *Cornea*, **21**(4), 393–9.

[61] Moorefield, E. C., McKee, E. E., Solchaga, L. *et al.* 2011. Cloned, CD117 selected human amniotic fluid stem cells are capable of modulating the immune response. *PLoS One*, **6**(10), e26535.

[62] Mulder, G. D., Lee, D. K. and Jeppesen, N. S. 2012. Comprehensive review of the clinical application of autologous mesenchymal stem cells in the treatment of chronic wounds and diabetic bone healing. *Int. Wound J.*, **9**(6), 595–600.

[63] Naito, H., Tojo, T., Kimura, M. *et al.* 2011. Engineering bioartificial tracheal tissue using hybrid fibroblast-mesenchymal stem cell cultures in collagen hydrogels. *Interact. Cardiovasc. Thorac. Surg.*, **12**(2), 156–61.

[64] Natesan, S., Baer, D. G., Walters, T. J., Babu, M. and Christy, R. J. 2010. Adipose-derived stem cell delivery into collagen gels using chitosan microspheres. *Tissue Eng. Part A*, **16**(4), 1369–84.

[65] Natesan, S., Zhang, G., Baer, D. G. *et al.* 2011. A bilayer construct controls adipose-derived stem cell differentiation into endothelial cells and pericytes without growth factor stimulation. *Tissue Eng. Part A*, **17**(7–8), 941–53.

[66] Navran, S. 2008. The application of low shear modeled microgravity to 3-D cell biology and tissue engineering. *Biotechnol. Annu. Rev.*, **14**, 275–96.

[67] Nguyen, L. H., Kudva, A. K., Guckert, N. L., Linse, K. D. and Roy, K. 2011. Unique biomaterial compositions direct bone marrow stem cells into specific chondrocytic phenotypes corresponding to the various zones of articular cartilage. *Biomaterials*, **32**(5), 1327–38.

[68] Nickerson, C. A. and Ott, C. M. 2004. A new dimension in modeling infectious disease. *ASM News*, **70**(4), 169–75.

[69] Nilsson, S. K. and Simmons, P. J. 2004. Transplantable stem cells: home to specific niches. *Curr. Opin. Hematol.*, **11**(2), 102–6.

[70] Nomi, M., Atala, A., Coppi, P. D. and Soker, S. 2002. Principals of neovascularization for tissue engineering. *Mol. Aspects Med.*, **23**(6), 463–83.

[71] Nomi, M., Miyake, H., Sugita, Y., Fujisawa, M. and Soker, S. 2006. Role of growth factors and endothelial cells in therapeutic angiogenesis and tissue engineering. *Curr. Stem Cell Res. Ther.*, **1**(3), 333–43.

[72] Nuttelman, C. R., Rice, M. A., Rydholm, A. E. *et al.* 2008. Macromolecular monomers for the synthesis of hydrogel niches and their application in cell encapsulation and tissue engineering. *Prog. Polym. Sci.*, **33**(2), 167–79.

[73] Nuttelman, C. R., Tripodi, M. C. and Anseth, K. S. 2005. Synthetic hydrogel niches that promote hMSC viability. *Matrix Biol.*, **24**(3), 208–18.

[74] Opara, E. C., Mirmalek-Sani, S. H., Khanna, O., Moya, M. L. and Brey, E. M. 2010. Design of a bioartificial pancreas. *J. Investig. Med.*, **58**(7), 831–7.

[75] Orive, G., De Castro, M., Kong, H. J. *et al.* 2009. Bioactive cell-hydrogel microcapsules for cell-based drug delivery. *J. Controll. Release*, **135**(3), 203–10.

[76] Peattie, R. A., Nayate, A. P., Firpo, M. A. *et al.* 2004. Stimulation of in vivo angiogenesis by cytokine-loaded hyaluronic acid hydrogel implants. *Biomaterials*, **25**(14), 2789–98.

[77] Peattie, R. A., Rieke, E. R., Hewett, E. M. *et al.* 2006. Dual growth factor-induced angiogenesis in vivo using hyaluronan hydrogel implants. *Biomaterials*, **27**(9), 1868–75.

[78] Pike, D. B., Cai, S., Pomraning, K. R. *et al.* 2006. Heparin-regulated release of growth factors in vitro and angiogenic response in vivo to implanted hyaluronan hydrogels containing VEGF and bFGF. *Biomaterials*, **27**(30), 5242–51.

[79] Poellmann, M. J., Harrell, P. A., King, W. P. and Wagoner Johnson, A. J. 2010. Geometric microenvironment directs cell morphology on topographically patterned hydrogel substrates. *Acta Biomater.*, **6**(9), 3514–23.

[80] Prestwich, G. D. and Kuo, J. W. 2008. Chemically-modified HA for therapy and regenerative medicine. *Curr. Pharm. Biotechnol.*, **9**(4), 242–5.

[81] Riley, C. M., Fuegy, P. W., Firpo, M. A. *et al.* 2006. Stimulation of in vivo angiogenesis using dual growth factor-loaded crosslinked glycosaminoglycan hydrogels. *Biomaterials*, **27**(35), 5935–43.

[82] Salinas, C. N., Cole, B. B., Kasko, A. M. and Anseth, K. S. 2007. Chondrogenic differentiation potential of human mesenchymal stem cells photoencapsulated within poly(ethylene glycol)-arginine-glycine-aspartic acid-serine thiol-methacrylate mixed-mode networks. *Tissue Eng.*, **13**(5), 1025–34.

[83] Santos, E., Zarate, J., Orive, G., Hernandez, R. M. and Pedraz, J. L. 2010. Biomaterials in cell microencapsulation. *Adv. Exp. Med. Biol.*, **670**, 5–21.

[84] Schiavinato, A., Finesso, M., Cortivo, R. and Abatangelo, G. 2002. Comparison of the effects of intra-articular injections of hyaluronan and its chemically cross-linked

derivative (Hylan G-F20) in normal rabbit knee joints. *Clin. Exp. Rheumatol.*, **20**(4), 445–54.

[85] Schmelzer, E., Triolo, F., Turner, M. E. *et al.* 2010. Three-dimensional perfusion bioreactor culture supports differentiation of human fetal liver cells. *Tissue Eng. Part A*, **16**(6), 2007–16.

[86] Serban, M. A., Liu, Y. and Prestwich, G. D. 2008. Effects of extracellular matrix analogues on primary human fibroblast behavior. *Acta Biomater.*, **4**(1), 67–75.

[87] Sharma, B., Williams, C. G., Khan, M., Manson, P. and Elisseeff, J. H. 2007. In vivo chondrogenesis of mesenchymal stem cells in a photopolymerized hydrogel. *Plast. Reconstr. Surg.*, **119**(1), 112–20.

[88] Skardal, A. 2010. *Hyaluronan and Gelatin Biomaterials for Bioprinting Engineered Tissues.* Salt Lake City, UT: Department of Bioengineering University of Utah.

[89] Skardal, A., Mack, D., Kapetanovic, E. *et al.* 2012. Bioprinted amniotic fluid-derived stem cells accelerate healing of large skin wounds. *Stem Cells Transl. Med.*, **1**(11), 792–802.

[90] Skardal, A., Mack, D. Atala, A. and Soker, S. 2013. Substrate elasticity controls cell proliferation, surface marker expression and motile phenotype in amniotic fluid-derived stem cells. *J. Mech. Behav. Biomed. Mater.*, **17**, 307–16.

[91] Skardal, A., Sarker, S. F., Crabbe, A., Nickerson, C. A. and Prestwich, G. D. 2010. The generation of 3-D tissue models based on hyaluronan hydrogel-coated microcarriers within a rotating wall vessel bioreactor. *Biomaterials*, **31**(32), 8426–35.

[92] Skardal, A., Zhang, J., McCoard, L., Oottamasathien, S. and Prestwich, G. D. 2010. Dynamically crosslinked gold nanoparticle–hyaluronan hydrogels. *Adv. Mater.*, **22** (42), 4736–40.

[93] Skardal, A., Zhang, J., McCoard, L. *et al.* 2010. Photocrosslinkable hyaluronan–gelatin hydrogels for two-step bioprinting. *Tissue Eng. Part A*, **16**(8), 2675–85.

[94] Skardal, A., Zhang, J. and Prestwich, G. D. 2010. Bioprinting vessel-like constructs using hyaluronan hydrogels crosslinked with tetrahedral polyethylene glycol tetracrylates. *Biomaterials*, **31**(24), 6173–81.

[95] Syedain, Z. H., Meier, L. A., Bjork, J. W., Lee, A. and Tranquillo, R. T. 2011. Implantable arterial grafts from human fibroblasts and fibrin using a multi-graft pulsed flow-stretch bioreactor with noninvasive strength monitoring. *Biomaterials*, **32**(3), 714–22.

[96] Tanentzapf, G., Devenport, D., Godt, D. and Brown, N. H. 2007. Integrin-dependent anchoring of a stem-cell niche. *Nature Cell Biol.*, **9**(12), 1413–18.

[97] Tigli, R. S., Cannizaro, C., Gumusderelioglu, M. and Kaplan, D. L. 2011. Chondrogenesis in perfusion bioreactors using porous silk scaffolds and hESC-derived MSCs. *J. Biomed. Mater. Res. A*, **96**(1), 21–8.

[98] Unsworth, B. R. and Lelkes, P. I. 1998. Growing tissues in microgravity. *Nature Med.*, **4**(8), 901–7.

[99] Vanderhooft, J. L., Alcoutlabi, M., Magda, J. J. and Prestwich, G. D. 2009. Rheological properties of cross-linked hyaluronan–gelatin hydrogels for tissue engineering. *Macromol. Biosci.*, **9**(1), 20–8.

[100] Vashi, A. V., Keramidaris, E., Abberton, K. M. *et al.* 2008. Adipose differentiation of bone marrow-derived mesenchymal stem cells using Pluronic F-127 hydrogel in vitro. *Biomaterials*, **29**(5), 573–9.

[101] Wang, D. A., Williams, C. G., Yang, F. *et al.* 2005. Bioresponsive phosphoester hydrogels for bone tissue engineering. *Tissue Eng.*, **11**(1-2), 201–13.

[102] Williams, C. G., Kim, T. K., Taboas, A. *et al.* 2003. In vitro chondrogenesis of bone marrow-derived mesenchymal stem cells in a photopolymerizing hydrogel. *Tissue Eng.*, **9**(4), 679–88.

[103] Yamamoto, K., Sokabe, T., Watabe, T. *et al.* 2005. Fluid shear stress induces differentiation of Flk-1-positive embryonic stem cells into vascular endothelial cells in vitro. *Am. J. Physiol. Heart Circ. Physiol.*, **288**(4), H1915–24.

[104] Zhang, J., Skardal, A. and Prestwich, G. D. 2008. Engineered extracellular matrices with cleavable crosslinkers for cell expansion and easy cell recovery. *Biomaterials*, **29**(34), 4521–31.

[105] Zhao, J., Zhang, N., Prestwich, G. D. and Wen, X. 2008. Recruitment of endogenous stem cells for tissue repair. *Macromol. Biosci.*, **8**(9), 836–42.

6

The hematopoietic stem cell niche

Aparna Venkatraman, Meng Zhao and Linheng Li

6.1 Introduction

Traditionally, the stem cell niche is defined as a specific anatomical location where stem cells reside and receive signals for its maintenance. Extrinsic signals from the surrounding environment communicate with intrinsic signals in the stem cells and regulate tissue regeneration during homeostasis and under conditions of stress. Extrinsic signals include membrane-bound signal and adhesion molecules and soluble signaling molecules, which regulate stem cell localization and maintenance of stemness. Historically, the stem cell niche was viewed as a single type of niche cell critical for maintaining stem cells. This dogma held good for invertebrates such as *C.elegans* and drosophila. However, in organisms such as mammals, the stem cell niche is far more complex than what was initially envisaged, especially if the niche is not a solid tissue, as in the hematopoietic system. With regard to HSC niche, there are several layers of complexity (summarized in Table 6.1).

- To begin with, bone marrow stromal cells are very heterogeneous. Even within the same cell type, it is not clear which developmental stage of these cells support stem cells.
- Additionally, advanced technology and sophisticated three-dimensional (3D) in-vivo imaging has revealed that many of the stromal cells which are niche components have overlapping locations. It is very likely that HSCs are surrounded on one side by a particular type of stromal cell, which provides adhesion molecules for localization and maintenance, and on the other side by another type of stromal cell that provides signals for stem cell behavior.
- Furthermore, HSCs exist in different states. Some are very dormant with low metabolism and divide infrequently (quiescent), while others are metabolically active and divide frequently (active) [1].
- Finally, non-stromal cells such as macrophages, along with bone marrow stromal cell components, have recently been gaining recognition as cells involved in regulating stem cell function.

Table 6.1 Summary of HSC niche complexity

Reasons for complexity in the niche
The bone marrow is not a solid tissue
The existence of HSCs in different states with similar immune phenotype
Individual niche cells have different developmental stages
Locations of niche cells overlap
Individual HSCs are surrounded by different niche cells
The involvement of non-stromal cells as niche cells

Owing to these many layers of complexity, in this chapter we first describe the role of individual stromal and non-stromal cell niche components in bone marrow. Second, we explain how different niche components synchronize and orchestrate stem cell activity. Third, we address the recent advances in technology which reveal a particular cell as a niche component.

6.2 Cellular components of the niche

Cellular components of the hematopoietic stem cell niche can be classified as stromal and non-stromal components.

6.2.1 Stromal components

The different cell types identified under this category include osteoblasts, osteoprogenitor cells, endothelial cells, mesenchymal cells, reticular cells, and adipocytes. For the sake of simplicity, these cellular components are classified, based on their location, as endosteal, vascular, and perivascular. However, with the hematopoietic system not being a solid tissue, signals emanating from the niche may be spatially and temporally compartmentalized.

6.2.1.1 The Endosteal niche

This niche comprises cells that are close to the inner bone surface: osteoblasts and osteoprogenitors.

6.2.1.1.1 Osteoblasts

These are mature bone cells present at the interface between bone and bone marrow. Osteoblasts are one of the earliest cell types to have gained recognition as a niche component for HSCs. In an in-vitro experiment, osteoblastic cells or cell lines co-cultured with HSCs were able to support hematopoiesis [2–4]. However, the formal proof of the involvement of osteoblasts as components of the HSC niche in vivo came from two complementary studies where genetic manipulation to augment osteoblast numbers increased HSC numbers, and selective osteoblast depletion disrupted hematopoiesis [5–8]. Static imaging identified a specific subset of osteoblast cells called SNO cells (spindle-shaped N-cadherin-positive osteoblasts or osteoprogenitor cells) as a potential niche cell [5]. However, the role of N-cadherin in the niche has been intensely debated since genetic deletion of N-cadherin in mice had only a very subtle phenotype in hematopoiesis [9]. Thus, it is likely that a certain degree of molecular redundancy exists, whereby other cadherins compensate for the lack of N-cadherin. Nevertheless, data from a recent study made it very clear that the N-cadherin-positive osteoblasts maintain HSCs in a quiescent state by dominant non-canonical *Wnt* signaling [10]. In that study, it was indeed found that Flamingo, an a-typical cadherin, is present at the interface between N-cadherin-positive osteoblasts and HSCs. Further studies are required in order to confirm the role of N-cadherin in this context, by deleting it from the niche in which the presence of Flamingo was reduced.

Once the cell type had been detected, the focus shifted to detecting molecular signals emanating from osteoblasts that are involved in localization and/or self-renewal of HSCs. Over the past decade such molecular signals have been identified, which built the case for the osteoblast being a functional niche component. Positive regulators in osteoblast include angiopoietin-1, N-cadherin, thrombopoietin, Jagged 1, calcium ions, ALCAM-1, and stromal derived factor-1 [6, 11–16]. In contrast, molecules identified as negative regulators of HSC numbers include osteopontin and dikkopf1 [17–20]. Among these signaling molecules, components of the Notch and *Wnt* signaling pathways were found to be expendable during normal homeostasis but important under certain stress conditions [21, 22]. However, non-canonical *Wnt* signaling from the niche cells has recently been recognized to play an important role in normal HSC homeostasis [10].

6.2.1.1.2 Osteoprogenitor cells

These immature osteoblasts are commonly referred to as osteoprogenitors or pre-osteoblasts. These osteoprogenitors are commonly found lining the mature osteoblasts or interspersed with them and thereby form an interface between the bone and the marrow. Since the number of osteoblasts present on the bone surface is always higher than the number of HSCs, it became apparent that there must be a specific subtype of osteoblasts constituting the potential niche component. As mentioned earlier, static imaging of bone marrow tissue sections revealed that the HSCs were in close proximity to SNO cells, but stem cells were not present close to mature osteoblasts [14]. Furthermore, ablation of osteoblasts via gancylcovir treatment in a transgenic mouse model did not decrease HSC number as expected, and instead decreased the overall bone marrow cellularity after prolonged time periods. This again suggested that other cellular components or a specific subset of cells within an osteoblast lineage could have niche regulatory roles [23, 24]. Functional proof that osteoprogenitors are niche components came from two independent studies. Osteoprogenitors isolated from mouse fetal long bones (CD45$^-$, CD105$^+$) or from human adult bone marrow (CD45$^-$, CD146$^+$), when transplanted under the kidney capsule or skin of immunodeficient mice, initiated ectopic HSC niche formation [25, 26]. Furthermore, in-vitro co-culture experiments demonstrated that HSCs co-cultured with osteoprogenitors had significantly higher engraftment than did osteoblasts in the long-term repopulation assay [27–29]. Finally, the formal proof of involvement of osteoprogenitors as niche components came from a recent in-vivo genetic model. Genetic deletion of the miRNA processing enzyme dicer in osteoprogenitors disrupted hematopoiesis, whereas the same deletion in mature osteoblasts had no such effect [30]. Overall these studies demonstrated unequivocally that osteoprogenitors are a potential niche cell type.

6.2.1.2 Vascular niche

This niche comprises endothelial cells that line the blood vessel.

6.2.1.2.1 Endothelial cells

These cells form an interface between the marrow and systemic circulation. At the embryonic stage of development, the origin of HSCs is closely associated with endothelial cells. HSCs originate in the yolk sac and aorta-gonad-mesonephros (AGM) region. During the second trimester of gestation, HSCs localize in the fetal liver and expand to form blood. By the end of this trimester, hematopoiesis is established in the bone marrow [31–33]. Since all these sites have no bone tissue other than the bone marrow, the vascular niche could be an alternative niche to the endosteal niche. This idea was supported by the discovery of the signaling lymphocyte activation molecule (SLAM) family of proteins, which mark HSCs with relatively high specificity. Static imaging using an antibody against the SLAM protein revealed a higher number of stem cells adjacent to sinusoids than adjacent to the endosteal region [34]. In one experiment, an antibody mediated in-vivo disruption of an endothelial cell marker (vascular endothelial growth factor receptor 2 or VEGFR 2) resulting in decreased engraftment of donor marrow cells into the recipient mice. In another experiment, adenoviral transfection of human umbilical vein endothelial cells (HUVECs), which constitutively activate AKT through recruitment of mTOR, led to secretion of specific angiogenic factors that maintain long-term HSCs. Conversely, transfection involving co-activation of AKT1 with the mitogen activated MAPK pathway up-regulated factors facilitating HSC proliferation and differentiation. A recent study involving conditional deletion of stem cell factor (*Scf*) in endothelial cells or leptin receptor expressing perivascular cells demonstrated a substantial decrease in HSC number [35]. However, the functional HSCs in this model were only partially affected, supporting the hypothesis that there exists a quiescent HSC population that was not affected by loss of SCF [36].

6.2.1.3 Perivascular niche

This niche comprises cells that are around the blood vessels: CXCL12-abundant reticular (CAR) cells and nestin$^+$ MSCs.

More than 60% of HSCs reside near the vasculature, but the molecular regulatory mechanism of these niches for HSC maintenance remains unclear [37]. Hence the search for molecular signals emanating from cells around the vessels began, leading to the discovery of the CAR and nestin$^+$ mesenchymal stem cells (MSCs) as potential niche components.

6.2.1.3.1 Chemokine ligand 12-abundant reticular cells (CAR)

These bi-potential adipo-osteogenic progenitors were identified in a mouse model where green fluorescent protein (GFP) was incorporated into the CXCL12 locus. CAR cells are present predominantly around the vessels and also close to the endosteum, though much less so. Immunohistochemical studies revealed that most of the putative HSCs are close to CAR cells. These cells are the predominant source of stromal derived factor-1 (CXCL12), which plays major roles in homing, retention, survival, and chemotaxis of HSCs in the bone marrow. The main receptor for CAR cells is CXCR4, which is present on HSCs. Conditional deletion of CXCR4 or selective ablation of CAR from an adult mouse led to a partial reduction in number of proliferating HSCs, suggesting that CAR cells mainly support active stem cells [38, 39].

6.2.1.3.2 Nestin$^+$ mesenchymal cells (MSCs)

These cells were identified in a transgenic mouse model in which GFP was driven by regulatory elements of the nestin promoter. Similarly to CAR cells, nestin-expressing stromal cells are predominantly perivascular but can occasionally be found close to the endosteum. These cells are closely associated with sympathetic nerve fibers that regulate HSC mobilization. Even though both express CXCL12, angiopoietin, and SCF, nestin$^+$ MSCs and CAR cells are still functionally different. Nestin$^+$ MSCs appear to be more primitive than CAR cells due to their bi-potential ability in vivo and tri-potential ability in vitro. It is very likely that nestin$^+$ MSCs overlapped partially with CAR cells. A recent study has demonstrated that *Scf*-expressing bone marrow stromal cells have very minimal nestin expression, suggesting that, despite overlapping in function, CAR cells could still be a different and potentially heterogeneous population [35].

Depletion of either of these cell types reduces the number of HSCs by ~50% in the bone marrow and increases HSC mobilization to the spleen [40]. However, it is unclear whether those HSCs near the vessel and those near the endosteal are in the same state or different states. Also, further investigation is needed to determine whether nestin$^+$ MSCs are required for long-term maintenance of quiescent stem cells. Overall, these studies convincingly demonstrate that ~50% of HSCs are held in the bone marrow by nestin$^+$ MSCs using the CXCL12–CXCR4 signaling axis.

6.2.2 Other stromal components: neural cells and adipocytes

6.2.2.1 Neural cells

Nerve cells innervating the bone marrow can transmit signals to stromal cells, which in turn can regulate HSC activity. HSCs circulating in and out of their bone marrow niches can be mediated by rhythmic secretion of noradrenaline from sympathetic nerve terminals and activation of the β_3-adrenergic receptor on stromal cells. Molecular events mediating HSC activity through nerves include degradation of Sp1 and down-regulation of CXCL12. This effect appears to be indirect, since it alters stromal cell number and function [41]. However, hematopoietic stem and progenitor cells (HSPCs) can also respond to signaling through dopaminergic and adrenergic receptors, indicating that direct neural signals can also regulate HSC activity [42, 43].

6.2.2.2 Adipocytes

These are lipid-containing cells derived from mesenchymal stromal cells. Recent studies have suggested that, apart from being space fillers, these cells can negatively regulate HSCs. In the bone marrow, adipocyte number increases with obesity, age, and stress or injury such as chemotherapy and irradiation. Comparing different regions of the mouse skeleton that vary in adiposity has revealed that HSC number and activity inversely correlate with adipocyte number. Additionally, genetic or pharmacological inhibition of adipocyte formation in adult mice accelerated marrow engraftment after irradiation compared with that in wild-type littermates or control mice not treated with the inhibitor [44]. Complementing these findings, obese ob/ob and db/db mice had impaired hematopoiesis [45, 46]. Collectively these results indicate that adipocytes have an inhibitory influence on HSC function and could be potential niche cells.

6.2.3 Non-stromal component

This niche comprises mature hematopoietic cells.

6.2.3.1 Macrophages

These mononuclear phagocytes have recently been reported to play a role in HSC retention and maintenance and hence could be a potential type of niche cell. Animal studies by two independent groups showed that depletion of monocytes and/or macrophages caused a mobilization of functional HSCs with repopulating capacity [47, 48]. Mechanistically, however, these groups had different results. Winkler *et al.* [48] observed a specific decrease in number of macrophages from endosteal stroma and associated loss of osteoblastic activity with a decrease in CXCL12. Chow *et al.* [47] observed a significant decrease in CXCL12 expression from isolated nestin^{+} MSCs, but their group did not observe any change in osteoblastic activity. Though the site for loss of CXCL12 is different with the two groups, overall it appears that monocytes and/or macrophages are positive regulators of CXCL12 expression and thereby indirectly help in retention of stem cells via CXCR4–CXCL12 signaling. Another indirect way in which macrophages regulate HSC homeostasis is by differentiating into osteoclasts. Activation of osteoclasts can cause egress of hematopoietic progenitors, and, conversely, inhibition of osteoclasts can prevent egress of hematopoietic progenitors into circulation [49].

6.3 Why do HSCs need multiple niches?

There are several possibilities that could explain why HSCs need different niche components. One of the most persuasive explanations is that HSCs exist in different states, namely active and quiescent, and the different niches help maintain these states. Static imaging of the SLAM family of proteins present in stem cells has revealed that around 60% of the HSCs are in the perivascular area and around 20% are in the endosteal region. This localization is corroborated by functional experiments showing that deletion of signals emanating from niche cells in the perivascular area results in ~50% loss of stem cells. Since depletion of CAR cells (present in the perivascular region) leads to a decrease in HSC cycling between

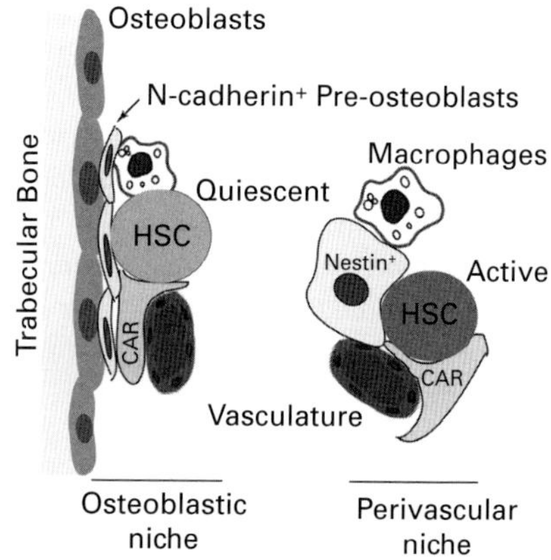

Figure 6.1 Hematopoietic stem cells (HSCs) reside both in osteoblastic and in vascular niches. Quiescent HSCs reside in trabecular bone, attached to N-cadherin^{+} pre-osteoblasts CXCL12-abundant reticular (CAR) cells and macrophages (osteomacs). Active HSCs are surrounded by perivascular cells, including CAR cells, nestin^{+} cells, endothelial cells, and CD169^{+} macrophages.

active and quiescent states, it is very likely that most of the HSCs in this region are in an active state. Hence, there is a high probability that niche cells present in the perivascular region (CAR cells, nestin^{+} MSCs) and macrophages support active stem cells. On the other hand, stem cells close to the endosteal zone are more quiescent and have a higher long-term engraftment potential [50]. It is not surprising that the endosteal niche supports more quiescent cells since this zone is more hypoxic, being away from active vascular diffusion. HSCs close to the endosteal niche are exposed to less oxygen and thereby have reduced generation of reactive oxygen species and DNA damage. Maintenance of the hypoxic state keeps stem cells in a low metabolic state and in quiescence [51, 52].

Another possibility is that stem cells may choose different niches as their fate changes (stem cells changing to more progenitor-like or differentiated cells). This could be because some of the signals, such as N-cadherin–N-cadherin homophilic binding and N-cadherin–β-catenin and thrombopoietin signaling, are unique to osteoprogenitors/osteoblasts and not present in other niche components. These unique signals may help stem cells maintain themselves in a specific state, such as, for example, the quiescent state, since cells close to the endosteal region have been proved to be quiescent. Alternatively, concentrations of signaling mediators could dictate stem cell fate. For example, signaling molecules such as CXCL12 are common to multiple niche cells, albeit at different concentrations. It is thus likely that HSCs require the same signaling molecules at different concentrations while altering their fate. Another possibility is that crosstalk between niches using similar signaling molecules could influence HSC fate and, additionally, multiple niche cells networking among themselves could maintain a specific state of the stem cell. Overall, it is now evident from these findings that the concept of "niche" has evolved from "one stem cell–one niche cell" to a broader paradigm encompassing different states and fates of stem cells and multicellular niche components.

6.4 Technology to visualize in-vivo location of HSCs

Functional studies prove the existence of the interaction between HSCs and their niches, but do not reveal their location. This is important, since many of the signals from stem cells are membrane-bound. Investigating the location of stem cells would help us further understand how niche components contribute to stem cell regulation. Earlier imaging studies were mainly dependent on two-dimensional (2D) static imaging in tissue sections using antibodies. However, it has become increasingly evident that HSCs exist in the 3D space and more sophisticated imaging is required in order to reveal the stem-cell–niche-cell interaction. In-vivo 3D imaging can resolve many of these issues and extend our understanding of stem cell behavior in homeostasis and stress. Two-photon intravital microscopy in combination with fluorescent probes enables the visualization of HSC–niche interactions at the single-cell level with sub-micrometer resolution in 3D. In 2009, two groups simultaneously developed this technology for visualization of HSCs in vivo. Linheng Li's group developed an ex-vivo real-time imaging technology to monitor the homing of purified HSCs labeled by GFP in the trabecular area of long bone. In this study, purified GFP-expressing HSCs were transplanted into irradiated recipient mice, and the sliced long bone with exposed marrow was imaged by two-photon microscopy in real time. This ex-vivo technique enabled visualization of HSC–niche interaction in real time for the first time [53]. David Scadden's group, using similar technology, imaged the calvarium bone marrow after transplanting HSCs labeled with lipophilic cyanine dyes [54]. Both groups successfully detected the endosteal location of HSCs in irradiated mice. This technique was then extended to identify another stem-cell-supporting component, namely regulatory T (T_{reg}) cells. T_{reg} cells co-localize with HSCs in the endosteal surface and provide an immune-privileged zone, thereby protecting HSCs from immune attack [55]. Though two-photon microscopic techniques reveal the exact location of stem cells, there are limitations due to the multiple steps required, which can influence the outcome of HSC–niche interaction. The first step is identification and sorting of stem cells from preferentially labeled bone marrow (e.g. from GFP transgenic mice) using a cocktail of antibodies (lin^-, $Sca1^{high}$, $c\text{-}kit^+$, $CD34^-$, $Flk2^-$, $CD150^{high}$), a multiparametric flow analyzer, and a sorter. Next, these sorted cells are transplanted into irradiated mice, and then imaging is carried out. The initial cell sorting under high pressure and the additional manipulation required before imaging could influence stem cell behavior and thus might not truly reflect the homeostatic or native conditions where stem cells reside.

6.5 Future outlook and challenges

One of the challenges with in-vivo imaging studies is that they heavily rely on bone marrow transplantation in irradiated mice. As mentioned earlier, the various steps involved in the process may lead to variations from the natural state and therefore an endogenous HSC fluorescence reporter would be the most desirable option for in-vivo visualization. However, such a specific HSC endogenous reporter has yet to be identified. Another challenge for stem cell in-vivo imaging is the imaging depth: currently the limit is about 150 μm, which restricts imaging of the upper half of the calvarium flat bone and exposed long bone. The ability to image the long bone in vivo, especially the trabecular area, would require advanced optical technology and new fluorescent probes/proteins excited by two-photon absorption at long wavelengths. Nevertheless, with the current available technology, understanding of HSC–niche interaction has taken a great leap forward.

REFERENCES

[1] Li, L. and Clevers, H. 2010. Coexistence of quiescent and active adult stem cells in mammals. *Science*, **327**, 542–5.

[2] Taichman, R. S. and Emerson, S. G. 1994. Human osteoblasts support hematopoiesis through the production of granulocyte colony-stimulating factor. *J. Exp. Med.*, **179**, 1677–82.

[3] Taichman, R. S. and Emerson, S. G. 1998. The role of osteoblasts in the hematopoietic microenvironment. *Stem Cells*, **16**, 7–15.

[4] Taichman, R. S., Reilly, M. J. and Emerson, S. G. 1996. Human osteoblasts support human hematopoietic progenitor cells in vitro bone marrow cultures. *Blood*, **87**, 518–24.

[5] Zhang, J., Niu, C., Ye, L. *et al.* 2003. Identification of the haematopoietic stem cell niche and control of the niche size. *Nature*, **425**, 836–41.

[6] Calvi, L. M., Adams, G. B., Weibrecht, K. W. *et al.* 2003. Osteoblastic cells regulate the haematopoietic stem cell niche. *Nature*, **425**, 841–6.

[7] Visnjic, D., Kalajzic, I., Gronowicz, G. *et al.* 2001. Conditional ablation of the osteoblast lineage in Col2.3deltatk transgenic mice. *J. Bone Miner. Res.*, **16**, 2222–31.

[8] Visnjic, D., Kalajzic, Z., Rowe, D. W. *et al.* 2004. Hematopoiesis is severely altered in mice with an induced osteoblast deficiency. *Blood*, **103**, 3258–64.

[9] Kiel, M. J., Acar, M., Radice, G. L. and Morrison, S. J. 2009. Hematopoietic stem cells do not depend on N-cadherin to regulate their maintenance. *Cell Stem Cell*, **4**(2), 170–179.

[10] Sugimura, R., He, X. C., Venkatraman, A. *et al.* 2012. Noncanonical wnt signaling maintains hematopoietic stem cells in the niche. *Cell*, **150**, 351–65.

[11] Jung, Y., Wang, J., Schneider, A. *et al.* 2006. Regulation of SDF-1 (CXCL12) production by osteoblasts; a possible mechanism for stem cell homing. *Bone*, **38**, 497–508.

[12] Arai, F., Hirao, A., Ohmura, M. *et al.* 2004. Tie2/angiopoietin-1 signaling regulates hematopoietic stem cell quiescence in the bone marrow niche. *Cell*, **118**, 149–61.

[13] Adams, G. B., Chabner, K. T., Alley, I. R. *et al.* 2006. Stem cell engraftment at the endosteal niche is specified by the calcium-sensing receptor. *Nature*, **439**, 599–603.

[14] Zhang, H., Li, X. J., Martin, D. B. and Aebersold, R. 2003. Identification and quantification of N-linked glycoproteins using hydrazide chemistry, stable isotope labeling and mass spectrometry. *Nature Biotechnol.*, **21**, 660–6.

[15] Qian, H., Buza-Vidas, N., Hyland, C. D. *et al.* 2007. Critical role of thrombopoietin in maintaining adult quiescent hematopoietic stem cells. *Cell Stem Cell*, **1**, 671–84.

[16] Yoshihara, H., Arai, F., Hosokawa, K. *et al.* 2007. Thrombopoietin/MPL signaling regulates hematopoietic stem cell quiescence and interaction with the osteoblastic niche. *Cell Stem Cell*, **1**, 685–97.

[17] Fleming, H. E., Janzen, V., Lo Celso, C. *et al.* 2008. Wnt signaling in the niche enforces hematopoietic stem cell quiescence and is necessary to preserve self-renewal in vivo. *Cell Stem Cell*, **2**, 274–83.

[18] Nilsson, S. K., Johnston, H. M., Whitty, G. A. *et al.* 2005. Osteopontin, a key component of the hematopoietic stem cell niche and regulator of primitive hematopoietic progenitor cells. *Blood*, **106**, 1232–9.

[19] Stier, S., Ko, Y., Forkert, R. *et al.* 2005. Osteopontin is a hematopoietic stem cell niche component that negatively regulates stem cell pool size. *J. Exp. Med.*, **201**, 1781–91.

[20] Nakamura, Y., Arai, F., Iwasaki, H. *et al.* 2010. Isolation and characterization of endosteal niche cell populations that regulate hematopoietic stem cells. *Blood*, **116**, 1422–32.

[21] Mancini, S. J., Mantei, N., Dumortier, A. *et al.* 2005. Jagged1-dependent Notch signaling is dispensable for hematopoietic stem cell self-renewal and differentiation. *Blood*, **105**, 2340–2.

[22] Staal, F. J. and Luis, T. C. 2010. Wnt signaling in hematopoiesis: crucial factors for self-renewal, proliferation, and cell fate decisions. *J. Cell Biochem.*, **109**, 844–9.

[23] Visnjic, D., Kalajzic, Z., Rowe, D. W. *et al.* 2004. Hematopoiesis is severely altered in mice with an induced osteoblast deficiency. *Blood*, **103**, 3258–64.

[24] Zhu, J., Garrett, R., Jung, Y. *et al.* 2007. Osteoblasts support B-lymphocyte commitment and differentiation from hematopoietic stem cells. *Blood*, **109**, 3706–12.

[25] Chan, C. K., Chen, C. C., Luppen, C. A. 2009. Endochondral ossification is required for haematopoietic stem-cell niche formation. *Nature*, **457**, 490–4.

[26] Sacchetti, B., Funari, A., Michienzi, S. *et al.* 2007. Self-renewing osteoprogenitors in bone marrow sinusoids can organize a hematopoietic microenvironment. *Cell*, **131**, 324–36.

[27] Chitteti, B. R., Cheng, Y. H., Poteat, B. *et al.* 2010. Impact of interactions of cellular components of the bone marrow microenvironment on hematopoietic stem and progenitor cell function. *Blood*, **115**, 3239–48.

[28] Chitteti, B. R., Cheng, Y. H., Streicher, D. A. *et al.* 2010. Osteoblast lineage cells expressing high levels of Runx2 enhance hematopoietic progenitor cell proliferation and function. *J. Cell Biochem.*, **111**, 284–94.

[29] Cheng, Y. H., Chitteti, B. R., Streicher, D. A. *et al.* 2011. Impact of osteoblast maturational status on their ability to enhance the hematopoietic function of stem and progenitor cells. *J. Bone Miner. Res.*, **26**(5), 1111–21.

[30] Raaijmakers, M. H., Mukherjee, S., Guo, S. *et al.* 2010. Bone progenitor dysfunction induces myelodysplasia and secondary leukaemia. *Nature*, **464**, 852–7.

[31] Cumano, A. and Godin, I. 2007. Ontogeny of the hematopoietic system. *Ann. Rev. Immunol.*, **25**, 745–85.

[32] Orkin, S. H. and Zon, L. I. 2008. SnapShot: hematopoiesis. *Cell*, **132**, 712.

[33] Orkin, S. H. and Zon, L. I. 2008. Hematopoiesis: an evolving paradigm for stem cell biology. *Cell*, **132**, 631–44.

[34] Kiel, M. J., Yilmaz, O. H., Iwashita, T., Terhorst, C. and Morrison, S. J. 2005. SLAM family receptors distinguish hematopoietic stem and progenitor cells and reveal endothelial niches for stem cells. *Cell*, **121**, 1109–21.

[35] Ding, L., Saunders, T. L., Enikolopov, G. and Morrison, S. J. 2012. Endothelial and perivascular cells maintain haematopoietic stem cells. *Nature*, **481**, 457–62.

[36] Broudy, V. C. 1997. Stem cell factor and hematopoiesis. *Blood*, **90**, 1345–64.

[37] Kiel, M. J., Yilmaz, O. H., Iwashita, T., Terhorst, C. and Morrison, S. J. 2005. SLAM family receptors distinguish hematopoietic stem and progenitor cells and reveal endothelial niches for stem cells. *Cell*, **121**, 1109–21.

[38] Sugiyama, T., Kohara, H., Noda, M. and Nagasawa, T. 2006. Maintenance of the hematopoietic stem cell pool by CXCL12-CXCR4 chemokine signaling in bone marrow stromal cell niches. *Immunity*, **25**, 977–88.

[39] Omatsu, Y., Sugiyama, T., Kohara, H. *et al.* 2010. The essential functions of adipo-osteogenic progenitors as the hematopoietic stem and progenitor cell niche. *Immunity*, **33**, 387–99.

[40] Mendez-Ferrer, S., Michurina, T. V., Ferraro, F. *et al.* 2010. Mesenchymal and haematopoietic stem cells form a unique bone marrow niche. *Nature*, **466**, 829–34.

[41] Mendez-Ferrer, S., Lucas, D., Battista, M. and Frenette, P. S. 2008. Haematopoietic stem cell release is regulated by circadian oscillations. *Nature*, **452**, 442–7.

[42] Spiegel, A., Kalinkovich, A., Shivtiel, S., Kollet, O. and Lapidot, T. 2008. Stem cell regulation via dynamic interactions of the nervous and immune systems with the microenvironment. *Cell Stem Cell*, **3**, 484–92.

[43] Spiegel, A., Shivtiel, S., Kalinkovich, A. *et al.* 2007. Catecholaminergic neurotransmitters regulate migration and repopulation of immature human CD34+ cells through Wnt signaling. *Nature Immunol.*, **8**, 1123–31.

[44] Naveiras, O., Nardi, V., Wenzel, P. L. *et al.* 2009. Bone-marrow adipocytes as negative regulators of the haematopoietic microenvironment. *Nature*, **460**, 259–63.

[45] Pietramaggiori, G., Scherer, S. S., Alperovich, M. *et al.* 2009. Improved cutaneous healing in diabetic mice exposed to healthy peripheral circulation. *J. Investigative Dermatol.*, **129**, 2265–74.

[46] Claycombe, K., King, L. E. and Fraker, P. J. 2008. A role for leptin in sustaining lymphopoiesis and myelopoiesis. *Proc. Nat. Acad. Sci. USA*, **105**, 2017–21.

[47] Chow, A., Lucas, D., Hidalgo, A. *et al.* 2011. Bone marrow CD169+ macrophages promote the retention of hematopoietic stem and progenitor cells in the mesenchymal stem cell niche. *J. Exp. Med.*, **208**, 261–71.

[48] Winkler, I. G., Sims, N. A., Pettit, A. R. *et al.* 2010. Bone marrow macrophages maintain hematopoietic stem cell (HSC) niches and their depletion mobilizes HSCs. *Blood*, **116**, 4815–28.

[49] Kollet, O., Dar, A., Shivtiel, S. *et al.* 2006. Osteoclasts degrade endosteal components and promote mobilization of hematopoietic progenitor cells. *Nature Med.*, **12**, 657–64.

[50] Grassinger, J., Haylock, D. N., Williams, B., Olsen, G. H. and Nilsson, S. K. 2010. Phenotypically identical hemopoietic stem cells isolated from different regions of bone marrow have different biologic potential. *Blood*, **116**, 3185–96.

[51] Simsek, T., Kocabas, F., Zheng, J. *et al.* 2010. The distinct metabolic profile of hematopoietic stem cells reflects their location in a hypoxic niche. *Cell Stem Cell*, **7**, 380–90.

[52] Mohyeldin, A., Garzon-Muvdi, T. and Quinones-Hinojosa, A. 2010. Oxygen in stem cell biology: a critical component of the stem cell niche. *Cell Stem Cell*, **7**, 150–61.

[53] Xie, Y., Yin, T., Wiegraebe, W. *et al.* 2009. Detection of functional haematopoietic stem cell niche using real-time imaging. *Nature*, **457**, 97–101.

[54] Lo Celso, C., Fleming, H. E., Wu, J. W. *et al.* 2009. Live-animal tracking of individual haematopoietic stem/progenitor cells in their niche. *Nature*, **457**, 92–6.

[55] Fujisaki, J., Wu, J., Carlson, A. L. *et al.* 2011. In vivo imaging of Treg cells providing immune privilege to the haematopoietic stem-cell niche. *Nature*, **474**, 216–19.

PART II

Porous scaffolds for regenerative medicine

7

Nanofibrous polymer scaffolds with designed pore structure for regeneration

Zhanpeng Zhang, Jeremy M. Holzwarth and Peter X. Ma

7.1 Introduction

Organ failure and tissue loss are challenging health issues due to the widespread occurrence of injuries, the lack of donated organs for transplantation, and the limitations of conventional artificial implants. The field of tissue engineering and regenerative medicine emerged to solve these issues by providing biological alternatives that restore, maintain, or improve tissue function for harvested tissues and organs [1–5]. In a typical tissue engineering approach, cells are grown in a three-dimensional (3D) biodegradable scaffold, which, ideally, should perform the structural and biochemical functions of the natural extracellular matrix (ECM), providing cells with topological and chemical cues as well as mechanical support until the cell-produced ECM takes over. Therefore, there is a set of key characteristics that the scaffold should have. First, adequate space or porosity with high interconnectivity is needed throughout the 3D scaffold in order to allow cell adhesion, migration, proliferation, and differentiation into the desired cell phenotypes for new tissue formation [6, 7]. A porous structure not only defines the initial void space available for cell seeding/ingrowth and new tissue formation, but also determines the mass transport pathways. Second, appropriate surface architecture is critical since this is where the cell–matrix interactions occur. In connective tissues, such as bone, skin, ligament, and tendon, the ECM consists primarily of proteoglycans and fibrous proteins, such as collagen. The fibrous architecture of collagen contributes to the mechanical stabilities of the ECM, and plays a vital role in cell attachment, proliferation, and differentiation [8]. Type I collagen is the most abundant type of collagen and forms nanofiber bundles with fiber diameter ranging from 50 to 500 nm. A nanofibrous (NF) surface is desired to mimic the natural ECM and is found to be advantageous in improving cell attachment, migration, proliferation, and differentiation [9]. Therefore, polymeric scaffolds with porous structure at the micrometer scale and fibrous architecture at the nanometer dimension should be promising candidates for tissue regeneration. Although it is not the focus of this chapter, chemical and biological functionalization of scaffolds can enhance cell–biomaterial interactions [10].

With the advancement in micro- and nanotechnology, material design can be controlled down to the micrometer and nanometer scales. In the micrometer range, well-controlled porous architecture could be obtained via particulate leaching and solid free-form techniques, while at the nanometer scale, self-assembly, electrospinning, and phase separation techniques can build the NF structure. Self-assembly provides a way to form NF structures from various molecules with possible bioactivity. Electrospinning, which has attracted growing interest over the last decade in scaffold fabrication, is capable of generating nanofibers from a variety of materials with controllable fiber morphology over a certain size range. Thermally induced phase separation (TIPS) is another widely used method for the fabrication of nanofibers and offers great flexibility in the 3D structural design: scaffolds ranging from NF mesh via injectable microspheres to 3D porous scaffolds with predesigned pore shape can be fabricated when TIPS is combined with other techniques. In this chapter, we will discuss self-assembly, electrospinning, and TIPS techniques that have been widely employed for the fabrication of NF scaffolds from a variety of materials.

7.2 Molecular self-assembly

By definition, molecular self-assembly is the spontaneous organization of individual molecules into structurally well-defined stable arrangements through preprogrammed non-covalent interactions. These include hydrogen bonds, van der Waals forces, hydrophobic interactions, and electrostatic interactions [11–14].

A prime example is ionic self-complementary oligopeptides, which are building blocks consisting of repeating ionic hydrophilic and hydrophobic amino acids that can self-assemble into nanofibers [15–17]. In water, these oligopeptides form a beta-sheet where two surfaces are present: a polar surface with charged ionic chains and a non-polar surface with alanines. Upon exposure to monovalent alkaline cations or under physiological conditions, the oligopeptides spontaneously assemble into hydrogels composed of interwoven nanofibers with a diameter of 10–20 nm and pores of 50–200 nm [15–17].

In addition to ionic self-complementary oligopeptides, peptide-amphiphiles (PAs) are widely employed for nanofiber assembly. Typically, PAs need to have a long alkyl tail (hydrophobic portion) and a peptide region (hydrophilic portion) to make the molecule amphiphilic [18, 19]. The self-assembly of these peptide-amphiphiles into nanofibers can be driven either by pH change or by the introduction of divalent ions (such as Ca^{2+}), which neutralize the electrostatic repulsion between molecules to allow the clustering of hydrophobic segments in the core and hydrophilic segments on the surface of the fibers in the aqueous environment. Under similar principles, synthetic diblock/triblock copolymers and dendrimers can self-assemble into nanofibrous structures [20–22].

Self-assembly provides several advantages for nanofiber fabrication, including a simple fabrication process, easy cell encapsulation in a hydrogel, and the injectability that allows *in situ* scaffold formation. However, self-assembled hydrogels often lack a stable 3D geometry, which is needed in many tissue regeneration scenarios, such as bone tissue regeneration. Other limitations include the choice of building blocks, which are currently limited to biological molecules, such as peptides, whose synthesis is often time-consuming and costly; the difficulty of controlling pore size and shape within the scaffold; and the significantly smaller fiber diameter (usually less than 10 nm) than that of collagen.

7.2.1 Electrospinning

Electrospinning was first developed in the early twentieth century, but was not translated to the field of tissue engineering to fabricate nanofibrous scaffolds until much more recently. The electrospinning setup includes a polymer solution or melt reservoir, a grounded collector, and a high-voltage electric field in between (Figure 7.1(a)). The electric field draws the polymer solution/melt from a tip to form the so-called "Taylor cone." When the voltage is high enough to overcome the surface tension of the polymer solution/melt, a charged jet will be shot out from the tip of the cone toward the grounded collector, along which the solvent evaporates/melt solidifies to form solid-state thin fibers. In addition to the basic setup, the electrospinning apparatus could have different configurations to organize fiber deposition. In one example, nanofibrous tubes were formed using a rotatory collector [23] (Figure 7.1(b)–(e)). In another example, patterning the collector with conducting polymers could lead to the formation of patterned electrospun fibers [24]. In addition, the dual-syringe system employed in co-axial electrospinning is capable of generating a core–shell structure within the nanofibers [25–29].

Electrospun nanofibrous scaffolds have been generated from a large variety of materials ranging from natural polymers, such as collagen [30], chitosan [31], and silk fibroin [20], to synthetic biodegradable macromolecules, including poly(glycolic acid) (PGA) [32, 33], poly(lactic acid) (PLA) [33], and their copolymers [33]. Different polymers can also be mixed for

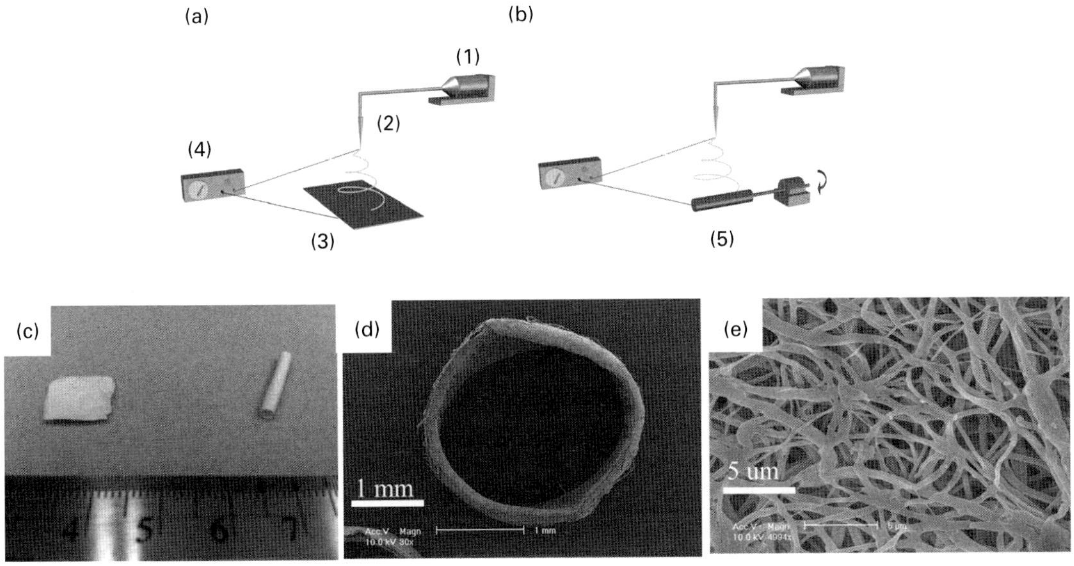

Figure 7.1 Schematic pictures of the electrospinning setup with (a) a plate grounded collector and (b) a mandrel-like grounded collector: (1) syringe containing polymer solution; (2) syringe needle; (3) grounded collection plate; (4) power supply; (5) rotator grounded collector. (c) The appearance of electrospun NF mesh and NF tube made using a plate collector and a rotator mandrel-like collector, respectively. (d) Cross-section of an electrospun PLLA/PCL tubular NF scaffold and (e) its inner surface. Images (c), (d), and (e) are from Peter X. Ma's lab.

electrospinning of blend nanofibers [32, 34, 35]. Recently, inorganic nanofibers were also created by electrospinning [36]. Besides the flexible material choice, the fiber morphology can also be controlled by adjusting the process parameters, which include applied voltage, solution concentration, polymer and solvent properties, and the distance between the polymer solution/melt and the collector. Depending on the materials used, fibers with diameters ranging from nanometer to micrometer scales can be created [37] (Figure 7.2).

It has been challenging to apply electrospinning in the fabrication of clinically relevant 3D constructs with designed pore structure. Although electrospinning can generate a network of open pores, the size of the pores is dependent on the fiber size and is, at best, a few microns. In addition, the shape of the pores cannot be well controlled. Various strategies have been employed in recent efforts to improve electrospun 3D scaffolds, including using dual fiber sizes [38] and combined porogen-leaching techniques [39]. A detailed discussion on electrospinning for tissue regeneration can be found in Chapter 8 in this book.

7.2.2 Thermally induced phase separation

7.2.2.1 Preparation of NF matrix

Phase separation is a thermodynamic process that involves a homogeneous multicomponent system, which tends to separate into multiple phases to lower the system's free energy. For polymer solutions, phase separation is made to occur either thermally or by adding a non-solvent, forming polymer-rich and polymer-lean phases. Upon solvent extraction, sublimation, or evaporation, the polymer-rich phase solidifies to form the skeleton of the polymer foam, while the polymer-lean phase becomes the open pores [2]. Different polymer–solvent systems, solution concentrations, and processing parameters, such as phase

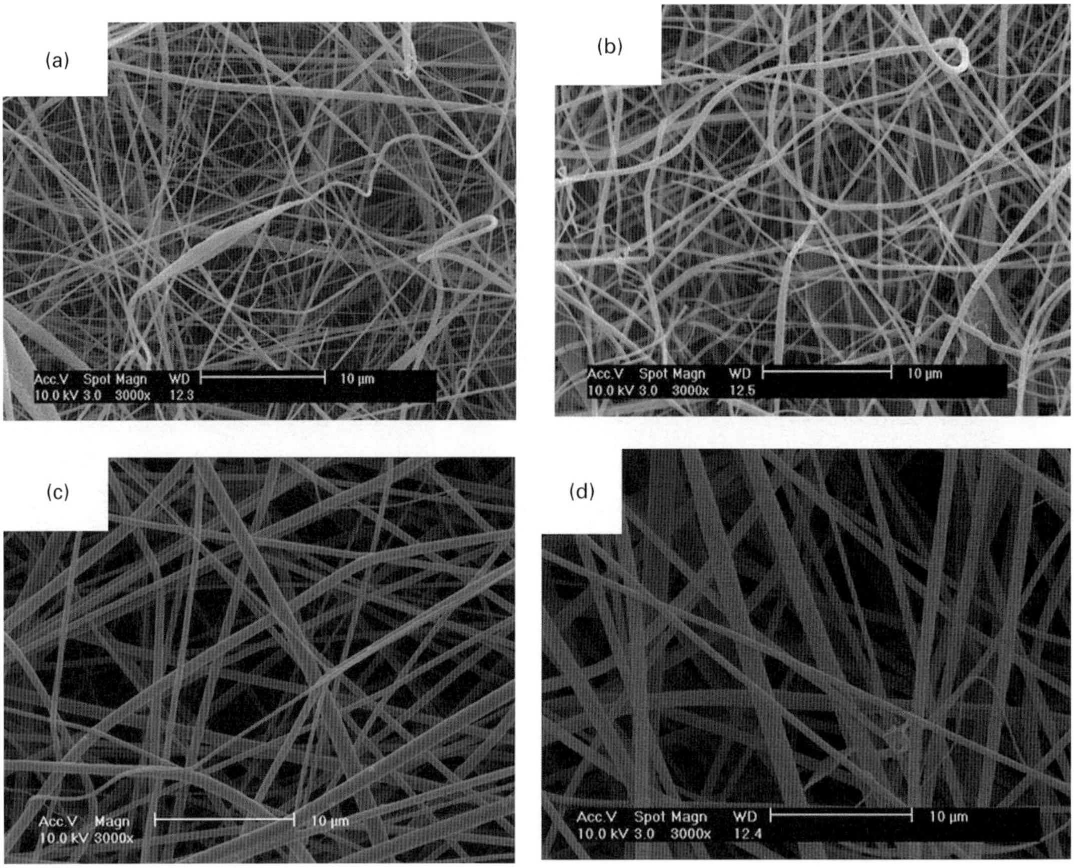

Figure 7.2 SEM images of nanofibers with different fiber diameters electrospun from various PLLA concentrations: (a) 6 wt%, (b) 8 wt%, (c) 10 wt%, and (d) 12 wt%. Reprinted from *Advanced Functional Materials*, volume 20, Chuanglong He, Guiyong Xiao, Xiaobing Jin, Chenghui Sun, Peter X. Ma, Electrodeposition on nanofibrous polymer scaffolds: rapid mineralization, tunable calcium phosphate composition and topography, pages 3568–3576, Copyright (2010), with permission from John Wiley & Sons.

separation temperature, can generate different pore structures for the scaffolds [40]. When phase separation is induced thermally, if the solvent crystallization temperature is higher than the phase separation temperature used, solid–liquid phase separation occurs, whereby the solvent crystallizes to form the pore shape after solvent sublimation. If the solvent crystallization temperature is lower than the phase separation temperature used, a liquid–liquid phase separation takes place as the temperature of the solution is decreased. Within certain polymer concentration and temperature ranges, the liquid–liquid phase separation follows a spinodal decomposition pathway and forms a bicontinuous pattern where both polymer-rich and polymer-lean regions are interconnected [40]. A typical TIPS technique to create NF structures involves five steps: polymer dissolution, liquid–liquid phase separation and gelation, solvent extraction, freezing, and freeze-drying [41–44]. For example, poly(L-lactic acid) (PLLA) is dissolved in a chosen solvent system and thermally induced to phase separate into nanofibers (Figures 7.3(a) and (b)). The chosen solvent system should have a low crystallization temperature in order to allow liquid–liquid phase

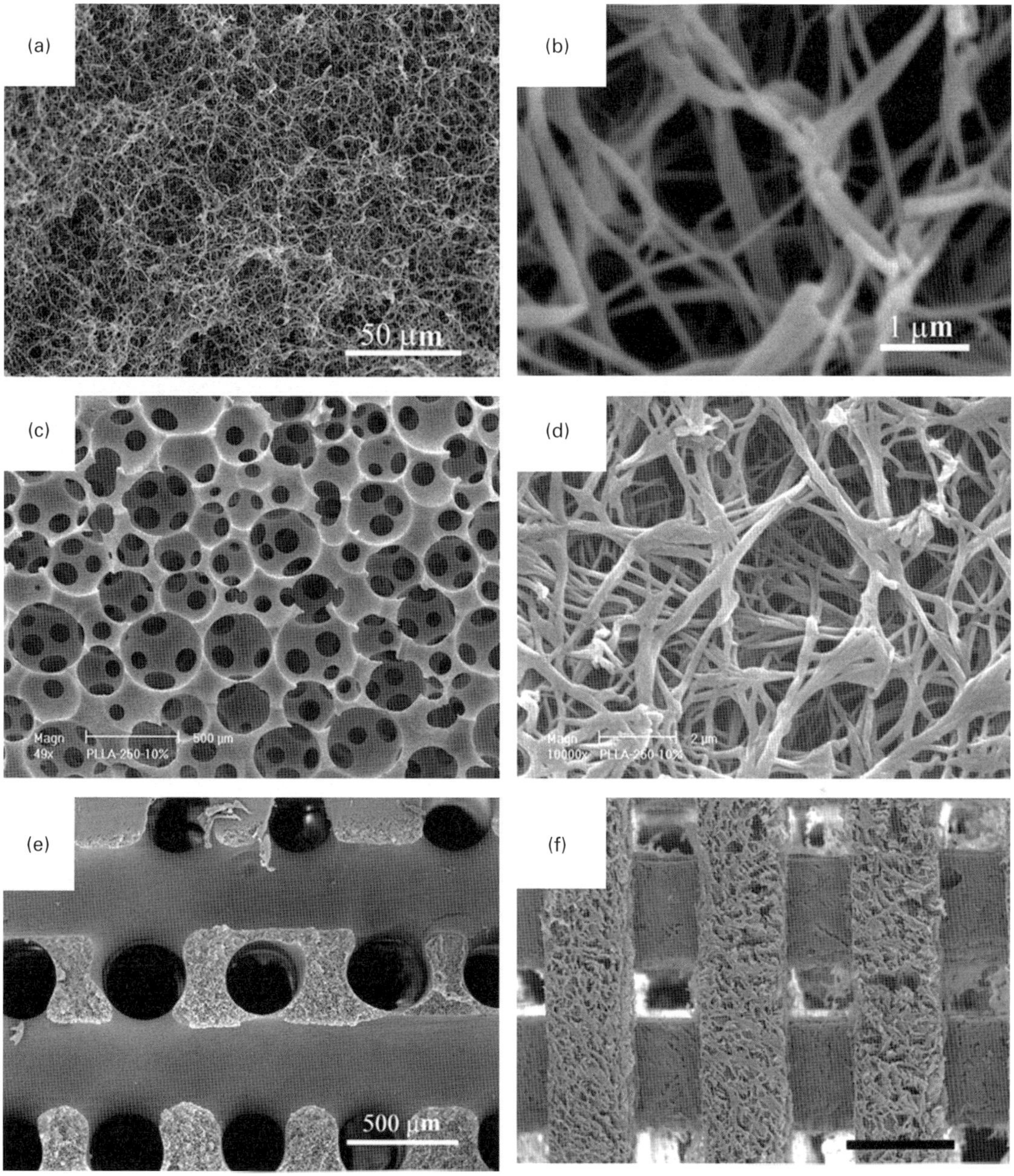

Figure 7.3 SEM images of a PLLA NF mesh prepared from 2.5% PLLA/THF solution at a phase separation temperature of 8 °C with magnification of (a) 500× and (b) 20,000×; (c) and (d) macroporous scaffolds prepared from sugar sphere template leaching and phase separation; (e) macroporous scaffolds prepared from sugar fiber template leaching and phase separation; and (f) macroporous scaffolds prepared from a solid free form (SFF) and phase separation. Images (a) and (b) reprinted from the *Journal of Biomedical Materials Research*, volume 46, Peter X. Ma and Ruiyun Zhang, Synthetic nano-scale extracellular matrix, pages 60–72, Copyright (1999), with permission from John Wiley & Sons. Images (c) and (d) reprinted from

separation, e.g. one could use tetrahydrofuran, dimethyl formamide, pyridine, tetrahydrofuran–methanol, dioxane–methanol, dioxane–water, dioxane–acetone, or dioxane–pyridine. Since PLLA is a semicrystalline polymer, the polymer can crystallize during the phase separation process to help stabilize the structure. After the removal of the solvent via extraction, sublimation, or evaporation, a 3D continuous NF PLLA structure with a porosity as high as 98.5% can be generated [43]. The diameter of the phase-separated nanofibers ranges from 50 to 500 nm, which is similar to that of natural collagen fibers. In addition, the surface-to-volume ratio of the NF scaffold is much higher than that of a conventional solid-wall scaffold, which makes the scaffold degrade significantly faster for tissue engineering applications [45].

In addition to PLLA, many other synthetic polymers and naturally derived polymers have also been fabricated into nanofibers by TIPS. For instance, a series of biodegradable amphiphilic poly(hydroxyalkyl (meth)acrylate)-graft-poly(L-lactic acid) (PHAA-g-PLLA) copolymers has been synthesized and fabricated into NF structures by TIPS [46]. These copolymers have functional groups that facilitate the conjugation of bioactive moieties and degrade faster than the PLLA homopolymer. In another example, gelatin was fabricated into highly porous NF matrices by TIPS using either ethanol–water or methanol–water mixtures [42]. Gelatin is a mixture of peptide chains from the hydrolysis of collagen, and thus essentially has the same chemical composition as collagen. As a benefit, the denaturing hydrolysis process eliminates any possible resident pathogens. Thus, the NF gelatin scaffold mimics ECM collagen both in chemical composition and in physical structure, and is advantageous in tissue engineering [42].

7.2.2.2 NF 3D scaffolds with anatomical shapes and predesigned macropores

Beyond creating ECM-like nanofibers from various materials, phase separation could also be easily combined with other techniques to provide additional architectural control at multiple scales. Several techniques, including particulate leaching and reverse solid free-form fabrication (SFF), have been combined with TIPS to construct macro/micropore/channel networks within the NF matrix [6, 42, 44, 47] (Figures 7.3(c)–(f)).

In one example, sugar spheres (with diameters in the range 150–500 μm) were assembled into a mold (negative replica) to fabricate NF scaffolds with interconnected spherical pores [47] (Figures 7.3(c) and (d)). In this process, water was used to extract the solvent from the system and to leach the sugar spheres to generate the predesigned spherical pore network. By use of different heat-treatment conditions, the microspheres were bonded with different-sized interconnections. Therefore, the average macropore size and the interconnectivity of the pores throughout the scaffold can be controlled. Similarly, sugar fibers were assembled as a geometric porogen 3D structure to build a tubular pore network [6] (Figure 7.3(e)). Furthermore, SFF fabrication was employed to construct a wax mold with computer-designed internal structural features. It was then used as a negative replica to fabricate NF scaffolds with interconnected microchannels [41] (Figure 7.3(f)). The ability to control the architecture at various size levels makes translation to the clinic easier, since a specifically designed scaffold may be the best approach to certain applications.

In clinical trials where patient-specific scaffold designs are needed, the 3D overall shapes of the fabricated scaffolds should be easily controlled to fill the defects. This

Caption for Figure 7.3 (*cont.*) the *Journal of Biomedical Materials Research* Part A, volume 78, Guobao Wei and Peter X. Ma, Macroporous and nanofibrous polymer scaffolds and polymer/bone-like apatite composite scaffolds generated by sugar spheres, pages 306–315, Copyright (2006), with permission from John Wiley & Sons. Image (e) reprinted from the *Journal of Biomedical Materials Research* Part A, volume 52, Ruiyun Zhang and Peter X. Ma, Synthetic nano-fibrillar extracellular matrices with predesigned macroporous architectures, pages 430–438, Copyright (2000), with permission from John Wiley & Sons. Image (f) reprinted from *Biomaterials*, volume 27, Victor J. Chen, Laura A. Smith, Peter X. Ma, Bone regeneration on computer-designed nano-fibrous scaffolds, pages 3973–3979, Copyright (2006), with permission from Elsevier.

(a) (b) (c) (d) (e)

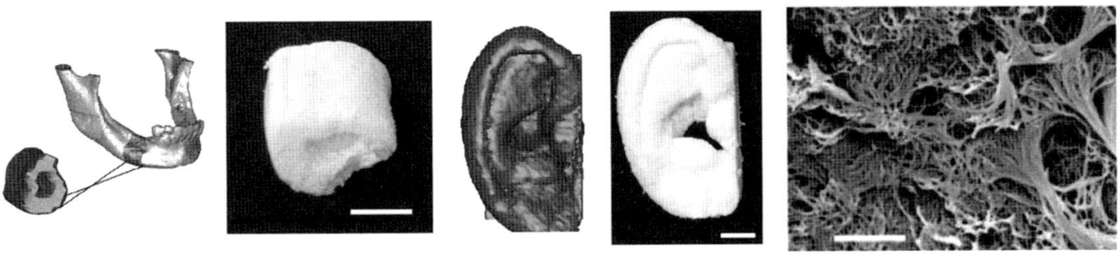

Figure 7.4 Scaffolds created from 3D reconstructions of computed-tomography (CT) scans or histological sections. (a) Human mandible reconstruction from CT scans (the dark-shaded segment shows the reversed image of the bone fragment to be engineered); (b) resulting NF scaffold of the mandible segment (scale bar: 10 mm); (c) human ear reconstruction from histological sections; (d) resulting NF scaffold of the human ear (scale bar: 10 mm); (e) the NF pore wall morphology (scale bar: 5 μm). Reprinted from *Biomaterials*, volume 27, Victor J. Chen, Laura A. Smith, Peter X. Ma, Bone regeneration on computer-designed nano-fibrous scaffolds, pages 3973–3979, Copyright (2006), with permission from Elsevier.

challenge was tackled by combining TIPS with computer-assisted design (CAD) and computer-assisted manufacture (CAM) [41]. This approach enables the design and fabrication of patient-specific scaffolds. Computed-tomography scans of histological sections of human anatomical parts were employed by CAD in designing and constructing the 3D shapes of the wax mold, thereby controlling the external shape of the resulting scaffolds. By combining particulate leaching and phase separation, NF scaffolds with predesigned pore structure as well as controlled 3D shapes, which include ear [41], human mandible segment [41], and hand digit bone [48], were successfully fabricated (Figure 7.4).

7.2.2.3 Preparation of injectable NF scaffolds

In addition to using CAD and CAM as described above, scaffolds capable of being injected are an alternative way to fill the defects accurately and with minimal surgical intervention, especially when the defect or wound is irregularly shaped. Microspheres are injectable and have been used as carriers to deliver cells for bone [49], cartilage [50], dermal [51], hepatic [52], and adipose [53] tissue regeneration. However, traditional microsphere fabrication techniques, such as emulsification [54] and emulsion polymerization [55], often lack control over the exterior and interior morphologies of the microspheres.

A novel methodology has been developed to fabricate injectable hollow microspheres with NF structures recently [56] (Figure 7.5). In this work, star-shaped PLLA (SS-PLLA) was synthesized using poly(amidoamine) dendrimers as initiators, dissolved in tetrahydrofuran, emulsified in glycerol under rigorous stirring, and quenched in liquid nitrogen to generate the NF hollow microspheres, where the NF structure formation was driven by TIPS (Figure 7.5(a)). Upon solvent extraction and freeze-drying, highly porous hollow microspheres with open pores on the NF shells were obtained without using any template (Figures 7.5(b) and (c)). When a linear PLLA was employed with the same process, NF microspheres without a hollow core structure were generated. Thus, the star-shaped polymer architecture was an important feature allowing the assembly of the NF hollow microspheres in this case. The novel NF hollow microspheres were examined as an injectable scaffold for cartilage regeneration both in vitro and in vivo [56]. The engineered cartilage was similar to native cartilage in structure, composition, and biomechanical properties, and fully filled a critical-sized osteochondral defect in rabbits with smooth integration with the host cartilage.

7.3 Stem cells and nanofibers

While the scaffold is a major component of tissue engineering, cells play a vital role in the regeneration process. The cell source must be chosen appropriately

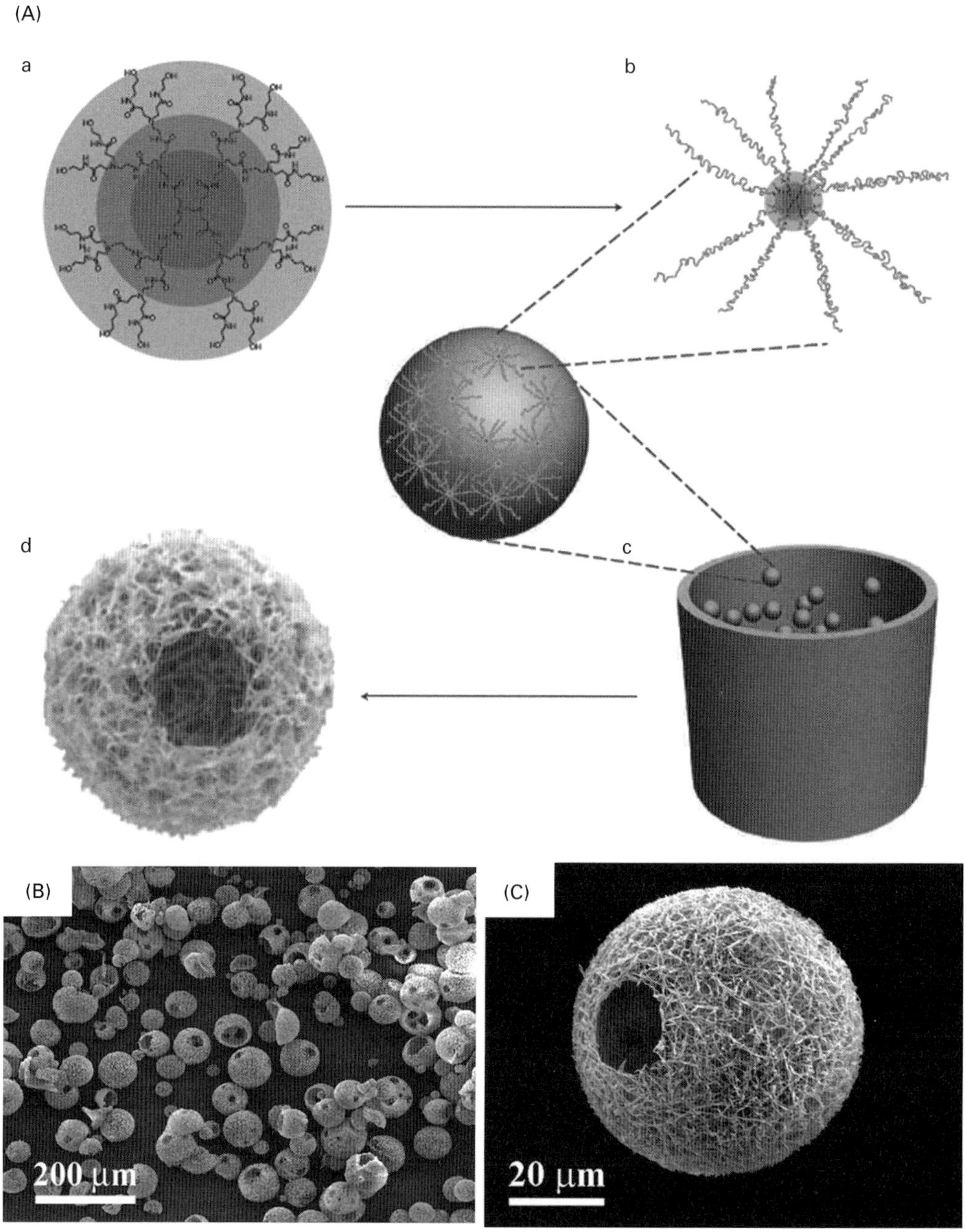

Figure 7.5 (A) A schematic diagram of SS-PLLA synthesis and nanofibrous hollow microsphere fabrication: a, PAMAM (G2) as an initiator for the synthesis of SS-PLLA; b, The SS-PLLA with coils representing the PLLA chains; c, preparation of SS-PLLA microspheres using a surfactant-free emulsification process; d, nanofibrous hollow microspheres were obtained after phase separation, solvent extraction, and freeze-drying. (B) SEM image of nanofibrous hollow microspheres fabricated from SS-PLLA, showing that almost every microsphere had one or more open holes on the shell. (C) SEM image of a representative nanofibrous hollow microsphere, showing the nanofibrous architecture and a hole of diameter approximately 20 μm on the microsphere shell. Reprinted from *Nature*, volume 10, Xiaohua Liu, Xiaobing Jin, Peter X. Ma, Nanofibrous hollow microspheres self-assembled from star-shaped polymers as injectable cell carriers for knee repair, pages 398–406, Copyright (2011), with permission from Nature Publishing Group.

for the application, but various stem cells have shown great promise. However, stem cells require a high level of control in order to guide their differentiation down the desired lineage. Along with growth factors and media conditions, substrate architecture, such as nanofibers, has been shown to assist in controlling their differentiation.

A recent study showed the ability of nanofibers to increase the chondrogenic differentiation of mesenchymal stem cells (MSCs) [57], a multipotent cell line usually derived from bone marrow and commonly used in bone and cartilage regeneration. MSCs were seeded on both flat and NF films and cultured in the presence of transforming growth factor β_1 (TGF-β_1). After 7 days, there was nearly a three-fold increase in expression of Sox-9, an early chondrogenic marker, in the cells on the nanofibers compared with that in the cells on the flat films. Similarly, human amniotic-fluid-derived stem cells (hAFSCs), a recently discovered cell line that falls in between MSCs and embryonic stem cells (ESCs), were cultured on NF and solid scaffolds in the presence of recombinant human bone morphogenic protein-7 (rhBMP-7) [58]. After 1 week, alkaline phosphatase activity, a marker of osteogenesis, was markedly higher on the nanofibrous scafoflds than on the control scaffolds without the NF feature. Both after 2 weeks and after 4 weeks, the calcium content on the NF scaffolds was significantly higher than that on the control scaffolds. Thus, the NF scaffolds induced higher levels of chondrogenic and osteogenic differentiation.

Compared with MSCs and AFSCs, ESCs are more immature stem cells, and are arguably the most difficult stem cells to control since they have the capability to undergo differentiation into every cell type in the body. Thus, using nanofibers to help control their fate is even more important. In a bone tissue regeneration application, mouse ESCs were cultured both on solid and on NF films under osteogenic conditions for 26 days [59]. Afterwards, there were elevated levels of osteocalcin and bone sialoprotein mRNA in the cells on the nanofibers compared with the levels in those on the solid film, illustrating the higher level of osteogenic differentiation promoted by the nanofibers.

In a separate application, electrospun nanofibers were used to promote the neural differentiation of neural stem cells, a more mature stem cell line. The cells were cultured on polyethersulfone nanofibers along with a flat tissue culture polystyrene surface (TCPS), both coated with laminin [60]. After 5 days, the cells were labeled for nestin, a neural progenitor marker and Tuj-1, a neuronal marker. There were more nestin-positive cells on the TCPS, indicating that many of the cells had not differentiated. However, there was a high percentage of Tuj-1-positive cells on the fibers (of diameter 283 nm), revealing that nanofibers can promote neuronal differentiation of the stem cells.

To further illustrate the advantages of NF scaffolds, their application was expanded to other tissue engineering applications. For instance, in dentin regeneration, a study compared the odontogenic differentiation of human dental pulp stem cells (hDPSCs) on NF and solid-walled PLLA scaffolds [61]. After 1, 2, and 3 weeks in odontogenic medium, alkaline phosphatase activity was greater on the NF scaffolds than on their solid-walled counterparts. Additionally, there were higher levels of osteocalcin and dentin sialophosphoprotein after 1, 2, and 4 weeks. In nucleus pulposus engineering, rabbit MSCs were used to generate nucleus-pulposus-like tissue [62]. In the presence of TGF-β_1 and 2% oxygen, cells seeded on an NF matrix for 2 weeks had higher levels of Sox-9, collagen type II, aggrecan, and HIF-1α, four markers for ECM production associated with nucleus pulposus, than did the cells seeded on a solid film.

It's clear that nanofibers are superior for the differentiation of a wide array of stem cells in a wide array of applications, but it is also important to elucidate their mechanism of action. It has been shown that nanofibers selectively adsorb certain serum proteins, such as fibronectin, vitronectin, and laminin [63]. These proteins have binding motifs for surface proteins, such as integrins, that help the cells adhere to the fiber and trigger intracellular signaling cascades. In fact, ESCs express the $\alpha_2\beta_1$ integrin, which is associated with collagen type I, and $\alpha_5\beta_1$ integrin, which is associated with fibronectin, at higher levels on NF matrices than they do on solid films [59]. Blocking either the α_2 or the

α_5 integrin subunit substantially inhibited mesodermal and osteogenic differentiation. Downstream, the osteogenic induction of nanofibers is associated with the RhoA–Rock signaling pathway [64]. Inhibition of ROCK, the RhoA effector, increases the expression of bone sialoprotein, and therefore the osteogenic differentiation.

7.4 Conclusions

Scaffolds are a critically important element in tissue engineering and regenerative medicine, and have been designed to deliver a synthetic microenvironment that not only provides physical support, but preferably also delivers bioactive stimuli in a 3D controlled manner. Molecular self-assembly, electrospinning, and TIPS techniques have produced ECM-mimicking nanofibers from various synthetic and naturally derived materials. Various fabrication technologies have been utilized or developed to engineer complex porous structures for such scaffolds. These diverse NF porous scaffolds have been shown to facilitate the regeneration of a variety of tissues, including bone, cartilage, and dentin. Although rapid progress has been made, significant challenges remain. More accurate and independent control over structural features and physical/biological properties of the NF porous scaffolds is needed in order to allow more systematic and quantitative studies on the relationships among structural characteristics, cell function, and tissue regeneration.

In addition to the scaffold, cells play a vital role in tissue regeneration by replacing the synthetic scaffold with natural ECM and functional tissue. Specifically, stem cells have shown great promise on account of their versatility. Pluripotent cells, such as ESCs, are capable of differentiating into a variety of cell types and able to proliferate extensively, which makes them great candidates for myriad applications. More mature stem cells, such as MSCs or progenitors, have the advantage of being simpler to differentiate down the desired lineage. These stem cells show even greater promise when seeded on nanofibers, which have been demonstrated to promote osteogenic, chondrogenic, neural, and odontogenic differentiation, among others. However, more work needs to be done to elucidate the interaction between these stem cells and NF scaffolds. A better understanding of the mechanism by which nanofibers modulate cell fate will allow more intelligent scaffold design and implementation. That will become more and more important as the field develops toward engineering high-level tissues and organs, requiring precise control of both scaffold architecture and cell behavior on numerous size scales. In summary, while the combination of advanced NF scaffolds with versatile stem cells has shown great promise, more work is needed if we are to reach the bright future of regenerative medicine.

ACKNOWLEDGEMENTS

The authors would like to acknowledge the financial support from the National Institutes of Health (NIDCR DE015384, DE017689 and DE022327: PXM), DOD (W81XWH-12-2-0008: PXM) and NSF (DMR-1206575: PXM). JMH was partially supported by the NIH/NIDCR Training Grant (T32 DE 007057) at the University of Michigan School of Dentistry.

REFERENCES

[1] Langer, R. and Vacanti, J. P. 1993. Tissue engineering. *Science*, **260**(5110), 920–6.

[2] Ma, P. X. 2004. Scaffolds for tissue fabrication. *Mater. Today*, **7**(5), 30–40.

[3] Ma, P. X. 2005. Tissue engineering. In *Encyclopedia of Polymer Science and Technology*, 3rd edition, ed. Kroschwitz, J. I., Vol. 12. Hoboken, NJ: John Wiley & Sons, Inc., pp. 261–91.

[4] Rice, M. A., Dodson, B. T., Arthur, J. A. and Anseth, K. S. 2005. Cell-based therapies and tissue engineering. *Otolaryngol. Clinics North America*, **38**(2), 199–214.

[5] Ma, P. X. 2008. Biomimetic materials for tissue engineering. *Adv. Drug Deliv. Rev.*, **60**(2), 184–98.

[6] Zhang, R. and Ma, P. X. 2000. Synthetic nano-fibrillar extracellular matrices with predesigned macroporous architectures. *J. Biomed. Mater. Res.*, **52**(2), 430–8.

[7] Ma, P. X. and Choi, J. W. 2001. Biodegradable polymer scaffolds with well-defined interconnected spherical pore network. *Tissue Eng.*, **7**(1), 23–33.

[8] Alberts, B., Johnson, A., Lewis, J. *et al.* 2002. *Molecular Biology of the Cell.* New York: Garland.

[9] Holzwarth, J. M. and Ma, P. X. 2011. Biomimetic nanofibrous scaffolds for bone tissue engineering. *Biomaterials*, **32**(36), 9622–9.

[10] Liu, X., Holzwarth, J. M. and Ma, P. X. 2012. Functionalized synthetic biodegradable polymer scaffolds for tissue engineering. *Macromol. Biosci.*, **12**(7), 911–19.

[11] Whitesides, G. M., Mathias, J. P. and Seto, C. T. 1991. Molecular self-assembly and nanochemistry: a chemical strategy for the synthesis of nanostructures. *Science*, **254**(5036), 1312–19.

[12] Lehn, J. M., 1993. Supramolecular chemistry. *Science*, **260**(5115), 1762–3.

[13] Ball, P. 1994. Polymers made to measure. *Nature*, **367**(6461), 323–4.

[14] Zhang, S. 2003. Fabrication of novel biomaterials through molecular self-assembly. *Nature Biotechnol.*, **21**(10), 1171–8.

[15] Zhang, S., Holmes, T., Lockshin, C. and Rich, A. 1993. Spontaneous assembly of a self-complementary oligopeptide to form a stable macroscopic membrane. *Proc. Nat. Acad. Sci. USA*, **90**(8), 3334–8.

[16] Zhang, S., Holmes, T. C., Dipersio, C. M. *et al.* 1995. Self-complementary oligopeptide matrices support mammalian cell attachment. *Biomaterials*, **16**(18), 1385–93.

[17] Holmes, T. C., de Lacalle, S., Su, X. *et al.* 2000. Extensive neurite outgrowth and active synapse formation on self-assembling peptide scaffolds. *Proc. Nat. Acad. Sci. USA*, **97**(12), 6728–33.

[18] Hartgerink, J. D., Beniash, E. and S. I. Stupp. 2001. Self-assembly and mineralization of peptide-amphiphile nanofibers. *Science*, **294**, 1684–8.

[19] Hartgerink, J. D., Beniash, E. and Stupp, S. I. 2002. Peptide-amphiphile nanofibers: a versatile scaffold for the preparation of self-assembling materials. *Proc. Nat. Acad. Sci. USA*, **99**(8), 5133–8.

[20] Yu, M., Nowak, A. P., Pochan, D. P. and Deming, T. J. 1999. Methylated mono- and diethyleneglycol functionalized polylysines: nonionic, alpha-helical, water-soluble polypeptides. *J. Am. Chem. Soc.*, **121**(51), 12210–11.

[21] Pochan, D. J., Pakstis, L., Ozbas, B., Nowak, A. P. and Deming, T. J. 2002. SANS and cryo-TEM study of self-assembled diblock copolypeptide hydrogels with rich nano- through microscale morphology. *Macromolecules*, **35**(14), 5358–60.

[22] Nowak, A. P., Breedveld, V., Pakstis, L. *et al.* 2002. Rapidly recovering hydrogel scaffolds from self-assembling diblock copolypeptide amphiphiles. *Nature*, **417**(6887), 424–8.

[23] Yang, F., Muragan, R., Wang, S. and Ramakrishna, S. 2005. Electrospinning of nano/micro scale poly(L-lactic acid) aligned fibers and their potential in neural tissue engineering. *Biomaterials*, **26**(15), 2603–10.

[24] Zhang, D. and Chang, J. 2007. Patterning of electrospun fibers using electroconductive templates. *Adv. Mater.*, **19**(21), 3664–7.

[25] Jiang, H., Hu, Y., Li, Y. *et al.* 2005. A facile technique to prepare biodegradable coaxial electrospun nanofibers for controlled release of bioactive agents. *J. Controlled Release*, **108**(2–3), 237–43.

[26] Zhang, Y. Z., Wang, X., Feng, Y. *et al.* 2006. Coaxial electrospinning of (fluorescein isothiocyanate-conjugated bovine serum albumin)-encapsulated poly(ε-caprolactone) nanofibers for sustained release. *Biomacromolecules*, **7**(4), 1049–57.

[27] Liao, I. C., Chew, S. Y. and Leong, K. W. 2006. Aligned core–shell nanofibers delivering bioactive proteins. *Nanomedicine*, **1**(4), 465–71.

[28] Jiang, H., Hu, Y., Zhao, P., Li, Y. and Zhu, K. 2006. Modulation of protein release from biodegradable core–shell structured fibers prepared by coaxial electrospinning. *J. Biomed. Mater. Res. Part B: Appl. Biomater.*, **79**(1), 50–7.

[29] Sun, Z. C., Zussman, E., Yarin, A. L., Wendorff, J. H. and Greiner, A. 2003. Compound core–shell polymer nanofibers by co-electrospinning. *Adv. Mater.*, **15**(22), 1929–32.

[30] Matthews, J. A., Wnek, G. E., Simpson, D. G. and Bowlin, G. L. 2002. Electrospinning of collagen nanofibers. *Biomacromolecules*, **3**(2), 232–8.

[31] Bhattarai, N., Edmondson, D., Veiseh, O., Matsen, F. A. and Zhang, M. 2005. Electrospun chitosan-based nanofibers and their cellular compatibility. *Biomaterials*, **26**(31), 6176–84.

[32] Park, K. E., Kang, H. K., Lee, S. J., Min, B. M. and Park, W. H. 2006. Biomimetic nanofibrous scaffolds: preparation and characterization of PGA/chitin blend nanofibers. *Biomacromolecules*, **7**(2), 635–43.

[33] Li, W. -J., Cooper, J. A. Jr., Mauck, R. L. and Tuan, R. S. 2006. Fabrication and characterization of six electrospun poly(α-hydroxy ester)-based fibrous scaffolds for tissue engineering applications. *Acta Biomater.*, **2**(4), 377–85.

[34] Jin, H. -J., Fridrikh, S. V., Rutledge, G. C. and Kaplan, D. L. 2002. Electrospinning *Bombyx mori* silk with poly(ethylene oxide). *Biomacromolecules*, **3**(6), 1233–9.

[35] Li, M., Mondrinos, M. J., Chen, X. *et al.* 2006. Co-electrospun poly(lactide-*co*-glycolide), gelatin, and elastin blends for tissue engineering scaffolds. *J. Biomed. Mater. Res. Part A*, **79**(4), 963–73.

[36] Kim, H. W., Kim, H. E. and Knowles, J. C. 2006. Production and potential of bioactive glass nanofibers as a next-generation biomaterial. *Adv. Functional Mater.*, **16**(12), 1529–35.

[37] He, C., Xiao, G., Jin, X., Sun, C. and Ma, P. X. 2010. Electrodeposition on nanofibrous polymer scaffolds: rapid mineralization, tunable calcium phosphate composition and topography. *Adv. Functional Mater.*, **20**(20), 3568–76.

[38] Tuzlakoğlu, K., Bolgen, N., Salgado, A. *et al.* 2005. Nano- and micro-fiber combined scaffolds: a new architecture for bone tissue engineering. *J. Mater. Sci.: Mater. Med.*, **16**(12), 1099–104.

[39] Nam, J., Huang, J., Agarwal, S. and Lannutti, J. 2007. Improved cellular infiltration in electrospun fiber via engineered porosity. *Tissue Eng.*, **13**(9), 2249–57.

[40] Zhang, R. and Ma, P. X. 2001. Processing of polymer scaffolds: phase separation. In *Methods of Tissue Engineering*, ed. Atala, A. and Lanza, R. P. San Diego, CA: Academic Press, pp. 715–724.

[41] Chen, V. J., Smith, L. A. and Ma, P. X. 2006. Bone regeneration on computer-designed nano-fibrous scaffolds. *Biomaterials*, **27**(21), 3973–9.

[42] Liu, X. and Ma, P. X. 2009. Phase separation, pore structure, and properties of nanofibrous gelatin scaffolds. *Biomaterials*, **30**(25), 4094–103.

[43] Ma, P. X. and Zhang, R. 1999. Synthetic nano-scale fibrous extracellular matrix. *J. Biomed. Mater. Res.*, **46**(1), 60–72.

[44] Chen, V. J. and Ma, P. X. 2004. Nano-fibrous poly(L-lactic acid) scaffolds with interconnected spherical macropores. *Biomaterials*, **25**(11), 2065–73.

[45] Chen, V. J. and Ma, P. X. 2006. The effect of surface area on the degradation rate of nano-fibrous poly(L-lactic acid) foams. *Biomaterials*, **27**(20), 3708–15.

[46] Liu, X. and Ma, P. X. 2010. The nanofibrous architecture of poly(L-lactic acid)-based functional copolymers. *Biomaterials*, **31**(2), 259–69.

[47] Wei, G. and Ma, P. X. 2006. Macroporous and nanofibrous polymer scaffolds and polymer/bone-like apatite composite scaffolds generated by sugar spheres. *J. Biomed. Mater. Res. Part A*, **78**(2), 306–15.

[48] Wang, P., Hu, J. and Ma, P. X. 2009. The engineering of patient-specific, anatomically shaped, digits. *Biomaterials*, **30**(14), 2735–40.

[49] Kang, S. W., Yang, H. S., Seo, S. W., Han, D. K. and Kim, B. S. 2008. Apatite-coated poly(lactic-*co*-glycolic acid) microspheres as an injectable scaffold for bone tissue engineering. *J. Biomed. Mater. Res. Part A*, **85**(3), 747–56.

[50] Mercier, N. R., Costantino, H. R., Tracy, M. A. and Bonassar, L. J. 2005. Poly(lactide-*co*-glycolide) microspheres as a moldable scaffold for cartilage tissue engineering. *Biomaterials*, **26**(14), 1945–52.

[51] Huss, F. R. M., Nyman, E., Bolin, J. S. C. and Kratz, G. 2010. Use of macroporous gelatine spheres as a biodegradable scaffold for guided tissue regeneration of healthy dermis in humans: an in vivo study. *J. Plast. Reconstr. Aesth. Surg.*, **63**(5), 848–57.

[52] Kawase, M., Michibayashi, N., Nakashima, Y. *et al.* 1997. Application of glutaraldehyde-crosslinked chitosan as a scaffold for hepatocyte attachment. *Biol. Pharm. Bull.*, **20**(6), 708–10.

[53] Chung, H. J. and Park, T. G. 2009. Injectable cellular aggregates prepared from biodegradable porous microspheres for adipose tissue engineering. *Tissue Eng. Part A*, **15**(6), 1391–1400.

[54] O'Donnell, P. B. and McGinity, J. W. 1997. Preparation of microspheres by the solvent evaporation technique. *Adv. Drug Delivery Rev.*, **28**(1), 25–42.

[55] Piirma, I. 1985. Colloids. In *Encyclopedia of Polymer Science and Engineering*, 2nd edn., ed. Mark, H. F. Bikales, N. M., Overberger, C. G., Menges, G. and Kroschwitz, J. I. New York: John Wiley and Sons, pp. 125–30.

[56] Liu, X., Jin, X. and Ma, P. X. 2011. Nanofibrous hollow microspheres self-assembled from star-shaped polymers as injectable cell carriers for knee repair. *Nature Mater.*, **10**(5), 398–406.

[57] Hu, J., Feng, K., Liu, X. and Ma, P. X. 2009. Chondrogenic and osteogenic differentiations of human bone marrow-derived mesenchymal stem cells on a nanofibrous scaffold with designed pore network. *Biomaterials*, **30**(28), 5061–7.

[58] Sun, H., Feng, K., Hu, J. *et al.* 2010. Osteogenic differentiation of human amniotic fluid-derived stem cells induced by bone morphogenetic protein-7 and enhanced by nanofibrous scaffolds. *Biomaterials*, **31**(6), 1133–9.

[59] Smith, L. A., Liu, X., Hu, J. and Ma, P. X. 2009. Enhancing osteogenic differentiation of mouse embryonic stem cells by nanofibers. *Tissue Eng.: Part A*, **15**(7), 1855–64.

[60] Christopherson, G. T., Song, H. and Mao, H. Q. 2008. The influence of fiber diameter of electrospun substrates on neural stem cell differentiation and proliferation. *Biomaterials*, **30**(4), 556–64.

[61] Wang, J., Ma, H., Jin, X. *et al.* 2011. The effect of scaffold architecture on odontogenic differentiation of human dental pulp stem cells. *Biomaterials*, **32**(31), 7822–30.

[62] Feng, G., Jin, X., Hu, J. *et al.* 2011. Effects of hypoxias and scaffold architecture on rabbit mesenchymal stem cell differentiation towards a nucleus pulposus-like phenotype. *Biomaterials*, **32**(32), 8182–9.

[63] Woo, K. M., Chen, V. J. and Ma, P. X. 2003. Nano-fibrous scaffolding architecture selectively enhances protein adsorption contributing to cell attachment. *J. Biomed. Mater. Res. Part A*, **67A**(2), 531–7.

[64] Hu, J., Liu, X. and Ma, P. X. 2008. Induction of osteoblast differentiation phenotype on poly(L-lactic acid) nanofibrous matrix. *Biomaterials*, **29**(28), 3815–21.

8

Electrospun micro/nanofibrous scaffolds

Vince Beachley and Xuejun Wen

8.1 Introduction

Polymer nanofibers have several properties that make them an extremely promising material in regenerative medicine. These favorable properties are derived from their high surface-area-to-volume ratios, their size relationship to that of cells, and their geometric similarity to natural extracellular matrix (ECM) fibers such as collagen. The literature in the field of tissue engineering generally defines nanofibers as those with diameters less than 1000 nm, while fibers larger than that are described as microfibers. The high surface-area-to-volume ratio of nanofibers allows them to interact with biomolecules at very high efficiency. In addition, nanofibers and microfibers are valuable in tissue engineering because their size is suitable for assembling complex three-dimensional (3D) architectures that can be perceived and populated by cells.

It has become increasingly apparent that cell behaviors are highly dependent on the physical environment. Substrate microstructure cues such as size, orientation, and dimensionality modulate cell behaviors ranging from attachment and morphology to differentiation and ECM production. Specifically, it has been shown that polymer nanofibrous structures can improve cell attachment; increase cell viability, proliferation, and ECM production; and predictably push cells toward specific morphologies and differentiation paths [1]. Researchers have been exploring ways of designing polymer nanofiber scaffolds that elicit desired cell responses for specific tissue engineering applications. The vast majority of these designs start with the electrospinning fabrication method. The electrospinning method is a simple and relatively inexpensive process, yet demonstrates amazing versatility in terms of the types of fibers and structures that can be fabricated. This chapter will introduce the basics of electrospinning and describe in detail strategies to make nanofiber structures for tissue engineering applications. These strategies will be focussed on electrospinning fibers with desired biofunctionality, electrospinning fiber arrays with uniaxial alignment, and methods of assembling individual fibers into 3D scaffolds conducive to cell population. It is our hope that the tools presented here can be used to design better electrospun scaffolds for applications in regenerative medicine.

8.2 Introduction to electrospinning

Electrospinning is an electrostatic method of fabricating polymer nanofibers that was discovered in the early 1900s. While this method has been known for a very long time, it has recently generated a vast amount of interest due to the emerging understanding of the applications of polymer nanofibers in fields such as tissue engineering. Solid nanofibers can be formed by an electrospinning apparatus from a polymer solution or melt. Many different types of polymers are compatible with this method, especially if they are soluble in some type of volatile organic solvent. Electrospinning is relatively simple to perform, but it is a very sensitive process, and many different variables must be correctly adjusted in order to obtain fibers with the desired morphology.

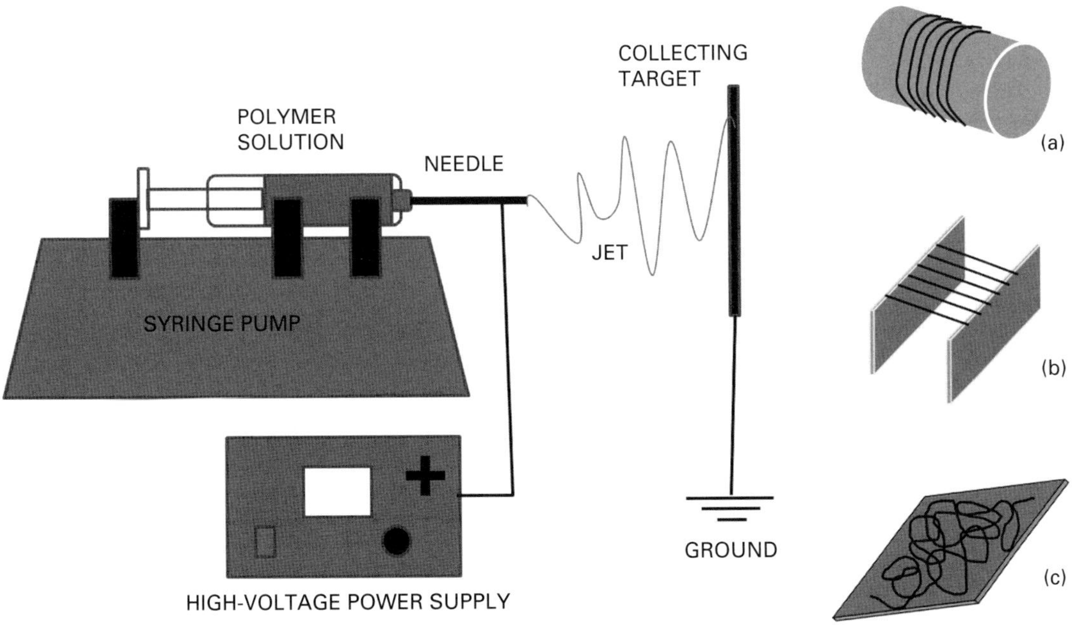

Figure 8.1 A schematic diagram of an electrospinning setup. The electrospinning jet is accelerated from the needle tip to the grounded collector by the electrostatic forces. The three most common collector types are (a) rotating mandrel, (b) static parallel plate, and (c) static flat plate. Aligned fiber orientations are possible for the rotating-mandrel and parallel-plate collectors.

8.2.1 Basic electrospinning setup

The basic electrospinning setup (Figure 8.1) consists of a polymer solution that is pumped through a cylindrical orifice, or spinneret (most commonly a blunt-tipped needle). High-voltage electrical potential is applied to the polymer solution to draw it out of the spinneret toward a collecting target placed several centimeters away from the orifice. Polymer solutions are commonly drawn into a syringe and connected to a syringe pump to move polymer solution to the needle tip at a steady rate. Generally, a high-voltage power source is directly connected to the orifice tip and a grounded target is placed several centimeters away to create the electrostatic potential necessary for jet initiation. Once the jet has been initiated, it travels toward the grounded target and solid nanofibers are deposited at the collection site. Many different types of collectors may be used to accumulate the deposited nanofibers. The most common geometries are a flat sheet, rotating mandrel, or parallel plate. Specific collector configurations will be discussed in more detail in subsequent sections.

8.2.2 Mechanisms

The driving force behind the electrospinning process is the electrostatic attraction of the polymer solution to the collecting target. The polymer solution is subject to competing forces within the capillary: an electrostatic force that pulls it out and toward the collecting target, and viscous forces that resist movement. When the electrostatic force becomes large enough to overcome the viscous force then the rounded meniscus adopts a conical shape, or Taylor cone, which ejects a liquid jet that is many times thinner than the diameter of the needle. As the jet travels toward the collecting target it is whipped about violently due to charge instabilities [2, 3]. Whipping motions further thin the liquid jet to nanoscale diameters, and the increasingly high surface-area-to-volume ratio facilitates the rapid evaporation of solvents and the formation of solid nanofibers at the collecting site.

8.2.3 Parameters

It is relatively simple to set up an electrospinning apparatus to produce nanofibers. However, the process involves many parameters and a high degree of randomness that can make it difficult to repeatably produce fibers with the desired characteristics. Several of the most important parameters in an electrospinning setup are discussed below.

8.2.3.1 Voltage

The electrostatic potential between the spinneret and the collector is the driving force for the electrospinning process. This potential is usually created by applying a positive charge to the spinneret while the collector remains grounded. However, an electrospinning jet can be initiated with several different configurations of positive/negative charge and ground between the needle and collecting target [4, 5]. A minimum voltage must be applied to produce an electric field strong enough to induce jet initiation. The voltage may be increased beyond that threshold to optimize electrospinning conditions. Increasing the applied voltage increases the electrostatic forces and whipping instabilities in the electrospinning jet, and it has been shown that increasing the applied voltage can result in uniform fibers with reduced bead formation and increased fiber diameter. Several groups have demonstrated that increased voltage results in increased fiber diameters due to an increased mass flow rate associated with a stronger electrostatic field [6, 7]. However, in some electrospinning configurations the fiber diameter may be reduced due to thinning effects that stronger electrostatic forces may have on the electrospinning jet [8].

8.2.3.2 Flow rate

Electrostatic forces pull polymer solution from the tip of the spinneret, but are not adequate to independently draw solution from a reservoir through a needle. A constant flow rate of solution through the needle must be maintained by an external force, such as a syringe pump. It is important that the flow rate remain consistent with a lack of air bubbles that may interrupt the electrospinning process. Increasing the flow rate has been shown to result in fibers with increased diameter [9].

8.2.3.3 Spinneret diameter

The spinneret diameter is not as important to fiber diameter as other factors such as solution properties, flow rate, and voltage. This is because the jet ejected from the needle is much smaller than the actual needle diameter due to the formation of the Taylor cone. However, small-diameter needles may require increased flow pressures and may be more subject to clogging, while large-diameter needles may be more susceptible to dripping or spitting.

8.2.3.4 Spinneret-to-collector distance

The distance between the spinneret and the collector has two effects on electrospinning. First, it changes the electric field strength. A higher voltage must be applied to produce the same electric field strength when the tip-to-collector distance is increased. The tip-to-collector distance also influences the time that it takes for the electrospinning jet to reach the collector. Thus, fiber size and morphology may be affected by the tip-to-collector distance because of whipping instabilities experienced during the jet path and the effect of solvent evaporation, which is more likely to be incomplete at shorter distances.

8.2.3.5 Solution properties

Solution properties are the most important parameter in electrospinning. A solution's viscosity and conductivity are determined by solvent properties, polymer properties, and any additives in the solution. The solution viscosity must be within an optimum range. If a solution is too viscous it is not possible for jet initiation to occur, but, if the solution is not viscous enough, then instabilities will cause the jet to break up into droplets. Solution viscosity varies for each polymer-solvent combination, but increasing polymer concentration results in increased solution viscosity. Within the spinnable range, it has been shown that increasing polymer solution viscosity may result in more uniform fibers (without beads) and increased fiber diameter [6, 9–11].

The solution conductivity determines the charge-carrying capacity of the jet, and thus highly conductive solutions are subject to greater electrostatic forces and instabilities [12]. The solution conductivity is dependent on the polymer and the solvent used, and it can be increased by adding substances such as NaCl and albumin (BSA) [13, 14]. Increasing the solution conductivity results in fibers with smaller diameters, and highly conductive solutions may be difficult to electrospin due to the instability of the jet [13, 14]. The conductivity of electrospinning solutions can also have a dramatic effect on fiber morphology. In one example, uniform fibers (without beads) were obtained by adding NaCl to increase the conductivity of a polymer solution [15].

8.3 Biofunctionalization of electrospun nanofibers

Electrospinning is an extremely versatile fabrication technology in tissue engineering because a wide variety of biocompatible polymer materials can be formed into fibers. Polymers with ideal mechanical properties, degradation properties, and biocompatibility may be selected for specific applications, or new types of polymer materials can be designed and synthesized to fit a specific need. In addition to advantages in material selection, electrospinning is suitable for several methods of nanofiber biofunctionalization. Highly biofunctional nanofibers can be electrospun from natural materials found in the ECM, and biomolecules such as growth factors, adhesion molecules, and drugs can be incorporated into the bulk of electrospun nanofibers or attached to their surface. Biofunctionalized electrospun nanofiber scaffolds can be designed with properties that are tailored to specific tissue engineering applications.

8.3.1 Electrospinning natural ECM molecules

Natural ECM molecules have a biomolecular complexity that is difficult to match in synthetic materials. These materials demonstrate excellent cell interactions and may promote improved attachment, proliferation, and differentiation. Several types of natural ECM molecules can be electrospun into nanofibers or mixed with synthetic materials in a polymer solution to form blended nanofibers. Blended nanofibers share improved mechanical properties and spinnability due to the synthetic component and enhanced bioactivity from the ECM component [16, 17].

8.3.1.1 Collagen

Types of soluble type I collagen can be dissolved in organic solvents, such as 1,1,1,3,3,3-hexafluoro-2-propanol (HFIP), and in aqueous acids. Pure bead-free collagen nanofibers have been electrospun from such solutions with diameters in the range 100–500 nm [18, 19]. The water-soluble collagen that is commonly electrospun must be crosslinked before it can be applied to in-vitro or in-vivo applications. Crosslinking agents that are commonly used include 1-ethyl-3-(3-dimethylaminopropyl) carbodiimide hydrochloride (EDC), glutaraldehyde vapor, 1,6-diisocyanatohexane, and genipin [18, 20, 21]. Blended collagen–synthetic-polymer nanofibers can be easily electrospun when the two materials are dissolved together in a common solvent [22]. Collagen was blended within polycaprolactone (PCL) nanofibers as well-distributed small spherical aggregates for low concentrations (10% wt/wt vs. PCL) and as large irregular shapes at higher concentrations (50% wt/wt vs. PCL) [23]. Synthetic nanofibers blended with collagen demonstrated improved bioactivity as shown by cell attachment, proliferation, and ECM production when compared with fibers without collagen incorporation [24, 25]. Blending collagen with synthetic polymers allows fabrication of collagen-containing nanofibers that have a range of morphologies, and mechanical and degradation properties that aren't possible with pure collagen fibers. Studies have shown that collagen is extensively denatured by the organic solvents commonly used in electrospinning, and it has been suggested that similar bioactivity could be obtained by electrospinning much more affordable gelatin [26]. However, results from several studies where electrospun collagen and gelatin were directly compared indicated that electrospun collagen may retain at least some increased bioactivity when compared with gelatin [24, 27, 28].

8.3.1.2 Gelatin

Gelatin can be dissolved in organic solvents, such as HFIP and 2,2,2-trifluoroethanol (TFE), and in aqueous acids. Pure gelatin nanofibers have been electrospun from such solutions with fiber diameters in the range 50–500 nm [18, 29]. Just like for collagen nanofibers, electrospun gelatin nanofibers must be crosslinked with agents such as EDC, glutaraldehyde vapor, 1,6-diisocyanatohexane, and genipin [18, 30]. Gelatin nanofiber blends can be electrospun with other polymers when they are dissolved in a single solution, and cells show improved bioactivity when cultured on synthetic nanofibers that have been blended with gelatin [24, 31–33]. Cell attachment and proliferation have been shown to increase systematically with increasing gelatin content in nanofiber blends [17], and blended gelatin–PCL nanofibers demonstrated enhanced neural differentiation compared with pure PCL fibers [32].

8.3.1.3 Elastin

Elastin and tropoelastin can be dissolved in HFIP or aqueous acids and electrospun into nanofibers with diameters ranging from 1 μm to several microns [18, 19, 21]. The morphology of electrospun elastin fibers has been observed as a ribbon-like shape, in contrast to the uniform circular cross-section observed for most other electrospun fibers. Electrospun elastin fibers must be crosslinked before use in hydrated conditions with crosslinking agents such as EDC, glutaraldehyde vapor, and 1,6-diisocyanatohexane [18, 19, 21]. Elastin has also been electrospun from solutions containing synthetic polymer materials to produce blended fibers [18, 34].

8.3.1.4 Chitosan

It is difficult to electrospin pure chitosan nanofibers because of properties such as their limited solubility, ionic character, and networks of strong hydrogen bonds [35]. There are some examples where chitosan fibers of high molecular weight (more formally, relative molecular mass) were electrospun from organic solvents and high-concentration acid solutions. The fiber diameters were in the range 60–330 nm [35–37]. Chitosan nanofibers have also been electrospun as blends when dissolved with low concentrations of polyethylene oxide (PEO, 10%) [38]. Blended fibers had diameters in the range 150–200 nm and demonstrated favorable bioactivity [38].

8.3.1.5 Dextran

Dextran fibers with a wide range of fiber diameters can be electrospun from aqueous solutions and organic solvents [14]. Dextran nanofibers must be crosslinked before they are used in an aqueous environment due to their high solubility. Photocrosslinked methacrylated dextran nanofibers were able to form a stable hydrogel under hydrated conditions [14]. Dextran has also been mixed with synthetic polymers in solutions to electrospin blended nanofibers, which demonstrated favorable bioactivity [39].

8.3.1.6 Fibrinogen

Fibrinogen has been dissolved in a solution containing HFIP and 10× minimal essential medium at a ratio of 9:1. Fibrinogen nanofibers with diameters in the range 80–700 nm were electrospun for these solutions [40]. Uncrosslinked fibrinogen nanofibers demonstrated the ability to maintain their structure in hydrated conditions and demonstrated favorable bioactivity in in-vitro culture conditions [41, 42]. The degradation rate of fibrinogen fibers can be slowed by adding protease inhibitors to cell culture media [41, 42].

8.3.1.7 Laminin

Laminin nanofibers with diameters in the range 90–300 nm and various degrees of bead composition were electrospun from solutions of purified laminin dissolved in HFIP [43]. Uncrosslinked laminin nanofibers were able to retain their structure under cell culture conditions and demonstrated favorable bioactivity.

8.3.1.8 Hyaluronic acid

Hyaluronic acid nanofibers dissolved in an acidic solution have been electrospun successfully. However, this requires a complex procedure whereby heated air is blown around the electrospinning jet [44]. Hyaluronic acid has also been electrospun from solutions mixed with PEO [45, 46]. Extraction of the PEO component resulted in pure hyaluraonic acid nanofibers with diameters of around 110 nm. Hyaluronic acid nanofiber scaffolds demonstrated favorable bioactivity in in-vitro experiments.

8.3.2 Surface biofunctionalization

Polymeric materials have immense versatility for surface modification. In tissue engineering applications, various adhesion molecules, growth factors, and drugs may be attached to promote desired cellular responses. Biomolecules can be added to the surface of electrospun nanofibers by physical absorption or with chemical bonds. The literature on polymer surface modifications is vast, so this section will discuss only work that is directly related to surface functionalizing electrospun nanofibers for biological applications. Many other polymer surface modification techniques may be applicable to electrospun nanofibers as long as no part of the protocol damages or destroys the relatively sensitive nanofiber structures.

8.3.2.1 Physical absorption

Physical absorption is the simplest method of nanofiber surface functionalization. When polymer nanofibers are incubated in solutions containing solubilized biomolecules they may adhere to the surface of the fibers due to electrostatic forces, hydrophobic interactions, hydrogen bonding, or van der Waals forces. Hydrophobic nanofiber scaffolds can be treated with air plasma to increase the efficiency of physical absorption. Air plasma makes the fibers more hydrophilic and promotes greater infiltration of water-soluble biomolecules. Plasma treatment may also cause etching and ablation damage to the fibers. Placing a sample at a distance downstream of the plasma source has been explored as a way to improve efficiency, while minimizing damage [47]. In certain cases plasma treatment may also be used to increase the efficiency of covalent grafting procedures described in the following section [48].

8.3.2.2 Covalent bonding

Biomolecules can be chemically bonded to exposed functional groups on the surface of electrospun nanofibers to provide a more efficient coating with greater long-term retention [49]. Covalent surface modification requires that (1) appropriate functional groups are exposed on the nanofiber surface, and (2) chemical reactions that bind the selected biomolecule to those functional groups are carried out.

8.3.2.2.1 Surface functional groups

Some polymers naturally contain functional groups. Treatment methods to add functional groups to the nanofiber surface may be available if a desired functional group is not present. Carboxyl and amine functional groups are most commonly utilized for covalent surface modification reactions with electrospun nanofibers. Carboxyl groups can be exposed on degradable polyesters such as PLLA and PCL by simple chemical treatments such as incubation with sodium hydroxide (NaOH) [50, 51]. Amine groups have been added to the surface of degradable polyester fibers with 1,6-hexanediamine-propanol solution or ethylenediamine (ED) treatments [52, 53]. Linker molecules can be used to tether appropriate functional groups to polymer nanofibers as well. Carboxyl groups were added to polymer nanofibers by grafting acrylic acid as a plasma treatment [54], and by grafting poly(acrylic acid) as a linker molecule with photopolymerization [55]. An amino terminated poly(ethylene glycol) (di-NH_2-PEG) was attached to free carboxyl groups as a way to add exposed amine groups to polymer nanofibers that contained free carboxyl groups [56]. Linker molecule properties such as length may have an effect on the cell response to the polymer surface, so it is important to consider different linker molecule properties when they are used to surface functionalize polymer nanofibers [55, 57, 58]. Functional groups can also be added to polymers by modifying the synthesis procedure. For example, a polyester block copolymer with free amine groups was synthesized by polymerizing PCL with PEG linkers that contained free amine groups [59]. A block copolymer of PLGA and amine-terminated PEG was mixed in a polymer solution with pure PLGA and electrospun [60]. This allowed additional control of the ratios of PLGA to di-NH_2-PEG in the blended nanofibers. The carboxyl group content of a methyl methacrylate (MMA) and acrylic acid (AA) copolymer could be controlled by varying the ratio of MMA to AA during synthesis [61].

8.3.2.2.2 Covalent attachment of biomolecules

Controlled chemical reactions are performed to attach desired biomolecules to appropriate exposed functional groups on the surface of polymer nanofibers. One of the most commonly referenced bonding reactions is that of 1-ethyl-3-(3-dimethylaminopropyl) carbodiimide hydrochloride (EDC) [27, 47, 48]. Carboxyl groups and primary amine groups can be activated for a bonding reaction when incubated with solubilized EDC. Addition of N-hydroxysuccinimide (NHS) to the reaction converts an unstable amine-reactive intermediate into an amine-reactive NHS ester and improves the efficiency of the bonding reaction [27, 48]. Other agents such as glutaraldehyde and 1-hydroxybenzole (HOBt) in combination with EDC have been utilized to bond biomolecules to polymer nanofibers [52, 59].

8.3.2.3 Examples of surface biofunctionalized nanofibers

Many different types of biomolecule have been attached to the surface of polymer nanofibers by physical absorption. Several groups have incubated nanofiber scaffolds in simulated body fluid (SBF), a solution containing ion concentrations similar to that of human plasma, to coat them with nanocrystalline apatites [62]. The incubation time and specific ion content of the solution can be adjusted to optimize the apatite surface coating [50, 51]. The bioactivity of hydroxyapatite coatings has been demonstrated by stimulation of osteogenic genes in osteoblastic cells cultured on coated nanofiber scaffolds [51]. Other biomolecules that have been attached to the surface of polymer nanofibers by physical absorption include collagen, laminin, and E-selectin [49, 63, 64]. Attachment of these biomolecules was confirmed by detecting enhanced cell attachment, spreading, viability, and phenotype preservation in cells cultured in vitro. The physical absorption method of surface functionalization has the advantage of being a very simple and gentle process that limits damage to fragile nanofiber structures. The major disadvantage of the physical absorption method is a relatively weak binding that may be inefficient and unstable.

Several examples of covalent surface functionalization of polymer nanofibers are available in the literature as well. Collagen and laminin were covalently attached to polymer nanofibers to enhance their bioactivity as neural tissue engineering scaffolds [49, 61]. Covalent attachment of fibronectin to nanofibers was confirmed by increased collagen synthesis in esophageal epithelial cells, and surface attachment of RGD peptide resulted in increased attachment and proliferation of fibroblasts [52, 60]. Covalent bonding provides much more efficient and stable surface attachment than does physical absorption. However, covalent bonding procedures may be complex and require the use of harsh chemicals that can damage polymer nanofibers and biomolecules. For example, covalent bonding may require the use of organic solvents that can deactivate biomolecules such as growth factors.

Physical absorption and covalent bonding processes can be used in combination to take advantage of the favorable properties of each method. For example, when carboxyl groups on polymer nanofibers are exposed by NaOH treatment prior to SBF incubation, the efficiency of hydroxyapatite coating by physical absorption is increased [50, 51]. An innovative method of attaching growth factors to polymer nanofibers was developed by incorporating covalent and physical absorption processes. Covalent bonding techniques are used to attach molecules such as heparin, followed by physical absorption of growth factors [27, 56]. The efficiency and stability of growth factor attachment is improved because covalently bound heparin acts as a reservoir to store, stabilize, and protect growth factors. Thus, strong growth factor attachment can be achieved without exposing them to harsh conditions that could deactivate their biofunctionality.

8.3.3 Bulk incorporation of biomolecules

Biomolecules can be directly incorporated into the bulk structure of nanofibers during electrospinning. Agents may be directly mixed into a polymer solution before electrospinning to form uniform fibers with embedded biomolecules, or a multisolution co-axial electrospinning setup may be utilized to embed biomolecules within shell fibers. Bulk biomolecule incorporation eliminates the need for secondary processing and bulk methods have demonstrated incorporation of greater amounts of biomolecule and increased bioactivity when compared with surface modification methods [49]. Biomolecules incorporated into the bulk of nanofibers may demonstrate extended release kinetics due to diffusion through pores, or release due to polymer degradation. The release profile of agents contained in nanofibers is commonly characterized by an initial burst followed by steady long-term release.

8.3.3.1 Adding biomolecules to a polymer solution

Many different agents may be added to a polymer solution to incorporate them into electrospun nanofibers. Biomolecules can be (1) directly dissolved in the polymer solution if a common solvent is available [65], (2) dissolved in a miscible solvent and suspended in the polymer solution [65–67], or (3) dissolved in an immiscible solvent and added to the polymer solution with agitation to form an emulsion [68–70]. Miscible solutions containing several components can be designed in order to best incorporate biomolecules into a polymer solution. For example, water-soluble heparin was incorporated into dichloromethane (DCM)-soluble PCL nanofibers using a three-component solution that contained methanol [71]. Water is miscible in methanol, which is miscible in DCM, so aqueous heparin could be suspended in the polymer solution as a stable uniform mixture by using methanol as an intermediary. Nanofibers electrospun from single-phase solutions have demonstrated a uniform distribution of biomolecules [65]. A uniform biomolecule distribution becomes more difficult to obtain for other types of solutions because the electrospinning process may be disturbed by polymer solutions containing miscible solvents or emulsions [68]. Thus, multiphase solutions may be more difficult to electrospin and biomolecule distribution may be aggregated [65, 70]. However, in some cases, an even biomolecule distribution has been observed in nanofibers electrospun from solutions containing miscible solvents [71]. Nanofibers electrospun from emulsion solutions formed by vortexing, sonication, or stirring have resulted in beadlike pockets and core–shell distributions [72–74]. The biomolecule incorporation efficiencies reported for different electrospinning systems vary widely. This is to be expected because of the immense variability that exists for different polymer materials, biomolecules, electrospinning parameters, and quantification methods. For example, heparin was electrospun from a miscible solution with an efficiency of 100% [71], for laminin directly blended in a PLLA solution an efficiency of 75% was demonstrated [49], and a polymer solution with nerve growth factor (NGF) added as an emulsion resulted in nanofibers with an efficiency of just 2.5% [68].

It is important to note that adding biomolecules to a polymer solution by any method may result in changes in the morphology of the resulting electrospun fibers. The electrospinning process is very sensitive to any changes in jet properties, such as viscosity and charge density, that may result from changes in the composition of the polymer solution [65, 66, 71]. The addition of increasing concentrations of retinoic acid to an electrospinning solution resulted in decreasing fiber diameters, and fiber diameters were observed to increase with increasing loading concentrations of bovine serum albumin (BSA) added to another

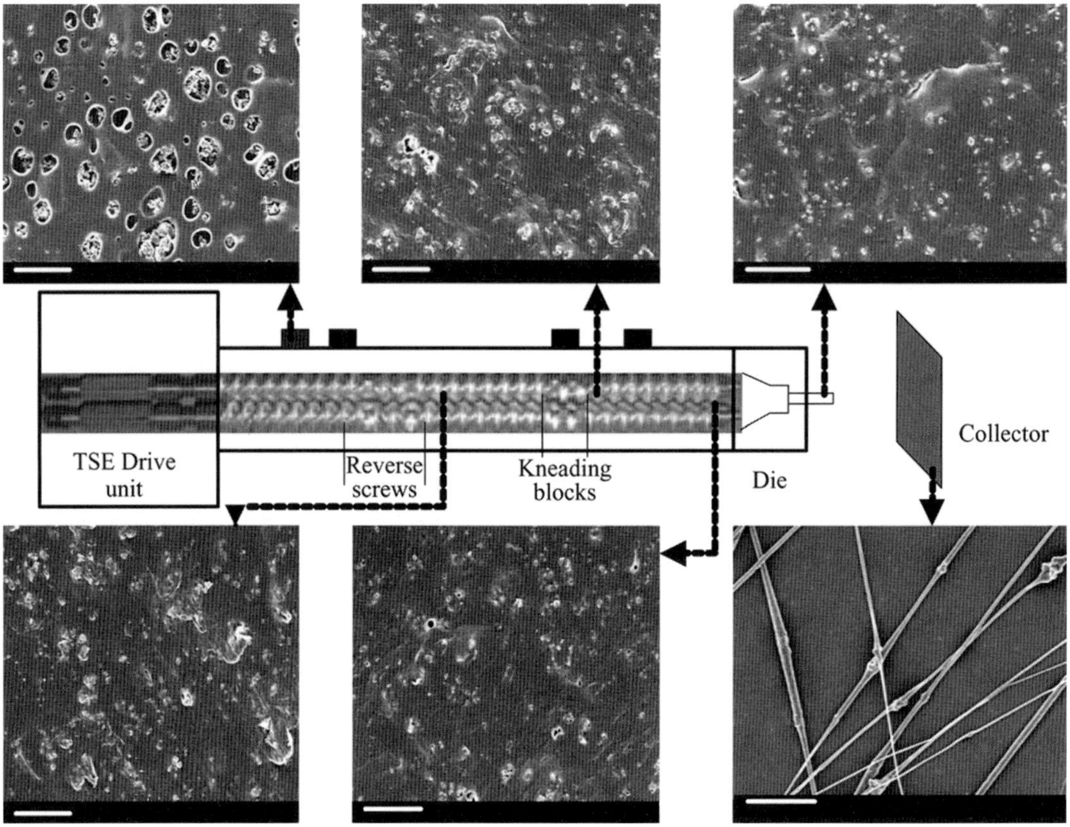

Figure 8.2 A schematic diagram of a twin screw extrusion/electrospinning device and images of nanoparticle distribution and resultant nanofibers (Scale bar = 20 μm) [77].

solution [65]. Morphological changes were accompanied by changes in mechanical properties in these fibers due to the inclusion of aggregates. Incorporation of retinoic acid into polymer nanofibers resulted in increased mechanical strength independent of fiber diameter, and increasing levels of BSA decreased the ductility of the resultant fibers for two different polymer types [65].

Direct biomolecule addition into electrospun nanofibers is a complex process, but the versatility of this method allows the incorporation of many different types of substances, including drugs, adhesion molecules, growth factors, antibiotics, vitamins, and DNA [49, 66–68, 71, 75]. Many different types of biomolecules are able to demonstrate sustained release from polymer fibers and retain at least some degree of bioactivity. Nanoparticles can even be mixed into a polymer solution as a dispersion and electrospun to form composite nanofibers with embedded particles [76, 77]. One group designed a special extruding device (Figure 8.2) to continuously break up nanoparticle aggregates with a polymer-solution–nanoparticle dispersion to maintain a uniform distribution [77].

8.3.3.1 Co-axial electrospinning

Another method of incorporating desired biomolecules into electrospun nanofibers is by a modified method known as co-axial electrospinning. Co-axial electrospinning utilizes a co-axial nozzle to form a jet from two or more different solutions simultaneously. The solutions are separately fed into a nozzle with concentric geometry where they are ejected as a two-phase liquid electrospinning jet. The inner phase is entirely surrounded by the outer phase. The resulting polymer fibers demonstrate a core–shell morphology, where one material makes up a solid filament core and a second material surrounds it in a concentric orientation [78]. Core–shell nanofibers offer several advantages in biomolecule loading. If a substance is electrospun within the inner core filament, then extended release of the substance is possible without the initial burst effect observed for electrospun nanofibers loaded with biomolecules by conventional methods. In addition, the biomolecules in the inner jet are minimally exposed to toxic solvents required in the formation of the outer shell material [79]. The flow rate of each solution can be controlled independently to promote uniform fiber formation and to adjust fiber diameter and the core-to-shell volume ratio.

Co-axial electrospinning is a versatile method that is capable of producing different types of nanofibers that cannot be made by conventional methods. Hollow nanofibers can be electrospun using this technique [80], and nanofibers can be formed from materials that cannot be directly electrospun. For example, nanofibers of poly(glycerol sebacate) were produced by electrospinning its precursors in the inner core of core–shell nanofibers [81]. Pure poly(glycerol sebacate) fibers remained after curing and removal of the shell materials.

8.4 Electrospinning aligned nanofiber structures

One of the inherent advantages of the electrospinning method is the ability to fabricate nanofibrous structures with uniaxially aligned morphologies. Several tissue types, including blood vessel, nerve, muscle, and connective tissue, depend on a highly aligned cellular and ECM organization for proper function. Aligned ECM nanofibers in blood vessels and connective tissue efficiently resist mechanical loads, muscles rely on organized cellular alignment to effectively generate forces, and well-aligned axons allow electrical signals to be quickly transferred throughout the body.

When cells are cultured on nanofibrous scaffolds in vitro, they adopt an elongated aligned morphology similar to that observed in natural tissues. Furthermore, elongated cells cultured on aligned substrates exhibit behaviors desirable in aligned tissue engineering. Cells cultured on aligned nanofibers have been shown to preferentially migrate in the direction of fiber alignment, deposit well-organized aligned ECM, and preferentially differentiate into phenotypes associated with aligned tissues. It is of the highest importance that tissue engineering scaffolds designed to regenerate aligned tissues have the ability to impart alignment on resident cells as a prerequisite for forming tissue with biomimetic organization and function. Challenges in aligned tissue engineering include optimization of substrate topographical cues to promote desired cell behaviors and designing scaffolds that utilize these cues within an architecture conductive to the development of tissue-like structures.

Some degree of aligned nanofiber fabrication is possible with several different methods of nanofiber production such as drawing, templating, micropatterning, fluid flow, and bacterial [82]. However, the vast majority of research and publications relating to aligned nanofiber scaffold fabrication relates to the electrospinning technique. This is most likely due to the immense versatility associated with the electrospinning method as well as a selection of different methods for inducing fiber alignment and aligned scaffold assembly. Most methods of collecting aligned nanofibers from an electrospinning jet are based on the rotating-mandrel technique or the parallel-plate technique. Fiber alignment is induced by high velocities and mechanical forces via the rotating-mandrel technique and the parallel-plate technique utilizes electrical forces to mediate fiber alignment. The specific arrangement of aligned fibers in structures collected by either of these techniques is influenced by the electrospinning parameters and the specific conditions associated with the collecting setup. While the rotating-mandrel and parallel-plate techniques are the basis of most aligned electrospun scaffold fabrication strategies, many modifications to these base methods have been utilized in an attempt to improve upon them. Modified collection methods have been applied to allow increased control over fiber alignment, length, precision placement, and 3D organization.

8.4.1 The rotating-mandrel method

The jet that is ejected as the result of a standard electrospinning process travels at a high velocity of up to several meters per second [83]. This high velocity results in an unpredictable random fiber orientation when a standard static collector is used. However, when the collection target is moved at a high speed it is possible to maintain a greater degree of control over nanofiber deposition. If a static collecting target is replaced by a grounded mandrel rotating at high speed it becomes possible to collect uniaxially aligned nanofibers from an electrospinning jet. The diameters of collecting mandrels are commonly a few centimeters or larger, and they are rotated at speeds up to several thousand revolutions per minute (rpm). High rotational velocities result in tangential velocities at the edges of the mandrel that may approach the velocity of the electrospinning jet. The tangential velocity is the most informative value in comparing results from studies conducted by different researchers because mandrel diameter varies widely between individual experiments. Aligned nanofibers are deposited on rotating mandrels as a circumferentially oriented uniaxially aligned mesh. It is possible to collect relatively thick aligned fiber meshes by this method, but the collection rate and the degree of alignment may decrease as the mat thickness increases due to insulating and repulsive effects exerted by previously deposited fibers [84].

The microstructure and orientation of nanofibers collected by a rotating mandrel are sensitive to the speed of the rotating collector. It can be logically predicted that the nanofiber alignment will be maximized when the tangential velocity of the rotating-mandrel collector precisely matches the velocity of the electrospinning jet [85]. Thus, the relationship between fiber orientation and mandrel diameter may be classified into three stages: (1) the mandrel velocity is too far below the jet velocity to initiate significant fiber alignment, (2) increasing mandrel velocity results in increasing fiber alignment up to an optimum speed, and (3) extreme velocities and resultant fiber fracture result in decreased fiber alignment [86]. Different setups have different jet velocities, mandrel diameters, polymer mechanical properties, and electrical properties, so the observed threshold mandrel velocity for fiber alignment varies significantly. For example, authors of several studies where various synthetic polymer nanofibers were electrospun observed an onset of fiber alignment at tangential mandrel velocities of around 3 m/s [87–90], while speeds up to 10 m/s [91] have been required in others. Experimental evidence confirms that fiber alignment generally improves as mandrel velocity is increased after the initial onset of fiber alignment [87–93]. However, fibers have been observed to break due to increasing tensile forces exerted by the mandrel as the rotation speed reaches a certain magnitude [91]. Fiber breakage results in reduced uniformity and alignment in resulting meshes [85]. Fiber fracture is dependent not only on the mandrel speed, but also on the material properties of the polymer jet. It has been shown that nanofibers electrospun from more brittle polymer materials are more likely to fracture at lower mandrel speeds [94]. More elastic polymers are less likely to fracture, but the tensile forces exerted by the rotating mandrel may result in a reduction in fiber diameter in deformable materials. The diameter of fibers collected on a rotating mandrel generally decreases with increasing mandrel velocity [87, 91–93, 95, 96]; however, in some circumstances, slight increases in fiber diameter have been observed [86, 97]. The magnitude of the reduction in fiber diameter associated with mandrel velocities in the range 5–15 m/s has been reported to be in the range 15%–40% [87, 91–93, 95, 96]. In addition to reductions in fiber diameter, the tensile forces exerted on the polymer jet by a rotating mandrel have been observed to influence the molecular orientation of deposited nanofibers [86, 97].

The rotating-mandrel method is a simple and effective way to collect aligned nanofibers from an electrospinning jet. Some general trends related to rotating-mandrel setups can be drawn from the literature and may be useful references in designing a specific experiment. In particular, the relationships of fiber alignment to tangential velocity and of polymer jet elasticity to fiber elongation and fracture have been found to be relatively consistent across several studies. However, due to the high level of variability involved with electrospinning different polymer solutions due to differences in viscosity, conductivity, voltage, feed rate, and rate of solvent evaporation, it may be difficult to precisely predict how any specific electrospinning system will respond.

8.4.2 The parallel-plate method

The parallel-plate method of collecting aligned nanofibers from an electrospinning jet utilizes electrostatic forces to induce fiber alignment. Because the electrospinning jet is highly charged, it will align in the presence of certain electric field configurations. The electric field that results from two grounded parallel plates placed below an electrospinning nozzle can exert forces on an electrospinning jet that cause it to align perpendicular to the plates. As the jet whips back and forth, aligned nanofibers are suspended across the plates in a perpendicular orientation, with one end adhering to each of the plates. An analysis of this phenomenon, which was first conducted by Li *et al.* [98] is shown in Figures 8.3(a)–(c). The electrical properties of the jet are increasingly important for electrospinning across parallel plates because electrostatic forces are responsible both for initiating jet formation and for guiding fiber alignment. Thus, many polymer solutions that are easily electrospun as random meshes are difficult to collect as aligned arrays across parallel plates because the properties of the solutions are not conducive to parallel-plate collection.

It may be hypothesized that a polymer solution must have physical and electrical properties within a critical range in order for parallel-plate electrospinning to be effective. Aligning forces are electrostatically mediated so their magnitude is dependent on the conductivity of the jet. Thus, when the conductivity is too low there might not be adequate electrical forces to stretch nanofibers across the gap between the plates. On the other hand, if the conductivity of a solution is too high this can result in high-velocity whipping motions that

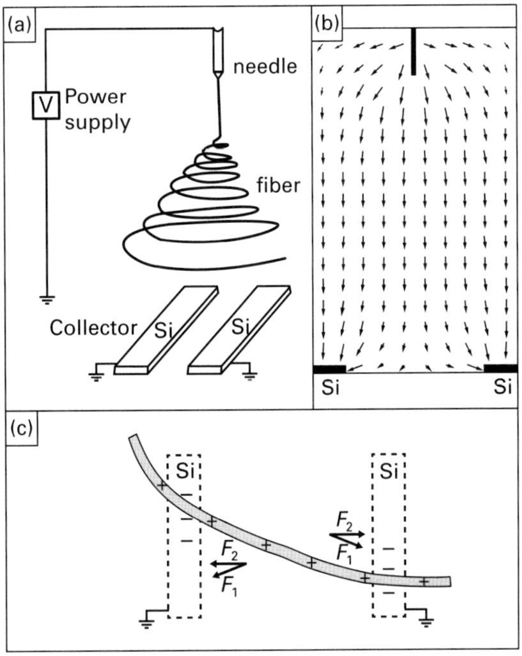

Figure 8.3 Schematic representations of (a) a parallel-plate electrospinning setup, (b) the resultant electric field, and (c) the forces acting on the jet [98].

cannot be adequately stabilized by the aligning electric field. In one study it was found that a polyelectrolyte solution (poly(phenylene vinylene), PPV) could not be electrospun in an aligned orientation across parallel plates. It was hypothesized that the high conductivity of the solution contributed to the formation of a highly unstable jet that could not be effectively controlled by aligning forces present at the collecting site [99]. Addition of a neutral polymer (polyvinyl pyrrolidone, PVP) allowed well-aligned nanofibers to be collected across the parallel plates (Figure 8.4). The authors of another study found that aligned fiber collection across parallel plates became ineffective when NaCl was added to a polymer solution [100]. It was hypothesized that this was due to instabilities in the electrospinning jet caused by the increased conductivity of the solution. In contrast, nanofibers electrospun from a melt were able to align across parallel plates only at short distances and oriented as a randomly aligned mesh when

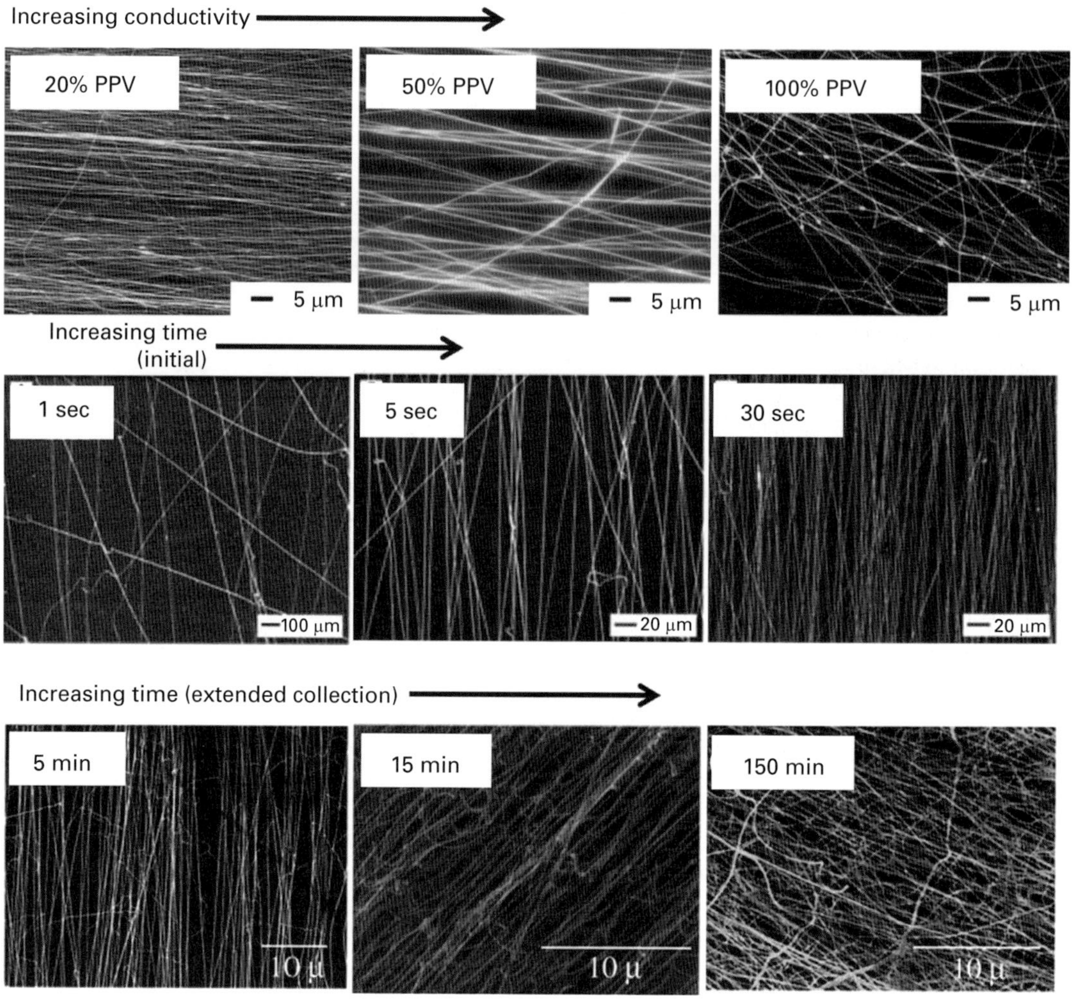

Figure 8.4 Images of nanofibers electrospun across parallel plates with conductivity (top [99]) or time (middle [103] and bottom [107]) increasing from left to right. Individual images are labeled for percentage PPV in a PPV:PVP polymer solution, or elapsed time from the onset of electrospinning. The images for initial (middle) and extended (bottom) collection times are taken from two different and unrelated investigations.

the distance between the plates was increased [101]. The forces exerted on the low-conductivity solution may have been too small to induce alignment in this case. Solution viscosity plays a role in jet stabilization, and increasing viscosity may help to stabilize an electrospinning jet to make parallel-plate electrospinning possible.

In addition to solution conductivity, the electrostatic forces present in an electrospinning setup are dependent on the applied voltage. When the applied voltage is increased the electric field is increased, and thus the electrostatic forces acting to align the jet are increased. However, when the voltage is increased the jet instability is generally also increased, which may disrupt fiber alignment and extension across the parallel plates. Therefore, optimal fiber alignment and extension across a parallel plate collector may correspond to a critical applied voltage that balances the magnitude of aligning forces and the resultant jet instabilities [102].

Another limitation to the parallel-plate method is that it may be difficult or impossible to collect extremely thin fibers. Parallel-plate collection is different from other methods in that the deposited fibers are suspended across the plates and must have the mechanical integrity required to support their weight. Extremely thin fibers, especially those of more brittle materials, have been observed to break under the force of their own weight or due to forces exerted by repulsive charge from the jet or other fibers [98]. One strategy to overcome this limitation is to place an electrically resistive substrate between the parallel plates to support deposited fibers [98]. This may also help to shield any conductive materials below the air gap that may attract undesirable randomly aligned fibers. Substrates such as quartz and polystyrene that have a bulk resistivity greater than 10^{22} Ω cm may be placed in between parallel plates with minimal influence on fiber quality. Random fiber deposition may occur when materials with bulk resistivity less than 10^{12} Ω cm, such as glass, are used [103, 104].

8.4.2.1 Charge retention

Solid nanofibers formed from an electrospun jet carry a significant charge. Fibers that contact a solid conductive collecting target are able to discharge immediately. Fibers suspended across parallel plates, however, may retain their charge because of their limited contact with the conductive surfaces [98]. The electric field at the collecting surface is constantly changing with increasing fiber density because charge builds up in the collecting area as successive fibers are deposited. Charge retention has important effects on fiber orientation and the rate of collection. The residual charge of fibers in the gap in low-density arrays initially results in an increase in alignment because parallel alignment represents the lowest energy state for an array of charged fibers [98, 103, 105]. This phenomenon is demonstrated in Figure 8.4, where improved alignment at several time points up to 30 s is observed [103]. Numerical models are in agreement with experimental evidence suggesting that residual charge has a positive effect on alignment at low fiber densities [106]. However, fiber alignment is impaired by the buildup of charge and material in the collection area as the fiber density increases over longer periods of time (Figure 8.4) [107]. The rate of fiber deposition may decrease as more fibers are deposited in the collection area, until charge repulsion finally results in a nearly complete cessation of fiber deposition. Because of the charge-repulsion effect it becomes difficult to fabricate thick layers of aligned fibers by the parallel-plate method [108].

8.4.2.2 Gap size

The length of distance in between the plates is an important parameter in parallel-plate nanofiber collection. Fiber alignment and array densities are significantly affected by the gap size. The strength of the electric field created by the plates decreases with increasing gap distance, which in turn decreases the draw of force stretching and aligning fibers across the plates. Therefore, it becomes increasingly difficult to collect aligned nanofibers by the parallel-plate method as the gap distance is increased [109]. Relatively long nanofibers (up to 50 cm) have been collected across parallel plates, but, as the gap distance becomes large, the fiber density and rate of collection tend to decrease with increasing gap distance until fiber collection ceases completely [8, 110]. Generally it is not feasible to collect dense aligned nanofiber arrays at larger gap sizes because decreasing electrostatic aligning forces are overcome by smaller charge-repulsion forces. The maximum fiber length in high-density aligned nanofiber arrays is usually limited to a few centimeters due to gap-size limitations. It has been observed that nanofiber arrays collected across parallel plates at distances from 3 to 6 cm were subject to significant reductions in fiber density as the gap size was increased [102, 105].

Fiber alignment is also affected by the gap distance. Fiber alignment may initially increase with increasing gap distance at shorter lengths, but then decrease with increasing gap distance at larger lengths. The critical length for maximum alignment has been reported to be 1 and 3 mm for two different electrospinning systems [102, 109]. However, the reported affects of gap distance on fiber alignment vary widely due to the many variations between individual electrospinning systems. For example, increased fiber alignment was been observed for increasing gap distances in the range 2–6 cm in one system [105], while a decrease in alignment with increasing gap distance in the range 0.5–2.5 cm was observed for a different system [100].

8.4.2.3 Effects of electrostatic forces on fiber diameter

The electrostatic field that aligns and elongates nanofibers across a parallel-plate collector exerts a mechanical tensile force similar to the force experienced by fibers collected on a rotating mandrel. Similarly to the case for rotating-mandrel collection, fibers collected across parallel plates may demonstrate reduced diameters when compared with fibers collected on a flat static surface. The magnitude of the force applied to fibers in a parallel-plate system is dependent on the strength of the electric field and on the electrical properties of the jet. It can be predicted that parallel-plate setups with high electric fields and more deformable materials will demonstrate more significant diameter reductions due to nanofiber stretching. In one example, the diameter of nanofibers collected across parallel plates decreased in relation to flat-plate collection with increasing concentration of doped carbon nanotubes [111]. It can be hypothesized that increasing the nanotube concentration increased the conductivity of the solution and thus the magnitude of the forces stretching the fibers across the parallel-plate collector. Observed reductions in fiber diameter across parallel plates were also especially pronounced for melt electrospinning, which may have been due to the deformability of the hot fibers [101].

8.4.3 Challenges in aligned nanofiber electrospinning

Aligned nanofiber arrays can easily be collected from an electrospinning jet with the rotating-mandrel and parallel-plate techniques. Each of these methods has specific advantages and limitations. The rotating-mandrel technique allows easy collection of large-area arrays, but highly aligned orientations may be difficult to obtain and high rotation speeds may lead to tightly wound structures and fractured fibers [108]. Aligned nanofiber arrays fabricated with the parallel-plate technique are easily transferable to other substrates, but fiber alignment is very sensitive to solution properties and there are limitations on maximum fiber density and fiber length [108]. Limitations associated with the two main methods of aligned nanofiber collection constrain the types of aligned nanofiber structures that can be assembled by electrospinning. In an attempt to expand the versatility of aligned nanofiber electrospinning, several innovative modifications have been made that address limitations of the two base methods. Modified collection techniques have demonstrated the ability to improve fiber alignment and control over placement, and increase continuous fiber length, mat density, and overall yield.

8.4.3.1 Focussing and guiding the electrospinning jet

The electrospinning jet can be difficult to control for static-plate collectors and aligned collection techniques. This results in deposition areas that may be undesirably large, with a lack of uniformity. Large deposition areas may result in wasted materials and make repeatable fabrication of precision nanofiber structures difficult. Generally the fiber-deposition area can be decreased by moving the electrospinning nozzle closer to the collecting target; however, this method alone might not adequately address limitations and can bring unwanted side effects [112]. Several innovative modifications to standard electrospinning techniques have been explored in order to bring greater control over the electrospinning jet in terms of controlling precise fiber placement and focussing the overall area of fiber deposition. Such technologies include the use of sharp-edged collectors, repulsive electric fields, and attractive oppositely charged counter-electrodes.

Confinement and general stabilization of the whipping motions of an electrospinning jet early in its trajectory can result in a more focussed fiber-deposition area. One method of jet stabilization is to utilize objects with the same charge as the jet to confine it. Charged objects such as rings, cylinders, and plates can be placed around an electrospinning jet to form an electrostatic barrier that confines the jet and results in a more focused and better-controlled fiber deposition at the collection site [113–115]. This method can be quite effective. In one instance, the fiber-deposition area for a randomly oriented nanofiber mesh was reduced from 7 cm to 1 cm in diameter with the addition of charged rings around the electrospinning jet [115].

Another method to focus the nanofiber deposition area is the use of a sharp-edged collector. Sharp-edged collectors confine nanofiber deposition by limiting the actual area available and by focussing the electric field at the surface of the collector [116]. Thin sharp-edged rotating disks have been used by several groups in place of rotating mandrels to collect focussed thin aligned nanofiber arrays. A similar technique involved wrapping a thin wire around spokes on a rotating mandrel [117]. In another variation of this method, a thin wire was wrapped around an insulating mandrel [118]. This method allowed simultaneous collection of multiple focussed aligned nanofiber arrays. Thin sharp-edged objects have also been applied to the parallel-plate technique. Focussed aligned nanofiber arrays were collected at lengths up to several centimeters when two steel blades were placed upright in a direction perpendicular to the standard parallel-plate configuration [110]. Sharp-edged plates in the standard parallel-plate configuration collected greater quantities of aligned fibers than did flat parallel plates [119].

Electrospinning jet deposition can be focussed and its location can be controlled when an oppositely charged counter-electrode is placed near the collecting area to attract the jet. Electrospinning systems that implement an attracting counter-electrode generally utilize a setup where a collecting mandrel is placed in between the electrospinning nozzle and the counter-electrode (Figures 8.5 and 8.6). Focussed narrow aligned fiber arrays have been deposited on rotating mandrels when attractive counter-electrodes were placed immediately behind or inside of the mandrel [120, 121]. The width of nanofiber deposition may decrease further with decreasing collector-to-spinneret distance and thus increasing field strength [112]. Parallel arrays of strip and sharp-edged bar counter-electrodes have also been utilized to focus aligned nanofiber deposition around a rotating mandrel [122, 123]. When both like and oppositely charged counter-electrodes are placed near the collecting area the electrospinning jet can be focussed even more effectively. Placement of two like-charged (same as the jet) electrodes on either side of an oppositely charged electrode (Figure 8.5) reduced the area of fiber deposition by up to 60% [85]. The attraction of an electrospinning jet to an attractive counter-electrode is strong enough that it can alter the direction of the jet even when it is not placed directly below the nozzle [120]. Thus, the specific placement of aligned nanofibers can be controlled when counter-electrodes are used effectively. An electrospinning setup shown in Figure 8.6 utilized an electrode placed off-center of the nozzle to pull the jet at an angular trajectory relative to the collecting mandrel [122]. This setup allowed deposition of aligned fibers oriented at a predictable angle about the circumference of the mandrel. Counter-electrodes are able to hone the electrospinning jet to a specific portion of a rotating mandrel, and lateral translation of either the counter-electrode or the mandrel makes dynamic control of fiber deposition patterns possible [121].

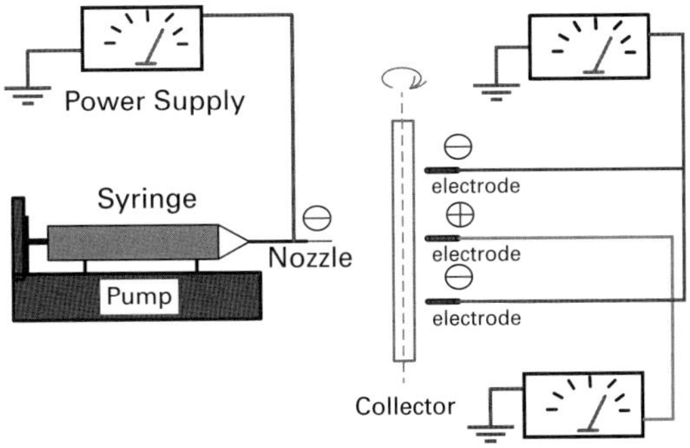

Figure 8.5 A schematic diagram of an electrospinning setup where attractive and repulsive counter-electrodes are implemented to focus the area of nanofiber deposition [85].

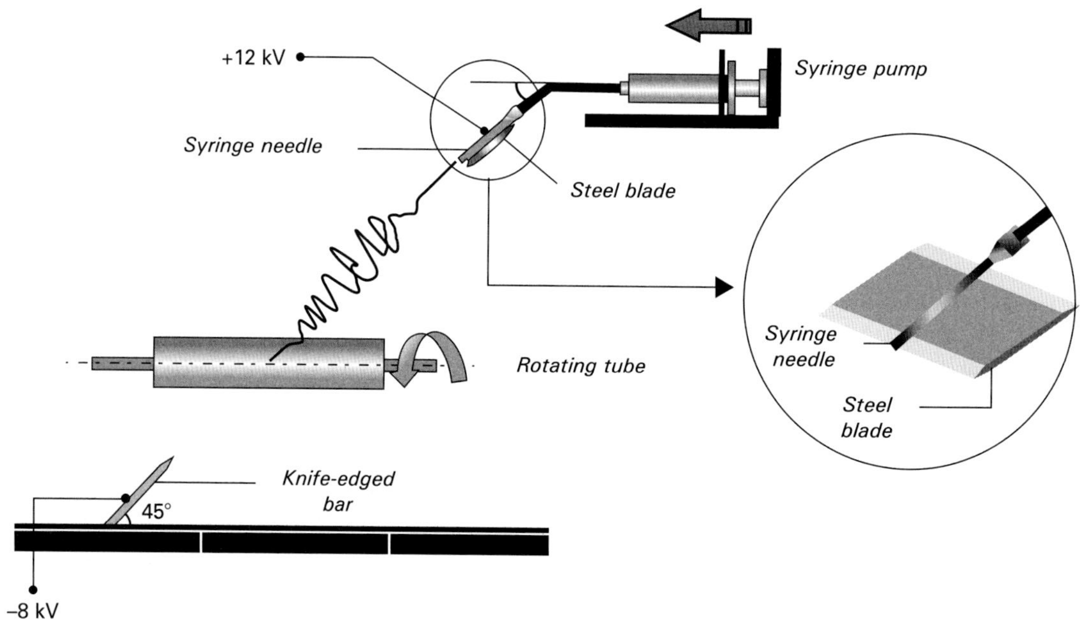

Figure 8.6 A schematic diagram of an electrospinning setup where an attractive counter-electrode is implemented to change the trajectory of an electrospinning jet. For this setup aligned nanofiber wrapped around the mandrel at a 45° angle [122].

8.4.3.2 Alignment

Many of the methods of focussing and steering the electrospinning jet described above also serve to improve fiber alignment due to geometrical constraints and increased electrostatic forces. Specific examples exist where each of the methods described above resulted in improved fiber alignment. A confining electric field applied by two like-charged plates focussed an electrospinning jet and resulted in observed increases in fiber alignment across a parallel-plate collector [113]. Thin-blade collectors leave little room for deposition of unaligned fibers, and the focussed electric field at the blade surface can improve fiber alignment independently of geometrical constraints [122]. Placement of attractive counter-electrodes behind a rotating-mandrel setup also can improve fiber array alignment. This allows well-aligned fiber collection at lower rotation speeds [85].

Several other methods have been developed to improve fiber alignment using alternating current (AC) potentials. When an alternating potential is applied to a parallel-plate collector, the attraction of the jet can be quickly transferred between the two plates. In this type of system, the jet is initially attracted to one of the two plates, but the jet moves to the other plate when the voltage is switched. High-frequency oscillation between the plates guides nanofiber deposition back and forth and results in improved alignment (Figure 8.7) [124–126]. The AC potential can be applied to one plate while the other remains grounded [124, 125], or high-voltage reed relays or switches can be used to alternatively charge and ground the two plates [126, 127]. This technique has been used with attractive and repulsive AC potentials in combination with ground [126, 127]. The frequency at which the potential is switched between the plates has an effect on the resulting fiber orientation, and an optimum frequency at which the fiber alignment is maximized may be determined [114, 124]. Interestingly, fiber alignment may also be improved when an AC potential is applied directly to the nozzle to initiate electrospinning in a standard rotating-mandrel setup. It was hypothesized

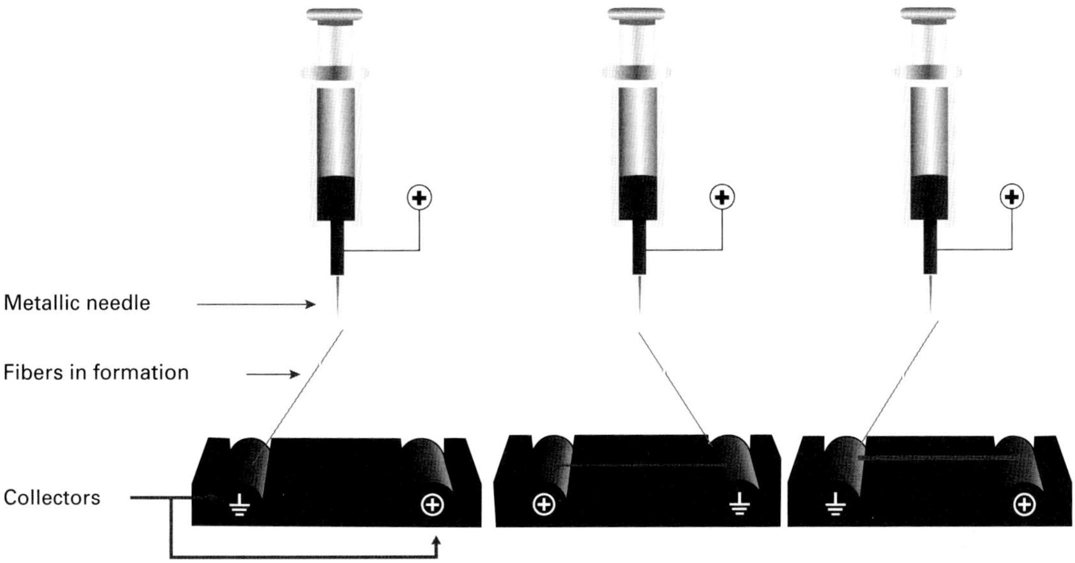

Figure 8.7 A schematic diagram of an electrospinning setup where an alternating electrical potential is applied to a parallel-plate setup to guide nanofiber deposition and improve fiber alignment [126].

that this effect was due to a more stable jet that results from decreased net charge compared with that for electrospinning initiated with direct current (DC) [128]. It was discovered that fiber alignment could be further improved with the addition of a bias DC potential to the AC potential [129].

8.4.3.3 Length

One of the advantages of the parallel-plate method is that single continuous nanofibers are suspended in air and can be easily transferred from the collecting device. The maximum length of these fibers is limited and methods of collecting longer fibers may extend the potential applications of this method. It has been demonstrated that very long fibers can be collected when large plates are used. Nanofibers up to 50 cm were collected across parallel plates that had dimensions of 30.5 cm × 7.5 cm × 0.7 cm, and it was hypothesized that it may be possible to collect even longer fibers with larger plates [8]. The length of collected fibers can also be increased by utilizing external forces. Nanofibers up to 25 cm in length were fabricated when an electrospinning jet was shot sideways such that one end adhered to a raised target and the other was pulled down by gravity where it adhered to a support [130]. Another similar setup utilized gas flow to pull the non-adhered end of long nanofibers (length >20 cm) toward an electrode [131].

8.4.3.4 Fiber density/scaffold thickness

One of the major challenges associated with the parallel-plate technique is the limitation on fiber density and scaffold thickness as discussed in Section 8.4.2.1. This limitation is due to repulsive forces caused by residual charge on deposited fibers that resist further fiber collection. One method of overcoming this limitation is to utilize non-electrical forces to overcome charge resistance in structure assembly. The addition of a magnetic field to attract fibers in a parallel-plate setup was sufficient to overcome repulsive charge forces and allow the assembly of thick aligned structures [132]. Another approach utilized mechanical forces to overcome repulsive forces and assemble successive low-density nanofiber arrays into thick aligned structures. This technique used mobile tracks to replace the static parallel plates and made it possible to assemble indefinitely thick structures [133].

8.4.3.5 Yield

It is important that electrospinning fabrication procedures have high yield for translation to industrial applications. The most straightforward method of scaling up electrospinning processes is through the use of multiple spinnerets [134–136]. Whenever multiple spinnerets are used it is important to consider interference between the spinnerets because the charged jets repel one another [137]. Another way to improve the yield in collection of aligned fibers is to move the collecting surface. Rotating mandrels are commonly translated normal to the electrospinning jet so that the area of aligned fiber deposition is increased [121, 136, 138]. A rotating-wire mandrel acts as several parallel-plate configurations that collect aligned fibers simultaneously [139]. Aligned fibers will collect in the air gaps between the spokes of the wire mandrel, and as it rotates each of the individual gaps is presented directly below the electrospinning nozzle. In a similar approach, fins were added to a rotating mandrel, and several suspended aligned fiber arrays were collected simultaneously [140]. Parallel plates have also been put directly into motion. Two parallel plates were replaced by conductive tracks that continuously pull deposited nanofibers down away from the collecting zone, thus allowing continuous production of aligned nanofiber arrays from a single nozzle [133].

8.5 Cell organization within electrospun nanofiber scaffolds

Tissue engineering scaffolds must be able to support appropriate cell types and promote desirable regenerative behaviors in those resident cells. Electrospinning technology has demonstrated a great amount of promise in tissue engineering and has generated widespread investigation, but electrospun nanofiber scaffolds face challenges that limit their potential success. One of the major challenges faced in applying this highly versatile fabrication method to tissue engineering is the difficulty of incorporating cells into the scaffolds. Cells may be introduced into nanofiber scaffolds during electrospinning, or through cell migration into the scaffolds. Strategies for promoting cell migration into electrospun scaffolds include physically assisted seeding methods and increasing scaffold porosity in order to promote cell migration.

8.5.1 Electrospinning with cells

Cells can be incorporated directly into nanofiber scaffolds in one step during electrospinning. Several methods of depositing cells within the nanofiber matrix have been investigated. In one design a charged ring on the surface of a cell culture medium was used as the electrospinning collecting target. Intermittent pipetting of a cell suspension over the collecting area resulted in a uniform cell distribution within nanofiber constructs [141]. A similar approach used electrostatic spraying to deliver a cell suspension to a grounded collecting target simultaneously with electrospinning [142]. This method also resulted in nanofiber constructs with uniform cell integration. Cells have even been encapsulated directly inside of polymer fibers. Fibroblasts and adipose-derived adult stem cells were mixed directly into an aqueous PVA solution and electrospun according to conventional methods [143]. The resultant fibers had a beaded morphology to surround the relatively large cells. Cells incorporated into electrospun scaffolds remained viable in all of the studies discussed above, and significant toxic effects were not observed.

8.5.2 Cell population through migration

Non-cellularized nanofiber scaffolds must be populated by cell migration through the pores of the structure and into the interior. Scaffold properties that determine the ability of a scaffold to promote cell infiltration include the porous architecture and any chemical or biological cues that are present within the scaffolds.

8.5.2.1 Mechanically assisted seeding

Natural cell migration into electrospun scaffolds in vitro can be assisted by externally applied mechanical forces, such as by application of a vacuum, flow perfusion, or centrifuging [144, 145]. These methods can be utilized to increase the sometimes very slow rates at which cells populate a matrix in vitro. Flow perfusion is useful for promoting quick cell infiltration into scaffolds with hydrodynamic forces, and it also improves nutrient transport deep within the scaffolds [145]. For this reason, flow perfusion may result in better cell viability deep within nanofiber scaffolds.

8.5.2.2 Cell permeability

A nanofiber scaffold must have adequate pore size and void space for cells to move about and occupy. Without this property, cells will be unable to migrate in naturally or with assisted seeding. Generally the pore size of randomly oriented electrospun scaffolds is directly related to the fiber diameter. Larger fiber diameters result in larger pores and thus increased permeability to cell infiltration [146]. The relationship between fiber size and scaffold pore size has been evaluated quantitatively for randomly oriented electrospun scaffolds with fiber diameters in the range 2–10 μm [145]. The resultant pore size for fibers of diameter 2 μm was 10 μm, and for 10-μm-diameter fiber scaffolds the pore size was increased to 40 μm. Despite large differences in pore size, the overall porosity was similar (85%–89%) for all fiber diameters, with the greatest overall porosity measured in scaffolds of smaller fiber diameter. The effect of pore size on cell infiltration was directly investigated by comparing 5-μm-fiber-diameter scaffolds with 5-μm-diameter scaffolds with a thin layer of electrospun 600-nm-diameter fibers on their surface. It was concluded that cell infiltration was severely limited by the 600-nm-fiber layer under static and flow-perfusion conditions [145]. Similar results were obtained in another study when cell migration into electrospun scaffolds with fiber diameters in the range 3.4–12.1 μm was measured over 3 days of culture [147]. It was observed that even the relatively large fibers of diameter 3.4 μm significantly impeded cell infiltration compared with the case of 12.1-μm scaffolds. The optimal pore size may vary for specific applications, but if cell infiltration is desired then the minimum pore size cannot be much smaller than the size of the migrating cells. Much of the potential of nanofiber scaffolds comes from their size, and small-diameter fibers in the nanoscale range (1–1000 nm) are generally desirable. However, randomly oriented nanofiber scaffolds with fiber diameters in the nanoscale range have poor cell-penetration properties. These contrasting requirements result in a tradeoff between scaffold pore size and fiber diameter that is a limiting factor for randomly oriented electrospun scaffolds in tissue engineering applications.

8.5.2.3 Strategies to improve cell permeability

Several innovative strategies have been developed to increase the pore size of electrospun nanofiber scaffolds without increasing the fiber diameters. These methods attempt to combine the desirable properties of nanoscale fiber diameters with increased pore size for cell penetration. Strategies include using composite structures, adding large pores, including sacrificial or cell-permeable materials within the mesh, and electrospinning into liquids.

8.5.2.3.1 Composite scaffolds

Several groups have fabricated composite nanofiber scaffolds that combine polymer nanofibers and much larger microfibers. These scaffolds combine the advantage of large pore size associated with larger fibers and the advantage of the high surface-area-to-volume ratio and improved cell interactions associated with nanofibers. Several different methods of microfiber fabrication have been combined with electrospinning to design such scaffolds. A starch-based scaffold composed of 160-μm fibers was fabricated by fiber bonding and nanofibers (of diameter 400 nm) were electrospun within the pores of the scaffold [148, 149]. The nanofibers provided structure for cells to migrate and span the large pores between microfibers. A similar scaffold was made up of microfibers fabricated by direct melt deposition and nanofibers that were electrospun [150].

Nanofibers have even been directly electrospun onto the surface of 30-μm microfibers [151]. Nanofiber-coated microfibers were subsequently formed into a highly porous scaffold. Exclusively electrospun composite scaffolds have been fabricated by modifying electrospinning conditions to form layers of microfibers (of diameter 5 μm) and layers of nanofibers (of diameter 400–500 nm) [145].

8.5.2.3.2 Pore formation with sacrificial materials

One strategy for improving cell infiltration into electrospun scaffolds is to create large pores by embedding particles within a nanofiber mesh and dissolving them out. An interconnecting porous network can promote cell infiltration deep within the scaffolds. Two different methods of salt leaching have been used to add large pores within nanofiber networks. Salt particles were crystallized within electrospun nanofiber (diameter 400 nm) scaffolds by soaking them in a saline solution followed by lyophilization [152]. Dissolution of the salt particles resulted in a mesh with 600–900-μm pores in contrast to the 1–2-μm porous structure of the original electrospun scaffold. Dry salt particles have also been directly incorporated into an electrospun mesh by depositing them in the collecting area at intervals during the electrospinning process [153]. The embedded salt particles were dissolved to form a porous network that promoted cell infiltration in in-vitro culture.

The addition of a large pore network to an electrospun mesh promotes cell migration into the scaffold, but cells still may be unable to migrate out of the large pores and into the nanofibrous architecture. Strategies that distribute smaller sacrificial materials within electrospun scaffolds have been developed in an attempt to increase the porosity of the nanfibrous architecture uniformly. It was found that, if the collecting target is cooled to −30 °C during ambient electrospinning, then ice crystals are formed within the resultant nanofiber meshes [154]. Removal of the embedded ice crystals by freeze drying results in a nanofiber mesh with pores around 100 times larger than those in conventional electrospun meshes. The pore size could be changed by adjusting the level of humidity, and larger pores promoted cell infiltration within nanofiber scaffolds. Soluble polymer materials have been directly electrospun within nanofiber scaffolds to increase pore size and cell infiltration. Composite aligned fiber scaffolds containing PCL and water-soluble PEO nanofibers were electrospun simultaneously into a uniform mesh [155]. The scaffold pore size increased with dissolution of PEO fibers in water, and it was demonstrated that cell infiltration into the scaffolds increased with increasing percentage of PEO fibers. While the authors of several studies utilizing sacrificial leaching methods have published promising results, others have observed limited improvements in cell infiltration [156]. It was hypothesized that this may be due to a collapse of the nanofiber structure that can occur after dissolution of the sacrificial component.

8.5.2.3.3 Cell-permeable materials

Cell-permeable materials can be combined with electrospun nanofibers in a composite structure. Hydrogels can be used as a spacer to increase the porosity of nanofibrous architecture and act as a barrier to collapse. Cells may be able to move through larger hydrogel-filled pores more easily than in conventional electrospun structures. Composite films containing nanofibers and protein matrix were fabricated by combining thin electrospun arrays with an aqueous gelatin solution [157]. The gelatin provided structural support for the fiber array and acted as an immobilizing spacer between individual nanofibers. Hydrogel was electrosprayed onto a collecting mandrel simultaneously with electrospinning in a one-step composite fabrication process [156]. Incorporation of hydrogel within the nanofiber matrix resulted in an increased depth of cell penetration in in-vitro culture experiments.

8.5.2.3.4 Suspension in liquids

Another strategy to increase the porosity of electrospun nanofiber scaffolds is to suspend nanofibers in liquid. One approach involved attaching lipase onto the surface of hydrophobic nanofibers followed by alcohol pre-treatment [158]. This process resulted in the dispersion of tightly packed nanofibers into a loosely entangled fiber mesh. Highly porous architecture could be maintained under aqueous conditions if the fibers remained hydrated during the washing procedures. Nanofibers can also be electrospun directly into liquids. Silk fibroin nanofibers formed a 3D structure when they were collected in a methanol bath, and that structure was maintained after hydration and freeze drying [159]. The increases in porosity in these scaffolds resulted in improved cell penetration. A dynamic-flow collecting system was designed to collect electrospun nanofiber yarns directly in water [160]. The PCL nanofiber yarns collected by this method were used to fabricate 3D networks of loosely dispersed nanofibers.

8.5.2.3.5 *Layer-by-layer assembly*

Cells can be cultured on small nanofiber scaffolds and then combined into a larger construct that will inherently contain cells throughout its thickness. A relatively large nanofiber cylinder (8 mm diameter, 3 mm height) was constructed by stacking 30 disks (8 mm diameter, 100 μm thickness) that had been cultured with cells [161]. This construct contained cells at each layer throughout its thickness; however, cell penetration into individual layers may still be a limitation. A similar strategy utilized much thinner layers to increase the overall percentage of the scaffold populated with cells. Very thin nanofiber sheets were collected on a wire ring (15 mm diameter, ~10 μm thickness) and cultured with cells. Cell–nanofiber sheets formed and then stacked up into constructs that appeared to have full-thickness cell composition [162]. Layer-by-layer assembly has also been achieved by stacking individual layers over a number of days as opposed to combining all of the cell-seeded pieces at one time [163].

8.6 Concluding remarks

Micro/nanofibrous scaffolds have tremendous potential in the field of regenerative medicine. Electrospinning is a simple and versatile method of fabricating such scaffolds. Both the biochemical composition and the geometrical structure of electrospun scaffolds can be modified for specific applications. However, fabricating electrospun scaffolds with ideal properties remains a challenge. Innovative research is currently being undertaken to address these challenges by identifying new techniques for biofunctionalizing electrospun fibers and assembling electrospun scaffolds with controlled fiber orientations and 3D cell incorporation. We hope that these advances will lead to the development of the next generation of nanofibrous scaffolds in regenerative medicine applications.

REFERENCES

[1] Beachley, V. and Wen, X. 2010. Polymer nanofibrous structures: fabrication, biofunctionalization, and cell interactions. *Prog. Polym. Sci.*, **35**(7), 868–892.

[2] Yarin, A., Koombhongse, S. and Reneker, D. 2001. Bending instability in electrospinning of nanofibers. *J. Appl. Phys.*, **89**(5), 3018.

[3] Shin, Y., Hohman, M. M., Brenner, M. P. and Rutledge, G. C. 2001. Electrospinning: a whipping fluid jet generates submicron polymer fibers. *Appl. Phys. Lett.*, **78**(8), 1149.

[4] Casper, C. L., Yamaguchi, N., Kiick, K. L. and Rabolt, J. F. 2005. Functionalizing electrospun fibers with biologically relevant macromolecules. *Biomacromolecules*, **6**(4), 1998–2007.

[5] Tong, H.-W. and Wang, M. 2011. Electrospinning of poly(hydroxybutyrate-*co*-hydroxyvalerate) fibrous tissue engineering scaffolds in two different electric fields. *Polymer Eng. Sci.*, **51**(7), 1325–38.

[6] Deitzel, J. M., Kleinmeyer, J., Harris, D. and Beck Tan, N. C. 2001. The effect of processing variables on the morphology of electrospun nanofibers and textiles. *Polymer*, **42**(1), 261–72.

[7] Meechaisue, C., Dubin, R., Supaphol, P., Hoven, V. P. and Kohn, J. 2006. Electrospun mat of tyrosine-derived polycarbonate fibers for potential use as tissue scaffolding material. *J. Biomater. Sci., Polymer Edition*, **17**(9), 1039–56.

[8] Beachley, V. and Wen, X. 2009. Effect of electrospinning parameters on the nanofiber diameter and length. *Mater. Sci. Eng. C Mater. Biol. Appl.*, **29**(3), 663–8.

[9] Megelski, S., Stephens, J. S., Chase, D. B. and Rabolt, J. F. 2002. Micro- and nanostructured surface morphology on electrospun polymer fibers. *Macromolecules*, **35**(22), 8456–66.

[10] Fong, H., Chun, I. and Reneker, D. H. 1999. Beaded nanofibers formed during electrospinning. *Polymer*, **40**(16), 4585–92.

[11] Demir, M. M., Yilgor, I., Yilgor, E. and Erman, B. 2002. Electrospinning of polyurethane fibers. *Polymer*, **43**(11), 3303–9.

[12] Hayati, I., Bailey, A. I. and Tadros, T. F. 1987. Investigations into the mechanisms of electrohydrodynamic spraying of liquids: I. Effect of electric field and the environment on pendant drops and factors affecting the formation of stable jets and atomization. *J. Colloid Interface Sci.*, **117**(1), 205–221.

[13] Zhang, C., Yuan, X., Wu, L., Han, Y. and Sheng, J. 2005. Study on morphology of electrospun poly(vinyl alcohol) mats. *Eur. Polymer J.*, **41**(3), 423–32.

[14] Jiang, H., Fang, D., Hsiao, B. S., Chu, B. and Chen, W. 2004. Optimization and characterization of dextran membranes prepared by electrospinning. *Biomacromolecules*, **5**(2), 326–33.

[15] Zong, X., Kim, K., Fang, D. *et al.* 2002. Structure and process relationship of electrospun bioabsorbable nanofiber membranes. *Polymer*, **43**(16), 4403–4412.

[16] Chen, F., Li, X., Mo, X. *et al.* 2008. Electrospun chitosan–P(LLA-CL) nanofibers for biomimetic extracellular matrix. *J. Biomater. Sci. Polymer Edition*, **19**(5), 677–91.

[17] Jeong, S. I., Lee, A. Y., Lee, Y. M. and Shin, H. 2008. Electrospun gelatin/poly(L-lactide-*co*-ε-caprolactone) nanofibers for mechanically functional tissue-engineering scaffolds. *J. Biomater. Sci. Polymer Edition*, **19**(3), 339–57.

[18] Li, M., Mondrinos, M. J., Ghandhi, M. R. *et al.*, 2005. Electrospun protein fibers as matrices for tissue engineering. *Biomaterials*, **26**(30), 5999–6008.

[19] Boland, E. D., Mondrinos, M. J., Gandhi, M. R. *et al.* 2004. Electrospinning collagen and elastin: preliminary vascular tissue engineering. *Frontiers Biosci.*, **9**, 1422–32.

[20] Rho, K. S., Jeong, L., Lee, G. *et al.* 2006. Electrospinning of collagen nanofibers: effects on the behavior of normal human keratinocytes and early-stage wound healing. *Biomaterials*, **27**(8), 1452–61.

[21] Buttafoco, L., Kolkman, N. G., Engbers-Buijtenhuijs, P. *et al.* 2006. Electrospinning of collagen and elastin for tissue engineering applications. *Biomaterials*, **27**(5), 724–34.

[22] Chen, Z. C., Ekaputra, A. K., Gauthaman, K. *et al.* 2008. In vitro and in vivo analysis of co-electrospun scaffolds made of medical grade poly(ε-caprolactone) and porcine collagen. *J. Biomater. Sci. Polymer Edition*, **19**(5), 693–707.

[23] Kwon, I. K. and Matsuda, T. 2005. Co-electrospun nanofiber fabrics of poly(L-lactide-*co*-ε-caprolactone) with type I collagen or heparin. *Biomacromolecules*, **6**(4), 2096–105.

[24] Han, I., Shim, K. J., Kim, J. Y. *et al.* 2007. Effect of poly(3-hydroxybutyrate-*co*-3-hydroxyvalerate) nanofiber matrices cocultured with hair follicular epithelial and dermal cells for biological wound dressing. *Artif. Organs*, **31**(11), 801–8.

[25] Meng, W., Kim, S. Y., Yuan, J. *et al.* 2007. Electrospun PHBV/collagen composite nanofibrous scaffolds for tissue engineering. *J. Biomater. Sci. Polymer Edition*, **18**(1), 81–94.

[26] Zeugolis, D. I., Panengad, P. P., Yew, E. S. *et al.* 2008. Electro-spinning of pure collagen nano-fibres – just an expensive way to make gelatin? *Biomaterials*, **29**(15), 2293–305.

[27] Casper, C. L., Yang, W., Farach-Carson, M. C. and Rabolt, J. F. 2007. Coating electrospun collagen and gelatin fibers with perlecan domain I for increased growth factor binding. *Biomacromolecules*, **8**(4), 1116–23.

[28] Gauthaman, K., Venugopal, J. R., Yee F. C. *et al.* 2009. Nanofibrous substrates support colony formation and maintain stemness of human embryonic stem cells. *J. Cell Molec. Med.*, **13**(9B), 3475–84.

[29] Song, J. H., Kim, H. E. and Kim, H. W. 2008. Production of electrospun gelatin nanofiber by water-based co-solvent approach. *J. Mater. Sci. Mater. Med.*, **19**(1), 95–102.

[30] Zhang, Y. Z., Venugopal, J., Huang, Z. M., Lim, C. T. and Ramakrishna, S. 2006. Crosslinking of the electrospun gelatin nanofibers. *Polymer*, **47**(8), 2911–17.

[31] Kim, H. W., Yu, H. S. and Lee, H. H. 2008. Nanofibrous matrices of poly(lactic acid) and gelatin polymeric blends for the improvement of cellular responses. *J. Biomed. Mater. Res. A*, **87**(1), 25–32.

[32] Ghasemi-Mobarakeh, L., Prabhakaran, M. P., Morshed, M., Nasr-Esfahani, M.-H. and Ramakrishna, S. 2008. Electrospun poly(ε-caprolactone)/gelatin nanofibrous scaffolds for nerve tissue engineering. *Biomaterials*, **29** (34), 4532–9.

[33] Meng, W., Xing, Z. C., Jung, K.-H. *et al.* 2008. Synthesis of gelatin-containing PHBV nanofiber mats for biomedical application. *J. Mater. Sci. Mater. Med.*, **19**(8), 2799–807.

[34] Stitzel, J., Liu, J., Lee, S. J. *et al.* 2006. Controlled fabrication of a biological vascular substitute. *Biomaterials*, **27**(7), 1088–94.

[35] Geng, X., Kwon, O. H. and Jang, J. 2005. Electrospinning of chitosan dissolved in concentrated acetic acid solution. *Biomaterials*, **26**(27), 5427–32.

[36] Ohkawa, K., Minato, K. I., Kumagai, G., Hayashi, S. and Yamamoto, H. 2006. Chitosan nanofiber. *Biomacromolecules*, **7**(11), 3291–4.

[37] Ohkawa, K., Cha, D., Kim, H., Nishida, A. and Yamamoto, H. 2004. Electrospinning of chitosan. *Macromolec. Rapid Commun.*, **25**, 1600–5.

[38] Chu, X. H., Shi, X. L., Feng, Z. Q., Gu, Z. Z. and Ding, Y. T. 2009. Chitosan nanofiber scaffold enhances hepatocyte adhesion and function. *Biotechnol. Lett.*, **31**(3), 347–52.

[39] Pan, H., Jiang, H. and Chen, W. 2006. Interaction of dermal fibroblasts with electrospun composite polymer scaffolds prepared from dextran and poly lactide-*co*-glycolide. *Biomaterials*, **27**(17), 3209–20.

[40] Wnek, G., Carr, M., Simpson, D. and Bowlin, G. 2003. Electrospinning of nanofiber fibrinogen structures. *Nano Lett.*, **3**(2), 213–16.

[41] McManus, M. C., Boland, E. D., Simpson, D. G., Barnes, C. P. and Bowlin, G. L. 2007. Electrospun fibrinogen: feasibility as a tissue engineering scaffold in a rat cell culture model. *J. Biomed. Mater. Res. A*, **81**(2), 299–309.

[42] McManus, M., Boland, E., Sell, S. *et al.* 2007. Electrospun nanofibre fibrinogen for urinary tract tissue reconstruction. *Biomed. Mater.*, **2**(4), 257–62.

[43] Neal, R. A., McClugage, S. G., Link, M. C. *et al.* 2009. Laminin nanofiber meshes that mimic morphological properties and bioactivity of basement membranes. *Tissue Eng. Part C Methods*, **15**(1), 11–21.

[44] Um, I. C., Fang, D., Hsiao, B. S., Okamoto, S. and Chu, B. 2004. Electro-spinning and electro-blowing of hyaluronic acid. *Biomacromolecules*, **5**(4), 1428–36.

[45] Ji, Y., Ghosh, K., Li, B. *et al.* 2006. Dual-syringe reactive electrospinning of cross-linked hyaluronic acid hydrogel nanofibers for tissue engineering applications. *Macromolec. Biosci.*, **6**(10), 811–17.

[46] Ji, Y., Ghosh, K., Xiao, Z. S. *et al.* 2006. Electrospun three-dimensional hyaluronic acid nanofibrous scaffolds. *Biomaterials*, **27**(20), 3782–92.

[47] Duan, Y., Wang, Z., Yan, W. *et al.* 2007. Preparation of collagen-coated electrospun nanofibers by remote plasma treatment and their biological properties. *J. Biomater. Sci. Polymer Edition*, **18**(9), 1153–64.

[48] Ma, Z., He, W., Yong, T. and Ramakrishna, S. 2005. Grafting of gelatin on electrospun poly(caprolactone) nanofibers to improve endothelial cell spreading and proliferation and to control cell orientation. *Tissue Eng.*, **11**(7–8), 1149–58.

[49] Koh, H. S., Yong, T., Chan, C. K. and Ramakrishna, S. 2008. Enhancement of neurite outgrowth using nanostructured scaffolds coupled with laminin. *Biomaterials*, **29**(26), 3574–82.

[50] Chen, J., Chu, B. and Hsiao, B. S. 2006. Mineralization of hydroxyapatite in electrospun nanofibrous poly(L-lactic acid) scaffolds. *J. Biomed. Mater. Res. A*, **79**(2), 307–17.

[51] Yu, H. S., Jang, J. H., Kim, T. I., Lee, H. H. and Kim, H. W. 2009. Apatite-mineralized polycaprolactone nanofibrous web as a bone tissue regeneration substrate. *J. Biomed. Mater. Res. A*, **88**(3), 747–54.

[52] Zhu, Y., Leong, M. F., Ong, W. F., Chan-Park, M. B. and Chian, K. S. 2007. Esophageal epithelium regeneration on fibronectin grafted poly(L-lactide-*co*-caprolactone) (PLLC) nanofiber scaffold. *Biomaterials*, **28**(5), 861–8.

[53] Nisbet, D. R., Yu, L. M. Y., Zahir, T., Forsythe, J. S. and Shoichet, M. S. 2008. Characterization of neural stem cells on electrospun poly(ε-caprolactone) submicron scaffolds: evaluating their potential in neural tissue engineering. *J. Biomater. Sci. Polymer Edition*, **19**(5), 623–34.

[54] Park, K., Ju, Y. M., Son, J. S., Ahn, K.-D. and Han, D. K. 2007. Surface modification of biodegradable electrospun nanofiber scaffolds and their interaction with fibroblasts. *J. Biomater. Sci. Polymer Edition*, **18**(4), 369–82.

[55] Chua, K. N., Chai, C., Lee, P. C. *et al.* 2007. Functional nanofiber scaffolds with different spacers modulate adhesion and expansion of cryopreserved umbilical cord blood hematopoietic stem/progenitor cells. *Exp. Hematol.*, **35**(5), 771–81.

[56] Patel, S., Kurpinski, K., Quigley, R. *et al.* 2007. Bioactive nanofibers: synergistic effects of nanotopography and chemical signaling on cell guidance. *Nano Lett.*, **7**(7), 2122–8.

[57] Bakowsky, U., Schumacher, G., Gege, C. *et al.* 2002. Cooperation between lateral ligand mobility and accessibility for receptor recognition in selectin-induced cell rolling. *Biochemistry*, **41**(14), 4704–12.

[58] Houseman, B. T. and Mrksich, M. 2001. The microenvironment of immobilized Arg-Gly-Asp peptides is an important determinant of cell adhesion. *Biomaterials*, **22**(9), 943–55.

[59] Choi, J. S., Leong, K. W. and Yoo, H. S. 2008. In vivo wound healing of diabetic ulcers using electrospun nanofibers immobilized with human epidermal growth factor (EGF). *Biomaterials*, **29**(5), 587–96.

[60] Kim, T. G. and Park, T. G. 2006. Biomimicking extracellular matrix: cell adhesive RGD peptide modified electrospun poly(D,L-lactic-*co*-glycolic acid) nanofiber mesh. *Tissue Eng.*, **12**(2), 221–33.

[61] Li, W., Guo, Y., Wang, H. *et al.* 2008. Electrospun nanofibers immobilized with collagen for neural stem cells culture. *J. Mater. Sci. Mater. Med.*, **19**(2), 847–54.

[62] Zhang, D., Chang, J. and Zeng, Y. 2008. Fabrication of fibrous poly(butylene succinate)/wollastonite/apatite composite scaffolds by electrospinning and biomimetic process. *J. Mater. Sci. Mater. Med.*, **19**(1), 443–9.

[63] He, W., Ma, Z., Yong, T., Teo, W. E. and Ramakrishna, S. 2005. Fabrication of collagen-coated biodegradable polymer nanofiber mesh and its potential for endothelial cells growth. *Biomaterials*, **26**(36), 7606–15.

[64] Ma, K., Chan, C. K., Liuo, S. *et al.* 2008. Electrospun nanofiber scaffolds for rapid and rich capture of bone marrow-derived hematopoietic stem cells. *Biomaterials*, **29**(13), 2096–103.

[65] Chew, S. Y., Hufnagel, T. C., Lim, C. T. and Leong, K. W. 2006. Mechanical properties of single electrospun drug-encapsulated nanofibres. *Nanotechnology*, **17**(15), 3880–91.

[66] Kim, K., Luu, Y. K., Chang, C. *et al.* 2004. Incorporation and controlled release of a hydrophilic antibiotic using poly(lactide-*co*-glycolide)-based electrospun nanofibrous scaffolds. *J. Control. Release*, **98**(1), 47–56.

[67] Luu, Y. K., Kim, K., Hsiao, B. S., Chu, B. and Hadjiargyrou, M. 2003. Development of a nanostructured DNA delivery scaffold via electrospinning of PLGA and PLA-PEG block copolymers. *J. Control. Release*, **89**(2), 341–53.

[68] Chew, S. Y., Wen, J., Yim, E. K. F. and Leong, K. W. 2005. Sustained release of proteins from electrospun biodegradable fibers. *Biomacromolecules*, **6**(4), 2017–24.

[69] Maretschek, S., Greiner, A. and Kissel, T. 2008. Electrospun biodegradable nanofiber nonwovens for controlled release of proteins. *J. Control. Release*, **127**(2), 180–7.

[70] Sanders, E. H., Kloefkorn, R., Bowlin, G. L., Simpson, D. G. and Wnek, G. E. 2003. Two-phase electrospinning from a single electrified jet: microencapsulation of aqueous reservoirs in poly(ethylene-*co*-vinylacetate) fibers. *Macromolecules*, **36**, 3803–5.

[71] Luong-Van, E., Grøndahl, L., Chua, K. N. *et al.* 2006. Controlled release of heparin from poly(ε-caprolactone) electrospun fibers. *Biomaterials*, **27**(9), 2042–50.

[72] Qi, H., Hu, P., Xu, I. and Wang, A. 2006. Encapsulation of drug reservoirs in fibers by emulsion electrospinning: morphology characterization and preliminary release assessment. *Biomacromolecules*, **7**(8), 2327–30.

[73] Li, X., Su, Y., He, C. *et al.* 2009. Sorbitan monooleate and poly(L-lactide-*co*-ε-caprolactone) electrospun nanofibers for endothelial cell interactions. *J. Biomed. Mater. Res. A*, **91**(3), 878–85.

[74] Yang, Y., Li, X., Qi, M., Zhou, S. and Weng, J. 2008. Release pattern and structural integrity of lysozyme encapsulated in core-sheath structured poly(DL-lactide) ultrafine fibers prepared by emulsion electrospinning. *Eur. J. Pharm. Biopharm.*, **69**(1), 106–16.

[75] Taepaiboon, P., Rungsardthong, U. and Supaphol, P. 2007. Vitamin-loaded electrospun cellulose acetate nanofiber mats as transdermal and dermal therapeutic agents of vitamin A acid and vitamin E. *Eur. J. Pharm. Biopharm.*, **67**(2), 387–97.

[76] Erisken, C., Kalyon, D. M. and Wang, H. 2008. Functionally graded electrospun polycaprolactone and beta-tricalcium phosphate nanocomposites for tissue engineering applications. *Biomaterials*, **29**(30), 4065–73.

[77] Erisken, C., Kalyon, D. M. and Wang, H. 2009. A hybrid twin screw extrusion/electrospinning method to process nanoparticle-incorporated electrospun nanofibres *Nanotechnology*, **19**(16), 165302.

[78] Sun, Z., Zussman, E., Yarin, E. L., Wendorff, J. H. and Greiner, A. 2003. Compound core-shell polymer nanofibers by co-electrospinning. *Adv. Mater.*, **15**(22), 1929–32.

[79] Zhang, Y. Z., Wang, X., Feng, Y. *et al.* 2006. Coaxial electrospinning of (fluorescein isothiocyanate-conjugated bovine serum albumin)-encapsulated poly(ε-caprolactone) nanofibers for sustained release. *Biomacromolecules*, **7**(4), 1049–57.

[80] Loscertales, I. G., Barrero, A., Márquez, M. *et al.* 2004. Electrically forced coaxial nanojets for one-step hollow nanofiber design. *J. Am. Chem. Soc.*, **126**(17), 5376–7.

[81] Yi, F. and LaVan, D. A. 2008. Poly(glycerol sebacate) nanofiber scaffolds by core/shell electrospinning. *Macromolec. Biosci.*, **8**(9), 803–6.

[82] Beachley, V., Katsanevakis, E., Zhang, N. and Wen, X. 2012. Highly aligned polymer nanofiber structures: fabrication and applications in tissue engineering. In *Biomedical Applications of Polymeric Nanofibers*, ed. Jayakumar, R. and Nair, S. Berlin: Springer, pp. 171–212.

[83] Reneker, D. H. and Chun, I. 1996. Nanometre diameter fibres of polymer, produced by electrospinning. *Nanotechnology*, **7**(3), 216–23.

[84] Yee, W. A., Kotaki, M., Liu, Y. and Lu, X. 2007. Morphology, polymorphism behavior and molecular orientation of electrospun poly(vinylidene fluoride) fibers. *Polymer*, **48**(2), 512–21.

[85] Wu, Y. Q., Carnell, L. A. and Clark, R. L. 2007. Control of electrospun mat width through the use of parallel auxiliary electrodes. *Polymer*, **48**(19), 5653–61.

[86] Edwards, M. D., Mitchell, G. R., Mohan, S. D. and Olley, R. H. 2010. Development of orientation during electrospinning of fibres of poly(ε-caprolactone). *Eur. Polymer J.*, **46**(6), 1175–83.

[87] Bashur, C. A., Dahlgren, L. A. and Goldstein, A. S. 2006. Effect of fiber diameter and orientation on fibroblast morphology and proliferation on electrospun poly(D, L-lactic-*co*-glycolic acid) meshes. *Biomaterials*, **27**(33), 5681–8.

[88] Wang, H. B., Mullins, M. E., Cregg, J. M. *et al.* 2009. Creation of highly aligned electrospun poly-L-lactic acid fibers for nerve regeneration applications. *J. Neural Eng.*, **6**(1), 016001.

[89] Aviss, K. J., Gough, J. E. and Downes, S. 2010. Aligned electrospun polymer fibres for skeletal muscle regeneration. *Eur. Cells Mater.*, **19**, 193–204.

[90] Courtney, T., Sacks, M. S., Stankus, S., Guan, J. and Wagner, W. R. 2006. Design and analysis of tissue engineering scaffolds that mimic soft tissue mechanical anisotropy. *Biomaterials*, **27**(19), 3631–8.

[91] Zhong, S., Teo, W. E., Zhu, X. *et al.* 2006. An aligned nanofibrous collagen scaffold by electrospinning and its effects on in vitro fibroblast culture. *J. Biomed. Mater. Res. A*, **79**(3), 456–63.

[92] Lee, J. Y., Bashur, C. A., Gomez, N., Goldstein, A. S. and Schmidt, C. E. 2010. Enhanced polarization of embryonic hippocampal neurons on micron scale electrospun fibers. *J. Biomed. Mater. Res. Part A*, **92**(4), 1398–406.

[93] Li, W. J., Mauck, R. L., Cooper, J. A., Yuan, X. and Tuan, R. S. 2007. Engineering controllable anisotropy in electrospun biodegradable nanofibrous scaffolds for musculoskeletal tissue engineering. *J. Biomech.*, **40**(8), 1686–93.

[94] Chan, K. H. K., Wong, S. Y., Tiju, W. C. *et al.* 2010. Morphologies and electrical properties of electrospun poly(R)-3-hydroxybutyrate-*co*-(R)-3-hydroxyvalerate/ multiwalled carbon nanotubes fibers. *J. Appl. Polymer Sci.*, **116**(2), 1030–5.

[95] Bashur, C. A., Shaffer, R. D., Dahlgren, L. A., Guelcher, S. A. and Goldstein, A. S. 2009. Effect of fiber diameter and alignment of electrospun polyurethane meshes on mesenchymal progenitor cells. *Tissue Eng. Part A*, **15**(9), 2435–45.

[96] Thomas, V., Jose, M. V., Chowdhury, S. *et al.* 2006. Mechano-morphological studies of aligned nanofibrous scaffolds of polycaprolactone fabricated by electrospinning. *J. Biomater. Sci. Polymer Edition*, **17**(9), 969–84.

[97] Jose, M. V., Steinert, B. W., Thomas, V. *et al.* 2007. Morphology and mechanical properties of Nylon 6/ MWNT nanofibers. *Polymer*, **48**(4), 1096–104.

[98] Li, D., Wang, Y. L. and Xia, Y. N. 2003. Electrospinning of polymeric and ceramic nanofibers as uniaxially aligned arrays. *Nano Lett.*, **3**(8), 1167–71.

[99] Xin, Y., Huang, Z., Chen, J. *et al.* 2008. Fabrication of well-aligned PPV/PVP nanofibers by electrospinning. *Mater. Lett.*, **62**(6–7), 991–3.

[100] Kuo, C. C., Wang, C. T. and Chen, W. C. 2008. Highly-aligned electrospun luminescent nanofibers prepared from polyfluorene/PMMA blends: fabrication, morphology, photophysical properties and sensory applications. *Macromolec. Mater. Eng.*, **293**(12), 999–1008.

[101] Dalton, P. D., Grafahrend, D., Klinkhammer, K., Klee, D. and Möller, M. 2007. Electrospinning of polymer melts: phenomenological observations. *Polymer*, **48**(23), 6823–33.

[102] Jalili, R., Morshed, M. and Ravandi, S. A. H. 2006. Fundamental parameters affecting electrospinning of PAN nanofibers as uniaxially aligned fibers. *J. Appl. Polymer Sci.*, **101**(6), 4350–7.

[103] Li, D., Wang, Y. L. and Xia, Y. N. 2004. Electrospinning nanofibers as uniaxially aligned arrays and layer-by-layer stacked films. *Adv. Mater.*, **16**(4), 361–6.

[104] Wray, L. S. and Orwin, E. J. 2009. Recreating the microenvironment of the native cornea for tissue engineering applications. *Tissue Eng. Part A*, **15**(7), 1463–72.

[105] Bazbouz, M. B. and Stylios, G. K. 2008. Alignment and optimization of nylon 6 nanofibers by electrospinning. *J. Appl. Polymer Sci.*, **107**(5), 3023–32.

[106] Liu, L. H. and Dzenis, Y. A. 2008. Analysis of the effects of the residual charge and gap size on electrospun nanofiber alignment in a gap method. *Nanotechnology*, **19**(35), 355307.

[107] Katta, P., Alessandro, M., Ramsier, R. and Chase, G. 2004. Continuous electrospinning of aligned polymer nanofibers onto a wire drum collector. *Nano Lett.*, **4**(11), 2215–18.

[108] Teo, W. E. and Ramakrishna, S. 2006. A review on electrospinning design and nanofibre assemblies. *Nanotechnology*, **17**, R89–106.

[109] Pokorny, M., Niedoba, K. and Velebny, V. 2010. Transversal electrostatic strength of patterned collector affecting alignment of electrospun nanofibers. *Appl. Phys. Lett.*, **96**(19), 193111.

[110] Teo, W. E. and Ramakrishna, S. 2005. Electrospun fibre bundle made of aligned nanofibres over two fixed points. *Nanotechnology*, **16**(9), 1878–84.

[111] Ayutsede, J., Gandhi, M., Sukigara, S. *et al.* 2006. Carbon nanotube reinforced *Bombyx mori* silk nanofibers by

the electrospinning process. *Biomacromolecules*, **7**(1), 208–14.

[112] Carnell, L. S., Siochi, E. J., Wincheski, R. A., Holloway, N. M. and Clark, R. L. 2009. Electric field effects on fiber alignment using an auxiliary electrode during electrospinning. *Scripta Mater.*, **60**(6), 359–61.

[113] Acharya, M., Arumugam, G. K. and Heiden, P. A. 2008. Dual electric field induced alignment of electrospun nanofibers. *Macromolec. Mater. Eng.*, **293**(8), 666–74.

[114] Kim, G. and Kim, W. 2006. Formation of oriented nanofibers using electrospinning. *Appl. Phys. Lett.*, **88**(23), 233101.

[115] Deitzel, J. M., Kleinmeyer, J. D., Hirvonen, J. K. and Beck Jan, N. C. 2001. Controlled deposition of electrospun poly(ethylene oxide) fibers. *Polymer*, **42**, 8163–70.

[116] Theron, A., Zussman, E. and Yarin, A. L. 2001. Electrostatic field-assisted alignment of electrospun nanofibres. *Nanotechnology*, **12**(3), 384–90.

[117] Yao, L., O'Brien, N., Windebank, A. and Pandit, A. 2009. Orienting neurite growth in electrospun fibrous neural conduits. *J. Biomed. Mater. Res. Part B – Appl. Biomater.*, **90**(2), 483–91.

[118] Bhattarai, N., Edmondson, D., Veiseh, O., Matsen, F. A. and Zhang, M. 2005. Electrospun chitosan-based nanofibers and their cellular compatibility. *Biomaterials*, **26** (31), 6176–84.

[119] Secasanu, V. P., Giardina, C. K. and Wang, Y. D. 2009. A novel electrospinning target to improve the yield of uniaxially aligned fibers. *Biotechnol. Progress*, **25**(4), 1169–75.

[120] Carnell, L. S., Siochi, E. J., Holloway, N. M. *et al.* 2008. Aligned mats from electrospun single fibers. *Macromolecules*, **41**(14), 5345–9.

[121] Sundaray, B., Subramanian, V. Natarajan, T. S. *et al.* 2004. Electrospinning of continuous aligned polymer fibers. *Appl. Phys. Lett.*, **84**(7), 1222–4.

[122] Teo, W. E., Kotaki, M., Mo, X. M. and Ramakrishna, S. 2005. Porous tubular structures with controlled fibre orientation using a modified electrospinning method. *Nanotechnology*, **16**(6), 918–24.

[123] Mo, X. M. and Weber, H. J. 2004. Electrospinning P (LLA-CL) nanofiber: a tubular scaffold fabrication with circumferential alignment. *Macromolec. Symp.*, **217**, 413–16.

[124] Lee, H., Yoon, H. and Kim, G. 2009. Highly oriented electrospun polycaprolactone micro/nanofibers prepared by a field-controllable electrode and rotating collector. *Appl. Phys. A – Mater. Sci. Processing*, **97**(3), 559–65.

[125] Kim, G. H. 2006. Electrospinning process using field-controllable electrodes. *J. Polymer Sci. Part B – Polymer Phys.*, **44**(10), 1426–33.

[126] Attout, A., Yunus, S. and Bertrand, P. 2008. Electrospinning and alignment of polyaniline-based nanowires and nanotubes. *Polymer Eng. Sci.*, **48**(9), 1661–6.

[127] Ishii, Y., Sakai, H. and Murata, H. 2008. A new electrospinning method to control the number and a diameter of uniaxially aligned polymer fibers. *Mater. Lett.*, **62**(19), 3370–2.

[128] Kessick, R., Fenn, J. and Tepper, G. 2004. The use of AC potentials in electrospraying and electrospinning processes. *Polymer*, **45**(9), 2981–4.

[129] Sarkar, S., Deevi, S. and Tepper, G. 2007. Biased AC electrospinning of aligned polymer nanofibers. *Macromolec. Rapid Commun.*, **28**(9), 1034–9.

[130] Rafique, J., Yu, J., Yu, J. L. *et al.* 2007. Electrospinning highly aligned long polymer nanofibers on large scale by using a tip collector. *Appl. Phys. Lett.*, **91**(6), 63–126.

[131] Zhou, W., Li, Z., Zhang, Q. *et al.* 2007. Gas flow-assisted alignment of super long electrospun nanofibers. *J. Nanosci. Nanotechnol.*, **7**(8), 2667–73.

[132] Liu, Y. Q., Zhang, X., Xia, Y. and Yang, H. 2010. Magnetic-field-assisted electrospinning of aligned straight and wavy polymeric nanofibers. *Adv. Mater.*, **22**(22), 2454–7.

[133] Beachley, V. and Wen, X. 2010. *Fabrication of Three-Dimensional Aligned Nanofiber Array.* Clemson, SC: Clemson University.

[134] Madhugiri, S., Dalton, A., Gutierrez, J., Ferraris, J. P. and Balkus, K. J. 2003. Electrospun MEH-PPV/SBA-15 composite nanofibers using a dual syringe method. *J. Am. Chem. Soc.*, **125**(47), 14531–8.

[135] Kidoaki, S., Kwon, I. K. and Matsuda, T. 2005. Mesoscopic spatial designs of nano- and microfiber meshes for tissue-engineering matrix and scaffold based on newly devised multilayering and mixing electrospinning techniques. *Biomaterials*, **26**(1), 37–46.

[136] Ding, B., Kimura, E., Sato, T., Fujita, S. and Shiratori, S. 2004. Fabrication of blend biodegradable nanofibrous nonwoven mats via multi-jet electrospinning. *Polymer*, **45**(6), 1895–1902.

[137] Theron, S. A., Yarin, A. L., Zussman, E. and Kroll, E. 2005. Multiple jets in electrospinning: experiment and modeling. *Polymer*, **46**(9), 2889–99.

[138] Chow, W. N., Simpson, D. G., Bigbee J. W. and Colello, R. J. 2007. Evaluating neuronal and glial growth on electrospun polarized matrices: bridging the gap in

percussive spinal cord injuries. *Neuron Glia Biol.*, **3**, 119–26.

[139] Yao, Y. F., Gu, Z. Z., Zhang, J. Z. *et al.* 2007. Fiber-oriented liquid crystal polarizers based on anisotropic electrospinning. *Adv. Mater.*, **19**(21), 3707–11.

[140] Afifi, A. M., Nakajima, H., Yamane, H., Kimura, Y. and Nakano, S. 2009. Fabrication of aligned poly(L-lactide) fibers by electrospinning and drawing. *Macromolec. Mater. Eng.*, **294**(10), 658–65.

[141] Yang, X., Shah, J. D. and Wang, H. 2009. Nanofiber enabled layer-by-layer approach toward three-dimensional tissue formation. *Tissue Eng. Part A*, **15**(4), 945–56.

[142] Stankus, J. J., Soletti, L., Fujimoto, K. *et al.* 2007. Fabrication of cell microintegrated blood vessel constructs through electrohydrodynamic atomization. *Biomaterials*, **28**(17), 2738–46.

[143] van Aalst, J. A., Reed, C. R., Han, L. *et al.* 2008. Cellular incorporation into electrospun nanofibers: retained viability, proliferation, and function in fibroblasts. *Ann. Plast. Surg.*, **60**(5), 577–83.

[144] Li, W. J., Jiang, Y. J. and Tuan, R. S. 2008. Cell-nanofiber-based cartilage tissue engineering using improved cell seeding, growth factor, and bioreactor technologies. *Tissue Eng Part A*, **14**(5), 639–48.

[145] Pham, Q. P., Sharma, U. and Mikos, A. G. 2006. Electrospun poly(ε-caprolactone) microfiber and multilayer nanofiber/microfiber scaffolds: characterization of scaffolds and measurement of cellular infiltration. *Biomacromolecules*, **7**(10), 2796–805.

[146] Eichhorn, S. J. and Sampson, W. W. 2005. Statistical geometry of pores and statistics of porous nanofibrous assemblies. *J. R. Soc. Interface*, **2**(4), 309–18.

[147] Balguid, A., Mol, A., van Marion, M. H. *et al.* 2009. Tailoring fiber diameter in electrospun poly(ε-caprolactone) scaffolds for optimal cellular infiltration in cardiovascular tissue engineering. *Tissue Eng. Part A*, **15**(2), 437–44.

[148] Tuzlakoğlu, K., Bolgen, N., Salgado, A. J. *et al.* 2005. Nano- and micro-fiber combined scaffolds: a new architecture for bone tissue engineering. *J. Mater. Sci. Mater. Med.*, **16**(12), 1099–104.

[149] Santos, M. I., Tuzlakoğlu, K., Fuchs, S. *et al.* 2008. Endothelial cell colonization and angiogenic potential of combined nano- and micro-fibrous scaffolds for bone tissue engineering. *Biomaterials*, **29**(32), 4306–13.

[150] Park, S. H., Kim, T. G., Kim, H. C., Yang, D. Y. and Park, T. G. 2008. Development of dual scale scaffolds via direct polymer melt deposition and electrospinning for applications in tissue regeneration. *Acta Biomater.*, **4**(5), 1198–207.

[151] Thorvaldsson, A., Stenhamre, H., Gatenholm, P. and Walkenström, P. 2008. Electrospinning of highly porous scaffolds for cartilage regeneration. *Biomacromolecules*, **9**(3), 1044–9.

[152] Ki, C. S., Park, S. Y., Kim, H. J. *et al.* 2008. Development of 3-D nanofibrous fibroin scaffold with high porosity by electrospinning: implications for bone regeneration. *Biotechnol. Lett.*, **30**(3), 405–10.

[153] Nam, J., Huang, Y., Agarwal, S. and Lannutti, J. 2007. Improved cellular infiltration in electrospun fiber via engineered porosity. *Tissue Eng.*, **13**(9), 2249–57.

[154] Leong, M. F., Rasheed, M. Z., Lim, T. C. and Chian, K. S. 2009. In vitro cell infiltration and in vivo cell infiltration and vascularization in a fibrous, highly porous poly(D,L-lactide) scaffold fabricated by cryogenic electrospinning technique. *J. Biomed. Mater. Res. A*, **91**(1), 231–40.

[155] Baker, B. M., Gee, A. O., Metter, R. B. *et al.* 2008. The potential to improve cell infiltration in composite fiber-aligned electrospun scaffolds by the selective removal of sacrificial fibers. *Biomaterials*, **29**(15), 2348–58.

[156] Ekaputra, A. K., Prestwich, G. D., Cool, S. M. and Hutmacher, D. W. 2008. Combining electrospun scaffolds with electrosprayed hydrogels leads to three-dimensional cellularization of hybrid constructs. *Biomacromolecules*, **9**(8), 2097–103.

[157] Beachley, V. and Wen, X. 2009. Fabrication of nanofiber reinforced protein structures for tissue engineering. *Mater. Sci. Eng. C Mater. Biol. Appl.*, **29** (8), 2448–53.

[158] Nair, S., Kim, J., Crawford, B. and Kim, S. H. 2007. Improving biocatalytic activity of enzyme-loaded nanofibers by dispersing entangled nanofiber structure. *Biomacromolecules*, **8**(4), 1266–70.

[159] Ki, C. S., Kim, J. W., Hyun, J. H. *et al.* 2007. Electrospun three-dimensional silk fibroin nanofibrous scaffold. *J. Appl. Polymer Sci.*, **106**(6), 3922–8.

[160] Teo, W. E., Liao, S., Chan, C. K., Ramakrishna, S. 2008. Remodeling of three-dimensional hierarchically organized nanofibrous assemblies. *Current Nanosci.*, **4**(4), 361–9.

[161] Srouji, S., Kizhner, T., Suss-Tobi, E., Livne, E. and Zussman, E. 2008. 3-D Nanofibrous electrospun multilayered construct is an alternative ECM mimicking scaffold. *J. Mater. Sci. Mater. Med.*, **19**(3), 1249–55.

[162] Ishii, O., Shin, M., Sueda, T. and Vacanti, J. P. 2005. In vitro tissue engineering of a cardiac graft using a degradable scaffold with an extracellular matrix-like topography. *J. Thorac. Cardiovasc. Surg.*, **130**(5), 1358–63.

[163] Inanç, B., Arslan, Y. E., Seker, S., Elçin, A. E. and Elçin, Y. M. 2009. Periodontal ligament cellular structures engineered with electrospun poly(DL-lactide-*co*-glycolide) nanofibrous membrane scaffolds. *J. Biomed. Mater. Res. A*, **90**(1), 186–95.

9

Biological scaffolds for regenerative medicine

Vineet Agrawal and Stephen F. Badylak

9.1 Introduction

The ideal biological scaffold would provide structural support appropriate for the tissue of interest, and an adhesion surface that maintains phenotypic cues suited to the tissue and has the ability to change as the functional requirements of the target tissue change. The extracellular matrix (ECM) is the aggregate product of cells that reside in a given tissue, organ, or microenvironment and has all of these characteristics. In addition to serving as structural support for the tissue, the ECM has numerous functional roles that it fulfills through site-specific ligands that serve as cell-attachment anchors, differentiation cues, and mediators of intracellular signaling pathways. Furthermore, the ECM is in a constant state of "dynamic reciprocity" with the resident cells of the given tissues or organ, which is manifested by the temporal change in composition and structure in response to the requirements and activity of the resident cells that reside within the ECM. Stated differently, the composition and structure of the matrix are optimized for each tissue and change in response to mechanical forces, biochemical milieu, oxygen requirements/concentration, pH, and gene expression, among other factors. The ECM also plays a central role in mammalian development, normal physiology, and the response to injury. For these reasons, if harvested and processed appropriately, the ECM has been shown to promote constructive, site-specific remodeling when used as a biological scaffold for regenerative medicine applications.

Beginning with a discussion of the components that comprise the extracellular matrix, the present chapter will review the use of extracellular matrix as a biological scaffold material in tissue engineering and regenerative medicine applications with a specific focus on the mechanisms by which such scaffolds promote functional restoration of tissue following injury.

9.2 Composition of the ECM

All components of the ECM are manufactured and secreted by the cells of each tissue. The ECM is composed of several distinct families of molecules, including glycosaminoglycans/proteoglycans, fibrillar proteins, and sequestered bioactive growth factors each in a particular three-dimensional (3D) structure that is unique to the tissues of origin (Figure 9.1). It may be useful to think of the ECM as a naturally occurring mixed polymer with a unique, tissue-specific structure and composition. Each component is discussed below in greater detail.

9.2.1 Glycosaminoglycans and proteoglycans

Glycosaminoglycans (GAGs) are linear polymers consisting of repeating hexosamine and uronic acid disaccharides. With the exception of hyaluronic acid, GAGs form complexes with a core linker protein to form proteoglycans (PGs). Amongst GAGs, there is remarkable diversity in the composition and structure of the caroboxyl, hydroxyl, and sulfate groups that comprise the individual GAGs (e.g. hyaluronic acid, heparan-sulfate, dermatin-sulfate, chondroitin-sulfate, and

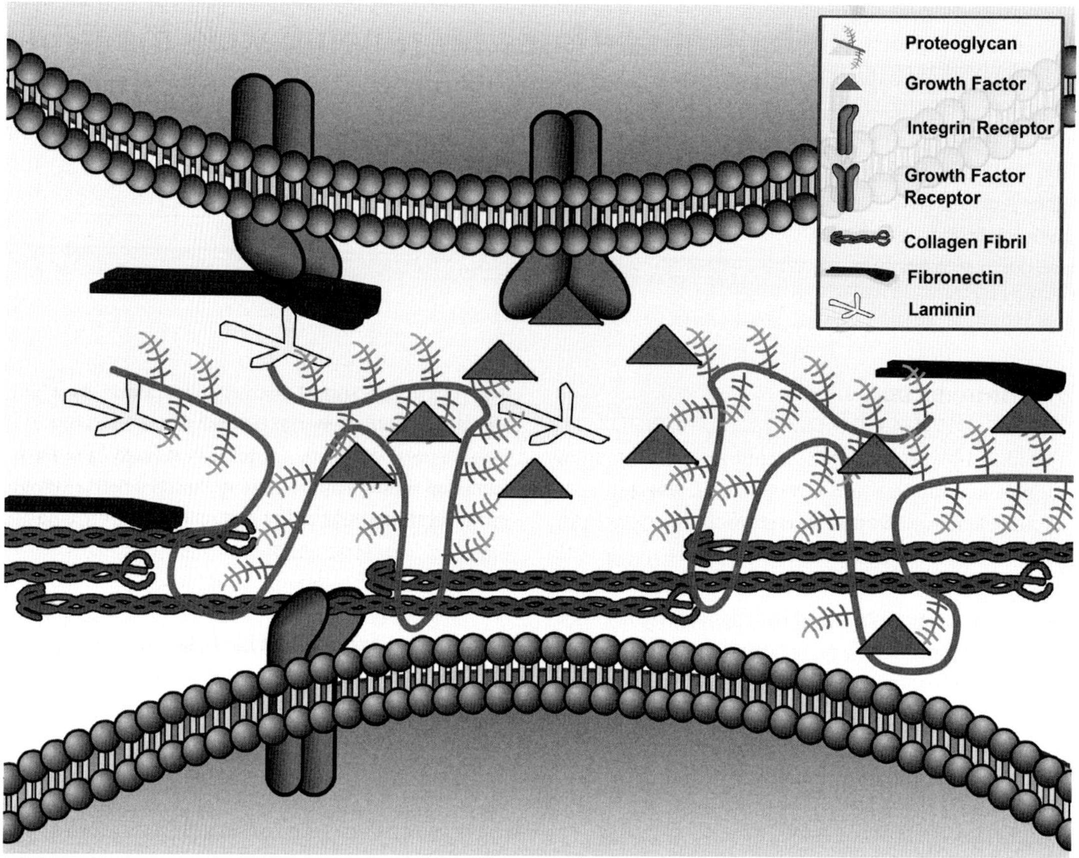

Figure 9.1 A schematic diagram of the major components of the extracellular matrix.

keratin-sulfate) [1]. However, a common property of many GAGs is their strong polyanionic charge that is thought to be responsible for the hydrophilic properties of PGs. The hydrophilic property of GAGs is responsible for attracting and retaining water within the interstitial spaces of the tissue, which is an important property for tissues such as articular cartilage where the retention of fluid is necessary for proper lubrication of joints.

Hyaluronic acid (HA) is the only non-sulfated GAG and is distinct from other GAGs in that it does not covalently link with core proteins to form proteoglycans. However, HA plays an important role in mediating cell phenotype and function [2], and has been used extensively both in preclinical and in clinical applications for tissue engineering and regenerative medicine [3]. Partially through its transmembrane receptor, CD44, HA is thought to a play a major role in the assembly of the pericellular matrix and subsequent propagation of cellular signals [4].

9.2.2 Fibrillar proteins

Fibrillar proteins comprise the most abundant family of proteins within the extracellular matrix. Fibrillar proteins are highly conserved from species to species. The traditional functions of fibrillar proteins include structural support for tissue and serving as a local substrate for cell adhesion.

More than 90% of the dry weight of ECM is represented by collagen, the most abundant of fibrillar proteins in the ECM. Collagen is also the most abundant protein in the body [5], comprising approximately 25%–30% of its total protein content. To date, over 28 different types of collagens and 49 distinct collagen α-chain gene products have been identified. The most common subtype of collagen is type I. Other collagen subtypes exist in much smaller quantities, although they play important roles in determining the structure–function relationships of the tissues in which they reside. For example, collagen type III plays an important role in maintaining the structure of submucosal tissues such as the urinary bladder and small intestine [6]. Collagen type IV is uniquely limited to the basement membrane of vascular and epithelial tissues [7], and plays an important role in mediating epithelial and endothelial cell attachment to the basement membrane. Type VI collagen is a relatively small, dumbbell-shaped molecule that plays a role in linking glycosaminoglycans to larger fibrillar proteins such as collagen type I [8]. Type VII collagen is found within the basement membrane of tissues and serves as an anchoring fibril to prevent overlying epithelial cells from shear stress [9].

Among the other fibrillar proteins, fibronectin and laminin are also thought to be important contributors to the biology and function of the extracellular matrix. Fibronectin is an abundant protein in ECM, second only to collagen in amount. Fibronectin is a dimeric molecule of 250,000-Da subunits and exists both in soluble and in insoluble forms. Fibronectin is found in the ECM of submucosal tissues, basement membranes, and interstitial tissues. Laminin is another structural component of the ECM, consisting of an 800-kD noncollagenous protein with a cross-shaped structure that allows simultaneous binding to collagen domains, heparin, and various cells within the tissue. This unique structure of laminin supports epithelial attachment to basement membranes and guidance of neural migration in development [10–12] and injury [13–15].

9.2.3 Growth factors and cytokines

Bound to the GAGs, PGs, and fibrillar proteins within the ECM are small bioactive factors. These sequestered factors include growth factors such as vascular endothelial growth factor (VEGF), members of the fibroblast growth factor (FGF) family, stromal-derived growth factor (SDF-1), epidermal growth factor (EGF), transforming growth factor β (TGF-β), keratinocyte growth factor (KGF), hepatocyte growth factor (HGF), platelet derived growth factor (PDGF), and bone morphogenetic protein (BMP) [16–18]. Because sequestered growth factors are secreted by the resident cells of each tissue, the exact type and amount of each within the ECM is highly tissue-dependent and related to the specific functional requirements of the tissue. These growth factors can play an important role in mediating the host response to injury, and thus the retention of such growth factors in the harvested ECM from decellularized tissue help provide a bioactive tissue remodeling response in vivo. For example, following a partial hepatectomy, rapid activation of plasminogen activators results in the cleavage and release of active HGF from the liver ECM [19]. Release of matrix-bound HGF is considered to be one of the factors that initiates the complex processes that eventually lead to functional regeneration of the liver following injury [20, 21].

9.3 Structure of ECM

The combination of GAGs, PGs, fibrillar proteins, and sequestered growth factors forms the extraordinarily complex structure of the extracellular matrix (Figure 9.1). The exact composition of the ECM can differ from tissue to tissue (or even within different regions of the same tissue) because the aggregate ECM product is the result of all 3D secreted proteins of the resident cells. For the same reason, the ultrastructure of the ECM varies based on the tissue of origin. These ultrastructural properties are thought to affect the local phenotype and function of cells interacting with the ECM.

The relationships of ECM ultrastructure to cell behavior have been thoroughly investigated in embryonic development. The structure and spatial organization of ECM change throughout development, beginning with changes as early as just after fertilization of the egg [22]. Additionally, changes in the ECM ultrastructure have been observed to correlate closely with developmental milestones such as myocardial precursor migration for cardiogenesis [23–25], migration of neural crests from the border of the neural plate and non-neural ectoderm [26, 27], and morphogenesis/maturation of glandular and endodermal gut tissue [27–29]. In adult tissue, specific structures within the ECM such as the basement membrane are an important physical barrier for cell invasion that eventually promote proper re-epethelialization following injury [30, 31]. The alignment and stiffness of collagen fibers and other proteins within the ECM can influence the morphology, alignment, and intrinsic gene expression of cells that interact with the matrix [32, 33].

At the macroscale, microscale, and even nanoscale levels, the topography and geometry of a substrate play an integral role in influencing the cell response to a substrate. It has recently been shown that the surface composition of ECM scaffolds prepared from various tissues is unique and tissue-specific [34, 35]. For this reason, the native ECM represents the ideal substrate for tissue engineering applications if it is prepared with minimal changes to structure and composition. Although recent advances in fabrication technology have allowed the fabrication of synthetic scaffolds to approximate physical properties of the ECM such as porosity and permeability, as discussed in subsequent sections, the complex 3D ultrastructure and ligand landscape of the ECM surface cannot yet be replicated in the laboratory setting.

9.4 Preparation of biological scaffolds composed of extracellular matrix

Biological scaffold materials composed of allogeneic and xenogeneic extracellular matrix (ECM) have been used in pre-clinical animal studies to facilitate constructive remodeling of a variety of tissues including esophagus [36–40], myocardium [41–44], blood vessels [45–47], urinary bladder [48–51], cartilage [52], and skeletal muscle [53–57]. When scaffolds are properly prepared and manufactured, the host response to ECM scaffolds includes rapid degradation of the scaffold [58–60], infiltration of the material by host cells [60, 61], modulation of the innate immune response to a pro-regenerative phenotype [62, 63], and eventual replacement of the scaffold by organized, site-appropriate, functional host tissue [51, 58, 64, 65]. The otherwise default response to injured tissue or non-degradable biomaterials consists of inflammation and the associated deposition of dense, connective tissue [66].

Table 9.1 A partial list of agents and methods currently used to decellularize tissues

Method	References
Mechanical/physical methods	
Mechanical agitation	[37, 47]
Freeze/thaw	[70]
Electroporation	[71]
Force/pressure	[72]
Non-biological chemical agents	
Alkaline/acidic solutions	[72, 73]
Hypertonic/hypotonic solutions	[74, 75]
Non-ionic agents	[70, 76]
Ionic agents	[77–79]
Zwitterionic agents	[80, 81]
Solvents (e.g. alcohols, acetone)	[82, 83]
Biological chemical agents	
Nucleases	[75]
Chelators (EGTA/EDTA)	[70]
Trypsin	[70, 84]
Dispase	[72, 85]

9.4.1 Preparation of ECM scaffolds

The method of production of scaffolds composed of ECM is a key determinant of the host response [63, 67], downstream remodeling, and eventual functionality. Decellularization of the source tissue typically requires the use of multiple modalities including physical, mechanical, chemical, and enzymatic methods [68]. Commonly used physical methods include freeze-thaw, force and pressure, and electroporation [69]. Table 9.1 shows a partial list of potential methods of decellularization.

The goal of tissue decellularization is to remove as many of the cellular components as possible while

Tissue	Protocol	Length
Small Intestine	Mechanical Agitation → 0.1% PAA, 1 h → PBS 15 min → dH_2O 30 min → PBS 15 min	Total ~5 h
Urinary Bladder	Mechanical Agitation → 0.1% PAA, 1 h → PBS 15 min → dH_2O 30 min → PBS 15 min	Total ~5 h
Trachea	dH_2O with antibiotics → 4% deoxycholate 4 h → DNase 3 h → dH_2O → dH_2O → PBS with antibiotics	Total ~8 h
Brain	PBS with antibiotics → Freeze–thaw −80 °C 4X → dH_2O 18 h → 4% SDS 1 h → DNase/NaCl 15 min → dH_2O 18 h → 4% SDS 1 h → DNase/NaCl 15 min	Total ~39 h
Liver	Freeze–thaw −80 °C 24 h → 0.02% Trypsin, 0.05% EGTA, 2 h → dH_2O 15 min → 2X PBS 15 min → TritonX-100, 0.05% EGTA, 1 h → dH_2O 15 min → 2X PBS 15 min → 0.1% PAA 1 h	Total ~60 h
Lung	0.1% SDS 2 h → 1% TritonX-100, 10 min → PBS with antibiotics, 72 h	Total ~74 h
Heart	10 μM adenosine 15 min → 1% SDS 12 h → 1% TritonX-100, 30 min → PBS with antibiotics, 124 h	Total ~137 h

Figure 9.2 A partial list of decellularization methods for the small intestine [47], urinary bladder [37], trachea [135], brain [136], liver [131, 137], lung [132], and heart [138] shows that the optimal decellularization methods depend upon the tissue of origin.

preserving the native ultrastructure and composition of the underlying ECM. Because each tissue has a unique composition of cellular and ECM material, the optimal method for decellularization differs according to the tissue of origin (Figures 9.2 and 9.3).

Even with optimal decellularization, it has been shown that cellular components known to elicit an adverse response are retained in small amounts within scaffolds. The two most well-studied components include the Galα_1-3Galβ_1-4GlcNAcβ-R (α-Gal) epitope and DNA. The α-Gal epitope is known to cause hyperacute rejection of organ transplants [70–73]. However, results from studies comparing allogeneic and xenogeneic α-Gal −/− porcine sources of ECM have shown that the resulting ECM scaffolds elicit no adverse effects upon tissue remodeling [74, 75]. Fragments of DNA have also been shown to remain in scaffolds at low amounts even after decellularization and terminal sterilization processes [18, 76, 77]. DNA fragments of size less than 200 bp generally do not elicit an adverse host response and inhibit tissue remodeling [67]. Additionally, the authors of recent studies have also

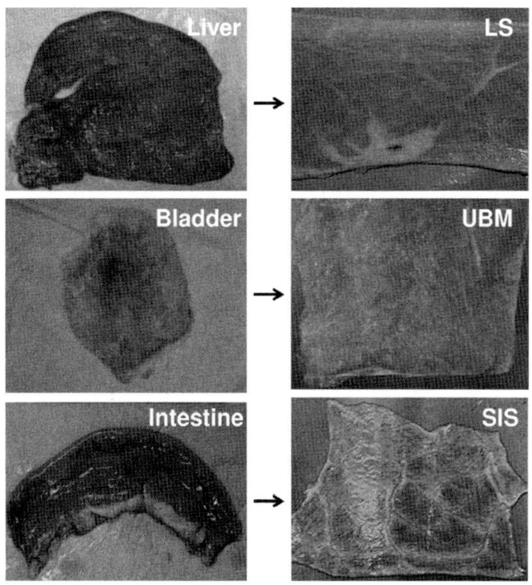

Figure 9.3 A macroscopic examination of three source tissues (liver, bladder, and intestine) before and after decellularization.

identified both intracellular and extracellular antigens ("damage- associated molecular patterns") such as HMGB1, S100, and LPS that are found in decellularized tissues at small levels [78, 79], but their role in mediating the host response to ECM scaffolds is only partially understood. This concept continues to be an intense area of current research.

9.4.2 Modification of ECM scaffolds

Optimal decellularization of a tissue or organ yields an ECM that maintains the composition and ultrastructure of the native tissue. Many tissues such as dermis, small intestine, and urinary bladder are configured as a sheet form prior to decellularization. Because many clinical applications require a 3D structure beyond the two-dimensional (2D) sheet-like form, it is often desirable or necessary to manufacture scaffolds into site-specific forms following the decellularization process.

Intact ECM scaffolds have been molded and vacuum pressed into shapes that include tubes [39], cones [80], and multilaminate sheets [81]. These scaffolds have been utilized in applications such as esophageal repair (tubular) [39], gastro-esophageal junction repair (cone-shaped) [80], and orthopedic applications (multilaminate sheets) [83]. Furthermore, ECM materials can be comminuted into a powder for various purposes [83], or subsequently solubilized to form a hydrogel [84–86]. The versatility of ECM scaffold configuration has enhanced the utility of such scaffolds for tissue engineering and regenerative medicine applications.

Some properties of the native ECM within the tissue/organ, such as the mechanical properties and the susceptibility to degradation, can be altered by chemical, physical, or enzymatic methods. For example, chemical crosslinking is used in the production of many commercially available ECM scaffolds to slow or prevent degradation and increase mechanical strength. Chemicals that are commonly used include carbodiimide and glutaraldehyde, but other chemicals such as genipin have also been used [87, 88]. While it may be desirable to increase the mechanical strength and retention of the ECM scaffold for certain applications, chemical modification invariably is associated with adverse effects upon the host response (i.e. biocompatibility becomes a problem) [61].

9.4.3 Commercial production of ECM scaffolds

ECM scaffolds composed of a single source of extracellular matrix, namely the porcine small intestinal submucosa, have been used in over one million patients [89]. ECM scaffolds are produced by numerous companies for use in a variety of human applications. These scaffolds are harvested from a variety of both allogeneic and xenogeneic tissues including dermis, urinary bladder, small intestine, pericardium, and cardiac valvular tissue. A partial list of commercial products, company, tissue source, format, and clinical application is provided in Table 9.2.

9.5 Mechanisms by which ECM scaffolds promote constructive remodeling

The mechanisms by which ECM scaffolds promote constructive tissue remodeling are still only partially understood, but include release of growth factors and cryptic peptides that promote endogenous stem cell recruitment, angiogenesis, and cell proliferation and differentiation at the site of ECM scaffold implantation. Modulation of the innate immune response has been shown to be a critical component of these functional outcomes.

9.5.1 The normal phases of wound healing in adult mammals

Wound healing in an adult mammal is a well-orchestrated integration of multiple systems within a host that results in quick closure of the wound so as to maintain the integrity of the barrier between the host and the outside world [90]. The phases of wound healing can broadly be divided into four phases (Figure 9.4). The coagulation phase is the initial response to injury. Immediately after injury, hemostasis occurs via local platelet aggregation, fibrin deposition, and activation of the coagulation cascade. The main purpose of this phase is to achieve

Table 9.2 A partial list of commercially available ECM scaffolds

Product	Company	Tissue source	Format	Application
AlloDerm	Lifecell	Human skin	Crosslinked	Soft tissue repair
AlloPatch®	Musculoskeletal Transplant Foundation	Human fascia lata	Crosslinked	Orthopedic applications
Axis™	Mentor	Human dermis	Natural	Pelvic organ prolapsed
CollaMend®	Bard	Porcine dermis	Crosslinked	Soft tissue repair
CuffPatch™	Arthrotek	Porcine small intestinal submucosa (SIS)	Crosslinked	Reinforcement of soft tissues
DurADAPT™	Pegasus Biologicals	Horse pericardium	Crosslinked	Dura repair
Dura-Guard®	Synovis Surgical	Bovine pericardium		Spinal and cranial repair
Durasis®	Cook SIS	Porcine SIS	Natural	Repair dura matter
Durepair®	TEI Biosciences	Fetal bovine skin	Natural	Repair of cranial or spinal dura
FasLata®	Bard	Cadaveric fascia lata	Natural	Soft tissue repair
Graft Jacket®	Wright Medical Tech	Human skin	Crosslinked	Foot ulcers
Oasis®	Healthpoint	Porcine SIS	Natural	Partial and full thickness wounds; superficial and second-degree burns
NeoForm	Mentor Worldwide LLC	Human dermis		Tendon, breast
OrthADAPT™	Pegasus Biologicals	Horse pericardium	Crosslinked	Reinforcement, repair and reconstruction of soft tissue in orthopedics
Pelvicol®	Bard	Porcine dermis	Crosslinked	Soft tissue repair
Peri-Guard®	Synovis Surgical	Bovine pericardium		Pericardial and soft tissue repair
Permacol™	Tissue Science Laboratories	Porcine skin	Crosslinked	Soft connective tissue repair
PriMatrix™	TEI Biosciences	Fetal bovine skin	Natural	Wound management
Restore™	DePuy	Porcine SIS	Natural	Reinforcement of soft tissues
Stratasis®	Cook SIS	Porcine SIS	Natural	Treatment of urinary incontinence
SurgiMend™	TEI Biosciences	Fetal bovine skin	Natural	Surgical repair of damaged or ruptured soft tissue membranes
Surgisis®	Cook SIS	Porcine SIS	Natural	Soft tissue repair and reinforcement
Suspend™	Mentor	Human fascia lata	Natural	Urethral sling
TissueMend®	TEI Biosciences	Fetal bovine skin	Natural	Surgical repair and reinforcement of soft tissue in rotator cuff
Vascu-Guard®	Synovis Surgical	Bovine pericardium		Reconstruction of blood vessels in neck, legs, and arms
Veritas®	Synovis Surgical	Bovine pericardium		Soft tissue repair
Xclma™	Molnlycke	ECM protein, PGA, water		Venous leg ulcers
Xenform™	TEI Biosciences	Fetal bovine skin	Natural	Abdominal and pelvic soft tissue applications
Zimmer®	Tissue Science Laboratories	Porcine dermis	Crosslinked	Orthopedic applications

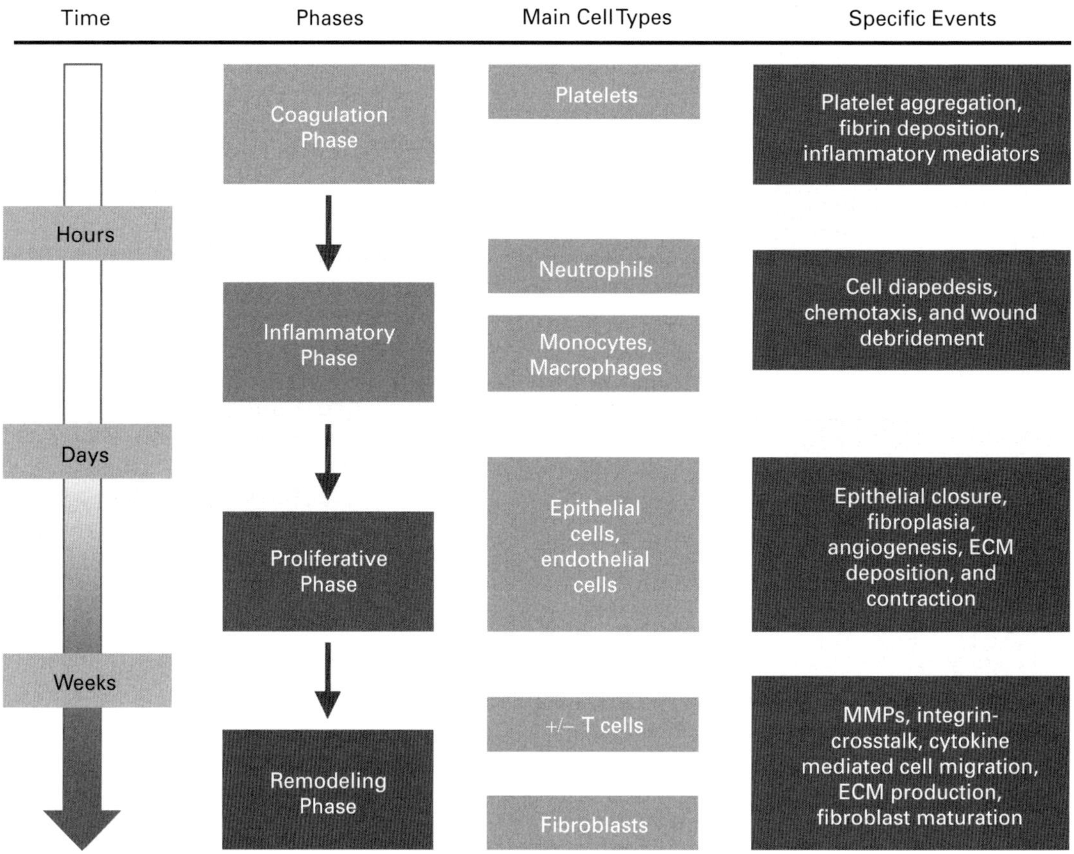

Figure 9.4 A schematic diagram outlining the phases of normal wound healing in adult mammals.

hemostasis and protect against pathogen colonization of the site of injury. This phase culminates in the eventual release of inflammatory cytokines and mediators that then recruit innate immune cells such as neutrophils and monocytes/macrophages to commence the inflammatory phase of wound healing. Neutrophils and monocytes/macrophages are recruited to the site of injury during the inflammatory phase, and they phagocytose cellular debris at a site of injury as well as release paracrine factors that then recruit other cell types [91].

This hemostasis phase eventually gives rise to the proliferative phase of wound healing in which re-epithelialization and angiogenesis occur via migration of epithelial and endothelial cells to the site of injury. Over the course of weeks, wound contraction occurs in the remodeling phase and the extracellular matrix at the site of injury is eventually replaced by ECM deposited by infiltrating fibroblasts and myofibroblasts at the site of injury. In some pathological cases, inflammatory cells such as T cells may be present at later time points after injury, this being a sign of an ongoing chronic inflammatory response that deviates from the normal wound healing response.

9.5.2 The phases of constructive remodeling following ECM scaffold implantation

While the coagulative phases and inflammatory phases still occur following implantation of an ECM

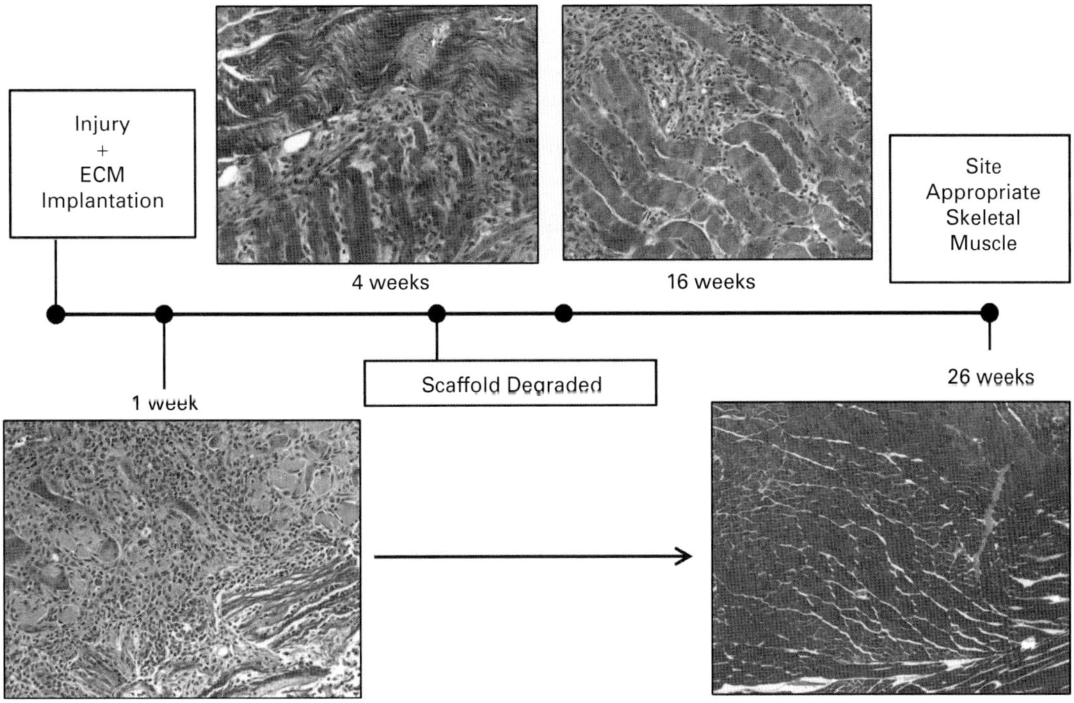

Figure 9.5 The time course of remodeling at a site of ECM scaffold implantation.

scaffold at a site of injury [64, 92], the overall time course of remodeling deviates significantly from the default wound healing response in the later proliferative and remodeling phases. The time course of remodeling has been well documented in a rodent model of abdominal wall injury [60–62, 93] (Figure 9.5). Immediately following excision of the native tissue and ECM implantation, the initial phase of wound healing occurs and results in the recruitment of neutrophils [64]. As early as 48 hours after ECM implantation, the mononuclear cell infiltrate dominates the remodeling site. This cell population can persist for weeks, constituting a distinct departure from the typical mammalian response to injury. Four weeks after injury, the site of ECM scaffold implantation has been replaced with dense, neo-connective tissue deposited by host cells that have infiltrated the scaffold. Importantly, the ECM scaffold is no longer present. Sixteen weeks after implantation, the site of ECM scaffold implantation is populated with vascular structures, small islands of immature muscular tissue (in sites where muscle tissue is appropriate), and growing nerve fibers that histologically co-localize with the small islands of muscle, i.e. the beginning of constructive remodeling. Of note, evidence of constructive remodeling is seen only *after* the scaffold has become no longer histologically identifiable. By 26 weeks after implantation, the site of ECM scaffold implantation has been replaced with site-appropriate, functional muscular tissue that is grossly indistinguishable from the surrounding native muscle [60–62, 93].

From this time-course analysis and other studies, the immune response, mechanotransduction at the site of injury, site-directed recruitment of differentiated and progenitor cells, and rapid degradation and release of bioactive peptides have all been identified as important factors in predicting the outcome of remodeling following implantation of an ECM scaffold.

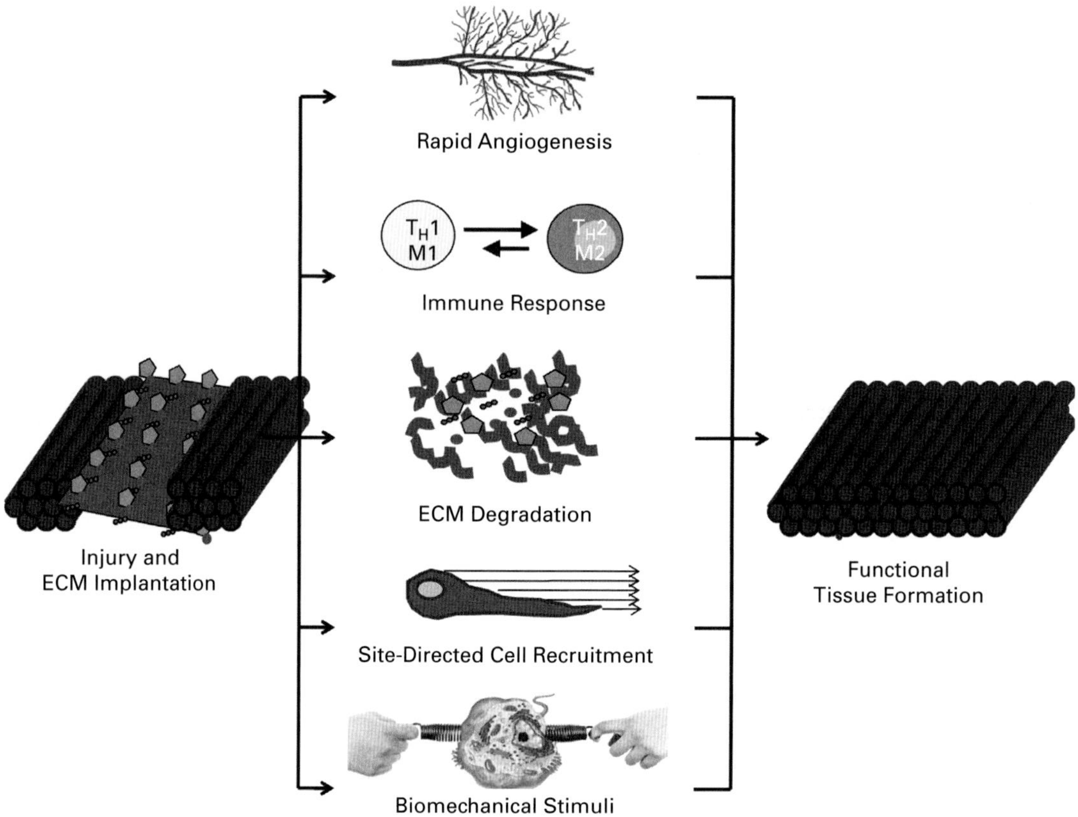

Figure 9.6 A schematic summary of mechanisms by which remodeling ECM scaffolds promote constructive remodeling.

9.5.3 The immune response to ECM scaffold implantation

Neutrophils, monocytes, macrophages, and T cells are found at a site of ECM implantation in vivo [60, 61, 64, 92, 94]. However, the persistence of mononuclear cells at the site of injury for weeks after ECM implantation markedly differs from the time course of normal wound healing at a site of injury. While such a sustained mononuclear response may be considered a chronic inflammatory response as seen in pathological conditions, the sustained mononuclear infiltration in response to ECM scaffold implantation eventually results in constructive remodeling [61], suggesting that mononuclear cells may play a role in mediating this process.

The beneficial effect of a sustained persistence of mononuclear macrophages at a site of ECM scaffold implantation is associated with the polarization of the local immune response toward a more anti-inflammatory, pro-wound-healing phenotype [62]. Immune cells such as T cells and monocytes/macrophages exhibit various phenotypes, or polarizations, that dictate their overall function at a site of injury. For example, T cells are broadly classified into pro-inflammatory (Th1), anti-inflammatory (Th2), or regulatory (Treg) T cells [95]. Likewise, macrophages can broadly be classified into pro-inflammatory M1 macrophages, pro-wound-healing M2 macrophages [96], and regulatory macrophages [97].

Decellularized and unmodified ECM scaffolds that promote constructive remodeling and functional restoration at a site of injury have been shown to elicit a dominant Th2 response in vivo [64].

ECM scaffolds also induce an early and sustained anti-inflammatory, M2 phenotype in the recruited monocytes and macrophages at the site of injury [61, 62]. Removal of the macrophages via depletion of circulating monocytes inhibits the constructive remodeling response to ECM scaffolds and results in fibrous encapsulation [60]. In each case with a poor remodeling outcome, the predominant phenotype of mononuclear phagocytes at the site of ECM implantation is the pro-inflammatory M1 phenotype [63, 94].

9.5.4 Mechanical stimulation and mechanotransduction at the site of ECM implantation

Previous studies have shown that the microenvironment in which the ECM scaffold is placed can influence the overall remodeling outcome. For example, an ECM scaffold derived from the porcine urinary bladder remodels into abdominal wall [63], bladder [98], trachea [99], or myocardium [41] when placed at each respective site of injury. One of the microenvironmental factors that contributes to this phenomenon is the local mechanical force that the ECM scaffold experiences at the site of injury. Via transduction of the biomechanical forces to local cells in contact with the scaffold [33, 100], physiological mechanical loads not only influence cell phenotype but also then promote site-appropriate tissue reconstruction at a site of injury and ECM scaffold implantation [98].

9.5.5 Rapid degradation of the ECM scaffold and release of bioactive peptides

One of the hallmarks of unmodified ECM scaffolds is their rapid degradation in vivo within 60–90 days after implantation [51, 59]. As discussed in the context of the time course of remodeling, the constructive remodeling response only occurs *after* the scaffold has been predominantly degraded. Inhibition of the degradation of the scaffold through any of a number of means, including chemical crosslinking [60, 61] and depletion of host phagocytic cells [60], results in a poor remodeling outcome in vivo. These observations in the time course of remodeling show that rapid degradation of ECM scaffolds is an important prerequisite for constructive remodeling at the site of injury. In fact, scaffold degradation may be the initiating event for all subsequent events at the site of injury that deviate from the normal wound healing response.

One mechanism by which rapid degradation of ECM scaffolds results in constructive remodeling is the release of bioactive cryptic peptides. In addition to the release of sequestered growth factors and cytokines in the ECM, local proteolysis of the ECM scaffolds results in enzymatic digestion of the structural proteins (i.e. collagen, fibronectin, and laminin) which comprise a majority of the ECM scaffold [6]. The resulting degradation products of ECM have been shown to possess novel bioactive properties that are not present in the parent ECM structural proteins. These peptides are called "matricryptic peptides" [101–112]. Antimicrobial activity has been attributed to such peptides in the form of defensins [112], cecropins [113, 114], and magainins [115]. Other matricryptic peptides have been shown to be able to regulate angiogenesis, with separate peptides possessing angiogenic and anti-angiogenic activity [105, 116]. Matricryptic peptides that modulate the local and systemic immune response by modulating phagocytic activity, gene expression, and chemotaxis of various immune cells have also been identified [117]. Within the context of tissue engineering, matricryptic peptides with mitogenic and chemotactic activity for other cell types such as endothelial, Schwann, and smooth muscle cells have been identified [105, 108, 116]. The sustained generation and release of these cryptic peptides from degrading ECM scaffolds is thought to be an important contributing factor to constructive remodeling in vivo.

9.5.6 Site-directed recruitment of progenitor cells

In addition to mononuclear macrophages and circulating immune cells [61, 62], circulating bone-marrow-derived cells are known to partially comprise the dense mononuclear infiltrate that populates the site of ECM implantation [61, 62, 109–111, 118–120]. Although the mechanisms underlying the site-directed accumulation of progenitor-like cells at the site of injury by ECM scaffolds are not well understood, it has been hypothesized that ECM scaffold degradation products may play a potential role in progenitor cell recruitment. In addition to possessing chemotactic properties for site-specific differentiated cells [108, 116], matricryptic peptides also possess chemotactic properties for various progenitor cells [94, 121–124]. These progenitor cells are thought to contribute to constructive remodeling of tissue at a site of ECM scaffold implantation through paracrine immunomodulatory effects [125] as well as through differentiation into functional, site-specific tissue [118, 119, 126].

9.5.7 Rapid angiogenesis

Angiogenesis is implicit in the success of regenerative medicine strategies because it provides the means for nourishment necessary for the anabolic process of tissue ingrowth. In the absence of angiogenesis, lack of sufficient nutrition may lead to failure of the biomaterials to integrate with the surrounding tissue and may eventually lead to necrotic death of the local tissue. However, ECM scaffolds that are not chemically or mechanically modified promote rapid angiogenesis within the 1–3 days following scaffold implantation [54, 61]. In addition to the presence of angiogenic growth factors such as VEGF and bFGF that are rapidly eluted from the scaffold [127], degradation of the scaffold results in sustained release of matricryptic peptides with the ability to regulate angiogenesis [105, 116].

9.6 Tissue engineering of complex tissues via whole organ decellularization

Most applications utilizing biological scaffolds composed of ECM have shown promise primarily for soft tissues [37–39, 41–51, 53–56]. In recent years, a promising approach for constructive remodeling of more complex, 3D structures has emerged. Utilizing anterograde and retrograde perfusion of decellularization agents in whole organs, complete decellularization of organs has been achieved to yield an intact 3D scaffold for tissue engineering of complex organs such as the heart, liver, kidney, and lung [128–134]. Utilizing a combination of these 3D matrices and either select progenitor cell populations or a combination of parenchymal cells, 3D organs have been re-engineered with at least short-term in-vivo function in pre-clinical animal models of orthotopic or heterotropic transplantation [129–132]. It is thought that 3D scaffolds that largely preserve the unique composition and ultrastructure are the ideal substrates for tissue engineering of these whole organs for implantation in vivo. This is an active area of current research efforts, and whole organ decellularization may be a viable strategy for the creation of new organs for transplantation into patients in the future.

9.7 Summary

In summary, the extracellular matrix is an ideal substrate for creating biomaterials for tissue engineering and regenerative medicine applications. When optimally decellularized and not chemically modified, the extracellular matrix largely retains the ultrastructure and composition of the native organ from which it is derived. For this reason, it functions as an inductive template for cell migration, proliferation, and differentiation at a site of injury. Implantation of biological scaffolds composed of extracellular matrix has resulted in constructive remodeling in multiple pre-clinical animal models and human clinical applications. The mechanisms underlying this process are thought to include (1) rapid angiogenesis into the site of injury, (2) local mechanical stimulation, (3) polarization of the host immune response toward a pro-regenerative response, (3) rapid degradation of the ECM scaffold, and (4) site-directed recruitment of differentiated and progenitor cells to the site of injury.

REFERENCES

[1] Rozario, T. and DeSimone, D. W. 2010. The extracellular matrix in development and morphogenesis: a dynamic view. *Dev. Biol.*, **341**(1), 126–40.

[2] Toole, B. P. 2001. Hyaluronan in morphogenesis. *Semin. Cell Dev. Biol.*, **12**(2), 79–87.

[3] Zheng Shu, X., Liu, Y., Palumbo, F. S., Luo, Y. and Prestwich, G. D. 2004. *In situ* crosslinkable hyaluronan hydrogels for tissue engineering. *Biomaterials*, **25**(7–8), 1339–48.

[4] Evanko, S. P., Angello, J. C. and Wight, T. N. 1999. Formation of hyaluronan- and versican-rich pericellular matrix is required for proliferation and migration of vascular smooth muscle cells. *Arterioscler. Thromb. Vasc. Biol.*, **19**(4), 1004–13.

[5] Di Lullo, G. A., Sweeney, S. M., Korkko, J., Ala-Kokko, L. and San Antonio, J. D. 2002. Mapping the ligand-binding sites and disease-associated mutations on the most abundant protein in the human, type I collagen. *J. Biol. Chem.*, **277**(6), 4223–31.

[6] Badylak, S. F. 2002. The extracellular matrix as a scaffold for tissue reconstruction. *Semin. Cell Dev. Biol.*, **13**(5), 377–83.

[7] Hahn, E., Wick, G., Pencev, D. and Timpl, R. 1980. Distribution of basement membrane proteins in normal and fibrotic human liver: collagen type IV, laminin, and fibronectin. *Gut*, **21**(1), 63–71.

[8] Munakata, H., Takagaki, K., Majima, M. and Endo, M. 1999. Interaction between collagens and glycosaminoglycans investigated using a surface plasmon resonance biosensor. *Glycobiology*, **9**(10), 1023–7.

[9] Sakai, L. Y., Keene, D. R., Morris, N. P. and Burgeson, R. E. 1986. Type VII collagen is a major structural component of anchoring fibrils. *J. Cell Biol.*, **103**(4), 1577–86.

[10] Rogers, S. L., Edson, K. J., Letourneau, P. and McLoon, S. C. 1986. Distribution of laminin in the developing peripheral nervous system of the chick. *Dev. Biol.*, **113**(2), 429–35.

[11] Zagris, N., Chung, A. E. and Stavridis, V. 2000. Differential expression of laminin genes in early chick embryo. *Int. J. Dev. Biol.*, **44**(7), 815–18.

[12] Wan, Y. J., Wu, T. C., Chung, A. E. and Damjanov, I. 1984. Monoclonal antibodies to laminin reveal the heterogeneity of basement membranes in the developing and adult mouse tissues. *J. Cell Biol.*, **98**(3), 971–9.

[13] Liesi, P., Kaakkola, S., Dahl, D. and Vaheri, A. 1984. Laminin is induced in astrocytes of adult brain by injury. *EMBO J.*, **3**(3), 683–6.

[14] Powell, S. K., Williams, C. C., Nomizu, M., Yamada, Y. and Kleinman, H. K. 1998. Laminin-like proteins are differentially regulated during cerebellar development and stimulate granule cell neurite outgrowth in vitro. *J. Neurosci. Res.*, **54**(2), 233–47.

[15] Fishman, R. B. and Hatten, M. E. 1993. Multiple receptor systems promote CNS neural migration. *J. Neurosci.*, **13**(8), 3485–95.

[16] Bonewald, L. F. 1999. Regulation and regulatory activities of transforming growth factor beta. *Crit. Rev. Eukaryot. Gene Expr.*, **9**(1), 33–44.

[17] Kagami, S., Kondo, S., Löster, K. *et al.* 1998. Collagen type I modulates the platelet-derived growth factor (PDGF) regulation of the growth and expression of β_1 integrins by rat mesangial cells. *Biochem. Biophys. Res. Commun.*, **252**(3), 728–32.

[18] Roberts, R., Gallagher, J., Spooncer, E. *et al.* 1988. Heparan sulphate bound growth factors: a mechanism for stromal cell mediated haemopoiesis. *Nature*, **332**(6162), 376–8.

[19] Stolz, D. B., Mars, W. M., Petersen, B. E., Kim, T.-H. and Michalopoulos, G. K. 1999. Growth factor signal transduction immediately after two-thirds partial hepatectomy in the rat. *Cancer Res.*, **59**(16), 3954–60.

[20] Michalopoulos, G. K. 1990. Liver regeneration: molecular mechanisms of growth control. *FASEB J.*, **4**(2), 176–87.

[21] Nakamura, T., Sakai, K. and Matsumoto, K. 2011. Hepatocyte growth factor twenty years on: much more than a growth factor. *J. Gastroenterol. Hepatol.*, **26**(Suppl. 1), 188–202.

[22] Rozario, T. and DeSimone, D. W. 2010. The extracellular matrix in development and morphogenesis: a dynamic view. *Dev. Biol.*, **341**(1), 126–40.

[23] Lockhart, M., Wirring, E., Phelps, A. and Wessels, A. 2011. Extracellular matrix and heart development. *Birth Defects Res. A Clin. Mol. Teratol.*, **91**(6), 535–50.

[24] Little, C. D. and Rongish, B. J. 1995. The extracellular matrix during heart development. *Experientia*, **51**(9–10), 873–82.

[25] Borg, T. K., Raso, D. S. and Terracio, L. 1990. Potential role of the extracellular matrix in postseptation development of the heart. *Ann. NY Acad. Sci.*, **588**, 87–92.

[26] Perris, R. and Perissinotto, D. 2000. Role of the extracellular matrix during neural crest cell migration. *Mech. Dev.*, **95**(1–2), 3–21.

[27] Werb, Z. and Chin, J. R. 1998. Extracellular matrix remodeling during morphogenesis. *Ann. NY Acad. Sci.*, **857**, 110–18.

[28] Rauch, U. and Schafer, K. H. 2003. The extracellular matrix and its role in cell migration and development of the enteric nervous system. *Eur. J. Pediatr. Surg.*, **13**(3), 158–62.

[29] Parikh, D. H., Tam, P. K., Van Velzen, D. and Edgar, D. 1992. Quantitative and qualitative analysis of the extracellular matrix protein, laminin, in Hirschsprung's disease. *J. Pediatr. Surg.*, **27**(8), 991–5; discussion 995–6.

[30] Margadant, C., Raymond, K., Kreft, M. *et al.* 2009. Integrin $\alpha_3\beta_1$ inhibits directional migration and wound re-epithelialization in the skin. *J. Cell Sci.*, **122**(Part 2), 278–88.

[31] Woodley, D. T., Bachmann, P. M. and O'Keefe, E. J. 1991. The role of matrix components in human keratinocyte re-epithelialization. *Prog. Clin. Biol. Res.*, **365**, 129–40.

[32] Karamichos, D., Brown, R. A. and Mudera, V. 2007. Collagen stiffness regulates cellular contraction and matrix remodeling gene expression. *J. Biomed. Mater. Res. A*, **83**(3), 887–94.

[33] Gilbert, T. W., Stewart-Akers, A. M., Sydeski, J. *et al.* 2007. Gene expression by fibroblasts seeded on small intestinal submucosa and subjected to cyclic stretching. *Tissue Eng.*, **13**(6), 1313–23.

[34] Barnes, C. A., Brison, J., Michel, R. *et al.* 2011. The surface molecular functionality of decellularized extracellular matrices. *Biomaterials*, **32**(1), 137–43.

[35] Brown, B. N., Barnes, C. A., Kasick, R. T. *et al.* 2010. Surface characterization of extracellular matrix scaffolds. *Biomaterials*, **31**(3), 428–37.

[36] Ackbar, R., Ainoedhofer, H., Gugatschka, M. and Saxena, A. K. 2012. Decellularized ovine esophageal mucosa for esophageal tissue engineering. *Technol. Health Care*, **20**(3), 215–23.

[37] Badylak, S., Meurling, S., Chen, M., Spievack, A. and Simmons-Byrd, A. 2000. Resorbable bioscaffold for esophageal repair in a dog model. *J. Pediatr. Surg.*, **35**(7), 1097–103.

[38] Lopes, M. F., Cabrita, A., Ilharco, J. *et al.* 2006. Esophageal replacement in rat using porcine intestinal submucosa as a patch or a tube-shaped graft. *Dis. Esophagus*, **19**(4), 254–9.

[39] Badylak, S. F., Vorp, D. A., Spievack, A. R. *et al.* 2005. Esophageal reconstruction with ECM and muscle tissue in a dog model. *J. Surg. Res.*, **128**(1), 87–97.

[40] Badylak, S. F., Tullius, R., Kokini, K. *et al.* 2011. Esophageal preservation in five male patients after endoscopic inner-layer circumferential resection in the setting of superficial cancer: a regenerative medicine approach with a biologic scaffold. *Tissue Eng. Part A*, **17**(11–12), 1643–50.

[41] Kochupura, P. V., Azeloğlu, E. U., Kelly, D. J. *et al.* 2005. Tissue-engineered myocardial patch derived from extracellular matrix provides regional mechanical function. *Circulation*, **112**(9 Suppl.), I144–9.

[42] Badylak, S. F., Kochupura, P. V., Cohen, I. S. *et al.* 2006. The use of extracellular matrix as an inductive scaffold for the partial replacement of functional myocardium. *Cell Transplant.*, **15**(Suppl. 1), S29–40.

[43] Robinson, K. A., Li, J., Mathison, M. *et al.* 2005. Extracellular matrix scaffold for cardiac repair. *Circulation*, **112**(9 Suppl.), I135–43.

[44] Ota, T., Taketani, S., Iwai, S. *et al.* 2007. Electromechanical characterization of a tissue-engineered myocardial patch derived from extracellular matrix. *J. Thorac. Cardiovasc. Surg.*, **133**(4), 979–85.

[45] Lantz, G. C., Badylak, S. F., Coffey, A. C., Geddes, L. A. and Sandusky, G. E. 1992. Small intestinal submucosa as a superior vena cava graft in the dog. *J. Surg. Res.*, **53**(2), 175–81.

[46] Badylak, S. F., Lantz, G. C., Coffey, A. *et al.* 1989. Small intestinal submucosa as a large-diameter vascular graft in the dog. *J. Surg. Res.*, **47**(1), 74–80.

[47] Lantz, G. C., Badylak, S. F., Coffey, A. C. *et al.* 1990. Small intestinal submucosa as a small-diameter arterial graft in the dog. *J. Invest. Surg.*, **3**(3), 217–27.

[48] Kropp, B. P., Eppley, B. L., Prevel, C. D. *et al.* 1995. Experimental assessment of small intestinal submucosa as a bladder wall substitute. *Urology*, **46**(3), 396–400.

[49] Kropp, B. P., Rippy, M. K., Badylak, S. F. *et al.* 1996. Regenerative urinary bladder augmentation using small intestinal submucosa: urodynamic and histopathologic assessment in long-term canine bladder augmentations. *J. Urol.*, **155**(6), 2098–104.

[50] Pope, J. C. IV, Davis, M. M., Smith, E. R. Jr. *et al.* 1997. The ontogeny of canine small intestinal submucosa regenerated bladder. *J. Urol.*, **158**(3, Part 2), 1105–10.

[51] Record, R. D., Hillegonds, D., Simmons, C. *et al.* 2001. In vivo degradation of ^{14}C-labeled small intestinal submucosa (SIS) when used for urinary bladder repair. *Biomaterials*, **22**(19), 2653–9.

[52] Schwarz, S., Koerber, L., Elsaesser, A. F. *et al.* 2012. decellularized cartilage matrix as a novel biomatrix for cartilage tissue-engineering applications. *Tissue Eng. Part A*, **18**(21–22), 2195–209.

[53] Clarke, K. M., Lantz, G. C., Salisbury, S. K. *et al.* 1996. Intestine submucosa and polypropylene mesh for abdominal wall repair in dogs. *J. Surg. Res.*, **60**(1), 107–14.

[54] Badylak, S. , F., Kokini, K., Tullius, B., Simmons-Byrd, A. and Morff, R. *et al.* 2002. Morphologic study of small intestinal submucosa as a body wall repair device. *J. Surg. Res.*, **103**(2), 190–202.

[55] Badylak, S. , F., Kokini, K., Tullius, B. and Whitson, B. 2001. Strength over time of a resorbable bioscaffold for

body wall repair in a dog model. *J. Surg. Res.*, **99**(2), 282–7.

[56] Prevel, C. D., Eppley, B. L., Summerlin, D. J. *et al.* 1995. Small intestinal submucosa: utilization for repair of rodent abdominal wall defects. *Ann. Plast. Surg.*, **35**(4), 374–80.

[57] Mase, V. J., Jr., Hsu, J. R., Wolf, S. E. *et al.* 2010. Clinical application of an acellular biologic scaffold for surgical repair of a large, traumatic quadriceps femoris muscle defect. *Orthopedics*, **33**(7), 511.

[58] Gilbert, T. W., Stewart-Akers, A. M. and Badylak, S. F. 2007. A quantitative method for evaluating the degradation of biologic scaffold materials. *Biomaterials*, **28**(2), 147–50.

[59] Gilbert, T. W., Stewart-Akers, A. M., Simmons-Byrd, A. and Badylak, S. F. 2007. Degradation and remodeling of small intestinal submucosa in canine Achilles tendon repair. *J. Bone Joint Surg. Am.*, **89**(3), 621–30.

[60] Valentin, J. E., Stewart-Akers, A. M., Gilbert, T. W. and Badylak, S. F. 2009. Macrophage participation in the degradation and remodeling of extracellular matrix scaffolds. *Tissue Eng. Part A*, **15**(7), 1687–94.

[61] Valentin, J. E., Badylak, J. S., McCabe, G. P. and Badylak, S. F. 2006. Extracellular matrix bioscaffolds for orthopaedic applications. A comparative histologic study. *J. Bone Joint Surg. Am.*, **88**(12), 2673–86.

[62] Badylak, S. F., Valentin, J. E., Ravindra, A. K., McCabe, G. P. and Stewart-Akers, A. M. 2008. Macrophage phenotype as a determinant of biologic scaffold remodeling. *Tissue Eng. Part A*, **14**(11), 1835–42.

[63] Brown, B. N., Valentin, J. E., Stewart-Akers, A. M., McCabe, G. P. and Badylak, S. F. 2009. Macrophage phenotype and remodeling outcomes in response to biologic scaffolds with and without a cellular component. *Biomaterials*, **30**(8), 1482–91.

[64] Allman, A. J., McPherson, T. B., Badylak, S. F. *et al.* 2001. Xenogeneic extracellular matrix grafts elicit a Th2-restricted immune response. *Transplantation*, **71**(11), 1631–40.

[65] Allman, A. J., McPherson, T. B., Merrill, L. C., Badylak, S. F. and Metzger, D. W. 2002. The Th2-restricted immune response to xenogeneic small intestinal submucosa does not influence systemic protective immunity to viral and bacterial pathogens. *Tissue Eng.*, **8**(1), 53–62.

[66] Turner, N. J. and Badylak, S. F. 2012. Regeneration of skeletal muscle. *Cell Tissue Res.*, **347**(3), 759–74.

[67] Gilbert, T. W., Freund, J. M. and Badylak, S. F. 2009. Quantification of DNA in biologic scaffold materials. *J. Surg. Res.*, **152**(1), 135–9.

[68] Gilbert, T. W., Sellaro, T. L. and Badylak, S. F. 2006. Decellularization of tissues and organs. *Biomaterials*, **27**(19), 3675–83.

[69] Crapo, P. M., Gilbert, T. W. and Badylak, S. F. 2011. An overview of tissue and whole organ decellularization processes. *Biomaterials*, **32**(12), 3233–43.

[70] Collins, B. H., Chari, R. S., Magee, J. C. *et al.* 1994. Mechanisms of injury in porcine livers perfused with blood of patients with fulminant hepatic failure. *Transplantation*, **58**(11), 1162–71.

[71] Cooper, D. K., Good, A. H., Koren, E. *et al.* 1993. Identification of ′-galactosyl and other carbohydrate epitopes that are bound by human anti-pig antibodies: relevance to discordant xenografting in man. *Transpl. Immunol.*, **1**(3), 198–205.

[72] Galili, U., Mandrell, R. E., Hamadeh, R. M. *et al.* 1985. Human natural anti-α-galactosyl IgG. II. The specific recognition of α (1–3)-linked galactose residues. *J. Exp. Med.*, **162**(2), 573–82.

[73] Oriol, R., Ye, Y., Koren, E. and Cooper, D. K. 1993. Carbohydrate antigens of pig tissues reacting with human natural antibodies as potential targets for hyperacute vascular rejection in pig-to-man organ xenotransplantation. *Transplantation*, **56**(6), 1433–42.

[74] Daly, K., Stewart-Akers, A. M., Hara, H. *et al.* 2009. Effect of the αGal epitope on the response to small intestinal submucosa extracellular matrix in a nonhuman primate model. *Tissue Eng. Part A*, **15**(12), 3877–88.

[75] Raeder, R. H., Badylak, S. F., Sheehan, C., Kallakury, B. and Metzger, D. W. 2002. Natural anti-galactose $\alpha_{1,3}$ galactose antibodies delay, but do not prevent the acceptance of extracellular matrix xenografts. *Transpl. Immunol.*, **10**(1), 15–24.

[76] Derwin, K. A., Baker, A. R., Spragg, R. K., Leigh, D. R. and Iannotti, J. P. 2006. Commercial extracellular matrix scaffolds for rotator cuff tendon repair. Biomechanical, biochemical, and cellular properties. *J. Bone Joint Surg. Am.*, **88**(12), 2665–72.

[77] Zheng, M. H., Chen, J., Kirilak, Y. *et al.* 2005. Porcine small intestine submucosa (SIS) is not an acellular collagenous matrix and contains porcine DNA: possible implications in human implantation. *J. Biomed. Mater. Res. B Appl. Biomater.*, **73**(1), 61–7.

[78] Daly, K. A., Liu, S. Agrawal , V. *et al.* 2012. Damage associated molecular patterns within xenogeneic biologic scaffolds and their effects on host remodeling. *Biomaterials*, **33**(1), 91–101.

[79] Daly, K. A., Liu, S., Agrawal, V. *et al.* 2012. The host response to endotoxin-contaminated dermal matrix. *Tissue Eng. Part A*, **18**(11–12), 1293–303.

[80] Nieponice, A., Gilbert, T. W. and Badylak, S. F. 2006. Reinforcement of esophageal anastomoses with an extracellular matrix scaffold in a canine model. *Ann. Thorac. Surg.*, **82**(6), 2050–8.

[81] Freytes, D. O., Badylak, S. F., Webster, T. J., Geddes, L. A. and Rundell, A. E. 2004. Biaxial strength of multi-laminated extracellular matrix scaffolds. *Biomaterials*, **25**(12), 2353–61.

[82] Dejardin, L. M., Arnoczky, S. P., Ewers, B. J., Haut, R. C. and Clarke, R. B. 2001. Tissue-engineered rotator cuff tendon using porcine small intestine submucosa. Histologic and mechanical evaluation in dogs. *Am. J. Sports Med.*, **29**(2), 175–84.

[83] Gilbert, T. W., Stolz, D. B., Biancaniello, F., Simmons-Byrd, A. and Badylak, S. F. 2005. Production and characterization of ECM powder: implications for tissue engineering applications. *Biomaterials*, **26**(12), 1431–5.

[84] Freytes, D. O., Martin, J., Velankar, S. S., Lee, A. S. and Badylak, S. F. 2008. Preparation and rheological characterization of a gel form of the porcine urinary bladder matrix. *Biomaterials*, **29**(11), 1630–7.

[85] Wolf, M. T., Daly, K. A., Brennan-Pierce, E. P. *et al.* 2012. A hydrogel derived from decellularized dermal extracellular matrix. *Biomaterials*, **33**(29), 7028–38.

[86] Seif-Naraghi, S. B., Horn, D., Schup-Magoffin, P. A. and Christman, K. L. 2012. Injectable extracellular matrix derived hydrogel provides a platform for enhanced retention and delivery of a heparin-binding growth factor. *Acta Biomater.*, **8**(10), 3695–703.

[87] Sung, H. W., Chang, W. H., Ma, C. Y. and Lee, M. H. 2003. Crosslinking of biological tissues using genipin and/or carbodiimide. *J. Biomed. Mater. Res. A*, **64**(3), 427–38.

[88] Sung, H. W., Chang, Y., Liang, I. L., Chang, W. H. and Chen, Y. C. 2000. Fixation of biological tissues with a naturally occurring crosslinking agent: fixation rate and effects of pH, temperature, and initial fixative concentration. *J. Biomed. Mater. Res.*, **52**(1), 77–87.

[89] Badylak, S. F. 2007. The extracellular matrix as a biologic scaffold material. *Biomaterials*, **28**(25), 3587–93.

[90] Falanga, V. 2005. Wound healing and its impairment in the diabetic foot. *Lancet*, **366**(9498), 1736–43.

[91] Lolmede, K., Campana, L., Vezzoli, M. *et al.* 2009. Inflammatory and alternatively activated human macrophages attract vessel-associated stem cells, relying on separate HMGB1- and MMP-9-dependent pathways. *J. Leukoc. Biol.*, **85**(5), 779–87.

[92] Wokalek, H. and Ruh, H. 1991. Time course of wound healing. *J. Biomater. Appl.*, **5**(4), 337–62.

[93] Valentin, J. E., Turner, N. J., Gilbert, T. W. and Badylak, S. F. 2010. Functional skeletal muscle formation with a biologic scaffold. *Biomaterials*, **31**(29), 7475–84.

[94] Crisan, M., Yap, S., Casteilla, L. *et al.* 2008. A perivascular origin for mesenchymal stem cells in multiple human organs. *Cell Stem Cell*, **3**(3), 301–13.

[95] Gatenby, P. A., Callard, R. E. and Basten, A. 1984. T cells, T cell subsets and immunoregulation. *Aust. NZ J. Med.*, **14**(1), 89–96.

[96] Mantovani, A., Sica, A., Sozzani, S. *et al.* 2004. The chemokine system in diverse forms of macrophage activation and polarization. *Trends Immunol.*, **25**(12), 677–86.

[97] Mosser, D. M. and Zhang, X. 2008. Activation of murine macrophages. In *Current Protocols in Immunology*. New York: John Wiley, Unit 14 2.

[98] Boruch, A. V., Nieponice, A., Qureshi, I. R., Gilbert, T. W. and Badylak, S. F. 2010. Constructive remodeling of biologic scaffolds is dependent on early exposure to physiologic bladder filling in a canine partial cystectomy model. *J. Surg. Res.*, **161**(2), 217–25.

[99] Gilbert, T. W., Gilbert, S., Madden, M., Reynolds, S. D. and Badylak, S. F. 2008. Morphologic assessment of extracellular matrix scaffolds for patch tracheoplasty in a canine model. *Ann. Thorac. Surg.*, **86**(3), 967–74; discussion 967–74.

[100] Androjna, C., Spragg, R. K. and Derwin, K. A. 2007. Mechanical conditioning of cell-seeded small intestine submucosa: a potential tissue-engineering strategy for tendon repair. *Tissue Eng.*, **13**(2), 233–43.

[101] Autelitano, D. J., Rajic, A., Smith, A. I. *et al.* 2006. The cryptome: a subset of the proteome, comprising cryptic peptides with distinct bioactivities. *Drug Discov. Today*, **11**(7–8), 306–14.

[102] Mukai, H., Seki, T., Nakano, H. *et al.* 2009. Mitocryptide-2: purification, identification, and characterization of a novel cryptide that activates neutrophils. *J. Immunol.*, **182**(8), 5072–80.

[103] Mukai, H., Hokari, Y., Seki, T. *et al.* 2008. Discovery of mitocryptide-1, a neutrophil-activating cryptide from healthy porcine heart. *J. Biol. Chem.*, **283**(45), 30596–605.

[104] Davis, G. E., Matricryptic sites control tissue injury responses in the cardiovascular system: relationships

to pattern recognition receptor regulated events. *J. Mol. Cell Cardiol.*, 48(3), 454–60.

[105] Davis, G. E., Bayless, K. J., Davis, M. J. and Meininger, G. A. 2000. Regulation of tissue injury responses by the exposure of matricryptic sites within extracellular matrix molecules. *Am. J. Pathol.*, **156**(5), 1489–98.

[106] Ng, J. H. and Ilag, L. L. 2006. Cryptic protein fragments as an emerging source of peptide drugs. *IDrugs*, **9**(5), 343–6.

[107] Pimenta, D. C. and Lebrun, I. 2007. Cryptides: buried secrets in proteins. *Peptides*, **28**(12), 2403–10.

[108] Agrawal, V., Brown, B. N., Beattie, A. J., Gilbert, T. W. and Badylak, S. F. 2009. Evidence of innervation following extracellular matrix scaffold-mediated remodelling of muscular tissues. *J. Tissue Eng. Regen. Med.*, **3** (8), 590–600.

[109] Agrawal, V., Johnson, S. A., Reing, J. *et al.* 2010. Epimorphic regeneration approach to tissue replacement in adult mammals. *Proc. Nat. Acad. Sci. USA*, **107**(8), 3351–5.

[110] Agrawal, V., Kelly, J., Tottey, S. *et al.* 2011. An isolated cryptic peptide influences osteogenesis and bone remodeling in an adult mammalian model of digit amputation. *Tissue Eng. Part A*, **17**(23–24), 3033–44.

[111] Agrawal, V., Tottey, S., Johnson, S. A. *et al.* 2011. Recruitment of progenitor cells by an extracellular matrix cryptic peptide in a mouse model of digit amputation. *Tissue Eng. Part A*, **17**(19–20), 2435–43.

[112] Ganz, T. 2003. Defensins: antimicrobial peptides of innate immunity. *Nature Rev. Immunol.*, **3**(9), 710–20.

[113] Moore, A. J., Beazley, W. D., Bibby, M. C. and Devine, D. A. 1996. Antimicrobial activity of cecropins. *J. Antimicrob. Chemother.*, **37**(6), 1077–89.

[114] Moore, A. J., Devine, D. A. and Bibby, M. C. 1994. Preliminary experimental anticancer activity of cecropins. *Pept. Res.*, **7**(5), 265–9.

[115] Berkowitz, B. A., Bevins, C. L. and Zasloff, M. A. 1990. Magainins: a new family of membrane-active host defense peptides. *Biochem. Pharmacol.*, **39**(4), 625–9.

[116] Li, F., Li, W., Johnson, S. *et al.* 2004. Low-molecular-weight peptides derived from extracellular matrix as chemoattractants for primary endothelial cells. *Endothelium*, **11**(3–4), 199–206.

[117] Adair-Kirk, T. L. and Senior, R. M. 2008. Fragments of extracellular matrix as mediators of inflammation. *Int. J. Biochem. Cell. Biol.*, **40**(6–7), 1101–10.

[118] Badylak, S. F., Park, K., Peppas, N., McCabe, G. and Yoder, M. 2001. Marrow-derived cells populate scaffolds composed of xenogeneic extracellular matrix. *Exp. Hematol.*, **29**(11), 1310–18.

[119] Zantop, T., Gilbert, T. W., Yoder, M. C. and Badylak, S. F. 2006. Extracellular matrix scaffolds are repopulated by bone marrow-derived cells in a mouse model of achilles tendon reconstruction. *J. Orthop. Res.*, **24**(6), 1299–309.

[120] Agrawal, V., Siu, B. F., Chao, H. *et al.* 2012. Partial characterization of the Sox2+ cell population in an adult murine model of digit amputation. *Tissue Eng. Part A*, **18**(13–14), 1454–63.

[121] Reing, J. E., Zhang, L., Myers-Irvin, J. *et al.* 2009. Degradation products of extracellular matrix affect cell migration and proliferation. *Tissue Eng. Part A*, **15**(3), 605–14.

[122] Clark, L. D., Clark, R. K. and Heber-Katz, E. 1998. A new murine model for mammalian wound repair and regeneration. *Clin. Immunol. Immunopathol.*, **88**(1), 35–45.

[123] Brennan, E. P., Tang, X. H., Stewart-Akers, A. M., Gudas, L. J. and Badylak, S. F. 2008. Chemoattractant activity of degradation products of fetal and adult skin extracellular matrix for keratinocyte progenitor cells. *J. Tissue Eng. Regen. Med.*, **2**(8), 491–8.

[124] Tottey, S., Corselli, M., Jeffries, E. M. *et al.* 2011. Extracellular matrix degradation products and low-oxygen conditions enhance the regenerative potential of perivascular stem cells. *Tissue Eng. Part A*, **17**(1–2), 37–44.

[125] Chen, P. M., Yen, M. L., Liu, K. J. *et al.* 2011. Immunomodulatory properties of human adult and fetal multipotent mesenchymal stem cells. *J. Biomed. Sci.*, **18**, 49.

[126] Becerra-Bayona, S., Guiza-Arguello, V., Qu, X., Munoz-Pinto, D. J. and Hahn, M. S. 2012. Influence of select extracellular matrix proteins on mesenchymal stem cell osteogenic commitment in 3D contexts. *Acta Biomater.*, **8**(12), 4397–404.

[127] Chun, S. Y., Lim, G. J., Kwon, T. G. *et al.* 2007. Identification and characterization of bioactive factors in bladder submucosa matrix. *Biomaterials*, **28**(29), 4251–6.

[128] Sullivan, D. C., Mirmalek-Sani, S. H., Deegan, D. B. *et al.* 2012. Decellularization methods of porcine kidneys for whole organ engineering using a high-throughput system. *Biomaterials*, **33**(31), 7756–64.

[129] Uygun, B. E., Soto-Gutierrez, A., Yagi, H. *et al.* 2010. Organ reengineering through development of a transplantable recellularized liver graft using decellularized liver matrix. *Nature Med.*, **16**(7), 814–20.

[130] Ott, H. C., Clippinger, B., Conrad, C. *et al.* 2010. Regeneration and orthotopic transplantation of a bioartificial lung. *Nature Med.*, **16**(8), 927–33.

[131] Soto-Gutierrez, A., Zhang, L., Medberry, C. *et al.* 2011. A whole-organ regenerative medicine approach for liver replacement. *Tissue Eng. Part C Methods*, **17**(6), 677–86.

[132] Petersen, T. H., Calle, E. A., Zhao, L. *et al.* 2010. Tissue-engineered lungs for in vivo implantation. *Science*, **329** (5991), 538–41.

[133] Orlando, G., Farney, A. C., Iskandar, S. S. *et al.* 2012. Production and implantation of renal extracellular matrix scaffolds from porcine kidneys as a platform for renal bioengineering investigations. *Ann. Surg.*, **256**(2), 363–70.

[134] Lu, H., Hoshiba, T., Kawazoe, N. and Chen G. 2012. Comparison of decellularization techniques for preparation of extracellular matrix scaffolds derived from three-dimensional cell culture. *J. Biomed. Mater. Res. A*, **100**(9), 2507–16.

[135] Baiguera, S., Jungebluth, P., Burns, A. *et al.* 2011. Tissue engineered human tracheas for in vivo implantation. *Biomaterials*, **31**(34), 8931–8.

[136] Ribatti, D., Conconi, M. T., Nico, B. *et al.* 2003. Angiogenic response induced by acellular brain scaffolds grafted onto the chick embryo chorioallantoic membrane. *Brain Res.*, **989**(1), 9–15.

[137] Evans, D. W., Moran, E. C., Baptista, P. M., Soker, S. and Sparks, J. L. 2013. Scale-dependent mechanical properties of native and decellularized liver tissue. *Biomech. Model. Mechanobiol.*, **12**(3), 569–80.

[138] Ott, H. C., Matthiesen, T. S., Goh, S. K. *et al.* 2008. Perfusion-decellularized matrix: using nature's platform to engineer a bioartificial heart. *Nature Med.*, **14**(2), 213–21.

10

Bioceramic scaffolds

Zhanwen Xiao, Zhe Wang, Bangcheng Yang and Xingdong Zhang

10.1 Introduction

Global demand for bone grafts has been increasing rapidly in recent years. In particular, an increase in the elderly population worldwide at an annual rate of more than 5% has led to a rapid increase in the bone-diseased population because the elderly suffer easily from osteoporotic fractures, degenerative scoliosis, and degenerative spondylolisthesis [1].

Bone is a complex biomineralized organ with an intricate hierarchical microstructure assembled through the deposition of apatite minerals on collagenous matrix [2], and is able to self-heal a small defect. However, the self-healing is less effective for a large defect. For this, bone grafting is required in orthopaedic surgery.

Bone grafting is a surgical procedure that introduces new bone or a substitution material (bone graft) into defects in bone or around broken bone to help bone healing. Depending on the source of bone grafts, they may be roughly divided into autologous bone grafts (autografts), allografts and artificial (synthetic) bone grafts. These bone grafts have their own particular advantages and drawbacks. Theoretically, an autograft should be the best choice because the bone graft is the patient's own bone, taken frequently from his/her hip bone or pelvis, which renders clear advantages such as a mechanical match with the damaged bone, excellent osteogenic potential, and immune safety [3]. Nevertheless, the principal disadvantage of using autograft bone is that the patient needs to bear additional chronic pain at the incision site, runs potential risks such as infection, additional blood loss, and morbidity, and must bear a longer operation duration and higher costs [4]. Therefore, the other approaches are becoming popular.

Allograft bone is taken from a bone tissue bank where lots of bones from donors (usually dead persons) have been stored frozen. As an alternative to autografting, allografting has distinct advantages, such as simplicity, avoidance of morbidity, and adequacy for of defects various sizes, but one also runs increasing risks of immune incompatibility, bacterial infection, and viral transmission, and it is less effective than autografting [5]. In that case, for large bone defects, artificial prosthetic appliances made of titanium or alumina have been chosen as bone substitutes in the hope of replacing autografting or allografting [6].

An artificial bone graft is commonly created in vitro by using a bone tissue engineering technique. The tissue-engineered bone graft is actually composed of bone cells, usually mesenchymal stem cells (MSCs) and a three-dimensional (3D) porous support (called a scaffold) that mimics bone structure and serves as a temporary matrix for bone cell proliferation, extracellular matrix deposition, and subsequent blood vessel ingrowth. In addition, bone morphogenic proteins (BMPs) are commonly introduced into the porous scaffold to differentiate the stem cells into the osteogenic lineage [7]. So far, there has been a growing body of clinical evidence to demonstrate that good bone repair, comparable to that of allograft bone, can be achieved. Thus, artificial bone grafting is believed to be a promising alternative to allografting and autografting [8–11]. The primary advantages of using synthetic bone grafts include the low risk of disease transmission and the fact that there will be no shortage of supply. Nevertheless, the disadvantages are also evident, such as poor mechanical strength and the need for exogenous growth factors.

More encouragingly, some bare ceramic scaffolds in which there are neither bone cells nor exogenous growth factors have recently been found to play an almost equally good role in bone grafting in comparison with engineered bone grafts when implanted into an animal's bone-defect sites [12–15] or even non-bone sites [16–20]. This phenomenon is called osteoinduction in which osteogenesis occurred. The naturally occurring process in a bone fracture healing process could also be seen in the implanted ceramic scaffolds, strongly implying that it is possible to realize bone grafting by directly implanting an appropriate bioceramic scaffold rather than the engineered bone graft.

In principle, an ideal bone tissue scaffold must be biocompatible, bioactive, biodegradable, and osteoinductive, but no bioceramic scaffold can meet all the requirements. Nevertheless, the latest in-vivo assays have shown that some advanced bioceramics such as bioglass and two-phase calcium phosphate (BCP) ceramics seem to be promising bone scaffold materials because they exhibited osteoinductive behavior both in non-bone and in bone locations [12–20]. For this reason, considerable effort has recently been directed toward understanding the interactions between the implants and host tissue.

10.2 Bioceramics

10.2.1 Definition of bioceramics

Bioceramics, by definition, are ceramic materials that have been specially developed for biomedicine applications such as bone fillers, implant coatings, and ceramic–polymer composite to repair or replace hard tissues such as the hip joint, auditory ossicle, and tooth root. Just like ordinary ceramics that consist of non-metallic inorganic solid materials, bioceramics are hard but brittle, wear-resistant, electrically and thermally insulating, and chemically stable. However, bioceramics differ from the common ceramics in several ways. Structurally, common ceramics are primarily crystalline, whereas bioceramics can be either crystalline or non-crystalline. Common ceramics do not have to be biocompatible, but bioceramics must be biocompatible due to the fact that a host's immune system always rejects a non-biocompatible foreign object. Thus, biocompatibility is a prerequisite for bioceramics.

Actually, all the existing bioceramics can meet the biocompatibility requirement, but there exist significant differences in degradability and bioactivity among them. Bioactivity here means the ability to integrate a foreign object into surrounding tissue so that a strong inosculation interface between the object and host tissue can form. The powerful interface can resist a relative displacement occurring between host tissue and the object implanted, thereby resulting in a high success rate in hard tissue restoration. Thus, the bioactivity is an important index for assessing and classifying bioceramics.

10.2.2 Classification of bioceramics

In general, bioceramics can be classified into bioinert and bioactive ceramics in terms of their bioactivities, and the bioactive ceramics can be further classified into two subtypes, of class A and class B, depending on the extent of bioactivity and whether the bioceramic can elicit both an intracellular and an extracellular response at its interface [21]. Furthermore, bioceramics may also be divided into less-degradable and biodegradable (bioresorbable) ceramics according to their biodegradation rate in an in-vivo environment. In addition, on the basis of the chemical composition, bioceramics can be further classified into silica-based, phosphate-based, and metallic-oxide-based bioceramics. Herein, we classify bioceramics into two classes according to the bioceramics' surface chemical reactivity with the physiological fluid.

10.2.2.1 Bioinert ceramics

The bioinert ceramics are characterized by a lack of a direct bonding to bone as implanted into the body. The bioinert bioceramics include alumina (Al_2O_3), zirconia (ZrO_2), silica, carbon fiber, and synthetic diamond. Among them, the common bioinert ceramics are zirconia and alumina. Alumina is the first bioinert ceramic to have been used for replacing the metallic femoral head of hip prostheses in 1972 [22]. Since then, alumina ceramics have been used for hip arthroplasty [23–25]. In practice, bioinert ceramics have been employed to fabricate high-strength, load-bearing hip prostheses and dental implants because of their good biocompatibility, high hardness, low friction coefficient, and excellent corrosion resistance. The high corrosion resistance (namely, chemical inertness) makes them hold up in the body for many years, but it is perhaps precisely this chemical inertness that often causes final failure of hip replacement because a non-adherent fibrous capsule forming on the prosthesis surface offers only a limited contact-bonding force that is not strong enough to withstand a big shear force from the movement of host tissue in spite of the presence of a mechanical interlock between the ceramic and the host tissue [21]. To improve the interface bonding force, considerable effort has been made to activate the bioinert ceramic surface by injecting elements or depositing porous coatings of bioactive ceramics onto the dense support [26]. In particular, the presence of porous structure (coating) on the dense implant surface allows tissue ingrowth, leading to a larger surface of contact with host tissue. Surface treatments have significantly strengthened the interface bond over the past decade.

10.2.2.2 Bioactive ceramics

Ever since the first bioactive ceramic (45S5 Bioglass®) was discovered by Hench *et al.* in 1969 [27, 28], efforts to understand the underlying activation mechanism and develop more bioactive ceramics have never stopped. So far, the known bioactive ceramics may be chemically divided into two big groups: one is silica-based ceramics including glasses and glass-ceramics with various compositions; the other is calcium phosphate (CaP)-based ceramics, including hydroxyapatite (HAP), tricalcium phosphate (TCP), and a mixture of HAP and TCP. The two groups of bioactive ceramics enjoy similar advantages (bioactivity and osteoconductivity) and suffer from the same disadvantage (brittleness). Thus most of them are often used for non-structural reconstructions, defeat-fillers, and coatings because their block form alone has been found to be too brittle for use in structural grafts.

10.3 Biological response to implanted bioceramics

All biomaterials are required to be biocompatible. Biocompatibility means that the implanted materials are non-toxic to living cells and also do not elicit any immune rejection reaction or coagulating reaction [29]. On the other hand, no matter how biocompatible an implanted object may be, once implanted, it is always identified as a foreign-body by the host tissue [30, 31], eliciting a cascade of biological events such as vascular exudation, cellular infiltration, acute inflammation, chronic inflammation and granulation tissue formation, foreign body reaction (FBR), and fibrous capsule formation. Among the events is a foreign-body reaction, which often results in the formation of an avascular fibrous capsule separating itself from the implant [31–34]. This is generally thought to result from the implant being too large relative to a macrophage to be phagocytosed. For this reason, the macrophages aggregating around the implant fuse to form larger foreign-body giant cells (FBGCs) composed of up to a few dozen individual macrophages, making an attempt to damage the implant through the release of reactive oxygen substances such as superoxides and oxygen free radicals, degradative enzymes, and acid into the interface between the giant cells and the implant surface [32, 35, 36]. In general, macrophages and foreign-body giant cells tend to remain at the implant surface until the implant is removed or isolated from the host tissue by fibrous capsule. The formation of the fibrous capsule is undesired for the implantation of bone graft replacements because the capsule serves as a physical barrier, resulting in not only loss of the implant's function, but also a loosening of the interface between the implant and host tissue due to the lack of strong direct bonding between them. Furthermore, the loosening interface, in turn, causes macrophage activation and a cyclic foreign-body reaction, resulting in long-lasting inflammation. As a result, a second surgical intervention is necessary in order to remove the implant from the body. Failure of bone grafting often occurred with artificial prosthetic devices such as alumina- and zirconia-based hips and joints before the 1970s.

Efforts directed toward preventing capsule formation around the implants were unsuccessful until the first bioglass (called 45S5 Bioglass®) was discovered by Hench and co-workers in 1969 [28, 37] not to provoke host tissue to form fibrous capsule and, instead, to be bonded with host tissue so strongly that the bioglass could not easily be removed from the surrounding tissue [29, 38]. This important discovery encouraged researchers to reconsider their understanding of the influence of the chemical properties of bioceramics on host tissues because, before the 1970s, chemically inert ceramics such as alumina and zirconia had been regarded as optimal materials from which to fabricate artificial prosthetic replacements for joints and dental implants due to the widely accepted belief that inert ceramics did not react with body fluids and host tissues to create any additional chemical product detrimental to the host tissues. Since then, the bioglasses have become a new class of biomaterials, and a new term that arose in the context of bioglasses, namely "bioactivity," has also become popular in the biomedical community. This indicates that the development and assessment of biomaterials has entered a new era.

10.4 Bone-like apatite formation

The formation of new bone tissue on the implanted biomaterials involves a complex biochemical cascade of molecular interactions. Hench pioneeringly proposed a mechanism consisting of 11 stages in chronological order to understand the complex biochemical process [29, 38, 39]. The process can also be roughly divided into two main stages. The first main stage is characterized by the formation of a layer of bone-like apatite on the implanted bioceramic surface through a series of surface physical–chemical reactions [40–42], and the other main stage involves an intricate biological self-healing process. The first and second main stages correspond to stages 1–5 and 6–11 in Hench's model, respectively. Thus, the first main stage becomes a key step toward success in artificial bone grafting. This point has been confirmed by the success with the first synthetic biomaterial (45S5 Bioglass®) [43, 44]. Therefore, to develop a desirable artificial bioceramic graft, it is essential to understand the underlying mechanism of the response for the bioglass's bioeffect.

A crucial characteristic of the bioglass is its ability to induce *in situ* formation of a layer of bone-like apatite on its surface when it comes into contact with living host tissues. The bone-like apatite was analyzed and found to be composed of calcium hydroxyl carbonate apatite (HCAP), which is equivalent in composition and structure to the major inorganic phase of natural bones [29, 41, 45]. Perhaps for just this reason, the neonatal apatite layer covering the bioglass tricks the immune system into acceptance of the implanted bioglass, causing the system to start a wound-healing procedure similar to that in the normal case without an implant [34]. As a result, the implanted bioglass forms a strong chemical bond with neogenesis bone tissues by means of the interfacial HCAP layer [29, 38]. The chemical bond may be derived from a wide range of chemical forces that include ionic, covalent, van der Waals, and hydrogen bonding, as well as London dispersion forces. Thus, whether or not there is a layer of bone-like apatite forming on an implanted biomaterial has become a direct criterion for assessing the biomaterial's bioactivity, although bioactivity is generally defined to be the ability to form chemical bonds between the implanted biomaterials and host tissues.

Regarding the formation of HCAP, Hench *et al.* proposed a widely accepted mechanism [29, 38, 41], which contains five sequential stages: (1) rapid exchange of Na ions in the glass with H ions in aqueous solution; (ii) loss of soluble silica and formation of silanols; (iii) condensation of silanols to form a hydrated silica gel; (iv) migration of calcium and phosphate ions to the silica-rich layer to form an amorphous calcium phosphate layer; and (v) incorporation of hydroxyl and carbonate from the solution and subsequent crystallization of the calcium phosphate layer to form HCAP. Because the HCAP plays crucial roles in triggering the bone healing procedure and creating chemical bonds between the implanted bioglass and host tissue, much effort has been devoted to investigating the factors influencing HCAP formation on bioceramics.

The formation of an apatite layer on bioceramics includes the nucleation of calcium phosphate (CaP), growth of CaP and crystallization of CaP. The nucleation is a rate-controlling step toward HCAP formation because, once nucleated, the apatite can grow spontaneously owing to the fact that the body fluid is highly supersaturated with respect to apatite sediments. For CaP precipitation, the nucleation mainly depends on the Ca and phosphate ion concentrations, pH, temperature and surface features of the solid onto which CaP will be deposited. Generally, regardless of whether the case is in vivo or in vitro, the temperature is always kept constant at 37 °C; and the ionic concentration product of calcium and phosphate ions in body fluid or acellular simulated body fluid (SBF) is higher than the solubility product constant K_{sp} of CaP. This means that the concentrations of calcium and phosphate ions are supersaturated with respect to CaP at neutral pH, namely there exists a thermodynamic driving force for CaP nucleation. However, in most cases, CaP does not necessarily precipitate because the precipitation–dissolution equilibrium of CaP is highly sensitive to the pH at the solid/solution interface; even at neutral pH, the free orthophosphate (PO_4^{3-}) ion concentration accounts for just a small fraction of the total number of phosphate ions in fluid or SBF, leading to a lower supersaturation level. Additionally, for the case in vivo, the inflammation reaction often causes an acidic microenvironment around the implant [45], where a smaller supersaturation level of CaP will decrease the nucleation probability of CaP, meaning that CaP precipitation hardly occurs.

Theoretically, an alkaline environment is always favorable for increasing the nucleation rate of CaP and for accelerating crystallization of CaP precipitate because an elevated pH can cause a significant increase both in thermodynamic and in kinetic driving forces for CaP nucleation [46], and also promote carbonatization of the CaP precipitation. Furthermore, the nucleation of carbonate-containing HAP is more kinetically favorable than that of stoichiometric HAP [46]. Therefore, the pH at the solid/solution interface is one of the most important factors determining the apatite formation. For instance, many bioglasses can cause the interface pH to increase from 7.4 to 8 or even 11, depending on the chemical composition of the bioglasses when in contact with SBF [47] due to the unavoidable surface exchange of Na^+ in bioglasses with H^+ in solution. As a result, an apatite layer can form on bioglass surfaces within a few hours' exposure to SBF solution. In contrast, bioglasses with high silica content, bioglass ceramics and CaP ceramics often need a longer immersion time in order to form apatite in SBF, which could be attributed to a slow and small increase in pH when they are in contact with SBF.

In addition to pH, a bioceramic's surface properties, including chemical and geometrical factors, also play important roles in controlling apatite formation. Sometimes, even if both ion supersaturation and pH criteria are satisfied, the nucleation of CaP does not necessarily occur due to a lack of very efficient nucleation centers that are essential to trigger a cascade precipitation of CaP. In general, the nucleation centers on a solid surface could be nanoscale geometrical sites, chemical groups with different charges, or both. Among the chemical groups on bioceramics is hydroxyl (—OH), which has been assumed to play a key role in modulating apatite formation on silica-based bioglass and glass ceramics [28, 38, 41, 48, 49]. A unique characteristic of silica-based ceramics is their ability to form a silica-rich gel layer on their surfaces as they come into contact with aqueous solutions. The silica gel has plenty of surface silanol groups, which can be partly deprotonated depending on pH to form $Si—O^-$ groups, leading to the formation of a negatively charged gel surface. Generally, a negatively charged surface is always favorable for heterogeneous nucleation, whereas nucleation will be inhibited on a positively charged surface [50]. Thus, the silica gel surface can drive Ca ions to accumulate and reach a high supersaturation level near the negatively charged sites, while phosphate ions in solution also migrate gradually toward the sites where Ca^{2+} ions accumulate due to Ca^{2+} neutralizing the negative charges on the gel surface. As a result, the nucleation of CaP is preferentially triggered [51–53].

Furthermore, the physical surface of a bioceramic is also a factor affecting CaP nucleation. The surface physical characteristics mainly include the surface topographic structure at micrometer and nanometer scale [54–56], the total surface exposed to SBF solution [56–59], and the degree of crystallization [60, 61], which have been shown to made a great impact on the CaP nucleation rate and final apatite crystalline structure. The influence on the apatite layer could be derived from surface dissolution reactions, which are primarily dependent on the crystalline state and total surface area exposed to aqueous solution. Generally, low crystallininity and large surface area can cause a rapid surface dissolution, leading to a rapid increase in surface ion concentrations and pH, and accelerating the nucleation and precipitation of CaP.

10.5 Osteoinductive potential of bioceramics

10.5.1 Osteoinduction and its importance for bone healing

Osteoinduction is a stimulating osteogenesis process in which primitive, undifferentiated, and pluripotent cells are somehow stimulated to develop into the bone-forming cell lineage [62], and is also essential for bone fracture healing [63, 64]. Actually, there are many undifferentiated cells in bone tissue and bone marrow, which can be recruited to the injured sites to form osteoprogenitor cells when stimulated by the right stimulants [65]. An early osteoinductive stimulant was found to be a demineralized bone matrix [66]. In order to find out why the demineralized bone matrix exhibits osteoinduction behavior, Urist *et al.* [67] digested the matrix by using bacterial collagenase and isolated a kind of glycoprotein from the digestive juice. The glycoprotein was called bone morphogenetic protein (BMP). It is believed to be naturally released in response to trauma and during bone remodeling. Nowadays, it is known that BMP is one of the transforming growth factor (TGF)-β family of growth factors, and at least 15 types of BMP [68, 69] have so far been identified, among which BMP-2 and BMP-7 seem to be particularly associated with osteoinduction. In addition to the native BMPs, additional external factors, such as stress, electrical signals, and implanted objects, may also be potentially direct or indirect bone-induction agents [16, 69, 70]. In particular, implanted bioceramic scaffolds are of interest for bone tissue repair and regeneration.

10.5.2 History of osteoinductive bioceramics

Of all bioactive ceramics, calcium phosphate and in particular hydroxyapatite ceramics have received more attention as bone graft substitutes due to their similarity to the mineral components of bone and teeth, and their excellent biocompatibility, bioactivity, osteoconductivity, and potential osteoinductivity. Osteoconductivity means an ability to favor migration of bone cells and vasculature toward the inside of a porous CaP scaffold. Generally, it is thought that CaP ceramics are osteoconductive rather than osteoinductive, but the classic view has been challenged by the latest experimental evidence from in-vivo animal assays.

In 1988, Heughebaert *et al.* [71] observed a bone-like substance occurring around a block of hydroxyapatite ceramic implanted in the soft tissue of hamsters. In 1990, Yamasaki [16] also observed bone formation around porous hydroxyapatite ceramics implanted in the subcutaneous tissues of a dog. In 1991, reliable histological evidence to demonstrate osteoinduction of CaP ceramics was first given by Ripamonti [70] and our group [72]. Moreover, subsequent results demonstrated that new bone that had originated from the osteoinduction could reinforce the mechanical strength of the implanted CaP ceramics, giving a strength reaching the level of natural bone. These studies indicated the osteoinductive potential of CaP ceramics. Nevertheless, in spite of this, the osteoinductive ability of CaP ceramic is still a matter of discussion because the limited data gathered on CaP ceramic's osteoinduction do not allow one to draw a conclusion. Therefore, it is crucial to study CaP ceramics' osteoinduction systematically on the basis of histological and cellular/molecular evidence. In addition, the biosafety and the potential clinical application of osteoinductive materials should be investigated extensively.

10.5.3 Experimental evidence of osteoinduction of porous CaP ceramics

To elucidate the osteoinduction of CaP ceramics, the histological and molecular genetic evidence for osteoinduction by CaP and features of CaP affecting the osteoinduction are presented below.

As mentioned above, osteoinduction involves at least two processes: recruiting undifferentiated MSCs and stimulating the cells to differentiate into bone-forming cells. This means that an osteoinductive material should play the double role of recruiting and stimulating undifferentiated MSCs, whatever direct or indirect roles it might play when implanted into the body. Thus, to examine whether a bioceramic is osteoinductive, two things have to be done. First, its recruitment role must be addressed by identifying the origin of undifferentiated MSCs gathering around the implanted bioceramic. Second, its osteogenic differentiation role must be also confirmed. However, it is hard to identify the origin of the MSCs gathering around an implanted bioceramic if the ceramic is implanted into a bone defect site due to the fact that there are many unmatured bone-forming cells in normal bone tissue. Therefore, to evaluate a bioceramic's ability to recruit undifferentiated MSCs, a widely accepted method is to implant a bioceramic into non-osseous (ectopic) sites of an animal, invoking an ectopic bone-formation model. This may be a strategy of killing two birds with one stone, since, if ectopic bone formation can be confirmed by histological evidence, the recruiting role and inductive differentiation role of the implanted ceramic can be verified simultaneously owing to the fact that non-osseous locations frequently lack bone cytokine stimulation and endogenous bone-forming cells. For this reason, ectopic bone-formation design has been widely used to evaluate the osteoinductive capacity of a biomaterial.

In ectopic bone-formation design, the selection of animal models in which to test a bioceramic's osteoinductivity is of importance because the selected model animal is expected to mimic the histological features and immunological responses observed in humans. Many experimental models have been developed, such as the mouse, hamster, rabbit, dog, pig, goat, and sheep, as well as monkey, but the efficacy of ectopic bone formation has been found to be dependent on animal species. For CaP ceramics, the osteoinductivity is in the order pig > dog > rabbit > rat [73]. However, from a practical and cost-based point of view, the mouse, rabbit, and dog are still often chosen as testing models. In addition, the influence of implantation location on the outcome is also a particularly important consideration. The common non-osseous locations include subcutaneous, intramuscular, and kidney capsule sites [74], but subcutaneous and intramuscular implantations are often chosen.

10.5.3.1 Histological evidence of ectopic bone formation

In the past decades, our [72, 75–77] and other groups [12, 62, 78–80] have given proofs of ectopic bone formation induced by CaP ceramics. To address the ectopic bone-formation process, below we give two typical examples, showing MSCs being recruited into inside the implanted CaP ceramic and the evolution of osteogenesis, respectively.

(1) *Occurrence of MSCs within porous CaP ceramic.* According to the assumption of biomaterial osteoinduction, if CaP ceramic is osteoinductive, after implantation into a non-osseous location of an animal, MSCs as an early indication of osteoinduction should be found around/inside the CaP scaffold. As expected, MSCs characterized by positive immunohistological staining were observed on TCP/HAP ceramics implanted into muscle of pigs, as shown in Figure 10.1. Moreover, TEM ultrastructural analysis also showed lots of polymorphous cells accumulating around the concave pits inside the CaP ceramics, indicating the possible existence of undifferentiated MSCs [81]. Besides that, collagen fibers and calcium phosphate secreted by the cells inside the ceramics were also observed, indicating the presence of osteoblasts [81]. Both results indicate that the

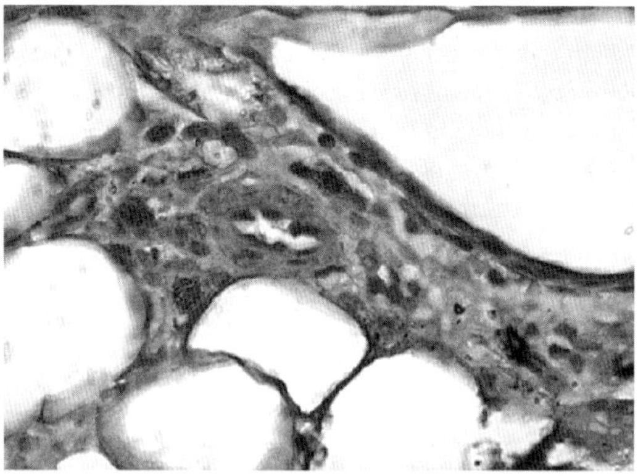

Figure 10.1 Immunohistochemical analyses showing the presence of MSCs inside the porous TCP/HAP ceramic.

muscle implantation of CaP ceramics causes the presence of MSCs inside the CaP scaffold and the generation of osteoblasts [81].

(2) *Evolution of osteogenesis within porous CaP ceramic.* Normal new bone formation can be realized by either intramembranous ossification or endochondral ossification. The intramembranous ossification occurs in flat bones of the skull and requires cartilage precursor. The endochondral osteogenesis is the most commonly occurring process, requiring hyaline cartilage as a precursor. However, ectopic bone (heterotopic ossification) formation is a process resulting in formation of bone in soft tissue where normal bone does not exist, so the process is atypical bone formation that can readily be confused with osteosarcoma and osteochondroma, even with calcification. Calcification is the formation of calcium-based salts and crystals within cells and tissue. Thus, it is essential to identify the events involved in ectopic bone formation caused by CaP implantation.

A typical osteogenesis process can be briefly described as follows, from our observation of histomorphological characteristics of new bone forming in porous TCP/HAP ceramics implanted in dog muscles. The implanted porous TCP/HAP ceramics were characterized by a phase composition of TCP/HAP = 35/65, a porosity of 60%, and an average pore size of 300 μm, and were sintered at 1100 °C [82]. Seven days after implantation, blood cells and loose fibrous tissue were observed inside the scaffold; blood capillaries and polymorphous cells were found to accumulate on the walls of the pores at day 21 (21d), and osteoids appeared at 30d; woven bone with obvious bone lacuna occurred at 45d, and osteoclasts were observed at 60d, demonstrating the occurrence of bone remodeling. Afterwards, the occurrence of bone marrow and a full Haversian system were observed at 90d and 180d [13], respectively. In the time-course analysis of histomorphology, all events related to new bone formation, including the occurrence of osteoblasts, osteoblast cell lining, osteocytes, osteoclasts, woven bone, lamina bone, and the Haversian system, were observed in the porous biphasic ceramics implanted into muscle of dogs, demonstrating that these CaP ceramics are osteoinductive. Meanwhile, no chondrocyte was found inside the ceramics, suggesting that the ectopic bone formation occurs via intramembranous ossification.

In addition, testing the variation in the volume of neo-bone formed with implantation time is also an alternative way to distinguish ectopic bone formation from osteosarcoma, osteochondroma, and calcification. In general, normal new bone volume increases with time during the initial phase, but the rate of increase gradually becomes slow and remains constant during the later phase. In practice, the occurrence of ectopic bone formation inside TCP/HAP ceramics implanted in a dog's muscle has shown that the change in volume of neo-bone with implantation time is similar to that of normal new-bone formation in the initial phase of the implantation, suggesting that the ectopic osteogenesis induced by TCP/HAP is not out of control, thus osteochondroma should be avoided.

In addition to muscle implantation in dogs, subcutaneous implantation has also been carried out to examine whether the CaP ceramics are osteoinductive. Our results showed that new bone tissue also appeared inside the porous TCP/HAP scaffold implanted, but the osteogenesis rate was slower than that of muscle implantation [74].

10.5.3.2 Molecular evidence of ectopic bone formation induced by CaP ceramics

Normal fracture healing processes are quite complex and involve a series of cellular and biochemical events. New bone formation requires the cooperation of bone-forming cells, including osteoblasts, osteocytes and lining cells. Of particular interest is the osteoblast that plays a key role in generating new bone matrix, osteoid, and mineral. The osteoblast originates primarily from osteoblastic differentiation of mesenchymal stem cells (MSCs), and the osteodifferentiation is regulated by many hormonal and autocrine/paracrine factors. Among the factors, bone morphogenetic proteins (BMPs) have been proven to play directly important roles in triggering osteogenetic differention of MSCs and osteoprogenitors, and proliferation, growth inhibition, and arrest of maturation of bone-forming cells, depending on the cellular microenvironment and the interactions with other regulatory factors [82]. For ectopic bone formation from intramuscular and subcutaneous sites, BMPs might derive either from the recruitment of blood circulation or from the secretion of non-osseous cells stimulated by ceramics [83, 84]. In some cases, even a lower dose of BMP can also induce differentiation of MSCs into osteoblasts [85].

In addition to BMPs, a crucial transcription factor called core binding factor alfa1 (Cbfa1) is essential for osteogenetic differentiation [86]. Interestingly, Cbfa1 expression has also been proved by the observation of positive expression of Cbfa1 antibody in MSCs inside CaP ceramics [85].

Normal osteogenesis follows its own time sequence to trigger designated events. At an early stage, an unmatured osteoblast secrets primarily collagen I matrix protein; at an intermediate stage, the osteoblast expresses alkaline phosphatase (ALP), which plays an important role in the calcification of cartilage and bone. At a later stage, the cell becomes fully differentiated and starts to successively secrete matrix proteins such as osteonectin (OCN), osteopontin (OPN), and bone sialoprotein (BSP). Finally, during the mineralization phase, the osteoblast expresses osteocalcin. Interestingly, the expression of bone matrix protein markers can also be identified in ectopic bone formation induced by CaP ceramics [81, 83].

Bone is a living tissue that needs to keep a dynamic balance between bone formation and bone resorption. In the dynamic balance, osteoclastogenesis is mediated through receptor activator of NFkB (RANK), receptor ligand RANKL, with osteoprotegerin (OPG) being a natural decoy receptor for RANKL. In other words, RANKL is a stimulator of differentiation of osteoclasts and OPG is an inhibitor of osteoclastogenesis. Thus, the expression of OPG mRNA and RANL mRNA should be characteristic of the normal bone remodeling cycle. To examine whether CaP ceramic affects the bone remodeling cycle, Saos-2 (human osteoblast-like cell line) was cultured on different CaP ceramics in vitro, and analysis on the expression of mRNA of RANKL/OPG in the culture systems indicated that CaP bioceramics did not deteriorate in terms of the normal expression of RANKL and OPG of Saos-2 [87, 88].

Briefly, on the basis of the histological and molecular evidence for osteogenic potential induced by CaP bioceramics, it is safe to say that CaP bioceramic exhibits not only osteoinductive capacity, but also positive effects on bone repair and regeneration. Besides, the known cellular and molecular events occurring in osteogenetic processes which are known from investigations on osteogenesis induced by bioceramics are summarized briefly in Figure 10.2.

10.5.4 Bioceramic scaffold structure-dependent osteoinductive potential

More evidence shows that not all kinds of bioceramics have osteoinductive potential. In fact, the osteoinductive potential of bioceramics strongly depends on their properties, including chemical composition and geometrical and mechanical characteristics. In principle, bioceramics, except for bioinert ceramics such as alumina and zirconia, have more or less osteoinductive potential depending on their surface chemical properties and porous inner architecture.

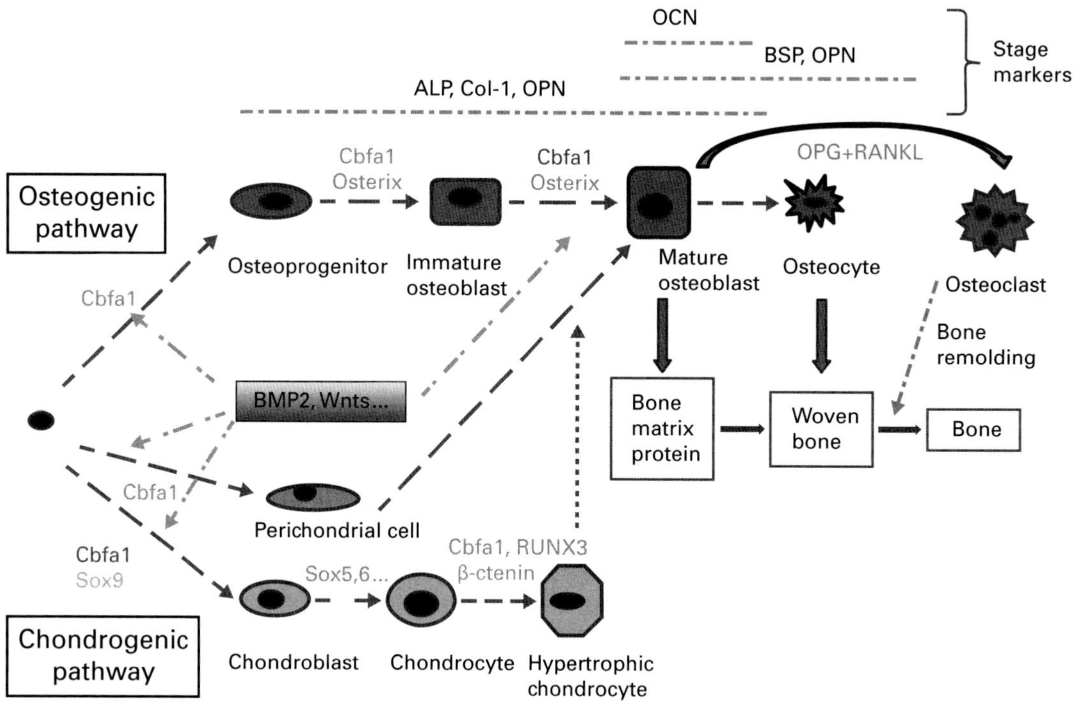

Figure 10.2 The molecular markers involved in osteogenesis.

10.5.4.1 Surface chemistry on osteoinduction

Bioactivity, defined as the ability of a biomaterial to bond chemically to host tissue by forming a layer of bone-like apatite at the interface between the biomaterial and the host tissue, is a prerequisite for osteoinductivity of a bioceramic. Assuming that a bone-like apatite layer can form on the biomaterial surface, the bioactivity is basically determined by its surface chemical properties, including what chemical elements make up the surface and the dissolubility of the surface in body fluid. If the biomaterial surface tends to be soluble in body fluid and, importantly, the dissolution product can induce apatite formation, the biomaterial can generally exhibit excellent bioactivity and even osteoinductivity. This is especially true for bioceramics, including crystalline ceramics and non-crysalline glasses, because their surfaces are often less dissoluble.

The surface solubility of a bioactive ceramic determines the formation rate of bone-like apatite. When a bioceramic surface starts to dissolve, the ion concentration and pH near the solid surface will deviate from those of the bulk fluid. For bioglass and CaP ceramics, their surface dissolution can increase the supersaturation of calcium phosphate through increasing the concentration of calcium and phosphate ions, or pH, leading to rapid nucleation and growth of apatite. Moreover, the surface dissolution of bioceramics also plays directly or indirectly a subtle role in regulating subsequent osteoinduction.

Among the most commonly used CaP ceramics, including tricalcium phosphate (TCP), hydroxyapatite (HAP), and their combinations such as biphasic calcium phosphate (BCP) ceramic, TCP is the most soluble, while HAP is less soluble, such that the dissolution rate of HAP is too low to achieve the optimal osteogenesis results, whereas the dissolution rate of β-TCP ceramics is too fast to retain temporary mechanical support for the desired period of time [76].

Therefore, to achieve an optimum surface solubility of CaP ceramics, a reasonable idea is to prepare a composite mixture consisting of HAP and TCP with different TCP/HAP mass ratios. The composite is called biphasic calcium phosphate (BCP) ceramic. The dissolution rate of BCP increases with increasing TCP/HAP mass ratio. Thus, the ratio of TCP/HAP not only affects the rate of bone-like apatite formation, but also regulates the outcome of osteogenesis.

Various mass ratios of TCP/HAP ranging from 0 to 10 have been investigated in animal models. On the basis of the amount of newly formed bone required, the optimal ratio of TCP/HAP ranges from 3:7 to 4:6 [89].

The surface dissolution rate of bioactive ceramics is closely associated with surface crystallization. The level of surface crystallization is mainly controlled by the temperature at which a ceramic is thermally processed. If a ceramic is sintered at a temperature higher than its crystallization temperature, fast surface crystallization and crystal growth will make the ceramic less soluble, leading to a significant decrease in bioactivity and subsequent osteoinduction. The effect of surface crystallization of bioactive ceramics on their osteogenesis has been widely confirmed irrespective of whether the ceramic is bioglass or a CaP bioceramic. For example, the famous 45S5 Bioglass® has been proven to be the most bioactive, but, when processed thermally at a temperature higher than its glass temperature, its bioactivity decreases significantly [85] or even vanishes [90]. In general, 45S5 Bioglass®-based glass powder is prone to crystallize at the desired sintering temperature, so it is hard to avoid surface crystallization and the occurrence of a new crystalline phase [85, 90]. Therefore, in addition to chemical composition, the thermal processing of bioglass is one of the key factors regulating its bioactivity and osteogensis.

Similarly, the bioactivity of HAP is also strongly dependent on the sintering temperature. For instance, HAP sintered at 1100 °C can induce significant osteogenesis, but this does not occur when it is sintered at 1200 °C [75–77]. Even BCP ceramics with identical mass ratios of TCP/HAP (3:7) exhibit a marked difference in osteogenesis rate when sintered at 1100 °C and 1200 °C: BCP sintered at 1100 °C needs 6 weeks, but BCP sintered at 1200 °C needs 12 weeks to reach a similar result. The difference in osteogenesis rate is assumed to be a consequence of the difference in their surface dissolution rates.

10.5.4.2 Three-dimensional microstructure on osteoinduction

In addition to the surface chemistry of bioceramics, the 3D porous architecture of bioceramics also plays a crucial role in enhancing osteoinduction and osteogenesis. A bioceramic's 3D porous architecture, as the name implies, is a complex porous scaffold, which is expected to mimic the framework of naturally occurring cancellous bone where there exist rich macropores, micropores, and microchannels that provide living space for bone tissue and blood vessel. Thus, an implanted bioceramic scaffold must possess plenty of inner pores that can be used for cell ingrowth and mass transfer; meanwhile, the scaffold must also be strong enough to prevent it from collapse within an expected time. In practice, it is difficult to prepare a bioceramic scaffold that can meet simultaneously the need for large porosity and high strength because high porosity is always accompanied by a decrease in the strength of the porous scaffold. Nevertheless, it is also possible to fabricate a porous bioceramic scaffold that can mimic structurally the cancellous bone characterized by open-shaped pores with a large size in the range of 500–600 μm [91], a compression strength of 2–20 MPa, and a porosity of 30%–90%. Therefore, much effort has been devoted to fabricating the desired porous bioceramic scaffold by using advanced design and preparation processing.

The microstructural parameters of porous bioceramic scaffolds include mainly porosity, pore size, pore shape and pore size distribution, and the pore-interconnected channel size. The basic function of a pore inside the scaffold is to accommodate ingrowth cells, while the role of the pore-interconnected channel is to allow body fluid, blood vessels, and cells to develop toward the center of the scaffold. Thus, an ideal scaffold should possess the largest possible inner surface in order to hold more cells. Actually, the influence of scaffold microstructure on bone regeneration is a consequence of complex actions occurring at the interface between host tissue and the external and inner surfaces of the scaffold because, when implanted, the porous scaffold acting as a part of the extracellular matrix plays multiple roles, including bonding chemically with host tissue by inducing apatite formation, stimulating cell migration toward the inner space of the scaffold, and offering a microenvironment for cell survival, proliferation, and differentiation. Therefore, it is unpractical to make accurate predictions about how bioceramic microstructures influence the resulting osteogenesis. However, on the basis of reported results, a general tendency for bioceramic microstructure to promote osteogenesis can be summarized as follows.

Porosity, defined as the percentage of void space in a solid, is an important parameter characterizing porous scaffolds for bone tissue engineering. High porosity means large specific surface area, which favors apatite nucleation and mechanical fixation between the scaffold and host bone tissue. High porosity (>80%) is believed to create significantly positive effects in terms of enhancing osteogenesis, but the positive effect does not necessarily take place because the low strength arising from an overly high porosity (>80%) often causes untimely collapse of the implanted scaffold. Therefore, for bioactive ceramic scaffolds, a porosity ranging from 40% to 70% is available for bone defect repair, depending on the implanted sites.

Pore type includes closed pores and open pores that include dead-end pores, interconnected pores, and passing pores. The interconnected pores and passing pores look like inner tunnels allowing mass transport, cell adhesion, and bone ingrowth. It is of particular importance that the interconnection channels offer a passageway for cell distribution and migration, blood vessel formation, and tissue migration. Thus, the number of open pores is directly related to bone formation. In general, the total porosity can be controlled in the range from 40% to 80%.

For a given porosity ranging from 40% to 70%, an optimal pore diameter is generally within the range 200–500 μm, and the pore-interconnected channel size is in the range 100–200 μm. Besides that, microporosity (pore diameter <10 μm) plays a crucial role in promoting osteogensis [85, 88, 89]. Micropores frequently appear on the wall surfaces of a macropore (>10 μm) and mainly result from the sintering process. Generally, the higher the sintering temperature, the lower the microporosity the bioceramic has, thereby resulting in a lower activity. For example, a CaP ceramic sintered at 1100 °C has a higher microporosity than that of one sintered at 1200 °C, thereby resulting in a significant difference in osteogenesis. It was found that the formation of new bone tissue occurred only for CaP ceramics sintered at 1100 °C 45 days after implantation, and no new bone formation was found in CaP ceramics sintered at 1200 °C until 90 days after implantation [20, 89, 92]. The difference in osteogenesis was attributed to the difference in microporosity between the two CaP ceramics. In spite of multiple factors affecting osteogenesis, higher microporosity is often accompanied by higher surface area, larger surface adsorption, a rapid surface dissolution rate, and proper topological stimuli. The exact mechanism of how the 3D structure influences the osteogenesis needs to be studied using relatively quantitative methods. Advanced 3D printing techniques will certainly play a crucial role here because modern 3D printers enable one to build almost anything imaginable, including complex human organs [93, 94].

10.6 Nano-bioceramics

A nano-bioceramic is a ceramic material that is composed of grains of diameter less than 100 nm. Like other nanomaterials, a nano-bioceramic is also believed to exhibit peculiar properties different from those of the same material at common microscale-grained dimensions. These properties, including higher fracture strength, large specific surface area, lots of grain boundaries and defects, as well as high surface energy, are assumed to be beneficial to improving its bioactivity, osteoinductive capacity, and biodegradability because of the enhanced surface dissolution rate and amount of surface adsorption and in particular selective adsorption of proteins that might

Table 10.1 Advantages and disadvantages of different sintering routes for ceramic fabrication [95]

Methods	Advantages	Disadvantages
Conventional muffle sintering	Inexpensive devices; high yield; suitable for conventional and large-size ceramic fabrication	Time- and energy-consuming; unsuitable for nanoceramic fabrication
Spark plasma sintering	Rapid process; low energy cost; suitable for nanoceramic fabrication	Expensive devices; low yield; difficult for large-size nanoceramic fabrication
Microwave sintering	Rapid process; low energy cost; suitable for nanoceramic fabrication	Expensive devices; low yield; difficult for large-size nanoceramic fabrication

promote recruitment of bone cells and osteoblastic differentiation of MSCs. Therefore, a better osteogenesis outcome is expected to be seen with nano-bioceramics.

10.6.1 Fabrication of porous CaP nanoceramic scaffolds

The preparation of a porous CaP nanoceramic scaffold is similar to that for a conventional porous ceramic scaffold except for the use of nanopowders and different sintering system. Nanopowders can readily be obtained by various techniques [95], but it has been a great challenge to sinter the nanopowders and still retain the nanoscale grains in the sintered solid because the melted nanoparticles easily merge with each other to become a big grain during sintering at elevated temperatures due to the high surface energy of nanoparticles. The longer the thermal processing time at high temperature, the larger the grains grow. Therefore, for preparation of nanoceramics, a rapid heating and cooling system is required for fast welding together of the particles and, almost simultaneously, to quickly cool the particles being welded together, otherwise the melted particles will merge with each other to become a big grain. Obviously, conventional means of thermal processing are hardly suitable for nanoceramic fabrication owing to their slow heating rate. For this reason, many techniques (Table 10.1) have been developed to prepare nanoceramics, for example, spark plasma sintering [96–98], microwave sintering [99–101], hot pressure sintering [102], and high-pressure sintering [103]. Among these techniques, microwave sintering is the most attractive technique for the fabrication of CaP nanoceramics because of its rapid heating rate, thereby leading to sintered CaP ceramic having fine grain size and improved mechanical strength.

10.6.2 Characteristics of CaP nano-bioceramic scaffolds

Microwave sintering offers two main advantages: shortening the sintering time and producing ceramics with nanoscale grain size. For example, with microwave sintering one needs only 20 minutes to sinter HAP ceramics, whereas with conventional sintering one needs at least two hours [104]. More importantly, microwave sintering enables ceramics to exhibit amazing features such as enhanced fracture strength and nanoscale surface topography. Figure 10.3 shows a clear difference in surface topography between HAP ceramics obtained by microwave sintering (A) and those produced by conventional sintering (B). The rich grain boundaries and nanopores of the nano-HAP ceramic possibly play some unpredicted but probably positive roles in regulating protein adsorption and cellular behavior.

To better elucidate the differences in structure and properties between the common porous CaP and porous nano-CaP bioceramics, Table 10.2 lists some parameters describing their features. As a whole, porous CaP nanoceramics not only retain the advantages of the porous structure, the amount of micropores, and a chemical composition similar to the conventional ones, but are also endowed with

Table 10.2 Physicochemical properties of CaP nano- and conventional ceramics

	nHAP	cHAP	nBCP	cBCP
Compressive strength (MPa)	2.6 ± 0.16	2.63 ± 0.13	2.4 ± 0.21	2.53 ± 0.23
Porosity (%)	75 ± 4	74 ± 5	75 ± 5	74 ± 3
Macropore size (μm)	248 ± 38	238 ± 46	348 ± 90	323 ± 95
Grain size (nm)	115 ± 21	731 ± 170	86 ± 20	768 ± 321
Composition	HAP; carbonate apatite	HAP	HAP (~60%); carbonate apatite (<1%); β-TCP (~40%)	β-TCP (~40%); HAP (~60%)
Crystallinity	Low	High	Low	High
Specific surface area ($m^2\ g^{-1}$)	4.5167	0.4838	9.6225	1.4129
Zeta potential in SBF (mV) (pH 7.4)	−5.66 ± 0.332	−2.94 ± 0.275	2.56 ± 0.2 to −3.74 ± 1.32[a]	−3.13 ± 0.25

[a] The zeta potential of nBCP always changes during measurement. The possible reason is fast surface reaction of nBCP in SBF. nHAP, nano-hydroxyapatite; cHAP, conventional hydroxyapatite; nBCP, nano-biphasic calcium phosphate; and cBCP, conventional biphasic calcium phosphate [95].

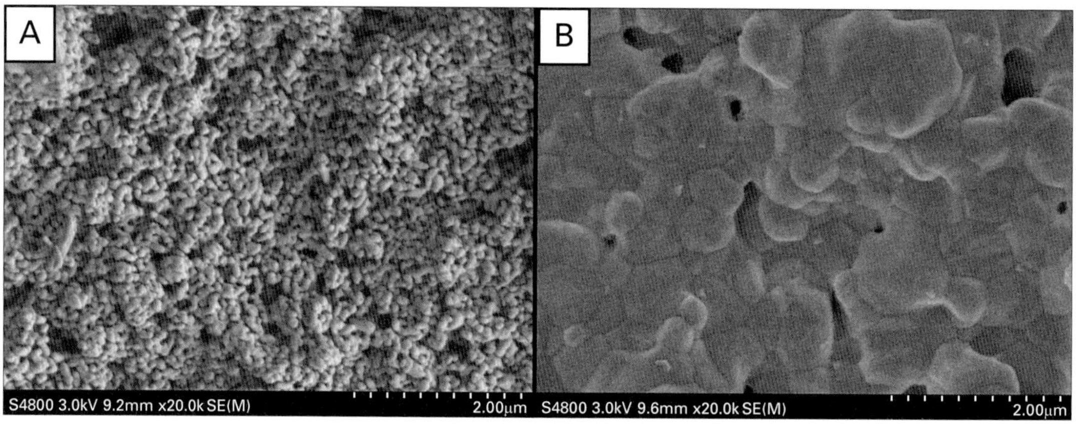

Figure 10.3 SEM images of fractured surface of porous (A) nano- and (B) conventional HAP ceramics.

nanoscale grains, a biomimetic component (carbonate apatite) and several times higher specific surface area (SSA) and lower crystallinity. These features of nanoceramics are expected to display unexpected excellent biological effects [105].

10.6.3 Biological performance of CaP nanoceramics

Almost all initial reactions between biomaterials and biological events always take place on the surface of the biomaterial. Thus, the surface properties of nanoceramics undoubtedly influence any important interactions with biological events occurring in the surroundings of the nanoceramics. The influence of the nanoceramic on biological events can be reflected by direct interactions between the nanoceramic and cells and also by indirect interactions between protein-coated nanoceramic and cells, or by a combination thereof. However, whatever route is taken, the outcome of a nanoceramic affecting biological events can be found by analyzing the events which happened.

10.6.3.1 Protein adsorption

On being implanted into the body, a bioceramic surface unavoidably comes into contact with body fluid, thereby causing adsorption to occur on its surface. The surface adsorption involves the accumulation of water, various ions, and proteins. Knowledge of protein adsorption on the CaP ceramic surface is crucial for designing and developing new bioceramics. Protein adsorption is a very complex process, which is driven by different protein–surface forces including van der Waals, hydrophobic, and electrostatic forces. The driving forces are frequently affected by factors including pH, ionic strength, and solid surface properties. In particular, the solid surface properties, including topography, surface energy, hydrophilicity, roughness, and surface charge have been found to affect significantly protein adsorption characteristics such as the amount of protein adsorbed and the kinds of protein adsorbed [106–108], and even result in competitive or selective protein adsorption [109, 110]. A consequence of the selective adsorption of proteins is that the biomaterial surface will be rich in some proteins and poor in others, which may trigger some biological pathways such as blood coagulation and a cell's biochemical cascade reactions. Perhaps this is the reason why nanostructured surfaces may enhance cell adhesion, proliferation, and differentiation [111, 112].

The selective adsorption of BMPs was assumed to be one of the most important factors responsible for the osteoinductivity of CaP ceramics. To understand the selective protein adsorption of CaP ceramics, bovine serum albumin (BSA) and lysozyme (LSZ) acting as model proteins were used to investigate their adsorption on porous CaP nanoceramics and conventional ones. The adsorption tests demonstrated that both types of CaP ceramic have strong abilities to adsorb BSA and LSZ proteins, but the nanoceramic can adsorb a higher amount of proteins than can the conventional one. Moreover, the small protein LSZ was found to be preferentially adsorbed on both CaP ceramics even when the BSA concentration was higher than that of LSZ, thereby indicating that CaP ceramics can selectively adsorb different proteins. The selective adsorption strongly depends on the properties of the CaP surface and protein itself, particularly on their surface charge characteristic.

At physiological pH (7.4), CaP ceramics have negatively charged surfaces, and BSA is also negatively charged (isoelectric point 5), whereas both LSZ and BMP-2 are positively charged, and their corresponding isoelectric points are 11 and 8.2. Furthermore, from the protein-dimension point of view, the molecular weights (more formally, relative molecular masses) of LSZ and BSA are 14.3 kDa and 66.5 kDa, respectively [113]; for the BMP-2 native dimer and monomer the molecular weight is 28–33 kDa and 14–17 kDa, respectively [114]. Taken together, BMP-2 in nature is more similar to LSA, thus leading to the postulation that a porous CaP implant likely adsorbs preferentially BMP-2 from the microenvironment within which it is placed; subsequently, the absorbed BMP-2 is released to induce osteodifferentiation and osteogenesis. Although it is difficult to find direct in-vivo evidence to support the hypothesis, its validity cannot be ruled out completely on the basis of findings regarding ectopic bone formation in animal modes and the success of bone tissue engineering where rhBMP-2 is embedded into CaP ceramic scaffolds before being implanted into the human body. Obviously, further investigation on this topic is required.

10.6.3.2 Bioeffect of nanoceramics

10.6.3.2.1 Cell adhesion and proliferation

Regardless of whether or not there are protein-adsorption layers on a material surface or what roles the adsorbed protein layers play, living cells can always sense and respond to the nanostructures of the implanted CaP scaffold. The cellular response to a nanostructured surface can be reflected in cellular behaviors, including cell morphology, adhesion, migration, proliferation, and differentiation. In some cases, the influence of nanostructured solid surfaces on cellular behavior even exceed that of surface chemistry [106]. Therefore, surface topography, particularly of nanostructured surfaces, has aroused increasing interest in discussions on bioactivity in recent years.

In comparison with smooth solid surfaces, nanostructured and microstructured surfaces have been

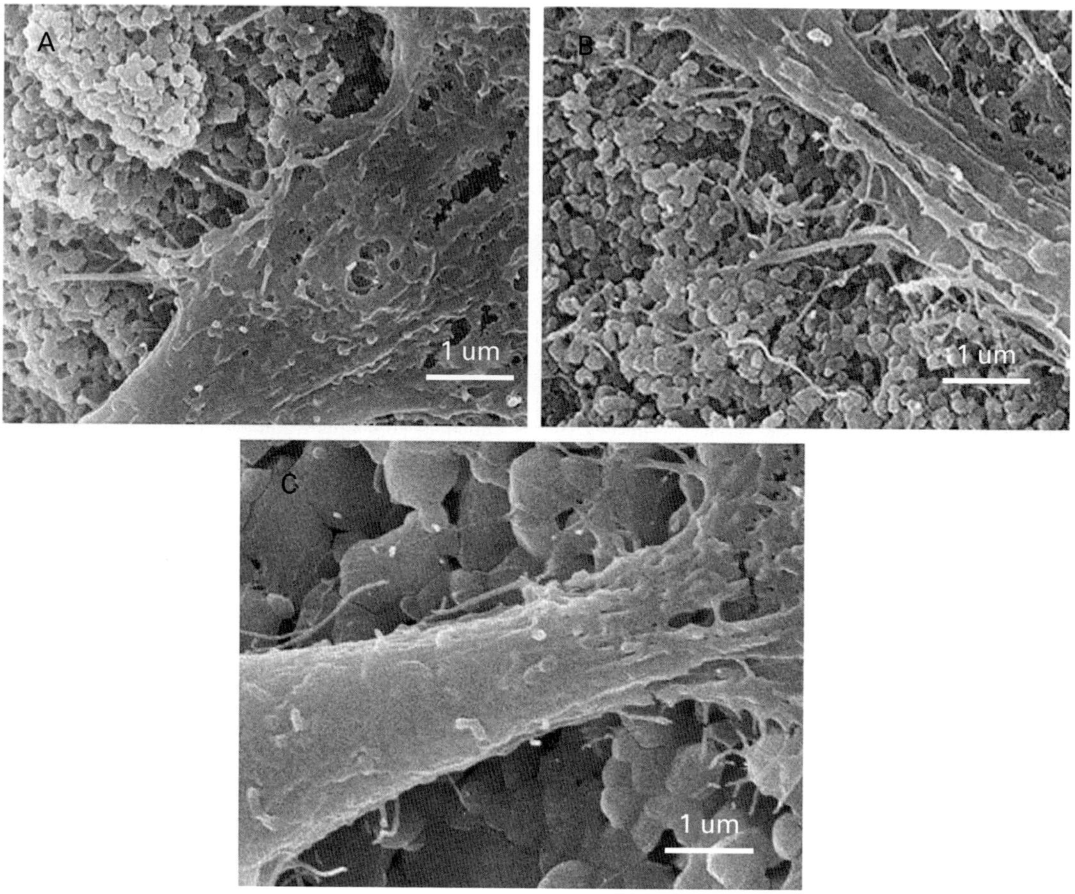

Figure 10.4 Cell adhesion on different CaP ceramics. The magnified SEM micrographs show the adhesion of rat osteoblasts after culture for 3 days on (A) nano-, (B) submicro-, and (C) conventional BCP ceramics. Reprinted from [118] with permission. The scale bars show 1 μm.

found to significantly enhance adhesion of osteoblasts [115]. Furthermore, a nanostructured surface has been proved to be more beneficial for improving bioactivity than a microstructured surface [116, 117]. The nano-enhanced bioeffect can even be observed in bioinert ceramics of alumina and titania when their surfaces are covered with crystal grains of their nanophase [106].

To gain more knowledge about how a living cell responds to a nanostructured surface on which it anchors, Figure 10.4 [118] shows straightforward information about this aspect. In this example, osteoblasts were respectively cultured on three types of CaP ceramics with nanoscale (A), sub-microscale (B) and microscale (C) grains on their surfaces for 3 days. It can be clearly seen from Figure 10.4 that, on the nanostructured surface (A), the osteoblast extended over a large area and developed a large number of filopodia at its periphery, looking like hundreds of protrusions radiating from the cell. In contrast, on microstructured surface (C), the osteoblast extended only over a limited area and developed few filopodia. This phenomenon clearly indicates that osteoblasts are highly sensitive to the size of surface geometric structures. In general, if a solid surface is favorable for cell growth, cells tend to extend their filopodia in order to achieve better sensing of their environment. Thus, the large numbers of filopodia appearing on the CaP nanoceramic surface (A) mean that the CaP nanoceramic are more beneficial for supporting osteoblast growth than is the conventional ceramic.

Similarly, a nanostructured bioceramic surface can also enhance cell proliferation. Moreover, the proliferation of osteoblasts is strongly dependent on the geometric size of surface nanostructures. On the whole, nanoceramics exhibit the most active effect on osteoblast proliferation and sub-microceramics come second, whereas conventional ceramics exhibit a higher proliferation rate than do ceramics with smooth surfaces [116–119].

The underlying mechanism of how surface nanogeometric structures impact adherent osteoblast behaviors is still unclear, but it can be interpreted in terms of a size-matching effect. When the size of surface geometric features, including pores, pillars, and grooves, matches well that of a filopodium (~80 nm in diameter), the nano-topographic surface may either present a special surface energy that is favorable for selective protein adsorption, or establish a special environment that can meet cellular requirements for mechanical, chemical, and spatial environments. As a result, surface nano-geometric structures may serve as cellular activators to enhance cellular functions. In general, the average size of geometric features on CaP nanoceramic did not exceed 100 nm, matching the 80-nm diameter of a filopodium; thus, CaP nanoceramic exhibited an excellent bioeffect. However, when the size of surface geometric structures far exceeds that of filopodia, the bioeffect of a nanostructured surface will decrease or even vanish.

10.6.3.2.2 Osteogenic gene expression and osteoinduction

As mentioned above, the authors of a number of studies have demonstrated that nanoceramics have potential ability to enhance adhesion and proliferation of osteoblasts, but a more important concern is whether the nano-geometric stimuli can further transfer to cellular downstream processes whereby gene expression and osteogenesis may be altered. For this reason, investigations on CaP nanoceramics [118] and nanostructured Ti surface [120, 121] have shown that surface nanostructures could up-regulate the level of osteogenics-related gene expression such as of BSP, OPN, OCN [121], and BMP-2 [95].

In order to examine whether surface nanostructures affect the resulting osteogenesis, ectopic bone formation was employed to compare the amount of new formed bone between nanoceramic and conventional CaP ceramics (BCP and HAP) that were implanted intramuscularly in dogs. In the intramuscular implantations, the histological analyses demonstrated that, 45 days after implantation, a small amount of new formed bone accompanied by fibrous, connective tissue, and capillaries had appeared within pores of CaP nanoceramics, but no bone tissue was detected in HAP ceramics. Ninety days after implantation, distinct differences in amount of newly formed bone can be identified by histological analysis (Figure 10.5). For porous BCP nanoceramics (A), one can see a large amount of newly formed bone tissues occurring inside the BCP nanoceramics, and some local regions of BCP nanoceramics had been replaced by newly formed bone characterized by typical lacunae and osteoblast lines. Moreover, the nearby bone tissues appear to integrate to form a whole mature bone, and the medullary cavities can be also seen inside the BCP nanoceramics. However, for the conventional BCP ceramics, new bone tissue can also be seen, but the amount of newly formed bone is far lower than that with the BCP nanoceramics (image B in Figure 10.5). Nevertheless, for the porous HAP ceramics (image C and D in Figures 10.5), no bone-related tissue was found except for the residual fibrous connective tissue and capillaries. These results indicate that nanoceramics can enhance ectopic osteogenesis, but the enhancement on osteogenesis is also dependent on the surface chemistry of the ceramics.

On the basis of the animal tests, it can be seen that BCP ceramics exhibit a higher osteogenic capacity than do HAP ceramics, and BCP nanoceramics show advanced osteogenesis stronger than that with conventional BCP ceramics. However, the nano-enhanced osteogenic effect has not been identified on HAP

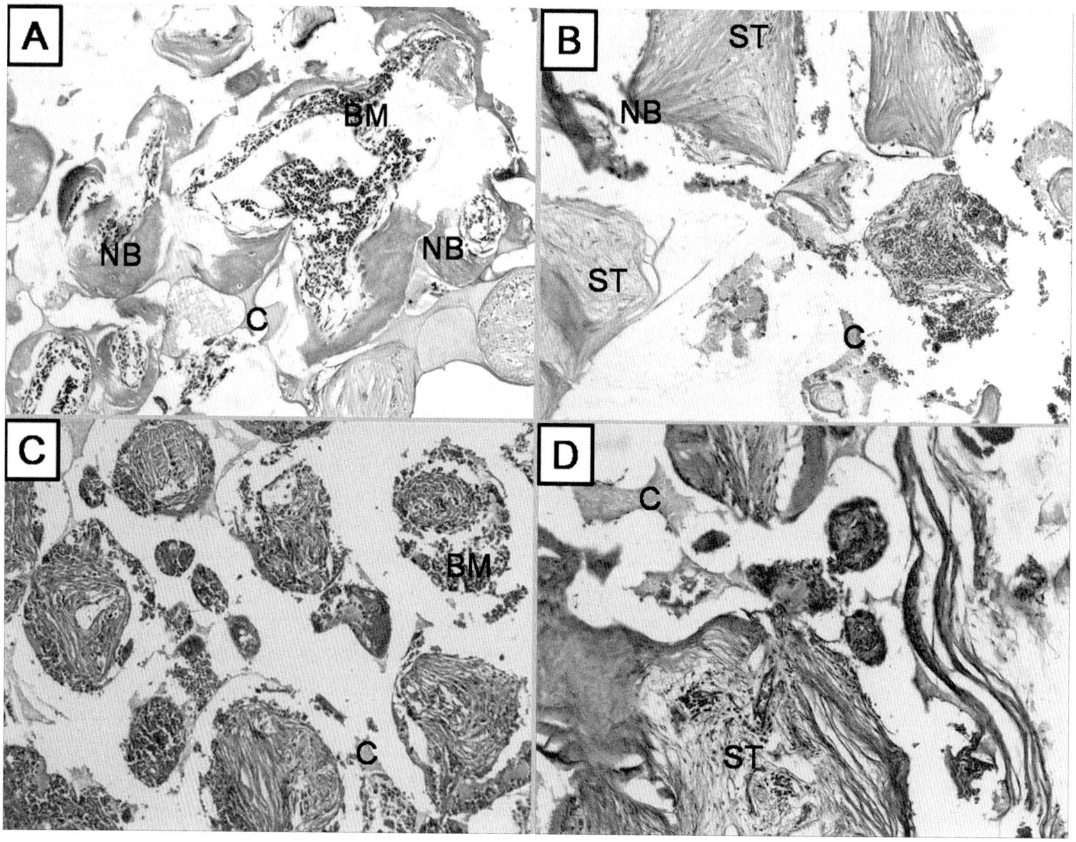

Figure 10.5 HE-stained histological slides of different CaP ceramics implanted intramuscularly in dogs for 90 days. These samples are (A) nBCP, (B) cBCP, (C) nHAP, and (D) cHAP; the photograph magnification is 200×. C, ceramics; NB, newly formed bone tissue; BM, bone marrow; ST, soft tissue.

nanoceramics. This result is likely due to the fact that HAP is less soluble than BCP. Therefore, the nano-enhanced bioeffect is dependent also on other factors such as surface chemistry.

Surface nanostructures affecting osteogenesis is a quite complex process that involves multiple steps: from protein adsorption to regulating adhesion, proliferation and differentiation, in which a cascade of biochemical reactions must take place. To help understand the complex process, Figure 10.6 [95] shows a concise flowchart to illustrate the possible steps occurring during osteogenesis. In brief, the CaP nanoceramics may selectively adsorb proteins on their surface, thereby enhancing cell adhesion, proliferation, and differentiation. Appropriate surface properties of CaP ceramics can lead to the release of critical concentrations of Ca^{2+} and PO_4^{3-} ions, inducing the formation of a bone-like layer on the CaP ceramics under the regulation of endogenous biological molecules [122]. Subsequently, the native bone healing procedure is triggered and subtly regulated by the presence of implanted bioceramics serving as a part of the extracellular matrix. In a few words, such an osteogenic mechanism is suitable not only for nanomaterials, but also for all bioceramics.

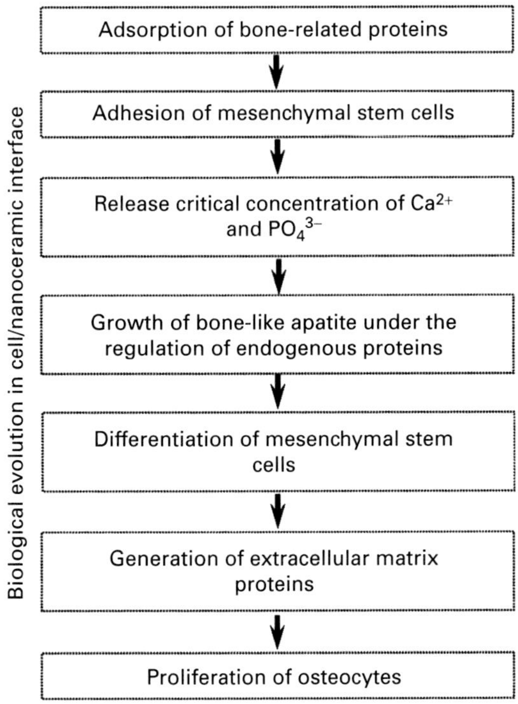

Figure 10.6 A proposed biological evolution of osteoinductivity [95].

10.6.4 Biosecurity and anticancer activity of the CaP nanoceramics

On the one hand, nano-bioceramics can exhibit amazingly positive bioeffects, such as enhanced adsorption, osteoinduction, and osteogenesis. On the other hand, they may also produce unpredicted negative bioeffects including inducing tumors and disturbing normal metabolism. Therefore, the biosecurity of nanomaterials, especially nano-biomaterials, has aroused much concern in recent years.

Biosecurity concerns relating to nanomaterials arise mainly because nanoparticles (of diameter <100 nm) can penetrate through bioshields (such as skin, vessel walls, and cell membranes) with little difficulty due to the numerous nanopores existing in the bioshield and the native pinocytosis of cells. Once nanoparticles have entered a blood vessel or come inside cells, the interactions among proteins, nanoparticles, and degradable products of nanoparticles certainly change the intracellular microenvironment, thereby altering normal cell behaviors [123]. The variation in molecular forces inside cells may have positive results, but can also cause negative results, depending on the bioenvironment and the properties of the nanoparticle. For example, nanoparticles (of diameter <200 nm) can gain access through the blood/brain barrier to cause brain diseases [124]; nanoparticles can penetrate through the lung/blood barrier, leading to a risk of disease [125].

10.6.4.1 Cytotoxicity of CaP nanoparticles

For implanted bioceramics, their huge size differs in nature from nanoparticles, but, due to erosion by bodily fluids and mechanical wear, bioceramic surface degradation may generate nanoparticles. The nanoparticles may diffuse into the surrounding tissues and also migrate to other organs through the circulation of bodily fluid. Although the common bioceramics are biocompatible in bulk form, nanoparticles of them may still show potentially negative bioeffects. For example, it has been found that CaP nanoparticles altered gene expression when they went into cells [126]. Hence, the cytotoxicity of CaP nanoparticles, especially HAP nanoparticles, has attracted much attention.

To evaluate the biosecurity of nanoparticles generated in vivo by biodegradation of bioceramic implants, cytotoxicity tests in vitro are generally used to mimic the situation in vivo by consideration of cell type, nanoparticle dosage, nanoparticle features, including chemical composition, surface charge, and geometric size or even shape.

Different types of cell may have different responses to the same nanoparticle. To examine the response of bone cells to HAP nanoparticles, Shi *et al.* selected three types of bone-related cells, namely MSCs, osteosarcoma cells of type U2OS and MG63 cells, to co-culture with varying concentrations of HAP nanoparticles [127, 128]. Their results showed that, at the same dosage of HAP nanoparticles, MSCs exhibited greater viability and proliferation, whereas growth of U2OS and MG63 cells was greatly inhibited, and many

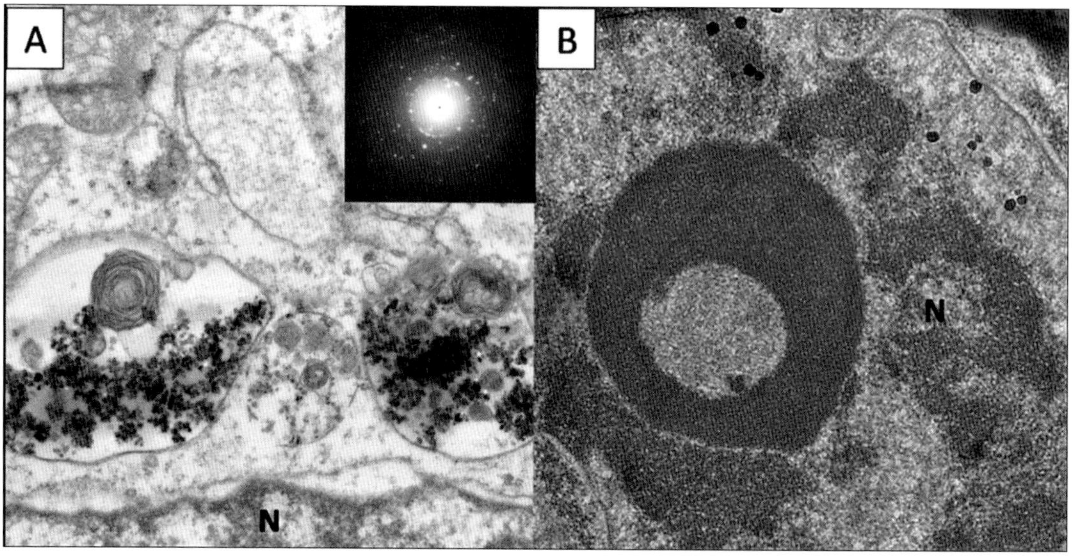

Figure 10.7 (A) TEM images of HAP-NPs in lysosomes. The inset shows the selected area electron diffraction patterns (SAED) of the particles, which confirmed the existence of HAP-NPs. (B) TEM images of MG63 co-cultured with 250 μg/ml HAP-NPs for 5 days, in which retrogressive change of nucleolus occurred, which formed the ring-shaped nucleoli; N, nucleus. Redrawn from [129] with permission.

of the U2OS and MG63 cells died by apoptosis. Moreover, apoptosis of osteosarcoma cells was found to depend on the HAP size because larger HAP nanoparticles (diameter 80 nm) were more effective in inducing apoptosis than were smaller ones (20 nm) [128]. TEM observations showed that HAP nanoparticles could enter both MG63 cells and normal osteoblasts.

To further examine cell-type-dependent cytotoxicity, both osteoblasts and MG63 cells were used to compare their responses to HAP nanoparticles [129]. Typical apoptosis was observed in the MG63 cells, especially under the culture condition of 250 μg/ml of nanoparticles for 5 days. In addition, the phenomenon of nanoparticles entering MG63 cells was also examined by TEM superstructure analysis [129]. When nanoparticles approach cells, the cell membrane starts to sink, and then the nanoparticles are engulfed by independent vesicles forming in the cells. Once they have entered the cells, most of the nanoparticles accumulate within the lysosomes (Figure 10.7, image A). Later, some nanoparticles enter the nucleus (B), leading to the occurrence of ring-shaped nucleoli. The abnormal shape of nuclei is an indication of apoptosis. In contrast, when nanoparticles entered osteoblasts, nanoparticles caused only a slight suppression of the proliferation of osteoblasts, and no adverse effect on the lysosome and the nucleus was observed, although the nanoparticles also appeared in cytoplasm and lysosomes of the osteoblasts.

10.6.4.2 Anticancer potential CaP nanoparticles

Nanoparticle-induced cytotoxicity has been found to be strongly dependent on the cell type tested. Interestingly, normal bone-forming cells such as osteoblasts and MSCs are less sensitive to nanoparticles, whereas non-normal bone-forming cells such as MG63 and osteosarcoma cells of type U2OS are highly sensitive to nanoparticles [127–129]. The exact reason for this phenomenon is unknown, but the phenomenon can be applied to inhibit or even kill tumor cells [130–133].

HAP nanoparticles have been used to test in-vitro nanoparticle-induced cytotoxicity to various normal and tumor cells. For example, a dosage of 150 μg/ml of HAP nanoparticles of diameter 50–60 nm was found to induce significant apoptosis of A375 cells, but little adverse influence on fibroblasts could be observed [134, 135]. Moreover, TEM images and EDS spectra also showed that HAP nanoparticles accumulated inside the nucleolus and vacuoles in cytoplasm of A375 cells, but, for fibroblasts, HAP nanoparticles were distributed mainly in cytoplasm rather than in the nucleolus. More interestingly, the results also indicated that nanoparticle size rather than morphology plays a crucial role in inducing apoptosis [134, 135].

The apoptosis effect of HAP nanoparticles on human hepatoma HepG2 cells was found to be dependent on the size of HAP nanoparticles [136]. HepG2 cells were used to test their response to different sizes of HAP nanoparticles (diameters in the range 20–180 nm), and the results showed that the antitumor activity and the induced apoptosis strongly depended on the size of the HAP nanoparticles, and the efficacies decreased in the order of 45 nm $>$ 26 nm $>$ 78 nm $>$ 175 nm. Optimal tumor cell inhibition efficiency was found for the HAP nanoparticles of diameter 45 nm at a concentration of 400 μg/ml.

The cytotoxicity of HAP nanoparticles is strongly correlated with their surface physicochemical properties. Human monocyte-derived macrophapges in vitro were employed to assess the influence of the surface properties of HAP nanoparticles on cytotoxicity [137]. In these tests, the HAP microparticles tested were synthesized by suspended gel preparation and a spray-drying method. It was found that HAP from suspended gel processing exhibited the strongest cytotoxicity over a large dose range (31–500 μg/ml), but, in contrast, the HAP from spray-drying processing could show cytotoxicity only at higher concentrations ($>$250 μg/ml). The toxicity of HAP nanoparticles is likely to be associated with the increased cytoplasmic calcium load derived from high surface loading of nanoparticles [137].

In summary, the biological risks, cytotoxicity, and anticancer activity of HAP nanoparticles are size- and dose-dependent. More interestingly, HAP nanoparticles have a unique ability to induce apoptosis of different cells selectively, which can lead them to act as tumor inhibitors or even tumor killers. This property should find applications in bone regenerative medicine.

10.7 Bioceramic coatings

The brittleness of bioceramics makes them unsuitable for load-bearing conditions, such as in a hip prosthesis, in a dental implant, and for repair of long bone defects. Biomedical metals, such as titanium metal and its alloys, stainless steel, and Co–Cr–Mo alloys have been widely used for this purpose because of their strength. The inertness of these metals makes them form bioinert bonding with the bony tissue. In order to improve the biological properties of biomedical devices made from metals, bioactive ceramics have been used as coatings on the metals' surfaces for the purpose of providing bioactive bonding between the devices and bony tissue.

In recent years, infections caused by medical devices have attracted many researchers to the idea of developing coatings with antibacterial properties. Some bioceramic coatings containing antibacterial components, such as Ag^+ and nano-titania, have been developed [138, 139].

Many kinds of bioceramic coating on metal surfaces have been developed with different methods, including plasma spraying bioceramic coatings [140], electrochemical bioceramic coatings [141], and biomimetic bioceramic coatings prepared with methods performed under normal atmospheric conditions [142].

10.7.1 Plasma spraying bioceramic coatings

The plasma spraying method is the main commercial method for bioceramic coating preparation. Since the 1980s, most commercial calcium phosphate coatings on titanium metal or Co–Cr alloy have been prepared with plasma spraying techniques. The plasma spraying method is a high-temperature process that involves injecting bioactive powder into a plasma flame at high temperature. The powder is heated and the surface of the powder particles is rendered molten in the plasma flame. The powder is sprayed at high pressure and velocity onto the metal device surface. The molten

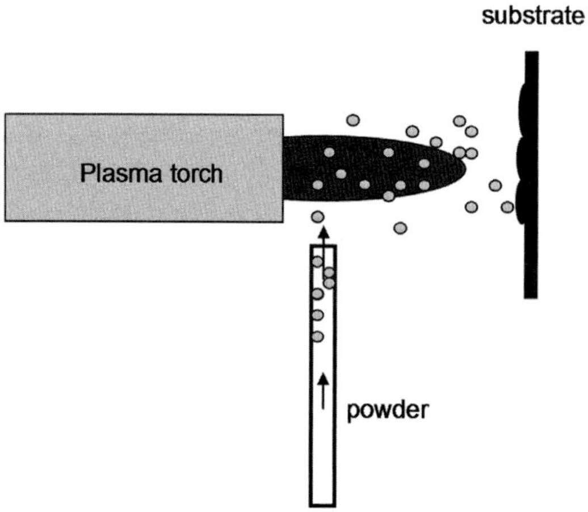

Figure 10.8 A schematic diagram of the plasma spraying system.

surface of the powder particles makes them plastic, and allows a dense and strongly adhesive coating to be formed on the metals (Figure 10.8). The plasma spraying method has been employed to prepare bioactive calcium phosphate, wollastonite, and titania coatings on titanium surfaces.

10.7.1.1 Plasma spraying of calcium phosphate ceramic coatings

Calcium phosphate is the most widely used bioactive ceramic in commercial clinical application. Hydroxyapatite (HAP), α-tricalcium phosphate (α-TCP), β-tricalcium phosphate (β-TCP), brushite (DCP), octacalcium phosphate (OCP), and tetracalcium phosphate (TCPM) have been used in medical devices. During the plasma spraying process, HAP powder is widely employed for the coating preparation. Owing to the high temperature, the thin outer layer of each HAP particle will inevitably undergo phase transitions. In order to get calcium phosphate coatings with optimized performance, many methods have been developed. For example, the phase and bonding strength of the coating could be controlled by varying the plasma spraying parameters, fixing the powder microstructure before deposition, or applying a bio-inert bonding coating between the calcium phosphate coating and the substrate.

The phase transition of the calcium phosphate coating might make the stability of the coating inadequate for clinical application, so some post-treatment methods to improve the stability of the coating have been applied. The most widely used method for this purpose is the water-vapor treatment [143]. In this process, the as-received coatings are subjected to high-temperature (about 120 °C) water-vapor treatment for 3 hours after the plasma spraying. After the treatment, the crystallinity of the coating could be significantly improved, and some calcium phosphate phase with a high dissolution rate could be transformed into HAP, which is the most stable phase in biological environments.

Huang *et al.* [144] recently reported an electrochemical post-treatment method. They immersed the as-received coating in NaOH electrolyte, and applied a positive voltage to the coating. The crystallinity of the coating was significantly improved, and the surface was also endowed with negative charge after the treatment, which significantly improved the performance of the coating. The treated coating could form bioactive bonding with bony tissue with higher push-out strength than that obtained when the coating was treated with the water-vapor method (Figure 10.9).

10.7.1.2 Plasma spraying of wollastonite coating

The CaO–SiO_2-based ceramics are bioactive, and could form bonding with the bony tissue. Wollastonite ($CaSiO_3$), a typical CaO–SiO_2 material, is mainly used for traditional ceramics. Many studies have proved that wollastonite can promote osteoblast proliferation and enhance alkaline phosphate (ALP) activities of the cells [145]. In-vivo studies showed that wollastonite could achieve chemical integration with living bone [146]. So it is also used for bioactive coating on metals.

The plasma spraying technique is used for preparation of wollastonite coatings on metal substrates [147]. The coating produced is not homogeneous, but has a rough surface structure. Because of the high temperature during the plasma spraying process, some decomposition of the wollastonite occurs, making the coating have compounds such as SiO_2 and CaO with the wollastonite as the main phase. It has been

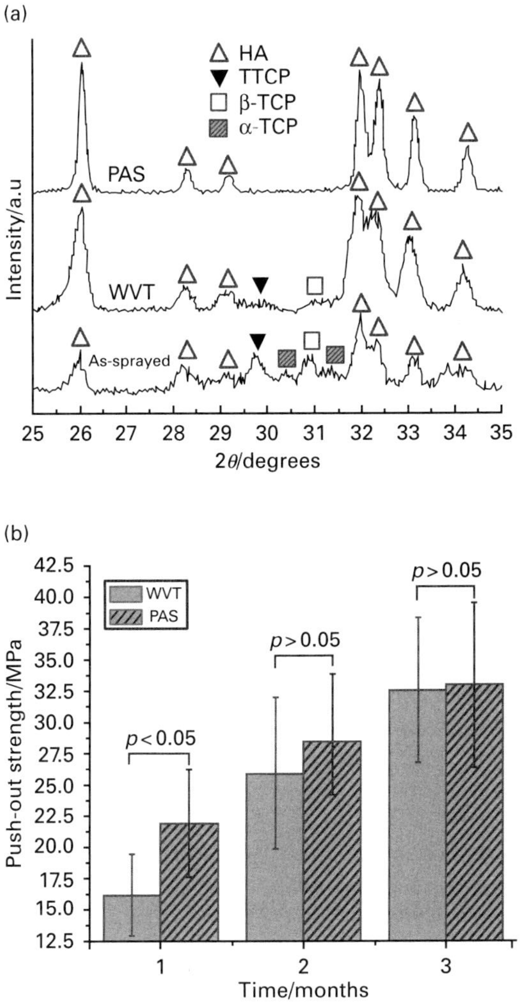

Figure 10.9 The crystallinities of coatings subjected to electrochemical treatment (PAS) and water-vapor treatment (WVT) (a), and their effects on push-out strength with the bony tissue in animal test (b). Reprinted from [144] with permission.

reported that the SiO_2 and CaO phases in the coating might be beneficial for the performance of the wollastonite coating in vivo.

Some other CaO–SiO_2 materials are also used for bioactive coating on metals. For example, dicalcium silicate (Ca_2SiO_4) [147] and diopside ($CaMgSi_2O_6$) [148] could also be sprayed onto a titanium metal substrate using a plasma spraying technique in order to get a bioactive coating.

10.7.1.3 Plasma spraying of titania coatings

Titania with nanostructure has been proved to be bioactive. Titania ceramics that could be used for biomaterials include anatase and rutile. Bulk nano-titania ceramics could induce a bioactive response in biological environments [149].

Some authors have reported that plasma-sprayed titania coatings have great bonding strength with the titanium metal substrate because their properties are homogeneous with those of the titanium metal surface. The overheated titania nano-powder during the plasma spraying process could form metallurgical bonding with the substrate. The high bonding strength has meant that it is widely used as the inter-layer for HAP coating preparation, whereby the bonding strength between the coating and the substrate is significantly improved [150].

During the plasma spraying process, if the crystal grain of the titania is controlled on the nano scale, the nano-titania coating could induce bone bonding in vivo. Some authors have tried to develop bioactive titania coatings with plasma spraying techniques.

10.7.1.4 Plasma spraying of antibacterial coatings

During the plasma spraying process, if Ag^+, Cu^{2+} or Zn^{2+} ions are added to the powder, the coating produced will contain these antibacterial ions. In a study reported by Fielding *et al.*, it was found that 2.0% Ag^+ is enough to endow the HAP coating with antibacterial properties [151].

In most cases, the addition of Ag^+, Zn^{2+}, and Cu^{2+} has no negative effect on the mechanical properties of the coating. However, the potential cytotoxic effect of these ions will induce negative effects on the biological performance of the coating. For example, 2.0% Ag^+ in HAP coatings will completely inhibit the ALP activity of osteoblasts [151]. For this reason, coatings containing antibacterial ions need further evaluation of their biosafety.

10.7.2 Electrochemical bioceramic coatings

In an electrochemical system, the metal substrate is used as an electrode (anode or cathode). Some particular ions (for example, Ca^{2+}, PO_4^{3-}, O^{2-}), or particles (HAP particles) in the electrolyte react with the metal substrate or are deposited on the metal substrate under suitable condition, to give bioactive bioceramic coatings. Many kinds of bioactive coatings, including calcium phosphate, titania, and bioactive composite coatings containing HAP could be prepared by electrochemical methods. In this chapter, we introduce the HAP coatings prepared by cathode electrodeposition, electrophoretic deposition, and bioactive titania coating and a titania/HAP composite coating prepared by anodic oxidation.

10.7.2.1 HAP coating prepared by cathode electrodeposition

In most studies, a solution of $NH_4H_2PO_4$ and $Ca(NO_3)_2$ is used as the electrolyte for preparation of HAP coatings by a cathode electrodeposition method. The metal substrate is connected to the cathode in the system. The HAP coating could be formed on the metal substrate by applying a suitable voltage (current) to the cathode [152].

The electrochemical reaction at the cathode surface has a great effect on the properties of the HAP coating. The decomposition of water at the cathode raises the pH near the electrode, whereupon Ca^{2+} and PO_4^{3-} ions are deposited on the substrate in the high pH environment to form the HAP coating. The Ca/P ratio of the HAP coating can be optimized by controlling the Ca/P ratio of the electrolyte. Most studies have shown that the structure of the HAP coating obtained by the cathode electrodeposition method is similar to that of the apatite in the bone. But the bonding strength with the metal substrate needs to be improved before it can be used in the clinic.

It is also very interesting to develop HAP coatings containing antibacterial ions by this method. In most cases, the antibacterial ions, such as Ag^+, Cu^{2+} or Zn^{2+} ions, are added to the electrolyte [152]. These ions will be co-deposited on the metal surface during the process. It is very easy to adjust the antibacterial ion concentration in the coating and the distribution of these ions in the coating is homogeneous.

10.7.2.2 HAP coatings prepared by electrophoretic deposition

HAP particles in a suspension system move to the cathode in an electric field under the influence of the electrophoretic effect because of the charges on the HAP particle surfaces. After the HAP particles have been deposited on the metal cathode, one has the HAP coating, which might have a great performance for clinical applications [153]. A main advantage of this coating is the limitless freedom regarding the shape of the substrate. We might get a HAP coating in the pore of a porous substrate by this method. The bonding strength of this coating might be improved by a different post-treatment.

10.7.2.3 Bioactive titania coatings prepared by anodic oxidation

In recent years, anodic oxidation has been employed to develop bioactive titania coatings on titanium metal surfaces. In a study by Yang *et al.* [154], titanium metal was immersed in H_2SO_4 electrolyte, and it was used as the anode in the electrochemical system. After a suitable voltage that could induce a spark discharge had been applied to the anode, a titania coating formed on the titanium metal surface. This coating is in the anatase and/or rutile phase with a porous structure. The coating could induce apatite formation in simulated bodily fluid, and formed bonding with the bony tissue (Figure 10.10).

The anodic oxidation method could be used also to form bioactive titania nanotubes on the titanium metal surface [155]. In most studies, fluoride-containing electrolytes are used for this purpose. After application to the titanium metal anode of a suitable voltage, titania nanotubes that are beneficial for the growth of osteoblasts could form on the metal surface.

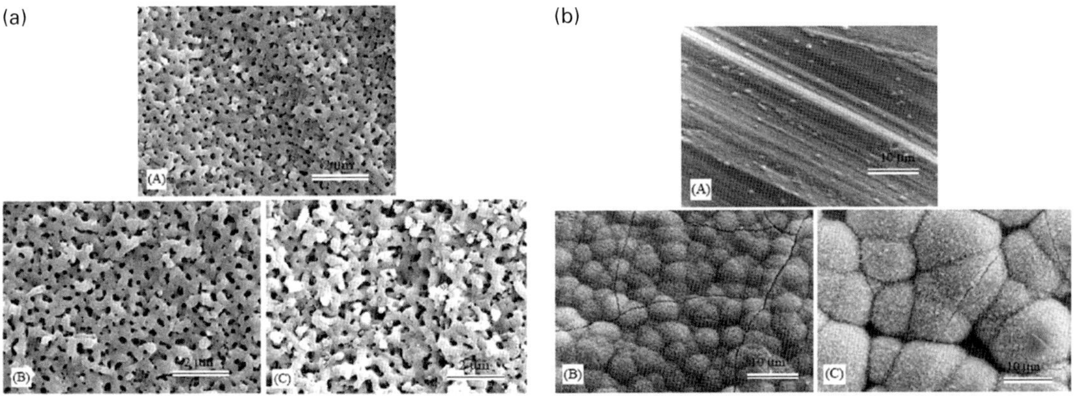

Figure 10.10 Porous titania coatings with anatase and/or rutile phase on titanium metal surfaces after anodic oxidation (a), and the apatite formed on the coating in SBF (b). Reprinted from [154] with permission.

10.7.2.4 Bioactive titania/HAP coatings prepared by anodic oxidation

Some investigators have developed bioactive titania coatings containing HAP by the anodic oxidation method. In these studies, an anode made with titanium metal substrate is treated at a suitable voltage or current in an electrolyte containing Ca and P ions, for example, sodium β-glycerophosphate and calcium acetate [156]. The oxide films obtained are subjected to further treatment to transform the Ca and P in the film into HAP. The final coating is composed of bioactive titania and HAP.

10.7.3 Biomimetic bioceramic coatings prepared under normal atmospheric conditions

Apatite coating could form on the metal surface in simulated bodily fluid after the metal had been subjected to suitable treatment. This apatite coating forms under normal atmospheric conditions, which makes its composition and structure more similar to that of the natural apatite in the bone. It is widely accepted that this coating is a biomimetic coating. For the purpose of obtaining biomimetic coatings, many methods have been developed in the past decades, including alkali-heat treatment [157], acid-alkali treatment [158], and anodic oxidation treatment [154].

It is well known that metal surfaces that have been subjected to different treatments contain some functional groups, such as Ti—OH, Ta—OH, or Si—OH, that are essential for the formation of a biomimetic apatite coating in the simulated bodily fluid. For example, titanium metal subjected to alikali-heat treatment induces apatite formation via the Ti—OH which comes from the hydrolysis of sodium titanate.

In this section, we have briefly introduced several bioceramic coatings. Actually, bioceramic coatings have become a most important field for biomaterials science. Some other methods, for example, the ion deposition method and the sol-gel method, are widely employed to get different kinds of coating. We recommend that readers refer to other references for further information on bioceramic coatings.

10.8 Conclusions

Bioceramics, especially bioactive ceramics, have played important roles in helping hard tissue to repair and regenerate. Although their clinical applications are primarily limited to filling and patching of small defects due to the lower mechanical strength of their porous blocks, this will undoubtedly be altered with advances in understanding of the interaction between implant and host tissue and fast progress in processing techniques such as 3D bioprinting.

Porous CaP ceramics have been proven to be osteoinductive even if implanted in non-osseous sites. The osteoinductivity results from the native wound-healing process that is mediated by the implanted CaP scaffold. The presence of the implanted CaP ceramic at the wound site surely somehow influences the normal wound-healing process, thereby promoting or suppressing the healing process toward osteogenetic differentiation, depending on the properties of the CaP ceramic. This may be the reason why CaP ceramic's osteogenetic potency is dependent on its properties, implantation site, and animal species. Unlike a tissue-engineered CaP implant that has been pre-filled with bone cells and growth factors prior to implantation, the porous CaP implant mentioned here has nothing inside it before it is implanted. Thus, after being implanted, the scaffold has to exert its own effect to adsorb growth factors and recruit cells from its surroundings, and guide wound healing toward osteogenesis. In this sense, there is a direct correlation between the CaP implant's performance and the rate and amount of new bone formation. However, the exact correlation is largely unknown and remains to be investigated.

According to the requirements of hard-tissue repair and regeneration, bioactive ceramic scaffolds, acting as temporary supports to provide a 3D niche for recruiting and accommodating cells related to bone formation until the newly formed bone tissue can maintain subsequent bone remodeling, are expected to have simultaneously three characters: osteoinductive potential, appropriate mechanical strength, and a desirable biodegradation rate. Unfortunately, none of the bioactive ceramics alone can meet all the needs. Fortunately, among the commonly bioactive ceramics, CaP ceramics are the most promising candidate material for fabricating synthetic bone grafts because BCP ceramic can largely satisfy two of the three needs, namely osteoinductivity and biodegradability. With regard to the mechanical strength of porous CaP implants, some commercially available porous CaP-based scaffolds can match the strength of cancellous bone; moreover, their strength can be further improved with the help of a combination of computer simulation, 3D design and printing, nanotechniques, and advanced thermal processing. Even if it is unrealistic to expect CaP implants to replace damaged hips in the very near future, CaP ceramic is also the preferred material used for bioactivation of titanium-based load-bearing devices. Therefore, further improvement in the strength of porous CaP scaffolds will be crucial to extending their applications from small-defect filling to large-defect grafting.

The porosity of a porous CaP scaffold plays complicated roles in the osteogenetic process. Superficially, high porosity is generally beneficial to osteogenesis, but, for porous HAP with the same porosity as BCP, the high porosity does not necessarily cause a favorable osteogenesis because it has been found that the porous HAP exhibited poorer osteogenesis than that of the BCP. Moreover, high porosity certainly results in a significant decrease in mechanical strength. Therefore, it is still necessary to achieve a balance between the osteogenesis and the mechanical strength by optimal design.

To increase the strength of existing CaP scaffolds, a key issue is to find optimal porous structures, in which a low macroporosity and a high density of pore-interconnected channels might be preferred because an excessively high macroporosity significantly decreases the strength but offers only a limited contribution to osteogenesis. To enhance the osteogenetic capacity of CaP scaffolds with low macroporosity, more attention should be paid to increasing the surface activity of the ceramic. For this purpose, the available means include increasing the number of concavities of sub-microscale size and the density of nano-geometric features on the inner surfaces of macropores, and increasing the rate of formation of bone-like apatite by modifying or doping the ceramic surface. Besides, to help design scaffold architecture, more attention should also be focussed on understanding the molecular, cellular, and genetic mechanisms underlying the osteogenesis process regulated by the CaP ceramic's surface properties, including chemical composition, Young's modulus, stiffness, and topographic features.

REFERENCES

[1] Mauck, K. F. and Clarke, B. L. 2006. Diagnosis, screening, prevention, and treatment of osteoporosis. *Mayo Clinic Proc.*, 662–72.

[2] Service, R. F. 2000 Tissue engineers build new bone. *Science*, **289**, 1498–500.

[3] LeGeros, R. Z. 2002. Properties of osteoconductive biomaterials: calcium phosphates. *Clin. Orthopaedics Related Res.*, **395**, 81–98.

[4] Banwart, J. C., Asher, M. A. and Hassanein, R. S. 1995. Iliac crest bone graft harvest donor site morbidity: a statistical evaluation. *Spine*, **20**, 1055.

[5] Costantino, P. D. and Friedman, C. D. 1994. Synthetic bone graft substitutes. *Otolaryngol. Clinics North America*, **27**, 1037.

[6] Damien, C. J. and Parsons, J. R. 1991. Bone graft and bone graft substitutes: a review of current technology and applications. *J. Appl. Biomater.*, **2**, 187–208.

[7] Langer, R. and Vacanti, J. P. 1993. Tissue engineering. *Science*, **260**, 920–6.

[8] Rose, F. R. A. J. and Oreffo, R. O. C. 2002. Bone tissue engineering: hope vs hype. *Biochem. Biophys. Res. Commun.*, **292**, 1–7.

[9] Crane, G. M., Ishaug, S. L. and Mikos, A. G. 1995. Bone tissue engineering. *Nature Med.*, **1**, 1322–4.

[10] Minuth, W. W., Sittinger, M. and Kloth, S. 1997. Tissue engineering: generation of differentiated artificial tissues for biomedical applications. *Cell Tissue Res.*, **291**, 1–11.

[11] Jones, J. and Hench, L. 2001. Biomedical materials for new millennium: perspective on the future. *Mater. Sci. Technol.*, **17**, 891–900.

[12] Ripamonti, U. 1996. Osteoinduction in porous hydroxyapatite implanted in heterotopic sites of different animal models. *Biomaterials*, **17**, 31–5.

[13] Yuan, H., Van Blitterswijk, C., De Groot, K. and De Bruijn, J. 2006. A comparison of bone formation in biphasic calcium phosphate (BCP) and hydroxyapatite (HA) implanted in muscle and bone of dogs at different time periods. *J. Biomed. Mater. Res. Part A*, **78**, 139–47.

[14] Fujibayashi, S., Shikata, J., Tanaka, C., Matsushita, M. and Nakamura, T. 2001. Lumbar posterolateral fusion with biphasic calcium phosphate ceramic. *J. Spinal Disorders Techniques*, **14**, 214–21.

[15] Kitsugi, T., Nakamura, T., Yamamura, T. *et al.* 1987. SEM-EPMA observation of three types of apatite-containing glass ceramics implanted in bone: the variance of a Ca-P-rich layer. *J. Biomed. Mater. Res.*, **21**, 1255–71.

[16] Yamasaki, H. 1990. Heterotopic bone formation around porous hydroxyapatite ceramics in the subcutis of dogs. *Jap. J. Oral Biol.*, **32**, 190–2.

[17] Yamasaki, H. and Sakai, H. 1992. Osteogenic response to porous hydroxyapatite ceramics under the skin of dogs. *Biomaterials*, **13**, 308–12.

[18] Yuan, H., Yang, Z., de Bruijn, J. D., de Groot, K. and Zhang, X. 2001. Material-dependent bone induction by calcium phosphate ceramics: a 2.5-year study in dog. *Biomaterials*, **22**, 2617–23.

[19] Yuan, H., Van Den Doel, M., Li, S. *et al.* 2002. A comparison of the osteoinductive potential of two calcium phosphate ceramics implanted intramuscularly in goats. *J. Mater. Sci.: Mater. Med.*, **13**, 1271–5.

[20] Yuan, H., Kurashina, K., de Bruijn, J. D. *et al.* 1999. A preliminary study on osteoinduction of two kinds of calcium phosphate ceramics. *Biomaterials*, **20**, 1799–806.

[21] Cao, W. and Hench, L. L. 1996. Bioactive materials. *Ceramics Int.*, **22**, 493–507.

[22] Boutin, P. 1972. Arthroplastie total de la hanche par prothèse en alumine frittée. *Rev. Chirurgie Orthopédique Réparatrice Appareil Moteur*, **58**, 229–246.

[23] Lusty, P., Tai, C., Sew-Hoy, R. *et al.* 2007. Third-generation alumina-on-alumina ceramic bearings in cementless total hip arthroplasty. *J. Bone Joint Surgery*, **89**, 2676–83.

[24] D'Antonio, J., Capello, W., Manley, M. and Bierbaum, B. 2000. New experience with alumina-on-alumina ceramic bearings for total hip arthroplasty. *J. Arthroplasty*, **17**, 390–7.

[25] Kim, Y.-H., Kim, J.-S., Choi, Y.-W. and Kwon, O.-R. 2009. Intermediate results of simultaneous alumina-on-alumina bearing and alumina-on-highly cross-linked polyethylene bearing total hip arthroplasties. *J. Arthroplasty*, **24**, 885–91.

[26] Klopčič, S. B., Kovač, J. and Kosmač, T. 2007. Apatite-forming ability of alumina and zirconia ceramics in a supersaturated Ca/P solution. *Biomolec. Eng.*, **24**, 467–71.

[27] Hench, L., Splinter, R., Allen, W. and Greenlee, T. 1971. Mechanisms of interfacial bonding between ceramics and bone. *J. Biomed. Mater. Res.*, **2**, 485.

[28] Hench, L. L. and Paschall, H. 1973. Direct chemical bond of bioactive glass-ceramic Materials to bone and muscle. *J. Biomed. Mater. Res.*, **7**, 25–42.

[29] Nuss, K. M. and von Rechenberg, B. 2008. Biocompatibility issues with modern implants in bone – a review for clinical orthopedics. *Open Orthopaedics J.*, **2**, 66.

[30] Cypher, T. J. and Grossman, J. P. 1996. Biological principles of bone graft healing. *J. Foot Ankle Surgery*, **35**, 413–17.

[31] Anderson, J. M., Rodriguez, A. and Chang, D. T. 2008. Foreign body reaction to biomaterials. *Seminars in Immunology: NIH Public Access*, p. 86.

[32] Anderson, J. M. 2001. Biological responses to materials. *Ann. Rev. Mater. Res.*, **31**, 81–110.

[33] Martin, P. and Leibovich, S. J. 2005. Inflammatory cells during wound repair: the good, the bad and the ugly. *Trends Cell Biol.*, **15**, 599–607.

[34] George Broughton, I., Janis, J. E. and Attinger, C. E. 2006. Wound healing: an overview. *Plastic Reconstructive Surgery*, **117**, 1e-S-32e-S.

[35] Fujiwara, N. and Kobayashi, K. 2005. Macrophages in inflammation. *Current Drug Targets – Inflammation Allergy*, **4**, 281–6.

[36] Luttikhuizen, D. T., Harmsen, M. C. and Luyn, M. J. V. 2006. Cellular and molecular dynamics in the foreign body reaction. *Tissue Eng.*, **12**, 1955–70.

[37] Hench, L. L. and West, J. K. 1996. Biological applications of bioactive glasses. *Life Chem. Rep.*, **13**, 187–241.

[38] Clark, A., Hench, L. and Paschall, H. 1976. The influence of surface chemistry on implant interface histology: a theoretical basis for implant materials selection. *J. Biomed. Mater. Res.*, **10**, 161–74.

[39] Hench, L. L. 1998. Bioceramics. *J. Am. Ceram. Soc.*, **81**, 1705–28.

[40] Hench, L. L. and Polak, J. M. 2002. Third-generation biomedical materials. *Science*, **295**, 1014–17.

[41] Rehman, I., Hench, L., Bonfield, W. and Smith, R. 1994. Analysis of surface layers on bioactive glasses. *Biomaterials*, **15**, 865–70.

[42] Varila, L., Fagerlund, S., Lehtonen, T., Tuominen, J. and Hupa, L. 2012. Surface reactions of bioactive glasses in buffered solutions. *J. Eur. Ceram. Soc.*, **32**, 2757–63.

[43] Hench, L. 2000. The challenge of orthopaedic materials. *Current Orthopaedics*, **14**, 7–15.

[44] Hench, L., Hench, J. W. and Greenspan, D. 2004. Bioglass: a short history and bibliography. *J. Australasian Ceram. Soc.*, **40**, 1–42.

[45] Park, S.-Y., Bae, D.-J., Kim, M.-J., Piao, M. L. and Kim, I.-S. 2012. Extracellular low pH modulates phosphatidylserine-dependent phagocytosis in macrophages by increasing stabilin-1 expression. *J. Biol. Chem.*, **287**, 11261–71.

[46] Lu, X. and Leng, Y. 2005. Theoretical analysis of calcium phosphate precipitation in simulated body fluid. *Biomaterials*, **26**, 1097–108.

[47] Zhang, D., Hupa, M. and Hupa, L. 2008. *In situ* pH within particle beds of bioactive glasses. *Acta Biomater.*, **4**, 1498–505.

[48] Damen, J. and Ten Cate, J. 1989. The effect of silicic acid on calcium phosphate precipitation. *J. Dental Res.*, **68**, 1355–9.

[49] Damen, J. and Ten Cate, J. 1992. Silica-induced precipitation of calcium phosphate in the presence of inhibitors of hydroxyapatite formation. *J. Dental Res.*, **71**, 453–7.

[50] Calvert, P. and Mann, S. 1997. The negative side of crystal growth. *Nature*, **386**, 127–9.

[51] Zhu, P., Masuda, Y. and Koumoto, K. 2004. The effect of surface charge on hydroxyapatite nucleation. *Biomaterials*, **25**, 3915–21.

[52] Lu, H. H., Pollack, S. R. and Ducheyne, P. 2000. Temporal zeta potential variations of 45S5 bioactive glass immersed in an electrolyte solution. *J. Biomed. Mater. Res.*, **51**, 80–7.

[53] Ohtsuki, C., Kokubo, T. and Yamamuro, T. 1992. Mechanism of apatite formation on $CaOSiO_2$–P_2O_5 glasses in a simulated body fluid. *J. Non-Cryst. Solids*, **143**, 84–92.

[54] Pereira, M. M., Clark, A. E. and Hench, L. L. 1995. Effect of texture on the rate of hydroxyapatite formation on gel-silica surface. *J. Am. Ceram. Soc.*, **78**, 2463–8.

[55] Li, P., Nakanishi, K., Kokubo, T. and de Groot, K. 1993. Induction and morphology of hydroxyapatite, precipitated from metastable simulated body fluids on sol-gel prepared silica. *Biomaterials*, **14**, 963–8.

[56] Salinas, A., Vallet-Regi, M. and Izquierdo-Barba, I. 2001. Biomimetic apatite deposition on calcium silicate gel glasses. *J. Sol-Gel Sci. Technol.*, **21**, 13–25.

[57] Li, R., Clark, A. and Hench, L. 1991. An investigation of bioactive glass powders by sol-gel processing. *J. Appl. Biomater.*, **2**, 231–9.

[58] Li, P., Ohtsuki, C., Kokubo, T. *et al.* 1992. Apatite formation induced by silica gel in a simulated body fluid. *J. Am. Ceram. Soc.*, **75**, 2094–7.

[59] Li, P., Kangasniemi, I., De Groot, K., Kokubo, T. and Yli-Urpo, A. 1994. Apatite crystallization from metastable calcium phosphate solution on sol-gel-prepared silica. *J. Non-Cryst. Solids*, **168**, 281–6.

[60] Guanabara, P. Jr., Rodrigues, A. and Peitl, O. 2004. Bioactivity study of glass-ceramics with various crystalline fractions obtained by controlled crystallization. *Mater. Sci. Eng. C*, **24**, 689–91.

[61] Klein, C., de Groot, K., Chen, W., Li, Y. and Zhang, X. 1994. Osseous substance formation induced in porous calcium phosphate ceramics in soft tissues. *Biomaterials*, **15**, 31–4.

[62] Albrektsson, T. and Johansson, C. 2001. Osteoinduction, osteoconduction and osseointegration. *European Spine J.*, **10**, S96–S101.

[63] Levander, G. 1938. A study of bone regeneration. *Surg. Gynecol. Obstet.*, **67**, 705–14.

[64] Urist, M. R. and McLean, F. C. 1952. Osteogenetic potency and new-bone formation by induction in transplants to the anterior chamber of the eye. *J. Bone Joint Surgery*, **34**, 443–75.

[65] Young, R. W. 1963. Nucleic acids, protein synthesis and bone. *Clin. Orthopaedics Related Res.*, **26**, 147–60.

[66] Urist, M. R. 1965. Bone: formation by autoinduction. *Science*, **150**, 893–9.

[67] Urist, M. R., Mikulski, A. and Lietze, A. 1979. Solubilized and insolubilized bone morphogenetic protein. *Proc. Nat. Acad. Sci. USA*, **76**, 1828–32.

[68] Dealler, S. 1981. Electrical phenomena associated with bones and fractures and the therapeutic use of electricity in fracture healing. *J. Med. Eng. Technol.*, **5**, 73–9.

[69] Yasuda, I. 1977. The classic fundamental aspects of fracture treatment. *Clin. Orthopaedics Related Res.*, **124**, 5–8.

[70] Ripamonti, U. 1991. The morphogenesis of bone in replicas of porous hydroxyapatite obtained from conversion of calcium carbonate exoskeletons of coral. *J. Bone Joint Surgery*, **73**, 692–703.

[71] Heughebaert, M., LeGeros, R., Gineste, M., Guilhem, A. and Bonel, G. 1988. Physicochemical characterization of deposits associated with HA ceramics implanted in nonosseous sites. *J. Biomed. Mater. Res.*, **22**, 257–68.

[72] Zhang, X., Zou, P. and Wu, C. 1991. A study of porous block HA ceramics and its osteogenesis. In *Bioceramics and the Human Body* ed. Ravaglioli, A. and Krajewski, A. Amsterdam: Elsevier Applied Science, pp. 408–15.

[73] Yuan, H., van Blitterswijk, C. A., de Groot, K. and de Bruijn, J. D. 2006. Cross-species comparison of ectopic bone formation in biphasic calcium phosphate (BCP) and hydroxyapatite (HA) scaffolds. *Tissue Eng.*, **12**, 1607–15.

[74] Scott, M. A., Levi, B., Askarinam, A. *et al.* 2011. Brief review of models of ectopic bone formation. *Stem Cells Development*, **21**, 655–67.

[75] Yang, Z., Yuan, H., Tong, W. *et al.* 1996. Osteogenesis in extraskeletally implanted porous calcium phosphate ceramics: variability among different kinds of animals. *Biomaterials*, **17**, 2131–7.

[76] Yuan, H., De Bruijn, J., Li, Y. *et al.* 2001. Bone formation induced by calcium phosphate ceramics in soft tissue of dogs: a comparative study between porous α-TCP and β-TCP. *J. Mater. Sci.: Mater. Med.*, **12**, 7–13.

[77] Yang, Z. J., Yuan, H., Zou, P. *et al.* 1997. Osteogenic responses to extraskeletally implanted synthetic porous calcium phosphate ceramics: an early stage histomorphological study in dogs. *J. Mater. Sci.: Mater. Med.*, **8**, 697–701.

[78] Ripamonti, U., Van den Heever, B. and Van Wyk, J. 1993. Expression of the osteogenic phenotype in porous hydroxyapatite implanted extraskeletally in baboons. *Matrix*, **13**, 491–502.

[79] Habibovic, P., Sees, T. M., van den Doel, M. A., van Blitterswijk, C. A. and de Groot, K. 2006. Osteoinduction by biomaterials – physicochemical and structural influences. *J. Biomed. Mater. Res. Part A*, **77**, 747–62.

[80] Habibovic, P. and de Groot, K. 2007. Osteoinductive biomaterials – properties and relevance in bone repair. *J. Tissue Eng. Regenerative Med.*, **1**, 25–32.

[81] Zhang, X. 2008. Osteoinduction and ostogenic genes expression regulated by Ca-P bioceramics. Biomaterials in Asia. In *Commemoration of the 1st Asian Biomaterials Congress*, Tsukuba, 2007. Singapore: World Scientific.

[82] Wang, E. A. 1993. Bone morphogenetic proteins (BMPs): therapeutic potential in healing bony defects. *Trends Biotechnol.*, **11**, 379–83.

[83] Qu, S., Guo, X., Weng, J. *et al.* 2004. Evaluation of the expression of collagen type I in porous calcium phosphate ceramics implanted in an extra-osseous site. *Biomaterials*, **25**, 659–67.

[84] Yuan, H., Zou, P., Yang, Z. *et al.* 1998. Bone morphogenetic protein and ceramic-induced osteogenesis. *J. Mater. Sci.: Mater. Med.*, **9**, 717–21.

[85] Peitl Filho, O. and Latorre, G. P. 1996. Effect of crystallization on apatite-layer formation of bioactive glass. *J. Biomed. Mater. Res.*, **30**, 509–14.

[86] Bellucci, D., Cannillo, V. and Sola, A. 2010. An overview of the effects of thermal processing on bioactive glasses. *Sci. Sintering*, **42**, 307–20.

[87] Wang, C., Duan, Y., Markovic, B. *et al.* 2004. Phenotypic expression of bone-related genes in osteoblasts grown on calcium phosphate ceramics with different phase compositions. *Biomaterials*, **25**, 2507–14.

[88] Wang, C., Duan, Y., Markovic, B. *et al.* 2004. Proliferation and bone-related gene expression of osteoblasts grown on hydroxyapatite ceramics sintered at different temperature. *Biomaterials*, **25**, 2949–56.

[89] Fan, H. S., Ikoma, T., Bao, C. *et al.* 2006. Surface characteristics and osteoinductivity of biphasic calcium phosphate ceramics with different sintering temperature. *Key Eng. Mater.*, **309**, 1299–302.

[90] Li, P., Yang, Q., Zhang, F. and Kokubo, T. 1992. The effect of residual glassy phase in a bioactive glass-ceramic on the formation of its surface apatite layer in vitro. *J. Mater. Sci.: Mater. Med.*, **3**, 452–6.

[91] Hench, L. L. 1993. *An Introduction to Bioceramics.* Singapore: World Scientific.

[92] Habibovic, P., Yuan, H., van der Valk, C. M. *et al.* 2005. 3D microenvironment as essential element for osteoinduction by biomaterials. *Biomaterials*, **26**, 3565–75.

[93] Hollister, S. J. 2005. Porous scaffold design for tissue engineering. *Nature Mater.*, **4**, 518–24.

[94] Chu, T.-M. G., Orton, D. G., Hollister, S. J., Feinberg, S. E. and Halloran, J. W. 2002. Mechanical and in vivo performance of hydroxyapatite implants with controlled architectures. *Biomaterials*, **23**, 1283–93.

[95] Hong, Y., Fan, H., Li, B. *et al.* 2010. Fabrication, biological effects, and medical applications of calcium phosphate nanoceramics. *Mater. Sci. Eng.: R: Reports*, **70**, 225–42.

[96] Gu, Y., Loh, N., Khor, K., Tor, S. and Cheang, P. 2002. Spark plasma sintering of hydroxyapatite powders. *Biomaterials*, **23**, 37–43.

[97] Xu, J., Khor, K., Gu, Y., Kumar, R. and Cheang, P. 2005. Radio frequency (rf) plasma spheroidized HA powders: powder characterization and spark plasma sintering behavior. *Biomaterials*, **26**, 2197–207.

[98] Li, W. and Gao, L. 2003. Fabrication of HAp–ZrO_2(3Y) nano-composite by SPS. *Biomaterials*, **24**, 937–40.

[99] Rameshbabu, N. and Rao, K. P. 2009. Microwave synthesis, characterization and in-vitro evaluation of nanostructured biphasic calcium phosphates. *Current Appl. Phys.*, **9**, S29–S31.

[100] Menezes, R. and Kiminami, R. 2008. Microwave sintering of alumina–zirconia nanocomposites. *J. Mater. Processing Technol.*, **203**, 513–17.

[101] Jalota, S., Tas, A. C. and Bhaduri, S. B. 2004. Microwave-assisted synthesis of calcium phosphate nanowhiskers. *J. Mater. Res.*, **19**, 1876.

[102] Li, P., Chen, I.-W. and Penner-Hahn, J. E. 1993. X-ray-absorption studies of zirconia polymorphs. II. Effect of Y_2O_3 dopant on ZrO_2 structure. *Phys. Rev. B*, **48**, 10074.

[103] Lu, B., Yi, D. Q., Yan, B. *et al.* 2005. High-pressure sintering and magnetic properties of $Fe_{86}Zr_{11-x}Nb_xB_3$ ($x = 5.5, 6$) amorphous alloys. *Trans. Nonferrous Metals Soc. China*, **15**, 828–33.

[104] Fang, Y., Agrawal, D. K., Roy, D. M. and Roy, R. 1994. Microwave sintering of hydroxyapatite ceramics. *J. Mater. Res.*, **9**, 180–7.

[105] Murugan, R. and Ramakrishna, S. 2006. Production of ultra-fine bioresorbable carbonated hydroxyapatite. *Acta Biomater.*, **2**, 201–6.

[106] Webster, T. J., Ergun, C., Doremus, R. H., Siegel, R. W. and Bizios, R. 2000. Specific proteins mediate enhanced osteoblast adhesion on nanophase ceramics. *J. Biomed. Mater. Res.*, **51**, 475–83.

[107] Lück, M., Paulke, B. R., Schröder, W., Blunk, T. and Müller, R. 1998. Analysis of plasma protein adsorption on polymeric nanoparticles with different surface characteristics. *J. Biomed. Mater. Res.*, **39**, 478–85.

[108] Lopes, M., Monteiro, F., Santos, J., Serro, A. and Saramago, B. 1999. Hydrophobicity, surface tension, and zeta potential measurements of glass-reinforced hydroxyapatite composites. *J. Biomed. Mater. Res.*, **45**, 370–5.

[109] Webster, T. J., Siegel, R. W. and Bizios, R. 1999. Osteoblast adhesion on nanophase ceramics. *Biomaterials*, **20**, 1221–7.

[110] Webster, T. J., Schadler, L. S., Siegel, R. W. and Bizios, R. 2001. Mechanisms of enhanced osteoblast adhesion on nanophase alumina involve vitronectin. *Tissue Eng.*, **7**, 291–301.

[111] Ma, P. X. and Zhang, R. 1999. Synthetic nano-scale fibrous extracellular matrix. *J. Biomed. Mater. Res.*, **46**, 60–72.

[112] Chen, V. J., Smith, L. A. and Ma, P. X. 2006. Bone regeneration on computer-designed nano-fibrous scaffolds. *Biomaterials*, **27**, 3973–9.

[113] Rezwan, K., Meier, L. P. and Gauckler, L. J. 2005. Lysozyme and bovine serum albumin adsorption on uncoated silica and AlOOH-coated silica particles: the influence of positively and negatively charged oxide surface coatings. *Biomaterials*, **26**, 4351–7.

[114] Abbatiello, S. and Porter, T. 1997. Anion-mediated precipitation of recombinant human bone morphogenetic protein (rhBMP-2) is dependent upon the heparin binding N-terminal region. *Protein Sci.*, **6**, 99.

[115] Wan, Y., Wang, Y., Liu, Z. *et al.* 2005. Adhesion and proliferation of OCT-1 osteoblast-like cells on micro- and nano-scale topography structured poly(L-lactide). *Biomaterials*, **26**, 4453–9.

[116] Guo, X., Gough, J. E., Xiao, P., Liu, J. and Shen, Z. 2007. Fabrication of nanostructured hydroxyapatite and analysis of human osteoblastic cellular response. *J. Biomed. Mater. Res. Part A*, **82**, 1022–32.

[117] Zhao, Y., Zhang, Y., Ning, F., Guo, D. and Xu, Z. 2007. Synthesis and cellular biocompatibility of two kinds of HAP with different nanocrystal morphology. *J. Biomed. Mater. Res. Part B: Appl. Biomater.*, **83**, 121–6.

[118] Li, B., Chen, X., Guo, B. *et al.* 2009. Fabrication and cellular biocompatibility of porous carbonated biphasic calcium phosphate ceramics with a nanostructure. *Acta Biomater.*, **5**, 134.

[119] Hansen, J. C., Yul Lim, J., Xu, L.-C. *et al.* 2007. Effect of surface nanoscale topography on elastic modulus of individual osteoblastic cells as determined by atomic force microscopy. *J. Biomech.*, **40**, 2865–71.

[120] Tambasco de Oliveira, P. and Nanci, A. 2004. Nanotexturing of titanium-based surfaces upregulates expression of bone sialoprotein and osteopontin by cultured osteogenic cells. *Biomaterials*, **25**, 403–13.

[121] Isa, Z. M., Schneider, G. B., Zaharias, R., Seabold, D. and Stanford, C. M. 2006. Effects of fluoride-modified titanium surfaces on osteoblast proliferation and gene expression. *Int. J. Oral Maxillofacial Implants*, **21**, 203.

[122] Lobel, K. and Hench, L. 1996. In-vitro protein interactions with a bioactive gel-glass. *J. Sol-Gel Sci. Technol.*, **7**, 69–76.

[123] Service, R. 2003. American Chemical Society meeting: nanomaterials show signs of toxicity. *Science*, **300**, 243.

[124] Tsuji, J. S., Maynard, A. D., Howard, P. C. *et al.* 2006. Research strategies for safety evaluation of nanomaterials, part IV: risk assessment of nanoparticles. *Toxicol. Sci.*, **89**, 42–50.

[125] Card, J. W., Zeldin, D. C., Bonner, J. C. and Nestmann, E. R. 2008. Pulmonary applications and toxicity of engineered nanoparticles. *Am. J. Physiol. – Lung Cellular Molec. Physiol.*, **295**, L400–11.

[126] Yuan, H., Li, Y., De Bruijn, J., De Groot, K. and Zhang, X. 2000. Tissue responses of calcium phosphate cement: a study in dogs. *Biomaterials*, **21**, 1283–90.

[127] Shi, Z., Huang, X., Liu, B. *et al.* 2010. Biological response of osteosarcoma cells to size-controlled nanostructured hydroxyapatite. *J. Biomater. Appl.*, **25**, 19–37.

[128] Shi, Z., Huang, X., Cai, Y., Tang, R. and Yang, D. 2009. Size effect of hydroxyapatite nanoparticles on proliferation and apoptosis of osteoblast-like cells. *Acta Biomater.*, **5**, 338–45.

[129] Qing, F., Wang, Z., Hong, Y. *et al.* 2012. Selective effects of hydroxyapatite nanoparticles on osteosarcoma cells and osteoblasts. *J. Mater. Sci.: Mater. Med.*, **23**, 2245–51.

[130] Aoki, H., Ogaki, M. and Kano, S. 1993. Effects of adriacin-absorbing hydroxyapatite-sol on Ca-9 cell growth. *Rep. Inst. Med. Dent. Eng.*, **27**, 39–44.

[131] Cao, X., Li, S., Zhang, R. and Yan, Y. 2003. Effect on the hepatocellular carcinoma cell proliferation and cell cycle treated with hydroxyapatite nanoparticles. *Chinese J. Cancer Prevention Treatment*, **10**, 256–8.

[132] Liu, Z.-S., Tang, S.-L. and Ai, Z.-L. 2003. Effects of hydroxyapatite nanoparticles on proliferation and apoptosis of human hepatoma BEL-7402 cells. *World J. Gastroenterol.*, **9**, 1968–71.

[133] Chen, X., Deng, C., Tang, S. and Zhang, M. 2007. Mitochondria-dependent apoptosis induced by nanoscale hydroxyapatite in human gastric cancer SGC-7901 cells. *Biol. Pharmaceutical Bull.*, **30**, 128–32.

[134] Li, B., Guo, B., Fan, H. and Zhang, X. 2008. Preparation of nano-hydroxyapatite particles with different morphology and their response to highly malignant melanoma cells in vitro. *Appl. Surf. Sci.*, **255**, 357–60.

[135] Guo, B., Li, B., Wang, X. L. *et al.* 2007. Effect of different hydroxyapatite particles on malignant melanoma cell behavior. *Key Eng. Mater.*, **342**, 761–4.

[136] Yuan, Y., Liu, C., Qian, J., Wang, J. and Zhang, Y. 2010. Size-mediated cytotoxicity and apoptosis of hydroxyapatite nanoparticles in human hepatoma HepG2 cells. *Biomaterials*, **31**, 730–40.

[137] Motskin, M., Wright, D., Muller, K. *et al.* 2009. Hydroxyapatite nano and microparticles: correlation of particle properties with cytotoxicity and biostability. *Biomaterials*, **30**, 3307–17.

[138] Zhang, P., Zhang, Z., Li, W. and Zhu, M. 2013. Antibacterial TiO_2 coating incorporating silver nanoparticles by microarc oxidation and ion implantation. *J. Nanomater.*, 1–8.

[139] Yang, B., Gan, L., Qu, Y. and Yue, C. 2010. Anti-inflammatory properties of bioactive titanium metals. *J. Biomed. Mater. Res. Part A*, **94**, 700–5.

[140] De Groot, K., Wolke, J. and Jansen, J. 1998. Calcium phosphate coatings for medical implants. *Proc. Inst. Mech. Eng., Part H: J. Eng. Med.*, **212**, 137–47.

[141] Wang, Y.-Q., Tao, J., Wang, L., He, P.-T. and Wang, T. 2008. HA coating on titanium with nanotubular anodized TiO_2 intermediate layer via electrochemical deposition. *Trans. Nonferrous Metals Soc. China*, **18**, 631–5.

[142] Jonášová, L., Müller, F. A., Helebrant, A., Strnad, J. and Greil, P. 2004. Biomimetic apatite formation on chemically treated titanium. *Biomaterials*, **25**, 1187–94.

[143] Cao, Y., Weng, J., Chen, J. *et al.* 1996. Water vapour-treated hydroxyapatite coatings after plasma spraying and their characteristics. *Biomaterials*, **17**, 419–24.

[144] Huang, Y., Qu, Y., Yang, B. *et al.* 2009. In vivo biological responses of plasma sprayed hydroxyapatite coatings

with an electric polarized treatment in alkaline solution. *Mater. Sci. Eng. C*, **29**, 2411–16.

[145] Ohgushi, H., Tamai, S., Dohi, Y. *et al.* 1996. In vitro bone formation by rat marrow cell culture. *J. Biomed. Mater. Res.*, **32**, 333–40.

[146] Wang, C., Xue, Y., Lin, K. *et al.* 2012. The enhancement of bone regeneration by a combination of osteoconductivity and osteostimulation using β-$CaSiO_3$/β-$Ca_3(PO_4)_2$ composite bioceramics. *Acta Biomater.*, **8**, 350–60.

[147] Cao, H. and Liu, X. 2013. Plasma-sprayed ceramic coatings for osseointegration. *Int. J. Appl. Ceram. Technol.*, **10**, 1–10.

[148] Xue, W., Liu, X., Zheng, X. and Ding, C. 2004. Plasma-sprayed diopside coatings for biomedical applications. *Surf. Coatings Technol.*, **185**, 340–5.

[149] Li, Z., Qu, Y., Zhang, X. and Yang, B. 2009. Bioactive nano-titania ceramics with biomechanical compatibility prepared by doping with piezoelectric $BaTiO_3$. *Acta Biomater.*, **5**, 2189–95.

[150] Heimann, R. B., Schürmann, N. and Müller, R. T. 2004. In vitro and in vivo performance of Ti_6Al_4V implants with plasma-sprayed osteoconductive hydroxyapatite–bioinert titania bond coat "duplex" systems: an experimental study in sheep. *J. Mater. Sci.: Mater. Med.*, **15**, 1045–52.

[151] Fielding, G. A., Roy, M., Bandyopadhyay, A. and Bose, S. 2012. Antibacterial and biological characteristics of silver containing and strontium doped plasma sprayed hydroxyapatite coatings. *Acta Biomater.*, **8**, 3144–52.

[152] Lin, D.-Y. and Wang, X.-X. 2010. Electrodeposition of hydroxyapatite coating on CoNiCrMo substrate in dilute solution. *Surf. Coatings Technol.*, **191**, 3205–13.

[153] Farnoush, H., Mohandesi, J. A. and Fatmehsari, D. H. 2013. Effect of particle size on the electrophoretic deposition of hydroxyapatite coatings: a kinetic study based on a statistical analysis. *Int. J. Appl. Ceram. Technol.*, **10**, 87–96.

[154] Yang, B., Uchida, M., Kim, H.-M., Zhang, X. and Kokubo, T. 2004. Preparation of bioactive titanium metal via anodic oxidation treatment. *Biomaterials*, **25**, 1003–10.

[155] Das, K., Bandyopadhyay, A. and Bose, S. 2008. Biocompatibility and *in situ* growth of TiO_2 nanotubes on Ti using different electrolyte chemistry. *J. Am. Ceram. Soc.*, **91**, 2808–14.

[156] Ishizawa, H. and Ogino, M. 1995. Characterization of thin hydroxyapatite layers formed on anodic titanium oxide films containing Ca and P by hydrothermal treatment. *J. Biomed. Mater. Res.*, **29**, 1071–9.

[157] Kim, H., Miyaji, F., Kokubo, T. and Nakamura, T. 1997. Effect of heat treatment on apatite-forming ability of Ti metal induced by alkali treatment. *J. Mater. Sci.: Mater. Med.*, **8**, 341–7.

[158] Zhao, C., Zhu, X., Yuan, T., Fan, H. and Zhang, X. 2010. Fabrication of biomimetic apatite coating on porous titanium and their osteointegration in femurs of dogs. *Mater. Sci. Eng. C*, **30**, 98–104.

11

Collagen-based tissue repair composite

Xiaoming Li and Fu-zhai Cui

11.1 Introduction

The most abundant proteins in the extracellular matrix are members of the collagen family. Collagen is composed largely of the amino acids glycine, proline, and hydroxyproline, which are often present as Gly–X–Y repeats (where X and Y are either proline or hydroxyproline). Tropocollagen is the subunit of collagen fibrils formed of three polypeptide strands (each offset by one amino acid), approximately 300 nm long and 1.5 nm in diameter. Each of the three parallel polypeptide strands is in a left-handed helical polyproline II-type coil with three residues to form a right-handed triple helix. The tropocollagen units assemble in a parallel, quarter-staggered arrangement. There is a 40-nm gap, also called the "hole zone," between the ends of each of these units, with 27 nm of overlap between adjacent units. The chemistry underlying the formation of these tissues is all quite similar; the fundamental differences depend on their hierarchical fibrillar architectures. More than 20 human collagens have been reported, many of which display a 67-nm periodicity, due to the axial packing of the individual collagen molecules [1, 2].

Collagens constitute an important family of proteins in the vertebrate body and serve as extracellular matrix molecules for many soft and hard connective tissues, including cornea, skin, tendon, cartilage, and bone [1, 3]. Collogen provides cellular recognition for regulating cell attachment and functions. Collagen favors cell adhesion that is normally found in joint tissues and those exogenous cells embedded in a collagen delivery device. Almost all of the connective tissues with collagen fibrils as the basic building blocks have remarkably similar chemistry at the macromolecular and fibrillar levels of structure. However, differentiation in the hierarchical structure takes place as these fibrils are arranged in the specific architecture required for the construction of special tissues each with unique functions, which is generally considered the function of other, non-collagen, molecules.

Up to now, 28 types of collagen have been identified in vertebrates. The five most common types are type I, found in dermis, tendon, ligaments, and bone (main component of bone); type II, found in cartilage (main component of cartilage); type III, which is the main component of reticular fibers, and is commonly found alongside type I in skin, blood vessels, and intestine; type IV, which forms bases of cell basement membrane; and type V, found in cell surfaces, hair, bone, dermis, cornea, and placenta. Among them, type I collagen and type II collagen are the most used for medical implants.

This chapter presents and discusses the research findings on collagen-based composite (CBC) for repair of bone, nucleus pulposus, cartilage, skin, vessel, and other tissues.

11.2 CBC for bone tissue repair

There is a great need for bone grafts to repair fractures and defects as a result of tumor reconstruction, chronic infection, or traumatic bone loss. Autologous bone grafting is widely accepted as the gold standard for the treatment of bone defects and non-unions.

Table 11.1 Mineralized collagen-based composites that have been approved for clinic use by the FDA and SFDA

	HEALOS DePuy Spine	Vitoss Orthovita	bongold Allgens	Mastergraft Medtronic	chronOs Synthes	CopiOs Zimmer	Mozaik Integra
Formulations							
Sponge	Yes	Yes	No	Yes	Yes	Yes	Yes
Putty	No	Yes	Yes	Yes	Yes	Yes	Yes
Injectable	Yes (HEALOS Fx)	Yes	Yes				
Granules	Yes (conduit)	Yes	Yes	Yes		Yes	Yes
Radiopaque	No	Yes	No	Yes	Yes	Yes	Yes
Compression resistance	No	Yes	Yes	Yes	Yes	No	Yes
Composition	30% Mineral, 70% collagen	80% Mineral, 20% collagen	50% Mineral, 50% collagen	80% Mineral, 20% collagen	80% Mineral, 20% collagen	70% Mineral 30% collagen	80% Mineral, 20% collagen
Approved by	FDA	FDA	SFDA	FDA	FDA	FDA	FDA
References	[119]	[120]	[121]	-	[122]	[123]	

However, the supply of autografts is limited and donor-site morbidity is a concern, as are the prolonged operation times required. An alternative is allogeneic bone grafts, which carry the potential risk of disease transmission and/or infection [4–7]. In order to avoid the problems associated with either autologous or allogeneic bone grafts, there is a continuing interest in the use of synthetic bone graft materials such as gels, demineralized human bone matrix, titanium alloy, polymers, calcium sulfates, bioactive glass, calcium phosphate cement and ceramics, and collagen-based materials [8–21]. However, collagen-based materials are the most interesting biomaterials because collagen is the main organic component in bone. Collagen can promote early mineralization and support new bone formation, while at the same time allowing its replacement by new bone [1, 2, 5, 6, 14–21]. Several mineralized collagen-based composites have been approved for specific clinic applications in bone repair by the Food and Drug Administration (FDA) in the USA and the State Food and Drug Administration (SFDA) in China (Table 11.1).

Recently, nano-hydroxyapatite (nano-HA)/collagen-based (nHAC) composites, inspired by research on natural bone, have received much attention. The composites are prepared by directly mixing the nano-HA and collagen. Nano-HA is sourced from modern ceramic technology, while collagen is purified from animal tissue and then used as a fixing agent for HA. The weak binding between HA and collagen gives them a poor cooperative effect in vivo for defect repair. The collagen degrades faster than HA, which remains in the original form. Furthermore, Caroline M. Curtin *et al.* recently found that the nHAC can offer a highly efficient non-viral gene delivery platform for stem-cell-mediated bone formation. The composite can act as gene-activated matrices for BMP2 delivery, which promotes a better transfection of mesenchymal stem cells (MSCs). Finally, these processes can enhance calcium production [22]. In addition, the properties of nHAC can be improved by adding some specific substances. The nano-hydroxyapatite/collagen/poly(L-lactide) (nHAC/PLA) composite is a representative nano-HA/collagen-based composite, which is commonly used for tissue repair due to its excellent biocompatibility. According to the studies undertaken by Cui and his colleagues, although poor handling properties were found in the tests, the biocompatibility and bone regeneration performance of nHAC/PLA were satisfactory in a critical box-shaped defect model in the mandible of rabbits. Moreover, when compared with nHAC/PLA, the biocompatibility of another nano-hydroxyapatite (nano-HA)/collagen-based composite exhibited a better performance when calcium sulfate hemihydrate was added [23].

Researchers have also tried to develop mimetic methods to prepare nano-HA/collagen composite. The natural bone is a representative example of a typical hierarchically ordered organization. Bone tissues are mainly constructed from nano-HA crystals and a collagen framework. These crystals form, resulting in a highly complex, but ordered mineral–organic composite material. Cui *et al.* have examined the initial mineralization stage in detail [24]. Sufficient evidence has been found from X-ray diffraction patterns to speculate that the amorphous–crystalline phase transformation occurs during the mineralization stage. It is conjectured that, before mineralization, carbonyl and carboxyl groups on the surface of collagen molecules chelate calcium ions and serve as nucleation sites for calcium phosphate [24]. The 40-nm gaps on the collagen are critical in mineralization, since they appear to be the site of mineral nucleation. The crystals appear to grow and proliferate from this area. The size of this gap also appears to constrain mineral growth. The commonly accepted model of higher-order aggregation suggests that five tropocollagen units align longitudinally (overlapping by about a quarter of the molecular length) into a collagen microfibril. After mixing with phosphate-containing neutralization buffer, amorphous calcium phosphates begin to form on the collagen surface, and this re-initiates the self-assembly of the collagen molecules. The calcium phosphate particles formed decrease in size during this process, eventually forming compact crystals. At the same time, the collagen molecules overlap to form local networks. At the end of this stage, the collagen molecules self-assemble into three-dimensional (3D) fibril networks, and the initially loose cluster structure rearranges into the more ordered structure of the gelation phase.

The term biomimetic process refers to a kind of microstructural processing technique that involves mimicry of a biological mechanism, or is inspired by a biological mechanism, in part or as a whole, which can also generate highly ordered hybrid compositions, complex texture, and ultrafine crystallite materials [25]. The co-precipitation of HA with collagen to produce a biodegradable nano-HA/collagen composite, was first reported in 1995 [26], and is a promising biomimetic route for making bone-substitute materials [26–29]. In order to bypass the problem of a surface barrier for continuous mineralization in between the collagen, collagen, or atelocollagen, a water-soluble form of collagen used in cosmetics and for culturing cells is first dispersed in an acidic solution, and then the co-precipitation is induced by increasing the pH or by the addition of mixing agents.

The direct nucleation of HA nanocrystals onto collagen fibers has been performed starting from an aqueous suspension made from a calcium solution and a phosphate solution together with collagen solution of pH 9–10 at room temperature. Solution conditions of high ion concentration and high pH were employed. The mineral content in the composites can be up to 60% by weight. Typically, the type I collagen sponge is presoaked with a highly basic PO_4^{3-}-containing solution, and is then immersed in a Ca^{2+}-containing solution to allow mineral deposition.

To ensure the quality of the final product it is necessary to control the Ca/P ratio in the reaction solution. One way to do this is to dissolve commercial calcium phosphate in acid; another is to add the Ca and P in a certain ratio into the solution, after which a reaction is induced. The composite product obtained is freeze-dried at -40 °C. The formation of nanocrystals of HA elegantly aligned with their *c*-axis preferentially oriented along the collagen fibers constitutes evidence that there exists a strong interaction between the HA and collagen phases. During this process, which mimics the mineralization of natural bone to a certain extent, the HA/collagen materials provide good properties, making them candidate bone repair scaffolds in orthopedic and maxillofacial surgery. Generally, nHAC is produced using this method, and remains in powder form. To support cell ingrowth, a small amount of poly(lactic acid) (PLA) polymer, a non-toxic, biodegradable material, is used as a scaffold material in tissue engineering. This material is compounded with the powder and 3D scaffolds (nHACP) can be prepared [30]. It has been proven that these materials are nanocomposites, in which nano-sized bone-like apatite is induced and uniformly embedded in collagen matrix. The self-organization of calcified collagen fibrils into fibers is also possible under certain conditions. This

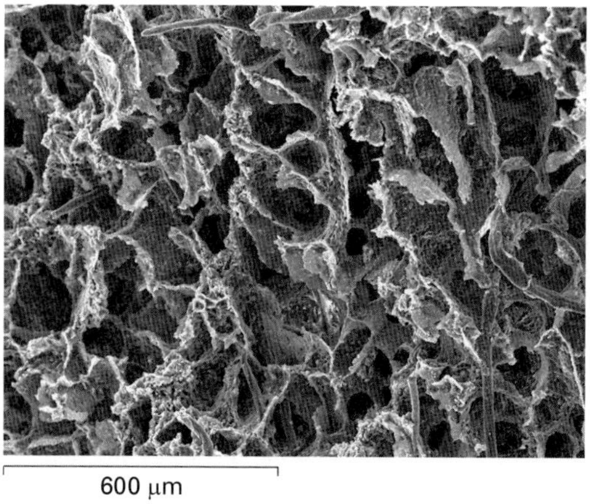

Figure 11.1 SEM micrographs of the nHACP/CHI composite (SEM, ×100). (Adapted with permission from [14]. Copyright 2005 John Wiley and Sons.)

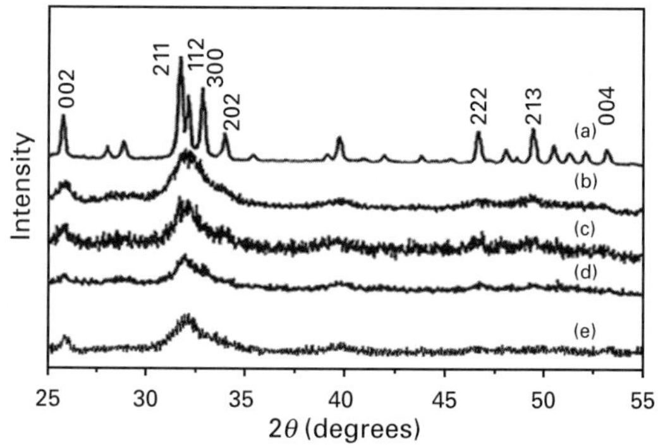

Figure 11.2 X-ray diffraction patterns of materials: (a) HA crystal; (b) nHAC; (c) nHAC/PLA; (d) natural bone; and (e) nHACP/CHI. (Adapted with permission from [14]. Copyright 2005 John Wiley and Sons.)

occurs since the mechanical rigidity of the porous nHACP is much lower than that of natural spongy bone. Moreover, as a scaffold material, PLA has several obvious weaknesses: fast biodegradation, acidic degradation byproducts, and hydrophobicity [31, 32]. As a kind of alkali, chitin can neutralize the acidity caused by PLA degradation and eliminate the inflammations, reduce the speed of hydrolyzation and prolong the existence of the material in the body. Considering the characteristics, Li *et al.* prepared a kind of porous nHACP/CHI scaffold by adding chitin fibres into the nHACP, with the expectation that adding chitin fibres would increase the strength of pure nHACP scaffolds [14, 33]. It was found that the addition of the chitin fibres improves not only the mechanical properties, but also the biocompatibility of the nHACP scaffolds. Figure 11.1 shows an SEM micrograph of the nHACP/CHI, for which the porosity is about 90% and the pore size is about 200 μm. As shown in Figure 11.2, the reinforced scaffold retains the characteristics of nHAC and resembles natural bone both in terms of its components and in crystal size. Cells attached and grew better on the reinforced scaffold than they did on the unreinforced scaffold. Moreover, it was determined from further in-vivo experiments that the nHACP/CHI scaffolds could completely repair a 40-mm defect in goat shank, giving it appropriate mechanical strength [5]. It was also shown that the nHACP and pure PLA could not repair this defect, although the mechanical properties and biocompatibility of nHACP are better than those of pure PLA [5]. Additionally, the chitin fibres, as a kind of amylose, may make the composition of the reinforced scaffold more similar to that of the natural bone because the organic components of natural bone comprise amyloses besides collagen.

Researchers have recently tried to use other materials besides collagen, such as bioactive glasses, to mimic the natural inorganic component of bone. Wang and his co-workers have tried using bioactive glasses (BGs) in the system $CaO\text{-}P_2O_5\text{-}SiO_2$, which is similar to the natural inorganic component of bone. It has been reported that this stimulates the formation, precipitation, and deposition of phosphate ions from the physiological solution and can result in enhanced bone/matrix interface strength. As a kind of phospholipid, phosphatidylserine (PS), with high affinity for calcium ions, has been shown to be able to form complexes with both Ca^{2+} and PO_4^{3-}, and nucleate hydroxyapatite formation [34, 35]. Considering the characteristics and enlightened by the concept of biomimicry, Xu *et al.* prepared a bioactive and bioresorbable composite scaffold by compounding bioactive glasses in the system $CaO\text{-}P_2O_5\text{-}SiO_2$ (58sBG), type I collagen, and PS [36]. SEM micrographs of the surface

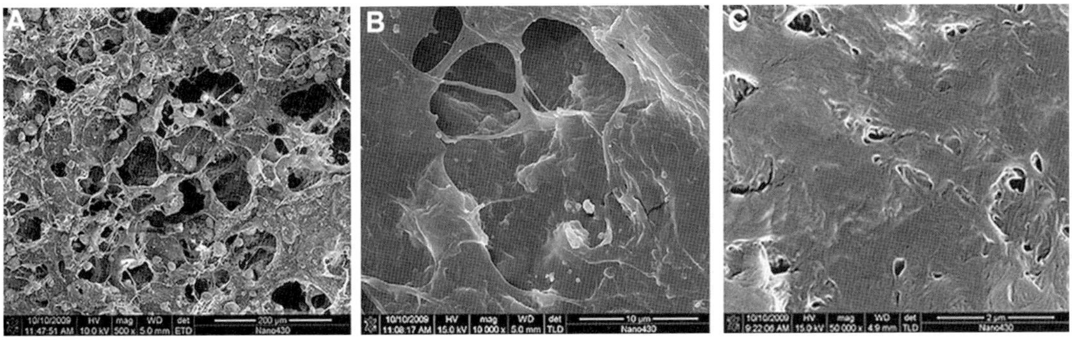

Figure 11.3 SEM micrographs of the surface morphology of BG–COL–PS scaffolds: (A) the cross-section of the scaffold with a structure of irregular interconnected pores ranging from several microns up to about 300 μm; (B) the microstructure of the scaffold; (C) the micropores located on the pore walls of macropores in the scaffold. (Adapted with permission from [36]. Copyright 2011 Elsevier Ltd.)

morphology and microstructure of the fabricated porous scaffolds are shown in Figure 11.3. The bioglass–collagen–phosphatidylserine (BG–COL–PS) composite scaffolds showed a structure of irregular interconnected pores, and the pore sizes of scaffolds mainly ranged from several microns up to about 300 μm (Figure 11.3, images A and B). The biphasic structure of the scaffold allowed micropores whose size was less than 2 μm (Figure 11.3 image C). Rat mesenchymal stem cells (rMSCs) grown on BG–COL–PS composite scaffolds exhibited a high degree of attachment, growth, and osteogenic differentiation. The in-vivo results suggest that the BG–COL–PS composite scaffolds exhibited biocompatibility and extensive osteoconductivity with host bone. Moreover, the BG–COL–PS with rMSC constructs dramatically enhanced the new bone formation. The data suggest that the BG–COL–PS scaffolds fulfilled the basic requirements of a bone tissue engineering scaffold, including satisfactory mechanical properties and good biocompatibility. Furthermore, the BG–COL–PS scaffolds also have the potential to be applied in orthopedic and reconstructive surgery.

11.3 CBC for nucleus pulposus tissue repair

The incidence of lower back pain (LBP) is second only to that of infections of the upper respiratory tract, which is also the predominant cause of disability [37]. Generally, disk degenerative disease (DDD) is considered to be the main cause of LBP [38–40]. Although various methods have been employed for the treatment of DDD, ranging from conservative management to invasive procedures such as diskectomy, spinal fusion, total disk replacement, and nucleus pulposus (NP) replacement [41], none of them can deal with the inherent loss of functional native disk tissue. Furthermore, the application of artificial disk replacement has been shown to be potentially the optimal therapy for DDD. However, further study is still needed because of the limitations associated with this technology [42]. Hence, biological implants with reasonable structure and function seem to be ideal candidates for restructuring the disk, and then treating DDD.

Since the research on tissue-engineered IVD has not made any big strides, the materials utilized still remain the same as in previous studies, such as collagen type I (CI) [41–44], poly-(D,L-lactide) [45], calcium polyphosphate substrate [46], alginate [47, 48], small-intestine submucosa (SIS) [49], HyA [50], chitosan [51], and a mixture of gelatin, 6-CS, and HyA [52]. However, collagen type II (CII), not CI, is the primary element of the ECM of native NP tissue under physiological conditions. As an ideal scaffold for tissue-engineered NP, it has a better ability to simultaneously provide the three principal components of the ECM of native NP, and then emulate the biological environment of local tissue in turn, so the system type II collagen (CII)-hyaluronate (HyA)-chondroitin-6-sulfate (6-CS) was investigated. Collagen type II is different from CI in regard to structure and hydrophilicity. Some works on injectable cell-seeded scaffolds using atelocollagen II gel have been reported [53, 54].

Gruber and his colleagues compared the biological functionality of collagen sponge, collagen gel, agarose, alginate, and fibrin gel formulations. They confirmed that collagen sponges provided the best microenvironment for ECM production and gene expression of disk cells because the sponge carrier system favored adhesion of cells. Additionally, the porosity of collagen sponges may favor diffusion of nutrients and waste products, and may also provide space for new cells and ECM. Although collagen gels could also support good cell growth, such constructs did not result in either abundant ECM production or ECM gene expression when compared with collagen sponges. Cell growth, ECM production, and gene expression in alginate, agarose, and fibrin microenvironments were inferior. Findings with alginate and agarose indicated that, compared with the collagen sponge carrier, disk cells assume a rounded shape in alginate or agarose, and cell divisions result in the formation of small colonies that lie within lacunar-like cavities in the carrier material. Additionally, less ECM production is seen, with discrete matrix accumulations between and around cells. Similar findings can be seen with fibrin gel. In addition, the same results have been obtained from cell proliferation assays and gene expression assays. Hence collagen sponge seems to be a more appropriate candidate for NP tissue engineering due to its more porous structure, compared with that of the collagen gel [55]. Recently, Li *et al.* [56] have prepared a porous crosslinked NP tissue engineering scaffold using the following method. First, CII was completely dissolved in hydrogen chloride (HCl) solution (pH 2–3) by stirring at 4 °C to a final concentration of 1.25% (wt/vol). The pH of the CII solution was adjusted to about 1–2. A solution of HyA (1.25% wt/vol) was prepared by dissolving HyA in distilled water and cooled to 4 °C. Then, the pre-cooled HyA solution was dripped into the prepared CII solution to a final ratio of 1–9 (by volume HyA to CII), which mimics the HyA-to-CII ratio in the native NP tissue, and stirred at 4 °C for 4 h. The mixed solution was centrifuged (at 3000 rpm, for 15 min) at 4 °C to remove air bubbles and then poured gently into culture dishes and frozen at −80 °C overnight. The CII/HyA sponge was constructed by lyophilizing the mixed solution for 24 h. The dried CII/HyA sponge was then immersed in ethanol containing 50 mM 2-morpholino-ethanesulfonic acid (pH 5.5) for some time at room temperature, and then incubated in 40% ethanol containing 50 mM MES, 24 mM EDC, 5 mM NHS, and 2% 6-CS (wt/vol) for 24 h at room temperature for crosslinking. The processed scaffold was washed twice with 0.1 M Na_2HPO_4 (pH 9.1), twice with 1 M NaCl, six times with 2 M NaCl, and finally ten times with ultra-pure water. The scaffold was finally lyophilized for 24 h. Figure 11.4 shows the structure of the scaffold, indicating that the scaffolds were acidophilic with a neatly arranged porous structure with a pore size of more than 100 μm and that sulfated GAGs were attached to the collagens. The fabricated 3D constructs possess similar composition to that of native NP, with improved mechanical stability, satisfactory water-binding capacity, and overall high porosity.

11.4 CBC for cartilage tissue repair

Articular cartilage is an important component of the musculoskeletal system and often suffers injuries (caused by trauma, disease, and age-related degeneration) that may result in unbearable pain and dysfunction [57–59]. The limited self-renewal capacity of human hyaline cartilage has been shown to stimulate development in autologous chondrocyte (AC) transplantation (ACT) for regeneration of articular cartilage. Strategies of ACT-like arthroplasty and mosaicplasty result in the formation of fibrocartilaginous tissue and further induce osteoarthritis formation. Cartilage tissue engineering provides a novel medical therapy for arthritis [60]. Many biomaterials, including naturally occurring and synthetic polymers and their combinations, have been extensively investigated as potential AC tissue engineering scaffolds both in vitro and in vivo [61–66].

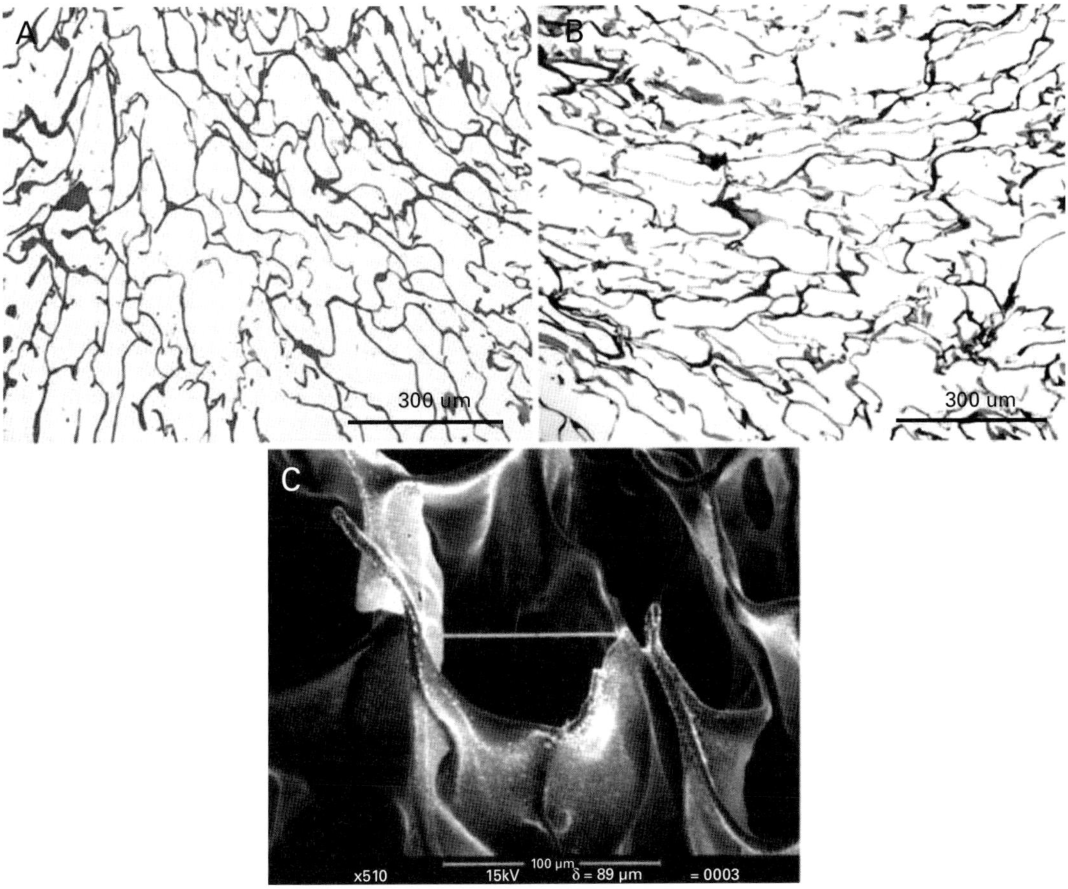

Figure 11.4 Microscopic observation of the scaffold: (a) porous structure of the scaffold (H&E, ×100); (b) GAG-attached scaffold (toluidine blue, ×100); (c) the ultrastructure of the scaffold (SEM, ×510). (Adapted with permission from [56]. Copyright 2010 Springer.)

It has been shown that the ECM is the key factor in maintaining chondrocytic phenotype and supporting chondrogenesis both in vitro and in vivo [67]. Therefore, as the main component of AC-specific ECM, collagen has been paid much more attention by scientists, and it can maintain the chondrocyte phenotype and production of glycosaminoglycans (GAGs) [68–70]. What is more, collagen also provides good biocompatibility and low antigenicity. Owing to these advantages, collagen would seem to be a potentially optimal biomaterial in tissue engineering [71]. However, its rapid degradation and poor mechanical properties also restrict its application in tissue engineering. To mitigate these disadvantages, researchers have investigated using crosslinking treatment or blending with other materials to synthesize biodegradable polymers, which have good mechanical strength and a controllable speed of degradation. Chemical and physical processes are two common methods for crosslinking collagen [72]. Both methods have advantages; however, since the physical methods cannot support crosslinking treatment as well as chemical methods can, researchers opt for chemical crosslinking treatment [73–75]. A wide range of reagents has been used for

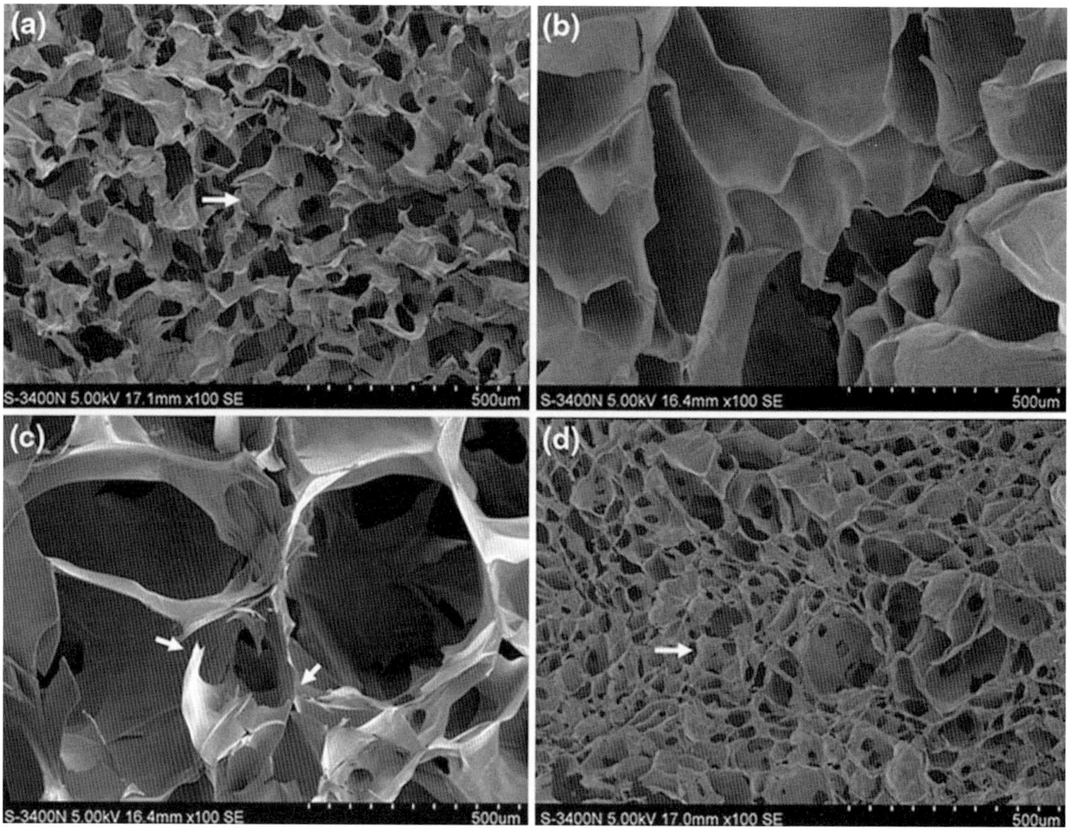

Figure 11.5 SEM of the scaffolds for cartilage tissue engineering. The pore wall of the uncrosslinked scaffold was paper-like (arrow), with a smaller pore size and porosity (a). With an increasing genipin concentration (b) and crosslinking temperature (c), the pore size became larger. At a temperature of 37 °C, the pores of the scaffold became broken and many fissures were formed on the surface of the pore walls (arrow, c). The pore size showed no changes with an increase of crosslinking time, and 12 h later the pore wall became thicker (arrow, d). (Adapted with permission from [86]. Copyright 2011 Springer.)

chemical crosslinking treatment, such as glutaraldehyde, formaldehyde, diisocyanate, diepoxide, and 1-ethyl-3-(3-dimethylaminopropyl) carbodiimide [74, 76, 77]. Furthermore, recently, genipin, a naturally occurring crosslinking reagent, has been employed for biomedical applications [78, 79], offering a new way for researchers to crosslink collagen-based materials. Sung *et al.* have discussed the use of genipin. According to them, compared with other reagents, such as glutaraldehyde and epoxy resin, genipin exhibits lower cytotoxicity and brings about potentially optimal crosslinking of cellular tissues and biomaterials containing primary amino groups [80–82].

Heretofore, chemical crosslinking treatments have been applied to some materials, including chondroitin sulfate (CS) and hyaluronan (HA), which are present in the cartilage ECM [60]. In addition to these materials, chitosan is another promising biodegradable material. Chitosan, which shares common structural characteristics with GAGs [83], has been used in various biomedical applications, such as wound healing, cartilage and bone regeneration, and drug delivery [84, 85]. It has been shown that GAGs play a crucial role in

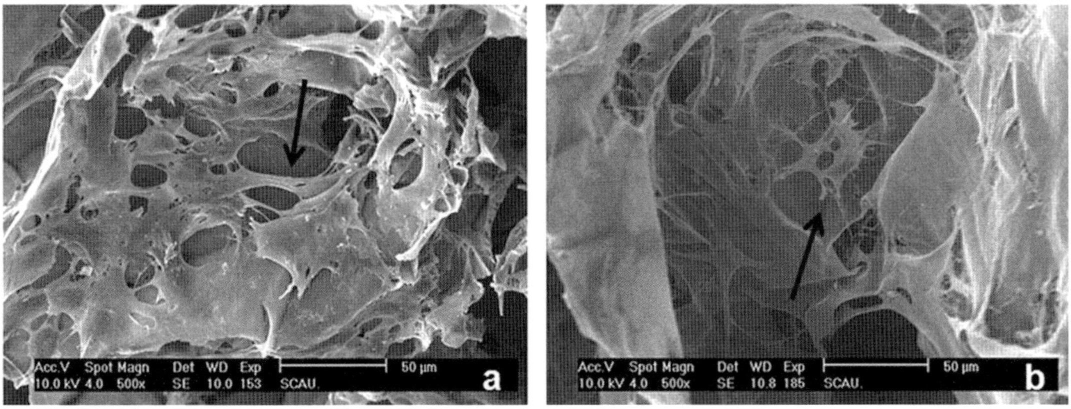

Figure 11.6 Morphology of chondrocytes seeded onto the surface of COL/Cht-50 scaffolds after 12 days of culturing; (a) on the surface of the scaffold; (b) inside the scaffold. (Adapted with permission from [57]. Copyright 2010 John Wiley and Sons.)

stimulation of chondrogenesis. In addition, there are close interactions between collagen and chitosan molecular chains. Considering these factors, adding chitosan in collagen may provide a promising candidate matrix for AC scaffolding [57]. The scaffold could be prepared by the published method as follows. First, solutions of collagen type II and chitosan were mixed in a certain ratio. Then these blends were frozen at −20 °C and lyophilized for 12 h in a freeze dryer to make pre-scaffolds. The pre-scaffolds were then crosslinked by immersion in ethanol containing genipin. After being crosslinked, the scaffolds were washed with distilled water and immersed in a saturated solution of glycine. When the color of the solution no longer changed, the scaffolds were removed and neutralized with 0.1 M Na_2HPO_4. The excess base was removed by repeated washing with distilled water until the matrix pH had returned to the physiological range (7.0–7.4) [86]. The scaffolds showed a 3D porous structure, the pores inside the scaffolds were interconnected in irregular patterns, and the pore size varied over a large range under different crosslinking conditions (Figure 11.5). As is shown by SEM images (Figure 11.6) of chondrocytes grown in the COL/Cht-50 scaffold (50% chitosan in collagen/chitosan scaffolds), 12 days after culturing the cells had spread around the pore walls of the scaffold; meanwhile, chondrocytes exhibited morphology just as fibroblastic and presented morphology in two-dimensional (2D) culture in the cell culture plates before seeding in the scaffold [57]. What is more, the extended lamellipodial protrusions provide the opportunity for the cells to come into contact with each other. It is indicated by the SEM images that the attachment and viability of chondrocytes can be enhanced by the genipin crosslinked collagen/chitosan scaffolds, which can also act as an appropriate 3D matrix for cartilage tissue engineering.

Recently, researchers tried to improve further the mechanical properties and plasticity of the scaffolds by compounding collagen and heavy polymers, because these polymers, such as poly(lactic acid) (PLA), poly(glycolic acid) (PGA), and their copolymer poly(lactic-*co*-glycolic acid) (PLGA), can easily be formed into designed shapes with relatively high mechanical strength. Chen and his colleagues developed hybrid structures of 3D scaffolds that combined the advantages of natural type I collagen and synthetic PLGA knitted mesh [87]. The mechanically strong PLGA mesh served as a skeleton, while the collagen microsponges facilitated cell seeding and tissue formation. The scaffolds were divided into three groups: (1) THIN, collagen microsponge formed in interstices of PLGA mesh; (2) SEMI, collagen microsponge formed on one side of PLGA mesh; and (3) SANDWICH, collagen sponge formed on both sides of PLGA mesh. Bovine chondrocytes were cultured in these scaffolds and transplanted subcutaneously into nude mice for 2, 4, and 8 weeks. All three groups of transplants showed homogeneous cell distribution, natural chondrocyte morphology, and abundant cartilaginous ECM deposition. Production of GAGs per DNA and the expression of type II collagen and aggrecan mRNA were much higher in the SEMI and SANDWICH groups than in the THIN group. When compared with native articular cartilage, the mechanical strength of the engineered cartilage reached 54.8% and 49.3% in terms of Young's modulus and 68.8% and 62.7% in terms of stiffness, respectively, in SEMI and SANDWICH. These scaffolds could be used for the tissue engineering of articular cartilage with adjustable thickness.

11.5 CBC for skin tissue repair

Skin tissue engineering requires biomaterials capable of recapitulating the structural architecture of unwounded skin. At present, skin tissue engineering scaffolds are mainly collagen-based. Honeycomb collagen scaffold is a unique product for various applications in the field of biomedical and tissue engineering. The specific honeycomb structure and the porosity of the honeycomb walls may allow transportation of nutrients to the cells and also removal of waste products as in a dynamic culture environment. Overall, the 3D environment of the honeycomb collagen scaffold may provide the natural ECM environment with the necessary mechanical support and biochemical interplay as in living systems for the formation of a dermal substitute. Furthermore, it was indicated by the study of George *et al.* [88] that honeycomb collagen scaffold is an efficient and suitable material for cell adherence, proliferation, and multiplication of human skin fibroblasts to form a dermal substitute, and that honeycomb collagen sheet is a mechanically stable, biocompatible, and biodegradable scaffold for dermal tissue engineering.

To combine the advantages of other materials, the dermal scaffolds have also been prepared as composites, consisting mostly of type I collagen fibers arranged in a reticular fashion [89]. Besides collagen, other components of the scaffold composite may include hyaluronic acid (HA), an important component of the ECM, which has been used as a viscoelastic biomaterial for medical purposes, in cosmetics because of its high water-retention capacity, and in drug delivery systems because of its biodegradability. HA exists in high concentrations during fetal skin development, is involved in cell migration and differentiation, and is the first macromolecule to appear in the ECM during wound healing [90, 91]. It has also been reported that the addition of HA promotes cell division in human fibroblasts by their passage through cell cycles when incorporated within a collagen matrix [92]. Given these advantages of HA, Park *et al.* fabricated porous collagenous matrix containing HA using a freeze-drying technique, and crosslinked the system with 1-ethyl-3-(3-dimethyl aminopropyl) carbodiimide (EDC) as scaffolds for dermal tissue regeneration [93]. Briefly, HA (relative molecular mass 120,000–150,000) as an aqueous solution was added to a 1% type I atelocollagen dispersion, to produce HA/collagen mixtures. The mixtures were homogenized at 8000 rpm for 3 min at 4 °C using a homogenizer, and the pH was adjusted to 7.4 by addition of drops of NaOH solution. The resulting slurry was poured into a polystyrene Petri dish, frozen at −70 °C, and lyophilized at −50 °C for 24 h. The dried porous collagen–HA matrices were immersed in EDC solution for 24 h to orient the crosslinking. The matrices produced were thoroughly washed in distilled water using a sonicator, and then relyophilized at −50 °C. They indicated that fetal human dermal fibroblasts adhered well to all of the collagen-based matrices as compared with the porous polyurethane matrix used as a control. A 3-(4,5-dimethylthiazolyl)-2,5-diphenyltetrazolium bromide-based proliferation test and the hematoxylin and eosin staining of a 2-week cultured matrix showed that the proliferation of fibroblasts was enhanced on a 9.6% HA-containing collagen matrix. No significant difference was found in terms of fibroblast migration into the various types of scaffolds as HA content was increased. In-vivo testing showed that dermis treated with collagen or collagen–HA matrix was thicker than the control, and that epithelial regeneration was accelerated and collagen synthesis increased. However, biosynthesis of collagens and other ECM proteins is the primary function of dermal fibroblasts. Type I and type III collagens are the major proteins in the dermal tissue, and their unique triple-helical structure provides mechanical stability and elasticity to the dermis. Therefore, it is necessary to note that the properties of the environment can strongly affect the behavior of fibroblasts [94], which play a crucial role in wound healing. Bell *et al.* [95] developed the collagen hydrogel in the system where physiological 3D contact exists between the scaffold and fibroblasts. Both chronic and acute wounds have been treated by application of the collagen hydrogel with keratinocyte sheets, named Apligraf® [96]. However, although this kind of biomaterial has shown several beneficial effects, it still cannot be the ideal permanent scaffold because of some defects, such as the low initial collagen concentration (0.66 mg/ml), poor mechanical properties [97], and sensitivity to metalloproteinases [98]. What is more, after culturing for 14 days, less than 3% of the initial surface of the collagen hydrogels had been colonized by cells. This value is in proportion to the cell density [95]. Reinforcement has been attempted in order to improve the mechanical properties, such as by using plastic compression [99]. The reinforced materials did indeed have better properties than the unreinforced materials, in that they were thinner, dried easier, or had a higher collagen concentration. However, this kind of material is still not an ideal one for the growth of cells and their delivery to the wound location. Recently, Helary and co-workers have developed concentrated collagen hydrogels (CCHs) obtained under controlled conditions [100]. Normal collagen hydrogels (NCHs) concentrated at 0.66 mg/ml including dermal fibroblasts (7.5 × 104 cells/hydrogel) at day one exhibited poor mechanical properties and could be handled only with difficulty, while CCHs at 3 mg/ml kept their original shape and were easily handled (Figure 11.7). Compared with NCH, the CCH contraction was delayed and smaller. At day 21, the surface area of CCHs at 3 mg/ml was 18 times greater than that of NCHs. Whatever the initial fibroblast density, CCHs favored cell growth that reached about 10 times the initial cell number at day 21; cell proliferation was inhibited in NCHs. Gelatinase A activities in CCHs were greater than in NCHs. According to studies

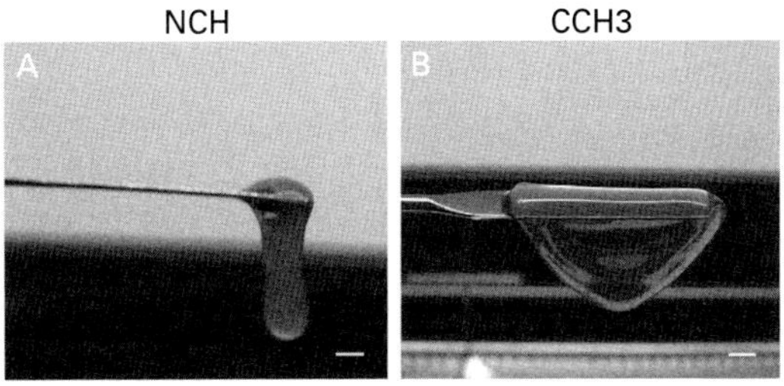

Figure 11.7 A macroscopic view of hydrogels. Handling of collagen hydrogels including dermal fibroblasts (7.5 × 104 cells/hydrogel) at day one. Normal collagen hydrogels (NCHs) concentrated at 0.66 mg/ml exhibited poor mechanical properties. Deposited on a spatula, they slipped, became deformed, and could be handled only with difficulty (A). Concentrated collagen hydrogels (CCHs) at 3 mg/ml kept their original shape and were easily handled (B). Bar: 5 mm. (Adapted with Permission from [100]. Copyright 2010 Elsevier Ltd.)

on rats in vivo, complete hydrolysis of NCHs had occurred by 15 days after implantation. In contrast, CCHs at 3 mg/ml were still present after 30 days. Moreover, CCHs showed cell colonization, neovascularization, and no severe inflammatory response. These results demonstrate that CCHs can be considered as new candidates for dermal substitution because they are easy to handle, do not contract drastically, favor cell growth, and can be quickly integrated in vivo.

11.6 CBC for vessel and other tissue repair

Providing mechanical and biological properties consistent with those of a native vessel is the overall goal of vascular tissue engineering. Various methods involving collagen as a primary scaffold constituent have been employed. In 1986, Weinberg and Bell [101] published a groundbreaking study in this field, using a collagen-based scaffold for blood vessel restructuring. Multiple layers of collagen integrated with a Dacron mesh were involved in an in-vitro model to provide the tensile strength required. In addition, smooth muscle cells were cultured in the graft and grown under dynamic conditions closely

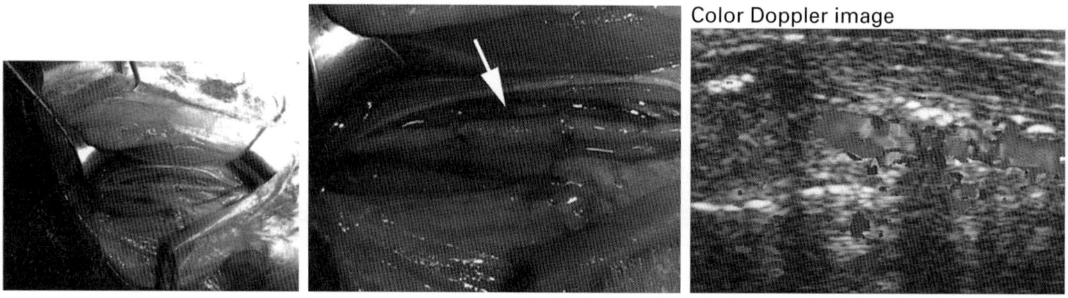

Figure 11.8 The multilayered oriented collagen tube transplanted as a blood vessel graft for the carotid artery of a rabbit. (Adapted with permission from [106]. Copyright 2012 MDPI.)

mimic king in-vivo conditions [102]. Endothelial cells were used to line the inner lumen. Also, for mechanical support, they added collagen, such as PGA and PLGA, to various polymeric materials. Decellularized vein has been used as a potential scaffold for vascular tissue engineering, which also can preserve ECM, which is deemed to the basement membrane structure, and has reasonable strength for vascular grafting [103]. Obviously, collagen, which is one of the main proteins forming vascular ECM, can not only play a significant role in these studies, but also provide potential candidate of scaffolds for tissue regeneration. To limit vessel distension, the elongation of large vessels under pressure is restricted by collagen fibers. In addition, it also transmits force around the vessel by providing attachment to smooth muscle cells [104, 105].

Collagen-based vascular grafts, however, are not without their limitations. In particular, many of these constructs possess inadequate mechanical properties to withstand hemodynamic pressures and shear stresses. Much effort has been invested over the years to discover suitable methods to augment the material strength. In 1986, Weinberg and Bell described the fabrication of tubular constructs that mimicked the structure of native arteries. The strength of these constructs consisting of fibroblast-seeded adventitia analogs, smooth-muscle-cell-seeded media analogs and endothelial cell intimal linings depended on the collagen concentration, initial cell density, and duration of culturing period [101]. Mechanical pulsatile conditioning has also been explored as a means of stimulating matrix production and fiber alignment [106–108]. While this cyclic conditioning has been associated with up to 200% increases in tensile strength, it has failed to produce constructs with sufficiently good mechanical properties for implantation. Recently, another group, led by Yoshihiro Isobe, synthesized a multilayered oriented collagen tube from rat-tail type I and porcine-skin type I collagen solutions, and transplanted it as a blood vessel graft for the carotid artery of a rabbit, as shown in Figure 11.8. A Doppler image of the graft is also shown in Figure 11.8 [106]. Sambanis and his colleagues presented the concept of a construct-sleeve hybrid (CSH) graft, which used a biological support to provide temporary reinforcement while cell-mediated remodeling of the construct occurs [109]. Support sleeves were fabricated from type I collagen gels and crosslinked with glutaraldehyde, ultraviolet, or dehydrothermal treatments. Collagen, Dulbecco's Modified Eagle's Medium, sodium hydroxide, and phosphate-buffered saline (pH 7.4) were combined on ice to produce a solution with a final collagen concentration of 2.0 mg/ml. The solutions were poured into glass test-tube molds of inner diameter 11.5 mm. Three-millimeter glass capillary tube mandrels fitted with rubber end stoppers (3.8 cm apart) were then inserted into the mold to form the inner lumen. The solutions were transferred to a 37-°C incubator and incubated for 1 h to ensure gelation of the collagen fibers. The acellular constructs were then removed from the test tubes and dehydrated under sterile conditions

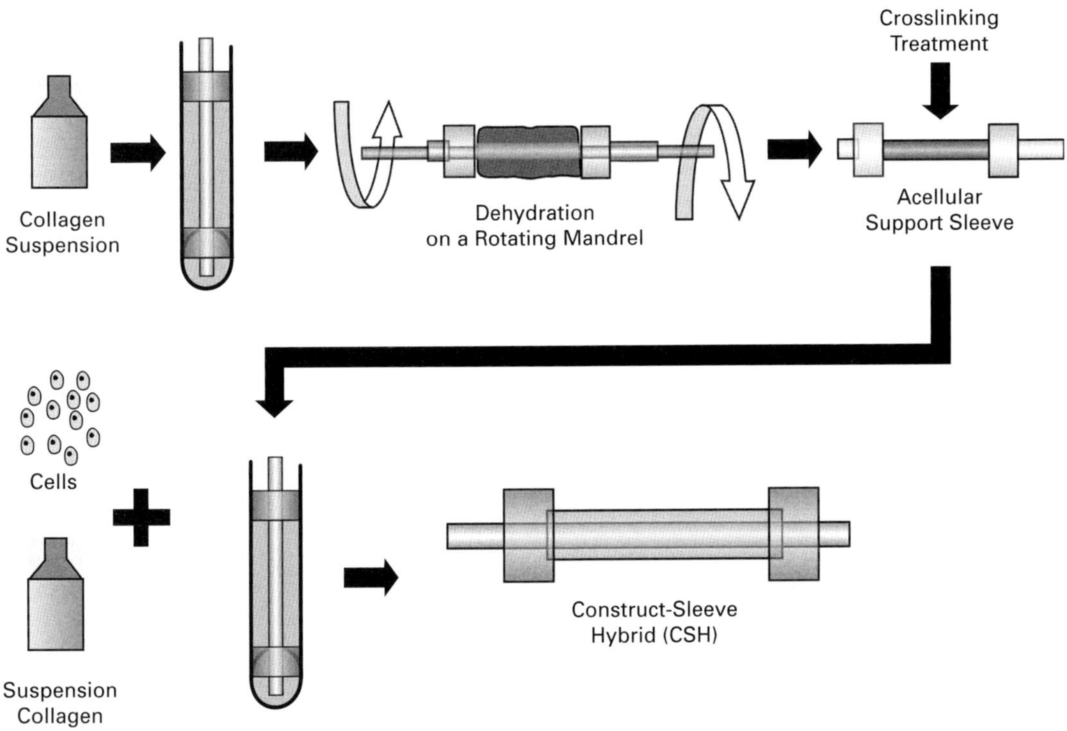

Figure 11.9 The CSH fabrication process. Gels were constructed from acid-soluble, type I collagen and dehydrated on a rotating mandrel to form acellular support sleeves. The sleeves were left as such or crosslinked with various crosslinking agents. They were then combined with cells in a second layer of collagen to form CSHs. (Adapted with permission from [109]. Copyright 2003 Elsevier Ltd.)

overnight on a rotating metal rod as shown in Figure 11.9. Uniaxial tensile testing of acellular sleeves revealed increased stiffness moduli and tensile stresses with crosslinking treatments. A second collagen layer, molded about the sleeve, containing cells created a CSH. For the culture in vitro, compared with unreinforced control structure, the mechanical strength of uncrosslinked (UnXL) and gutaraldehyde-treated (Glut) CHSs is significantly greater (20.4-fold and 121-fold increases in ultimate stress, respectively). Similarly, the peak pressures exhibited during burst testing were 100 and 650 mmHg in the UnXL and Glut CSHs, respectively. Construct compaction, cell viability, and histological examination demonstrated that the function of most cells remained unimpaired with the incorporation of the biological support sleeve.

Various organs have a 3D tubular structure, including the ureter, urethra, bile duct, intestine, esophagus, and trachea, besides blood vessels. Flat scaffolds may be sutured into tubes using a variety of techniques [110], though the preparation of pre-tubularized collagen scaffolds may facilitate the surgical procedure. Koens and co-workers recently explored several methodologies for the construction of collagenous tubular scaffolds, since collagen is the most abundant protein in the ECM of these organs [111]. The homogenized and deaerated collagen suspension was cast in a polystyrene mold. A spacer was placed to keep the mandrel in place and the construct was frozen at −20 °C (freezer), −80 °C (dry ice/ethanol), or −196 °C (liquid nitrogen), and subsequently lyophilized (Zirbus) resulting in tubular collagen scaffolds (Figure 11.10).

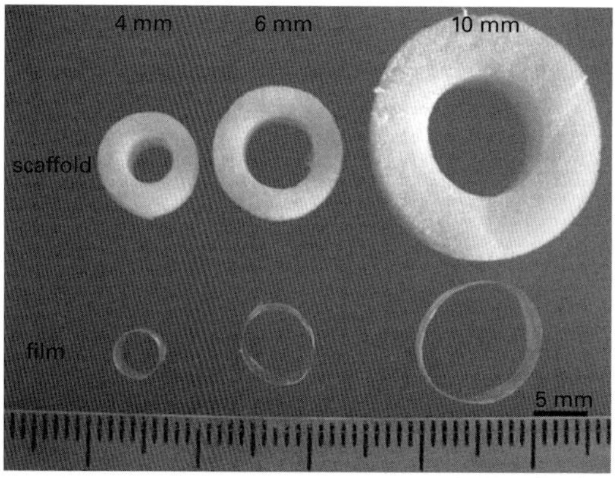

Figure 11.10 A macroscopic view of tubular collagenous scaffolds (−20 °C freezing) and films (air-drying) with inner diameters of 4, 6, and 10 mm. (Adapted with permission from [111]. Copyright 2011 Mary Ann Liebert, Inc.)

Typically, the basic tubular scaffolds prepared were up to 5 cm in length. Longer collagen scaffolds (11–12 cm) were made by preparing scaffolds in a custom-made two-segment mold with an inner diameter of 14 mm (Figure 11.11). One end of the mold was closed by a polystyrene cap with a centered hole, and a stainless steel mandrel (diameter 6 mm) was placed through the cap. The mold was filled with a homogenized and deaerated 0.8% (wt/vol) collagen suspension in 0.25 M acetic acid, after which the other end of the mold was closed, thus fixing the mandrel. The complete system was frozen at −20 °C for 16 h. Subsequently, caps were removed and the frozen mold was lyophilized. Next, the two mold segments and mandrel were removed, resulting in a long tubular scaffold.

Besides the above application, collagen-based materials have been used to repair other tissues. Amniotic membrane (AM) forms an excellent substrate for the clinical expansion of corneal epithelial stem cells for ocular surface reconstruction. Yet, as a natural biological product, AM presents significant inter- and intra-sample differences in structure, transparency, and chemical composition [112, 113], and is not routinely characterized before clinical use. Most importantly, since AM is tissue-derived, its physical and biological properties cannot be easily manipulated, so it lacks the scalability of an engineered polymer construct. To improve the surgical outcome of ocular surface reconstruction, researchers are experimenting with alternative scaffolds to replace AM. These alternative substrates are mainly collagen-based [114–117], since collagen is the major protein constituent of the corneal ECM, comprising 70% of the dry weight. Because, in its purified form, collagen forms a weakly crosslinked thermogel, for corneal tissue engineering applications, covalent intermolecular crosslinks between collagen molecules in macromolecular fibrils using appropriate biocompatible molecules are essential, meaning that one needs to develop stable materials with a high degree of mechanical integrity. The most commonly used crosslinkers include glutaraldehyde, hexamethylene diisocyanate, and acyl azide [116]. In addition, collagen-based materials have been used for treating gaps in spinal cord injury as well. Recently, R. H. Cholas *et al.* have undertaken a series of studies to investigate collagen implants alone and incorporating select therapeutic agents in a 5-mm full-resection gap model in the rat spinal cord. According to the results, collagen-based materials played a significant role in the treatment of spinal cord injury: they favorably align the reparative tissue with the long axis of the spinal cord; potentially reduce the formation of fluid-filled cysts; serve as a delivery vehicle for neural stem cells and the gene for glial-cell-line-derived neurotropic factor; and impede the collapse of musculature and connective tissue into the defect [118].

11.7 Conclusion

Collagen-based composites have been widely used as tissue repair materials owing to the fact that collagens have excellent biocompatibility, an appropriate biodegradation rate, and low immunogenicity, and constitute an important and prevalent family of proteins in the vertebrate body. The development of biomimetic fabrication of novel tissue repair materials depends on progress in research into the structure of natural tissue. Although there have been some obvious achievements in terms of the insight into natural tissues which has been gained, there are still many open questions regarding the formation of the

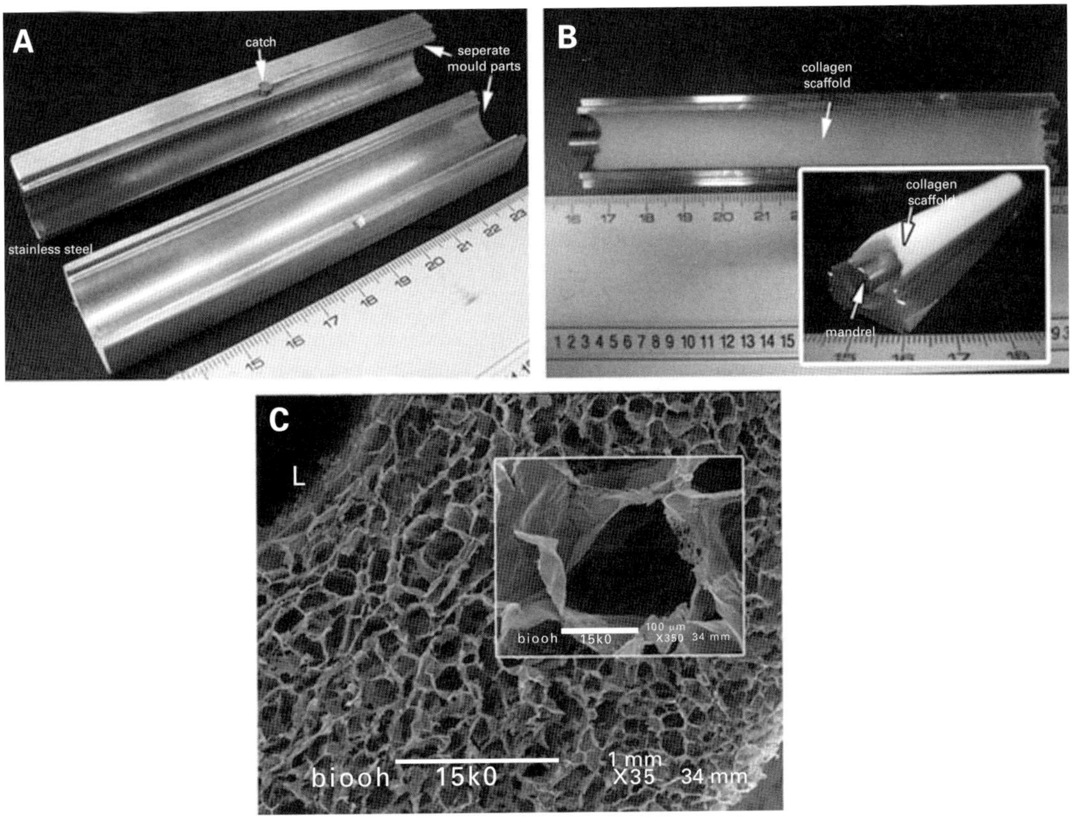

Figure 11.11 Construction of long tubular scaffolds (~10 cm) using a two-segment stainless steel mold, showing a macroscopic view without (A) and with (B) a tubular scaffold around a 6-mm-diameter stainless steel mandrel (see the inset in B for a close-up). The mold has two open ends, facilitating freeze-drying, and can be segmented into two separate longitudinal parts to improve scaffold removal. Electron microscopic images of scaffold's cross section at low (C, bar represents 1 mm) and high (C, inset, bar represents 100 μm) magnification display a highly porous structure. (Adapted with permission from [111]. Copyright 2011 Mary Ann Liebert, Inc.)

hierarchical nanostructure. When it comes to the fabrication of composites mimicking natural tissues from nanometer to the micrometer dimensions, there are many key issues, including control of morphology, incorporation of foreign ions, interaction with biomolecules, and assembly of the organic and inorganic phases, which are still not well understood. A better understanding of the formation mechanism of natural tissues will lead to improved collagen-based biomaterials that can be used as substitutes for various tissue regeneration processes. Furthermore, we should pay much more attention to design, preparation, and research methods. From a biological point of view, significant improvements have been realized with regard to investigative research tools, and in our understanding of the mechanisms involved in tissue and organ regeneration. Accordingly, the materials design and fabrication capabilities and processing technologies need to keep up with those advances.

ACKNOWLEDGEMENTS

The authors acknowledge the financial support from the National Natural Science Foundation of China (grants 31000431 and 50830102), the Beijing Nova

Program (grants 2010B011) and the Program for New Century Excellent Talents (NCET) in University from the Ministry of Education of China.

REFERENCES

[1] Cui, F. Z., Li, Y. and Ge, J. 2007. Self-assembly of mineralized collagen composites. *Mater. Sci. Eng. R – Reports*, **57**, 1–27.

[2] Prockop, D. J. and Kivirikko, K. I. 1995. Collagens: molecular biology, diseases, and potentials for therapy. *Ann. Rev. Biochem.*, **64**, 403–34.

[3] Palmer, L. C., Newcomb, C. J., Kaltz, S. R., Spoerke, E. D. and Stupp, S. I. 2008. Biomimetic systems for hydroxyapatite mineralization inspired by bone and enamel. *Chem. Rev.*, **108**, 4754–83.

[4] Banwart, J. C., Asher, M. A. and Hassanein, R. S. 1995. Iliac crest bone graft harvest donor site morbidity. A statistical evaluation. *Spine*, **20**(9), 1055–60.

[5] Li, X. M., Feng, Q. L., Liu, X. H., Dong, W. and Cui, F. Z. 2006. Collagen-based implants reinforced by chitin fibres in a goat shank bone defect model. *Biomaterials*, **27**, 1917–23.

[6] Liu, X. H., Li, X. M., Fan, Y. B. *et al.* 2010. Repairing goat tibia segmental bone defect using scaffold cultured with mesenchymal stem cells. *J. Biomed. Mater. Res. Part B*, **94**, 44–52.

[7] Younger, E. M. and Chapman, M. W. 1989. Morbidity at bone graft donor sites. *J. Orthop. Trauma*, **3**, 192–5.

[8] Gil-Albarova, J., Salinas, A. J., Bueno-Lozano, A. L. *et al.* 2005. The in vivo behaviour of a sol–gel glass and a glass-ceramic during critical diaphyseal bone defects healing. *Biomaterials*, **26**, 4374–82.

[9] Supronowicz, P., Gill, E., Trujillo, A. *et al.* 2011. Human adipose-derived side population stem cells cultured on demineralized bone matrix for bone tissue engineering. *Tissue Eng. Part A*, **17**, 789–98.

[10] Sargeant, T. D., Guler, M. O., Oppenheimer, S. M. *et al.* 2008. Hybrid bone implants: self-assembly of peptide amphiphile nanofibers within porous titanium. *Biomaterials*, **29**, 161–71.

[11] Winn, S. R. and Hollinger, J. O. 2000. An osteogenic cell culture system to evaluate the cytocompatibility of Osteoset (R), a calcium sulfate bone void filler. *Biomaterials*, **21**, 2413–25.

[12] Jones, J. R., Ehrenfried, L. M. and Hench, L. L. 2006. Optimising bioactive glass scaffolds for bone tissue engineering. *Biomaterials*, **27**, 964–73.

[13] Levengood, S. K. L., Polak, S. J., Wheeler, M. B. *et al.* 2010. Multiscale osteointegration as a new paradigm for the design of calcium phosphate scaffolds for bone regeneration. *Biomaterials*, **31**, 3552–63.

[14] Li, X. M., Feng, Q. L., Jiao, Y. F. and Cui, F. Z. 2005. Collagen-based scaffolds reinforced by chitosan fibres for bone tissue engineering. *Polymer Int.*, **54**, 1034–40.

[15] Li, X. M., Liu, X. H., Dong, W. *et al.* 2009. In vitro evaluation of porous poly(L-lactic acid) scaffold reinforced by chitin fibers. *J. Biomed. Mater. Res. Part B*, **90**, 503–9.

[16] Rezwan, K., Chen, Q. Z., Blaker, J. J. and Boccaccini, A. R. 2006. Biodegradable and bioactive porous polymer/inorganic composite scaffolds for bone tissue engineering. *Biomaterials*, **27**, 3413–31.

[17] Li, X. M., Van Blitterswijk, C. A., Feng, Q. L., Cui, F. Z. and Watari, F. 2008. The effect of calcium phosphate microstructure on bone-related cells in vitro. *Biomaterials*, **29**, 3306–16.

[18] Ooms, E. M., Wolke, J. G. C., van de Heuvel, M. T., Jeschke, B. and Jansen, J. A. 2003. Histological evaluation of the bone response to calcium phosphate cement implanted in cortical bone. *Biomaterials*, **24**, 989–1000.

[19] Fellah, B. H., Gauthier, O., Weiss, P., Chappard, D. and Layrolle, P. 2008. Osteogenicity of biphasic calcium phosphate ceramics and bone autograft in a goat model. *Biomaterials*, **29**, 1177–88.

[20] Liao, S. S., Cui, F. Z., Zhang, W. and Feng, Q. L. 2004. Hierarchically biomimetic bone scaffold materials: nano-HA/collagen/PLA composite. *J. Biomed. Mater. Res. Part B*, **69**, 158–65.

[21] Liao, S. S. and Cui, F. Z. 2004. In vitro and in vivo degradation of mineralized collagen-based composite scaffold: nanohydroxyapatite/collagen/poly(L-lactide). *Tissue Eng.*, **10**, 73–8.

[22] Curtin, C. M., Cunniffe, G. M., Lyons, F. G. *et al.* 2012. Innovative collagen nano-hydroxyapatite scaffolds offer a highly efficient non-viral gene delivery platform for stem cell-mediated bone formation. *Adv. Mater.*, **24**, 749–54.

[23] Liu, X., Liu, H. Y., Lian, X. J. *et al.* 2013. Osteogenesis of mineralized collagen bone graft modified by PLA and calcium sulfate hemihydrate: in vivo study. *J. Biomater. Appl.*, **28**(1), 12–19.

[24] Zhang, W., Huang, Z. L., Liao, S. S. and Cui, F. Z. 2003. Nucleation sites of calcium phosphate crystals during collagen mineralization. *J. Am. Ceram. Soc.*, **86**, 1052–4.

[25] Green, D., Walsh, D., Mann, S. and Oreffo, R. O. C. 2002. The potential of biomimesis in bone tissue engineering:

lessons from the design and synthesis of invertebrate skeletons. *Bone*, **30**, 810–15.

[26] Wang, R. Z., Cui, F. Z., Lu, H. B., Wen, H. B. and Li, H. D. 1995. Synthesis of nanophase hydroxyapatite/collagen composite. *J. Mater. Sci. Lett.*, **14**, 490–2.

[27] Du, C., Cui, F. Z., Zhang, W. *et al.* 2000. Formation of calcium phosphate/collagen composites through mineralization of collagen matrix. *J. Biomed. Mater. Res.*, **50**, 518–27.

[28] Kikuchi, M., Itoh, S., Ichinose, S., Shinomiya, K. and Tanaka, J. 2001. Self-organization mechanism in a bone-like hydroxyapatite/collagen nanocomposite synthesized in vitro and its biological reaction in vivo. *Biomaterials*, **22**, 1705–11.

[29] Rhee, S. H., Lee, J. D. and Tanaka, J. 2003. Nucleation of hydroxyapatite crystal through chemical interaction with collagen. *J. Am. Ceram. Soc.*, **83**, 2890–2.

[30] Liao, S. S., Cui, F. Z., Zhang, W. and Feng, Q. L. 2004. Hierarchically biomimetic bone scaffold materials: nano-HA/collagen/PLA composite. *J. Biomed. Mater. Res. Part B*, **69**, 158–65.

[31] Smith, R., Torres, A. and Li, S. M. 1987. Screening of microorganisms for biodegradation of poly(lactic-acid) and lactic acid-containing polymers. *J. Biomed. Mater. Res.*, **21**, 991–8.

[32] Tormala, R., Lemoine, D. and Francois, C. 1991. Stability study of nanoparticles of poly(ε-caprolactone), poly(D, L-lactide) and poly(D, L-lactide-coglycolide). *J. Biomed. Mater. Res.*, **25**, 1–10

[33] Li, X. M., Feng, Q. L., Wang, W. J. and Cui, F. Z. 2006. Chemical characteristics and cytocompatibility of collagen-based scaffold reinforced by chitin fibers for bone tissue engineering. *J. Biomed. Mater. Res. Part B*, **77**, 219–26.

[34] Merolli, A. and Santin, M. 2009. Role of phosphatidylserine in bone repair and its technological exploitation. *Molecules*, **14**, 5367–81.

[35] Genge, B. R., Wu, L. N. and Wuthier, R. E. 2008. Mineralization of annexin-5-containing lipid calcium-phosphate complexes: modulation by varying lipid composition and incubation with cartilage collagens. *J. Biol. Chem.*, **283**, 9737–48.

[36] Xu, C. X., Su, P. Q., Chen, X. F. *et al.* 2011. Biocompatibility and osteogenesis of biomimetic bioglass–collagen–phosphatidylserine composite scaffolds for bone tissue engineering. *Biomaterials*, **32**, 1051–8.

[37] Andersson, G. B., Schultz, A., Nathan, A. and Irstam, L. 1981. Roentgenographic measurement of lumbar intervertebral disc height. *Spine*, **6**, 154–8.

[38] Yasuma, T., Koh, S., Okamura, T. and Yamauchi, Y. 1990. Histological changes in aging lumbar intervertebral discs. Their role in protrusions and prolapses. *J. Bone Joint Surg. Am.*, **72**, 220–9.

[39] Kuslich, S. D., Ulstrom, C. L. and Michael, C. J. 1991. The tissue origin of low back pain and sciatica: a report of pain response to tissue stimulation during operations on the lumbar spine using local anesthesia. *Orthop. Clin. North Am.*, **22**, 181–7.

[40] Schwarzer, A. C., Aprill, C. N., Derby, R. *et al.* 1995. The prevalence and clinical features of internal disc disruption in patients with chronic low back pain. *Spine*, **20**, 1878–83.

[41] An, H., Boden, S. D., Kang, J. *et al.* 2003. Summary statement: emerging techniques for treatment of degenerative lumbar disc disease. *Spine*, **28**, S24–5.

[42] Huang, R. C. and Sandhu, H. S. 2004. The current status of lumbar total disc replacement. *Orthop. Clin. North Am.*, **35**, 33–42.

[43] Rong, Y., Sugumaran, G., Silbert, J. E. *et al.* 2002. Proteoglycans synthesized by canine intervertebral disc cells grown in a type I collagen–glycosaminoglycan matrix. *Tissue Eng.*, **8**, 1037–47.

[44] Sato, M., Kikuchi, M., Ishihara, M. *et al.* 2003. Tissue engineering of the intervertebral disc with cultured annulus fibrosus cells using atelocollagen honeycomb-shaped scaffold with a membrane seal (ACHMS scaffold). *Med. Biol. Eng. Comput.*, **41**, 365–71.

[45] Brown, R. Q., Mount, A. and Burg, K. J. 2005. Evaluation of polymer scaffolds to be used in a composite injectable system for intervertebral disc tissue engineering. *J. Biomed. Mater. Res. Part A*, **74**, 32–9.

[46] Seguin, C. A., Grynpas, M. D., Pilliar, R. M. *et al.* 2004. Tissue engineered nucleus pulposus tissue formed on a porous calcium polyphosphate substrate. *Spine*, **29**, 1299–306

[47] Chiba, K., Andersson, G. B., Masuda, K. *et al.* 1997. Metabolism of the extracellular matrix formed by intervertebral disc cells cultured in alginate. *Spine*, **22**, 2885–93.

[48] Baer, A. E., Wang, J. Y., Kraus, V. B. *et al.* 2001. Collagen gene expression and mechanical properties of intervertebral disc cell-alginate cultures. *J. Orthop. Res.*, **19**, 2–10.

[49] Le Visage, C., Yang, S. H., Kadakia, L. *et al.* 2006. Small intestinal submucosa as a potential bioscaffold for intervertebral disc regeneration. *Spine*, **31**, 2423–30.

[50] Crevensten, G., Walsh, A. J., Ananthakrishnan, D. *et al.* 2004. Intervertebral disc cell therapy for regeneration:

mesenchymal stem cell implantation in rat intervertebral discs. *Ann. Biomed. Eng.*, **32**, 430–4.

[51] Roughley, P., Hoemann, C., DesRosiers, E. *et al.* 2006. The potential of chitosan-based gels containing intervertebral disc cells for nucleus pulposus supplementation. *Biomaterials*, **27**, 388–96.

[52] Yang, S. H., Chen, P. Q., Chen, Y. F. *et al.* 2005. An in vitro study on regeneration of human nucleus pulposus by using gelatin/chondroitin-6-sulfate/hyaluronan tri-copolymer scaffold. *Artif. Organs*, **29**, 806–14.

[53] Sakai, D., Mochida, J., Iwashina, T. *et al.* 2006. Atelocollagen for culture of human nucleus pulposus cells forming nucleus pulposus-like tissue in vitro: influence on the proliferation and proteoglycan production of HNPSV-1 cells. *Biomaterials*, **27**, 346–53.

[54] Halloran, D. O., Grad, S., Stoddart, M. *et al.* 2008. An injectable cross-linked scaffold for nucleus pulposus regeneration. *Biomaterials*, **29**, 438–47.

[55] Gruber, H. E., Leslie, K., Ingram, J. *et al.* 2004. Cell-based tissue engineering for the intervertebral disc: in vitro studies of human disc cell gene expression and matrix production within selected cell carriers. *Spine J.*, **4**, 44–55.

[56] Li, C. Q., Huang, B., Luo, G. *et al.* 2010. Construction of collagen II/hyaluronate/chondroitin-6-sulfate tri-copolymer scaffold for nucleus pulposus tissue engineering and preliminary analysis of its physico-chemical properties and biocompatibility. *J. Mater. Sci. Mater. Med.*, **21**, 741–51.

[57] Yan, L. P., Wang, Y. J., Ren, L. *et al.* 2010. Genipin-cross-linked collagen/chitosan biomimetic scaffolds for articular cartilage tissue engineering applications. *J. Biomed. Mater. Res. Part A*, **95**, 465–75.

[58] Chang, K. Y., Hung, L. H., Chu, I. M., Ko, C. S. and Lee, Y. D. 2010. The application of type II collagen and chondroitin sulfate grafted PCL porous scaffold in cartilage tissue engineering. *J. Biomed. Mater. Res. Part A*, **92**, 712–23.

[59] Gross, A. E. 2003. Cartilage resurfacing: filling defects. *J. Arthroplasty*, **18**, 14–17.

[60] Ko, C. S., Huang, J. P., Huang, C. W. and Chu, I. M. 2009. Type II collagen-chondroitin sulfate-hyaluronan scaffold cross-linked by genipin for cartilage tissue engineering. *J. Biosci. Bioeng.*, **107**, 177–82.

[61] Li, Z.,Yao, S. J., Alini, M. and Stoddart,M. J. 2010. Chondrogenesis of human bone marrow mesenchymal stem cells in fibrin-polyurethane composites is modulated by frequency and amplitude of dynamic compression and shear stress. *Tissue Eng. Part A*, **16**, 575–84.

[62] Oliveira, J. T., Crawford, A., Mundy, J. M. *et al.* 2007. A cartilage tissue engineering approach combining starch-polycaprolactone fibre mesh scaffolds with bovine articular chondrocytes. *J. Mater. Sci. Mater. Med.*, **18**, 295–302.

[63] Moutos, F. T., Freed, L. E. and Guilak, F. 2007. A biomimetic three-dimensional woven composite scaffold for functional tissue engineering of cartilage. *Nature Mater.*, **6**, 162–7.

[64] Malafaya, P. B., Pedro, A. J., Peterbauer, A. *et al.* 2005. Chitosan particles agglomerated scaffolds for cartilage and osteochondral tissue engineering approaches with adipose tissue derived stem cells. *J. Mater. Sci. Mater. Med.*, **16**, 1077–85.

[65] Iwasaki, N., Yamane, S. T., Majima, T. *et al.* 2004. Feasibility of polysaccharide hybrid materials for scaffolds in cartilage tissue engineering: evaluation of chondrocyte adhesion to polyion complex fibers prepared from alginate and chitosan. *Biomacromolecules*, **5**, 828–33.

[66] Griffon, D. J., Sedighi, M. R., Schaeffer, D. V., Eurell, J. A. and Johnson, A. L. 2006. Chitosan scaffolds: interconnective pore size and cartilage engineering. *Acta Biomater.*, **2**, 313–20.

[67] Minas, T. and Nehrer, S. 1997. Current concepts in the treatment of articular cartilage defects. *Orthopedics*, **20**, 525–38.

[68] Hunter, C. J., Imler, S. M., Malaviya, P., Nerem, R. M. and Levenston, M. E. 2002. Mechanical compression alters gene expression and extracellular matrix synthesis by chondrocytes cultured in collagen I gels. *Biomaterials*, **23**, 1249–59.

[69] Nehrer, S., Breinan, H. A., Ramappa, A. *et al.* 1997. Canine chondrocytes seeded in type I and type II collagen implants investigated in vitro. *J. Biomed. Mater. Res.* **38**, 95–104.

[70] Wakitani, S., Goto, T., Young, R. G. *et al.* 1998. Repair of large full-thickness articular cartilage defects with allograft articular chondrocytes embedded in a collagen gel. *Tissue Eng.*, **4**, 429–44.

[71] Lee, C. H., Singla, A. and Lee, Y. 2001. Biomedical applications of collagen. *Int. J. Pharmacol.*, **221**, 1–22.

[72] Ma, L., Gao, C. Y., Mao, Z. W. *et al.* 2003. Collagen/chitosan porous scaffolds with improved biostability for skin tissue engineering. *Biomaterials*, **24**, 4833–41.

[73] Weadock, K. S., Miller, E. J., Bellincampi, L. D., Zawadsky, J. P. and Dunn, M. G. 2004. Physical cross-linking of collagen fibers: comparison of ultraviolet irradiation and dehydrothermal treatment. *J. Biomed. Mater. Res.*, **29**, 1373–9.

[74] Lynn, A. K., Yannas, I. V. and Bonfield, W. 2004. Antigenicity and immunogenicity of collagen. *J. Biomed. Mater. Res. B Appl. Biomater.*, **71**, 343–54.

[75] Liu, B. C., Harrell, R., Davis, R. H., Dresden, M. H. and Spira, M. 1989. The effect of gamma-irradiation on injectable human amnion collagen. *J. Biomed. Mater. Res.*, **23**, 833–44.

[76] Ma, L., Gao, C. Y., Mao, Z. W. *et al.* 2003. Thermal dehydration treatment and glutaraldehyde cross-linking to increase the biostability of collagen–chitosan porous scaffolds used as dermal equivalent. *J. Biomater. Sci. Polymer Edition*, **14**, 861–74.

[77] Park, S. N., Park, J. C., Kim, H. O., Song, M. J. and Suh, H. 2002. Characterization of porous collagen/hyaluronic acid scaffold modified by 1-ethyl-3-(3-dimethylamino-propyl)carbodiimide cross-linking. *Biomaterials*, **23**, 1205–12.

[78] Chiono, V., Pulieri, E., Vozzi, G. *et al.* 2008. Genipin-crosslinked chitosan/gelatin blends for biomedical applications. *J. Mater. Sci. Mater. Med.*, **19**, 889–98.

[79] Yuan, Y., Chesnutt, B. M., Utturkar, G. *et al.* 2007. The effect of cross-linking of chitosan microspheres with genipin on protein release. *Carbohydr. Polymers*, **68**, 561–7.

[80] Huang, L. L. H., Sung, H. W., Tsai, C. C. and Huang, D. M. 1998. Biocompatibility study of a biological tissue fixed with a naturally occurring crosslinking reagent. *J. Biomed. Mater. Res.*, **42**, 568–76.

[81] Liang, H. C., Chang, W. H., Lin, K. J. and Sung, H. W. 2003. Genipin-crosslinked gelatin microspheres as a drug carrier for intramuscular administration: in vitro and in vivo studies. *J. Biomed. Mater. Res. Part A*, **65**, 271–82.

[82] Mi, F. L., Tan, Y. C., Liang, H. F. and Sung, H. W. 2002. In vivo biocompatibility and degradability of a novel injectable-chitosan-based implant. *Biomaterials*, **23**, 181–91.

[83] Di Martino, A., Sittinger, M. and Risbud, M. V. 2005. Chitosan: a versatile biopolymer for orthopaedic tissue-engineering. *Biomaterials*, **26**, 5983–90.

[84] Silva, S. S., Motta, A., Rodrigues, M. T. *et al.* 2008. Novel genipin-cross-linked chitosan/silk fibroin sponges for cartilage engineering strategies. *Biomacromolecules*, **9**, 2764–74.

[85] Malafaya, P. B., Santos, T. C., Van Griensven, M. and Reis, R. L. 2008. Morphology, mechanical characterization and in vivo neo vascularization of chitosan particle aggregated scaffolds architectures. *Biomaterials*, **29**, 3914–26.

[86] Bi, L., Cao, Z., Hu, Y. Y. *et al.* 2011. Effects of different cross-linking conditions on the properties of genipin-cross-linked chitosan/collagen scaffolds for cartilage tissue engineering. *J. Mater. Sci. Mater. Med.*, **22**, 51–62.

[87] Dai, W. D., Kawazoe, N., Lin, X. T., Dong, J. and Chen, G. P. 2010. The influence of structural design of PLGA/collagen hybrid scaffolds in cartilage tissue engineering. *Biomaterials*, **31**, 2141–52.

[88] George, J., Onodera, J. and Miyata, T. 2008. Biodegradable honeycomb collagen scaffold for dermal tissue engineering. *J. Biomed. Mater. Res. Part A*, **87**, 1103–11.

[89] Wong, V. W., Rustad, K. C., Galvez, M. G. *et al.* 2011. Engineered pullulan–collagen composite dermal hydrogels improve early cutaneous wound healing. *Tissue Eng. Part A*, **17**, 631–44.

[90] Ruiz-Cardona, L., Sanzgiri, Y. D., Benedetti, L. M., Stella, V. J. and Topp, E. M. 1996. Application of benzyl hyaluronate membranes as potential wound dressings: evaluation of water vapour and gas permeabilities. *Biomaterials*, **17**, 1639–43.

[91] Alexander, S. A. and Donoff, R. B. 1980. The glycosaminoglycans of open wounds. *J. Surg. Res.* **29**, 422–9.

[92] Greco, R. M., Iocono, J. A. and Ehrlich, H. P. 1998. Hyaluronic acid stimulates human fibroblast proliferation within a collagen matrix. *J. Cell Physiol.*, **177**, 465–73.

[93] Park, S. N., Lee, H. J., Lee, K. H. and Suh, H. 2003. Biological characterization of EDC-crosslinked collagen–hyaluronic acid matrix in dermal tissue restoration. *Biomaterials*, **24**, 1631–41.

[94] Wong, T., McGrath, J. A. and Navsaria, H. 2007. The role of fibroblasts in tissue engineering and regeneration. *Br. J. Dermatol.*, **156**, 1149–55.

[95] Bell, E., Ivarsson, B. and Merrill, C. 1979. Production of a tissue-like structure by contraction of collagen lattices by human fibroblasts of different proliferative potential in vitro. *Proc. Nat. Acad. Sci. USA*, **76**, 1274–8.

[96] Wilkins, L. M., Watson, S. R., Prosky, S. J., Meunier, S. F. and Parenteau, N. L. 1994. Development of a bilayered living skin construct for clinical applications. *Biotechnol. Bioeng.*, **43**, 747–56.

[97] Brown, R. A. and Phillips, J. B. 2007. Cell responses to biomimetic protein scaffolds used in tissue repair and engineering. *Int. Rev. Cytol.*, **262**, 75–150.

[98] Fringer, J. and Grinnell, F. 2003. Fibroblast quiescence in floating collagen matrices: decrease in serum activation of MEK and Raf but not Ras. *J. Biol. Chem.*, **278**, 20612–17.

[99] Brown, R. A., Wiseman, M., Chuo, C. B., Cheema, U. and Nazhat, S. N. 2005. Ultrarapid engineering of biomimetic materials and tissues: fabrication of nano- and

microstructures by plastic compression. *Adv. Functional Mater.*, **15**, 1762–70.

[100] Helary, C., Bataille, I., Abed, A. *et al.* 2010. Concentrated collagen hydrogels as dermal substitutes. *Biomaterials*, **31**, 481–90.

[101] Weinberg, C. B. and Bell, E. 1986. A blood vessel model constructed from collagen and cultured vascular cells. *Science*, **231**, 397–400.

[102] Niklason, L. E. and Langer, R. S. 1997. Advances in tissue engineering of blood vessels and other tissues. *Transplant Immunol.*, **5**, 303–506.

[103] Schaner, P. J., Martin, N. D., Tulenko, T. N. *et al.* 2004. Decellularized vein as a potential scaffold for vascular tissue engineering. *J. Vasc. Surg.*, **40**, 146–53.

[104] Bou-Gharios, G., Ponticos, M., Rajkumar, V. and Abraham, D. 2004. Extracellular matrix in vascular networks. *Cell Prolif.*, **37**, 207–20.

[105] Boccafoschi, F., Habermehl, J., Vesentini, S. and Mantovani, D. 2005. Biological performances of collagen-based scaffolds for vascular tissue engineering. *Biomaterials*, **26**, 7410–17.

[106] Isobe, Y., Kosaka, T., Kuwahara, G. *et al.* 2012. Oriented collagen scaffolds for tissue engineering. *Materials*, **5**, 501–11.

[107] Seliktar, D., Black, R. A., Vito, R. P. and Nerem, R. M. 2000. Dynamic mechanical conditioning of collagen-gel blood vessel constructs induces remodeling in vitro. *Ann. Biomed. Eng.*, **28**(4), 351–62.

[108] Kanda, K. and Matsuda, T. 1994. Mechanical stress-induced orientation and ultrastructural change of smooth muscle cells cultured in three-dimensional collagen lattices. *Cell Transplant.*, **3**(6), 481–92.

[109] Berglund, J. D., Mohseni, M. M., Nerem, R. M. and Sambanis, A. 2003. A biological hybrid model for collagen-based tissue engineered vascular constructs. *Biomaterials*, **24**, 1241–54.

[110] Soltysiak, P., Hollwarth, M. E. and Saxena, A. K. 2010. Comparison of suturing techniques in the formation of collagen scaffold tubes for composite tubular organ tissue engineering. *Biomed. Mater. Eng.*, **20**, 1–11.

[111] Koens, M. J. W., Geutjes, P. J., Faraj, K. A. *et al.* 2011. Organ-specific tubular and collagen-based composite scaffolds. *Tissue Eng. Part C – Methods*, **17**, 327–35.

[112] Lei, Q., Xueyi, Y., Xin, W. *et al.* 2009. Reconstruction of corneal epithelium with cryopreserved corneal limbal stem cells in rabbit model. *Vet. J.*, **179**, 392–400.

[113] Connon, C., Kawasaki, S., Liles, M. *et al.* 2006. Gene expression and immunolocalisation of a calcium activated chloride channel during the stratification of cultivated and developing corneal epithelium. *Cell Tissue Res.*, **323**, 177–82.

[114] Cen, L., Liu, W., Cui, L., Zhang, W. and Cao, Y. 2008. Collagen tissue engineering: development of novel biomaterials and applications. *Pediatr. Res.*, **63**, 492–6.

[115] Duan, X. and Sheardown, H. 2007. Incorporation of cell-adhesion peptides into collagen scaffolds promotes corneal epithelial stratification. *J. Biomater. Sci. Polymer Edition*, **18**, 701–11.

[116] Duan, X. and Sheardown, H. 2006. Dendrimer cross-linked collagen as a corneal tissue engineering scaffold: mechanical properties and corneal epithelial cell interactions. *Biomaterials*, **27**, 4608–17.

[117] Zhong, S., Teo, W. E., Zhu, X. *et al.* 2005. Formation of collagen-glycosaminoglycan blended nanofibrous scaffolds and their biological properties. *Biomacromolecules*, **6**, 2998–3004.

[118] Cholas, R. H., Hsu, H.-P. and Spector, M. 2012. The reparative response to cross-linked collagen-based scaffolds in a rat spinal cord gap model. *Biomaterials*, **33**, 2050–9.

[119] http://www.medcompare.com/details/20376/Healos-Bone-Graft-Replacement.html.

[120] http://www.orthovita.com/vitoss/medialinks.aspx.

[121] http://www.allgensmed.com.

[122] http://www.synthes.com/sites/NA/products/Biomaterials/BoneVoidFillersSpine/Pages/chronOS_Spine.aspx.

[123] http://www.zimmer.com/web/enUS/pdf/CopiOs_Bone_Void_Filler_Brochure_97-1103-102-00_12_2007_FOR_USE_IN_THE_US_ONLY.pdf.

12

Polymer/ceramic composite scaffolds for tissue regeneration

Ian O. Smith, Melanie J. Gupte and Peter X. Ma

12.1 Biomimetics: nature provides the template

Where does a tissue engineer look for inspiration? What is the gold standard to which we hold our designs? Since antiquity, humankind has looked at the world around it for clues as to how we can improve our quality of life, and the gaze of the tissue engineer finds its way there as well. The metamorphosis of this inspiration into technology for the improvement of humankind is the mission of the engineer.

Complex structures are often found performing incredible feats in nature [1]. For example, brachiopod and mollusk shells are subjects of current study, due to their amazingly strong, layered structure [2, 3]. This natural composite structure is being used as inspiration for tissue-engineered structures for cortical bone. This is an example of nature-as-inspiration by utilizing composite material systems for bone tissue engineering scaffold design, an area of great success already, with potential for further advancement. The human body provides a model where collagen fibers are mineralized in a precise manner, resulting in a network of ceramic nanoscale crystals interspersed with an organic mesh. This leads to a hierarchical structure comprising these components and creating bone tissue, which through its complexity derives requisite qualities such as strength, toughness, fatigue life, and nutrient transfer [4]. This example is a common one, but not the only one. In fact, any scaffold design that incorporates one or more aspects of the naturally occurring extracellular matrix (ECM) is biomimetic by definition. In fact, in a broader sense so is any engineering design that borrows from nature. "What has fins like a whale, skin like a lizard and eyes like a moth? The future of engineering." Tom Mueller's question posed in *National Geographic* no doubt ignites a sense of wonderment resulting in brainstorming sessions about countless unsolved engineering problems, but we must focus. Within the scope of this chapter, we will focus on biomedical engineering, and more specifically polymer/ceramic composite scaffold design for use in tissue regeneration.

12.2 Today's tissue engineering: a brief synopsis

In their 2002 article in *Science*, Hench and Polak described a "third generation" of biomaterials where design invoked a desired cellular response and allowed the body to "heal itself" [5]. While this particular article may have been overtaken by the speed of biomedical research, this description is still very appropriate, especially in tissue engineering. It is as Langer and Vacanti describe in their seminal article on the subject: tissue engineering is an interdisciplinary field in which we develop materials to restore, maintain or improve tissue function [6]. For example, bone tissue engineering combines an artificial ECM, pre-osteoblastic cells, and factors that promote eventual tissue growth [7]. This approach fits well into the current thrust of tissue engineering research [8].

12.3 Composites: from dawn to the edge of tissue engineering technology

Through an understanding of the ECM and associated tissues, engineers have derived a design for tissue engineering scaffolds composed of polymers combined with ceramic crystals, polymer microspheres for drug and factor release, and even advanced nano-engineered structures to mimic biological structure and phenomena, in order to better provide the biological cues necessary for cellular/tissue response and incorporation.

One of the most widely used models for an artificial ECM is the polymer/ceramic composite system. Crystalline ceramics and amorphous materials have long been studied as potential candidates for bone tissue engineering applications [9–17]. For example, calcium phosphate (CaP) ceramics, including hydroxyapatite (HA), have attracted interest due to their similarity to bone mineral, their inherent biocompatibility, and their exceptional osteoconductivity. Hydroxyapatite exhibits a strong propensity for attracting osteoblasts but possesses a low resorption rate in vivo and is not mechanically strong, especially in highly porous forms. This is a disadvantage because porosity is a necessity for tissue ingrowth/regeneration [18].

How then does one get around these issues inherent to the material? Quite simply, as engineers, we get creative. Polymer scaffolds have also been investigated at length as candidates for artificial ECM. Natural and synthetic polymeric materials have been fabricated into scaffold structures, and some, such as poly(lactic acid) [14] and poly(lactic-*co*-glycolic acid) (PLGA), exhibit properties that make them attractive options. These properties include their ability to be formed into desired structures using such techniques as thermally induced phase separation and electrospinning, their mechanical properties, and resorbability. Polymers including these, along with polyamide, polycaprolactone, polyethylene, gelatin, chitosan, and collagen, have been fabricated into composite scaffold structures that incorporate HA [19–29]. These combinations allow the scaffold system to maintain many of the positive aspects of HA, while alleviating some of the negative features. Advantages of pairing HA with natural and/or synthetic polymers include improved control of design parameters such as porosity, degradability, and mechanical properties compared with pure HA scaffolds. Porosities greater than 90% are possible, whereas the scaffold porosity of pure HA is usually less than 70%. On a different scale, the addition of HA crystals to natural polymer scaffolds has been shown to improve mechanical properties compared with polymer control scaffolds and the presence of an HA component reduces adverse effects associated with the degradation of some synthetic polymers, including pH imbalance [29].

Again we come to a question of "how?" How do we incorporate HA crystals into a polymer scaffold? Even more importantly, how do we do so without having an adverse effect on the until-now successful method of forming such scaffolds? This question has been the subject of much work over the last decade, much of which has been completed by many, including our group, at the University of Michigan. Zhang and Ma began in straightforward fashion by simply mixing a ceramic component into a polymer solution prior to subjecting it to thermally induced phase separation (TIPS) [29]. While this technique met with significant success, it does not ideally control pore size and shape (Figure 12.1). Other issues that came to light while studying this method were the "locking up" of HA crystals within the bulk of the scaffold (whereas cell–biomaterial interaction occurs at the surface), and a lack of a desirable level of osteoconductivity shown by scaffolds fabricated using this particular TIPS method.

At around the same time as this early research was going on, the same group was attempting another approach to HA incorporation. Rather than mixing the HA component into the polymer solution prior to scaffold fabrication, they chose to take advantage of the surface properties of PLLA and "grow" HA onto already-existing polymer scaffolds, through a biomimetic process involving submersion in simulated body fluid (SBF) [30]. This was indeed successful, and apatite crystals similar to those present in bone were found along the surfaces of scaffold pores and their nature verified with SEM, XRD EDS, and FTIR (Figure 12.2).

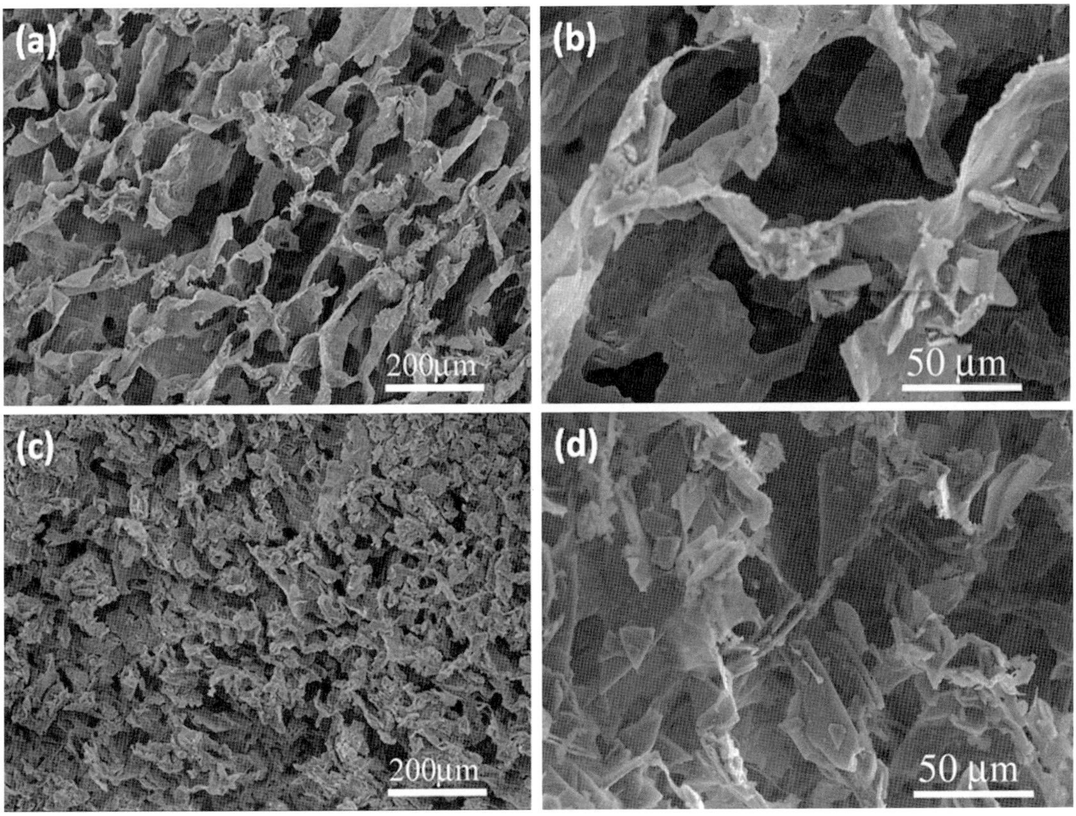

Figure 12.1 SEM micrographs of PLLA/HAP foams prepared from 2.5% (wt/vol) PLLA/HAP/dioxane mixtures with different HAP contents (quenching temperature 18 °C). Original magnifications: (a) PLLA/HAP: 70/30, ×100; (b) PLLA/HAP: 70/30, ×500; (c) PLLA/HAP: 30/70, ×100; (d) PLLA/HAP: 30/70, ×500. (Reprinted from [29], Zhang. R. and Ma, P. Poly(α-hydroxyl acids) hydroxyapatite porous composites for bone-tissue engineering. I. Preparation and morphology. *J. Biomed. Mater. Res.* 1999, **44**(4), 446–55, ©1999 with permission from John Wiley & Sons, Inc.)

This path of investigation would continue, although at first not aggressively. Rather, research would focus for a number of years on improvements in the structure of the underlying polymer scaffold, before eventually returning to the concept of apatite growth via a biomimetic method. The images in Figure 12.3 show one such refinement of scaffold structure by combining TIPS processing with the use of a sugar microsphere fugitive phase to yield a fibrous scaffold (Figure 12.3(a)) incorporating an interconnected network of pores (Figure 12.3(b)), mimicking the ECM and allowing a path for tissue ingrowth similar to the bone trabeculae [31].

This approach in which one incorporates nanofibrous elements into polymer scaffolds leads us back to the earlier example of incorporating HA through a biomimetic growth approach. Ideally, we would include apatite crystals similar to those that occur naturally during mineralization of the collagen fibers of the ECM. This combined approach yields a scaffold that mimics the mineralized extracellular matrix, or ECM. Nanofibrous polymer scaffolds consist of synthetic nanofibers, which can be made on a similar size scale to naturally occurring collagen I fibers (50–500 nm), which are native to the ECM and may have a role in bone formation. A matrix of these fibers serves

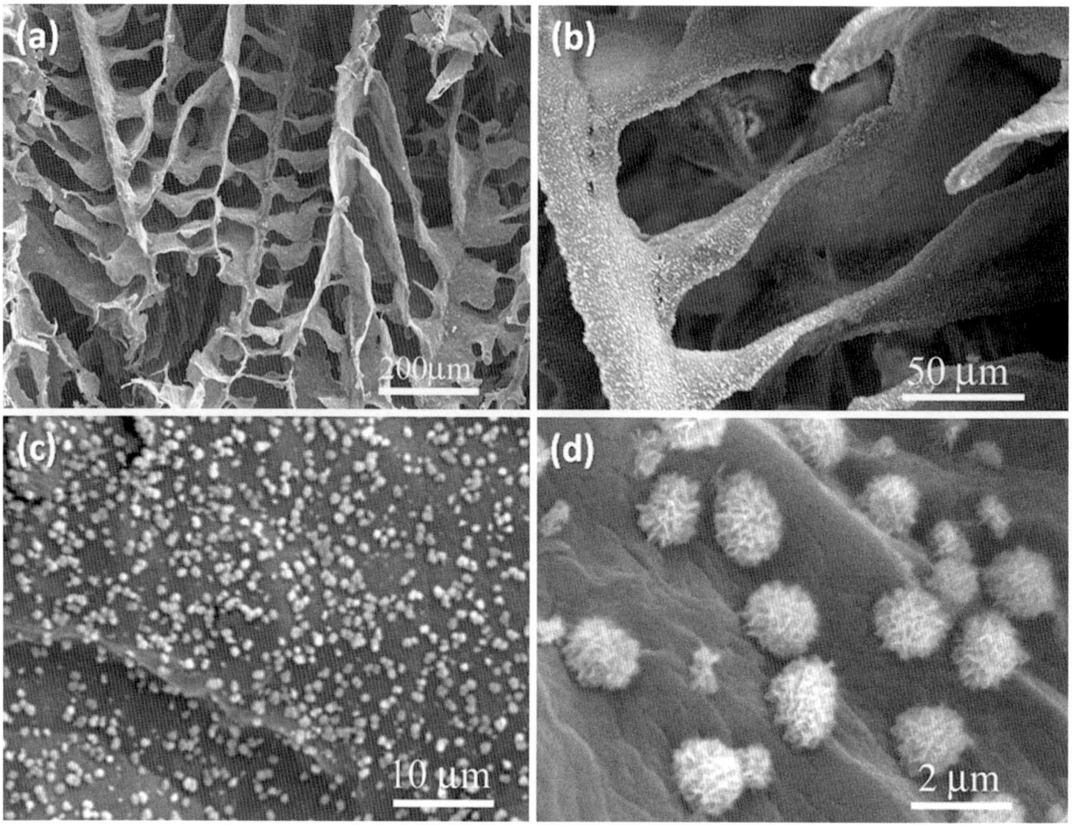

Figure 12.2 SEM micrographs of a PLLA foam incubated in simulated body fluid (SBF) for 30 days: original magnifications (a) ×100, (b) ×500, (c) ×2000, and (d) ×10,000. (Reprinted from [30], Zhang, R.Y. and Ma, P. X. Porous poly(L-lactic acid)/apatite composites created by biomimetic process. *J. Biomed. Mater. Res.* 1999, **45**(4), 285–93, ©1999 with permission from John Wiley & Sons, Inc.)

as a site for the nucleation of apatite crystals during the formation of woven bone.

Currently, the most common technique for forming polymer "nanofibers" is electrospinning [32, 33], which is accomplished by using an electric field to draw a thin stream of a polymer solution toward a collector. With this method, researchers have created fibers using PLLA, PLGA, PVA, gelatin, collagen, and other materials [32–38]. While effective for forming nano-scale fibers, this technique produces a roughly two-dimensional (2D) construct. Attempts to use electrospinning techniques to fabricate three-dimensional (3D) scaffolds have not successfully incorporated well-defined macroporosity and/or interconnectivity, which are necessary components in tissue engineering scaffolds. Using TIPS combined with sugar spheres is a novel and effective technique to create nanofibrous, interconnected, macroporous polymer scaffolds for tissue engineering that overcome the limitations of electrospinning. However, electrospinning has met with some success with low volume fractions of HA through mineralization, and more limited success at higher fractions with biomimetic crystalline architecture [34, 36, 39].

While SBF incubation is a well-established technique to deposit HA on polymer scaffolds, a faster

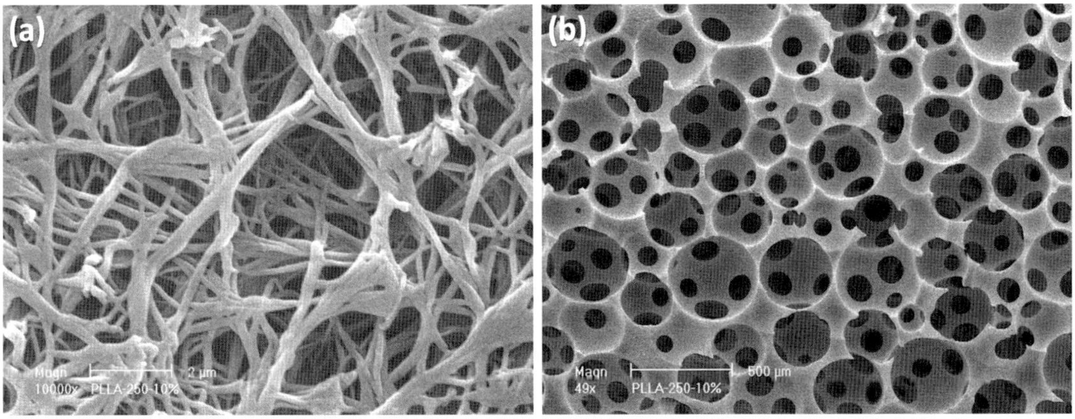

Figure 12.3 A 3D macroporous and nanofibrous PLLA scaffold built from sugar spheres/TIPS at (a) high (×10,000) and (b) low (×50) magnification. (Reprinted from [31], Wei, G. and Ma, P. X. Macroporous and nanofibrous polymer scaffolds and polymer/bone-like apatite composite scaffolds generated by sugar spheres. *J. Biomed. Mater. Res.* 2006, **78A**, 306–15, ©2006 with permission from John Wiley & Sons, Inc.)

method would be more desirable. Recently, a method has been developed that uses electrodeposition to grow HA crystals in just 30 minutes onto 2D films [40] or 3D scaffolds [41], prepared by electrospinning or TIPS. This method was initially used to coat titanium dental implants [42]. For electrodeposition, polymer substrates are adhered to a voltage-supplied electrode and submerged in an electrolyte containing both calcium and phosphate (Figure 12.4(a)). After 30 minutes, much faster than the 1–2-week SBF method, flower-shaped crystals are formed on the substrate. The deposited crystals consist of a combination of hydroxyapatite, dicalcium phosphate dihydrate (DCPD), and octacalcium phosphate (OCT), since it is common to obtain multiple mineral phases with any mineralization method. While the mechanism behind electrodeposition still requires some investigation, the process is tunable using temperature, pH, voltage, deposition time, and electrolyte composition to alter the crystal topography, calcium-to-phosphate ratio, size, and amount [40]. For example, increasing the polymer concentration (i.e. fiber diameter) or deposition time increases the amount of minerals deposited (Figure 12.4(b)). The morphology also changes from flower-like to flake-like when the deposition time is increased from 15 mins to 60 mins (Figures 4(c)–(e)).

It must be noted that PLLA and HA are by no means the only components utilized when designing a composite tissue engineering scaffold, as work by Cai, Jiang, Khang, Liu, Verma, Wang, and Wu, among others, details [43–49]. Other techniques instead of biomineralization have also been attempted for the enhancement of electrospun constructs, with positive bone and cartilage response, including the incorporation of tricalcium phosphate [50], carbon nanotubes [51], rosette nanotubes [52], bioactive glass [53], and even osteoblasts [54]. Furthermore, bone regeneration has also been performed without a traditional scaffold. For example, injectable versions similar to the materials discussed have been developed [55, 56]. While this chapter focusses on bone and cartilage tissue regeneration through the mimicking of the ECM, it should be noted that there are other applications for composite scaffold materials in tissue regeneration, most notably drug and growth factor delivery [57–62].

12.4 The intended goal: mineralized composites regulate stem cell differentiation

Now that we have explored the fabrication of various types of composite scaffolds, we have to ask "What is

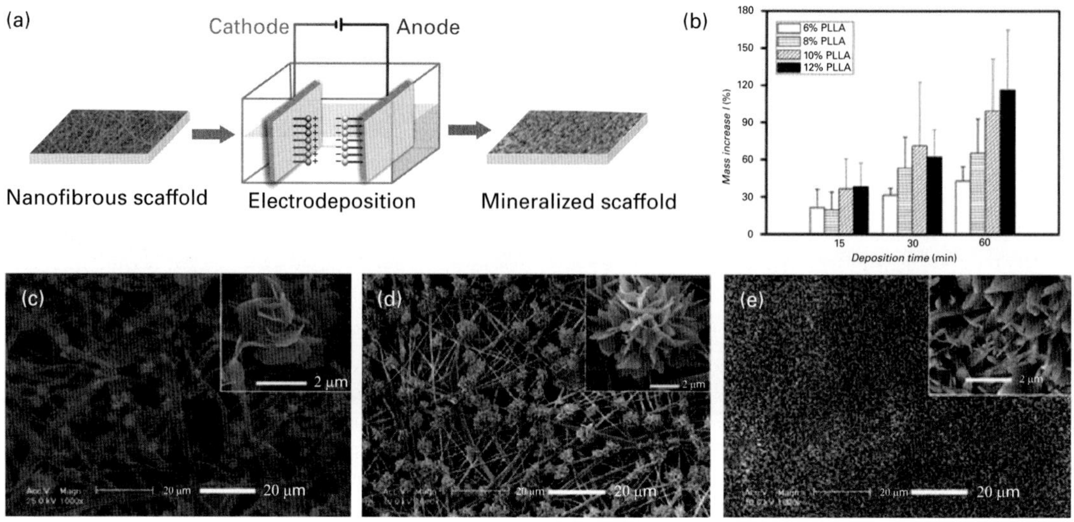

Figure 12.4 (a) Electrodeposition apparatus: as a nanofibrous scaffold is placed on the cathode and submerged in electrolyte, minerals are deposited on the scaffold when voltage is applied. (b) Mass increases as both polymer concentration (i.e. fiber diameter) and deposition time are increased. In (c)–(e) we show SEM micrographs of crystals' varied shapes after deposition at 3 V and 60 °C for durations of electrospinning of (c) on electrospun PLLA nanofibrous film 15 mins, (d) 30 mins, and (e) 60 mins, with insets of higher magnification. (Reprinted from [40], He, C., Xiao, G., Jin, X., Sun, C. and Ma, P. X. Electrodeposition on nanofibrous polymer scaffolds: rapid mineralization, tunable calcium phosphate composition and topography. *Adv. Functional Mater.*, 2010, **20**(20), 3568–76, ©2010 with permission from John Wiley & Sons, Inc.)

the point of developing composite scaffolds while pure polymer scaffolds are already widely used?" In addition to the improved mechanical properties mentioned earlier, one very important motivation is to control stem cell differentiation in regenerative medicine. Stem cells are a common cell source due to their availability and potential to form multiple tissue types [63], as compared with primary cell sources such as osteoblasts and chondrocytes. While growth factors and other differentiation-enhancing proteins can be added to cell culture media to control differentiation in vitro, this method cannot be used in vivo. Animal studies are essential to tissue engineering research because it is often only in vivo that true mechanisms behind tissue formation are uncovered. Once scaffolds have been implanted in vivo, often into mice or rats subcutaneously, they must stand alone to form the intended tissue. Therefore, by adhering minerals or drug delivery vehicles, for example, directly onto scaffolds, differentiation of stem cells (either migrated from the host or seeded on the scaffold prior to implantation) can be enhanced. While there are many types of composite scaffold, we will focus on biodegradable polymer/hydroxyapatite composite scaffolds because their biological effects on tissue formation have been thoroughly investigated.

When HA is added to a scaffold, first it can encourage cell adhesion and proliferation. Cell adhesion to the scaffold is important in preventing cell death and creating cell morphology similar to that in vivo. Calcium phosphate, of which HA is one type, may improve cell attachment, with each granule serving as a cell-attachment point [64]. Nanofibers then allow pre-osteoblasts to achieve a preferred 3D elongated shape on nanofiber films rather than the overly spread morphology achieved on flat films [65]. This suggests that a composite scaffold with nanofibers and HA may synergistically improve the cell microenvironment. Following adhesion, cell proliferation is essential for tissue formation and may also be enhanced by HA [37, 64].

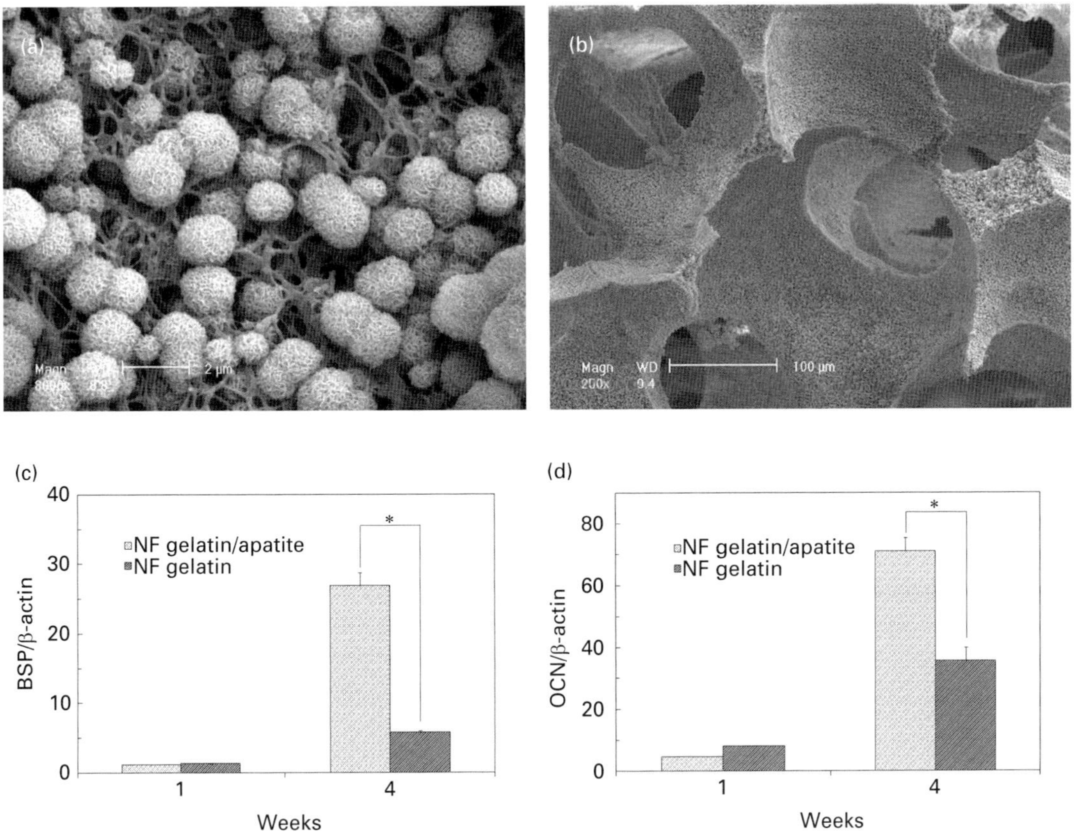

Figure 12.5 A phase-separated nanofibrous apatite/gelatin scaffold improves MC3T3-E1 differentiation. (a) SEM image at high magnification shows significant apatite presence. (b) Low magnification shows that apatite does not block pore interconnections of scaffold. Real-time PCR for (c) bone sialoprotein (BSP) and (d) osteocalcein (OCN) at 1 and 4 weeks of culture on gelatin or gelatin/apatite scaffold. * $p < 0.05$. (Reprinted from [46], Liu, X., Smith, L.A., Hu, J. and Ma, P. X. Biomimetic nanofibrous gelatin/apatite composite scaffolds for bone tissue engineering. *Biomaterials*, 2009, **30**, 2252–8, ©2009 with permission from Elsevier.)

Once stem cells greatly proliferate, they must differentiate into the desired mature cell type. It has been widely shown that HA improves osteogenic differentiation of numerous stem cell types, including embryonic stem cells [66], iPS cells [67], and bone-marrow-derived mesenchymal stem cells [68, 69]. Hydroxyapatite has also been shown to facilitate the differentiation of pre-osteoblasts [46] and enhance osteoblast function [70]. The positive effect of HA on osteogenic differentiation is marked by increased bone marker gene expression, collagen type I deposition, mineralization, and alkaline phosphatase activity. Owing to these effects, biomaterials containing HA can successfully support bone tissue formation. For example, Liu *et al.* showed that HA on a nanofibrous gelatin scaffold adheres to the nanofibers (Figure 12.5(a)) without blocking the interconnected porous structure (Figure 12.5(b)). When seeded with MC3T3-E1 pre-osteoblasts, HA significantly enhanced gene expression of bone sialoprotein (Figure 12.5(c)) and osteocalcein (Figure 12.5(d)) at four weeks [46]. Therefore, this composite scaffold improves osteogenic differentiation of pre-osteoblasts using both apatite minerals and nanofiber architecture.

Hydroxyapatite has been used to stimulate not only osteogenic differentiation but also chondrogenic differentiation. Human MSCs can be differentiated on a PLLA/HA electrospun scaffold to the chondrogenic lineage in vitro [38]. In vivo, a porous hydroxyapatite scaffold combined with BMP-2 release has successfully repaired articular cartilage defects in a rabbit model using recruited host stem cells [71]. However, more often, HA or tricalcium phosphate (TCP) is incorporated in biphasic scaffolds for osteochondral repair, mainly for the calcified cartilage and subchondral bone layers. Though HA does support chondrocyte growth and facilitate cartilage regeneration, these biphasic studies mainly concerned bone formation [72, 73]. Thus, the role HA plays in stem cell differentiation for cartilage formation needs further study.

But how exactly can nano-scale mineral crystals on a nanofibrous polymer scaffold biologically direct stem cells to a desired lineage? Nanofibers of the scaffold themselves enhance several stem cell behaviors: adhesion, proliferation, and differentiation. The suggested mechanisms behind these positive nanofiber effects include increased integrin expression [74], increased protein adsorption [75], and modified signaling pathways through paxillin, focal adhesion kinase, RhoA, and Rac [65, 76, 77]. While the mechanisms behind the cellular response to HA still require further investigation, a few mechanisms have been proposed. One suggested mechanism is that HA increases protein absorption, most significantly fibronectin and vitronectin absorption, through the integrin–FAK–Akt pathway, which then suppresses apoptosis [78]. This hypothesis was established through observation of MC3T3-E1 pre-osteoblasts on a 3D PLLA/hydroxyapatite composite scaffold in comparison with those on a pure PLLA scaffold. Because this study used pre-osteoblasts, the mechanism for stem cell differentiation must still be elucidated. Results from another study also implicate an FAK pathway using MC3T3-E1 pre-osteoblasts by showing activation of ERK in response to 2D hydroxyapatite disks [79]. To better simulate the in-vivo environment, 3D studies are warranted.

The HA composite scaffold model reveals that composite scaffolds can be highly useful in promoting cell adhesion and proliferation, and, more importantly, stem cell differentiation. Therefore, biodegradable polymer/bioceramic composite scaffolds may continue to be an integral tool in solving tissue-engineering challenges.

12.5 The right track? The future of composites for tissue regeneration

Tissue engineering is a fast-paced field that benefits from advances in other disciplines, such as biology, materials science, and medicine. As biologists make new molecular and cellular discoveries, they can inspire biomimetic scaffold design. As material scientists find new ways to manipulate polymers and other materials on the micro- and nano-scales, we can not only use them but also combine them to form composite scaffolds. As physicians enhance micro-surgery techniques, we can use tissue-engineered solutions to repair a patient's tissue function without invasive procedures.

With all this impressive progress, scaffold design remains critical to the advancement of tissue engineering and regenerative medicine. This is especially true in the realm of bone and dentin regeneration, since both of these tissues are required to withstand significant mechanical loads. By combining the fabrication of interconnected porous and nanofibrous scaffolds with methods of incorporating biomimetic ceramics, we can fabricate a composite scaffold that mimics the mineralized collagen fibers found in the native ECM of hard tissues. Polymer/ceramic scaffolds can successfully provide essential biological cues to enhance cell adhesion, proliferation, and differentiation for hard-tissue formation.

Bone regeneration research has made great strides but still requires future work. While polymer/ceramic scaffolds improve osteogenic differentiation of multiple stem cell types, the ceramic component effect must be clarified, especially in a 3D scaffold system. More importantly, the mechanisms behind how apatite enhances stem cell differentiation need to be elucidated in more depth because the limited mechanistic studies so far have used only differentiated cells.

Lastly, new composite scaffold fabrication techniques are needed in order to create a more native crystal topography. Through a better understanding of the cellular processes, as well as the development of new scaffold fabrication techniques, we can build better composite scaffolds for functional mineralized tissue regeneration.

ACKNOWLEDGEMENTS

The authors would like to acknowledge the financial support from the National Institutes of Health (NIDCR DE015384, DE017689 and DE022327: PXM), DOD (W81XWH-12-2-0008: PXM), and NSF (DMR-1206575: PXM). MJG was partially supported by a fellowship from the NIH/NIDCR Training Grant (T32 DE 007057).

REFERENCES

[1] Green, D. W. 2008. Tissue bionics: examples in biomimetic tissue engineering. *Biomed. Mater.*, **3**, 034010.

[2] Evans, J. S. 2008. "Tuning in" to mollusk shell nacre- and prismatic-associated protein terminal sequences. Implications for biomineralization and the construction of high performance inorganic–organic composites. *Chem. Rev.*, **108**(11), 4455–62.

[3] Schmahl, W. W., Greisshaber, E., Merkel, C. *et al.* 2008. Hierarchical fibre composite structure and micromechanical properties of phosphatic and calcitic brachiopod shell biomaterials: an overview. *Mineral. Mag.*, **72**(2), 541–62.

[4] Marquis, M. E., Lord, E., Bergeron, E. *et al.* 2009. Bone cells-biomaterials interactions. *Frontiers Biosci.*, **14**, 1023–67.

[5] Hench, L. L. and Polak, J. M. 2002. Third-generation biomedical materials. *Science*, **295**(5557), 1014–17.

[6] Langer, R. and Vacanti, J. P. 1993. Tissue engineering. *Science*, **260**(5110), 920–6.

[7] Wei, G. and Ma, P. X. 2004. Structure and properties of nano-hydroxyapatite/polymer composite scaffolds for bone tissue engineering. *Biomaterials*, **25**, 4749–57.

[8] Giannoudis, P. V., Dinopoulos, H. and Tsiridis, E. 2005. Bone substitutes: an update. *Injury, Int. J. Care Injured*, **36**(Suppl.), S20–7.

[9] Blaker, J. J., Nazhat, S. N., Maquet, V. and Boccaccini, A. R. 2011. Long-term in vitro degradation of PDLLA/bioglass bone scaffolds in acellular simulated body fluid. *Acta Biomater.*, **7**, 829–40.

[10] Francis, L., Meng, D., Knowles, J. C., Roy, I. and Boccaccini, A. R. 2010. Multi-functional P(3HB) microsphere/45S5 Bioglass-based composite scaffolds for bone tissue engineering. *Acta Biomater.*, **6**, 2773–86.

[11] Hajiali, H., Karbasi, S., Hosseinalipour, M. and Rezaie, H. R. 2010. Preparation of a novel biodegradable nanocomposite scaffold based on poly(3-hydroxybutyrate)/bioglass nanoparticles for bone tissue engineering. *J. Mater. Sci.: Mater. Med.*, **21**, 2125–32.

[12] Hench, L. L. 1998. Bioceramics. *J. Am. Ceram. Soc.*, **81**(7), 1705–28.

[13] Kundu, B., Soundrapandian, C., Nandi, S. K. *et al.* 2010. Development of new localized drug delivery system based on ceftriaxone–sulbactam composite drug impregnated porous hydroxyapatite: a systematic approach for in vitro and in vivo animal trial. *Pharm. Res.*, **27**, 1659–76.

[14] Milan, J., Planell, J. A. and Lacroix, D. 2009. Computational modelling of the mechanical environment of osteogenesis within a polylactic acid–calcium phosphate glass scaffold. *Biomaterials*, **30**(25), 4219–26.

[15] Misra, S. K., Ansari, T. I., Valappil, S. P. *et al.* 2010. Poly(3-hydroxybutyrate) multifunctional composite scaffolds for tissue engineering applications. *Biomaterials*, **31**, 2806–15.

[16] Xu, C., Su, P., Wang, Y. *et al.* 2010. A novel biomimetic composite scaffold hybridized with mesenchymal stem cells in repair of rat bone defects models. *J. Biomed. Mater. Res. Part A*, **95**(2), 495–503.

[17] Xu, C., Su, P., Chen, X. *et al.* 2011. Biocompatibility and osteogenesis of biomimetic Bioglass–collagen–phosphatidylserine composite scaffolds for bone tissue engineering. *Biomaterials*, **32**, 1051–8.

[18] Hing, K. A., Wilson, L. F. and Buckland, T. 2007. Comparative performance of three ceramic bone graft substitutes. *Spine J.*, **7**, 475–90.

[19] Douglas, T., Pamula, E., Hauk, D. *et al.* 2009. Porous polymer/hydroxyapatite scaffolds: characterization and biocompatibility investigations. *J. Mater. Sci.: Mater. Med.*, **20**, 1909–15.

[20] Henriksen, S. S., Ding, M., Vinther Juhl, M., Theilgaard, N. and Overgaard, S. 2011. Mechanical strength of ceramic scaffolds reinforced with biopolymers is comparable to that of human bone. *J. Mater. Sci.: Mater. Med.*, **22**, 1111–18.

[21] Khan, Y., El-Amin, S. F. and Laurencin, C. T. 2006. In vitro and in vivo evaluation of a novel polymer–ceramic composite scaffold for bone tissue engineering. In *28th IEEE EMBS Annual International Conference*, New York.

[22] Kim, S., Ahn, K. M., Park, M. S. *et al.* 2007. A poly(lactide-*co*-glycolide)/hydroxyapatite composite scaffold with enhanced osteoconductivity. *J. Biomed. Mater. Res. Part A*, **80**, 206–15.

[23] Kim, S.-S., Park, M. S., Gwak, S.-J., Choi, C. Y. and Kim, B.-S. 2006. Accelerated bonelike apatite growth on porous polymer/ceramic composite scaffolds in vitro. *Tissue Eng.*, **12**(10), 2997–3006.

[24] Kim, S., Park, M. S., Jeon, O., Choi, C. Y. and Kim, B.-S. 2006. Poly(lactide-*co*-glycolide)/hydroxyapatite composite scaffolds for bone tissue engineering. *Biomaterials*, **27**, 1399–409.

[25] Leong, N. L., Jiang, J. and Lu, H. H. 2006. Polymer–ceramic composite scaffold induces osteogenic differentiation of human mesenchymal stem cells. In *28th IEEE EMBS Annual International Conference*, New York.

[26] Qing, L. V., Nair, L. and Laurencin, C. T. 2008. Fabrication, characterization, and in vitro evaluation of poly (lactic acid glycolic acid)/nano-hydroxyapatite composite microsphere-based scaffolds for bone tissue engineering in rotating bioreactors. *J. Biomed. Mater. Res. Part A*, **91**, 679–91.

[27] Qiu, X., Hong, Z., Hu, J. *et al.* 2005. Hydroxyapatite surface modified by L-lactic acid and its subsequent grafting polymerization of L-lactide. *Biomacromolecules*, **6**, 1193–9.

[28] Scaglione, S., Lazzarini, E., Ilengo, C. and Quarto, R. 2010. A composite material model for improved bone formation. *J. Tissue Eng. Regen. Med.*, **4**, 505–13.

[29] Zhang, R. and Ma, P. 1999. Poly(α-hydroxyl acids) hydroxyapatite porous composites for bone-tissue engineering. I. Preparation and morphology. *J. Biomed. Mater. Res.*, **44**(4), 446–55.

[30] Zhang, R. Y. and Ma, P. X. 1999. Porous poly(L-lactic acid)/apatite composites created by biomimetic process. *J. Biomed. Mater. Res.*, **45**(4), 285–93.

[31] Wei, G. and Ma, P. X. 2006. Macroporous and nanofibrous polymer scaffolds and polymer/bone-like apatite composite scaffolds generated by sugar spheres. *J. Biomed. Mater. Res. Part A*, **78**, 306–15.

[32] Liu, X. H. and Ma, P. X. 2004. Polymeric scaffolds for bone tissue engineering. *Ann. Biomed. Eng.*, **32**(3), 477–86.

[33] Ma, P. X. 2008. Biomimetic materials for tissue engineering. *Adv. Drug Deliv. Rev.*, **60**, 184–98.

[34] Yang, D., Jin, Y., Zhou, Y. *et al.* 2008. In situ mineralization of hydroxyapatite on electrospun chitosan-based nanofibrous scaffolds. *Macromol. Biosci.*, **8**, 239–46.

[35] Chen, F., Tang, Q. L., Zhu, Y. J. *et al.* 2010. Hydroxyapatite nanorods/poly(vinyl pyrolidone) composite nanofibers, arrays and three-dimensional fabrics: electrospun preparation and transformation to hydroxyapatite nanostructures. *Acta Biomater.*, **6**, 3013–20.

[36] Song, J., Kim, H.-E. and Kim, H.-W. 2008. Electrospun fibrous web of collagen–apatite precipitated nanocomposite for bone regeneration. *J. Mater. Sci.: Mater. Med.*, **19**(8), 2925–32.

[37] Li, X. R., Xie, J. W., Yuan, X. Y. and Xia, Y. N. 2008. Coating electrospun poly(ε-caprolactone) fibers with gelatin and calcium phosphate and their use as biomimetic scaffolds for bone tissue engineering. *Langmuir*, **24**(24), 14145–50.

[38] Spadaccio, C., Rainer, A., Trombetta, M. *et al.* 2009. Poly-L-lactic acid/hydroxyapatite electrospun nanocomposites induce chondrogenic differentiation of human MSC. *Ann. Biomed. Eng.*, **37**(7), 1376–89.

[39] Chen, J., Chu, B. and Hsiao, B. S. 2006. Mineralization of hydroxyapatite in electrospun nanofibrous poly(L-lactic acid) scaffolds. *J. Biomed. Mater. Res. Part A*, **79**, 307–17.

[40] He, C., Xiao, G., Jin, X., Sun, C. and Ma, P. X. 2010. Electrodeposition on nanofibrous polymer scaffolds: rapid mineralization, tunable calcium phosphate composition and topography. *Adv. Functional Mater.*, **20**(20), 3568–76.

[41] He, C., Zhang, F., Cao, L. *et al.* 2012. Rapid mineralization of porous gelatin scaffolds by electrodeposition for bone tissue engineering. *J. Mater. Chem.*, **22**(5), 2111–19.

[42] Vijayaraghavan, T. V. and Bensalem, A. 1995. Hydroxyapatite (HA) coating by electrodeposition on α-Ti and α-β-Ti alloys. *J. Dental Res.*, **74**, 474.

[43] Cai, Z., Zhang, T., Di, L. *et al.* 2011. Morphological and histological analysis on the in vivo degradation of poly(propylene fumarate)/(calcium sulfate/β-tricalcium phosphate). *Biomed. Microdevices*, **13**(4), 623–31.

[44] Jiang, J., Tang, A., Ateshian, G. A. *et al.* 2010. Bioactive stratified polymer ceramic–hydrogel scaffold for integrative osteochondral repair. *Ann. Biomed. Eng.*, **38**(6), 2183–96.

[45] Khang, D., Kim, S. Y., Liu-Snyder, P. *et al.* 2007. Enhanced fibronectin adsorption on carbon nanotube/poly(carbonate) urethane: independent role of surface nano-roughness and associated surface energy. *Biomaterials*, **28**, 4756–68.

[46] Liu, X., Smith, L. A., Hu, J. and Ma, P. X. 2009. Biomimetic nanofibrous gelatin/apatite composite scaffolds for bone tissue engineering. *Biomaterials*, **30**, 2252–8.

[47] Verma, D., Katti, K. S. and Katti, D. R. 2008. Effect of biopolymers on structure of hydroxyapatite and interfacial interactions in biomimetically synthesized hydroxyapatite/biopolymer nanocomposites. *Ann. Biomed. Eng.*, **36**(6), 1024–32.

[48] Wang, H., Li, Y., Zuo, Y. *et al.* 2007. Biocompatibility and osteogenesis of biomimetic nano-hydroxyapatite/polyamide composite scaffolds for bone tissue engineering. *Biomaterials*, **28**(22), 3338–48.

[49] Wu, Y., Jiang, W., Wen, X *et al.* 2010. A novel calcium phosphate ceramic–magnetic nanoparticle composite as a potential bone substitute. *Biomed. Mater.*, **5**, 015001.

[50] Li, X., Yao, C., Sun, F. *et al.* 2008. Conjugate electrospinning of continuous nanofiber yarn of poly(L-lactide)/nanotricalcium phosphate nanocomposite. *J. Appl. Polymer Sci.*, **107**, 3756–64.

[51] Mei, F., Zhong, J., Yang, X. *et al.* 2007. Improved biological characteristics of poly(L-lactic acid) electrospun membrane by incorporation of multiwalled carbon nanotubes/hydroxyapatite nanoparticles. *Biomacromolecules*, **8**, 3729–35.

[52] Chen, Y., Bilgen, B., Pareta, R. A. *et al.* 2010. Self-assembled rosette nanotube/hydrogel composites for cartilage tissue engineering. *Tissue Eng. Part C*, **16**(6), 1233–43.

[53] Kim, H. W., Lee, H. H. and Chun, G. S. 2007. Bioactivity and osteoblast responses of novel biomedical nanocomposites of bioactive glass nanofiber filled poly(lactic acid). *J. Biomed. Mater. Res. Part A*, **85**, 651–63.

[54] Venugopal, J. R., Low, S., Choon, A. T., Kumar, A. B. and Ramakrishna, S. 2008. Nanobioengineered electrospun composite nanofibers and osteoblasts for bone regeneration. *Artificial Organs*, **35**(5), 388–97.

[55] Huang, Z., Tian, J., Yu, B., Xu, Y. and Feng, Q. 2009. A bone-like nano-hydroxyapatite/collagen loaded injectable scaffold. *Biomed. Mater.*, **4**, 055005.

[56] Kang, S. W., Yang, H. S., Seo, S. W., Han, D. K. and Kim, B. S. 2008. Apatite-coated poly(lactic-*co*-glycolic acid) microspheres as an injectable scaffold for bone tissue engineering. *J. Biomed. Mater. Res. Part A*, **85**, 747–56.

[57] Feng, K., Sun, H., Bradley, M. A. *et al.* 2010. Novel antibacterial nanofibrous PLLA scaffolds. *J. Controlled Release*, **146**(3), 363–9.

[58] Kundu, B., Nandi, S. K., Dasgupta, S. *et al.* 2011. Macro-to-micro porous special bioactive glass and ceftriaxone–sulbactam composite drug delivery system for treatment of chronic osteomyelitis: an investigation through in vitro and in vivo animal trial. *J. Mater. Sci.: Mater. Med.*, **22**, 705–20.

[59] Niu, X., Feng, Q., Wang, M., Guo, X. and Zheng, Q. 2009. Porous nano-HA/collagen/PLLA scaffold containing chitosan microspheres for controlled delivery of synthetic peptide derived from BMP-2. *J. Controlled Release*, **134**, 111–17.

[60] Wang, X., Oyane, A., Tsurushima, H. *et al.* 2011. BMP-2 and ALP gene expression induced by a BMP-2 gene–fibronectin–apatite composite layer. *Biomed. Mater.*, **6**, 045004.

[61] Wei, G., Jin, Q., Giannobile, W. V. and Ma, P. X. 2007. The enhancement of osteogenesis by nano-fibrous scaffolds incorporating rhBMP-7 nanospheres. *Biomaterials*, **28** (12), 2087–96.

[62] Zhu, M., Wang, H., Liu, J. *et al.* 2011. A mesoporous silica nanoparticulate/β-TCP/BG composite drug delivery system for osteoarticular tuberculosis therapy. *Biomaterials*, **32** 1986–95.

[63] Pittenger, M., Mackay, A., Beck, S. *et al.* 1999. Multilineage potential of adult human mesenchymal stem cells. *Science*, **284**(5411), 143–7.

[64] Eyckmans, J., Roberts, S. J., Schrooten, J. and Luyten, F. P. 2010. A clinically relevant model of osteoinduction: a process requiring calcium phosphate and BMP/Wnt signalling. *J. Cellular Molec. Medicine*, **14**(6b), 1845–56.

[65] Hu, J., Liu, X. and Ma, P. X. 2008. Induction of osteoblast differentiation phenotype on poly(L-lactic acid) nanofibrous matrix. *Biomaterials*, **29**(28), 3815–21.

[66] Garreta, E., Gasset, D., Semino, C. and Borrós, S. 2007. Fabrication of a three-dimensional nanostructured biomaterial for tissue engineering of bone. *Biomolec. Eng.*, **24**(1), 75–80.

[67] D'Angelo, F., Armentano, I., Cacciotti, I. *et al.* 2012. Tuning multi/pluri-potent stem cell fate by electrospun poly(L-lactic acid)-calcium-deficient hydroxyapatite nanocomposite mats. *Biomacromolecules*, **13**(5), 1350–60.

[68] Lao, L., Zhu, Y., Zhang, Y. *et al.* 2012. Mineralization of collagen-coated electrospun poly(lactide-*co*-glycolide) nanofibrous mesh to enhance growth and differentiation of osteoblasts and bone marrow mesenchymal stem cells. *Adv. Eng. Mater.*, **14**(4), B123–37.

[69] Polini, A., Pisignano, D., Parodi, M., Quarto, R. and Scaglione, S. 2011. Osteoinduction of human mesenchymal stem cells by bioactive composite scaffolds without supplemental osteogenic growth factors. *PLoS One*, **6**(10), e26211.

[70] Ngiam, M., Liao, S., Patil, A. J. *et al.* 2009. The fabrication of nano-hydroxyapatite on PLGA and PLGA/collagen

nanofibrous composite scaffolds and their effects in osteoblastic behavior for bone tissue engineering. *Bone*, **45**(1), 4–16.

[71] Tamai, N., Myoui, A., Hirao, M. *et al.* 2005. A new biotechnology for articular cartilage repair: subchondral implantation of a composite of interconnected porous hydroxyapatite, synthetic polymer (PLA-PEG), and bone morphogenetic protein-2 (rhBMP-2). *Osteoarthritis Cartilage*, **13**(5), 405–17.

[72] Ito, Y., Adachi, N., Nakamae, A., Yanada, S. and Ochi, M. 2008. Transplantation of tissue-engineered osteochondral plug using cultured chondrocytes and interconnected porous calcium hydroxyapatite ceramic cylindrical plugs to treat osteochondral defects in a rabbit model. *Artificial Organs*, **32**(1), 36–44.

[73] Tanaka, T., Komaki, H., Chazono, M. and Fujii, K. 2005. Use of a biphasic graft constructed with chondrocytes overlying a β-tricalcium phosphate block in the treatment of rabbit osteochondral defects. *Tissue Eng.*, **11**(1–2), 331–9.

[74] Smith, L., Liu, X., Hu, J., Wang, P. and Ma, P. X. 2009. Enhancing osteogenic differentiation of mouse embryonic stem cells by nanofibers. *Tissue Eng.: Part A*, **15**(7), 1855–64.

[75] Woo, K. M., Chen, V. J. and Ma, P. X. 2003. Nano-fibrous scaffolding architecture selectively enhances protein adsorption contributing to cell attachment. *J. Biomed. Mater. Res. Part A*, **67**(2), 531–7.

[76] Nur-E-Kamal, A., Ahmed, I., Kamal, J., Schindler, M. and Meiners, S. 2006. Three-dimensional nanofibrillar surfaces promote self-renewal in mouse embryonic stem Cells, *Stem Cells*, **24**(2), 426–33.

[77] Woo, K., Jun, J., Chen, V. *et al.* 2007. Nano-fibrous scaffolding promotes osteoblast differentiation and biomineralization. *Biomaterials*, **28**(2), 335–43.

[78] Woo, K., Seo, J., Zhang, R. and Ma, P. 2007. Suppression of apoptosis by enhanced protein adsorption on polymer/hydroxyapatite composite scaffolds. *Biomaterials*, **28**(16), 2622–30.

[79] Song, J. H., Kim, J. H., Park, S. *et al.* 2008. Signaling responses of osteoblast cells to hydroxyapatite: the activation of ERK and SOX9. *J. Bone Miner. Metab*, **26**(2), 138–42.

13

Computer-aided tissue engineering for modeling and fabrication of three-dimensional tissue scaffolds

Qudus Hamid, Chengyang Wang, Jessica Snyder and Wei Sun

13.1 Introduction

The need for replacement organs and tissue substitutes is on the rise. At present, there is an insufficient amount of tissue replacements for failed or damaged organs, due to the lack of donors. In the USA alone, over twenty million patients per year suffer from some form of tissue- and/or organ-related malady, and are awaiting a replacement. The financial cost of health care for these patients has been estimated to be over $400 billion annually [1, 2]. Computer-aided tissue engineered substitutes are one of the most promising applications of tissue replacements to address this issue. These tissue arrays are fabricated using techniques from a variety of science and engineering disciplines to create the optimum tissue replacement (in terms of the targeted functionality). Additionally, these tissue constructs play a vital role as pre-formed extracellular matrices to which cells can readily attach, whereupon they can rapidly multiply and form new tissue [3, 4]. In recent decades, scientists have proven that these fields are evolving into one of the most promising therapeutic approaches in regenerative medicine [5–9].

Three-dimensional tissue scaffolds are designed with a preferred internal architecture, wherein porosity and material connectivity provide the required structural integrity, mass transport, and comprehensive microenvironment for cell and tissue growth. A literature survey has shown that cell survival and proliferation within the tissue scaffold are dependent on oxygen, vital molecules, and the micro-architecture of the scaffolds [10, 11]. The complexity of tissue scaffolds requires novel approaches and computational algorithms to match the desired criteria for internal architecture, permeability, pore size, and connectivity. The dynamics of a tissue scaffold is governed by its structural and topological configuration defined by porosity, pore interconnectivity, tortuosity, and scaffold material permeability and diffusivity [12–14]. The scaffold tortuosity characterizes the diffusion path length of fluid molecules through the scaffold, which shapes the internal architecture of the scaffold and plays a major role in tissue growth and proliferation [15–19]. Many cells respond more favorably to a three-dimensional (3D) microenvironment (than to a two-dimensional (2D) microenvironment) with intricate intracellular architectures where the cell's morphological shape, behavior, and gene expression are richer, more robust, and more similar to in-vivo responses [20–22].

Computer-aided tissue engineering (CATE) utilizes computer technologies and biological informatics to design and model biological substitutes that restore, maintain, or improve tissue functions [23]. CATE technologies can produce tissue arrays with precision, accuracy, repeatability, and close mimicry (biological, mechanical, and chemical) of the targeted organ or tissue. The tissue constructs developed utilize data from several computer-aided technologies (computer-aided design (CAD), computer-aided engineering (CAE), and computer-aided manufacturing (CAM)) and medical imagery (radiography, magnetic resonance imaging (MRI), fiduciary markers, tomography, and ultrasound) [24–26]. CATE applications are categorized into three major components: (1) computer-aided tissue modeling and biomodeling, (2) scaffold informatics and biomimetic design, and (3) biomanufacturing for tissue and organ regeneration [27]. CATE has emerged as a leader for generating biomimetic tissue scaffolds from synthetic and natural polymers. CATE fabrication devices can produce complex biological architecture well into the micron and nano range [28–30]. For a tissue-engineered substitute to become successful, it must be designed to address its sole function. Given the functionality of the targeted organ, the appropriate device and materials will be chosen to construct the optimal chemical, mechanical, and biological cues within the desired tissue scaffold [31–36]. Before the tissue scaffold is fabricated, much work is done with the biomodel of the scaffold. With the biomodel one investigates the targeted organ and develops an engineered replica that can be fabricated. Owing to the complexity of tissues, it is very difficult to fabricate the exact architecture of the targeted organ. Instead, a model is developed to have mechanical, chemical, and biological features similar to those of the targeted tissue [37–41].

13.2 Overview of computer-aided tissue engineering

Figure 13.1 gives an overview of CATE [26]. The first component of CATE is computer-aided tissue modeling and biomodeling. This component is the investigative stage, where medical data are processed using various types of qualitative and quantitative anatomic, biophysical, CAD-based, and biomedical physical modeling. The computer-aided tissue modeling and biomodeling category of CATE focusses on the medical imagery/data and exact or defined geometry, volumetric representation, morphology, mechanics, deformation, kinematics, a contour-based model, and surface information. The second component of CATE, scaffold informatics and biomimetic design, builds from the first component of CATE. Data obtained from the first component are used to develop biomimetic design, multiscale models for biological systems, and scaffold informatics and models. Scaffold informatics and biomimetic design data enable researchers to classify tissue morphology, characterize cell/tissue morphology, design a framework for

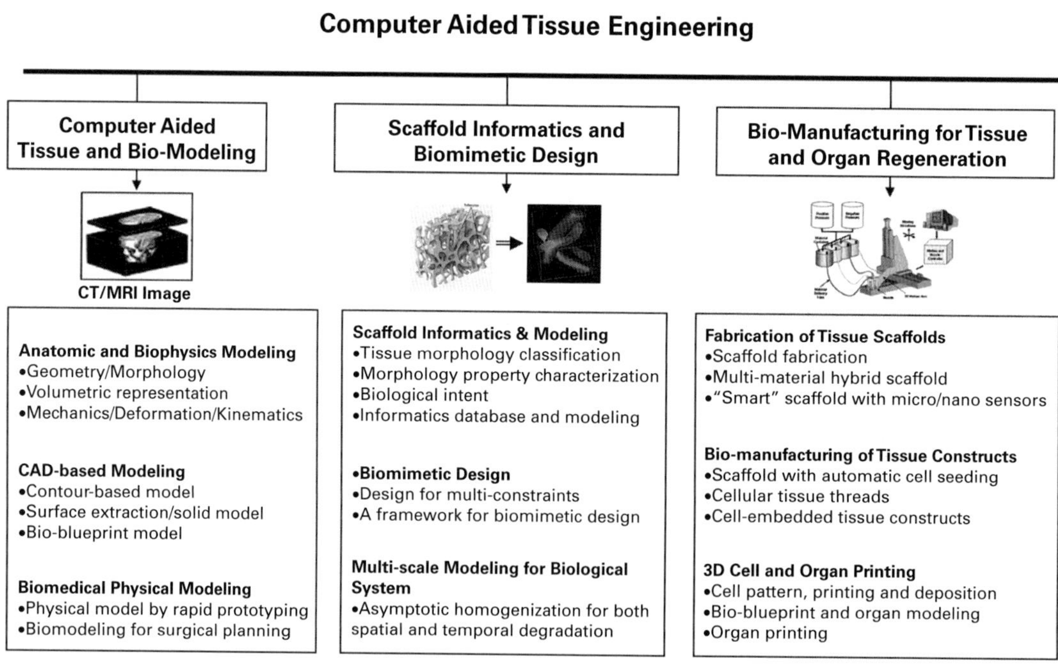

Figure 13.1 An overview of computer-aided tissue engineering.

biomimetic design, and develop an asymptotic homogenization for spatial and temporal degradation. The final component of CATE focusses on the biomanufacturing approaches for tissue and organ generation. This category develops tissue scaffold fabrication methods, which include, but are not limited to, scaffold fabrication, multimaterial hybrid scaffolds, scaffolds with automatic cell seeding, cells embedded within tissue constructs, cell patterning, cell printing, and organ printing. Together, these three components define the CATE approach.

13.2.1 Computer-aided tissue modeling and biomodeling

Humans have occupied the Earth for over one million years. During this period, the human body has evolved throughout time to sustain life [42]. Researchers are constantly conducting analysis to understand human anatomy and physiological needs. A better understanding of the human body, along with its tissues and organs, will enable scientists to develop tissue substitutes to replace damaged and/or failed tissue organs [43]. With the use of non-invasive medical imaging technologies, such as radiography, MRI, fiduciary markers, tomography, and ultrasound, it is simple to acquire medical informatics of organs and tissue. Each of these non-invasive medical imaging techniques generates medical data using various approaches and is used to gather information on different types of tissues [44–48]. For example, the MRI device acquires its images by first aligning the atoms within the body with the use of a magnetic field. Then the MRI systematically alters the magnetization by application of a radio frequency. This process is targeted at various locations and the device is rotated at different speeds to gain "layer-by-layer" information or "slices" of information [49]. This information can later be combined to produce multilayered (sometimes referred to as 3D) imagery. The MRI technique can gather information on bones and tissues. On the other hand, X-ray radiography is primarily used to capture information on dense materials, such as bone, in the form of 2D images, and provides very limited information for the reconstruction of a tissue [50].

The data generated from the medical imaging devices can be manipulated to construct a 3D model. These models provide adequate information for the development of a biomodel for the reconstruction of the targeted organ. The data gathered from the medical imaging device are raw images that possess a very limited amount of information in their original form. The raw images can be manipulated with the use of computer-aided reconstruction software [24, 25]. The computer-aided reconstruction software will convert the raw medical images into 3D voxel models that are CAD/CAM/CAE-friendly. In addition to reconstruction, these types of software aid in medical diagnosis [51], surgical planning [52], biomedical implants [53], and tissue engineering scaffold development [54, 55].

13.2.2 Scaffold informatics and biomimetic design

Researchers continue to advance the techniques of scaffold fabrication due to the vast development of imaging, optical microscopy, sensing, and characterization technologies. Advanced information about the architectural and mechanical support can be gathered from medical imagery [56]. The optimal design for a tissue scaffold would be one that possesses similar mechanics to that of the targeted organ. One major factor that influences the success of a tissue scaffold is the topology of the scaffold. In order for cells to proliferate and differentiate into mature cells, they must first attach to the substrate. Cell attachment is often influenced by the topology of the substrate. If the substrate does not have the surface chemistry the targeted cells require, they would not attach to that substrate; hence, that tissue scaffold would be useless [57, 58]. Secondary to the scaffold's topology are its mechanical properties. As mentioned previously, the mechanical properties partly define the functionality of the organ and are primarily responsible for the structural support of the organ. Some tissue scaffolds are designed to house the seeded cells and then biodegrade as the cell proliferates and differentiates into the targeted cells [59, 60]. At this point the mature cells will degrade the biomaterial completely, leaving the architecture of cells, which was once constructed from biomaterials [61].

Apart from designing the scaffold to meet biomimetic constraints, the tissue scaffold can be developed and analyzed to create a predictive model. For instance, if a model requires a particular tensile and/or compressive strength, a model with the desired architecture (based on the biological analysis of the targeted organ) can be developed (with the use of computer-aided technologies) and the predictive model would determine which biomaterial would best meet the desired constraints [37, 62–64]. In addition, given the biological, chemical, and mechanical constraints, a model can be developed and analyzed with computer-aided technologies to investigate the success rate of that tissue scaffold. These tissue models utilize CAD/CAM/CAE applications to optimize the chemical, biological, and mechanical properties within the desired tissue substitute [65].

13.2.3 Biomanufacturing for tissue and organ regeneration

Biomanufacturing is completely different from conventional manufacturing techniques. Conventional manufacturing techniques would utilize a raw stock material, from which mills, drills, and cutting tools would remove material to obtain the desired model. Biomanufacturing does not build tissue constructs with the use of mills, drills, and cutters [66, 67]. Instead, tissue scaffolds are biomanufactured by (1) layer-by-layer fabrication [4, 68, 69], (2) solid free-form fabrication [70, 71], or (3) photolithography [72–74]. Depending on the complexity and the desired material, the appropriate fabrication technique is chosen. Other important factors that determine the appropriate manufacturing techniques are the porosity, interconnectivity, and transport properties for nutrients that would enable the ingrowth of new cells and cell-tissue formation.

Layer-by-layer manufacturing utilizes CAD/CAM technologies to fabricate tissue constructs. CAD software would develop the 3D model of the targeted organ. The 3D model would then be converted to the appropriate file type and uploaded to the biomanufacturing device. Layer-by-layer manufacturing devices use ".stl" files to fabricate the tissue construct. The ".stl" file divides the 3D model into layers. The biomanufacturing device would fabricate each layer, one after another. Layers are usually fabricated directly above the previous layer and, at the end of the fabrication process, a 3D tissue construct is produced [75].

Solid free-form (SFF) biomanufacturing devices have the ability to move in 3D space. These devices usually consist of three or more motion arms that enable the material delivery system to fabricate the desired tissue construct. Most of the tissue constructs fabricated from SFF technologies are porous features, mainly because the material delivery component of these devices produces a filament or droplet feature from its nozzle or printing head. CAD and CAM technologies are used with SFF devices. CAD is utilized in the developed of the tissue model, while CAM technologies are used to manufacture the tissue construct. Unlike layer-by-layer manufacturing techniques, SFF does not require its CAM files to be in the ".stl" format. All SFF biomanufacturing devices use various CAM files. The data taken from the CAM files are the coordinates, mass, volume, and toolpath of the fabrication head.

Photolithographic biomanufacturing uses the layer-by-layer manufacturing approach to fabricate its tissue constructs. The materials used with this manufacturing technique are sensitive to light: when the material is exposed to light, it would change from a liquid to a solid. One approach of fabricating tissue constructs with photosensitive material is to add a small volume of the photosensitive material within a Petri dish; then light (the type of light is determined by the material's sensitivity) is used to produce the desired layer. More material is added and the process is repeated until the modeled tissue construct has been fabricated. The light in this manufacturing process can be stationary and the "mask" with the desired pattern is placed between the light and the substrate. In addition, the light can be placed on one or more motion arms where the motion arm(s) would move the light in a defined toolpath that would allow the fabrication of the desired layer. The second approach is to create a mold with the photosensitive material using the layer-by-layer approach. The mold is then utilized to produce the desired tissue construct. This method is used when the desired tissue construct has to be fabricated with a specific material that is not photosensitive.

13.3 CATE-assisted biomodeling and biomimetic design

Tissue substitutes are designed to be replicas of actual tissue organs. Researchers gather information about the tissue organ by conducting a biological investigation of the targeted organ and developing a biomodel. The biomodel presents biological, chemical, mechanical, physical, and structural information of the tissue organ. Each biomodel can be developed independently, and can later be combined with other biomodels. Owing to the limitations of software and computational power, only one biomodel is developed at a time. Biomodels are derived from non-invasive medical images. From the medical images, CAD applications are utilized to reconstruct a 3D model. The 3D model is later manipulated to produce the desired CAD model for tissue scaffold design and fabrication [76]. The design requirements and solutions investigated during the development of a tissue scaffold are listed in Table 13.1[24]. Figure 13.2 illustrates the difference in Young's modulus of a scaffold fabricated from L-polyglycolide (L-PGA), L-polylactic acid (L-PLA), and hydroxyapatite (HA) [77].

13.3.1 Non-invasive medical imaging processes

The development of a biomodel begins with non-invasive medical images. Non-invasive medical images can be captured with several medical imaging techniques, including, but not limited to, computed tomography (CT) and MRI. The former produces closely spaced axial slices of a patient's anatomy. When the CT slices are rejoined in the appropriate manner, the result fully describes the volume of the tissue. In CT imagery, a 3D image of an X-ray-absorbing object is reconstructed from a series of 2D cross-sectional images. During the progressive scan, an X-ray beam penetrates the object. As the tissue is penetrated, the transmitted beam intensity is measured by an array of detectors. Each such "projection" is obtained at a slightly different angle as the scanner rotates about the object. Each CT slice image is computed of tiny picture elements (pixels). Each pixel, in turn, is a small volume element (voxel) of patient tissue sampled by the CT scanner [78]. When compared with the other medical imaging techniques for generating an anatomical model of a physical part,

Table 13.1 Biomodeling design requirements and possible solutions [24]

Properties	Design requirements	Possible design solutions
Mechanical	Scaffold structural integrity	Biomaterial selection
	Internal architectural stability	Internal architecture
	Scaffold strength and stiffness	Porosity and pore distribution
		Fabrication method
Geometrical	Anatomical fitting	Scaffold external geometry
Manufacturing	Process ability	Advanced manufacturing using SFF-based techniques
	Process effect	
Biological	Cell loading, distribution, and nutrition	Process-controlled algorithms using appropriate process planning instructions
	Cell attachment and ingrowth	Biomaterial selection
	Cell-tissue aggregation and formation	Preferred internal architecture and layout
		Pore size and interconnectivity
		Vasculature

only CT can non-destructively dimension internal and external surfaces [79–81]. However, CT scanning, which is used only to create a mirror-image model of any organ, could not be ethically justified because of the dose of radiation administered (approximately 30–40 mGy) [82].

MRI has become increasingly popular owing to its ability to show subtle differences in soft tissue anatomy without the harmful effects of ionizing radiation associated with CT. MRI scanning is a non-invasive alternative that projects a 3D image of the soft tissues together with bone [37]. MRI has proven itself invaluable in visualizing pathology in soft tissue, especially in neurological, musculoskeletal, and vascular diseases [78]. A disadvantage of using MRI is the length of time that a patient is required to be exposed and remain motionless during scanning [83]. Table 13.2 summarizes a comparison of the basic imaging characteristics commonly used in producing 3D reconstruction CT and MRI. Figure 13.3 compares X-ray, CT, and MRI images.

13.3.2 Three-dimensional reconstruction

The images captured with CT or MRI devices are 2D images. Without the third dimension it becomes very difficult to examine and analyze the tissue(s). In order to properly visualize the tissue as a whole, multiple

Table 13.2 A comparison of characteristics of computed tomography and magnetic resonance imaging [78]

Characteristic	Computed tomography	Magnetic resonance imaging
Matrix size (pixels)	512 × 512	256 × 256
Voxel (mm)	0.5 × 0.5 × 2.0	0.5 × 0.5 × 1.5 (gap)
Density resolution	4096 levels (12 bit)	128 levels (16 bit)
Signal-to-noise ratio	High	Moderate
Segmentation	Threshold	Complex
Protocol	Simple (radiation)	Complex (benign)

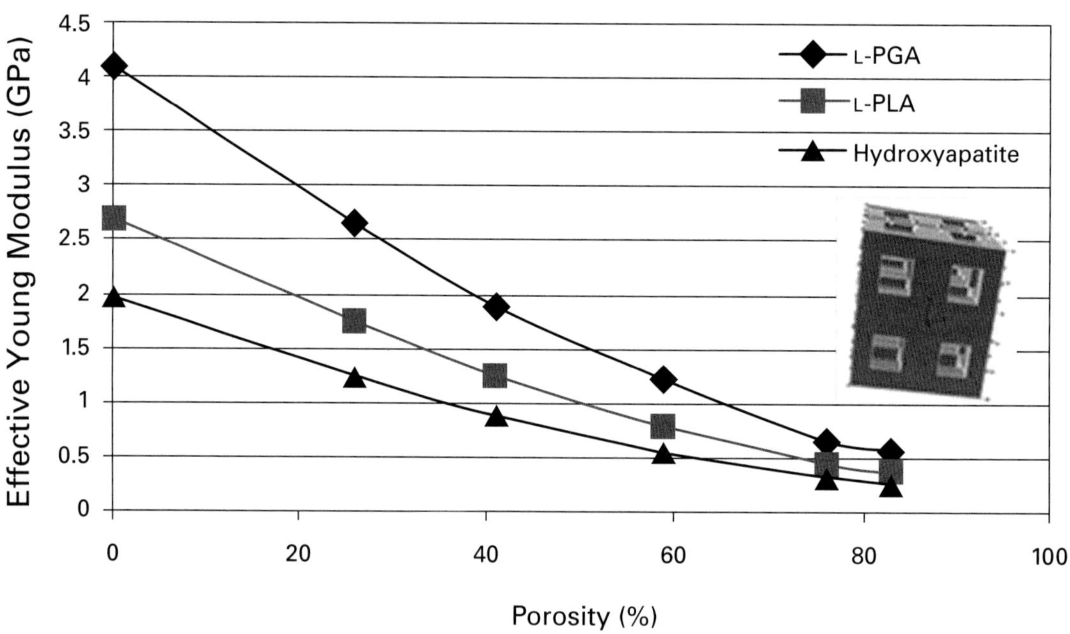

Figure 13.2 Mechanical properties' variation with biopolymers and porosity. (Reprinted from Sun, W., Starly, B., Darling, A. and Gomez, C. 2004. Computer-aided tissue engineering: biomimetic modeling and design of tissue scaffolds. *Biotechnol. Appl. Biochem.*, **39**, 49–58 [77].)

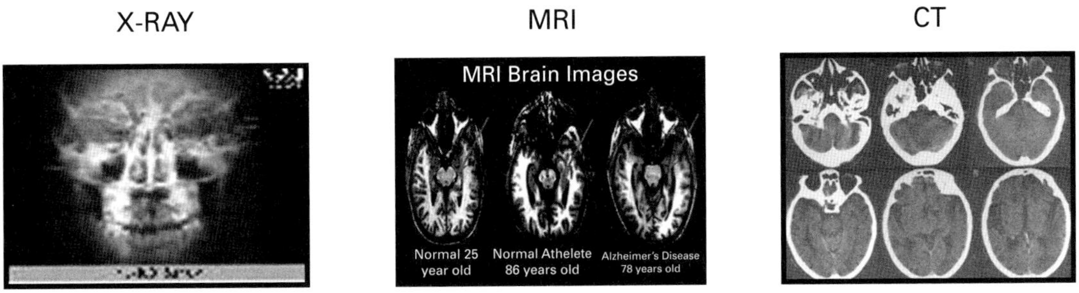

Figure 13.3 X-ray, MRI, and CT images.

views and slices are displayed at the same time. This method is very difficult for researchers, doctors, and surgeons to employ [84–87]. With the aided help of CAD software, it is possible to reconstruct the slices of information into a 3D model. Three-dimensional reconstruction (3DR) will enable researchers to directly study the tissue by displaying the 3D anatomical images or models. This newly constructed feature can be manipulated in terms of orientation, wireframe models, hidden wireframe models, surface/shaded models, and solid models with or without reflectivity, variable lighting, and transparency. With a 3DR model, volumes and surface conditions may be determined.

The process of constructing a 3D model from a set of CT scans usually begins with the isolation of an area of interest. To convert a set of 2D scans to a 3D model, all surfaces must be bounded to make a closed structure, and all edges within the area of interest must be defined. The roadmap which defines the process of 3DR is illustrated in Figure 13.4. In addition to the roadmap, listed below are the following benefits and issues with 3DR models [23].

(i) Visualization and understanding of the anatomical boundaries of structures in three dimensions, particularly those that are hidden, for example, an individual nerve fiber from within a buddle.
(ii) Intensity measurement: 3D models are considerably better than 2D models because there is no section thickness artifact. Although the use of 3D models improves the quantification of intensity, it also introduces a new set of problems.
(iii) The localization of entities, for example, dopamine-containing neurons in the human mid-brain [88]. Co-localization studies of antigens by immunocytochemical techniques also fall into this category.
(iv) The analysis of the distribution of the components: this can be at a tissue level, for example, lymphoma deposits in bone marrow trephines [89, 90] at a cellular level.
(v) Spatial quantitation, such as object counting; tissue density histograms, for example, the 3D distribution of tissue/cell numbers in different regions of the brain [88]; and determination of volumes occupied by reconstructed structures.
(vi) The examination of the relationships between components, such as whether they are connected or not, for example, neurons in the cortex [91] or notochordal tissue in embryos [92, 93].

The reconstructed 3D models yield novel views of patient anatomy while retaining the image voxel intensities that can be used for volume rendering, volumetric representation, and 3D image representation. These 3D images lead to the generation of anatomic models that are used for contour-based generation and 3D shaded surface representation of CAD-based medical models. The generation of the 3D models is not a simple task; several visualization or computation errors may arise during the generation process. Whenever an issue arises during the reconstruction process, a prototype model is developed with additive/constructive processes, as opposed to subtractive processes. Many applications have been developed in recent decades to utilize 3DR models to aid in medical diagnosis [51], surgical planning [52], biomedical implantation [53], and tissue engineering scaffold

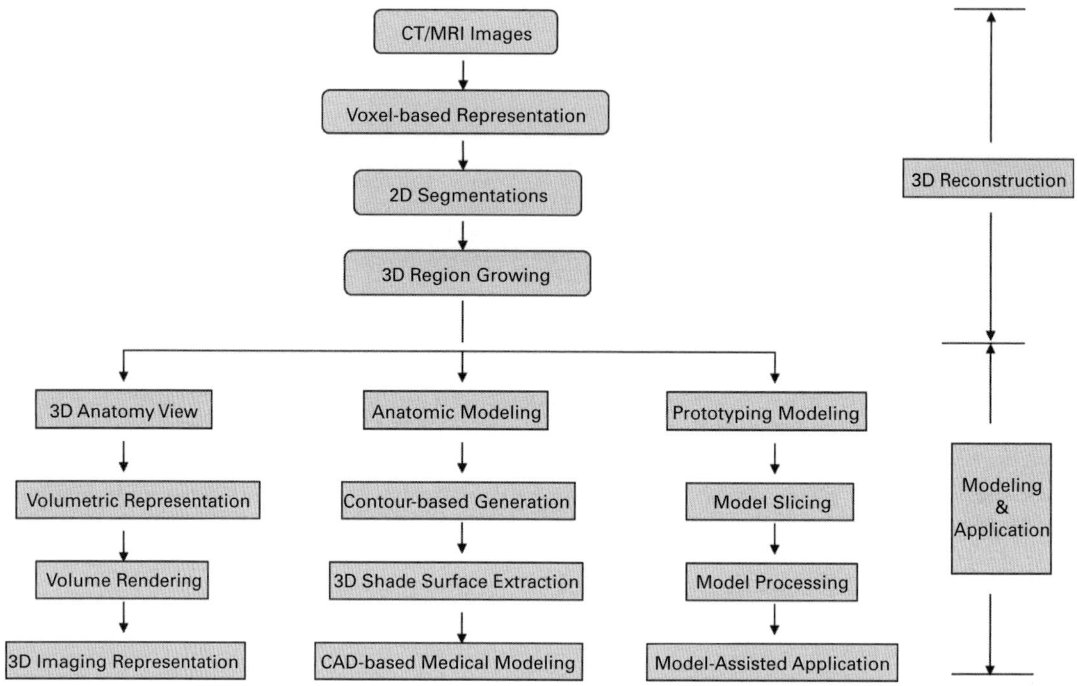

Figure 13.4 A three-dimensional reconstruction roadmap. (Reprinted from Sun W. and Lal, P. 2002. Recent development on computer aided tissue engineering – a review. *Computer Methods Programs Biomed.*, **67**, 85–103 [23].)

development [54, 55]. Figure 13.5 shows a screenshot of the reconstruction process in Materialise Mimics software and Figure 13.6 shows a realistic model of the inner organs from the visible human data (an imaging representation) [94].

13.3.3 Three-dimensional tissue scaffold design

The biomodel developed will identify the appropriate mechanical, chemical, and biological constraints that are needed to produce the optimal tissue construct. Owing to complexities within the targeted organ, and limitations of manufacturing and biological technologies, it is not possible to design a tissue scaffold that is identical to the targeted organ. Instead, a 3D tissue scaffold will be developed to meet the desired constraints of the targeted organ. Figure 13.7 shows an example of the complex architecture within the targeted organ and the equivalent scaffold design [95]. To properly define the properties of the tissue construct, the biomodel developed will be fully analyzed with the use of CAE applications. Figure 13.8 illustrates the development process of a tissue scaffold for the femur. As shown in Figure 13.8, the biomodel will be developed into several different CAD models: a CAD-based curve model and a non-uniform rational B-spline (NURBS)-based solid model. These models are then quantified in terms of their mechanical properties using a finite-element analysis (FEA) model, stress/deformation analysis, and a prosthesis design. Depending on the application, a prosthesis model can be developed for comparative purposes. Tissue substitutes are typically designed to be better than a prosthesis replacement.

The behavior of the cells and biological functions of the tissue influence the scaffold's micro-architecture. For cells to effectively attach, proliferate, and differentiate on the scaffold, the design must allow nutrients to travel throughout the scaffold. It has been found that

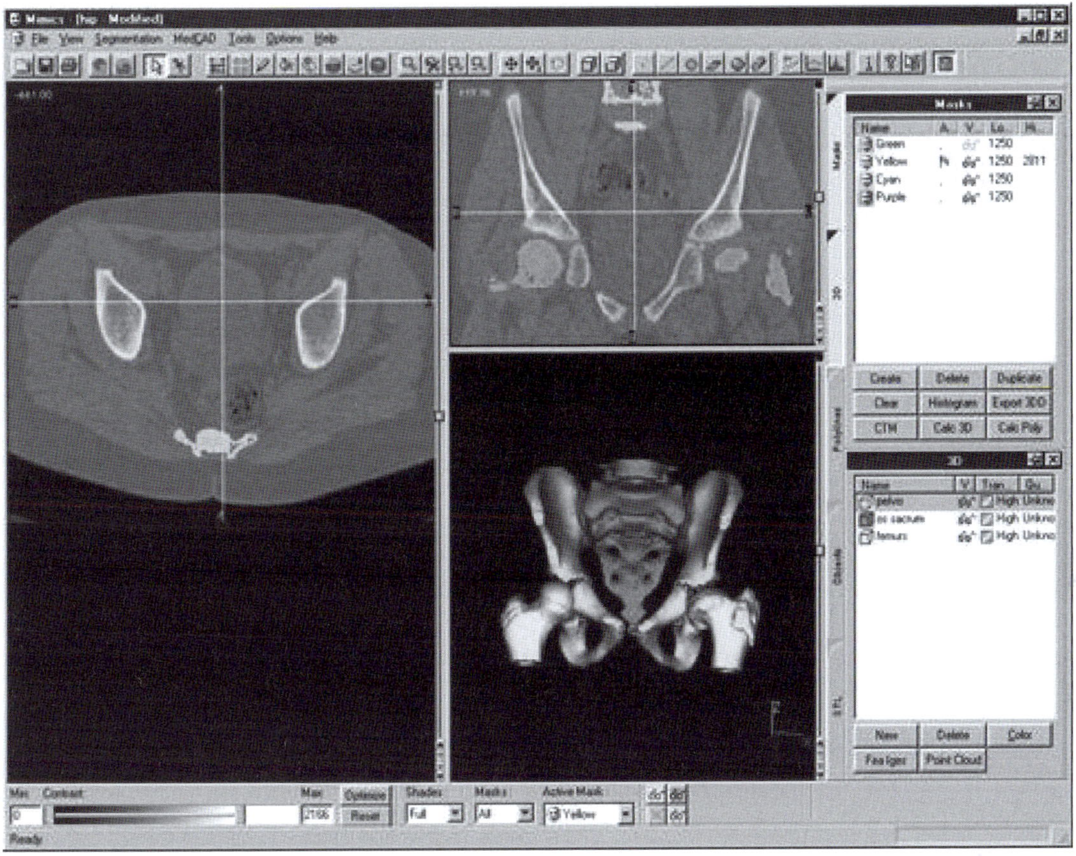

Figure 13.5 A screenshot of a 3DR process on Materialise Mimics.

cells can be enticed to migrate and grow along the direction of the designed microstruts, channel, and/or pores [96–98]. Mechanical forces such as shear stresses are experienced by the attached cell; these forces are influenced by the architectural design of the tissue scaffold. The architecture design plays an important role in the final effective mechanical, transport, and biological properties of the scaffold. The critical role the architectural support has for the targeted model is illustrated in Figure 13.9(b). As can be seen in Figure 13.9(b), different architectures are chosen to represent various parts of the femur, this is due to the transport, mechanical, and biological properties each scaffold design possesses. The femur as a whole has one function; however, various components of the femur have their own responsibility to ensure that the femur performs accordingly. Apart from the functionality, the internal architecture of the femur (actual) varies (this is shown in the 3D reconstruction of the femur, Figure 13.9(a)), which supports the theory of different architectural scaffold design for different components of the femur.

13.4 Additive manufacturing and fabrication by precision extrusion deposition

13.4.1 Precision extrusion deposition

The precision extrusion deposition (PED) device has three major components: the material delivery system,

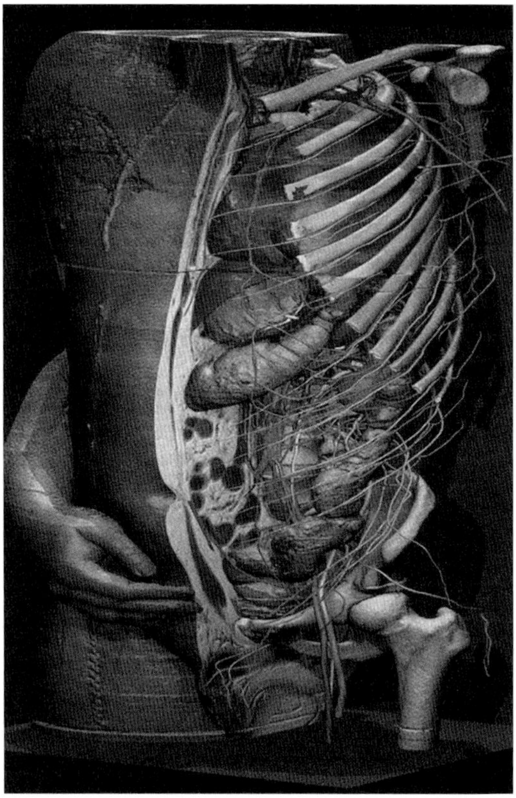

Figure 13.6 A realistic model of the inner organs from the visible human data. (Reprinted from Hohne, K. H., Pflesser, B., Pommert, A. *et al.* 2000. A realistic model of the inner organs from the visible human data. In *Med. Image Computing Computer-Assisted Intervention - Miccai 2000*, pp. 776–785 [94].)

3D motion, and computer-aided modeling. The material delivery component has interchangeable nozzles, two heating elements, and a precision drive screw. The heating element heats the material to the processing temperature, while the precision screw drives the material through the material delivery chamber to the nozzle for extrusion. A schematic view of the material delivery system, along with its temperature gradient, is shown in Figure 13.10. The 3D motion is governed by a set of linear servo motors that permits the PED to move in the $\pm X$, $\pm Y$, and $\pm Z$ directions. The computer-aided modeling component of the PED enables its user to model 3D structures accordingly [24, 25, 30].

As shown in Figure 13.10, there are two heating elements that control the temperature along the material delivery chamber. The top heating element (heating element 1), located at the inlet of the chamber, is typically set at a higher temperature in comparison to the bottom heating element (heating element 2) located at the nozzle [24, 25]. The primary goal of heating element 1 is to heat the biopolymer until it changes the polymer's phase from a solid phase to a liquid-like phase. The second heating element maintains the biopolymer's viscosity through the chamber until it is extruded. Heating element 1 has a higher temperature than heating element 2 because it takes more energy to change the biopolymer's phase from solid to liquid than to maintain the liquid phase. In addition to the phase change, the first heating element is also responsible for setting the appropriate viscosity that allows extrusion of cylindrical filaments [30].

The velocity, acceleration, and deceleration of the X, Y, and Z axes are independent of each other. However, the extrusion speed (sometimes referred to as the fourth axis) of the material delivery system is proportional to the velocity of the motion. Depending on the viscosity of the working material, the proportional gain must be adjusted accordingly to produce a smooth flow (no overflow or underflow of materials) of filaments as the PED builds the 3D structures. The proportional gain is the speed of the extrusion screw; the speed is proportional to the velocity of the X, Y, and Z linear slides. The working temperature of the material delivery chamber is optimized to maintain the proper viscosity for extrusion. The appropriate viscosity for extrusion is determined by the material's mechanical properties and the micronozzle diameter. Additionally, the motion velocities of the X, Y, and Z linear slides are optimized to ensure that there is no stretching or clumping of the extruded filament. The appropriate velocities eliminate the possibility of deformation.

In terms of the material delivery system, the two heating elements are regulated at their respective desired working temperatures, and then the polymer is inserted at the inlet (as shown in Figure 13.10(c), the inlet is located above the top heating element).

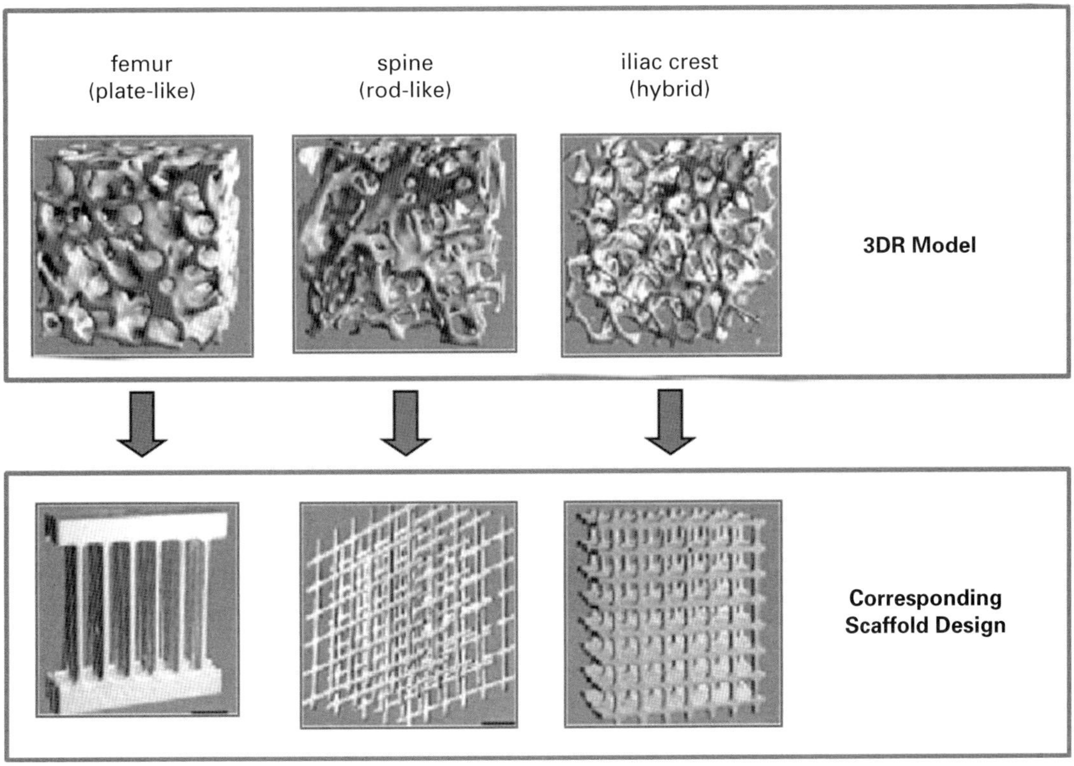

Figure 13.7 Corresponding scaffold models for various internal bone geometry. (Reprinted from Folch, A., Mezzour, S., Düring, M. *et al.* 2000. Stacks of microfabricated structures as scaffolds for cell culture and tissue engineering. *Biomed. Microdevices*, **2**, 207–214 [95].)

Polymers need to be in the form of small pellets of volume no greater than 15 mm^3 for extrusion. Once the polymer has been inserted, the (computer-controlled) rotational screw within the material delivery chamber transports the polymer pellet toward the nozzle for extrusion. While the polymer pellet is moving through the chamber, the heat would melt the polymer to its appropriate viscosity. Pellets are continuously fed in until the fabrication process has been completed. Commercially available polymers that can be utilized in the PED include, but are not limited to, polyglycolide (PGA), poly(lactic acid) (PLA), polycaprolactone (PCL), hydroxyapatite (HA), and polystyrene. Each polymer is unique in terms of its mechanical properties and biodegradability. Depending on the target organ/tissue, one or more of these polymers may be utilized to fabricate porous 3D scaffolds.

13.4.2 Assisting cooling device

In the case of high-temperature extrusion, the demand for a device that would fabricate scaffolds from high-melting-point biopolymers has increased significantly. This would require a device that has the ability to be integrated onto the PED and cool the extruded filaments as they are extruded. This device should not manipulate the material delivery chamber's temperature, induce rapid cooling, or deform the extruded filament's geometry in any shape or form. The assisted cooling (AC) device uses, but is not limited to, nitrogen (gaseous), air, oxygen, chilled water, and culture

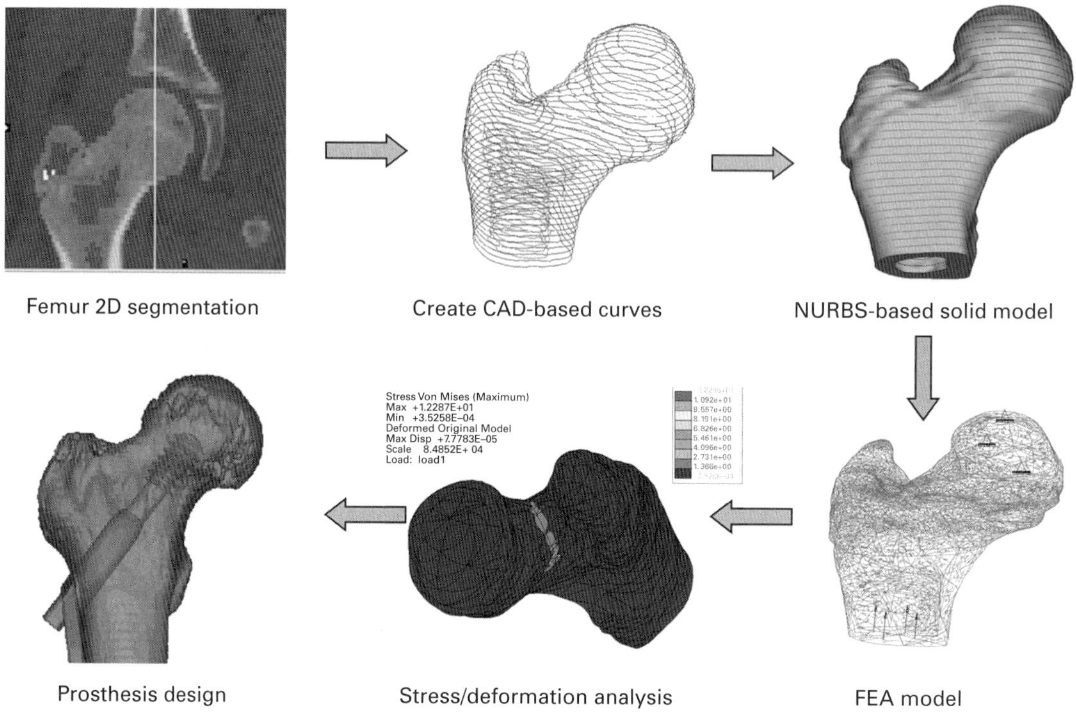

Figure 13.8 CAD-based anatomic modeling and finite-element simulation of a human femur.

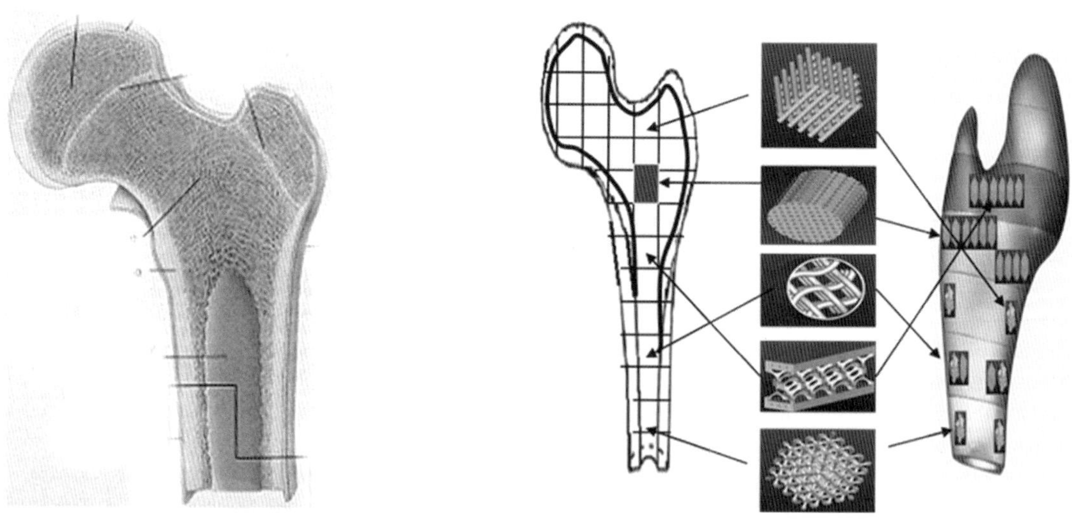

Figure 13.9 (a) Three-dimensional reconstruction of a femur. (b) Various scaffold designs for different components of the femur.

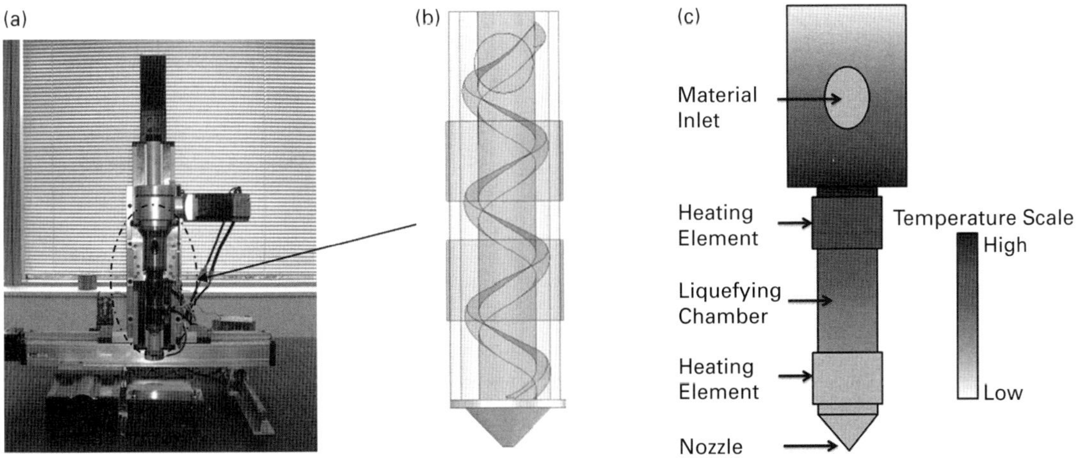

Figure 13.10 (a) A front view of the PED. (b) A schematic view of the material delivery chamber. (c) The temperature gradient of the material delivery chamber where the top heating element has a higher working temperature than the lower heating element.

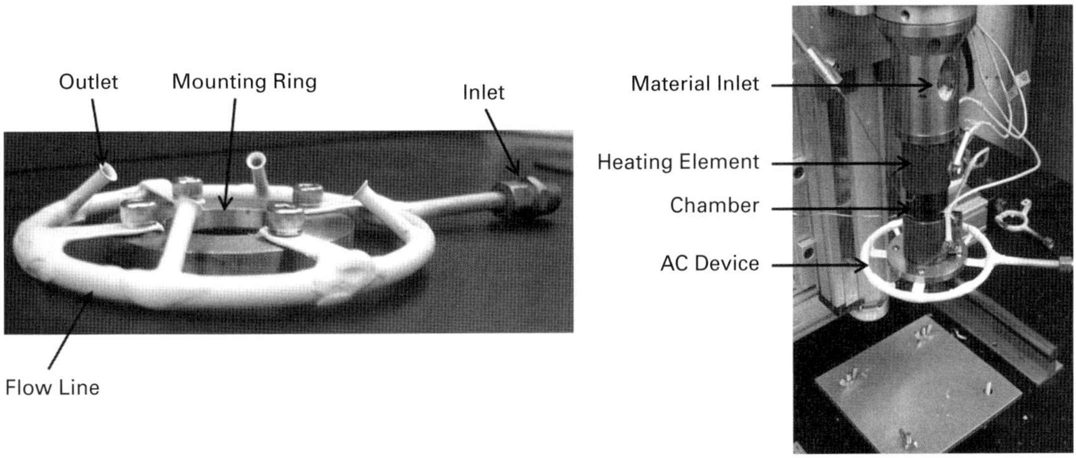

Figure 13.11 (a) The assisted cooling device. (b) The assisted cooling device integrated into the material delivery chamber of the precision extrusion deposition device.

medium to cool the filaments as they are extruded from the nozzle via convective and conductive cooling. As shown in Figure 13.11, the AC device will be mounted near the nozzle of the PED. Heat from the material delivery chamber of the PED has no influence on the AC working medium. The AC has four cooling points located on each quadrant on the flow line, this allows cooling in each direction of motion on the *X–Y* plane. The integration of the AC device in the material delivery chamber allows complete 3D cooling as scaffolds are fabricated [30]. Since the cooling medium is held at a constant temperature, it is the flow rate of the cooling medium that affects the extruded polymer. If the flow rate is high the polymer will be cooling rapidly, causing the filaments to break as they are patterned into a scaffold. If the rate is low, then the polymers will not dissipate a sufficient amount of heat and the filament will deform (become flat) and will create a porous scaffold. Optimization of the cooling medium's flow rate will reduce filament deformation and allow the fabrication of porous 3D scaffolds [99].

13.4.3 Biomaterials for tissue engineering applications

Biomaterials for tissue engineering applications are classified into two categories: (1) natural biopolymer and (2) synthetic biopolymers. Natural biopolymers are polymers that occur in nature and can be extracted and synthesized. Examples of natural biopolymers include, but are not limited to, gelatin, alginate, and collagen. On the other hand, synthetic biopolymers are polymers that are biocompatible (low levels of cytotoxicity) and made by scientists and engineers. Examples of synthetic biopolymers include, but are not limited to, polylactic acid (PLA), hydroxyapatite (HA), and polystyrene.

An important aspect of scaffold fabrication is the selection of the ideal biomaterial. Apart from the architectural design, the material used for the scaffold fabrication has a bearing on the mechanical, chemical, and biological properties. In terms of the mechanical properties, the Young modulus of the scaffold is affected by the material. For some scaffolds, the tensile and compressive strengths are essential for that scaffold to be successful. For example, if a scaffold is made from a low-compressive-strength material and is placed in a highly compressive environment, the scaffold will collapse and fail. It has also been shown that the mechanical properties have some effect on the cell's abilities to attach and proliferate. The chemical and biological properties influence the cell's ability to attach, proliferate, and differentiate. A biomaterial may be biocompatible in its raw/stock (unprocessed) form; however, once processed its properties can change (depending on the manufacturing techniques). Some manufacturing processes can change the material's toxicity level, making it difficult for cells to attach and proliferate. In additional to toxicity, surface properties can be modified. Surface modification can lead to a smooth or rough surface condition or it can change the degree of hydrophilicity or hydrophobicity of the biomaterial. Section 5.3 showcases an investigation of the degree of cytotoxicity within a scaffold.

13.4.4 Toolpath definition

Once the desired scaffold design has been developed, that model is converted into an ".stl" file and loaded into the PED database. In-house software called "Layered Manufacturing" reads the import.stl file and defines the optimal toolpath to fabricate the desired scaffold. The Layered Manufacturing application communicates directly with all the controllers on the PED system and uploads the predefined toolpath. Once initiated, the controllers read the predefined toolpath and fabricate the scaffold accordingly. Figure 13.12 is a screenshot of the in-house software with a sample scaffold preloaded within its database [25]. In addition to the in-house software, the PED uses Parker's commercially available Motion Planner software. Parker's Motion Planner software does not permit the use of a 3D model (CAD-based model). The only way to fabricate a scaffold with Motion Planner is to write a script that defines the toolpath, and directly upload to the controllers. For unpretentious scaffold designs this is a simple task; however, for very complex models, it is very difficult to write a script to define the toolpath. Writing scripts that define the toolpath of the PED usually takes a very long time when compared with developing a 3D model.

13.4.5 Scaffold fabrication

To demonstrate the PED capabilities of fabricating a 3D scaffold from a CAD-based model, a fairly simple model is designed and fabricated. The model developed has the mechanical geometry of a 0°/90° filament orientation (illustrated in Figure 13.13). CAD applications were utilized to develop the database for this model, and CAM applications were utilized to develop the fabrication protocols/procedures. The CAM model (.stl) is uploaded in the Layered Manufacturing database, which defines a toolpath. Process parameters such as the heating element temperature, motion velocity, and extrusion speed are predefined at their respective optimal settings. At the state of equilibrium, the toolpath is loaded onto the PED controllers for scaffold fabrication.

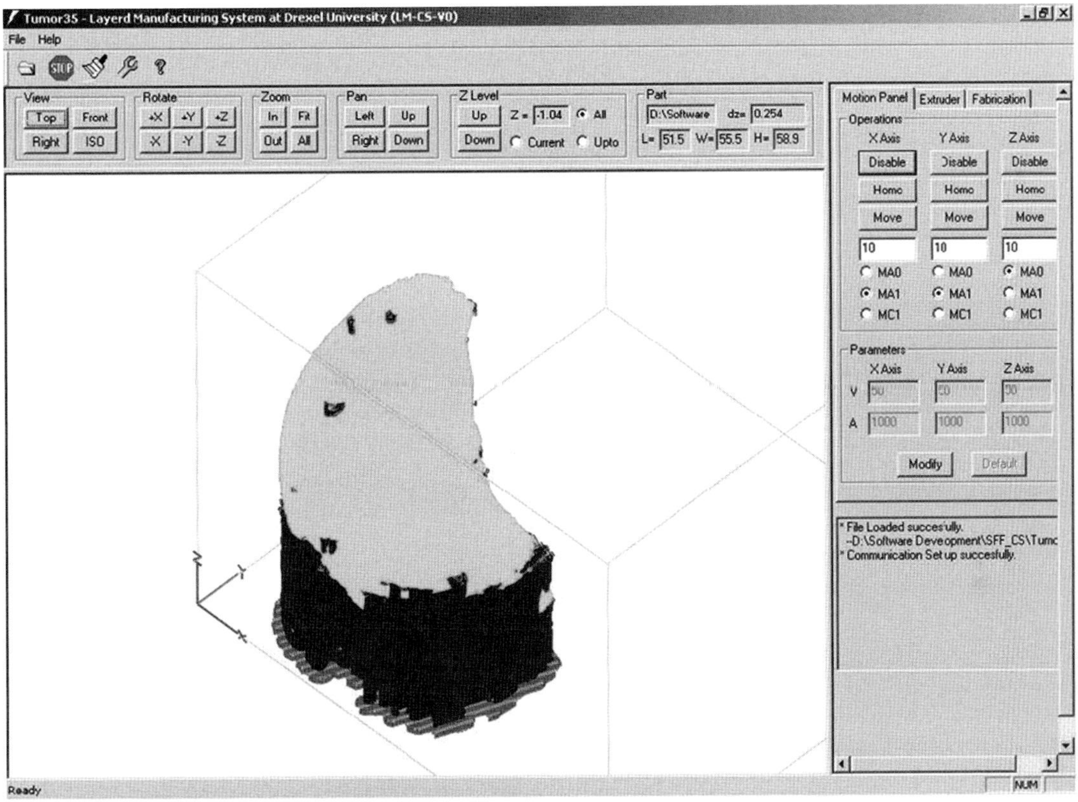

Figure 13.12 A screenshot of the Layered Manufacturing software for the PED system.

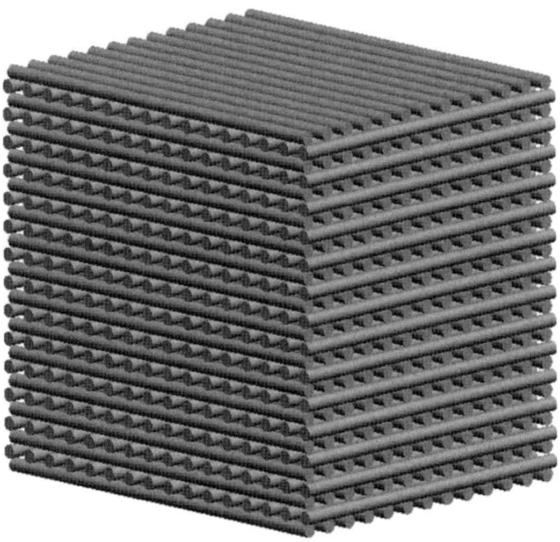

Figure 13.13 The modeled 0°/90° filament orientation scaffold.

Optimal temperature settings are essential for scaffold fabrication. If the temperature is too high, the polymer will be too liquid-like and may catch fire. If the temperature is too low, the polymer will be solid-like and will not extrude through the micro-nozzles [99]. To have a consistent flow of filaments for scaffold fabrication, the process parameters for the motion velocity must be optimized. Slow flow rates of the polymer through the material chamber require slow motion velocities for the *X*, *Y*, and *Z* axes, while high flow rates require faster motion velocities. For demonstration purposes, experiments conducted in this chapter utilized three scaffolds with varying porosity. The process parameters utilized for the fabrication of these PGA-based polymer scaffolds (listed in Table 13.3 [30]) are as follows: (1) heating element 1, 220 °C; (2) heating element 2,

Table 13.3 Properties of modeled three-dimensional uniform-porosity scaffolds

Scaffold feature	Scaffold 1	Scaffold 2	Scaffold 2
Filament orientation	0°/90°	0°/90°	0°/90°
Filament size (μm)	350	350	350
Pore size (μm)	200	350	500
Dimensions (L × W × H) (mm)	10 × 10 × 5	10 × 10 × 5	10 × 10 × 5
Porosity (%)	51.53	62.30	67.69

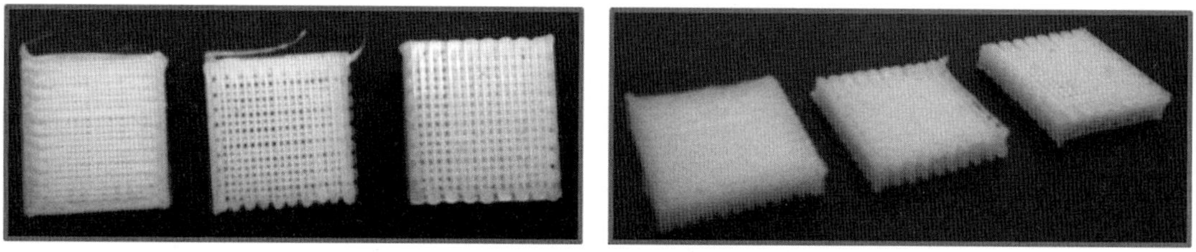

Figure 13.14 Top view (left) and isometric view (right) of scaffolds 1, 2, and 3.

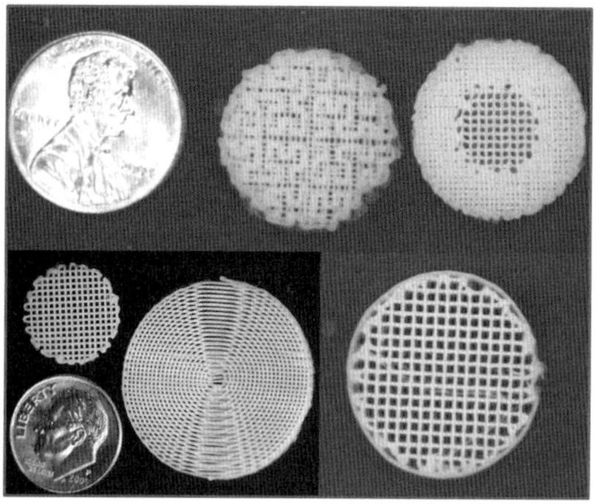

Figure 13.15 Various scaffold architectures fabricated with the PED. (Reprinted from Starly, B. 2006. Biomimetic design and fabrication of tissue engineered scaffolds using computer aided tissue engineering. Ph.D. Dissertation Mechanical Engineering and Mechanics, Drexel University, Philadelphia, PA, USA [24, 25, 100].)

200 °C; (3) AC medium, nitrogen; (4) AC flow rate, 0.03 kg/s; (5) applied cooling temperature of nitrogen from outlet of AC device, 16 °C; (6) proportional gain of extrusion screw, 1.25; and (7) motion velocity of linear arms, 2 mm/s. The varying porosity showcases how a design influences the success of a tissue scaffold. Figure 13.14 shows scaffold 1, 2, and 3 directly after the fabrication process. Figure 13.15 shows samples of scaffold fabricated from the PED with different type of architectural design [24, 25, 100].

The microstructural form and internal morphology of the refined fabricated scaffolds were evaluated using an FEI/Philips XL-30 field emission environmental scanning electron microscope (SEM). The images were taken using beam intensities of 5 kV and 10 kV and gaseous secondary-electron detectors of pressure 1.3 Torr. Before scaffolds were characterized for architectural integrity, appropriate preparation was conducted by first freezing in liquid nitrogen for approximately 5 minutes, and then scaffolds were removed and immediately sectioned using a sharp straight razor. Sectioned scaffolds allowed SEM characterization of the internal architecture. Visualization of the internal architecture illustrates the interconnectivity, filament formation, porosity, and structural integrity of the fabricated scaffolds (shown in Figure 13.16). SEM images were taken of each scaffold type (scaffold 1, 2, and 3), shown in Figure 13.17.

13.5 Characterization of PED fabricated three-dimensional tissue scaffold

Biological investigations allow researchers to monitor the cell's behavior while characterizing the scaffold's influence on the cell. Several biological investigations may be carried out to gain conclusive data about the future of a tissue substitute. These biological investigations include, but are not limited to, cytotoxicity analysis, cell–scaffold interaction, mineralization, morphological analysis, and various types of enzyme-linked immunosorbent assay (ELISA). To showcase how these investigations are characterized, scaffolds 1, 2, and 3 will undergo a series of biological investigations. The timeline of biological investigations can vary from 24 hours to years.

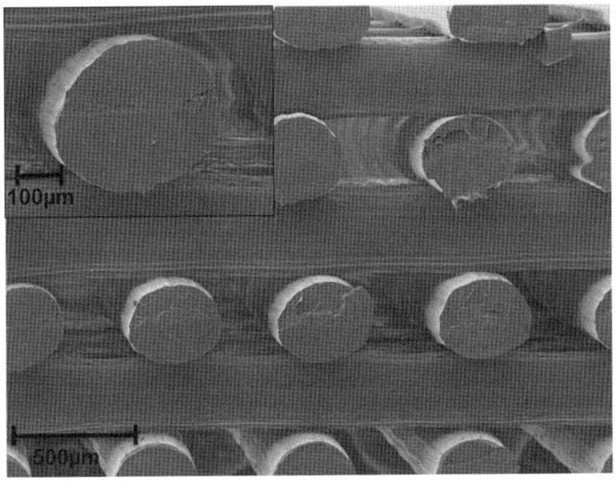

Figure 13.16 SEM image showing the internal architecture, porosity, and interconnectivity.

13.5.1 Qualitative cell growth within porous tissue scaffold

Cell growth can be observed on some scaffold with the use of an optical microscope (light must be about to pass through the scaffold). Researchers use this technique to qualitatively check for cell growth and for possible contamination that may arise due to human errors and/or impurities within the scaffold. Figure 13.18 provides a snapshot of the 7F2 cell line on scaffolds 1, 2, and 3 on sequences of images labeled A, B, and C, respectively, on days 0, 3, 5, 7, 14, and 21 on images labeled 1, 2, 3, 4, 5, and 6 respectively. As can be seen on the snapshots, cells are continuously growing and closing the pores within the scaffolds.

13.5.2 Fluorometric calibration

When it comes to biological investigations, many assays require a calibration curve. This curve is later used to characterize raw data and make use of the information obtained from the investigation(s). An example of a calibration curve that is used in the biological characterization of scaffolds 1, 2, and 3 is a fluorometric calibration curve. This calibration was conducted with the Alamar Blue assay (Serotec), which studies the cell's metabolic activity. This curve will be used later to determine the actual cell number in the proliferation study.

The protocol was as follows. A cell-laden scaffold was removed from the culture plates, washed twice, and placed into a new culture plate to which

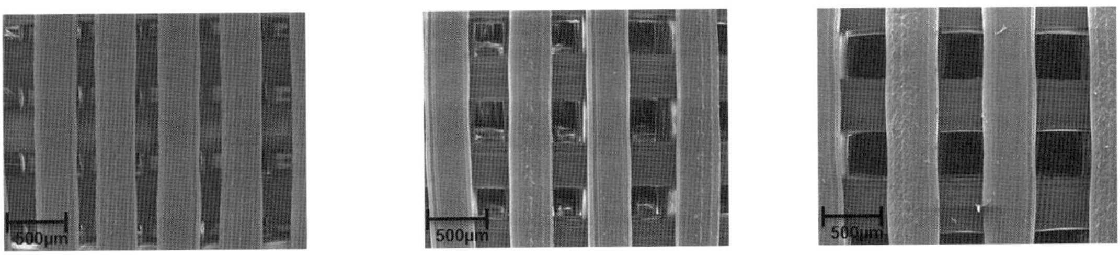

Figure 13.17 SEM images of scaffold 1 (left), and scaffold 2 (center), and scaffold 3 (right) showing the filament orientation. (Reprinted from Hamid, Q., Snyder, J., Wang, C. *et al.* 2011. Fabrication of three-dimensional scaffolds using precision extrusion deposition with an assisted cooling device. *Biofabrication*, **3**, 034109 [30].)

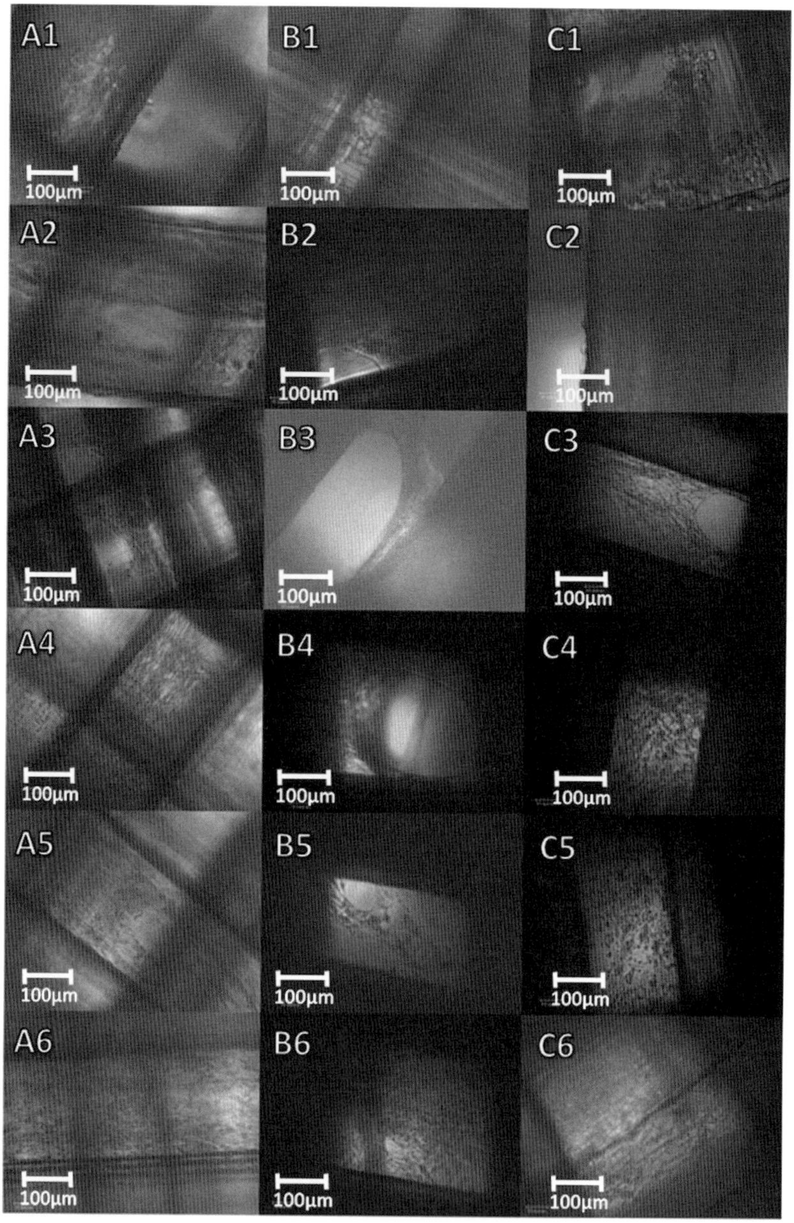

Figure 13.18 Snapshots of the 7F2 cell line on scaffolds 1, 2, and 3 on images labeled A, B, and C, respectively, on days 0, 3, 5, 7, 14, and 21 on images labeled 1, 2, 3, 4, 5, and 6 respectively. (Reprinted from Hamid, Q., Snyder, J., Wang, C. *et al.* 2011. Fabrication of three-dimensional scaffolds using precision extrusion deposition with an assisted cooling device. *Biofabrication*. **3**, 034109 [30].)

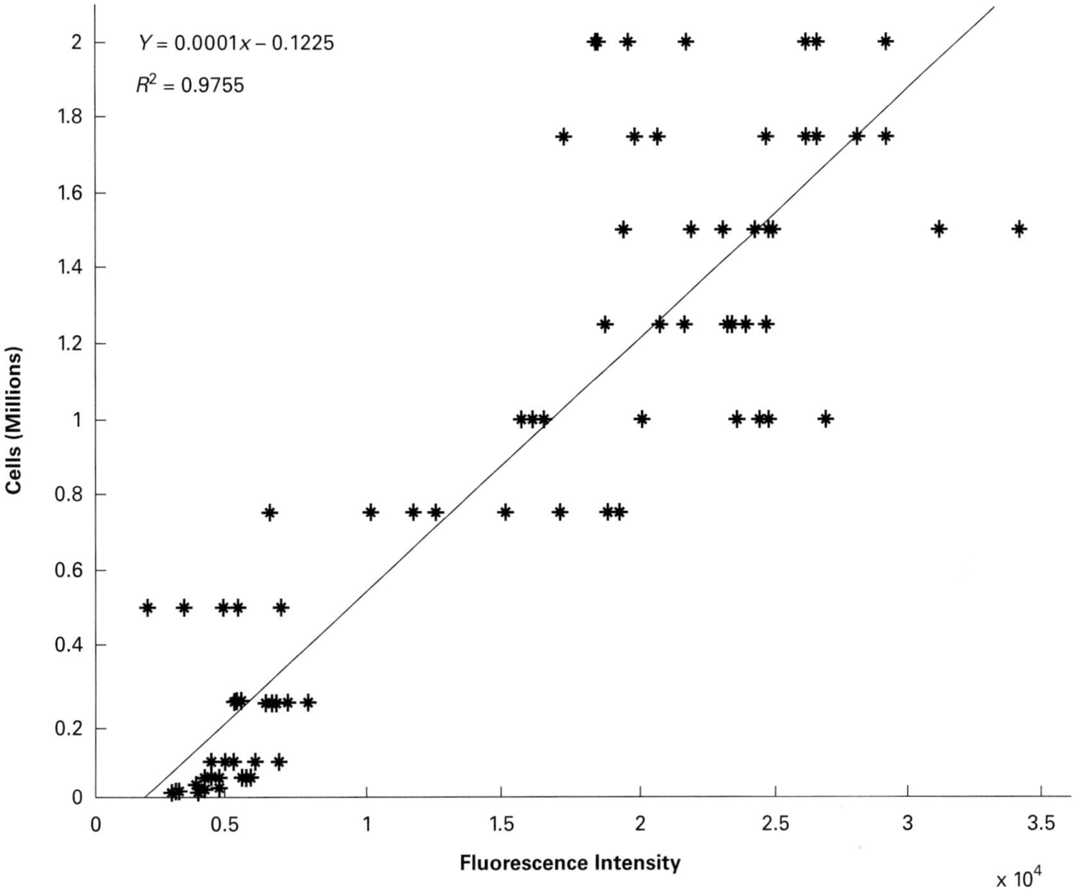

Figure 13.19 The 7F2 cell line calibration curve.

1 ml of fresh medium had been added. Then 10% Alamar Blue was added to the culture plate, which was incubated for four hours. The resulting 1 ml of solution was removed from the culture plate and placed into the microplate reader, whose excitation and emission wavelengths were 535 nm and 590 nm, respectively. This study was conducted on days 3, 5, 7, 11, 14, and 21. A cell number was obtained through a calibration curve determined by correlating a known cell number with the fluorescence intensity of the solution (Figure 13.19).

13.5.3 Cytotoxicity analysis

The toxicity level of the biomaterial used to fabricate the scaffold can change during the manufacturing processes. Many researchers would conduct cytotoxicity analysis to investigate the toxicities within the fabricated scaffold. Many cytotoxicity kits are available for this type of investigation. For this biological investigation, a MarkerGene™Live:Dead/Cytoxicity Assay Kit was used to analyze the cytotoxicity of the scaffolds. The manufacturer's protocols were followed to create the working Live:Dead solution from the propidium

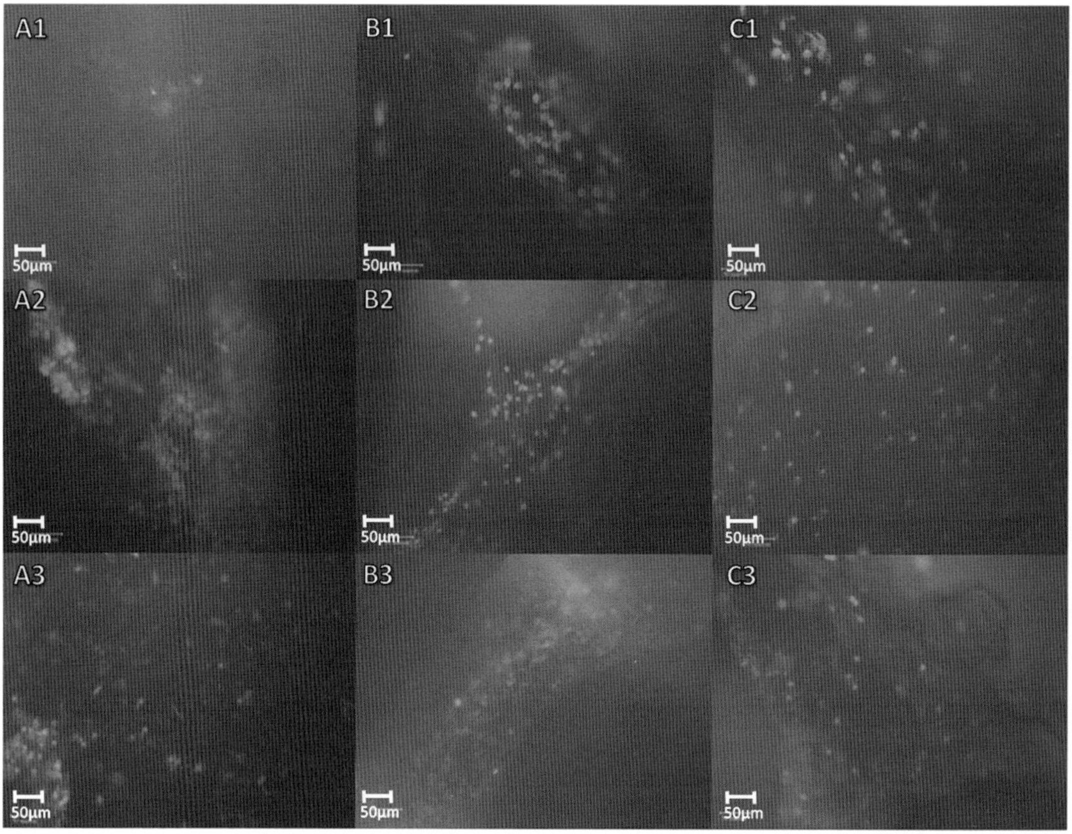

Figure 13.20 A1, A2, and A3 are fluorescence images of scaffold 1 on days 7, 14, and 21, respectively. B1, B2, and B3 are fluorescence images of scaffold 2 on days 7, 14, and 21, respectively. C1, C2, and C3 are fluorescence images of scaffold 3 on days 7, 14, and 21, respectively.

iodide solution and the carboxyfluorescein di-acetate solution. According to the manufacture's protocol; the carboxyfluorescein dye is retained within live cells, producing a green fluorescence, while cells with damaged membranes allow the entrance of propidium iodide, which undergoes a fluorescence enhancement upon binding to nucleic acids, promoting a red fluorescence in dead cells.

For this investigation, it is beneficial to obtain both quantitative and qualitative data. As can be seen in Figure 13.20 (qualitative data), live (green) and dead (red) cells are found within the scaffolds (live cells greatly outnumber the dead cells). Images A1, A2, and A3 are fluorescence images of scaffold 1 on days 7, 14, and 21, respectively; images B1, B2, and B3 are fluorescence images of scaffold 2 on days 7, 14, and 21, respectively; and images C1, C2, and C3 are fluorescence images of scaffold 3 on days 7, 14, and 21, respectively. Quantitative data are typically obtained with the use of a microplate reader. Data for these experimental analyses were obtained with the use of the GENios microplate reader from TECAN (North Carolina, USA). With the use of the manufacturer's recommended values of the appropriate excitation and emission wavelengths, quantitative data were obtained for scaffolds 1, 2, and 3 from day 7 to day 21 (Figure 13.21 shows the results). The qualitative and quantitative data demonstrate that the fabrication

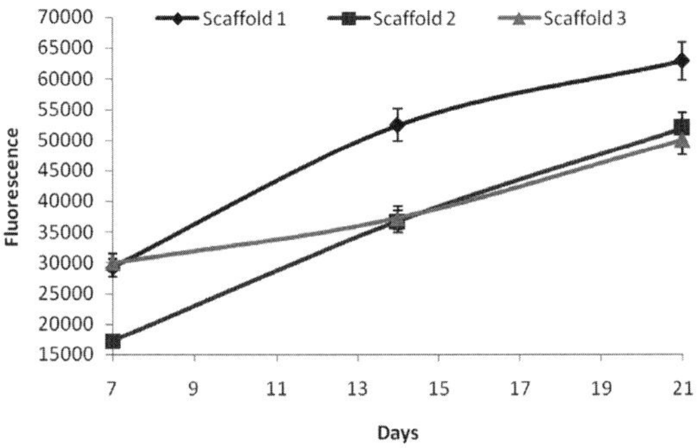

Figure 13.21 Quantitative results of the Live:Dead study of cells on scaffolds 1, 2, and 3.

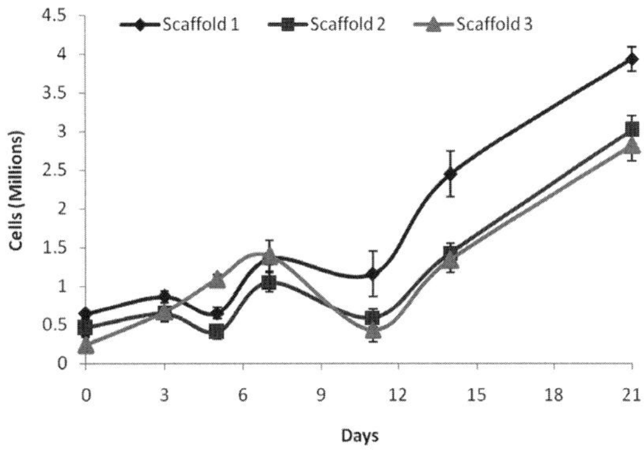

Figure 13.22 Proliferation of cells within scaffolds 1, 2, and 3.

process does not change the cytotoxicity level of the polymer in such a way as to hinder the success of these tissue scaffolds.

13.5.4 Cell–scaffold interactions

The direct interactions between cells play an important role in the development and function of multicellular organisms [101]. It is important that cells maintain this interaction within scaffolds, since, without cell–cell interaction within the scaffolds, cells cannot proliferate and differentiate into the mature cells that are essential for functional tissues.

The protocol was as follows. Harvested 7F2 cells were seeded onto scaffolds 1, 2, and 3 for a period of 21 days. The proliferation characterizations were conducted on days 0, 3, 5, 7, 11, 14, and 21. During each characterization process, the cell-laden scaffold was removed from the culture plates, washed twice, and placed into a new culture plate, to which 1 ml of fresh medium had been added. Then 10% Alamar Blue was added to the culture plate, which was incubated for four hours. The resulting 1 ml of solution was removed from the culture plate and placed into the microplate reader, whose excitation and emission wavelengths were 535 nm and 590 nm, respectively.

As seen in Figure 13.22, cells on scaffolds 1, 2, and 3 proliferated over the 21-day period. Cells on scaffold 1 showed the highest level of proliferation; this may have occurred due to the high surface area (in comparison with scaffolds 2 and 3) of the scaffold. Scaffold 3 had the longest active proliferation, which may have been due to the enormous pore size (in comparison with scaffolds 1 and 2) of the scaffold, since the large pores provided more "empty space" for cells to grow. The size of the pores on the scaffolds was directly correlated to the number of cells that become attached to the scaffold during the initial seeding process. Scaffold 1 retained the greatest amount of cells (60%), followed by scaffold 2 (43%) and scaffold 3 (23%). Scaffolds 1 and 2 showed similar proliferation trends in that there would be a decrease in number of cells on days 5 and 11 and on day 11 all scaffolds showed a proliferation trend which meant that there was a decrease in cell number. The decrease in cell number may be due to the inability of Alamar Blue to react with the cells trapped within the mineralized matrix, to the lack of nutrients getting to the cells deep within the scaffold, or to pores being closed up by proliferated cells and preventing nutrients from getting to other cells on the scaffolds. The data collected also revealed a great increase in number of cells after there is a decline in cell number, which may be due to the extracellular matrix (ECM) created by cells on the scaffold. At the end of the 21-day study, all scaffolds demonstrated an increased proliferation trend from day 14 to day 21.

13.5.5 Enzyme-linked immunosorbent assay

Enzyme-linked immunosorbent assays (ELISAs) are used for several biological investigations, including, but not limited to, screening for antibodies, antigen expression by cells, and surface antigens in serum or supernatants from antibody-secreting hybridomas. In ELISA assays one usually immobilizes cells at the bottom of the wells (microtitration plates) by passive adsorption, by use of poly-L-lysine and crosslinking with glutaraldehyde, or using by cell-specific capture antibodies. Once immobilized, the samples are typically incubated with enzyme-labeled antibodies, followed by substrate. The quantity of antigen expressed by the cell is said to be proportional to the amount of hydrolyzed substrate [102, 103].

13.5.5.1 Alkaline phosphatase activity

Alkaline phosphatase (ALP) is a protein found in all body tissues. Tissues with particularly high amounts of ALP include the liver, bile ducts, and bone [104–106]. The ALP activity is characterized by a hydrolase enzyme. The hydrolase enzyme removes the phosphate group from the cells. The characterization quantifies the amount of ALP enzymes present in the sample [107].

The protocol was as follows. Scaffolds were removed from culture plates and washed twice with 1× phosphate-buffered saline (PBS). The washed scaffolds were then submerged into 1 ml of 1% Triton X100 solution (Fisher) for cell lysis. Scaffolds were incubated for one hour and then centrifuged for 10 minutes at 1000 rpm. The ALP activity was calculated by the *p*-nitro phenyl phosphate (*p*-NPP) method. An ALP ready solution (Millipore) was utilized in these studies, in which 200 μl of ALP solution was added to 700 μl of supernatant and incubated for 45 minutes. The absorbance of this mixture was taken at 405 nm every minute for 60 minutes using the microplate reader. The absorbance collected was converted to International Units per liter (IU/l) using the conversion calculations provided by the manufacturer. This study was conducted at time points of 7, 14, and 21 days for scaffolds 1, 2, and 3. As seen in Figure 13.23, there is an up-regulation of ALP from day 7 to day 21 on scaffolds 1, 2, and 3. Scaffolds 2 and 3 have just about the same amount of alkaline phosphatase throughout the study while scaffold 1 had a slightly greater amount of alkaline phosphatase.

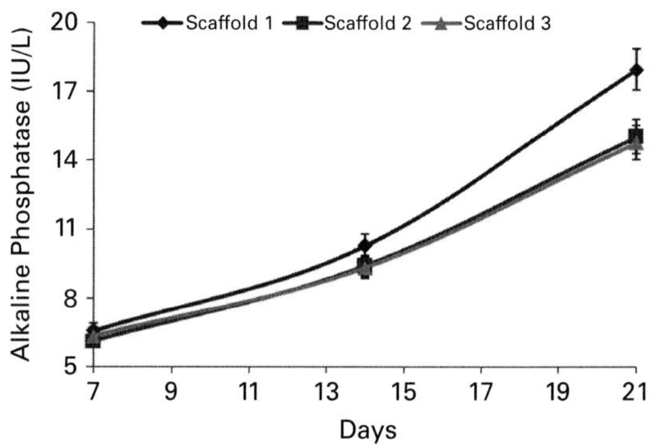

Figure 13.23 Alkaline phosphatase activity for scaffolds 1, 2, and 3.

13.5.5.2 Calcium production

Calcium is a mineral that is produced and stored by mature bone cells. A calcium production assay is used to characterize the cell's maturity level and ability to produce and/or store calcium. This assay can be utilized to show that the cells have not differentiated, or vice versa. Depending on the application and the desired outcome regarding the cells within the scaffold, this characterization assay can provide evidence of whether the desired results/outcomes have been achieved [108–110].

The protocol was as follows. Calcium levels in the cell-laden scaffolds 1, 2, and 3 were characterized on days 7, 14, and 21 with a Calcium Test Kit (Stanbio Laboratories, Texas, USA). Scaffolds were washed twice with 1 × PBS. The washed scaffolds were submerged in a cell lysis solution (0.5 ml Triton X100 with 0.5 ml trichloroacetic acid), incubated for one hour, and then centrifuged for 10 minutes at 1000 rpm. Characterizations were conducted according to the manufacturer's protocol; 10 μl of supernatant was added to the calcium test working solution (500 μl 2-amino, 2-methyl, 1-propanol (base reagent) with 500 μl *o*-cresolphthalin (color reagent)). Absorbance measurements were taken at 550 nm with a microplate reader. A standard absorbance was also taken for conversion of absorbance to mg/dl. As can be seen in Figure 13.24, there was an up-regulation of calcium from day 7 to day 21 on scaffolds 1, 2, and 3. Even though scaffold 1 had the lowest amount of calcium on day 7, at the end of the study, scaffold 1 had the greatest amount of calcium, while scaffolds 2 and 3 had just about the same amount of calcium throughout the study.

13.5.6 Morphological characterizations

The morphology (shape) of a cell is defined by its elemental structural properties. The morphology of the cells enables researchers to investigate how the tissue scaffold influences the physical properties of the cell. Growth conditions can vary the morphology of cells within the tissue scaffold. It has been shown that the mechanical properties of a tissue scaffold can change the physical/morphological properties of a cell [111–113].

The protocol was as follows. Some SEM images were obtained on day 21 to illustrate the cell morphology within scaffolds 1, 2, and 3. On day 21, scaffolds 1, 2, and 3 were removed from cell culture medium and washed twice with 1× PBS. Each scaffold was fixed with 4% glutaraldehyde (Sigma Aldrich, USA) for two hours. Each scaffold was then subjected to dehydration by submerging each scaffold for 10 minutes through a series of dilutions of ethanol (20%, 50%, 70%, 90%, 95%, and 100%). Scaffolds were then refrigerated at 4 °C for 24 hours. Prior to SEM characterization, each scaffold was coated with approximately 10–20 nm of platinum. As illustrated in Figure 13.25; on day 21, each scaffold has a significant amount of cells on the filament and within the pores. In addition, as the pore size increases, the spread of cells within the pores becomes less dense. Figure 13.26 is a 1000× magnification of the cells within the scaffolds. Each scaffold illustrates the same cell morphology shown in Figure 13.26.

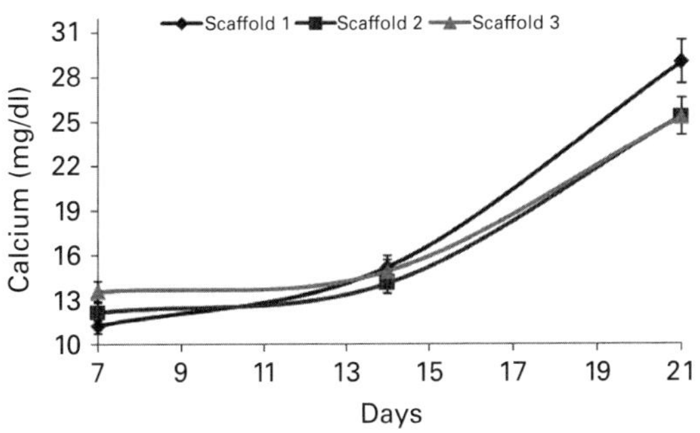

Figure 13.24 Calicum production for scaffolds 1, 2, and 3.

13.6 Summary and conclusions

The science and engineering of creating functional tissues and organs for transplantation integrates a variety of scientific and engineering disciplines to produce physiological "replacement parts" for the development of viable substitutes, which restore, maintain, or improve the function of human tissues. CATE technologies can be used to produce tissue arrays with precision, accuracy, repeatability, and close mimicry (biological, mechanical, and chemical) of the targeted organ or tissue. Tissue constructs can be developed utilizing data from several computer-aided technologies (computer-aided design (CAD),

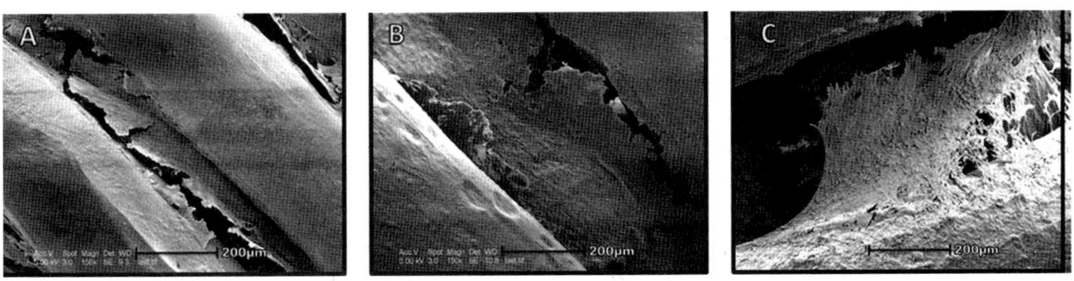

Figure 13.25 Cell morphology on day 21 for scaffolds 1 (A), 2 (B), and 3 (C).

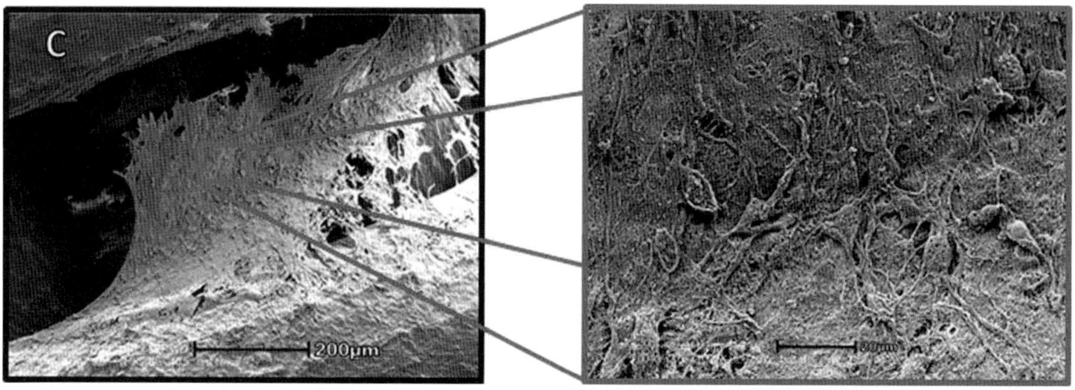

Figure 13.26 A magnified view of the cell morphology.

computer-aided engineering (CAE), and computer-aided manufacturing (CAM)) and types of medical imaging (radiography, magnetic resonance imaging (MRI), fiduciary markers, tomography, and ultrasound) [24, 25]. CATE applications are categorized into three major components: (1) computer-aided tissue modeling and biomodeling, (2) scaffold informatics and biomimetic design, and (3) biomanufacturing for tissue and organ regeneration. Non-invasive medical imagery has become significantly popular in the CATE fields. With faster computer systems, medical imagery technologies have the capabilities to gather more information with higher resolution. This information allows researchers to further investigate the mechanical and physiological orientation of a tissue organ. Advance understanding of the composition of a tissue organ will enable scientists to develop with more accuracy tissue scaffolds that allow closer mimicry of the targeted organ. Additionally, faster and smarter computing technologies will lead to the development of more sophisticated fabricating devices. Devices with advanced computing technologies can fabricate tissue scaffold with higher accuracy and precision.

Three-dimensional tissue constructs are developed from models generated from CATE technologies for the representation of tissue microstructure. This includes constructing a knowledge base for characterizing morphologies and correlating tissue scaffold properties, specifically by developing new primitives to model and represent tissue morphologies. These primitives are used to design scaffold structural geometries in 3D solid models and CAD formats. Additionally, the biomimetic design provides a theoretical, computational, and engineering framework of tissue scaffolds and replacements. These systematic approaches for designing tissue scaffolds are subjected to multiple anatomical, mechanical and biological constraints, and, concurrently, one can develop an interface database to transfer the intricate scaffold design information toward application to scaffold fabrication. Finally, quantitative engineering models enable researchers to predict the scaffold's geometry and porosity, the tortuosity of nutrient transport, and cell growth behavior as a function of the process parameters, the scaffold materials, and the selection of 3D scaffold configurations.

ACKNOWLEDGEMENT

Advanced Technologies and Regenerative Medicine (ATRM), LLC, a Johnson and Johnson Company are acknowledged for support of this project.

REFERENCES

[1] Merion, R. M. 2010. 2009 SRTR report on the state of transplantation preface. *Am. J. Transplantation*, **10**, 959–60.

[2] Klein, A. S., Messersmith, E. E., Ratner, L. E. *et al.* 2010. Organ donation and utilization in the United States, 1999-2008. *Am. J. Transplantation*, **10**, pp. 973–86.

[3] Zeltinger, J., Sherwood, J. K., Graham, D. A., Mueller, R. and Griffith, L. G. 2001. Effect of pore size and void fraction on cellular adhesion, proliferation, and matrix deposition. *Tissue Eng.*, **7**, pp. 557–72.

[4] Zein, I., Hutmacher, D. W., Tan, K. C. and Teoh, S. H. 2002. Fused deposition modeling of novel scaffold architectures for tissue engineering applications. *Biomaterials*, **23**, 1169–85.

[5] Shor, L., Guceri, S., Wen, X. J., Gandhi, M. and Sun, W. 2007. Fabrication of three-dimensional polycaprolactone/hydroxyapatite tissue scaffolds and osteoblast-scaffold interactions in vitro. *Biomaterials*, **28**, 5291–7.

[6] Hansbrough, J. F., Dore, C. and Hansbrough, W. B. 1992. Clinical trials of a living dermal tissue replacement placed beneath meshed, split-thickness skin grafts on excised burn wounds. *J. Burn Care Rehabil.*, **13**, 519–29.

[7] Bostman, O., Paivarinta, U., Partio, E. *et al.* 1992. Degradation and tissue replacement of an absorbable polyglycolide screw in the fixation of rabbit femoral osteotomies. *J. Bone Joint Surg. Am.*, **74**, 1021–31.

[8] Eschenhagen, T., Didie, M., Munzel, F. *et al.* 2002, 3D engineered heart tissue for replacement therapy. *Basic Res. Cardiol.*, **97**(Suppl. 1), I146–52.

[9] Eppley, B. L., Kilgo, M. and Coleman, J. J. 3rd. 2002. Cranial reconstruction with computer-generated hard-tissue replacement patient-matched implants: indications, surgical technique, and long-term follow-up. *Plastic Reconstructive Surgery*, **109**, 864–71.

[10] Maquet, V. and Jerome, R. 1997. Design of macroporous biodegradable polymer scaffolds for cell transplantation. *Mater. Sci. Forum*, **250**, 15–42.

[11] Wake, M. C., Partick, C. W. Jr. and Mikos, A. G. 1994. Pore morphology effects on the fibrovascular tissue growth in porous polymers. *Cell Transplant.*, **3**, 339–47.

[12] Mikos, A. G., Thorsen, A. J., Czerwonka, L. A. *et al.* 1994. Preparation and characterization of poly(L-lactic acid) foams. *Polymer*, **35**, 1068–77.

[13] Ratner, B. D. 1996. *Biomaterials Science: An Introduction to Materials in Medicine*. San Diego, CA: Academic Press.

[14] Rajeev, A. J. 2000. The manufacturing techniques of various drug loaded biodegradable poly(lactide-*co*-glycolide) (PLGA) devices. *Biomaterials*, **21**, 2475–90.

[15] Zalc, J. M., Reyes, S. C. and Iglesia, E. 2004. The effects of diffusion mechanism and void structure on transport rates and tortuosity factors in complex porous structures. *Chem. Eng. Sci.*, **59**, 2947–60.

[16] Hrabe, J., Hrabetova, S. and Segeth, K. 2004. A model of effective diffusion and tortuosity in the extracellular space of the brain. *Biophys. J.*, **87**, 1606–17.

[17] Shuler M. L. and Kargi, F. 2002. *Bioprocess Engineering: Basic Concepts*, 2nd edn. Upper Saddle River, NJ: Prentice Hall.

[18] Turing, A. M. 1990. The chemical basis of morphogenesis. 1953. *Bull. Math. Biol.*, **52**, 153–97; discussion 119–52.

[19] Botchwey, E. A., Dupree, M. A., Pollack, S. R., Levine, E. M. and Laurencin, C. T. 2003. Tissue engineered bone: measurement of nutrient transport in three-dimensional matrices. *J. Biomed. Mater. Res. Part A*, **67**, 357–67.

[20] Albrecht, D. R., Tsang, V. L., Sah, R. L. and Bhatia, S. N. 2005. Photo- and electropatterning of hydrogel-encapsulated living cell arrays. *Lab Chip*, **5**, 111–18.

[21] Abbott, A. 2003. Cell culture: biology's new dimension. *Nature*, **424**, 870–2.

[22] Benya, P. D. and Shaffer, J. D. 1982. Dedifferentiated chondrocytes reexpress the differentiated collagen phenotype when cultured in agarose gels. *Cell*, **30**, 215–24.

[23] Sun, W. and Lal, P. 2002. Recent development on computer aided tissue engineering – a review. *Computer Methods Programs Biomedicine*, **67**, 85–103.

[24] Starly, B. 2006. *Biomimetic Design and Fabrication of Tissue Engineered Scaffolds using Computer Aided Tissue Engineering*. Ph.D. Dissertation, Mechanical Engineering and Mechanics, Drexel University, Philadelphia, PA, USA.

[25] Shor, L. 2008. *Novel Fabrication Development for the Application of Polycaprolactone and Composite Polycaprolactone/Hydroxyapotote Scaffolds for Bone Tissue Engineering*, Ph.D. Dissertation, Mechanical Engineering and Mechanics, Drexel University, Philadelphia, PA, USA.

[26] Starly, B. and Sun, W. 2007. *Biomimetic Design and Fabrication of Tissue Engineered Scaffolds*. Saarbrücken: VDM Verlag.

[27] Sun, W., Darling, A., Starly, B. and Nam, J. 2004. Computer-aided tissue engineering: overview, scope and challenges. *Biotechnol. Appl. Biochem.*, **39**, 29–47.

[28] Ito, A., Takizawa, Y., Honda, H. *et al.* 2004. Tissue engineering using magnetite nanoparticles and magnetic force: heterotypic layers of cocultured hepatocytes and endothelial cells. *Tissue Eng.*, **10**, 833–40.

[29] Yang, S. F., Leong, K. F., Du, Z. H. and Chua, C. K. 2002. The design of scaffolds for use in tissue engineering. Part II. Rapid prototyping techniques. *Tissue Eng.*, **8**, 1-11.

[30] Hamid, Q., Snyder, J., Wang, C. *et al.* 2011. Fabrication of three-dimensional scaffolds using precision extrusion deposition with an assisted cooling device. *Biofabrication*, **3**, 034109.

[31] Burstein, A. H., Reilly, D. T. and Martens, M. 1976. Aging of bone tissue: mechanical properties. *J. Bone Joint Surg. Am.*, **58**, 82-6.

[32] Miller, K. and Chinzei, K. 2002. Mechanical properties of brain tissue in tension. *J. Biomech.*, **35**, 483-90.

[33] Martin, I., Obradovic, B., Treppo, S. *et al.* 2000. Modulation of the mechanical properties of tissue engineered cartilage. *Biorheology*, **37**, 141-7.

[34] Suchanek, W. and Yoshimura, M. 1998. Processing and properties of hydroxyapatite-based biomaterials for use as hard tissue replacement implants. *J. Mater. Res.*, **13**, 94-117.

[35] Hollister, S. J., Maddox, R. D. and Taboas, J. M. 2002. Optimal design and fabrication of scaffolds to mimic tissue properties and satisfy biological constraints. *Biomaterials*, **23**, 4095-103.

[36] Grabow, N., Schmohl, K., Khosravi, A. *et al.* 2004. Mechanical and structural properties of a novel hybrid heart valve scaffold for tissue engineering. *Artif. Organs.*, **28**, 971-9.

[37] Sun, W., Starly, B., Nam, J. and Darling, A. 2005. Bio-CAD modeling and its applications in computer-aided tissue engineering. *Computer-Aided Design*, **37**, 1097-114.

[38] Ma, P. X. 2008. Biomimetic materials for tissue engineering. *Adv. Drug Delivery Rev.*, **60**, 184-98.

[39] Giannatsis, J. and Dedoussis, V. 2009. Additive fabrication technologies applied to medicine and health care: a review. *Int. J. Adv. Manufacturing Technol.*, **40**, 116-27.

[40] Staudenmaier, R., Naumann, A. and Aigner, J. 2000. Ear reconstruction supported by a stereolithographic model. *Plastic Reconstructive Surgery*, **106**, 511-12.

[41] Lohfeld, S., Barron, V. and McHugh, P. E. 2005. Biomodels of bone: a review. *Ann. Biomed. Eng.*, **33**, 1295-311.

[42] Cavalli-Sforza, L. L., Piazza, A., Menozzi, P. and Mountain, J. 1988. Reconstruction of human evolution: bringing together genetic, archaeological, and linguistic data. *Proc. Nat. Acad. Sci. USA*, **85**, 6002-6.

[43] Zubal, I. G., Harrell, C. R., Smith, E. O. *et al.* 1994. Computerized three-dimensional segmented human anatomy. *Med. Phys.*, **21**, 299-302.

[44] Kirkwood, R. N., Culham, E. G. and Costigan, P. 1999. Radiographic and non-invasive determination of the hip joint center location: effect on hip joint moments. *Clin. Biomech. (Bristol, Avon)*, **14**, 227-35.

[45] Zhao, M., Beauregard, D. A., Loizou, L., Davletov, B. and Brindle, K. M. 2001. Non-invasive detection of apoptosis using magnetic resonance imaging and a targeted contrast agent. *Nature Med.*, **7**, 1241-4.

[46] Strangman, G., Boas, D. A. and Sutton, J. P. 2002. Non-invasive neuroimaging using near-infrared light. *Biol. Psychiatry*, **52**, 679-93.

[47] Nieman, K., Rensing, B. J., van Geuns, R. J. M. *et al.* 2002. Non-invasive coronary angiography with multi-slice spiral computed tomography: impact of heart rate. *Heart*, **88**, 470-4.

[48] Tardy, Y., Meister, J. J., Perret, F., Brunner, H. R. and Arditi, M. 1991. Non-invasive estimate of the mechanical properties of peripheral arteries from ultrasonic and photoplethysmographic measurements. *Clin. Phys. Physiol. Meas.*, **12**, 39-54.

[49] Lee, D. C. and Carroll, T. J. 2010. Magnetic Resonance Imaging. In *Practical Signal and Image Processing in Clinical Cardiology*, ed. Goldberger, J. J. and Ng, J. London: Springer, pp. 251-73.

[50] Davis, G. R. and Wong, F. S. 1996. X-ray microtomography of bones and teeth. *Physiol. Measurement*, **17**, 121-46.

[51] Jan, S. V., Salvia, P., Feipel, W. *et al.* 2006. In vivo registration of both electrogoniometry and medical imaging: development and application on the ankle joint complex. *IEEE Trans. Biomed. Eng.*, **53**, 759-62.

[52] Piatt, J. H., Starly, B., Sun, W. and Faerber, E. 2006. Application of computer-assisted design in craniofacial reconstructive surgery using a commercial image guidance system - technical note. *J. Neurosurgery*, **104**, 64-7.

[53] Evans, P., Starly, B. and Sun, W. 2006. Computer-aided tissue engineering for the design and evaluation of lumbar-spin arthroplasty. *Computer-Aided Design Appl.*, **3**, 771-8.

[54] Hollister, S. J., Maddox, R. D. and Taboas, J. M. 2002. Optimal design and fabrication of scaffolds to mimic tissue properties and satisfy biological constraints. *Biomaterials*, **23**, 4095-103.

[55] Hutmacher, D. W., Sittinger, M. and Risbud, M. V. 2004. Scaffold-based tissue engineering: rationale for computer-aided design and solid free-form fabrication systems. *Trends Biotechnol.*, **22**, 354-62.

[56] Sun, W., Starly, B., Darling, A. and Gomez, C. 2004. Computer-aided tissue engineering: application to

biomimetic modelling and design of tissue scaffolds. *Biotechnol. Appl. Biochem.*, **39**, 49–58.

[57] Yildirim, E. D., Ayan, H., Vasilets, V. N. *et al.* 2008. Effect of dielectric barrier discharge plasma on the attachment and proliferation of osteoblasts cultured over poly(ε-caprolactone) scaffolds. *Plasma Processes Polymers*, **5**, 58–66.

[58] Yildirim, E. D., Besunder, R., Pappas, D. *et al.* 2010. Accelerated differentiation of osteoblast cells on polycaprolactone scaffolds driven by a combined effect of protein coating and plasma modification. *Biofabrication*, **2**, 014109.

[59] Fang, Z., Starly, B. and Sun, W. 2005. Computer-aided characterization for effective mechanical properties of porous tissue scaffolds. *Computer-Aided Design*, **37**, 65–72.

[60] Wei, G. B. and Ma, P. X. 2004. Structure and properties of nano-hydroxyapatite/polymer composite scaffolds for bone tissue engineering. *Biomaterials*, **25**, 4749–57.

[61] Kuo, C. K. and Ma, P. X. 2001. Ionically crosslinked alginate hydrogels as scaffolds for tissue engineering: part 1. Structure, gelation rate and mechanical properties. *Biomaterials*, **22**, 511–21.

[62] Williams, J. M., Adewunmi, A., Schek, R. M. *et al.* 2005. Bone tissue engineering using polycaprolactone scaffolds fabricated via selective laser sintering. *Biomaterials*, **26**, 4817–27.

[63] Jaecques, S. V. N., Van Oosterwyck, H., Muraru, L. *et al.* 2004. Individualised, micro CT-based finite element modelling as a tool for biomechanical analysis related to tissue engineering of bone. *Biomaterials*, **25**, 1683–96.

[64] Lacroix, D., Chateau, A., Ginebra, M. P. and Planell, J. A. 2006. Micro-finite element models of bone tissue-engineering scaffolds. *Biomaterials*, **27**, 5326–34.

[65] Woodfield, T. B. F., Malda, J., de Wijn, J. *et al.* 2004. Design of porous scaffolds for cartilage tissue engineering using a three-dimensional fiber-deposition technique. *Biomaterials*, **25**, 4149–61.

[66] Sun, W., Yan, Y. N., Lin, F. and Spector, M. 2006. Biomanufacturing: a US-China National Science Foundation-sponsored workshop. *Tissue Eng.*, **12**, 1169–81.

[67] Weigel, T., Schinkel, G. and Lendlein, A. 2006. Design and preparation of polymeric scaffolds for tissue engineering. *Expert Rev. Med. Devices*, **3**, 835–51.

[68] Tang, Z. Y., Wang, Y., Podsiadlo, P. and Kotov, N. A. 2007. Biomedical applications of layer-by-layer assembly: from biomimetics to tissue engineering (vol 18, pg 3203, 2006). *Adv. Mater.*, **19**, 906–906.

[69] Yan, Y. N., Xiong, Z., Hu, Y. Y. *et al.* 2003. Layered manufacturing of tissue engineering scaffolds via multi-nozzle deposition. *Mater. Lett.*, **57**, 2623–8.

[70] Hutmacher, D. W., Sittinger, M. and Risbud, M. V. 2004. Scaffold-based tissue engineering: rationale for computer-aided design and solid free-form fabrication systems. *Trends Biotechnol.*, **22**, 354–62.

[71] Yarlagadda, P. K. D. V., Chandrasekharan, M. and Shyan, J. Y. M. 2005. Recent advances and current developments in tissue scaffolding. *Biomed. Mater. Eng.*, **15**, 159–77.

[72] Bryant, S. J., Cuy, J. L., Hauch, K. D. and Ratner, B. D. 2007. Photo-patterning of porous hydrogels for tissue engineering. *Biomaterials*, **28**, 2978–86.

[73] Dong, Y. X., Yong, T., Liao, S., Chan, C. K. and Ramakrishna, S. 2008. Degradation of electrospun nanofiber scaffold by short wave length ultraviolet radiation treatment and its potential applications in tissue engineering. *Tissue Eng. Part A*, **14**, 1321–9.

[74] Zhang, H., Hutmacher, D. W., Chollet, F., Poo, A. N. and Burdet, E. 2005. Microrobotics and MEMS-based fabrication techniques for scaffold-based tissue engineering. *Macromolec. Biosci.*, **5**, 477–89.

[75] Starly, B., Lau, A., Sun, W., Lau, W. and Bradbury, T. 2005. Direct slicing of STEP based NURBS models for layered manufacturing. *Computer-Aided Design*, **37**, 387–97.

[76] Starly, B., Lau, W., Bradbury, T. and Sun, W. 2006. Internal architecture design and freeform fabrication of tissue replacement structures. *Computer-Aided Design*, **38**, 115–24.

[77] Sun, W., Starly, B., Darling, A. and Gomez, C. 2004. Computer-aided tissue engineering: biomimetic modeling and design of tissue scaffolds. *J. Biotechnol. Appl. Biochem.*, **39**, 49–58.

[78] Mankovich, N. J., Samson, D., Pratt, W., Lew, D. and Beumer, J. 3rd. 1994. Surgical planning using three-dimensional imaging and computer modeling. *Otolaryngol. Clin. North Am.*, **27**, 875–89.

[79] Alair, G. 1998, Reverse engineering: from CT to CAD. In *Rapid Prototyping and Manufacturing '98*, Dearborn, MI.

[80] Yancey, R. 1998, Integration of reverse engineering, solid modeling, and rapid prototyping technologies for the production of net shape investment cast tooling. In *Rapid Prototyping and Manufacturing '98*, Dearborn, MI.

[81] Mankovich, N. J., Robertson, D. R. and Cheeseman, A. M. 1990. Three-dimensional image display in medicine. *J. Digital Imaging*, **3**, 69–80.

[82] Brenner, D. J. and Hall, E. J. 2007. Computed tomography – an increasing source of radiation exposure. *N. Engl. J. Med.*, **357**, 2277–84.

[83] USDHH Services 2011. *MRI (Magnetic Resonance Imaging)*. Available at http://www.fda.gov/RadiationEmittingProducts/RadiationEmittingProductsandProcedures/MedicalImaging/ucm200086.htm#u.

[84] Weibel, E. R. and Elias, H. 1967. Quantitative methods in morphology: Quantitative Methoden in der Morphologie. *Am. J. Med. Sci.*, **254**, 917.

[85] Marko, M., Leith, A. and Parsons, D. 1988. Three-dimensional reconstruction of cells from serial sections and whole-cell mounts using multilevel contouring of stereo micrographs. *J. Electron Microsc. Techn.*, **9**, 395–411.

[86] Vannier, M. W., Marsh, J. L. and Warren, J. O. 1984. Three dimensional CT reconstruction images for craniofacial surgical planning and evaluation. *Radiology*, **150**, 179–84.

[87] Chow, L. C. and Sommer, F. G. 2001. Multidetector CT urography with abdominal compression and three-dimensional reconstruction. *AJR Am. J. Roentgenol.*, **177**, 849–55.

[88] Woodward, W. 1983. *Brain and Heart Analysis Using a Micro-computer*. London: Morgan-Grampian.

[89] Salisbury, J. R. and Deverell, M. H. 1994, Three-dimensional reconstructions of benign lymphoid aggregates in bone marrow trephines. In *Eighth International Symposium on Diagnostic Quantitative Pathology*, Amsterdam.

[90] Salisbury, J. R. and Whimster, W. F. 1994. Progress in computer-generated 3-dimensional reconstruction – reply. *J. Pathol.*, **172**, 87.

[91] Rydmark, M., Jansson, T., Berthold, C. H. and Gustavsson, T. 1992. Computer-assisted realignment of light micrograph images from consecutive section series of cat cerebral cortex. *J. Microsc.*, **165**, 29–47.

[92] Salisbury, J. R. 1992. *Some Studies on the Human Fetal Notochord and on Chordomas*. M.D., University of London.

[93] Salisbury, J. R., Deverell, M. H., Cookson, M. J. and Whimster, W. F. 1993. Three-dimensional reconstruction of human embryonic notochords: clue to the pathogenesis of chordoma. *J. Pathol.*, **171**, 59–62.

[94] Hohne, K. H., Pflesser, B., Pommert, A. *et al.* 2000. A realistic model of the inner organs from the visible human data. In *Medical Image Computing and Computer-Assisted Intervention – Miccai 2000*, pp. 776–85.

[95] Folch, A., Mezzour, S., Düring, M. *et al.* 2000. Stacks of microfabricated structures as scaffolds for cell culture and tissue engineering. *Biomed. Microdevices*, **2**, 207–14.

[96] Taguchi, T., Xu, L. M., Kobayashi, H. *et al.* 2005. Encapsulation of chondrocytes in injectable alkali-treated collagen gels prepared using poly(ethylene glycol)-based 4-armed star polymer. *Biomaterials*, **26**, 1247–52.

[97] Malda, J., Martens, D. E., Tramper, J., van Blitterswijk, C. A. and Riesle, J. 2003. Cartilage tissue engineering: controversy in the effect of oxygen. *Crit. Rev. Biotechnol.*, **23**, 175–94.

[98] Miot, S., Woodfield, T., Daniels, A. U. *et al.* 2005. Effects of scaffold composition and architecture on human nasal chondrocyte redifferentiation and cartilaginous matrix deposition. *Biomaterials*, **26**, 2479–89.

[99] Rauwendall, C. 2001. *Polymer Extrusion*, 4th edn. Cincinnati, OH: Hanser Gardner Publications.

[100] Yildirim, E. D. 2010. *Plasma and Protein Surface Functionalization for Three-dimensional Polycaprolactone Tissue Scaffolds*, Ph.D. Dissertation Mechanical Engineering and Mechanics, Drexel University, Philadelphia, PA, USA.

[101] Cooper, G. M. and Hausman, R. E. 2009. *The Cell: A Molecular Approach*, 5th edn. Sunderland, MA: Sinauer Associates, Inc.

[102] Sedgwick, J. D. and Czerkinsky, C. 1992. Detection of cell-surface molecules, secreted products of single cells and cellular proliferation by enzyme-immunoassay. *J. Immunol. Methods*, **150**, 159–75.

[103] Paulie, S., Perlmann, H. and Perlmann, P. 2001. Enzyme-linked immunosorbent assay. In *eLS*. New York: John Wiley & Sons, Ltd.

[104] Goldman, L. and Ausiello, D. 2007. *Cecil Medicine*, 23rd edn. Philadelphia, PA: Saunders Elsevier.

[105] Feldman, M., Friedman, L. S. and Brandt, L. J. 2010. *Sleisenger and Fortran's Gastrointestinal and Liver Disease*, 9th edn. Philadelphia, PA: Saunders Elsevier.

[106] Chang, R. and Sun, W. 2009. *Biofabrication of Three-Dimensional Liver Cell-Embedded Tissue Constructs for in vitro Drug Metabolism Models*: LAP Saarbrücken: Lambert Academic Publishing.

[107] Berstine, E. G., Hooper, M. L., Grandchamp, S. and Ephrussi, B. 1973. Alkaline phosphatase activity in mouse teratoma. *Proc. Nat. Acad. Sci. USA*, **70**, 3899–903.

[108] McCullen, S. D., Zhu, Y., Bernacki, S. H. *et al.* 2009. Electrospun composite poly(L-lactic acid)/tricalcium

phosphate scaffolds induce proliferation and osteogenic differentiation of human adipose-derived stem cells. *Biomed. Mater.*, **4**(3), 035002.

[109] Shor, L., Güçeri, S., Chang, R. *et al.* 2009. Precision extruding deposition (PED) fabrication of polycaprolactone (PCL) scaffolds for bone tissue engineering. *Biofabrication*, **1**(1), 015003.

[110] Rosland, G. V., Svendsen, A., Torsvik, A. *et al.* 2009. Long-term cultures of bone marrow-derived human mesenchymal stem cells frequently undergo spontaneous malignant transformation. *Cancer Res.*, **69**, 5331–9.

[111] Nettles, D. L., Elder, S. H. and Gilbert, J. A. 2002. Potential use of chitosan as a cell scaffold material for cartilage tissue engineering. *Tissue Eng.*, **8**, 1009–16.

[112] VandeVord, P. J., Matthew, H. W. T., DeSilva, S. P. *et al.* 2002. Evaluation of the biocompatibility of a chitosan scaffold in mice. *J. Biomed. Mater. Res.*, **59**, 585–90.

[113] Xu, C. Y., Inai, R., Kotaki, M. and Ramakrishna, S. 2004. Aligned biodegradable nanofibrous structure: a potential scaffold for blood vessel engineering. *Biomaterials*, **25**, 877–86.

PART III

Hydrogel scaffolds for regenerative medicine

14

Polysaccharide hydrogels for regenerative medicine applications

Jacob A. Simson and Jennifer H. Elisseeff

14.1 Introduction

This chapter begins by reviewing the structure and origin of polysaccharides commonly used in hydrogels and then moves on to a brief discussion of the role of structural polysaccharides throughout tissues in the body. Common chemical modification techniques are discussed, followed by approaches used to crosslink polysaccharides into insoluble hydrogels. The authors will also describe recent research approaches for polysaccharide hydrogel materials as scaffolds for tissue engineering, vehicles for drug delivery, and tissue adhesives. The goal of this chapter is to provide the reader with an overview of the exciting potential of polysaccharide-based hydrogels in medicine.

14.2 Structure and origin of common polysaccharides

Polysaccharides are large linear or branched carbohydrate molecules composed of repeating monomer units. They can perform structurally, as in the extracellular matrix of animals and cell walls of plants [1], or provide energy storage capacity in the instances of glycogen and starch [2]. Every organism on the planet has the ability to produce polysaccharides. Solubilities of polysaccharides in water vary depending on the chemical structure [3]. Monomer units often contain chemical groups that can be functionalized chemically in order to modify their material properties. Important structural polysaccharides in the human body are known as glycosaminoglycans (GAGs), which are anionic, linear polysaccharides composed of repeating disaccharide units. The repeat unit is comprised of a hexosamine and either a hexose or hexuronic acid.

14.2.1 Hyaluronic acid

Hyaluronic acid (HA), also known as hyaluronate or hyaluronan, is a GAG consisting of repeating units of the disaccharide (1–4)-β-D-glucuronic acid linked to (1–3)-β-N-acetyl-D-glucosamine (GlcNAc) [4]. It can be derived using bacterial fermentation or harvested from animal tissue, the latter bringing a risk of cross-species infection [5]. It is a highly hydrophilic molecule with hydroxyl, carboxylic acid, and N-acetyl functionalities. It can range in molecular weight (more formally, relative molecular mass) from 10 kDa up to 10 MDa [6]. It is synthesized by HA synthases at the cell membrane and excreted into the extracellular space [7].

14.2.2 Chondroitin sulfate

Chondroitin sulfate (CS) is the most prevalent GAG in the human body [8]. It is composed of alternating glucuronic acid and N-acetyl galactosamine (GalNAc). It exists in several forms with varying sulfation patterns and biological activities [9]. Most commonly, CS is sulfated at the carbon 4 or carbon 6 of GalNAc, and less frequently at the carbon 2 of glucuronic acid. When used for biomaterials, CS is often harvested from bovine trachea or shark cartilage [10]. The molecule is highly hydrophilic due to its hydroxyl, carboxylic acid,

N-acetyl, and sulfate functionalities. Its molecular weight typically ranges from 6 kDa to 50 kDa [11].

14.2.3 Heparin

Heparin is a hydrophilic GAG molecule so highly sulfated that it has the most negative charge of any biological molecule [12]. The heparin chemical structure is variable depending on the tissue of origin, but the most common disaccharide repeating units are 2-O-sulfated iduronic acid (IdoA(2S)) linked to 6-O-sulfated, N-sulfated glucosamine (GlcNS(6S)) [13]. It contains hydroxyl, carboxylic acid, and sulfate functional groups. Molecular weights range from 5 kDa to 30 kDa [14]. Heparin is derived from mucosal tissues of animals, including bovine lung and porcine intestine [15].

14.2.4 Chitosan

Chitosan is a semi-crystalline, hydrophobic, linear, cationic polysaccharide GAG analog. The molecular structure is composed of β-(1-4)-linked D-glucosamine with variable and random N-acetyl glucosamine (GlcNAc) residues, ranging from 50 kDa to 1 MDa [16]. Having a structure similar to GAGs, chitosan seems to mimic their behavior [17]. Functionalities include hydroxyl and N-acetyl groups. It is derived from chitin, a structural component of arthropod exoskeleton and the second most abundant natural biopolymer on Earth. To produce chitosan, deacetylation is performed on the chitin polymer. The degree of crystallinity is dependent on the degree of deacetylation, with the lowest degree of crystallinity, and consequently highest solubility, occurring at 50% deacetylation. Chitosan has a pK_a near 6.3, and becomes soluble at pH levels below this pK_a [18].

14.2.5 Alginate

Alginate, or alginic acid, is an anionic linear polysaccharide derived from cell walls of brown algae. It is highly hydrophilic, consisting of β-D-mannuronic acid (M) and α-L-glucuronic acid (G). The monomers are grouped into either homopolymeric M or G blocks, or heteropolymeric MG blocks. Molecular weights range from 10 kDa to 1 MDa [19]. Alginate contains hydroxyl and carboxylic acid functionalities. Human enzymes don't have the capability to degrade the polysaccharide [20], though there are reports of degradability in the literature [21]. Additionally, human cells do not naturally adhere to the alginate molecule [22], but it can be modified to promote cell adhesion [23].

14.2.6 Dextran

Dextran is a cheap, readily available branched polysaccharide polymer. It is comprised entirely of glucose, bound linearly via α-1-6 linkages, and branched primarily via α-1-3 bonds, but also less frequently by α-1-2 and α-1-4 bonds [24]. It is highly hydrophilic, containing only hydroxyl functionalities. Dextran is derived from certain lactic acid bacteria, which produce it from sucrose molecules. Molecular weights are on the order of 10 kDa to 1 MDa [25]. Dextran does not support protein adsorption or non-specific cell binding [26], and is degradable by human enzymes [27].

14.3 Role of polysaccharides in tissues throughout the body

Polysaccharides are key components of tissues throughout the body. They serve various roles including structural support [28], signaling [29], lubrication [30], and anticoagulation [31]. Most typically, these polysaccharides are in the form of GAGs and proteoglycans (PGs). Proteoglycans consist of a protein core glycosylated by one or more GAG molecules O-linked through serine residues [32]. In tissue extracellular matrix (ECM), the PGs work in concert with proteins to provide mechanical integrity to the tissue. They can also sequester growth factors and present them to cells or modulate their bioactivity. Proteoglycan functions depend on tissue of interest.

14.3.1 Cartilage

Cartilage tissue plays important lubricating and structural roles throughout the body. Articular cartilage lines the surface of diarthroidal joints such as knees, hips, and shoulders, and helps to reduce friction on joint surfaces. It is composed of a type II collagen protein matrix interspersed with PG matrix. The protein matrix provides tensile integrity, while the PG matrix provides compressive strength. The predominant GAGs are CS and HA. Chondroitin sulfate chains are a crucial component of the PG aggrecan, which consists of a protein core linked to as many as 100 CS molecules [33]. The aggrecan molecules are linked to HA, creating an extensive, highly hydrated PG matrix that provides the incompressible nature of articular cartilage [34]. By the same mechanism, the presence of aggrecan provides incompressible character to meniscus [35] and intervertebral disk cartilage [36]. Additionally, HA is a major component of synovial fluid, which bathes cartilage with the purpose of lubrication [37].

14.3.2 Bone

Bone is a specialized tissue providing the body with support, protection, and mineral storage. It is composed of an inorganic matrix deposited within organic matrix. Bone tissue is comprised by less than 1% GAGs, of which greater than 90% is CS [38] with smaller contributions from HA and another GAG, dermatan sulfate [39]. The homeostasis of bone depends primarily on the balance of osteoclast and osteoblast activity of bone resorption and bone production, respectively. GAGs in the ECM play a role in modulating the activity of these cells. Both HA and CS inhibit osteoclast formation [40, 41] and resorption activity [42], and CS stimulates osteoblast differentiation, matrix synthesis, and mineralization [43] but inhibits proliferation [44]. Thus, though GAGs comprise only a small portion of bone matrix, their presence may play a large role in maintaining ECM homeostasis.

14.3.3 Skin

Skin, a vital organ to human survival, covers the body, providing a barrier to pathogens, regulating water and temperature homeostasis, and serving as a sensory organ. To permit motion, skin must be a relatively flexible and elastic tissue, thus GAGs are a crucial component of its ECM in addition to an array of collagenous and elastic proteins. Though GAGs contribute less than 0.3% of skin dry weight, their high affinity for water controls the volume and elasticity of the tissue [45]. The main GAG molecules residing in skin are HA and CS, with the former accounting for 75% of dermal GAGs [45]. In addition to providing the structural integrity needed by skin, GAGs also are essential in signaling for skin processes. In wounded skin, GAGs bind and present growth factors to direct inflammatory cells where their actions are needed, and even the presence of GAG fragments themselves can act as a signal for wound repair [46, 47]. In fetal wound healing, where scarring does not occur, HA is present in higher levels, suggesting that this GAG may be able to be leveraged in biomaterials to achieve better healing results [48].

14.3.4 Nerve

The ECM of nerve tissue contains relatively small amounts of fibrous proteins and high amounts of GAGs [49]. Hyaluronic acid plays a critical role in the migration of cells during the development of the nervous system [50]. Once matured, the predominant GAG molecule in neural ECM is CS. As in cartilage, CS is complexed into proteoglycans (PGs) and the resultant CSPG complex is aggregated with HA. The ECM in the nervous system is concentrated around special neurons into regions known as perineural nets [51]. The presence of CSPG in neural nets has been shown to effect neural plasticity, in that the removal of CS via the bacterial enzyme chondroitinase ABC results in the reopening of plasticity and the further development of neural networks [52]. Additionally, CS plays a critical role in the inability of damaged nerves to regain functionality. It is the main axonal inhibitory component in glial scarring [53]. The CS GAG plays a primary role in stabilizing the established neural network, but is disruptive of neurogenesis, and such information should be carefully considered when devising regenerative techniques.

14.3.5 Cornea

The cornea is a specialized transparent tissue in the eye that functions to focus light onto the retina. The structure and arrangement of ECM fibers is critical to maintain the transparency of the cornea. The stromal layer, comprising nearly 90% of corneal thickness, is composed of many layers of regularly spaced, uniformly sized type I collagen fibers in a parallel arrangement. GAGs reside in the interfibrillar spaces and play a key role in the assembly and organization of these collagen fibrils [54]. Dermatan sulfate and keratan sulfate are the predominant GAGs in the corneal stroma. Animals with gene deficiencies for keratan sulfate-rich lumican proteoglycans have opaque corneas [55]. Additionally, while not present in large amounts in healthy cornea, HA plays a key role in corneal development. As the cornea matures, HA synthesis decreases and keratan sulfate becomes more prevalent [56]. A similar trend has been noted in corneal healing, suggesting that corneal wound healing follows a process similar to cornea genesis [54].

14.3.6 Vasculature

GAGs play a significant role in vascular development and mature vessel function. Levels of HA are elevated in developing capillaries, where it is critical to the high activity of endothelial cell migration and proliferation [57]. With the maturation of vessels, cells decrease HA production and begin to produce sulfated GAGs, primarily heparin sulfate (HS) in addition to CS and dermatan sulfate [58, 59]. It is known that HS plays a key role in the antithrombotic nature of blood. Being closely related to heparin, HS is expressed heavily on the vessel wall, acting to inhibit the activity of antithrombin-III, preventing the coagulation of blood in vivo. Chondroitin Sulfate is present in the vessel ECM mainly in the form of versican, biglycan, and decorin PGs. Versican is known to affect cell adhesion, promote proliferation, and affect cell migration [60]. These PGs also may have an effect on matrix assembly. Chondroitin Sulfate chains on versican have been found to inhibit elastin fiber assembly [61], and biglycan and decorin are involved in regulating collagen fibrillogenesis [62].

14.4 Methods for crosslinking polysaccharides

Many of the important polysaccharides in human tissues are highly conserved among mammalian species. Other polysaccharides of interest can be generated in high quantities from lower-level organisms. The high abundance, biologically natural origin, and critical role in the human body of polysaccharides make them well suited for use in biomedical applications. The most frequent application of polysaccharides in biomaterials is in the form of hydrogels. A hydrogel is an insoluble network of hydrophilic molecules crosslinked by either physical or chemical means. The hydrogels hold large amounts of water and allow mass transport of small molecules such as nutrients, metabolic waste, and growth factors. Typically, cytocompatible crosslinking methods are employed so that cells can be suspended in the precursor solution and encapsulated in the resultant hydrogel with high viability. Synthetic polymers can be used in conjunction with polysaccharides to tune hydrogel parameters such as cell and protein adhesion, mechanical stiffness, and the pH and temperature of gelation.

14.4.1 Physical crosslinking methods

Temperature-driven solubility differences can be employed to physically crosslink polymeric materials into hydrogels via a phenomenon known as the lower critical solution temperature (LCST). Polymers that exhibit a thermo-responsive behavior are composed of hydrophilic and hydrophobic domains. Below this temperature, the hydrophilic domains of the polymer are extended and interacting with the aqueous solvent, allowing them to be dissolved. Above the critical temperature, the hydrophilic chains become dehydrated and collapse, revealing the hydrophobic domains to the aqueous solvent, greatly reducing the solubility of the polymer, and resulting in a physically crosslinked hydrogel. This phenomenon is favorable when designing injectible biomaterials. The biomaterial can be prepared ex vivo, mixing the dissolved polymer with cells or growth factors of interest below the LCST, then injected into the body where the temperature is above the critical temperature, resulting in the spontaneous generation of a hydrogel. Chitosan, dextran, and HA have been combined with synthetic thermoresponsive polymers to produce biosynthetic hydrogels for a variety of biomedical applications [63–66].

Leveraging the existence of ionic interactions can also form hydrogels. The polysaccharide alginate can be crosslinked physically into a hydrogel using divalent cations. When Ca^{2+} is added to a solution of sodium alginate, these cations displace the sodium cations and the alginate molecules are crosslinked into an insoluble calcium alginate hydrogel. Crosslinking occurs primarily between carboxylic acid functional groups on constituents in the "G" block of the polymer chains. Using Ba^{2+} or Sr^{2+} in place of Ca^{2+} resulted in hydrogels with higher stiffness and lower diffusivity [67]. Another method to ionically crosslink polysaccharide hydrogels is via formation of polyelectrolyte complexes. The combination of a polyanion (CS, HA, heparin, dextran, or alginate) with a polycation (chitosan or polylysine) can result in the formation of an insoluble hydrogel [68, 69].

14.4.2 Chemical crosslinking methods

The presence of chemical functional groups on polysaccharides provides engineers with a tool by which these materials can be chemically crosslinked into insoluble hydrogels. One commonly used method for crosslinking hydrophilic polymers into hydrogels is by way of photoinitiated radical crosslinking of acrylate groups. In this technique, a small photoinitiator molecule is activated by ultraviolet radiation in the presence of acrylate functional groups. The initiator molecule radicalizes the acrylate group, which can then react with other acrylate groups, setting off a chain reaction. By using multifunctional polymer molecules, a crosslinked matrix can be formed. While this technique was pioneered using synthetic polymers, it can also be applied to functionalized polysaccharides [70–72]. The limitation of using a photoinitiated system is that light penetration through tissue is a limiting factor for polymerizing injectible hydrogel matrices. Alternative methods for crosslinking that do not depend on light to initiate the chemical reaction are not restricted by depth of implant.

A simple chemical reaction that can be used to form hydrogels is known as click chemistry. The most common click chemistry reaction involves the combination of an azide group with an alkyne group to form a five-membered ring [73]. Since it can be performed under conditions that are generally cell-friendly, click chemistry can be used for cell encapsulation applications. However, the presence of the requisite catalyst Cu can produce reactive oxygen species, which can be toxic to nearby cells [74]. By functionalizing polysaccharides with azide and alkyne groups, this technique can be applied to generate naturally derived hydrogels [75].

Two common addition reactions applied to crosslink hydrogels are the Schiff-base and Michael reactions. The Schiff-base reaction occurs between a primary amine and a carbonyl group to form a stable imine crosslinking bond. Carbonyl and amine groups can be added onto common polysaccharides simply using carbodiimide chemistry, and the modified polysaccharides can be used for *in situ* formation of biodegradable hydrogels [76]. The Michael addition reaction is a base-catalyzed nucleophilic attack on a vinyl group. As with the Schiff-base reactions, simple chemistry can be used to functionalize the polysaccharides with the appropriate functional groups necessary for the Michael addition, which can then be combined to form injectible hydrogels [77].

Condensation reactions can also be utilized to crosslink a polymer network. A simple method to permit condensation reactions is through the use of N-hydroxysuccinimide (NHS) or closely related molecules. The NHS can be used to activate carboxylic acid functional groups, making them susceptible to nucleophilic attack. In the case of amine attack, the resulting amide crosslinking bond formed is highly stable in aqueous solutions, creating a hydrolytically stable polymer network [78]. Such chemistry allows the NHS-activated molecule to be suitable for hydrogel formation, but also makes it a candidate as a tissue adhesive, since it can react with primary amines located on proteins in the body.

An alternative method for crosslinking involves the use of enzymes to form stable intermolecular bonds. Examples of enzymatic crosslinking include the use of horseradish peroxidase (HRP) and tyrosinase [79–81]. On phenol-grafted HA and chitosan, HRP can crosslink the phenol groups with the use of hydrogen peroxide. Tyrosinase can oxidize tyrosyl residues on gelatin into quinones, which then crosslink with a nucleophile on the polysaccharide backbone. These enzyme-based crosslinking reactions can occur as quickly as within 10 seconds, or take as long as a half hour, depending on polymer and reactive group concentration.

14.5 Polysaccharide scaffolds for tissue engineering

The adult healing response to traumatic injuries results in replacement of the tissue defect with scar tissue. This type of healing can be useful in protecting an individual from infection, but it does not restore the full functionality of the original tissue. Tissue engineering is an approach that attempts to prevent the deposition of scar tissue in the defect space and promote the healing of the tissue of interest. Often this approach involves the implantation of a scaffold material to modulate the response of surrounding cells and tissue. In some cases, the scaffold contains fully differentiated or progenitor cells to aid in the healing process. The choice of material plays a major role in eliciting the desired healing response.

14.5.1 Cartilage repair

One of the most commonly targeted tissues for tissue engineering is articular cartilage [79, 82–85]. Articular cartilage lacks an intrinsic healing capability, and thus existing defects continue to degenerate, which can eventually progress to osteoarthritis (OA) of the joint. One current therapy to treat cartilage lesions is known as autologous chondrocyte implantation (ACI). Much of the current research in the articular cartilage field is in the development of scaffold materials to deliver chondrocytes or their mesenchymal stem cell (MSC) progenitors. These scaffolds serve to improve surgical handling, prevent cell leakage away from the defect site, and direct cell differentiation and matrix production.

The inclusion of an appropriate polysaccharide into a hydrogel scaffold can help to direct appropriate cell differentiation and tissue production. Varghese and colleagues investigated the effect of CS on the chondrogenesis of goat MSCs encapsulated in CS–PEG hydrogels. Here CS and PEG were acrylated and photocrosslinked. In the CS-containing hydrogels, MSCs self-aggregated into clumps, mimicking the action of mesenchymal condensation in limb bud formation. Additionally, the expression of cadherin 11, a cell surface molecule postulated to be critical to MSC condensation, increased during early stages in the CS–PEG hydrogel, whereas expression remained low in the PEG gel at all time points. In CS–PEG, gene expression of the important cartilage matrix molecules aggrecan, versican, and type II collagen and cartilage transcription factor Sox-9 were elevated at all time points investigated (through 42 days) compared with the PEG gels. Tissue production in the CS–PEG was far more extensive, with cell aggregrates growing so large that they protruded out of the hydrogel. Elevated production of type II collagen in CS–PEG compared with that in PEG alone was confirmed by immunohistochemistry.

Human trials for cartilage repair have been performed with CS, alginate, HA, and chitosan-based hydrogels. ChonDux® is a CS–PEG material used in conjunction with microfracture surgery. A cartilage defect is primed with a CS bioadhesive, subjected to the microfracture procedure, and filled with a PEG hydrogel. The ChonDux® system traps the mesenchymal clot, and has been shown to improve cartilage repair in animals [86] and in early results from a human trial in Europe. CARTIPATCH® is an agarose–alginate scaffold seeded with chondrocytes expanded in monolayer for augmentation of the ACI procedure. Expanded cells were encapsulated into a pre-formed hydrogel, which was implanted into the chondral or osteochondral defect space in the femoral chondyle. Two-year follow-up magnetic residence imaging (MRI) indicated that the average defect size decreased from 2.7 cm^2 to 0.4 cm^2, and cartilage repair in patients with lesions of size greater than 3 cm^2 was better than that in patients with smaller lesions. ICRS scoring during arthroscopic examination resulted in a mean score of 10 out of a maximum of 12. Follow-up biopsy showed that the regenerated tissue was predominantly hyaline. Hyaff 11® is a HA-based product that has been used in clinical trials. Glucuronic acid moieties are esterified with benzyl alcohol, significantly reducing the hydrophilicity of the molecule and causing it to gel. The scaffold is cultured with encapsulated human chondrocytes for two weeks, and is then implanted into the articular cartilage defect. Treated animals develop hyaline-like repair tissue that is integrated well with surrounding cartilage. In human clinical trials, patients administered this treatment recovered faster than did those treated with a collagen-based cell delivery scaffold [87] and experienced a reduction in pain in addition to an improvement in knee function [88]. BST-CarGel® is a chitosan blood-clot material designed to improve cartilage tissue repair after a microfracture procedure [89]. In a rabbit microfracture model, the chitosan-treated defects showed improved vascularity and remodeling of subchondral bone, which resulted in a wider area of bone and cartilage repair than with microfracture alone. When applied to sheep microfracture, the CarGel product resulted in repair of relatively mature cartilage tissue, with superficial, transitional, and radial zones separated from bone by a tidemark [90]. Early results from human trials indicate improvements in pain, stiffness, and function.

14.5.2 Bone repair

Bone voids can result from traumatic injury or disease. For small voids, bone autograft is the gold standard, but there is a limited supply of bone for autografting, and donor site morbidity is associated with this procedure. In the case of craniofacial bone defects, there is an aesthetic goal of avoiding scarring, so an injectible regenerative product could be advantageous. A study found that delivery of osteocyte progenitor MSC cells suspended in chitosan hydrogels resulted in bone regeneration about twice that of the non-filled control [91]. Another material investigated for craniofacial application used RGD-modified alginate as a scaffold to modulate bone healing [92]. Osteoblast adhesion and preosteoblast differentiation were improved in vitro by the presence of RGD. In-vivo culture of osteoblast seeded alginate gels showed good bone formation, improved by the presence of RGD. Another study investigated the ability of apatite-coated HA to differentiate osteoblast precursors and stimulate bone regeneration [93]. Alkaline phosphatase (ALP) activity was increased nearly 10-fold for mouse osteoblastic cells compared with those seeded on a collagen sponge. Repair of cranial rat defect was about 1.5 times that of the collagen sponge control, and twice that of the sham.

14.5.3 Skin repair

GAGs played an important role in the development of early skin regeneration products [94]. Burn victims are the primary candidates for engineered skin. A skin graft must be properly permeable to water to prevent both dehydration and pooling of fluid under the material. It should also be pliable to allow the patient to move around without damaging the graft. Hydrogels are an attractive option to serve these purposes, and, while most attempts have utilized collagen, a variety of polysaccharide designs have been pursued. A photopolymerized dextran–PEG hydrogel was applied to a mouse skin defect, and healing was compared with that achieved using Integra®, the industry gold standard for treating burns, and untreated control [95]. Only in the dextran hydrogel-treated samples was there full regeneration of skin appendages. Inhibition of cytokines associated with scarring and reduction in wound size were achieved by applying an alginate hydrogel to a full-thickness skin wound in a rat model [96]. A human trial for diabetic ulcer healing was attempted with an HA graft material [97]. The HA scaffold is cultured with autologous dermal fibroblasts and keratinocytes. Compared with standard care for diabetic foot ulcers, those receiving the HA grafts were 3.65 times as likely to have their wounds heal.

14.5.4 Nerve repair

Nerve healing is limited by the formation of a glial scar. In order to facilitate functional tissue healing, fibroblast invasion and scar deposition has to be prevented, and axon bridging across the defect must be promoted. The current gold standard is the use of nerve autograft, but obvious drawbacks to this are donor site morbidity and the limited supply of donor tissue. Many attempts at tissue engineering of artificial nerves with polysaccharide biomaterials have been documented. One group demonstrated in-vitro differentiation of neural progenitor cells (NPCs) encapsulated in a photocrosslinkable chitosan hydrogel upon exposure to pro-neural rat interferon-γ [98]. In designing biomaterials for nerve regeneration, one has to consider hydrogel mechanics, as substrate stiffness can affect progenitor differentiation lineage and tissue development [99]. An attempt to culture rat and human neurons on a divalently crosslinked alginate hydrogel revealed that neurite outgrowth occurred rapidly only in gels with low stiffness due to minimal crosslinking. Another group investigated the use of a HA–polylysine polyelectrolyte complex to stimulate nerve regeneration in a central nervous system (CNS) injury model [100]. The presence of the hydrogel reduced scarring compared with control and stimulated some axonal sprouting into the defect space. The inclusion of an inhibitory pathway antagonist for regeneration improved healing further.

14.5.5 Vascular repair

Vasculature is critical to the delivery of nutrients and oxygen and the removal of metabolic waste, and nearly all tissue is vascularized. When designing tissue-engineered matrices, we should consider not only the structure and function of that specialized organ, but also the vasculature needed to keep that tissue alive. Choosing scaffolds that facilitate vascular growth may be beneficial. One group investigating bone repair found that the presence of HA in their scaffold material enhanced the degree of vasculature in a regenerating bone marrow cavity [101]. Low-molecular-weight HA (35 kDa) was more effective at stimulating the generation of blood vessels than was high-molecular-weight HA (10^4–10^7 Da). Another group found that a PEG–dextran hydrogel used for skin grafting was well vascularized [95]. In addition to engineering a material that will develop vasculature, there is also a need for engineering stand-alone blood vessels. A dextran–gelatin hydrogel with mechanical properties suitable for vascular engineering was created using Schiff-base reaction and photoinitiated crosslinking [102]. This material supported spreading of endothelial cells in two dimensions and spreading and proliferation of smooth muscle cells for two weeks in culture. In another study, rat vena cavae were replaced with an HA tubular scaffold and samples were collected for histological analysis at 30, 60, and 90 days [103]. After one month, a new vessel had regenerated within the HA implant, and after three 3 months the HA had completely degraded.

14.6 Polysaccharide hydrogels as drug delivery vehicles

The field of regenerative medicine relies widely on the use of growth factors to stimulate and direct cellular processes such as differentiation, proliferation, and tissue production [104–106]. There are various growth factors available to stimulate different types of tissue regeneration. Transforming growth factor-β (TGF-β), bone morphogenic proteins (BMP), vascular endothelial growth factor (VEGF), and neurotrophic growth factor (NGF) stimulate formation of cartilage, bone, vascular, and neural tissues, respectively. The high cost of recombinant growth factors is a critical drawback to their use as an affordable treatment. An alternative approach to use of recombinant growth factors that has gained popularity in orthopedics is the application of platelet-rich plasma (PRP) and bone marrow aspirate [107–109]. The aim of using these materials is to concentrate an autologous supply of growth factors and progenitor cells in the hopes of leveraging the body's natural healing capabilities. Platelets contain seven growth factors that are fundamental to initiating the tissue healing process [110]. The PRP and bone marrow can be obtained intraoperatively with minimally invasive techniques during a surgical procedure, avoiding the high costs associated with artificially producing proteins.

The efficacy of a growth factor delivery system depends on the ability to deliver the drugs at a moderate level over an extended period of time. An implantable system must be loaded with a sufficient level of growth factor that can be released slowly with an appropriate profile. The natural ability to interact with growth factors makes polysaccharides an attractive material to use for a sustained-release system. Additionally, hydrogels offer the benefit of a localized delivery of growth factor. In certain applications it is critical that the growth factor be delivered very specifically. For instance, in the application of BMP-2 to bone in vertebral regeneration, non-specific delivery of the growth factor to the spinal canal resulted in ectopic bone formation and caused complications [111]. Various polysaccharide hydrogel materials have been investigated for their potential to serve as local drug delivery vehicles.

14.6.1 Delivery of recombinant growth factors

BMP-2-loaded hydrogels have demonstrated the ability to enhance bone repair in animal models. One such model involved chitosan BMP-2 delivery to a rat cranial bone graft [112]. Chitosan hydrogels were applied to cranial allograft and implanted into a critical defect in the cranium. At an early time point (day 2), the animals with BMP-2-loaded chitosan-coated allograft had better morphological repair than did those with the gold standard autograft control. At day 14, the BMP/chitosan allograft sample was indistinguishable with respect to morphological repair from the autograft sample, both of which showed superior healing than was found for the allograft alone and allograft/chitosan animals without BMP-2 loaded into the hydrogel. Another group delivered BMP-2 to a critical-sized femoral segmental defect in a rat using a hybrid poly(caprolactone) fiber-alginate hydrogel [113]. The BMP-2-loaded samples exhibited complete fusion of bone with good integration between old and new tissue, whereas growth-factor-deficient specimen regenerated only sparse bone in the defect space. The torsional strength and stiffness of the new bone were about three-quarters that of native tissue.

The natural growth factor binding activity of heparin can be leveraged to prolong growth factor release profiles from hydrogels. One group investigated how incorporating heparin into an alginate hydrogel would affect the release of several growth factors [114]. Methacrylated heparin was mixed with methacrylated alginate and dissolved growth factors, and then photopolymerized into hydrogels. The release profiles of heparin binding growth factors TGF-β, VEGF, BMP-2, and fibroblast growth factor (FGF-2) from unmodified alginate and heparin–alginate hydrogels were investigated in vitro. For all growth factors, nearly all of the loaded protein was released with in 4–7 days from the unmodified alginate hydrogels. In comparison, heparin–alginate hydrogels released these factors for a duration of more than 3 weeks. The maintenance of growth factor activity was confirmed in vitro and in vivo. In vitro, released VEGF increased the proliferation of human umbilical vein endothelial cells (HUVECs), and released BMP-2 increased the ALP activity of preosteoblasts. In vivo, subcutaneously implanted BMP-2-loaded heparin–alginate gels induced nearly twice as much peripheral bone formation as did the BMP-2-loaded alginate gels.

NGF is critical to the stimulation of nerve regeneration. One interesting approach to NGF delivery was through a heparin–fibrin composite hydrogel [115]. A heparin-binding peptide was crosslinked into the fibrin matrix during gelation, and heparin present in the solution was sequestered to the binding domain, creating the fibrin–polysaccharide composite gel. In vivo, the heparin-binding peptide would also act to concentrate endogenous heparin. NGF has an affinity for heparin, and forms a growth factor–hydrogel complex. The hydrogel was delivered into a sciatic nerve defect within a silicon nerve guidance conduit, and compared with nerve isograft, NGF-free fibrin hydrogel, and empty controls. The NGF-loaded hydrogels resulted in neural tissue repair at about 80% of the level of the nerve isograft, twice as high as for the NGF-free fibrin matrix, and three times the level of the empty conduit. Another polysaccharide approach to controlled delivery of NGF was through a chitosan–CS polyelectrolyte complex [116]. Encapsulated NGF was released quickly in the first 10 days, then at a much slower rate over the following two months. NGF-loaded scaffolds had regenerated nerve with a larger axon diameter and statistically identical conduction velocity as nerve autograft control.

14.6.2 Delivery of autologous growth factors

The delivery of autologous growth factors in the form of PRP or bone marrow is technologically very undeveloped. Currently, surgeons will use thrombin to activate the platelets in PRP just prior to spraying or injecting at the biological site of interest [117]. This method does little to localize the growth factors or control the rate of their release [110]. Only a few investigators have explored the use of polysaccharide hydrogels to deliver autologous growth factors. In one case, alginate hydrogel particles were investigated as a delivery vehicle for PRP-derived growth factors [118]. The release profile of PDGF, TGF-β, and IGF from two types of PRP-alginate carriers produced by different methods, namely using beads and capsules, was investigated. Beads had an average diameter of 1.9 mm, while capsules were 4.2 mm in diameter. Carrier type affected release of growth factors – TGF-β was released in greater quantity from the beads, while PDGF and IGF were released in greater quantity from the capsules. The bioactivity of the released growth factors was investigated by applying the releasate to human osteoblast-like cells cultured in vitro in monolayer. The proliferation and activity of ALP, a bone marker, were measured. At day 3, factors released from the beads had increased proliferation compared with control, while at day 14 factors from the capsules had had this effect. Factors released from the capsules were found to have an effect on ALP activity.

One other group investigated the possibility of delivering PRP using chitosan, but found that the incorporation of chitosan either alone or with PRP disrupted the regeneration of bone in a rabbit cranial defect model [119]. It was suggested that, since the chitosan was in the form of a sponge, lysozymes were less capable of breaking down the material and that perhaps chitosan in a hydrogel form could have resulted in enhanced bone repair.

14.7 Polysaccharide-based tissue adhesives

Current clinically available tissue adhesives include fibrin sealant and cyanoacrylates. Fibrin, being a naturally derived material, has the advantage of being biocompatible and supporting tissue regeneration, but it has disadvantages of short residence time and weak mechanical bonding. Cyanoacrylates, on the other hand, have the benefit of a very high adhesive strength, but cannot be used for many biomedical applications due to their cytotoxic chemistry and degradation products. There is a need for tissue adhesive materials with tunable biodegradation, robust mechanical properties, and tissue-friendly application and degradation chemistries. Polysaccharide biomaterials offer an opportunity to develop this next generation of tissue adhesives.

Chondroitin sulfate has been modified to serve as a tissue and biomaterial adhesive [78, 86, 120]. Wang and colleagues modified CS to serve as a tissue primer to bond hydrogel materials to a tissue surface [86]. Here CS was treated with glycidyl methacrylate and periodate to form a methacrylated-CS-aldehyde. When applied to tissue, the aldehyde groups on the molecule reacted with primary amines to bind the CS-adhesive to the tissue. Subsequently, poly(ethylene glycol) diacrylate (PEGDA) was applied and crosslinked by photoinitiation, resulting in a tissue-bound hydrogel. Studies were performed to investigate the integration of newly formed cartilage from encapsulated chondrocytes with existing cartilage tissue. Cartilage-bound cell-seeded hydrogels were cultured both in vitro and in vivo. In both cases, the production of sulfated GAGs and type II collagen by cells in the hydrogel resembled neocartilage, and the integration of neocartilage with cartilage tissue remained strong after 5 weeks in culture. Advanced tissue development and proteoglycan deposition occurred when CS-adhesive was present.

Strehin and colleagues developed a CS-derivative that can serve both as a bulk hydrogel and as tissue adhesive [78, 120]. Carboxylic acid groups on the CS were activated with NHS, allowing the material to react both with an aminated PEG to form a CS–PEG hydrogel and with primary amines on proteins on a tissue surface, gluing the hydrogel to the tissue. This two-component adhesive reacts spontaneously without the need for external photopolymerization. Adjusting the CS-NHS concentration and the pH of the reaction solution modulated the mechanical properties. The high viability (greater than 95%) of encapsulated bovine chondrocytes confirmed the reaction cytocompatibility. Mechanical testing demonstrated an adhesive strength greater than 10 times that of fibrin glue when applied to bovine cartilage explants. Also importantly, degradation of the CS–PEG hydrogel by chondroitanase-ABC enzyme demonstrated the ability for human enzymes to process the material. Lastly, the subcutaneous implantation of PEG and CS–PEG hydrogels in rats revealed the anti-inflammatory nature of the CS component by resolution of the inflammation response by 2 weeks, which persisted for longer than 4 weeks in the presence of PEG-alone gels. More recently, our group has begun to experiment with the application of the CS-adhesive to deliver intraoperative biologics by combining it with blood, bone marrow, and platelet-rich plasma. We have shown these materials to form hydrogels and support cell migration, tissue production, and tissue adhesion.

Recently, nature has inspired the use of catecholamines, small molecules employed by mussels to adhere to solids in wet environments, to mediate tissue adhesion. Hyaluronic acid and chitosan have been modified with catechol derivatives, which react with thiol and amine functional groups via Michael addition [63, 64]. Dopamine-conjugated HA was reacted with thiolated pluronics to form a crosslinked hydrogel. The gel demonstrates an LCST phase transition, which can be tuned to occur between 19 and 29 °C, depending on the pluronic concentration. Remaining unreacted catechol groups on the HA backbone can react with free amines and thiols on tissue. The adhesion strength to mouse skin was measured at 7 kPa. The same chemistry is used for a chitosan–catechol adhesive. Chitosan functionalized with catechol groups reacted with thiolated pluronics. Again, the occurrence of an LCST phase transition was demonstrated, between 26 and 29 °C. The hydrogels were degraded more than 50% in vitro and in vivo over a period of about 25 days. Adhesive strength measured on mouse skin was 15 kPa. The chitosan adhesive was found to reduce blood loss from a lacerated liver by 80% compared with untreated control.

Periodate was used to oxidize glucopyranose rings on dextran to produce a dextran–aldehyde corneal tissue adhesive [121, 122]. Here 20%–50% of the rings were oxidized. The aldehydes on dextran were reacted with amines on PEG via Schiff-base chemistry to form a hydrogel, and unreacted aldehydes were free to react with corneal-derived amines. It was found that using star PEG rather than linear PEG increased the swelling ratio and reduced the degradation rate. Increasing the number of PEG arms and amines per arm also increased the adhesive residence time. When applied to seal a rabbit corneal defect, the material was gone after 7 days. After degradation in vivo, the corneal burst pressure reached 120 mm Hg, indicating that full tissue healing had occurred. The burst pressures from in-vitro tests exceeded those for sutures. The adhesive strength ranged from 6 to 14 kPa and could be increased by increasing the dextran content of the polymer. The adhesive displayed less than half the cytotoxicity of cyanoacrylate when both were applied to rat 3T3 fibroblast cells in a monolayer.

14.8 Conclusion

Regenerative medicine approaches using polysaccharides are being developed to repair injury models for various types of human tissues. These approaches include the use of scaffolds for directing tissue formation and cell migration, releasing protein drugs for stimulation of endogenous tissue production, and reapproximating displaced tissue to facilitate interfacial healing. This chapter has been a brief summary of polysaccharide structure and function, methods for crosslinking polysaccharide biomaterials, and current research investigating the application of these biomaterials for regenerative tissue techniques.

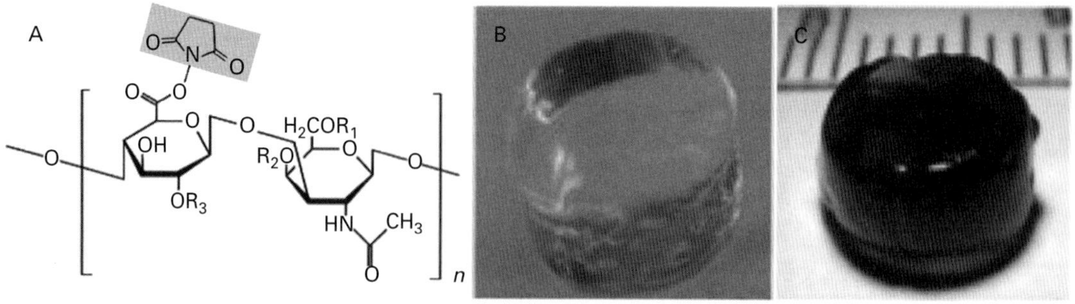

Figure 14.1 Chondroitin sulfate tissue adhesive hydrogel developed in our lab. (A) Molecular structure of the NHS-activated chondroitin sulfate polysaccharide. (B) The CS-PEG hydrogel formed by reacting CS–NHS with aminated six-arm polyethylene glycol. (C) The CS-bone-marrow hydrogel formed by reacting CS–NHS with bovine bone marrow.

ACKNOWLEDGEMENT

This work was supported by DOD W81XWH-11-2-0022.

REFERENCES

[1] Buckeridge, M. S. 2010. Seed cell wall storage polysaccharides: models to understand cell wall biosynthesis and degradation. *Plant Physiol.*, **154**(3), 1017–23.

[2] Robyt, J. F. 2001. *Polysaccharides: Energy Storage*. In *eLS*. New York: John Wiley & Sons, Ltd.

[3] Whistler, R. L. 1973. *Solubility of Polysaccharides and Their Behavior in Solution, in Carbohydrates in Solution*. Washington, DC: American Chemical Society, pp. 242–55.

[4] Hadler, N. M. and Napier, M. A. 1977. Structure of hyaluronic acid in synovial fluid and its influence on the movement of solutes. *Semin Arthritis Rheum.*, **7**(2), 141–52.

[5] Chong, B. F., Blank, L. M., McLaughlin, R., Nielsen, L. K. 2005. Microbial hyaluronic acid production. *Appl. Microbiol. Biotechnol.*, **66**(4), 341–51.

[6] Shimada, E. and Matsumura, G. 1975. Viscosity and molecular weight of hyaluronic acids. *J. Biochem.*, **78**(3), 513–17.

[7] Schulz, T., Schumacher, U. and Prehm, P. 2007. Hyaluronan export by the ABC transporter MRP5 and its modulation by intracellular cGMP. *J. Biol. Chem.*, **282**(29), 20999–1004.

[8] Gandhi, N. S. and Mancera, R. L. 2008. The structure of glycosaminoglycans and their interactions with proteins. *Chem. Biol. Drug Des.*, **72**(6), 455–82.

[9] Nandini, C. D. and Sugahara, K. 2006. Role of the sulfation pattern of chondroitin sulfate in its biological activities and in the binding of growth factors. *Adv. Pharmacol.*, **53**, 253–79.

[10] Desaire, H., Sirich, T. L. and Leary, J. A. 2001. Evidence of block and randomly sequenced chondroitin polysaccharides: sequential enzymatic digestion and quantification using ion trap tandem mass spectrometry. *Anal. Chem.*, **73**(15), 3513–20.

[11] Barnhill, J. G., Fye, C. L., Williams, D. W. *et al.* 2006. Chondroitin product selection for the glucosamine/chondroitin arthritis intervention trial. *J. Am. Pharm. Assoc.*, **46**(1), 14–24.

[12] Cox, M. N. and Lehninger, D. 2004. *Principles of Biochemistry*. New York: Freeman.

[13] Gatti, G., Casu, B., Hamer, G. K. and Perlin, A. S. 1979. Studies on the conformation of heparin by ^{1}H and ^{13}C NMR spectroscopy. *Macromolecules*, **12**(5), 1001–7.

[14] Triplett, D. A. 1979. Heparin: biochemistry, therapy, and laboratory monitoring. *Ther. Drug Monit.*, **1**(2), 173–97.

[15] Linhardt, R. J. and Gunay, N. S. 1999. Production and chemical processing of low molecular weight heparins. *Semin. Thromb. Hemost.*, **25**(Suppl. 3), 5–16.

[16] Suh, J. K. and Matthew, H. W. 2000. Application of chitosan-based polysaccharide biomaterials in cartilage tissue engineering: a review. *Biomaterials*, **21**(24), 2589–98.

[17] Chandy, T. and Sharma, C. P. 1990. Chitosan – as a biomaterial. *Biomater. Artif. Cells Artif. Organs*, **18**(1), 1–24.

[18] Kumar, G., Smith, P. J. and Payne, G. F. 1999. Enzymatic grafting of a natural product onto chitosan to confer water solubility under basic conditions. *Biotechnol. Bioeng.*, **63**(2), 154–65.

[19] Baldwin, A. D. and Kiick, K. L. 2010. Polysaccharide-modified synthetic polymeric biomaterials. *Biopolymers*, **94**(1), 128–40.

[20] Lansdown, A. B. and Payne, M. J. 1994. An evaluation of the local reaction and biodegradation of calcium sodium alginate (Kaltostat) following subcutaneous implantation in the rat. *J. R. Coll. Surg. Edinb.*, **39**(5), 284–8.

[21] Gilchrist, T. and Martin, A. M. 1983. Wound treatment with Sorbsan - an alginate fibre dressing. *Biomaterials*, **4**(4), 317–20.

[22] Augst, A. D., Kong, H. J. and Mooney, D. J. 2006. Alginate hydrogels as biomaterials. *Macromol. Biosci.*, **6**(8), 623–33.

[23] Rowley, J. A., Madlambayan, G. and Mooney, D. J. 1999. Alginate hydrogels as synthetic extracellular matrix materials. *Biomaterials*, **20**(1), 45–53.

[24] Naessens, M., Cerdobbel, A., Soetaert, W. and Vandamme, E. J. 2005. Leuconostoc dextransucrase and dextran: production, properties and applications. *J. Chem. Technol. Biotechnol.*, **80**(8), 845–60.

[25] Kamath, K. R. and Park, K. 1995. Study on the release of invertase from enzymatically degradable dextran hydrogels. *Polymer Gels Networks*, **3**(3), 243–54.

[26] Massia, S. P., Stark, J. and Letbetter, D. S. 2000. Surface-immobilized dextran limits cell adhesion and spreading. *Biomaterials*, **21**(22), 2253–61.

[27] Franssen, O., van Ooijen, R. D., de Boer, D., Maes, R. A. A. and Hennink, W. E. 1999. Enzymatic degradation of cross-linked dextrans. *Macromolecules*, **32**(9), 2896–902.

[28] Kiani, C., Chen, L., Wu, Y. J., Yee, A. J. and Yang, B. B. 2002. Structure and function of aggrecan. *Cell Res.*, **12**(1), 19–32.

[29] Fthenou, E., Zafiropoulos, A., Tsatsakis, A. *et al.* 2006. Chondroitin sulfate A chains enhance platelet derived growth factor-mediated signalling in fibrosarcoma cells. *Int. J. Biochem. Cell Biol.*, **38**(12), 2141–50.

[30] Swann, D. A., Radin, E. L., Nazimiec, M. *et al.* 1974. Role of hyaluronic acid in joint lubrication. *Ann. Rheum. Dis.*, **33**(4), 318–26.

[31] Damus, P. S., Hicks, M. and Rosenberg, R. D. 1973. Anticoagulant action of heparin. *Nature*, **246**(5432), 355–7.

[32] Lindahl, U. and Roden, L. 1966. The chondroitin 4-sulfate-protein linkage. *J. Biol. Chem.*, **241**(9), 2113–19.

[33] Doege, K. J., Sasaki, M., Kimura, T. and Yamada, Y. 1991. Complete coding sequence and deduced primary structure of the human cartilage large aggregating proteoglycan, aggrecan. Human-specific repeats, and additional alternatively spliced forms. *J. Biol. Chem.*, **266**(2), 894–902.

[34] Mow, V. C., Radcliffe, A. and Poole, A. R. 1992. Cartilage and diarthrodial joints as paradigms for hierarchical materials and structures. *Biomaterials*, **13**, 67–97.

[35] Sanchez-Adams, J., Willard, V. P. and Athanasiou, K. A. 2011. Regional variation in the mechanical role of knee meniscus glycosaminoglycans. *J. Appl. Physiol.*, **111**(6), 1590–6.

[36] Le Maitre, C. L., Pockert, A., Buttle, D. J., Freemont, A. J. and Hoyland J. A. 2007. Matrix synthesis and degradation in human intervertebral disc degeneration. *Biochem. Soc. Trans.*, **35**(Part 4), 652–5.

[37] Lapčík, L. Jr., Lapčík, L., De Smedt, S., Demeester, J. and Chabrecek, P. 1998. Hyaluronan: preparation, structure, properties, and applications. *Chem. Rev.*, **98**(8), 2663–84.

[38] van der Harst, M. R., Brama, P. A., van de Lest, C. H. *et al.* 2004. An integral biochemical analysis of the main constituents of articular cartilage, subchondral and trabecular bone. *Osteoarthritis Cartilage*, **12**(9), 752–61.

[39] Prince, C. W. and Navia, J. M. 1983. Glycosaminoglycan alterations in rat bone due to growth and fluorosis. *J. Nutr.*, **113**(8), 1576–82.

[40] Miyazaki, T., Miyauchi, S., Tawada, A., Anada, T. and Matsuzaka, S. 2010. Effect of chondroitin sulfate-E on the osteoclastic differentiation of RAW264 cells. *Dent. Mater. J.*, **29**(4), 403–10.

[41] Fujii, Y., Fujii, K., Nakano, K. and Tanaka, Y. 2003. Crosslinking of CD44 on human osteoblastic cells upregulates ICAM-1 and VCAM-1. *FEBS Lett.*, **539**(1–3), 45–50.

[42] Pivetta, E., Scapolan, M., Wassermann, B. *et al.* 2011. Blood-derived human osteoclast resorption activity is impaired by hyaluronan–CD44 engagement via a p38-dependent mechanism. *J. Cell Physiol.*, **226**(3), 769–79.

[43] Miyazaki, T., Miyauchi, S., Tawada A. *et al.* 2008. Over-sulfated chondroitin sulfate-E binds to BMP-4 and enhances osteoblast differentiation. *J. Cell Physiol.*, **217**(3), 769–77.

[44] Nikitovic, D., Zafiropoulos, A., Tzanakakis, G. N., Karamanos, N. K. and Tsatsakis, A. M. 2005. Effects of glycosaminoglycans on cell proliferation of normal osteoblasts and human osteosarcoma cells depend on their type and fine chemical compositions. *Anticancer Res.*, **25**(4), 2851–6.

[45] Bernstein, E. F., Underhill, C. B., Hahn, P. J., Brown, D. B. and Uitto, J. 1996. Chronic sun exposure alters both the content and distribution of dermal glycosaminoglycans. *Br. J. Dermatol.*, **135**(2), 255–62.

[46] Witt, D. P. and Lander, A. D. 1994. Differential binding of chemokines to glycosaminoglycan subpopulations. *Curr. Biol.*, **4**(5), 394–400.

[47] Termeer, C., Benedix, F., Sleeman, J. *et al.* 2002. Oligosaccharides of hyaluronan activate dendritic cells via toll-like receptor 4. *J. Exp. Med.*, **195**(1), 99–111.

[48] West, D. C., Shaw, D. M., Lorenz, P., Adzick, N. S. and Longaker, M. T. 1997. Fibrotic healing of adult and late gestation fetal wounds correlates with increased hyaluronidase activity and removal of hyaluronan. *Int. J. Biochem. Cell Biol.*, **29**(1), 201–10.

[49] Novak, U. and Kaye, A. H. 2000. Extracellular matrix and the brain: components and function. *J. Clin. Neurosci.*, **7**(4), 280–90.

[50] Pratt, R. M., Larsen, M. A. and Johnston, M. C. 1975. Migration of cranial neural crest cells in a cell-free hyaluronate-rich matrix. *Dev. Biol.*, **44**(2), 298–305.

[51] Yamaguchi, Y. 2000. Lecticans: organizers of the brain extracellular matrix. *Cell Mol. Life Sci.*, **57**(2), 276–89.

[52] Prabhakar, V., Capila, I., Bosques, C. J., Pojasek, K. and Sasisekharan, R. 2005. Chondroitinase ABC I from *Proteus vulgaris*: cloning, recombinant expression and active site identification. *Biochem. J.*, **386**(Part 1), 103–12.

[53] Silver, J. and Miller, J. H. 2004. Regeneration beyond the glial scar. *Nature Rev. Neurosci.*, **5**(2), 146–56.

[54] Hassell, J. R., Cintron, C., Kublin, C. and Newsome, D. A. 1983. Proteoglycan changes during restoration of transparency in corneal scars. *Arch. Biochem. Biophys.*, **222**(2), 362–9.

[55] Chakravarti, S., Petroll, W. M., Hassell, J. R. *et al.* 2000. Corneal opacity in lumican-null mice: defects in collagen fibril structure and packing in the posterior stroma. *Invest. Ophthalmol. Vis. Sci.*, **41**(11), 3365–73.

[56] Hart, G. W. 1976. Biosynthesis of glycosaminoglycans during corneal development. *J. Biol. Chem.*, **251**(21), 6513–21.

[57] Trochon, V., Mabilat, C., Bertrand, P. *et al.* 1996. Evidence of involvement of CD44 in endothelial cell proliferation, migration and angiogenesis in vitro. *Int. J. Cancer*, **66**(5), 664–8.

[58] Ausprunk, D. H. 1982. Synthesis of glycoproteins by endothelial cells in embryonic blood vessels. *Dev. Biol.*, **90**(1), 79–90.

[59] Ofosu, F. A., Modi, G. J., Smith, L. M. *et al.* 1984. Heparan sulfate and dermatan sulfate inhibit the generation of thrombin activity in plasma by complementary pathways. *Blood*, **64**(3), 742–7.

[60] Wight, T. N. 2002. Versican: a versatile extracellular matrix proteoglycan in cell biology. *Curr. Opin. Cell Biol.*, **14**(5), 617–23.

[61] Hinek, A., Wrenn, D. S., Mecham, R. P. and Barondes, S. H. 1988. The elastin receptor: a galactoside-binding protein. *Science*, **239**(4847), 1539–41.

[62] Hocking, A. M., Shinomura, T. and McQuillan, D. J. 1998. Leucine-rich repeat glycoproteins of the extracellular matrix. *Matrix Biol.*, **17**(1), 1–19.

[63] Lee, Y., Chung, H. J., Yeo, S. *et al.* 2010. Thermo-sensitive, injectable, and tissue adhesive sol–gel transition hyaluronic acid/pluronic composite hydrogels prepared from bio-inspired catechol–thiol reaction. *Soft Matter*, **6**(5), 977–83.

[64] Ryu, J. H., Lee, Y., Kong, W. H. *et al.* 2011. Catechol-functionalized chitosan/pluronic hydrogels for tissue adhesives and hemostatic materials. *Biomacromolecules*, **12**(7), 2653–9.

[65] Bhattarai, N., Ramay, H. R., Gunn, J., Matsen, F. A. and Zhang, M. 2005. PEG-grafted chitosan as an injectable thermosensitive hydrogel for sustained protein release. *J. Control. Release*, **103**(3), 609–24.

[66] Huang, X., Zhang, Y., Donahue, H. J. and Lowe, T. L. 2007. Porous thermoresponsive-co-biodegradable hydrogels as tissue-engineering scaffolds for 3-dimensional in vitro culture of chondrocytes. *Tissue Eng.*, **13**(11), 2645–52.

[67] Mørch, Y. A., Donati, I., Strand, B. L. and Skjåk-Braek, G. 2006. Effect of Ca^{2+}, Ba^{2+}, and Sr^{2+} on alginate microbeads. *Biomacromolecules*, **7**(5), 1471–80.

[68] Hoffman, A. S. 2002. Hydrogels for biomedical applications. *Adv. Drug Deliv. Rev.*, **54**(1), 3–12.

[69] Denuzière, A., Ferrier, D., Damour, O. and Domard, A. 1998. Chitosan–chondroitin sulfate and chitosan–hyaluronate polyelectrolyte complexes: biological properties. *Biomaterials*, **19**(14), 1275–85.

[70] Villanueva, I., Gladem, S. K., Kessler, J. and Bryant, S. K. 2010. Dynamic loading stimulates chondrocyte biosynthesis when encapsulated in charged hydrogels prepared from poly(ethylene glycol) and chondroitin sulfate. *Matrix Biol.*, **29**(1), 51–62.

[71] Gerecht, S., Burdick, J. A., Ferreira, L. S. *et al.* 2007. Hyaluronic acid hydrogel for controlled self-renewal and differentiation of human embryonic stem cells. *Proc. Nat. Acad. Sci. USA*, **104**(27), 11298–303.

[72] Zhang, Y. and Chu, C. C. 2001. Biodegradable dextran–polylactide hydrogel network and its controlled release of albumin. *J. Biomed. Mater. Res.*, **54**(1), 1–11.

[73] Kolb, H. C., Finn, M. G. and Sharpless, K. B. 2001. Click chemistry: diverse chemical function from a few good reactions. *Angew. Chem. Int. Ed. Engl.*, **40**(11), 2004–21.

[74] Manzl, C., Enrich, J., Ebner, H., Dallinger, R. and Krumschnabel, G. 2004. Copper-induced formation of reactive oxygen species causes cell death and disruption of calcium homeostasis in trout hepatocytes. *Toxicology*, **196**(1–2), 57–64.

[75] Hu, X., Li, D., Zhou, F. and Gao, C. 2011. Biological hydrogel synthesized from hyaluronic acid, gelatin and chondroitin sulfate by click chemistry. *Acta Biomater.*, **7**(4), 1618–26.

[76] Tan, H., Rubin, J. P. and Marra, K. G. 2009. Injectable *in situ* forming biodegradable chitosan–hyaluronic acid based hydrogels for cartilage tissue engineering. *Biomaterials*, **30**(13), 2499–506.

[77] Hiemstra, C., Aa, L. J., Zhong, Z., Dijkstra, P. J. and Feijen, J. 2007. Rapidly *in situ*-forming degradable hydrogels from dextran thiols through Michael addition. *Biomacromolecules*, **8**(5), 1548–56.

[78] Strehin, I., Ambrose, W. M., Schein, O., Salahuddin, A. and Elisseeff, A. 2009. Synthesis and characterization of a chondroitin sulfate–polyethylene glycol corneal adhesive. *J. Cataract Refract. Surg.*, **35**(3), 567–76.

[79] Jin, R., Moreira Teixeira, L. S., Dijkstra, P. J. 2009. Injectable chitosan-based hydrogels for cartilage tissue engineering. *Biomaterials*, **30**(13), 2544–51.

[80] Chen, T., Embree, H. D., Brown, E. M., Taylor, M. M. and Payne, G. F. 2003. Enzyme-catalyzed gel formation of gelatin and chitosan: potential for *in situ* applications. *Biomaterials*, **24**(17), 2831–41.

[81] Kurisawa, M., Chung, J. E., Yang, Y. Y., Gao, S. J. and Uyama, H. 2005. Injectable biodegradable hydrogels composed of hyaluronic acid–tyramine conjugates for drug delivery and tissue engineering. *Chem. Commun.*, (34), 4312–14.

[82] Ko, C. S., Huang, J. P., Huang, C. W. and Chu, I. M. 2009. Type II collagen–chondroitin sulfate–hyaluronan scaffold cross-linked by genipin for cartilage tissue engineering. *J. Biosci. Bioeng.*, **107**(2), 177–82.

[83] Selmi, T. A., Verdonk, P., Chambat, P. *et al.* 2008. Autologous chondrocyte implantation in a novel alginate–agarose hydrogel: outcome at two years. *J. Bone Joint Surg. Br.*, **90**(5), 597–604.

[84] Varghese, S., Hwang, N. S., Canver, A. C. *et al.* 2008. Chondroitin sulfate based niches for chondrogenic differentiation of mesenchymal stem cells. *Matrix Biol.*, **27**(1), 12–21.

[85] Jin, R., Teixeira, L. S., Dijkstra, P. J. *et al.* 2010. Enzymatically-crosslinked injectable hydrogels based on biomimetic dextran–hyaluronic acid conjugates for cartilage tissue engineering. *Biomaterials*, **31**(11), 3103–13.

[86] Wang, D. A., Varghese, S., Sharma, B. *et al.* 2007. Multifunctional chondroitin sulphate for cartilage tissue-biomaterial integration. *Nature Mater.*, **6**(5), 385–92.

[87] Kon, E., Gobbi, A., Filardo, G. *et al.* 2011. Second-generation autologous chondrocyte implantation: results in patients older than 40 years. *Am. J. Sports Med.*, **39**(8), 1668–75.

[88] Nehrer, S., Domayer, S., Dorotka, R. *et al.* 2006. Three-year clinical outcome after chondrocyte transplantation using a hyaluronan matrix for cartilage repair. *Eur. J. Radiol.*, **57**(1), 3–8.

[89] Buschmann, M. D. H., Hoemann, C. D., Hurtig, M. B. and Shive, M. S. 2007. Cartilage repair with chitosan–glycerol phosphate-stabilized blood clots. In *Cartilage Repair Strategies*, ed. Williams R. J. III. Totowa, NJ: Humana Press.

[90] Shive, M. S., Hoemann, C. D., Restrepo, A. *et al.* 2006. BST-CarGel: *in situ* chondroinduction for cartilage repair. *Operative Techniques Orthopaedics*, **16**(4), 8.

[91] Stephan, S. J., Tholpady, S. S., Gross, B. *et al.* 2010. Injectable tissue-engineered bone repair of a rat calvarial defect. *Laryngoscope*, **120**(5), 895–901.

[92] Alsberg, E., Anderson, K. W., Albeiruti, A., Franceschi, R. T. and Mooney, D. J. 2001. Cell-interactive alginate hydrogels for bone tissue engineering. *J. Dent. Res.*, **80**(11), 2025–9.

[93] Tanaka, K., Goto, T., Miyazaki, T. *et al.* 2011. Apatite-coated hyaluronan for bone regeneration. *J. Dent. Res.*, **90**(7), 906–11.

[94] Yannas, I. V. and Burke, J. F. 1980. Design of an artificial skin. I. Basic design principles. *J. Biomed. Mater. Res.*, **14**(1), 65–81.

[95] Sun, G., Zhang, X., Shen, Y. I. *et al.* 2011. Dextran hydrogel scaffolds enhance angiogenic responses and promote complete skin regeneration during burn wound healing. *Proc. Nat. Acad. Sci. USA*, **108**(52), 20976–81.

[96] Lee, W. R., Park, J. H., Kim, K. H. *et al.* 2009. The biological effects of topical alginate treatment in an animal model of skin wound healing. *Wound Repair Regen.*, **17**(4), 505–10.

[97] Uccioli, L., Giurato, L., Ruotolo, V. *et al.* 2011. Two-step autologous grafting using HYAFF scaffolds in treating difficult diabetic foot ulcers: results of a multicenter, randomized controlled clinical trial with long-term follow-up. *Int. J. Low Extrem. Wounds*, **10**(2), 80–5.

[98] Leipzig, N. D., Giurato, L., Ruotolo, V. *et al.* 2011. Differentiation of neural stem cells in three-dimensional

growth factor-immobilized chitosan hydrogel scaffolds. *Biomaterials*, **32**(1), 57–64.

[99] Park, J. S., Chu, J. S., Tsou, A. D. *et al.* 2011. The effect of matrix stiffness on the differentiation of mesenchymal stem cells in response to TGF-β. *Biomaterials*, **32**(16), 3921–30.

[100] Wei, Y. T., He, Y., Xu, C. L. *et al.* 2010. Hyaluronic acid hydrogel modified with nogo-66 receptor antibody and poly-L-lysine to promote axon regrowth after spinal cord injury. *J. Biomed. Mater. Res. B Appl. Biomater.*, **95**(1), 110–17.

[101] Raines, A. L., Sunwoo, M., Gertzmann, A. A. *et al.* 2011. Hyaluronic acid stimulates neovascularization during the regeneration of bone marrow after ablation. *J. Biomed. Mater. Res. Part A*, **96**(3), 575–83.

[102] Liu, Y. and Chan-Park, M. B. 2009. Hydrogel based on interpenetrating polymer networks of dextran and gelatin for vascular tissue engineering. *Biomaterials*, **30**(2), 196–207.

[103] Pandis, L., Zavan, B., Abatangelo, B. *et al.* 2010. Hyaluronan-based scaffold for in vivo regeneration of the rat vena cava: preliminary results in an animal model. *J. Biomed. Mater. Res. Part A*, **93**(4), 1289–96.

[104] Re'em, T., Kaminer-Israeli, Y., Ruvinov, E. and Cohen, S. 2012. Chondrogenesis of hMSC in affinity-bound TGF-β scaffolds. *Biomaterials*, **33**(3), 751–61.

[105] Lee, K. W., Yoon, J. J., Lee J. H. *et al.* 2004. Sustained release of vascular endothelial growth factor from calcium-induced alginate hydrogels reinforced by heparin and chitosan. *Transplant. Proc.*, **36**(8), 2464–5.

[106] Ruvinov, E., Leor, J. and Cohen, S. 2011. The promotion of myocardial repair by the sequential delivery of IGF-1 and HGF from an injectable alginate biomaterial in a model of acute myocardial infarction. *Biomaterials*, **32**(2), 565–78.

[107] Sánchez, M., Anitua, E., Azofra, J. *et al.* 2007. Comparison of surgically repaired Achilles tendon tears using platelet-rich fibrin matrices. *Am. J. Sports Med.*, **35**(2), 245–51.

[108] Fortier, L. A., Potter, H. G., Rickey, E. J. *et al.* 2010. Concentrated bone marrow aspirate improves full-thickness cartilage repair compared with microfracture in the equine model. *J. Bone Joint Surg. Am.*, **92**(10), 1927–37.

[109] Gobbi, A., Karnatzikos, G., Scotti, C. 2011. One-step cartilage repair with bone marrow aspirate concentrated cells and collagen matrix in full-thickness knee cartilage lesions: results at 2-year follow-up. *Cartilage*, **2**(3), 14.

[110] Marx, R. E. 2001. Platelet-rich plasma (PRP): what is PRP and what is not PRP? *Implant. Dent.*, **10**(4), 225–8.

[111] Wong, D. A., Kumar, A., Jatana, S., Ghiselli, G. and Wong, K. 2008. Neurologic impairment from ectopic bone in the lumbar canal: a potential complication of off-label PLIF/TLIF use of bone morphogenetic protein-2 (BMP-2). *Spine J.*, **8**(6), 1011–18.

[112] Canter, H. I., Vargel, I., Korkusuz, P. *et al.* 2010. Effect of use of slow release of bone morphogenetic protein-2 and transforming growth factor-β-2 in a chitosan gel matrix on cranial bone graft survival in experimental cranial critical size defect model. *Ann. Plast. Surg.*, **64**(3), 342–50.

[113] Kolambkar, Y. M., Dupont, K. M., Boerckel, J. D. *et al.* 2011. An alginate-based hybrid system for growth factor delivery in the functional repair of large bone defects. *Biomaterials*, **32**(1), 65–74.

[114] Jeon, O., Powell, C., Solorio, L. D., Krebs, M. D. and Alsberg, E. 2011. Affinity-based growth factor delivery using biodegradable, photocrosslinked heparin-alginate hydrogels. *J. Control. Release*, **154**(3), 258–66.

[115] Wood, M. D., Moore, A. M., Hunter, D. A. *et al.* 2009. Affinity-based release of glial-derived neurotrophic factor from fibrin matrices enhances sciatic nerve regeneration. *Acta Biomater.*, **5**(4), 959–68.

[116] Xu, H., Yan, Y. and Li, S. 2011. PDLLA/chondroitin sulfate/chitosan/NGF conduits for peripheral nerve regeneration. *Biomaterials*, **32**(20), 4506–16.

[117] Marx, R. E., Carlson, E. R., Eichstaedt, R. M. *et al.* 1998. Platelet-rich plasma: growth factor enhancement for bone grafts. *Oral Surg. Oral Med. Oral Pathol. Oral Radiol. Endod.*, **85**(6), 638–46.

[118] Lu, H. H., Vo, J. M., Chin, H. S. *et al.* 2008. Controlled delivery of platelet-rich plasma-derived growth factors for bone formation. *J. Biomed. Mater. Res. Part A*, **86**(4), 1128–36.

[119] Oktay, E. O., Demiralp, B., Demiralp, B. *et al.* 2010. Effects of platelet-rich plasma and chitosan combination on bone regeneration in experimental rabbit cranial defects. *J. Oral Implantol.*, **36**(3), 175–84.

[120] Strehin, I., Nahas, Z., Arora, K., Nguyen, T. and Elisseeff, J. 2010. A versatile pH sensitive chondroitin sulfate-PEG tissue adhesive and hydrogel. *Biomaterials*, **31**(10), 2788–97.

[121] Chenault, H. K., Bhatia, S. K., Dimaio, W. G. *et al.* 2011. Sealing and healing of clear corneal incisions with an improved dextran aldehyde-PEG amine tissue adhesive. *Curr. Eye Res.*, **36**(11), 997–1004.

[122] Artzi, N., Shazly, T., Crespo, C. *et al.* 2009. Characterization of star adhesive sealants based on PEG/dextran hydrogels. *Macromolec. Biosci.*, **9**(8), 754–65.

Functionalized poly(ethylene glycol) hydrogels for controlling stem cell fate

Chien-Chi Lin

15.1 Introduction

An emerging trend in tissue engineering and regenerative medicine is the design of scaffolds that recapitulate a stem cell's extracellular microenvironment, or "niche" (Cushing and Anseth 2007; Tibbitt and Anseth 2009). While the exact constituents of a stem cell niche are not well characterized, it is generally believed that morphogens, immobilized extracellular matrix (ECM) components, cell–cell interactions, and matrix elasticity are the major determinants that direct stem cell self-renewal or differentiation (Lutolf and Hubbell 2005). Research over the years has accumulated fundamental knowledge about stem cell biology in vitro. Most of the results were obtained from experiments conducting on flat, rigid, and two-dimensional (2D) tissue culture polystyrene (TCPS). These 2D environments, however, might not truly reproduce what a stem cell experiences in vivo, where relevant biological and biophysical cues are produced in a far more complex and spatially and temporally regulated manner. In fact, results from numerous studies have demonstrated that, compared with cell culture on TCPS, stem cells behave differently when cultured in three-dimensional (3D) matrices (Liu and Roy 2005; Ingber *et al.* 2006; Lee *et al.* 2008b; Lund *et al.* 2009).

Artificial matrices of synthetic or natural origins have been developed for culturing stem cells in 3D (Lee *et al.* 2008b; Lund *et al.* 2009). While natural ECM components, such as collagen and laminin, provide intrinsic biological recognition sites for cell attachment and migration, these natural matrices are ill-defined and poorly controlled with respect to their compositions and mechanical properties, respectively. Furthermore, one cannot afford to overlook the immunogenicity problems associated with allogenic or xenogenic materials, since this significantly limits the clinical translatability/relevance of stem-cell-based therapy. Matrices fabricated from synthetic polymers, on the other hand, provide well-defined and user-controllable chemical and physical properties (Nuttelman *et al.* 2008). The use of synthetic matrices, however, is not without challenges, insofar as synthetic polymers usually lack biological motifs for cellular recognition. Hence, significant efforts have been dedicated to fabricating synthetic polymeric scaffolds functionalized with biomimetic motifs that permit cellular interaction.

In general, synthetic polymers for regenerative medicine applications are prepared in one of the following three forms: porous scaffolds, fibrous scaffolds, and hydrogels (Lee *et al.* 2008b). The focus of this chapter is on hydrogels fabricated from poly(ethylene glycol) (PEG), with emphasis on synthetic approaches to functionalize PEG hydrogels for controlling stem cell fate in 3D. The PEG-based macromers constitute a class of synthetic polymers that possess many favorable properties, namely tissue-like elasticity, high water content, solute permeability, and biocompatibility. While the backbone of the PEG macromer ($[CH_2CH_2O]_n$) does not contain any biological recognition sites, the chemistry used to fabricate PEG-based hydrogels allows facile conjugation of bioactive molecules during gel crosslinking. Various chemistries have been developed for the conjugation of bioactive molecules into a PEG hydrogel to render the otherwise inert gels bioactive, including, but not limited to, homopolymerization of acrylates; thiol–acrylate, thiol–vinylsulfone, and thiol–ene polymerizations; and orthogonal "click" chemistry such as azide–alkyne Huisgen cycloaddition reactions. With these concepts in mind, this chapter will discuss (1) synthetic methods to create functionalized PEG hydrogels; (2) the utility of these hydrogels to permit and/or promote survival, self-renewal, and differentiation of stem/progenitor cells; (3) applications of functionalized PEG hydrogels in cartilage, bone, cardiovascular, and neural tissue engineering; and (4) the challenges of, and outlook for, functionalized PEG hydrogels in regenerative medicine.

15.2 PEG hydrogel chemistry and engineering

15.2.1 Chain growth and mixed-mode polymerizations

PEG hydrogels can be synthesized from chain-growth polymerizations using a variety of macromers (Nuttelman *et al.* 2008). Figure 15.1 illustrates commonly used macromers with PEG backbones and terminal vinyl groups (acrylates or methacrylates). The propagation of radicals by these vinyl groups results in a crosslinked hydrogel network. Among these macromers, PEG diacrylate (PEGDA) and PEG dimethacrylate (PEGDMA) have been widely used to fabricate hydrogels for controlled release, tissue engineering, and regenerative medicine applications. While hydrogels formed from crosslinking of PEGDA or PEGDMA are non-degradable on therapeutically relevant time scales, hydrolytic or enzymatic degradable segments can be easily incorporated into the macromer backbone (Figure 15.2). The "stealth" property of PEG makes these hydrogels "inert" to attachment of cells and adhesion/absorption of biomolecules, such as proteins. Thus, functional groups must be covalently incorporated within PEG hydrogels to impart bioactivity. This can be easily achieved through co-polymerizing monoacrylate-terminated peptides/proteins (Hern and Hubbell 1998). A widely used conjugation scheme is depicted in Figure 15.3(a), where acrylate groups can be introduced to peptides/proteins via reactions between primary amines and the N-hydroxysuccinimide (NHS) moiety on a bi-functional crosslinker, such as acryl–PEG–NHS (Hern and Hubbell 1998).

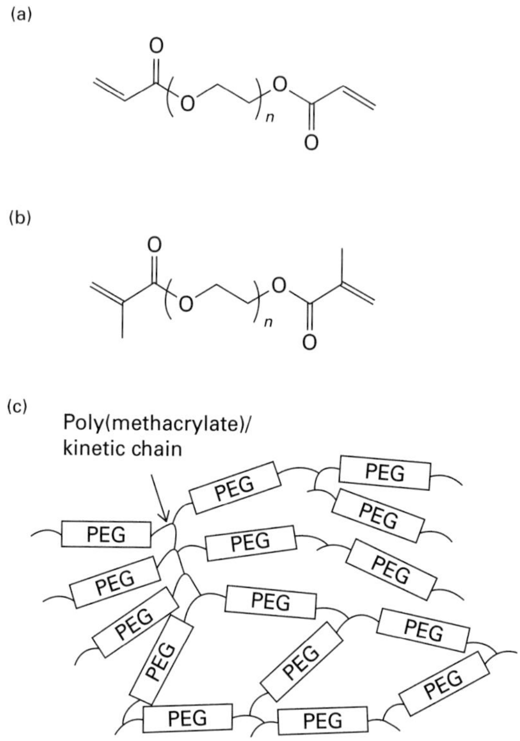

Figure 15.1 (a) The chemical structure of poly(ethylene glycol) diacrylate (PEGDA). (b) The chemical structure of PEG dimethacrylate (PEGDM). (c) A schematic representation of PEG hydrogels formed by chain-growth polymerization of PEGDA or PEGDM (the arrow indicates a poly(meth acrylate) kinetic chain).

Peptides or proteins with one or more sulfhydryl groups can also be covalently incorporated into PEG hydrogels through a mixed-mode photopolymerization (Salinas and Anseth 2008a). Figure 15.3(b) illustrates the mechanism of mixed-mode thiol–acrylate polymerization and incorporation of biomolecules, such as peptides. In principle, the polymerization mechanism shifts toward step-growth crosslinking when a higher-thiol-containing molecule is used (Rydholm *et al.* 2005). The major benefit of this scheme is that thiol-containing peptide mimetics can be easily incorporated into PEG hydrogels without additional

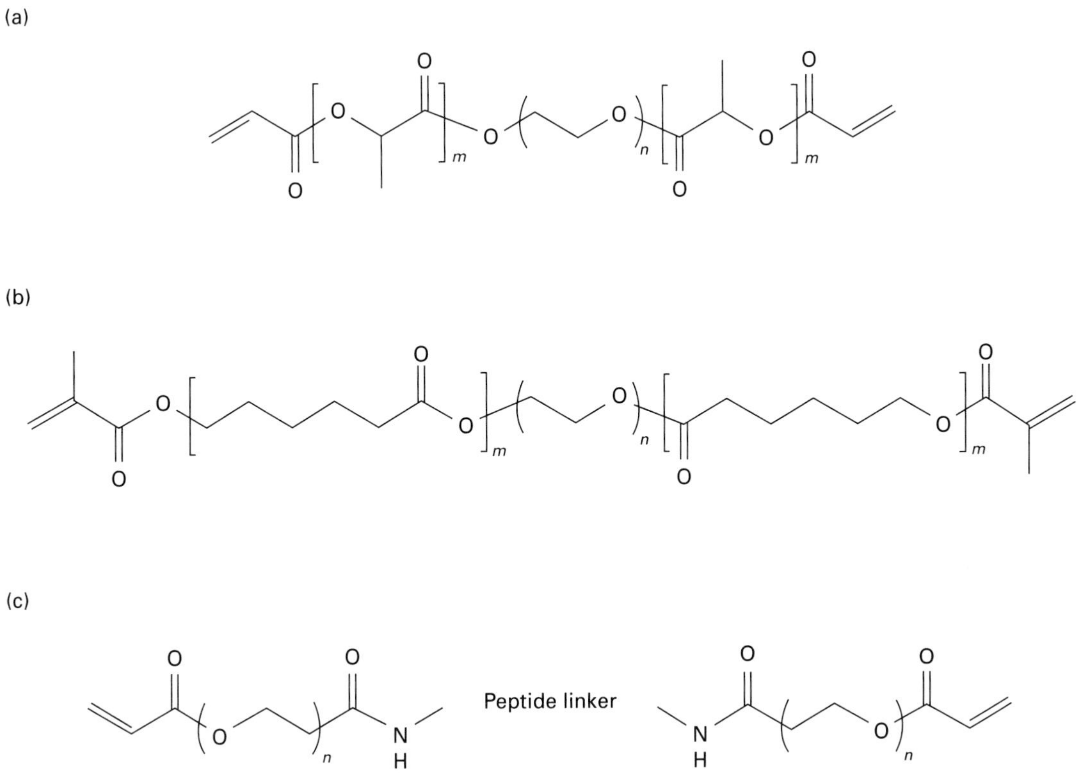

Figure 15.2 The chemical structures of (a) PLA-PEG-PLA, (b) PCL-PEG-PCL, and (c) PEG-peptide-PEG. All macromers bear diacrylates for crosslinking to form hydrogels.

modification. However, mixed-mode polymerizations can cause steric hindrance (rendering sites not accessible for biological interactions) for some peptides due to their close proximity to the polyacrylate kinetic chains (Figure 15.3(b)). Peptides with additional spacers inserted between the cysteine and bioactive motifs have been used to increase affinity binding of soluble proteins (Lin *et al.* 2010) or to enhance mesenchymal stem cell viability in PEG hydrogels (Salinas and Anseth 2008c).

15.2.2 Step growth polymerizations

15.2.2.1 Michael-type addition

Step-growth polymerizations create hydrogels with homogeneous network structure and with better mechanical properties than those of chain-growth polymerized gels with similar crosslinking densities (Figure 15.4) (Lutolf and Hubbell 2003b; Fairbanks *et al.* 2009). Step-growth PEG hydrogels prepared from Michael-type addition reactions have been used widely in tissue engineering and regenerative medicine applications. The formation of Michael-addition hydrogels is typically achieved through base-catalyzed nucleophilic addition between multifunctional PEG-vinylsulfone (Figure 15.5A) or PEG-acrylate with bis-cysteine peptide crosslinkers (Lutolf and Hubbell 2003a; Lutolf *et al.* 2003). The use of matrix metalloprotinases (MMPs)-sensitive peptide linkers (e.g. C̲GPQG↓IWGQC̲, where underlines indicate added cysteines for crosslinking while the arrow indicates the enzyme cleavage site) permits cell-mediated local gel degradation, which facilitates cellular activities, such as migration,

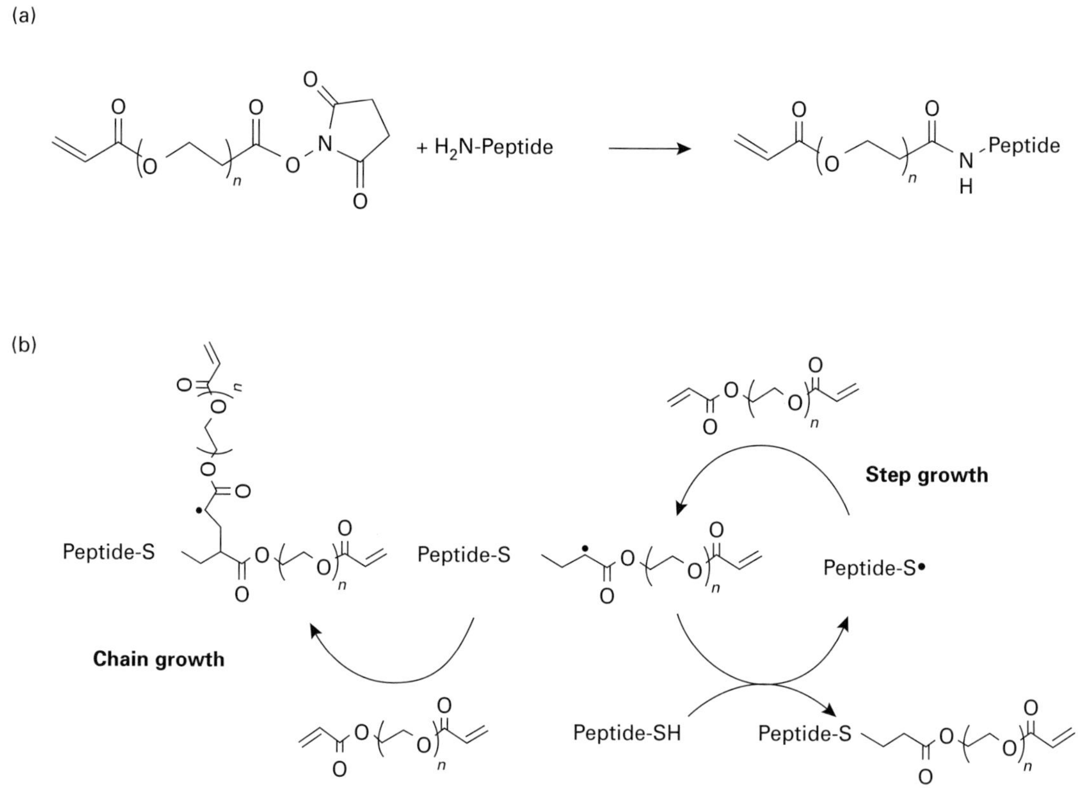

Figure 15.3 (a) Peptide acrylation with acryl-PEG-NHS. (b) Mixed-mode photo-polymerization to incorporate cysteine-containing peptides in PEGDA hydrogels.

proliferation, and differentiation. Bioactive motifs including cell-adhesive ligands (e.g. fibronectin-derived peptide Arg–Gly–Asp or RGD) are incorporated within these hydrogels through conjugating mono-cysteine-containing peptides with functionalized PEG macromers (e.g. vinylsulfone) during network crosslinking.

15.2.2.2 Thiol–norbornene photopolymerization

A radical-mediated, step-growth photopolymerization scheme, termed thiol–norbornene or thiol–ene photopolymerization, has also been developed to form hydrogels (Fairbanks *et al.* 2009). In this scheme, norbornene-functionalized multi-arm PEG macromers (Figure 15.5(b)) react with thiol-containing peptides via step-growth photopolymerization to form hydrogels. Compared with Michael-type conjugation hydrogels, thiol–ene polymerizations produce hydrogels with faster gelation kinetics (gel points within seconds) and lower degrees of network defects. Owing to its photoinitiated crosslinking, the thiol–ene reaction also permits spatial–temporal control over gelation kinetics. The incorporation of pendent bioactive motifs is similar to that described in the previous section, whereby mono-cysteine peptides are incorporated during network formation.

15.2.2.3 Orthogonal "click" chemistry

In addition to Michael-type and thiol–ene reactions, other orthogonal reactions or click chemistries have

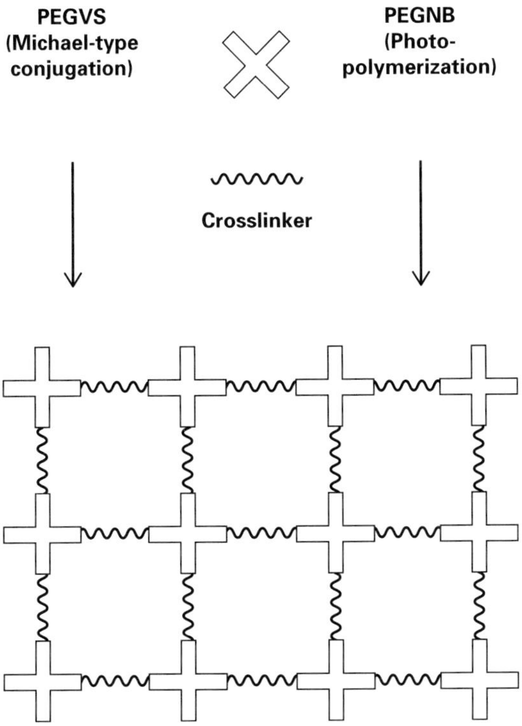

Figure 15.4 A schematic representation of PEG hydrogels formed by step-growth polymerization. PEG-vinylsulfone (PEGVS) or PEG-norbornene (PEGNB) reacts with bis-cysteine-containing peptide crosslinker via Michael-type conjugation or radical-mediated thiol–ene photo-polymerization, respectively, to form an idealized hydrogel network. (See Figure 15.5 for the chemical structures of PEGVS and PEGNB.)

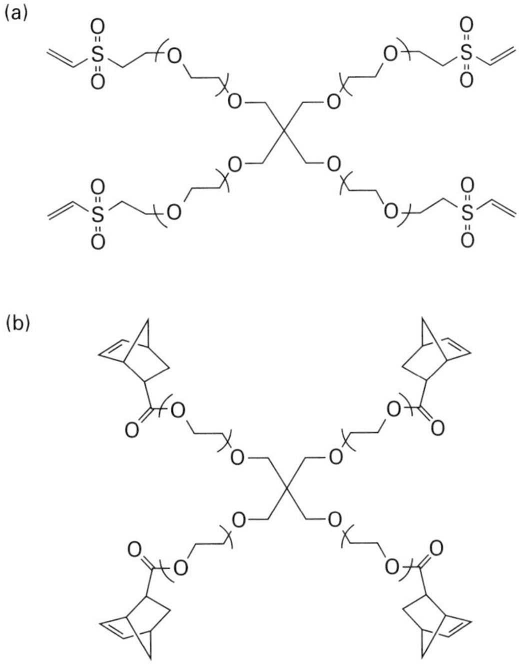

Figure 15.5 The chemical structures of (a) four-arm PEG-vinylsulfone (PEGVS) and (b) four-arm PEG-norbornene (PEGNB).

been developed to form PEG-based hydrogels, such as copper-catalyzed azide–alkyne cycloaddition (CuAAC) (Polizzotti *et al.* 2008), a metal-free cyclooctyne–azide click reaction (DeForest *et al.* 2009, 2010), native chemical ligation (Hu *et al.* 2009, 2010), and Diels–Alder reaction (Rimmer *et al.* 1999; Wei *et al.* 2010). The major advantage of these chemoselective chemistries is that initiator is not required for initiating gel crosslinking (except for CuAAC, where cytotoxic copper is used as a catalyst). To functionalize these "click" hydrogels, the same crosslinking motifs (e.g. alkyne, azide, thioester, etc.) as are used to crosslink gels are conjugated on the bioactive components for covalent immobilization during gel crosslinking.

15.2.3 *In situ* modulation of PEG hydrogel properties

While the methods described above have proven useful in controlling initial gel formulations to improve cell survival, most of them do not permit dynamic modification of gel bioactivity for spatiotemporally directing cell fate processes. During morphogenesis, stem cells receive complex biophysical and biochemical signals from the extracellular matrix. To mimic these delicately orchestrated events, research efforts have focussed on designing hydrogels that permit spatial–temporal modification of gel structural and functional properties. The first biomaterial strategy to demonstrate the feasibility of spatial–temporal control of bioconjugation was an agarose hydrogel system developed by Shoichet *et al.* Briefly, a photolabile motif (2-nitrobenzyl-protected cysteine) was incorporated into the hydrogels to guide 3D cell growth and migration (Luo and Shoichet 2004). Upon UV exposure, the 2-nitrobenzyl group is cleaved, leaving a free sulphydryl group for further conjugation with maleimide-terminated molecules. Using this technique, biomolecules (e.g. RGDS) can be patterned in 3D to guide cell migration in defined regions. While this is an elegant design, no "*in situ*" (i.e. in the presence of cells) modification is permitted, potentially due to the use of the cytotoxic maleimide group.

Anseth and her colleagues have made significant advancements in dynamically tunable hydrogels exploiting similar chemistries (Kloxin *et al.* 2009). In this system, a photolabile nitrobenzyl group was incorporated in crosslinkable PEG macromers or peptide termini. Hydrogels were formed via redox crosslinking, and the gel crosslinking density can be subsequently tuned in a spatial–temporal manner by controlling the dosage of UV light exposure. When the photolabile group was incorporated into PEG macromers, the network properties (e.g. elasticity, permeability, etc.) of such hydrogels can be altered using light exposure. On the other hand, when the photolabile group was incorporated on pendent peptide motifs, these peptides can be liberated with light. More importantly, the modification of hydrogel structural or functional properties can be performed in the presence of cells. Photolabile hydrogels have been used to control cell morphology and potentially can be used to direct stem cell differentiation (Kloxin *et al.* 2009, 2010).

Another approach to control the presentation of bioactive motifs is through photoconjugation of bioactive peptides, such as RGD, into hydrogels formed via orthogonal click chemistry. For instance, Polizzotti *et al.* synthesized "click" PEG hydrogels by reacting alkyne-functionalized PEG macromers with azide-terminated peptides (Polizzotti *et al.* 2008). One unique feature of this hydrogel platform was the incorporation of a lysine with an Aloc-protected side chain in the azide-terminated peptide crosslinker. Following the azide–alkyne click reactions to form hydrogels, thiol-containing bioactive peptides can be patterned within the pre-formed hydrogels through the allyl ester motif on the Aloc-protected lysine. One disadvantage of this chemistry is the use of cytotoxic metal catalyst that precludes *in situ* cell encapsulation. DeForest *et al.* (2009, 2010) further improved this gel platform by replacing the alkyne functionality with a cyclooctyne group that had originally been developed by the Bertozzi group (Baskin *et al.* 2007). This metal-free click chemistry retains the ability to photoconjugate bioactive peptide motifs while allowing *in situ* encapsulation of cells within hydrogels.

The biochemical properties of step-growth thiol–ene hydrogels can also be modified following network polymerization (Fairbanks *et al.* 2009). This was achieved by utilizing an excess amount of ene functionality during network crosslinking. Owing to the step-growth nature of the reaction, the excess amount of ene groups will remain available for further reactions to introduce sulphydryl-group-containing bioactive functionalities within cell-laden hydrogels. The Anseth group used this approach to pattern RGDS peptides in 3D and to control adhesion of fibroblasts within defined regions in a PEG hydrogel (Fairbanks *et al.* 2009). The spatial–temporal modification of hydrogel properties in the presence of cells may be useful to direct stem cell differentiation in discrete patterns.

15.3 Functionalized PEG hydrogels for directing stem and progenitor cell fate

15.3.1 Incorporating ECM components in PEG hydrogels to control stem cell fate in 3D

PEG hydrogels offer a "blank slate" for studying the influence of defined ECM components on stem cell fate processes. An intuitive approach to constructing a bioactive and instructive artificial ECM is to use components derived from natural ECM, including laminin, fibronectin, and collagen. It has been shown that the presence of fibronectin promotes stem cell attachment to otherwise non-adhesive hydrogels (Jongpaiboonkit *et al.* 2009), while laminin and collagen are crucial ECM proteins that maintain survival and potency of embryonic stem cells (Baskin *et al.*

2007; Lee *et al.* 2010) and mesenchymal stem cells (MSC) (Hwang *et al.* 2010). The most common method of incorporating these matrix proteins in hydrogels is through physical entrapment (i.e. forming hydrogels in the presence of soluble matrix proteins). The large molecular weights (more formally, relative molecular masses) ($>$100 kDa) of these matrix proteins prohibit their rapid diffusion from the permeable gels. Entrapped ECM components such as collagen and laminin have been shown to promote the survival and function of pancreatic β-cells (Weber *et al.* 2008) and enhance the differentiation of insulin-secretion cells from progenitor cells in PEG hydrogels (Mason *et al.* 2009; Mason and Mahoney 2010).

In addition to physical entrapment, ECM proteins such as fibronectin have been "PEGylated" with PEG diacrylate (PEGDA) through Michael-type addition and subsequently crosslinked into hydrogels via chain-growth photopolymerizations (Almany and Seliktar 2005; Dikovsky *et al.* 2006; Gonen-Wadmany *et al.* 2007). These gels have been used as 3D culture platforms for hESC-derived cardiomyocytes and rat neonatal cardiac cells (Shapira-Schweitzer *et al.* 2009). One downside of this approach is that the ECM proteins were denatured using reducing agents to expose internal cysteine residues for PEGylation. Thus, care must be taken to achieve well-tuned reaction conditions for maintaining the bioactivity of the ECM components (Gonen-Wadmany *et al.* 2011).

While large ECM molecules possess multiple epitopes for cell recognition, they are also prone to denaturation due to the sensitive nature of protein tertiary/quaternary structures. To increase the stability of biological motifs, oligopeptides derived from ECM proteins have been incorporated into bioinert hydrogels (Hern and Hubbell 1998). The most notable example is the use of fibronectin-derived peptide, Arg–Gly–Asp (RGD). Since its discovery in the 1980s (Pierschbacher and Ruoslahti 1984), the RGD sequence has been widely used in promoting integrin-mediated cell adhesion. In synthetic biomaterials such as the PEG hydrogels described here, the covalent incorporation of RGD peptide within the gel matrix is becoming a common practice to improve cell viability. To covalently conjugate RGD (or other bioactive peptides) within PEG hydrogels, Hern and Hubbell used N-hydroxysuccinimidyl-activated esters (either directly linked to acrylic acid or with a PEG spacer) to introduce an acrylate moiety to the N-terminal α-amine of the peptide (Hern and Hubbell 1998). These acrylated peptides are subsequently co-polymerized with PEGDA to render the otherwise inert PEG hydogels cell-adhesive or bioactive. This approach is extremely useful in promoting the survival and osteogenic differentiation of encapsulated hMSCs (Nuttelman *et al.* 2005).

Recent advances in bioconjugation chemistry have provided diverse schemes for easy and efficient incorporation of peptides in PEG hydrogels. As described earlier in this chapter, Anseth's group has utilized mixed-mode thiol–acrylate photopolymerizations to covalently conjugate cysteine-containing peptides within PEG hydogels (Salinas and Anseth 2008a, 2008c). This approach has been used to create adhesive PEG hydrogels for promoting the survival and directed differentiation (osteogenic, chondrogenic, and adipogenic differentiation) of hMSC (Salinas and Anseth 2008a, 2008c).

In addition to RGD, other peptide motifs derived from ECM components have shown potential for directing stem/progenitor cell fate processes in 3D. For example, Elisseeff and colleagues designed PEG hydrogels incorporating collagen-mimetic peptide (CMP) for chondrogenic differentiation of MSC (Lee *et al.* 2006, 2008a). In this approach, CMP was acrylated using acryloyl–PEG–NHS and subsequently conjugated within PEGDA hydrogels using chain-growth photopolymerization. The MSCs encapsulated in CMP/PEG hydrogels showed higher expression of chondrogenic markers and secreted more glycosaminoglycans (GAGs) and collagen-II (Lee *et al.* 2006). Different CMP sequences (e.g. GFOGER) were conjugated to PEG hydrogels via Michael-type conjugation to enhance chondrogenic differentiation of hMSC (Liu *et al.* 2010).

15.3.2 Affinity PEG hydrogels for controlling stem/progenitor cell fate in 3D

Researchers are often inspired by the diverse functions of the ECM when designing artificial hydrogel matrices for directing stem cell fate (Lutolf and Hubbell 2005). In addition to providing integrin-binding sites for cell attachment, the ECM also serves as a reservoir for growth factors. During embryogenesis, the ECM regulates the availability and bioactivity of growth factors and creates complex morphogen gradients to guide stem cell development, including migration, proliferation, and differentiation. The ability of the ECM to preserve bioactive growth factors stems from its high water content and the presence of charged polysaccharides, such as heparin sulfate proteoglycan, that can sequester and regulate the release of growth factors. Inspired by this mechanism, heparin has been used extensively to regulate the delivery of growth factors from synthetic or natural hydrogel matrices. Sakiyama-Elbert and Hubbell pioneered the development of heparin-functionalized fibrin matrices for controlled delivery of several growth factors critical in tissue morphogenesis, such as nerve growth factor (NGF) (Sakiyama-Elbert and Hubbell 2000a) and basic fibroblast growth factor (bFGF) (Sakiyama-Elbert and Hubbell 2000b). In this approach, heparin was sequestered by an affinity peptide that was enzymatically crosslinked within the fibrin matrix. The sequestered heparin then binds to soluble growth factors. The release of growth factor was regulated by heparin–growth-factor and heparin–peptide affinity, as well as fibrin matrix degradation.

Affinity-based sequestration of heparin in a degradable matrix could lead to unexpected complications after heparin was released from the matrix, since heparin is an anti-coagulant and could cause thrombocytopenia. Alternatively, heparin could be covalently incorporated within a permissive PEG hydrogel network for regulating the survival, function, and morphogenesis of stem and progenitor cells. The hydroxyl groups on heparin sulfate can be modified with methacrylate groups using methacrylic anhydride (Benoit *et al.* 2007), yielding methacrylated heparin that can be co-polymerized with PEG dimethacrylate. Immobilized heparin has been shown to regulate the activation of valvular interstitial cells (VICs) (Cushing *et al.* 2007). The interactions of immobilized or soluble heparin with other growth factors (e.g. bFGF or TGF-β) have been shown to have diverse effects on the differentiation and phenotypes of VICs. In addition to its effect on vascular cells, immobilized heparin also increased the adhesion and survival of hMSCs in PEG hydrogels (Benoit *et al.* 2007). The interplay between heparin and bone morphogenic protein 2 (BMP-2) has also been shown to increase osteogenic differentiation of encapsulated hMSCs (Benoit *et al.* 2007).

The use of heparin to regulate growth factor delivery has inspired many excellent bioactive hydrogel platforms. The binding of heparin to growth factors, however, is mostly based on non-specific electrostatic interactions. This non-specificity may cause unwanted interactions with other proteins when the heparin-containing hydogel matrices are implanted in vivo. To overcome this potential complication, small affinity binders, such as oligopeptides, with specific affinity for growth factors have been identified and incorporated within PEG hydrogels. Many affinity peptide sequences have been used for sequestering growth factors and are potentially useful in biomaterial and stem cell applications, such as KRTGQYKL for bFGF (Lin and Anseth 2009), sulfated tetrapeptide $SY(SO_3)DY(SO_3)$ for VEGF (Maynard and Hubbell 2005), and 12-mer consensus peptides identified from a phage-display library for NGF (Willerth *et al.* 2007).

In addition to affinity-based binding of growth factors, peptide sequences identified from cytokine receptor binding motifs have been incorporated in PEG hydrogels to regulate cytokine-induced cell damage. For example, WP9QY, a tumor necrosis factor-α (TNF-α) antagonist, has been covalently immobilized in PEG hydrogels for maintaining the osteogenic differentiation potential of hMSCs (Lin *et al.* 2009). Furthermore, an interleukin-1β (IL-1β) receptor binding peptide agonist has been used to protect pancreatic β-cells against IL-1β (Su *et al.* 2010). Similar approaches may have significant implication in vivo for encapsulated stem cells, since the inflammatory response to implanted biomaterials is inevitable.

15.3.3 Incorporating bioactive components in PEG hydrogels for controlling stem cell fate in 3D

The biomimetic approaches outlined in the above sections focussed on incorporating native ECM components within bio-inert PEG hydrogels. In addition to immobilized motifs, other bioactive molecules also play pivotal roles in tissue morphogenesis. Innovative research has focussed on the immobilization of growth factors to direct cell fate processes in 3D. For example, vascular endothelial growth factor (VEGF) has been covalently immobilized within PEG hydrogels for improving angiogenesis in vivo and in vitro. West and colleagues have developed a series of biomimetic PEG hydrogels immobilized with VEGF (Leslie-Barbick *et al.* 2009, 2011a, 2011b) or some other cell surface receptor (e.g. ephrin-A1) (Moon *et al.* 2007; Saik *et al.* 2011a) to promote tubule formation from the encapsulated endothelial cells. The chemistry for growth factor immobilization is similar to that for immobilizing peptides. Growth factors can be acrylated or thiolated for chain-growth or mixed-mode polymerizations and incorporated into PEG hydrogels during cell encapsulation. Other robust bioconjugation techniques (e.g. EDC/NHS chemistry for carboxylate–amine conjugation) can also be used to pre-conjugate growth factors on polymer chains prior to incorporation within cell-laden hydrogels. The bivalent binding affinity of VEGF to heparin has also been used to assemble PEG hydrogels and release VEGF upon competitive cell surface receptor binding (Nie *et al.* 2007; Yamaguchi *et al.* 2007). Immobilizing growth factors on surfaces or within hydrogels has proven beneficial in guiding cell migration, a critical step toward complex tissue organization.

In addition to VEGF, BMP-2 is another important component that has great influence in stem cell differentiation. While most investigators have utilized BMP-2 in soluble form, biomimetic BMP-2 peptides have recently been utilized to promote osteogenic differentiation of mesenchymal stem cells. For example, Murphy *et al.* designed modular peptide growth factor that contains a mineral-binding domain and a BMP-2 mimetic sequence (Lee *et al.* 2009; Lee and Murphy 2010). This design allows the modular peptide growth factor to simultaneously interact with stem cells and biomaterial surfaces. Jabbari and colleagues synthesized an azide-containing BMP-mimetic peptide for orthogonal conjugation onto PEG hydrogel substrates for promoting osteogenic differentiation of marrow stromal cells (He *et al.* 2008).

Dexamethasone, a potent osteogenic differentiation cue, has been routinely added in osteogenic culture media for differentiation of stem/progenitor cells into osteoblasts. Anseth and co-workers developed dexamethasone-functionalized PEG hydrogels for enhancing osteogenic differentiation of MSCs (Nuttelman *et al.* 2006). The synthetic approach employed to immobilize releasable dexamethasone within PEG hydrogels involved three-step synthesis. PEG–monomethacrylate (PEGMMA) was first reacted with D,L-lactide through a ring opening polymerization to yield PEGMMA–Lac, which was subsequently reacted with succinic anhydride to produce PEGMMA–Lac–Suc. Dexamethasone was then coupled to PEGMMA–Lac–Suc using standard diisopropylcarbodiimide (DCC) coupling. Depending on the number of lactide groups incorporated, the rate of dexamethasone release can be tuned. That the released dexamethasone was bioactive was demonstrated by confirming its ability to induce a high level of osteogeneic differentiation. Similar synthetic approaches have been utilized to incorporate releasable fluvastatin to affect MSCs, where fluvastatin increases MSC BMP2 production, resulting in autocrine signaling and osteogenic differentiation (Benoit *et al.* 2006).

15.3.4 Instructive microenvironment for stem/progenitor cell development

During development, stem/progenitor cells constantly remodel their extracellular environment. The ECM contains complex mesh of fibrous proteins such as collagen, laminin, and glycosaminoglycans (GAGs). Proteolysis is one mechanism by which cells "clear" their path for spreading, migration, or proliferation. Inspired by this approach, biomaterial scientists have developed a variety of matrices capable of instructing cellular development. For example, Hubbell and Lutolf have demonstrated the usefulness of this gel platform in understanding basic cell biology and as scaffolding materials for tissue regeneration. Specifically, Michael-type addition was used to crosslink multi-arm PEG–vinylsulfone macromers with bis-cysteine-containing MMP-sensitive peptides (Lutolf *et al.* 2003a, 2003b). Cell-adhesive ligands such as RGD were conjugated within the hydrogel network to allow for cell adhesion. Cells embedded within these MMP-sensitive hydrogels were able to locally remodel the matrix due to the secretion of various MMPs (e.g. MMP-1, -2, -3, -7, -8, -9, -13, and -14). It has also been shown that these cell-instructive PEG hydrogels enhanced bone regeneration, new vessel formation, and cardiomyoprogenitor cell differentiation (Kraehenbuehl *et al.* 2008).

A relatively new technique to construct cell-instructive hydrogels is the use of thiol–norbornene photopolymerization (Fairbanks *et al.* 2009), which produces a similar network structure to that obtained with the Michael-type hydrogels. In addition to the spatial and temporal control over gelation kinetics, a unique feature of thiol–norbornene photopolymerization is that it permits the conjugation of bioactive motifs dynamically using a secondary thiol–ene photo-click reaction and in the presence of cells. This technique facilitates the design of synthetic matrices to mimic the dynamic nature of ECM, from which to guide cell morphogenesis in 3D.

Another important guidance cue that stem cells receive during development is morphogen gradients. It is challenging to mimic this complex spatial and temporal presentation of growth factors in synthetic matrices. Degradable polymeric microparticles loaded with growth factors could be easily entrapped within cell-laden hydogels due to their large size (on the order of micrometers) compared with the mesh size of typical hydrogels (on the order of nanometers). Upon the degradation of the microparticles and release of entrapped growth factors, cells could be differentiated down specific lineages. These microparticles could also be distributed in a spatially regulated manner, from which to generate a growth factor concentration gradient for directing cell migration or differentiation.

Recently, bioconjugation techniques have been developed to immobilize growth factor gradients within hydrogels. These immobilized growth factors have been found in some cases to be more potent than their soluble form. Angiogenic growth factors, such as platelet-derived growth factor (PDGF), bFGF, and VEGF, have been immobilized within PEG hydrogels to promote angiogenesis (Zieris *et al.* 2010; Saik *et al.* 2011b). Laser scanning lithography has been used to spatially pattern RGDS and VEGF on the surface of PEG hydrogels for guiding endothelial cell adhesion and tubule formation (Leslie-Barbick *et al.* 2011b). Using a gradient maker, West and colleagues developed PEG hydrogels with an immobilized bFGF gradient capable of inducing smooth muscle cell migration (DeLong *et al.* 2005). To covalently immobilize bFGF, protein acrylation was achieved using acryl–PEG–NHS, a technique identical to that used to acrylate oligopeptides. These techniques potentially can be used to create 3D patterns within hydrogels for promoting cellular processes in a spatially and temporally regulated manner.

While spatially patterned hydrogel microenvironments are useful to control cell morphogenesis, this level of control is limited and cannot entirely recapitulate the dynamic nature of a stem cell niche. To dynamically modulate hydrogel biochemical and biomechanical properties to guide cell morphogenesis, a system must have the ability to present or remove certain signals during cell development. In other words, a temporal regulation of hydrogel biochemical and biophysical properties holds the key to truly recapitulate stem cell development. In this regard, the Anseth group has pioneered the development of dynamic hydrogels as artificial stem cell niches. In one example, RGD motifs were removed in a cell-dependent manner due to the addition of an MMP-sensitive peptide linker between RGD and the crosslinking site (e.g. acrylate or cysteine) (Salinas and Anseth 2008a). This technique is particularly useful in promoting chondrogenesis since persistent integrin binding has been shown to inhibit chondrogenic differentiation of MSCs (Salinas and Anseth 2008b). Recently, a photolabile nitrobenzo group was introduced in between the acrylate and polymer backbone or acrylate and pendent peptide to create dynamic hydrogel systems capable of decreasing gel crosslinking density or removing/releasing bioactive peptide to guide cell development (Kloxin *et al.* 2009, 2010).

15.4 Functionalized PEG hydrogels for stem-cell-mediated tissue regeneration

15.4.1 Cartilage and bone regeneration

Functionalized PEG hydrogels have been used for cartilage and bone regeneration for over a decade. MSCs, ESCs, and adult chondrocytes have all been encapsulated in functionalized PEG hydrogels for regenerating damaged bone or cartilage. Some applications have made significant progress and are in pre-clinical trials. PEG hydrogels are particularly useful in cartilage regeneration due to their high water content and tunable gel elasticity that mimics the native articular cartilage microenvironment. PEG hydrogels functionalized with the RGD motif have been used to encapsulate and guide chondrogenesis of MSCs and ESCs both in vitro and in vivo. One challenge facing chondrogenesis of stem cells in functionalized PEG hydrogels is regeneration of the osteochondral interface. While it may be challenging to achieve using a single hydrogel composition, a recent example illustrated the possibility of engineering articular cartilage constructs including the osteochondral interface using multilayer PEG-based hydrogels (Nguyen *et al.* 2011). In this example, hydrogel layers containing different compositions were, to some degree, reminiscent of the native articular cartilage microenvironment (chondroitin sulfate and MMP-sensitive peptide in the top layer or the superficial zone; chondroitin sulfate in the middle layer or the transitional zone; hyaluronic acid in the bottom layer or the deep zone). The encapsulated MSCs were differentiated to have different characteristics due to the variations in biochemical and biomechanical properties of the layered hydrogels.

Bone tissue engineering has also benefited from the development of functionalized PEG hydrogels. MSCs encapsulated in functionalized PEG hydrogels can be easily directed down the osteogenic lineage. However, a significant challenge facing functionalized PEG hydrogels designed for bone tissue engineering is how to tether the gel degradation profile while retaining preferred functionalities and structural integrity to achieve maximum bone healing. It has been shown that healing of bone defects was hindered when PEG hydrogels were non-degradable (Rizzi *et al.* 2006; Terella *et al.* 2010). Furthermore, many degradable hydrogels produce acidic degradation products, which causes unwanted inflammation that further delays proper bone healing. Cyclic acetal-modified PEG hydrogels, which produce neutral degradation products, have recently been demonstrated to support bone marrow stromal stem cell survival for osteogenic differentiation (Kaihara *et al.* 2009).

15.4.2 Cardiovascular regeneration and angiogenesis

The tunable elasticity of PEG hydrogels makes them suitable materials for cardiovascular tissue engineering applications. Recently developed hydrogel chemistries and engineering approaches have proven useful in studying vascular progenitor cell biology. For example, altering the matrix stiffness (by changing the hydrogel crosslinking density or locally modulating gel degradation) resulted in changes of valvular interstitial cell (VIC) morphogenesis (Ingber *et al.* 2006; Kloxin *et al.* 2010). While VICs underwent myofibroblastic differentiation on stiffer substrates (32 kPa), they were de-differentiated to fibroblastic phenotypes when substrate stiffness was decreased (to 7 kPa) *in situ*. This unique example demonstrated real-time cell phenotype modulation using proper hydrogel matrices. In another example, PEGylated fibronectin was incorporated within chain-growth-photopolymerized PEG hydrogels for cardiomyocyte encapsulation. The effects of cell density and matrix stiffness were studied to promote spontaneous cardiomyocyte contraction (Shapira-Schweitzer and Seliktar 2007).

Functionalized PEG hydrogels are important matrices for studying and promoting angiogenesis. West and colleagues developed biomimetic PEG hydrogels formed by chain-growth photopolymerization. These hydrogels were MMP-degradable and were immobilized with biomimetic motifs such as RGD, growth factors (PDGF, VEGF, etc.), and EphA receptor binding ligand (ephrinA1) (Moon *et al.* 2007; Leslie-Barbick *et al.* 2009, 2011a, 2011b; Saik, *et al.* 2011a, 2011b). Vascular endothelial cells formed vascular networks within these biomimetic PEG hydrogels. Notably, the newly formed vasculatures were more stable when smooth muscle cells were co-encapsulated within hydrogels (Moon *et al.* 2010), demonstrating the importance of multicellular interactions (cell-matrix and cell–cell interactions) for promoting angiogenesis.

15.4.3 Neural regeneration

PEG hydrogels are good material candidates for neural tissue engineering because their mechanical properties can be easily tuned (by changing macromer concentrations) to match the requirement of a low modulus (a few hundred Pa) for promoting neural stem/progenitor cell proliferation (Banerjee *et al.* 2009; Lampe *et al.* 2010). Similarly to other cell types, the survival and proliferation of neural cells also depends upon the conjugation of functional motifs within hydrogels. Thus, it is critical to simultaneously maintain soft material properties while allowing facile conjugation of bioactive ligands in chemically cross-linked hydrogels. Werner and colleagues recently synthesized star-PEG–heparin hydrogels with independently tuned gel modulus and heparin content for studying in vitro and in vivo neuronal cell adhesion and differentiation (Freudenberg *et al.* 2009). The gelation was achieved by standard EDC/NHS chemistry that conjugates amine groups on multi-arm PEG and carboxylic acid groups on heparin. Additional bioactive motifs, such as the cell-adhesive ligand RGD, were conjugated to heparin using the same chemistry. Heparin was used not only for crosslinking the hydrogels, but also for binding to growth factors, including bFGF and VEGF. It was found that the presence of RGD supported primary attachment and colony growth of mouse neural stem cells (NSCs), while heparin-mediated bFGF release maintained NSCs in an undifferentiated state. The biocompatibility of this hybrid star-PEG–heparin hydrogel has been demonstrated in rats by transplanting the gel into the brain parenchyma, with the goal of using this approach to treat neurodegenerative diseases such as Parkinson's disease. Only a minimal inflammatory response was observed. Although the use of EDC/NHS chemistry prohibits *in situ* cell encapsulation, the modular nature of this PEG hydrogel sheds light on future hydrogel design for decoupling of multiple biophysical and biochemical properties.

15.5 Challenges and future outlook

Functionalized PEG hydrogels have proven valuable in various tissue engineering and regenerative medicine applications. However, challenges exist and researchers have begun to address these important issues. First, while the main purpose of incorporating bioactive motifs within PEG hydrogels is to direct stem/progenitor cell morphogenesis, these bioactive motifs (e.g. RGDS) may interact with inflammatory and immune cells in vivo. For example, recent reports have identified the effect of immobilized RGD ligand on inflammation (Lynn *et al.* 2010, 2011). Implanted PEG hydrogels immobilized with RGD motifs appeared to elicit a strong early inflammatory response, which was evidenced by persistent (over 2 weeks after implantation) infiltration of macrophages (Lynn *et al.* 2011). If the surface-exposed bioactive ligands adversely affect the inflammatory response, it may be difficult to achieve desired stem cell morphogenesis. Given the high permeability of PEG hydrogels, one must also consider the effect of host-mediated soluble immune mediators such as cytokines and chemokines. To address this issue, appropriate animal studies are required. From the perspective of polymer science and engineering, the discovery of diverse and cytocompatible polymerization mechanisms may improve the efficacy of functionalized PEG hydrogels to regulate host immune response for enhancing stem cell differentiation.

Another challenge facing tissue engineering using functionalized PEG hydrogels stems from the delicate balance between biophysical and biochemical cues, as well as intricate cellular interactions. Thus, it is critical to be able to independently control multiple biophysical and biochemical properties, from which to decouple the influence of specific extracellular signals on cellular development. Traditional 2D culture utilizes a reductionist approach to identify the effect of individual biochemical signals. When PEG hydrogels are employed for 3D cell culture, this approach becomes a major challenge because multiple material properties are linked (e.g. elasticity and permeability), and it is often difficult to decouple them. Research in new polymer chemistry and bioconjugation techniques, such as bio-orthogonal "click" reactions, may offer new tools for creating innovative hydrogel platforms for constructing an artificial stem cell niche for fundamental cell biology and regenerative medicine applications.

REFERENCES

Almany, L. and Seliktar, D. 2005. Biosynthetic hydrogel scaffolds made from fibrinogen and polyethylene glycol for 3D cell cultures. *Biomaterials*, **26**(15), 2467–77.

Banerjee, A., Arha, M., Choudhary, S. *et al.* (2009. The influence of hydrogel modulus on the proliferation and differentiation of encapsulated neural stem cells. *Biomaterials*, **30**(27), 4695–99.

Baskin, J. M., Prescher, J. A., Laughlin, S. T. *et al.* 2007. Copper-free click chemistry for dynamic in vivo imaging. *Proc. Nat. Acad. Sci. USA*, **104**(43), 16793–7.

Benoit, D. S. W., Durney, A. R. and Anseth, K. S. 2007. The effect of heparin-functionalized PEG hydrogels on three-dimensional human mesenchymal stem cell osteogenic differentiation. *Biomaterials*, **28**(1), 66–77.

Benoit, D. S. W., Nuttelman, C. R., Collins, S. D. and Anseth, K. S. 2006. Synthesis and characterization of a fluvastatin-releasing hydrogel delivery system to modulate hMSC differentiation and function for bone regeneration. *Biomaterials*, **27**(36), 6102–10.

Cushing, M. C. and Anseth, K. S. 2007. Hydrogel cell cultures. *Science*, **316**(5828), 1133–4.

Cushing, M. C., Liao, J. T., Jaeggli, M. P. and Anseth, K. S. 2007. Material-based regulation of the myofibroblast phenotype. *Biomaterials*, **28**(23), 3378–87.

DeForest, C. A., Polizzotti, B. D. and Anseth K. S. 2009. Sequential click reactions for synthesizing and patterning three-dimensional cell microenvironments. *Nature Mater.*, **8**(8), 659–64.

DeForest, C. A., Sims, E. A. and Anseth, K. S. 2010. Peptide-functionalized click hydrogels with independently tunable mechanics and chemical functionality for 3D cell culture. *Chem. Mater.*, **22**(16), 4783–90.

DeLong, S. A., Moon, J. J. and West, J. L. 2005. Covalently immobilized gradients of bFGF on hydrogel scaffolds for directed cell migration. *Biomaterials*, **26**(16), 3227–34.

Dikovsky, D., Bianco-Peled, H. and Seliktar, D. 2006. The effect of structural alterations of PEG-fibrinogen hydrogel scaffolds on 3-D cellular morphology and cellular migration. *Biomaterials*, **27**(8), 1496–506.

Fairbanks, B. D., Schwartz, M. P., Halevi, A. E. *et al.* 2009. A versatile synthetic extracellular matrix mimic via thiol-norbornene photopolymerization. *Adv. Mater.*, **21**(48), 5005–10.

Freudenberg, U., Hermann, A., Welzel, P. B. *et al.* 2009. A star-PEG-heparin hydrogel platform to aid cell replacement therapies for neurodegenerative diseases. *Biomaterials*, **30**(28), 5049–60.

Gonen-Wadmany, M., Goldshmid, R. and Seliktar, D. 2011. Biological and mechanical implications of PEGylating proteins into hydrogel biomaterials. *Biomaterials*, **32**(26), 6025–33.

Gonen-Wadmany, M., Oss-Ronen, L. and Seliktar, D. 2007. Protein-polymer conjugates for forming photopolymerizable biomimetic hydrogels for tissue engineering. *Biomaterials*, **28**(26), 3876–86.

He, X. Z., Ma, J. Y. and Jabbari, E. 2008. Effect of grafting RGD and BMP-2 protein-derived peptides to a hydrogel substrate on osteogenic differentiation of marrow stromal cells. *Langmuir*, **24**(21), 12508–16.

Hern, D. L. and Hubbell, J. A. 1998. Incorporation of adhesion peptides into nonadhesive hydrogels useful for tissue resurfacing. *J. Biomed. Mater. Res.*, **39**(2), 266–76.

Hu, B. H., Su, J. and Messersmith, P. B. 2009. Hydrogels cross-linked by native chemical ligation. *Biomacromolecules*, **10**(8), 2194–200.

Hwang, N. S., Varghese, S., Lee, H. J., Zhang, Z. and Elisseeff, J. 2010. Regulation of osteogenic and chondrogenic differentiation of mesenchymal stem cells in PEG-ECM hydrogels. *Cell Tissue Res.*, **344**(3), 499–509.

Ingber, D. E., Mow, V. C., Butter, D. *et al.* 2006. Tissue engineering and developmental biology: going biomimetic. *Tissue Eng.*, **12**(12), 3265–83.

Jongpaiboonkit, L., King, W. J., Lyons, G. E. *et al.* 2009. Screening for 3D environments that support human mesenchymal stem cell viability using hydrogel arrays. *Tissue Eng. Part A*, **15**(2), 343–53.

Kaihara, S., Matsumura, S. and Fisher, J. P. 2009. Cellular responses to degradable cyclic acetal modified PEG hydrogels. *J. Biomed. Mater. Res. Part A*, **90**(3), 863–73.

Kloxin, A. M., Benton, J. A. and Anseth, K. S. 2010. *In situ* elasticity modulation with dynamic substrates to direct cell phenotype. *Biomaterials*, **31**(1), 1–8.

Kloxin, A. M., Kasko, A. M., Salinas, C. N. and Anseth, K. S. 2009. Photodegradable hydrogels for dynamic tuning of physical and chemical properties. *Science*, **324**(5923), 59–63.

Kraehenbuehl, T. P., Zammaretti, P., Van der Vlies, A. J. 2008. Three-dimensional extracellular matrix-directed cardio-progenitor differentiation: systematic modulation of a synthetic cell-responsive PEG-hydrogel. *Biomaterials*, **29**(18), 2757–66.

Lampe, K. J., Mooney, R. G., Bjugstad, K. B. and Mahoney, M. J. 2010. Effect of macromer weight percent on neural cell growth in 2D and 3D nondegradable PEG hydrogel culture. *J. Biomed. Mater. Res. Part A*, **94**(4), 1162–71.

Lee, H. J., Lee, J. S., Chansakul, T. *et al.* 2006. Collagen mimetic peptide-conjugated photopolymerizable PEG hydrogel. *Biomaterials*, **27**(30), 5268–76.

Lee, H. J., Yu, C., Chansakul, T. *et al.* 2008a. Enhanced chondrogenesis of mesenchymal stem cells in collagen mimetic peptide-mediated microenvironment. *Tissue Eng. Part A*, **14**(11), 1843–51.

Lee, J., Cuddihy, M. J. and Kotov, N. A. 2008b. Three-dimensional cell culture matrices: state of the art. *Tissue Eng. Part B - Rev.*, **14**(1), 61–86.

Lee, J. S. and Murphy, W. L. 2010. Modular peptides promote human mesenchymal stem cell differentiation on biomaterial surfaces. *Acta Biomater.*, **6**(1), 21–8.

Lee, J. S., Lee, J. S., Wagoner-Johnson, A. and Murphy, W. L. 2009. Modular peptide growth factors for substrate-mediated stem cell differentiation. *Angewandte Chem. Int. Edition Engl.*, **48**(34), 6266–9.

Lee, S. T., Yun, J. I., Jo, Y. S. *et al.* 2010. Engineering integrin signaling for promoting embryonic stem cell self-renewal in a precisely defined niche. *Biomaterials*, **31**(6), 1219–26.

Leslie-Barbick, J. E., Moon, J. J. and West, J. L. 2009. Covalently-immobilized vascular endothelial growth factor promotes endothelial cell tubulogenesis in poly(ethylene glycol) diacrylate hydrogels. *J. Biomater. Sci. - Polymer Edition*, **20**(12), 1763–79.

Leslie-Barbick, J. E., Saik, J. E., Gould, D. J., Dickinson, M. E. and West, J. L. 2011a. The promotion of microvasculature formation in poly(ethylene glycol) diacrylate hydrogels by an immobilized VEGF-mimetic peptide. *Biomaterials*, **32**(25), 5782–9.

Leslie-Barbick, J. E., Shen, C., Chen C. S. and West, J. 2011b. Micron-scale spatially patterned, covalently immobilized vascular endothelial growth factor on hydrogels accelerates endothelial tubulogenesis and increases cellular angiogenic responses. *Tissue Eng. Part A*, **17**(1–2), 221–9.

Lin, C. C. and Anseth, K. S. 2009. Controlling affinity binding with peptide-functionalized poly(ethylene glycol) hydrogels. *Adv. Functional Mater.*, **19**(14), 2325–31.

Lin, C. C., Boyer, P. D., Aimetti, A. A. and Anseth, K. S. 2010. Regulating MCP-1 diffusion in affinity hydrogels for enhancing immuno-isolation. *J. Controlled Release*, **142**(3), 384–91.

Lin, C. C., Metters, A. T. and Anseth, K. S. 2009. Functional PEG–peptide hydrogels to modulate local inflammation induced by the pro-inflammatory cytokine TNF alpha. *Biomaterials*, **30**(28), 4907–14.

Liu, H. and Roy, K. 2005. Biomimetic three-dimensional cultures significantly increase hematopoietic differentiation efficacy of embryonic stem cells. *Tissue Eng.*, **11**(1–2), 319–30.

Liu, S. Q., Tian, Q. A., Hedrick, J. L. *et al.* 2010. Biomimetic hydrogels for chondrogenic differentiation of human mesenchymal stem cells to neocartilage. *Biomaterials*, **31**(28), 7298–307.

Lund, A. W., Yener, B., Stegemann, J. P. and Plopper, G. E. 2009. The natural and engineered 3D microenvironment as a regulatory cue during stem cell fate determination. *Tissue Eng. Part B - Rev.*, **15**(3), 371–80.

Luo, Y. and Shoichet, M. S. 2004. A photolabile hydrogel for guided three-dimensional cell growth and migration. *Nature Mater.*, **3**(4), 249–53.

Lutolf, M. P. and Hubbell J. A., 2003. Synthesis and physicochemical characterization of end-linked poly(ethylene glycol)-co-peptide hydrogels formed by Michael-type addition. *Biomacromolecules*, **4**(3), 713–22.

Lutolf, M. P. and Hubbell, J. A. 2005. Synthetic biomaterials as instructive extracellular microenvironments for morphogenesis in tissue engineering. *Nature Biotechnol.*, **23**(1), 47–55.

Lutolf, M. P., Lauer-Fields, J. L., Schmoekel, H. G. *et al.* 2003a. Synthetic matrix metalloproteinase-sensitive hydrogels for the conduction of tissue regeneration: engineering cell-invasion characteristics. *Proc. Nat. Acad. Sci. USA*, **100**(9), 5413–18.

Lutolf, M. P., Raeber, G. P., Zisch, A. H., Tirelli, N. and Hubbell, J. A. 2003b. Cell-responsive synthetic hydrogels. *Adv. Mater.* **15**(11), 888–92.

Lynn, A. D., Blakney, A. K., Kyriakides, T. R. and Bryant, S. J. 2011. Temporal progression of the host response to implanted poly(ethylene glycol)-based hydrogels. *J. Biomed. Mater. Res. Part A*, **96**(4), 621–31.

Lynn, A. D., Kyriakides, T. R. and Bryant, S. J. 2010. Characterization of the in vitro macrophage response and in vivo host response to poly(ethylene glycol)-based hydrogels. *J. Biomed. Mater. Res. Part A*, **93**(3), 941–53.

Mason, M. N., Arnold, C. A. and Mahoney, M. J. 2009. Entrapped collagen type 1 promotes differentiation of embryonic pancreatic precursor cells into glucose-responsive β-cells when cultured in three-dimensional PEG hydrogels. *Tissue Eng. Part A*, **15**(12), 3799–808.

Mason, M. N. and Mahoney, M. J. 2010. Inhibition of γ-secretase activity promotes differentiation of embryonic pancreatic precursor cells into functional islet-like clusters in poly(ethylene glycol) hydrogel culture. *Tissue Eng. Part A*, **16**(8), 2593–603.

Maynard, H. D. and Hubbell, J. A. 2005. Discovery of a sulfated tetrapeptide that binds to vascular endothelial growth factor. *Acta Biomater.*, **1**(4), 451–9.

Moon, J. J., Lee, S. H. and West, J. L. 2007. Synthetic biomimetic hydrogels incorporated with Ephrin-A1 for therapeutic angiogenesis. *Biomacromolecules*, **8**(1), 42–9.

Moon, J. J., Saik, J. E., Poché, R. A. *et al.* 2010. Biomimetic hydrogels with pro-angiogenic properties. *Biomaterials*, **31**(14), 3840–7.

Nguyen, L. H., Kudva, A. K., Saxena, N. S. and Roy, K. 2011. Engineering articular cartilage with spatially-varying matrix composition and mechanical properties from a single stem cell population using a multi-layered hydrogel. *Biomaterials*, **32**(29), 6946–52.

Nie, T., Baldwin, A., Yamaguchi, N. and Kiick, K. L. 2007. Production of heparin-functionalized hydrogels for the development of responsive and controlled growth factor delivery systems. *J. Controlled Release* **122**(3): 287–296.

Nuttelman, C. R., Rice, M. A., Rydholm, A. E. *et al.* 2008. Macromolecular monomers for the synthesis of hydrogel niches and their application in cell encapsulation and tissue engineering. *Prog. Polymer Sci.*, **33**(2), 167–79.

Nuttelman, C. R., Tripodi, M. C. and Anseth, K. S. 2005. Synthetic hydrogel niches that promote hMSC viability. *Matrix Biol.*, **24**(3), 208–18.

Nuttelman, C. R., Tripodi, M. C. and Anseth, K. S. 2006. Dexamethasone-functionalized gels induce osteogenic differentiation of encapsulated hMSCs. *J. Biomed. Mater. Res. Part A*, **76**(1), 183–95.

Pierschbacher, M. D. and Ruoslahti, E. 1984. Cell attachment activity of fibronectin can be duplicated by small synthetic fragments of the molecule. *Nature*, **309**, 30–3.

Polizzotti, B. D., Fairbanks, B. D. and Anseth, K. S. 2008. Three-dimensional biochemical patterning of click-based composite hydrogels via thiolene photopolymerization. *Biomacromolecules*, **9**(4), 1084–7.

Rimmer, S., Tattersall, P., Ebdon, J. R. and Fullwood, N. J. 1999. New strategies for the synthesis of amphiphilic networks. *Reactive Functional Polymers*, **41**(1–3), 177–84.

Rizzi, S. C., Ehrbar, M., Halstenberg, S. *et al.* 2006. Recombinant protein-co-PEG networks as cell-adhesive and proteolytically degradable hydrogel matrixes. Part II: biofunctional characteristics. *Biomacromolecules*, **7**(11), 3019–29.

Rydholm, A. E., Bowman, C. N. and Anseth, K. S. 2005. Degradable thiol–acrylate photopolymers: polymerization and degradation behavior of an *in situ* forming biomaterial. *Biomaterials*, **26**(22), 4495–506.

Saik, J. E., Gould, D. J., Keswani, A. H., Dickinson, M. E. and West, J. L. 2011a. Biomimetic hydrogels with immobilized ephrinA1 for therapeutic angiogenesis. *Biomacromolecules*, **12**(7), 2715–22.

Saik, J. E., Gould, D. J., Watkins, E. M., Dickinson, M. E. and West, J. L. 2011b. Covalently immobilized platelet-derived growth factor-BB promotes antiogenesis in biomimetic poly(ethylene glycol) hydrogels. *Acta Biomater.*, **7**(1), 133–43.

Sakiyama-Elbert, S. E. and Hubbell, J. A. 2000a. Controlled release of nerve growth factor from a heparin-containing fibrin-based cell ingrowth matrix. *J. Controlled Release*, **69**(1), 149–58.

Sakiyama-Elbert, S. E. and Hubbell, J. A. 2000b. Development of fibrin derivatives for controlled release of heparin-binding growth factors. *J. Controlled Release*, **65**(3), 389–402.

Salinas, C. N. and Anseth, K. S. 2008a. Mixed mode thiol-acrylate photopolymerizations for the synthesis of PEG–peptide hydrogels. *Macromolecules*, **41**(16), 6019–26.

Salinas, C. N. and Anseth, K. S. 2008b. The enhancement of chondrogenic differentiation of human mesenchymal stem cells by enzymatically regulated RGD functionalities. *Biomaterials*, **29**(15), 2370–7.

Salinas, C. N. and Anseth, K. S. 2008c. The influence of the RGD peptide motif and its contextual presentation in PEG gels on human mesenchymal stem cell viability. *J. Tissue Eng. Regen. Med.*, **2**(5), 296–304.

Shapira-Schweitzer, K., Habib, M., Gepstein, L. and Seliktar, D. 2009. A photopolymerizable hydrogel for 3-D culture of human embryonic stem cell-derived cardiomyocytes and rat neonatal cardiac cells. *J. Molec. Cellular Cardiol.*, **46**(2), 213–24.

Shapira-Schweitzer, K. and Seliktar, D. 2007. Matrix stiffness affects spontaneous contraction of cardiomyocytes cultured within a PEGylated fibrinogen biomaterial. *Acta Biomater.*, **3**(1), 33–41.

Su, J., Hu, B. H., Lowe, W. L. Jr., Kaufman, D. B. and Messersmith, P. B. 2010. Anti-inflammatory peptide-functionalized hydrogels for insulin-secreting cell encapsulation. *Biomaterials*, **31**(2), 308–14.

Terella, A., Mariner, P., Brown, N., Anseth, K. and Streubel, S. O. 2010. Repair of a calvarial defect with biofactor and stem cell-embedded polyethylene glycol scaffold. *Arch. Facial Plastic Surg.*, **12**(3), 166–71.

Tibbitt, M. W. and Anseth, K. S. 2009. Hydrogels as extracellular matrix mimics for 3D cell culture. *Biotechnol. Bioeng.*, **103**(4), 655–63.

Weber, L. M., Hayda, K. N., Haskins, K. and Anseth, K. S. 2008. Cell–matrix interactions improve β-cell survival and insulin secretion in three-dimensional culture. *Tissue Eng. Part A*, **14**(12), 1959–68.

Wei, H. -L., Yang, Z., Chen, Y. *et al.* 2010. Characterisation of N-vinyl-2-pyrrolidone-based hydrogels prepared by a Diels–Alder click reaction in water. *Eur. Polymer J.*, **46**(5), 1032–9.

Willerth, S. M., Johnson, P. J., Maxwell, D. J. *et al.* 2007. Rationally designed peptides for controlled release of nerve growth factor from fibrin matrices. *J. Biomed. Mater. Res. Part A*, **80**(1), 13–23.

Yamaguchi, N., Zhang, L., Chae, B.-S. *et al.* 2007. Growth factor mediated assembly of cell receptor-responsive hydrogels. *J. Am. Chem. Soc.*, **129**(11), 3040–1.

Zieris, A., Prokoph, S., Levental, K. R. *et al.* 2010. FGF-2 and VEGF functionalization of starPEG-heparin hydrogels to modulate biomolecular and physical cues of angiogenesis. *Biomaterials*, **31**(31), 7985–94.

16

Fumarate-based hydrogels in regenerative medicine applications

Steven Lu, Kyobum Kim, Johnny Lam, F. Kurtis Kasper and Antonios G. Mikos

16.1 Introduction

Hydrogels are an excellent scaffold structure for numerous applications in tissue engineering and regenerative medicine. In particular, they can be used as cell and drug carriers to deliver such therapeutic components directly and locally [1]. Hydrogels can be injected and crosslinked *in situ*, reducing the need for risky invasive surgeries [2]. In addition, hydrogels can mimic the natural extracellular matrix (ECM) environment, and allow one to control cellular and tissue functions as well as the transport of nutrients and bioactive molecules [3, 4].

Fumarate-based hydrogels are synthetic polymers, allowing flexible control of physical, mechanical, and degradative properties for a desired application [4]. Fumaric acid, the fundamental component of these hydrogel scaffolds, is an unsaturated organic acid that is commonly found in the human body and can be metabolized through the Krebs cycle [5–7]. Polymer chains that contain fumarate units crosslink easily via the unsaturated double bonds and degrade through hydrolysis of the ester bonds in the fumarate group [6–9]. Furthermore, the biodegradable nature of these hydrogels allows neotissue ingrowth and eliminates the need for further surgery to remove the implanted scaffold [5, 10].

Current research on fumarate-based hydrogels as tissue engineering scaffolds for regenerative medicine applications includes poly(propylene fumarate-*co*-ethylene glycol) (P(PF-*co*-EG)), oligo(poly(ethylene glycol) fumarate) (OPF), and poly(lactide-*co*-ethylene oxide-*co*-fumarate) (PLEOF). These hydrogel scaffolds have been well characterized, with a number of in-vitro and/or in-vivo studies proving them to be non-cytotoxic to, and biocompatible with, surrounding tissues [11–14]. In addition, the ease in crosslinking modulation of fumarate-based hydrogels is a testament to their versatility. As biodegradable and biocompatible materials, each hydrogel has its unique physical and mechanical properties that can be tailored to meet the needs of specific regenerative medicine applications, including drug delivery and regeneration of bone, cartilage, and nerve tissue. This chapter will illustrate the chemistry and characterization behind these fumarate-based hydrogels in addition to their applications in regenerative medicine.

16.2 Poly(propylene fumarate-*co*-ethylene glycol) hydrogel

Macroporous hydrogels based on poly(propylene fumarate-*co*-ethylene glycol) (P(PF-*co*-EG)) have been investigated over the past decade for use as an injectable, biodegradable scaffolding material for the modulation of cellular behavior [15–17].

16.2.1 Chemistry

P(PF-*co*-EG) is a block copolymer of poly(propylene fumarate) (PPF) and poly(ethylene glycol) (PEG). It is formed via a multistep reaction that begins with the synthesis of PPF, a biodegradable polyester previously characterized and investigated for applications in orthopaedic and craniofacial tissue engineering [18–21].

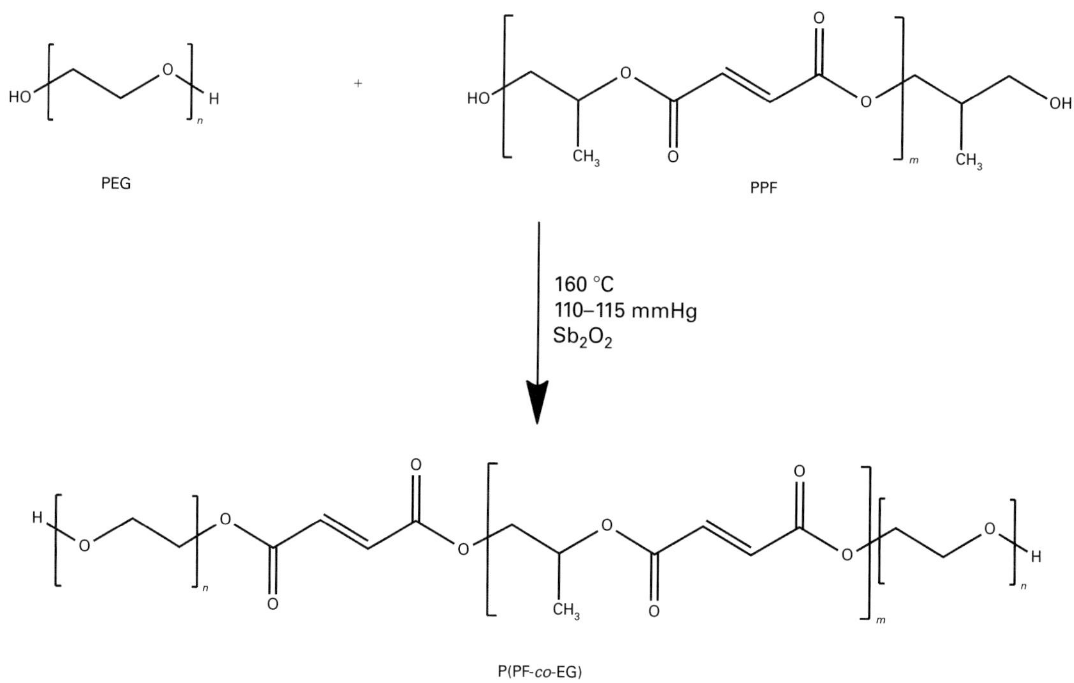

Figure 16.1 The transesterification reaction between PEG and PPF to form the copolymer P(PF-*co*-EG).

First, diethyl fumarate and propylene glycol are reacted in the presence of catalytic zinc chloride to create bis(2-hydroxypropyl) fumarate, a diester intermediate. The intermediate can then be transesterified under vacuum to yield a linear unsaturated form of PPF [22]. Once PPF has been obtained, it can be reacted with methoxy poly(ethylene glycol) to form the P(PF-*co*-EG) copolymer via a transesterification reaction as seen in Figure 16.1 [8, 23].

Owing to the presence of fumarate double bonds in the PPF blocks, P(PF-*co*-EG) is a highly unsaturated copolymer. As a result of this intrinsic property, the raw copolymer material can undergo crosslinking to produce amphiphilic hydrogels [11]. The amphiphilic nature of P(PF-*co*-EG) also permits the copolymer to undergo reversible thermal gelation via changes in intermolecular behavior upon fluctuations in temperature [8]. The thermal initiation system for crosslinking can leverage a crosslinker, such as poly(ethylene glycol) diacrylate (PEG-DA), in combination with a radical initiator (e.g. the redox radical initiators ammonium persulfate (APS) and ascorbic acid (AA)) [24]. Sodium bicarbonate can be added to the reaction to interact with AA to generate carbon dioxide gas. The generated gas allows the production of highly porous hydrogel materials that can be highly functionalized [25, 26].

16.2.2 Characterization

16.2.2.1 Swelling and degradation

P(PF-*co*-EG) consists of alternating hydrophobic PPF and hydrophilic PEG polymer blocks. Owing to the hydrophilic nature of the PEG component, P(PF-*co*-EG) materials can retain water to form amphiphilic hydrogels after crosslinking. By altering the amounts of the hydrophilic and hydrophobic components, the swelling properties of P(PF-*co*-EG) hydrogels can be tuned [16]. Indeed, previous studies on swelling have demonstrated that equilibrium swelling ratios of P(PF-*co*-EG) hydrogels are greater with higher amounts of PEG and smaller with higher amounts of PPF [16].

Additionally, physical properties such as compressive and tensile moduli can be modulated by adjusting the PPF:PEG ratio [16]. Because PPF retains the bulk structural integrity, higher amounts of PPF are correlated with materials of greater mechanical strength.

With regard to the degradation characteristics of P(PF-*co*-EG) hydrogels, the authors of several studies have observed the mechanism by which these amphiphilic hydrogels degrade [11, 26]. Owing to the presence of hydrolytically cleavable ester bonds in PPF, P(PF-*co*-EG) hydrogels are expected to undergo bulk degradation following the absorption of water. Typically, bulk degrading materials maintain their shape and volume but lose mechanical strength as their internal polymeric networks undergo hydrolysis. Indeed, the gradual loss of mechanical strength over time as manifested by decreases in complex dynamic flexural and tensile moduli was observed both under in-vitro and under in-vivo conditions [11, 26].

Like the swelling properties, the degradation rate of P(PF-*co*-EG) can be altered as well. For instance, greater amounts of mass loss are observed in hydrogels with higher PPF content [11]. Although PPF is responsible for a majority of the mechanical strength attributed to P(PF-*co*-EG) hydrogels, the ester linkages make it most susceptible to hydrolytic cleavage [26]. As a result, increasing the weight percentage of PPF initially increases the tensile strength of the hydrogel but ultimately increases the rate of bulk degradation. Since the current system uses PEG-DA as the crosslinker, the crosslinking density can be modified by changing the P(PF-*co*-EG):PEG-DA ratio to also affect the degradation of P(PF-*co*-EG) hydrogels. Purportedly, smaller P(PF-*co*-EG):PEG-DA ratios, or higher crosslinking densities, result in slower degradation [26]. This is because more ester linkages need to be cleaved in hydrogels with greater crosslinking densities, ultimately leading to a slower degradation rate. Unlike other polyester scaffolds, however, the degradation of P(PF-*co*-EG) hydrogels is not heavily influenced by porosity [26].

16.2.2.2 Cytocompatibility and biocompatibility

Investigations of the in-vitro cytotoxicity and in-vivo biocompatibility of P(PF-*co*-EG) hydrogels revealed favorable biological responses. Specifically, cytotoxicity was evaluated by exposing monolayer endothelial cell cultures to leachable materials from P(PF-*co*-EG) hydrogel films and then measuring their levels of viability and proliferation [27]. As determined by an MTT assay, the viability of monolayers exposed to gel compositions with high PEG amounts was not significantly different from that of negative controls [27]. Since P(PF-*co*-EG)-based hydrogels are intended to be injectable and to be used for biodegradable applications within the body, in-vivo biocompatibility is also crucial. A cage implant system was employed as the in-vivo model to assess biocompatibility [27]. Briefly, dehydrated gel films were placed inside sterilized small cylindrical cages and implanted subcutaneously into Sprague–Dawley rats [27]. Biochemical and histological analyses of exudates and extracted copolymer films revealed that the biocompatibility of P(PF-*co*-EG) hydrogels is dependent on the copolymer composition. In particular, increasing amounts of uncrosslinked PPF elicited more toxic responses in vivo [27]. Hence, cytotoxicity and inflammation can be attenuated with higher weight percentages or molecular weights (MWs; more formally, relative molecular masses) of the PEG component. Overall, P(PF-*co*-EG) hydrogels exhibited excellent biocompatibility upon implantation, demonstrating their suitability as effective tissue engineering scaffolds.

16.2.2.3 Modification with biomimetic peptides

With regard to biocompatibility, P(PF-*co*-EG) hydrogels were able to accommodate varying levels of cell adhesion. Copolymer modifications brought about by changing the amount of PEG can influence the physicochemical properties of hydrogels and thus cell adhesion. Tanahashi *et al.* reported that the adhesion of smooth muscle cells and human endothelial cells was dependent on the hydrophilicity of the hydrogels; less hydrophilic P(PF-*co*-EG) hydrogels elicited smaller amounts of cell adhesion [17]. However, cells bound to macroporous P(PF-*co*-EG) hydrogels alone do not display any morphological signs of activity [17]. In order to affect changes in cellular behavior,

ECM adhesion peptides such as the arginine–glycine–aspartic acid (RGD) sequence have been incorporated into the bulk macroporous hydrogel, imparting properties that are biomimetic of the natural ECM [15]. Adhesion and migration assays studying the behavior of bone marrow stromal cells, also referred to as mesenchymal stem cells (MSCs), on macroporous P(PF-*co*-EG) hydrogels demonstrated that cell-specific binding can be achieved and that the cells bound are biologically active [15]. For instance, marrow-derived osteoblasts have been shown to bind, spread, and migrate on RGD-functionalized P(PF-*co*-EG) hydrogels, revealing the ability of these scaffolds to activate anchorage-dependent behaviors in this particular cell type [15]. On incorporating RGD peptide sequences into P(PF-*co*-EG) copolymers using PEG spacers and PEG blocks of specific MWs, only cell types with receptors for the RGD sequence are selected for binding. Additionally, biomimetic P(PF-*co*-EG) hydrogels can sustain the differentiation of progenitor cells [15]. Utilizing RGD-functionalized P(PF-*co*-EG) hydrogels as three-dimensional (3D) scaffolds for culture of bone marrow-derived MSCs, the biomimetic hydrogel was used as a vehicle for osteoblastic differentiation [28]. One can imagine the utility of such technologies for the ex-vivo modulation of bone-marrow-derived MSCs to develop cell-inspired therapeutics for orthopedic tissue engineering applications.

Another way P(PF-*co*-EG) hydrogels were modified involved the tethering of positively charged agmatine to the PEG copolymer blocks [29]. Agmatine is a compound naturally synthesized from the amino acid arginine and is naturally metabolized by the body to form putrecine and urea [29]. Its cationic properties can be used to enhance the adhesion of vascular smooth muscle cells via the adsorption of anionic ECM molecules. Interestingly, P(PF-*co*-EG) hydrogels modified in the bulk with agmatine possess the ability to accommodate cell binding while maintaining high levels of hydrophilicity [30]. This property, together with the ability for these cationic hydrogels to biodegrade, makes agmatine-modified P(PF-*co*-EG) hydrogels very suitable for cell carrier applications in tissue engineering.

16.2.2.4 Thermoreversibility

Hydrogels based on certain compositions of P(PF-*co*-EG) copolymers possess thermoreversible properties. Such thermoreversible behavior, as indicated by the presence of a lower critical solution temperature (LCST), arises from the amphiphilic nature of the P(PF-*co*-EG) copolymers. Behravesh *et al.* reported the appearance of LCSTs for P(PF-*co*-EG) copolymer solutions that were synthesized using PEG of low MWs [8]. Indeed, the block length of the PEG components in the copolymer played a crucial role in determining the LCST and the sol–gel transition temperature. Copolymers comprising PEG with high MWs do not necessarily exhibit any thermoreversible properties due to their high hydrophilicity. P(PF-*co*-EG) hydrogels have been formulated to achieve LCSTs near room temperature (25 °C) and sol–gel transition temperatures near body temperature (35 °C) [24, 25]. These properties make P(PF-*co*-EG) hydrogels advantageous for the minimally invasive delivery of cells or other therapeutics for tissue engineering applications. Furthermore, these hydrogels can also be chemically crosslinked. Utilizing a water-soluble redox initiator system that incorporates a basic and an acidic initiator, macroporous P(PF-*co*-EG) hydrogels can be formed *in situ* to produce biodegradable scaffolds that can be functionalized for desired bioactivities [25].

16.2.3 Regenerative medicine applications

16.2.3.1 Bone regeneration

Using several in-vitro models, P(PF-*co*-EG)-based hydrogels have been investigated for potential applications in bone tissue engineering [15, 17, 28]. The authors of one such study seeded marrow-derived osteoblasts on biomimetic P(PF-*co*-EG) hydrogels and observed their subsequent adhesion and migration [15]. From the results, incorporating RGDS into P(PF-*co*-EG) hydrogels permitted the adhesion of up to 84% of the initial seeding density of marrow-derived osteoblasts [15]. Using a megacolony migration assay, Behravesh *et al.* detected increasing cell surface area coverage that occurred as a result of cell migration on

RGD rather than from proliferation of cells [15]. By employing such behavior, it becomes feasible to apply biomimetic P(PF-*co*-EG)-based hydrogels for the guided regeneration of orthopaedic or dental tissues. Cells would mechanistically bind to implanted biomimetic scaffolds and migrate according to biological cues (like RGD peptides) engineered to therapeutically direct these cells to the defect site. It was also demonstrated that MSCs seeded on P(PF-*co*-EG)-based hydrogels could undergo osteoblastic differentiation when treated with osteogenically conditioned media [28]. Specifically, MSCs seeded in macroporous 3D P(PF-*co*-EG) hydrogels exhibited substantial calcium deposition [28]. Using macroporous P(PF-*co*-EG) hydrogels that are biomimetic of the bone environment, marrow-derived progenitor cells may be harvested from patients with minimal donor site morbidity and expanded ex vivo for subsequent autologous cellular therapies.

16.2.3.2 Cartilage regeneration

Injectable and thermoreversible P(PF-*co*-EG)-based hydrogels have also been investigated for cartilage regeneration. Owing to the hydrophilicity of the PEG blocks, synthetic scaffolds based on P(PF-*co*-EG) copolymers inherently retain water to yield water-laden materials. Such properties are biomimetic of natural cartilage tissues. In an effort to assess the potential of applying P(PF-*co*-EG) hydrogels for cartilage regeneration, Fisher *et al.* encapsulated bovine articular chondrocytes within thermoreversibly gelled P(PF-*co*-EG) hydrogels and examined their viability [31]. Accordingly, the chondrocytes maintained satisfactory levels of proteoglycan and collagen type II synthesis. The proliferation of these cells was also increased with the addition of bone morphogenetic protein-7 [31].

16.3 Oligo(poly(ethylene glycol) fumarate) hydrogel

While P(PF-*co*-EG) showed promise as a hydrogel scaffold for regenerative medicine applications, oligo(poly(ethylene glycol) fumarate) (OPF) macromers were developed for the fabrication of hydrogels with improved control over hydrogel parameters. P(PF-*co*-EG) macromers contain multiple PPF blocks, with each PPF block comprising several fumarate groups [16, 22, 24]. However, these multiple fumarate groups can result in varying MW between crosslinks and mesh sizes in fabricated hydrogel networks [24]. OPF macromers consist of fumarate groups separated by PEG chains of defined MW. As a result, hydrogels with different mesh sizes can be easily fabricated by varying the MW of the PEG employed in the synthesis of the macromer [9]. OPF hydrogels with tailored and controlled physical properties have great potential in a myriad of tissue engineering applications.

16.3.1 Chemistry

OPF macromers consist of alternating units of fumarate groups and PEG chains, with the macromers capped by end PEG chains [6]. These macromers are synthesized in a one-pot reaction, as shown in Figure 16.2, through the addition of distilled fumaryl chloride (FuCl) and triethylamine (TEA) dropwise to distilled PEG in a PEG:FuCl molar ratio of 1:0.9. The molar ratio of FuCl to TEA is chosen to be 1:2 in order to remove chlorine atoms from the ends of FuCl

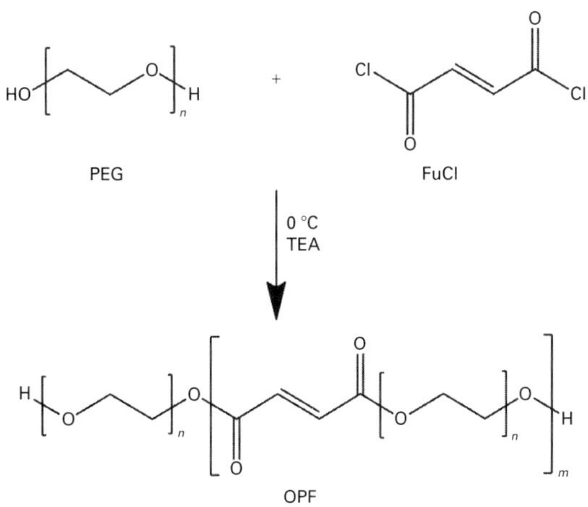

Figure 16.2 The synthesis of the OPF macromer from PEG and FuCl.

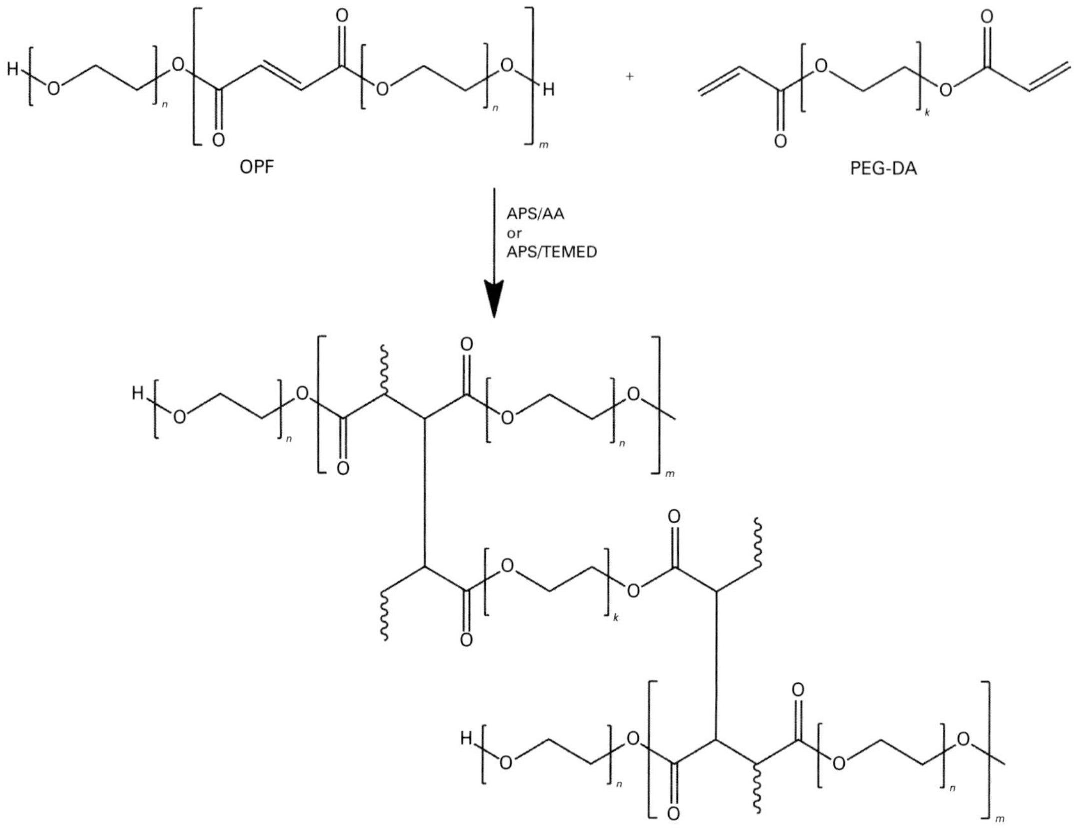

Figure 16.3 Chemical crosslinking of OPF with PEG-DA in the presence of initiators to form a hydrogel.

molecules. Upon completion of the reaction, the mixture is filtered, purified, and dried to obtain the macromer in powdered form [6].

Macromers of OPF have been crosslinked in a variety of ways to form hydrogels through its fumarate groups. Crosslinking can occur by radical polymerization through photoinitiation or thermal initiation. Photocrosslinking has been achieved with a commercialized photoinitiator such as Irgacure 2959 and *N*-vinylpyrrolidone (NVP) as a comonomer [32]. Thermal crosslinking has been implemented in the presence of either APS and AA or APS and *N,N,N′,N′*-tetramethylethylenediamine (TEMED) as shown in Figure 16.3. While both initiator systems have been used previously, the APS/TEMED initiator mix remains near neutral pH whereas the APS/AA system is acidic [13, 33]. Poly(ethylene glycol) diacrylate and *N,N′*-methylene bisacrylamide (BISAM) have been used as crosslinkers in combination with the initiator systems just described to form OPF hydrogels [9, 34].

16.3.2 Characterization

16.3.2.1 Swelling and degradation

Numerous swelling and degradation studies have been performed to investigate changes in physical properties as the OPF macromer length is varied [2, 9, 12]. Since OPF macromers consist of alternating units of fumarate groups and PEG chains, it is expected that incorporating longer PEG chains into the macromers would increase the hydrophilicity of the hydrogels, and thus greater swelling would occur. As the PEG chain MW increased from 1000 to 35,000, equilibrium swelling of chemically crosslinked hydrogels increased [9, 35, 36]. In addition, the MW between crosslinks (M_c) and mesh size (ξ) also increased as the initial PEG MW in OPF macromers increased [9].

As mentioned previously, degradation of OPF hydrogels is induced by cleavage of ester bonds within the polymer network by hydrolysis. The degree of degradation is extrapolated through mass-loss and swelling-ratio data over time and has been shown to be a function of PEG chain length in OPF macromers as well as crosslinking density [12]. There is an inverse relationship between crosslinking density and mass loss with greater mass loss occurring over time with a lower crosslinking density [12, 35].

When OPF hydrogels were crosslinked through photoinitiation, increasing the concentration of the comonomer NVP decreased the swelling ratio [32]. Over a period of 21 days, a significant increase in sol fraction for low NVP concentrations in comparison with high NVP concentrations was also seen [32].

Composite OPF hydrogels that have their own distinct swelling and degradation characteristics have also been fabricated. Composite hydrogels comprising OPF and gelatin microparticles (GMPs) have been investigated using GMPs as growth-factor (GF)-delivery vehicles and an enzymaticaly digestible porogen [34]. On comparing OPF hydrogels and OPF–GMP composite hydrogels, no significant difference in swelling ratio and mass loss was observed by day 28 in PBS [2]. However, a significant increase in swelling ratio of composite hydrogels over that of simple hydrogels was observed by day 28 in collagenase–PBS [2]. This increase in degradation highlights the potential enzymatic effects of an in-vivo environment on OPF–GMP composite hydrogels.

Mixed-mode OPF hydrogels crosslinked with PEG-dithiol produced hydrogels with distinct degradation and swelling properties. Hydrogels containing 20 wt% PEG-dithiol had greater swelling and smaller degradation times than did OPF hydrogels containing 10 wt% PEG-dithiol and 0 wt% PEG-dithiol [37].

16.3.2.2 Cytocompatibility and biocompatibility

Before utilizing OPF hydrogels in tissue engineering, their in-vitro cytotoxicity and in-vivo biocompatibility need to be investigated. The cytotoxicities of hydrogel constituents including the linear macromer, crosslinking agents, and initiators were examined. In addition, leachable substances from crosslinked hydrogels (i.e. the sol fraction) were tested. While OPF macromers were found to be non-cytotoxic with no significant difference between high- and low-MW OPF macromers, shorter-chain PEG-DA was more cytotoxic than longer-chain PEG-DA [13]. Unreacted leachable components from crosslinked hydrogels were also found to be non-cytotoxic [13]. Also, the chemical initiators used to fabricate crosslinked hydrogels exhibited favorable cytocompatibility at concentrations relevant to hydrogel formation [13, 38].

Since the intended applications for OPF hydrogels include injectable scaffolds, studies investigating in-vivo biocompatibility are essential. Research on the bone and soft tissue behavior of OPF hydrogels in rabbit models gave positive results [12, 39]. Cranial and subcutaneous implants resulted in formation of a thin fibrous capsule regardless of varying hydrogel fabrication parameters [12]. Also, in-vivo degradation products from hydrogels with PEG of MW 8000 elicited a minor inflammatory response, whereas hydrogels with PEG of MW 1000 underwent limited degradation [12]. Overall, minimal cytotoxicity and favorable biocompatibility establish OPF hydrogels as excellent synthetic scaffolds for tissue engineering applications.

16.3.2.3 Modification with biomimetic peptides

OPF hydrogels have been functionalized with biomimetic peptides with the intent to modulate cellular functions in guided tissue regeneration [40]. These peptides, including RGD and osteopontin-derived peptide (ODP), were incorporated into OPF hydrogels through bulk modification and it was demonstrated that altering peptide type and concentration for use in specific applications can be achieved [41, 42]. In a comparison between hydrogels modified with ODP or Gly–Arg–Gly–Asp–Ser (GRGDS), osteoblasts migrated faster on ODP modified hydrogels [43]. Also, the migration rate increased with increasing peptide concentration. In addition, bone-marrow-derived MSCs showed greater alkaline phosphatase (ALP) activity and greater osteopontin (OPN) secretion on ODP-modified hydrogels than on RGD-modified hydrogels [44]. These peptide-modification techniques support the versatility of OPF hydrogels to enhance cellular functions and direct tissue-specific regeneration.

16.3.3 Regenerative medicine applications

16.3.3.1 Bone regeneration

In a number of experiments, OPF hydrogels have been used as biomaterial scaffolds to support osteogenic differentiation of bone-marrow-derived MSCs. In particular, OPF hydrogels modified with RGD and ODP peptides exhibited greater OPN production and calcium deposition by seeded bone-marrow-derived MSCs in than did unmodified hydrogels [42]. In addition, bone-marrow-derived MSC adhesion, migration, and differentiation into osteoblasts were regulated by the concentration of incorporated adhesion peptides [43, 44]. Encapsulated bone-marrow-derived MSCs also exhibited osteogenic differentiation when cultured in osteogenic media with greater OPN and calcium deposition in hydrogels with greater swelling [1, 33]. Similarly, OPF gels with greater pore sizes exhibited enhanced osteogenic differentiation of bone-marrow-derived MSCs [45].

16.3.3.2 Cartilage regeneration

Besides osteogenesis, OPF hydrogels have been used to mimic a native articular cartilage environment to support cartilage tissue formation. The authors of several in-vitro studies investigated chondrogenesis of encapsulated cells in hydrogels through a myriad of cell and GF combinations. By combining marrow-derived MSCs or chondrocytes with transforming growth factor-β_1 (TGF-β_1) released from GMPs, greater chondrogenesis was observed with the release of TGF-β_1 than in the absence of TGF-β_1 [46, 47]. An insulin-like growth factor-1 (IGF-1) and TGF-β_1 dual-growth-factor-release system was also investigated with encapsulated MSCs. Results showed up-regulation of chondrocyte-specific genes for MSCs with TGF-β_1 and promotion of cell aggregation with IGF-1 [48]. The physical properties of OPF hydrogels also affect chondrogenesis, with a larger mesh size correlating to a larger PEG chain in OPF macromers increasing chondrogenesis of encapsulated MSCs [35]. In addition, in a hydrogel co-culture system utilizing osteogenic cells in the bottom layer and MSCs in the top layer of bilayered OPF constructs, there was a synergistic effect between the two layers that promoted chondrogenesis in the top layer [49, 50]. In-vivo studies utilizing OPF hydrogels to repair a full-thickness osteochondral defect have also been carried out. In these experiments, successful regeneration of subchondral tissue was seen on employing OPF hydrogel scaffolds [51–53]. In addition, OPF hydrogels comprising GFs, including IGF-1 and TGF-β_1, as well as MSCs show great potential for the repair of cartilage tissue.

16.3.3.3 Tendon/ligament regeneration

In a series of studies delivering fibroblasts for tendon/ligament regeneration, OPF-based hydrogels were used as a template biomaterial to investigate cellular responses from mechanical stimuli [37, 54, 55]. Fibroblasts harvested from cruciate ligaments and patellar tendons of bovine knee joints have been encapsulated in OPF–PEG-DA–PEG-dithiol mixed-mode hydrogels [37]. This research revealed that incorporation of 20 wt% PEG-dithiol can promote cell clustering and aggregation within hydrogel environments. Additionally, the differentiation of encapsulated human MSCs in OPF hydrogels into fibroblasts can be induced under cyclic tensile culture conditions [54]. Up-regulated expression levels of tenascin-C, collagen type I, and collagen type III were exhibited over 21 days in the presence of mechanical stimuli. In another study the spatial controllability of photolithographically patterned OPF hydrogels with high spatial fidelity and thickness was investigated [55]. By utilizing serial steps of photocrosslinking and lamination in a simple, inexpensive microfluidic device, tissue-scale (1–2 mm in thickness) OPF hydrogels encapsulating multiple primary cell types could be patterned with high spatial control.

16.3.3.4 Lens regeneration

One of the recent investigations of OPF hydrogels for tissue engineering applications concerned pigment epithelial cell encapsulation for lens regeneration [56]. Newt iris pigment epithelial cells were encapsulated in OPF hydrogels for implantation into lentectomized newts in vivo. Histological examination after 30 days indicated that encapsulated cells in hydrogel beads (1 mm in diameter) trans-differentiated into lens tissues. This was confirmed by lens fiber tissue formation without adverse side effects by hydrogel degradation [56].

16.3.3.5 Nerve tissue regeneration

Fumarate-based biomaterials have also been investigated for spinal cord and nerve regeneration in neural tissue engineering [57–60]. In order to overcome the drawbacks of autologous nerve grafts for the treatment of segmental peripheral nerve defects, such as malfunction in donor nerve site and size mismatch between a nerve graft and an implanted site, various hydrogel systems have recently been investigated [57]. Among these degradable synthetic biomaterials, OPF hydrogels produced with the aid of electrically charged reagents have been developed for preliminary applications in neural tissue engineering [57, 59]. By copolymerization with [2-(methacryloyloxy) ethyl]-trimethylammonium chloride (MAETAC), OPF hydrogels can be positively charged to support dorsal root ganglion neuron attachment and differentiation in a MAETAC monomer amount-dependent manner [57]. Another study concerned the incorporation of an electrically conductive polymer, polypyrrole (PPy) [59]. In order to achieve high conductivity in a nerve guidance conduit and to stabilize the positive charge, three anions were incorporated within the OPF–PPy hydrogel system, namely naphthalene sulfonic acid, docecyl benzene sulfonic acid, and dioctyl sulfosuccinate. This composite hydrogel system was not cytotoxic to PS12 cells over 7 days in vitro. More importantly, neurite extension analysis after 24 hours indicated that OPF–PPy hydrogels with naphthalene sulfonic acid promoted PS12 cell attachment and neurite length extension [59]. These recent results demonstrate the potential use of electrically conductive fumarate-based hydrogel composites for nerve regeneration [58, 60].

16.3.3.6 Delivery of bioactive molecules

The delivery of bioactive molecules from OPF hydrogel composites has been researched for medicinal and regenerative applications. Using an OPF hydrogel carrier composite, the delivery of a chemotherapeutic anticancer drug, doxorubicin (Dox), was investigated [61]. An ionic monomer, sodium methacrylate, was crosslinked with OPF to form negatively charged hydrogels, which could then couple with positively charged Dox through electrostatic interactions. This research demonstrated that the release kinetics of Dox from OPF hydrogels depended on the charge density of the hydrogel as well as the ionic strength of the surrounding environment [61]. In addition, released Dox maintained its anticancer activity against MG63 cells. Precise control of the concentration of drug incorporated could be achieved by modulation of the OPF hydrogel chemical composition, subsequent changes in polyelectrolyte properties, and interactions with the ionic strength and pH of the surrounding environment [61].

With the aid of poly(lactic-*co*-glycolic acid) (PLGA) microparticles, therapeutic proteins and drugs can be delivered in vivo in a controlled manner using OPF hydrogel platforms [62]. One such therapeutic protein, dibutyryl cyclic adenosine monophosphate (dbcAMP), has been encapsulated within PLGA microparticles in OPF hydrogels for spinal cord transection studies [62]. This study demonstrated that sustained delivery of dbcAMP reduced capillary formation and the volume of cyst and scar formation in the presence of Schwann cells and MSCs. A functional recovery of motor skills in an animal model was significantly improved when dbcAMP was delivered with only MSCs [62].

Therapeutic proteins have also been released from OPF hydrogels and OPF–GMP composites. Owing to innate charge differences, IGF-1 and TGF-β_1 with isoelectric points (IEPs) of 7.5 and 9.5, respectively, can bind to acidic GMPs with an IEP of 5.0 through ionic complexation at physiologic pH [63]. On complexing TGF-β_1 to GMPs, burst release of the GF was reduced in comparison with release from simple OPF hydrogels. Dual GF delivery systems using OPF–GMP composites have also been employed, with no deleterious effects of one GF release on the other [63]. Such systems offer spatial and temporal control of GF release for regenerative medicine applications [47–49].

Plasmid DNA can also be delivered using OPF hydrogels [64, 65] and OPF–GMP composites [66–68]. The release of plasmid DNA from an OPF hydrogel can be controlled by the PEG chain MW and subsequent degradation profile of the hydrogel [65, 66]. A study involving co-encapsulation of plasmid DNA and cells in OPF hydrogels demonstrated that bone tumor cells in hydrogels could be transfected by plasmid DNA encoding green fluorescent protein (GFP) and the transfected cells continuously expressed GFP protein over 21 days [64]. In the same study, estrogen receptor (ER)-negative human fetal osteoblasts were transfected by plasmid DNA encoding ER, and increased ALP activity and estrogen-dependent luciferase activities with the estrogen treatment were seen [64]. When plasmid DNA–GMP complexes were encapsulated in OPF hydrogels, a sustained release of plasmid DNA over 42 days was observed in mice in vivo relative to a direct injection of DNA solution and the delivery of non-embedded DNA [67]. In another study the potential of OPF composite hydrogels encapsulating plasmid DNA encoding human bone morphogenetic protein-2 (BMP-2) complexed to GMPs to enhance bone regeneration in a critical-sized rat cranial defect model was investigated [68].

16.4 Poly(lactide-*co*-ethylene oxide-*co*-fumarate) hydrogel

In addition to OPF, another fumarate-based hydrogel has been developed with controlled physical properties as an alternative for specific regenerative medicine applications. Poly(lactide-*co*-ethylene oxide-*co*-fumarate) (PLEOF) comprises an ultra-low-MW poly(L-lactide) (PLA) block that offers greater tunability of the fabricated hydrogel water content and degradation rate [69]. Preliminary studies show that PLEOF hydrogels have potential as a fumarate-based tissue-engineered scaffold with such added modifications.

16.4.1 Chemistry

PLEOF is also a PEG-based terpolymer modified using a fumarate unit to control crosslinkability [7]. *In situ* crosslinkable PLEOF macromers can be synthesized with PLA (produced by ring-opening polymerization of L-lactide with diethylene glycol as an initiator), PEG blocks, and FuCl by a condensation polymerization as shown in Figure 16.4 [7, 69]. The degradation products of the terpolymer include lactic acid and fumaric acid that can be metabolized, as well as PEG, which can be excreted by the body [7].

For the crosslinking reaction, BISAM was used as a crosslinker, while an acidic initiator, APS, and a basic radical catalyst, TEMED, were utilized for a neutral redox initiation [7]. The crosslinking properties of PLEOF hydrogels are dependent on the concentrations of the initiator and the accelerator. Increasing the APS and TEMED concentrations increased the rate of the crosslinking reaction, decreased the gelation time, and increased the ultimate storage modulus of PLEOF hydrogels [7]. Increasing the concentration of BISAM also increased the ultimate modulus of the gels [7]. An increase in the crosslinking density of PLEOF hydrogels was achieved by increasing the density of fumarate groups in PLEOF [7, 14]. In addition to chemical crosslinking, PLEOF can also be photocrosslinked with the aid of NVP, a photoinitiator, and UV radiation [69]. Like P(PF-*co*-EG) and OPF macromers, PLEOF precursor chains can be crosslinked through the C=C double bond in the fumarate group. The crosslinking density and degradation of photocrosslinked PLEOF hydrogels were dependent on the composition (e.g. the NVP concentration, PLA:PEG ratio, and PLEOF concentration) as well as the duration and intensity of UV irradiation [69].

In addition to chemically crosslinked hydrogels using BISAM, a peptide crosslinker was investigated in order to develop both hydrolytically and

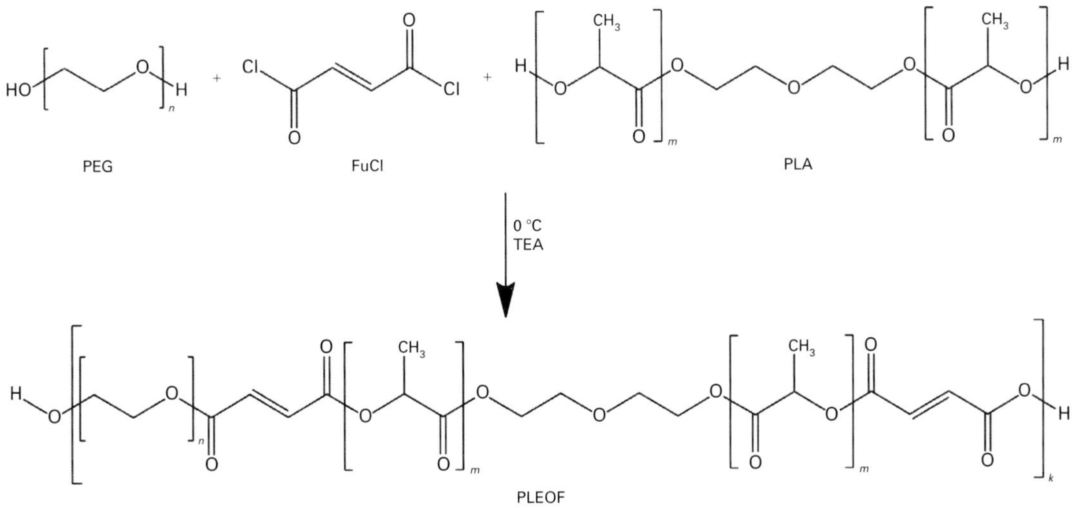

Figure 16.4 Synthesis of a PLEOF macromer between PEG, FuCl, and ultra-low-molecular-weight PLA.

enzymatically degradable PLEOF hydrogels [14]. In this study, the matrix metalloproteinase (MMP)-13 degradable peptide sequence QPQGLAK with acrylate end-groups functioned as the crosslinker polymerized with PLEOF macromers. Peptide-crosslinked PLEOF hydrogels had higher water content and sol fraction than did BISAM-crosslinked hydrogels due to the relatively higher MW of the peptide crosslinker [14]. Using both peptide and BISAM crosslinkers, the degradation rate of PLEOF hydrogels was modulated by the ratio of the two crosslinkers, the amount of MMP-13 needed to cleave the peptide sequences, and the incubation time of exposure to MMP-13 [14].

16.4.2 Characterization

A number of studies have been done to characterize the physical properties of this versatile terpolymer macromer. The swelling ratio of PLEOF can be adjusted by varying the ratio of hydrophobic PLA blocks to hydrophilic PEG blocks as well as the PEG chain length [69, 70]. In addition, the degradation rate is controlled by the ratio of PLA to PEG blocks and the hydrogel mesh size is modified through the density of fumarate groups in the terpolymer [7]. In experiments with photocrosslinked PLEOF hydrogels, hydrogels with greater PLA:PEG ratios exhibited less swelling and a greater sol fraction. Degradation experiments indicated that the PLA:PEG block ratio, and ultimately the ratio of lactide to fumarate units, affected the degradation rate of PLEOF hydrogels [69].

The cytocompatibility of PLEOF hydrogels was also tested with MSCs. MSCs cultured in a medium containing BISAM crosslinker had markedly lower cell viability than did those cultured in medium containing a peptide crosslinker [14]. The peptide-crosslinked hydrogel network was shown to be cytocompatible with encapsulated MSCs (e.g. 90% viability), however, the sol fraction exhibited some adverse effects (e.g. 65% viability) [14].

16.4.3 Regenerative medicine applications

16.4.3.1 Bone regeneration

Incorporation of peptides into PLEOF hydrogels can enhance their osteoconductivity [71]. In order to conjugate various bioactive peptides in PLEOF hydrogels, acrylamide-terminated RGD peptides were first crosslinked with fumarate groups in PLEOF macromers and PEGylated peptides derived from BMP-2 were grafted to the hydrogel surface by specific click chemistry between the azide group of the peptides and the propargyl group of the hydrogels [71]. Osteoblastic differentiation of encapsulated MSCs was observed in peptide-modified PLEOF hydrogels [14]. MSCs seeded onto hydrogels conjugated with both RGD and BMP-2 derived peptides exhibited increased ALP activity and mineralization over 21 days of in-vitro culture compared with hydrogels with single incorporation of either RGD or BMP-derived peptides [71]. Specifically, calcium deposition on PLEOF hydrogels with both peptides was significantly higher than that on solely RGD or BMP-2 derived peptide-grafted hydrogels.

Hydroxyapatite (HA) nanoparticles have also been incorporated for the fabrication of PLEOF nanocomposite hydrogels [72–74]. Interaction between HA nanoparticles with uncrosslinked PLEOF macromer chains [73] or incorporated peptides [72] influenced the viscoelastic properties of PLEOF composite hydrogels. Moreover, PLEOF–HA hydrogels conjugated with RGD peptides were utilized to coat electrospun PLA fiber meshes to form multilayered fiber-reinforced laminated composite hydrogels [74]. In this study, MSCs seeded onto laminated PLEOF hydrogels with incorporation of HA and RGD peptide conjugation exhibited enhanced osteoblastic differentiation, as evidenced by the expression of OPN and osteocalcin marker genes, and mineralization over 21 days of in-vitro culture.

16.4.3.2 Delivery of bioactive molecules

Recently, the release kinetics of stromal-derived factor-1α (SDF-1α) from PLEOF hydrogels and its effect on the migration of MSCs were investigated [70]. Increasing the PLA content in PLEOF macromers resulted in a decreased mesh size, increased SDF-1α loading efficiency, and sustained release of SDF-1α [70]. In addition, the migration rate of MSCs was dependent on the release kinetics of SDF-1α from the PLEOF hydrogels.

16.5 Conclusion

The multitude of human tissues, each uniquely developed with specific function, calls for versatile tissue-engineered scaffolds with tailored and controlled properties. The synthetic hydrogels described here have been conceived to possess fumarate units. These fumarate units contain double bonds that allow the formation of a crosslinked network, and ester groups that potentiate these hydrogels to degrade hydrolytically into biocompatible elements. P(PF-*co*-EG), OPF, and PLEOF have been synthesized with their own distinct physical properties and the development of these fumarate-based biomaterials has led to hydrogels with further adaptability over their physicochemical properties for regeneration of specific tissue types. Future developments can illustrate the robust potential of these fumarate-based hydrogels as injectable, biodegradable, and biocompatible tissue-engineered scaffolds.

ACKNOWLEDGEMENT

This work was supported by the US National Institutes of Health (R01-AR048756, AGM, FKK).

REFERENCES

[1] Temenoff, J. S., Park, H., Jabbari, E. *et al.* 2004. In vitro osteogenic differentiation of marrow stromal cells encapsulated in biodegradable hydrogels. *J. Biomed. Mater. Res. A*, **70**, 235–44.

[2] Holland, T. A., Tessmar, J. K., Tabata, Y. and Mikos, A. G. 2004. Transforming growth factor-beta 1 release from oligo(poly(ethylene glycol) fumarate) hydrogels in conditions that model the cartilage wound healing environment. *J. Control. Release*, **94**, 101–14.

[3] Lee, K. Y. and Mooney, D. J. 2001. Hydrogels for tissue engineering. *Chem. Rev.*, **101**, 1869–79.

[4] Drury, J. L. and Mooney, D. J. 2003. Hydrogels for tissue engineering: scaffold design variables and applications. *Biomaterials*. **24**, 4337–51.

[5] Temenoff, J. S., Kasper, F. K. and Mikos, A. G. 2007. Fumarate-based macromers as scaffolds for tissue engineering applications. In *Topics in Tissue Engineering*, ed. Ashammakhi, N., Reis, R. L. and Chiellini, E. Oulu: Expertissue E-Book, pp. 6.1–6.16.

[6] Jo, S., Shin, H., Shung, A. K., Fisher, J. P. and Mikos, A. G. 2001. Synthesis and characterization of oligo(poly(ethylene glycol) fumarate) macromer. *Macromolecules*, **34**, 2839–44.

[7] Sarvestani, A. S., He, X. and Jabbari, E. 2007. Viscoelastic characterization and modeling of gelation kinetics of injectable *in situ* cross-linkable poly(lactide-*co*-ethylene oxide-*co*-fumarate) hydrogels. *Biomacromolecules*, **8**, 406–15.

[8] Behravesh, E., Shung, A. K., Jo, S. and Mikos, A. G. 2002. Synthesis and characterization of triblock copolymers of methoxy poly(ethylene glycol) and poly(propylene fumarate). *Biomacromolecules*, **3**, 153–8.

[9] Temenoff, J. S., Athanasiou, K. A., LeBaron, R. G. and Mikos, A. G. 2002. Effect of poly(ethylene glycol) molecular weight on tensile and swelling properties of oligo(poly(ethylene glycol) fumarate) hydrogels for cartilage tissue engineering. *J. Biomed. Mater. Res.*, **59**, 429–37.

[10] Temenoff, J. S. and Mikos, A. G. 2000. Injectable biodegradable materials for orthopedic tissue engineering. *Biomaterials*, **21**, 2405–12.

[11] Suggs, L. J., Krishnan, R. S., Garcia, C. A. *et al.* 1998. In vitro and in vivo degradation of poly(propylene fumarate-co-ethylene glycol) hydrogels. *J. Biomed. Mater. Res.*, **42**, 312–20.

[12] Shin, H., Ruhe, P. Quinten, Mikos, A. G. and Jansen, J. A. 2003. In vivo bone and soft tissue response to injectable, biodegradable oligo(poly(ethylene glycol) fumarate) hydrogels. *Biomaterials*, **24**, 3201–11.

[13] Shin, H., Temenoff, J. S. and Mikos, A. G. 2003. In vitro cytotoxicity of unsaturated oligo[poly(ethylene glycol) fumarate] macromers and their cross-linked hydrogels. *Biomacromolecules*, **4**, 552–60.

[14] He, X. and Jabbari, E. 2007. Material properties and cytocompatibility of injectable MMP degradable poly (lactide ethylene oxide fumarate) hydrogel as a carrier for marrow stromal cells. *Biomacromolecules*. **8**, 780–92.

[15] Behravesh, E., Zygourakis, K. and Mikos, A. G. 2003. Adhesion and migration of marrow-derived osteoblasts on injectable *in situ* crosslinkable poly(propylene fumarate-*co*-ethylene glycol)-based hydrogels with a covalently linked RGDS peptide. *J. Biomed. Mater. Res. A*, **65**, 260–70.

[16] Suggs, L. J., Kao, E. Y., Palombo, L. L. *et al.* 1998. Preparation and characterization of poly(propylene fumarate-*co*-ethylene glycol) hydrogels. *J. Biomater. Sci. Polymer Edition*, **9**, 653–66.

[17] Tanahashi, K. and Mikos, A. G. 2002. Cell adhesion on poly(propylene fumarate-*co*-ethylene glycol) hydrogels. *J. Biomed. Mater. Res.*, **62**, 558–66.

[18] Fisher, J. P., Holland, T. A., Dean, D., Engel, P. S. and Mikos, A. G. 2001. Synthesis and properties of photocross-linked poly(propylene fumarate) scaffolds. *J. Biomater. Sci. Polymer Edition*, **12**, 673–87.

[19] Fisher, J. P., Vehof, J. W., Dean, D. *et al.* 2002. Soft and hard tissue response to photocrosslinked poly(propylene fumarate) scaffolds in a rabbit model, *J. Biomed. Mater. Res.*, **59**, 547–56.

[20] Timmer, M. D., Carter, C., Ambrose, C. G. and Mikos, A. G. 2003. Fabrication of poly(propylene fumarate)-based orthopaedic implants by photo-crosslinking through transparent silicone molds. *Biomaterials*, **24**, 4707–14.

[21] Kim, K., Dean, D., Lu, A., Mikos, A. G. and Fisher, J. P. 2011. Early osteogenic signal expression of rat bone marrow stromal cells is influenced by both hydroxyapatite nanoparticle content and initial cell seeding density in biodegradable nanocomposite scaffolds. *Acta Biomater.*, **7**, 1249–64.

[22] Kasper, F. K., Tanahashi, K., Fisher, J. P. and Mikos, A. G. 2009. Synthesis of poly(propylene fumarate). *Nature Protoc.*, **4**, 518–25.

[23] Suggs, L. J., Payne, R. G., Yaszemski, M. J., Alemany, L. B. and Mikos, A. G. 1997. Synthesis and characterization of a block copolymer consisting of poly(propylene fumarate) and poly(ethylene glycol). *Macromolecules*, **30**, 4318–23.

[24] Shung, A. K., Behravesh, E., Jo, S. and Mikos, A. G. 2003. Crosslinking characteristics of and cell adhesion to an injectable poly(propylene fumarate-*co*-ethylene glycol) hydrogel using a water-soluble crosslinking system. *Tissue Eng.*, **9**, 243–54.

[25] Behravesh, E., Jo, S., Zygourakis, K. and Mikos, A. G. 2002. Synthesis of *in situ* cross-linkable macroporous biodegradable poly(propylene fumarate-*co*-ethylene glycol) hydrogels. *Biomacromolecules*, **3**, 374–81.

[26] Behravesh, E., Timmer, M. D., Lemoine, J. J., Liebschner, M. A. and Mikos, A. G. 2002. Evaluation of the in vitro degradation of macroporous hydrogels using gravimetry, confined compression testing, and microcomputed tomography. *Biomacromolecules*, **3**, 1263–70.

[27] Suggs, L. J., Shive, M. S., Garcia, C. A., Anderson, J. M. and Mikos, A. G. 1999. In vitro cytotoxicity and in vivo biocompatibility of poly(propylene fumarate-*co*-ethylene glycol) hydrogels. *J. Biomed. Mater. Res.*, **46**, 22–32.

[28] Behravesh, E. and Mikos, A. G. 2003. Three-dimensional culture of differentiating marrow stromal osteoblasts in biomimetic poly(propylene fumarate-*co*-ethylene glycol)-based macroporous hydrogels. *J. Biomed. Mater. Res. A*, **66**, 698–706.

[29] Tanahashi, K., Jo, S. and Mikos, A. G. 2002. Synthesis and characterization of biodegradable cationic poly(propylene fumarate-*co*-ethylene glycol) copolymer hydrogels modified with agmatine for enhanced cell adhesion. *Biomacromolecules*, **3**, 1030–7.

[30] Tanahashi, K. and Mikos, A. G. 2003. Effect of hydrophilicity and agmatine modification on degradation of poly(propylene fumarate-*co*-ethylene glycol) hydrogels. *J. Biomed. Mater. Res. A*, **67**, 1148–54.

[31] Fisher, J. P., Jo, S., Mikos, A. G. and Reddi, A. H. 2004. Thermoreversible hydrogel scaffolds for articular cartilage engineering. *J. Biomed. Mater. Res. A*, **71**, 268–74.

[32] Dadsetan, M., Szatkowski, J. P., Yaszemski, M. J. and Lu, L. 2007. Characterization of photo-cross-linked oligo[poly(ethylene glycol) fumarate] hydrogels for cartilage tissue engineering. *Biomacromolecules*, **8**, 1702–9.

[33] Temenoff, J. S., Park, H., Jabbari, E. *et al.* 2004. Thermally cross-linked oligo(poly(ethylene glycol) fumarate) hydrogels support osteogenic differentiation of encapsulated marrow stromal cells in vitro. *Biomacromolecules*, **5**, 5–10.

[34] Holland, T. A., Tabata, Y. and Mikos, A. G. 2003. In vitro release of transforming growth factor-beta 1 from gelatin microparticles encapsulated in biodegradable, injectable oligo(poly(ethylene glycol) fumarate) hydrogels. *J. Control. Release*, **91**, 299–313.

[35] Park, H., Guo, X., Temenoff, J. S. *et al.* 2009. Effect of swelling ratio of injectable hydrogel composites on chondrogenic differentiation of encapsulated rabbit marrow mesenchymal stem cells in vitro. *Biomacromolecules*, **10**, 541–6.

[36] Temenoff, J. S., Steinbis, E. S. and Mikos, A. G. 2003. Effect of drying history on swelling properties and cell attachment to oligo(poly(ethylene glycol) fumarate) hydrogels for guided tissue regeneration applications. *J. Biomater. Sci. Polymer Edition*, **14**, 989–1004.

[37] Brink, K. S., Yang, P. J. and Temenoff, J. S. 2009. Degradative properties and cytocompatibility of a mixed-mode hydrogel containing oligo[poly(ethylene glycol)fumarate] and poly(ethylene glycol)dithiol. *Acta Biomater.*, **5**, 570–9.

[38] Temenoff, J. S., Shin, H., Conway, D. E., Engel, P. S. and Mikos, A. G. 2003. In vitro cytotoxicity of redox radical initiators for cross-linking of oligo(poly(ethylene glycol) fumarate) macromers. *Biomacromolecules*, **4**, 1605–13.

[39] Fisher, J. P., Lalani, Z., Bossano, C. M. *et al.* 2004. Effect of biomaterial properties on bone healing in a rabbit tooth extraction socket model. *J. Biomed. Mater. Res. A*, **68**, 428–38.

[40] Jo, S., Shin, H. and Mikos, A. G. 2001. Modification of oligo(poly(ethylene glycol) fumarate) macromer with a GRGD peptide for the preparation of functionalized polymer networks. *Biomacromolecules*, **2**, 255–61.

[41] Shin, H., Jo, S. and Mikos, A. G. 2002. Modulation of marrow stromal osteoblast adhesion on biomimetic oligo[poly(ethylene glycol) fumarate] hydrogels modified with Arg-Gly-Asp peptides and a poly(ethyleneglycol) spacer. *J. Biomed. Mater. Res.*, **61**, 169–79.

[42] Shin, H., Zygourakis, K., Farach-Carson, M. C., Yaszemski, M. J. and Mikos, A. G. 2004. Modulation of differentiation and mineralization of marrow stromal cells cultured on biomimetic hydrogels modified with Arg-Gly-Asp containing peptides. *J. Biomed. Mater. Res. A*, **69**, 535–43.

[43] Shin, H., Zygourakis, K., Farach-Carson, M. C., Yaszemski, M. J. and Mikos, A. G. 2004. Attachment, proliferation, and migration of marrow stromal osteoblasts cultured on biomimetic hydrogels modified with an osteopontin-derived peptide. *Biomaterials*, **25**, 895–906.

[44] Shin, H., Temenoff, J. S., Bowden, G. C. *et al.* 2005. Osteogenic differentiation of rat bone marrow stromal cells cultured on Arg-Gly-Asp modified hydrogels without dexamethasone and beta-glycerol phosphate. *Biomaterials*, **26**, 3645–54.

[45] Dadsetan, M., Hefferan, T. E., Szatkowski, J. P. *et al.* 2008. Effect of hydrogel porosity on marrow stromal cell phenotypic expression. *Biomaterials*, **29**, 2193–202.

[46] Park, H., Temenoff, J. S., Holland, T. A., Tabata, Y. and Mikos, A. G. 2005. Delivery of TGF-β_1 and chondrocytes via injectable, biodegradable hydrogels for cartilage tissue engineering applications. *Biomaterials*, **26**, 7095–103.

[47] Park, H., Temenoff, J. S., Tabata, Y., Caplan, A. I. and Mikos, A. G. 2007. Injectable biodegradable hydrogel composites for rabbit marrow mesenchymal stem cell and growth factor delivery for cartilage tissue engineering. *Biomaterials*, **28**, 3217–27.

[48] Park, H., Temenoff, J. S., Tabata, Y. *et al.* 2009. Effect of dual growth factor delivery on chondrogenic differentiation of rabbit marrow mesenchymal stem cells encapsulated in injectable hydrogel composites. *J. Biomed. Mater. Res. A*, **88**, 889–97.

[49] Guo, X., Liao, J., Park, H. *et al.* 2010. Effects of TGF-β_3 and preculture period of osteogenic cells on the chondrogenic differentiation of rabbit marrow mesenchymal stem cells encapsulated in a bilayered hydrogel composite. *Acta Biomater.*, **6**, 2920–31.

[50] Guo, X., Park, H., Liu, G. *et al.* 2009. In vitro generation of an osteochondral construct using injectable hydrogel composites encapsulating rabbit marrow mesenchymal stem cells. *Biomaterials*, **30**, 2741–52.

[51] Holland, T. A., Bodde, E. W., Baggett, L. S. *et al.* 2005. Osteochondral repair in the rabbit model utilizing bilayered, degradable oligo(poly(ethylene glycol) fumarate) hydrogel scaffolds. *J. Biomed. Mater. Res. A*, **75**, 156–67.

[52] Holland, T. A., Bodde, E. W., Cuijpers, V. M. *et al.* 2007. Degradable hydrogel scaffolds for in vivo delivery of single and dual growth factors in cartilage repair. *Osteoarthritis Cartilage*, **15**, 187–97.

[53] Guo, X., Park, H., Young, S. *et al.* 2010. Repair of osteochondral defects with biodegradable hydrogel composites encapsulating marrow mesenchymal stem cells in a rabbit model. *Acta Biomater.*, **6**, 39–47.

[54] Doroski, D. M., Levenston, M. E. and Temenoff, J. S. 2010. Cyclic tensile culture promotes fibroblastic differentiation of marrow stromal cells encapsulated in poly(ethylene glycol)-based hydrogels. *Tissue Eng. Part A*, **16**, 3457–66.

[55] Hammoudi, T. M., Lu, H. and Temenoff, J. S. 2010. Long-term spatially defined coculture within three-dimensional photopatterned hydrogels. *Tissue Eng. Part C Methods*, **16**, 1621–8.

[56] Zhang, M. W., Park, H., Guo, X. *et al.* 2010. Adapting biodegradable oligo(poly(ethylene glycol) fumarate) hydrogels for pigment epithelial cell encapsulation and lens regeneration. *Tissue Eng. Part C Methods*, **16**, 261–7.

[57] Dadsetan, M., Knight, A. M., Lu, L., Windebank, A. J. and Yaszemski, M. J. 2009. Stimulation of neurite outgrowth using positively charged hydrogels. *Biomaterials*, **30**, 3874–81.

[58] Runge, M. B., Dadsetan, M., Baltrusaitis, J. *et al.* 2010. The development of electrically conductive polycaprolactone fumarate-polypyrrole composite materials for nerve regeneration. *Biomaterials*, **31**, 5916–26.

[59] Runge, M. B., Dadsetan, M., Baltrusaitis, J. *et al.* 2010. Development of electrically conductive oligo(polyethylene glycol) fumarate-polypyrrole hydrogels for nerve regeneration. *Biomacromolecules*, **11**, 2845–53.

[60] Wang, S., Yaszemski, M. J., Knight, A. M. *et al.* 2009. Photo-crosslinked poly(ε-caprolactone fumarate) networks for guided peripheral nerve regeneration: material properties and preliminary biological evaluations. *Acta Biomater.*, **5**, 1531–42.

[61] Dadsetan, M., Liu, Z., Pumberger, M. *et al.* 2010. A stimuli-responsive hydrogel for doxorubicin delivery. *Biomaterials*, **31**, 8051–62.

[62] Rooney, G. E., Knight, A. M., Madigan, N. N. *et al.* 2011. Sustained delivery of dibutyryl cyclic adenosine monophosphate to the transected spinal cord via oligo[(polyethylene glycol) fumarate] hydrogels. *Tissue Eng. Part A*, **17**, 1287–302.

[63] Holland, T. A., Tabata, Y. and Mikos, A. G. 2005. Dual growth factor delivery from degradable oligo(poly(ethylene glycol) fumarate) hydrogel scaffolds for cartilage tissue engineering. *J. Control. Release*, **101**, 111–25.

[64] Dadsetan, M., Szatkowski, J. P., Shogren, K. L., Yaszemski, M. J. and Maran, A. 2009. Hydrogel-mediated DNA delivery confers estrogenic response in nonresponsive osteoblast cells. *J. Biomed. Mater. Res. A*, **91**, 1170–7.

[65] Kasper, F. K., Seidlits, S. K., Tang, A. *et al.* 2005. In vitro release of plasmid DNA from oligo(poly(ethylene glycol) fumarate) hydrogels. *J. Control. Release*, **104**, 521–39.

[66] Kasper, F. K., Jerkins, E., Tanahashi, K. *et al.* 2006. Characterization of DNA release from composites of oligo(poly(ethylene glycol) fumarate) and cationized gelatin microspheres in vitro. *J. Biomed. Mater. Res. A*, **78**, 823–35.

[67] Kasper, F. K., Kushibiki, T., Kimura, Y., Mikos, A. G. and Tabata, Y. 2005. In vivo release of plasmid DNA from composites of oligo(poly(ethylene glycol)fumarate) and cationized gelatin microspheres. *J. Control. Release*, **107**, 547–61.

[68] Kasper, F. K., Young, S., Tanahashi, K. *et al.* 2006. Evaluation of bone regeneration by DNA release from composites of oligo(poly(ethylene glycol) fumarate) and cationized gelatin microspheres in a critical-sized calvarial defect. *J. Biomed. Mater. Res. A*, **78**, 335–42.

[69] Sarvestani, A. S., Xu, W. J., He, X. Z. and Jabbari, E. 2007. Gelation and degradation characteristics of in situ photo-crosslinked poly(L-lactid-*co*-ethylene oxide-*co*-fumarate) hydrogels. *Polymer*, **48**, 7113–20.

[70] He, X., Ma, J. and Jabbari, E. 2010. Migration of marrow stromal cells in response to sustained release of stromal-derived factor-1α from poly(lactide ethylene oxide fumarate) hydrogels. *Int. J. Pharm.*, **390**, 107–16.

[71] He, X., Ma, J. and Jabbari, E. 2008. Effect of grafting RGD and BMP-2 protein-derived peptides to a hydrogel substrate on osteogenic differentiation of marrow stromal cells. *Langmuir*, **24**, 12508–16.

[72] Sarvestani, A. S., He, X. and Jabbari, E. 2007. Effect of osteonectin-derived peptide on the viscoelasticity of hydrogel/apatite nanocomposite scaffolds. *Biopolymers*, **85**, 370–8.

[73] Sarvestani, A. S. and Jabbari, E. 2006. Modeling and experimental investigation of rheological properties of injectable poly(lactide ethylene oxide fumarate)/hydroxyapatite nanocomposites. *Biomacromolecules*, **7**, 1573–80.

[74] Xu, W., Ma, J. and Jabbari, E. 2010. Material properties and osteogenic differentiation of marrow stromal cells on fiber-reinforced laminated hydrogel nanocomposites. *Acta Biomater.*, **6**, 1992–2002.

17

Hydrogel scaffolds for regenerative medicine

Edward A. Sander, Erin D. Grassl and Robert T. Tranquillo

17.1 Introduction

Some strategies in tissue engineering and regenerative medicine (TERM) rely on the use of an appropriate biomaterial to guide and foster tissue repair and regeneration. Collagen-based materials are perhaps the most widely investigated of these biomaterials because collagen is the primary structural protein responsible for tissue integrity in most tissues [1]. Collagen gels offer several advantages as a scaffolding material, including the ability to deliver a homogeneous distribution of entrapped cells into a specific geometry and excellent biocompatibility and transport properties [2]. However, collagen does have some disadvantages, including suppression of cell proliferation and protein synthesis [3, 4], issues that can limit the quality of the engineered tissue produced.

An alternative biopolymer that shares similar properties to collagen is fibrin. Fibrin is a natural biopolymer involved in the wound-healing process, and it forms the provisional matrix of a clot. It rapidly polymerizes to form a biocompatible and biodegradable fibrous scaffold that promotes cell proliferation and ECM synthesis. Another attractive property of fibrin is that its precursor (fibrinogen) can be extracted from the patient's blood, making it an autologous material. In this chapter we will review the properties of fibrin and fibrin-based engineered tissues and how these materials are being incorporated into TERM technologies.

17.2 Structure and formation

17.2.1 In-vivo formation

A provisional fibrin fiber matrix forms naturally when blood clots. During the clotting process, the proteolytic enzyme thrombin converts fibrinogen into monomeric fibrin, which then self-assembles into fibrin fibrils or filaments that can be further strengthened by cross-linking via transglutaminases. The resultant mechanical properties and functionality of the clot are intimately dependent on the structure and organization of the fibrin matrix. Many factors are known to affect the self-assembly process and the resulting fibrin network structure. In this section, we briefly describe the general structural features of the monomer fibrinogen and its assembly into a network of fibrin fibers, recognizing that many details are not addressed, and direct the interested reader to in-depth reviews of clot formation and fibrin assembly by others [5–7]. In addition, we have elected to use standardized fibrin nomenclature when possible [8].

Fibrinogen is a 340-kDa glycoprotein produced by hepatocytes that circulates in the plasma [9]. It consists of two identical subunits, each of which contains three distinct polypeptide chains (the Aα chain, Bβ chain, and γ chain), that are disulfide-linked into a 45-nm-long protein [5, 6, 10] (Figure 17.1). The chains fold to produce a pair of outer globular D regions that are connected to a central E region by coiled-coil connectors [8]. The C-termini of the γ chain and Bβ chain form

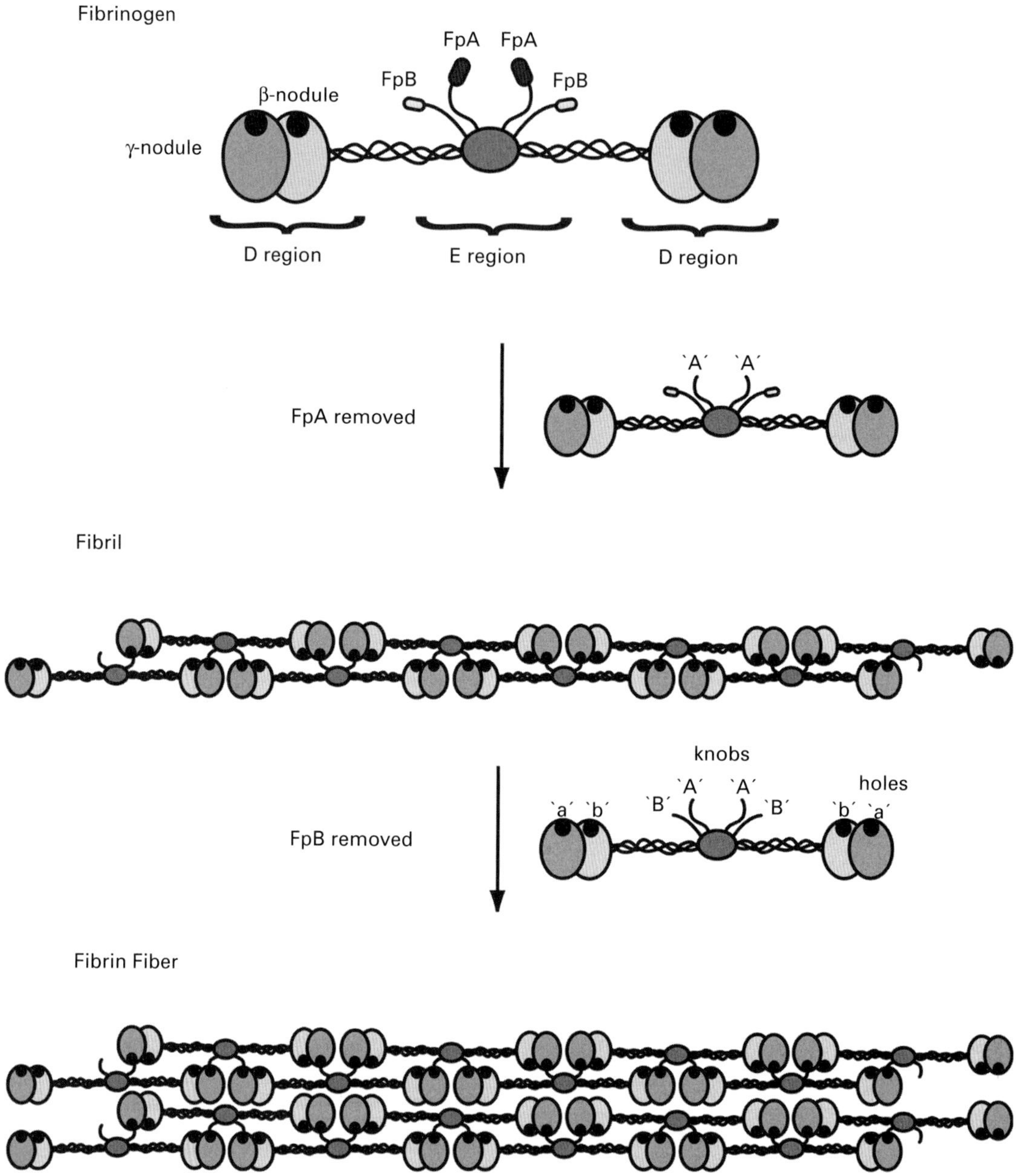

Figure 17.1 A schematic representation of fibrinogen and its assembly into higher-order structures. The fibrinogen monomer contains three regions consisting of two flanking D regions connected to a central E region. The E region contains the fibrinopeptide pairs A and B (FpA and FpB, respectively), which are cleaved by thrombin to form fibrin. The remaining knobs "A" and "B" associate with the complementary "a" and "b" holes located on the γ- and β-nodules in the D region, respectively, and in the process assemble first into fibrils and then into larger fibers. The A:a associations are necessary for fibril formation. The B:b associations also contribute to the assembly process, but these interactions are intentionally not shown due to uncertainty in how those associations form. Adapted from [16].

a γ nodule and a β nodule in the D region. Each nodule contains a hole involved in fibrin assembly [7]; the "a" hole [11] and "b" hole [12], respectively. The central E region contains fibrinopeptide pairs A and B (FpA and FpB).

During fibrin polymerization, the protease thrombin hydrolytically cleaves FpA and FpB - FpB is cleaved at a slower rate than FpA [13] - and the remaining knobs "A" and "B" in the E region associate with the complementary holes "a" and "b" in the D region of adjacent fibrin monomers, forming so-called A:a and B:b knob-hole interactions [7, 14]. Without A:a interactions fibrin cannot assemble into fibrils [15]. The role of B:b interactions has not been clarified, but they are thought to promote lateral aggregation [16, 17]. Other components of fibrin not discussed here, such as the αC domain, are also thought to contribute to self-assembly and to the tensile properties of the fiber [6, 18, 19]. It is through these non-covalent interactions that fibrin monomers self-assemble first into half-staggered, double-stranded fibrils (or protofibrils) [20]. These fibrils further associate laterally into larger fibrin fibers, typically 10–200 nm in diameter [7, 21–23]. The fibers are twisted [24] and organize themselves into interconnected and branched networks [5]. Two modes of branching have been identified: bilateral and equilateral junctions [25, 26]. Bilateral junctions form as lateral associations between double-stranded fibrils. Equilateral junctions form when three fibrin monomers interact with each other. These junctions are more prevalent when the rate of fibrinopeptide cleavage is reduced [5], and appear to be the most often encountered form of fiber branching [22, 27].

Fibrin is further crosslinked by activated transglutaminase factor XIIIa. Factor XIII is activated by thrombin into factor XIIIa, which can also crosslink other proteins, including fibronectin and collagen [28]. Factor XIIIa catalyzes the formation of one γ-glutamyl-ε-lysyl crosslink between the D domains of adjacent fibrin monomers, thereby producing γ–γ dimers [5]. Other crosslinks are also formed, such as between the Aα chains or between Aα chains and γ chains [28]. These crosslinks stabilize the fiber and prevent protofibrils from sliding past each other when stretched [29].

17.2.2 In-vitro formation

For in-vitro applications, fibrin gels (sometimes referred to as clots) are typically prepared by combining solutions of fibrinogen and thrombin. Calcium chloride is also usually added because calcium ions (Ca^{2+}) are an important co-factor for thrombin activity and increase the rate of self-assembly with concentration. Both fibrinogen and thrombin are most commonly obtained via purification from human [30–32], porcine [33], or bovine [31] platelet-rich plasma. Recombinant technologies are also emerging as a potential source for fibrinogen [18] and thrombin [18, 34], offering some advantages over plasma-purified proteins, particularly in terms of immunogenicity/disease transmission and availability. Regardless of the source, when fibrinogen, thrombin, and Ca^{2+} are mixed together a gel quickly forms. This gel consists of a solid fiber network and an interstitial fluid, which is often the tissue culture medium being used in the application. It is the combination of this network structure, which accounts for less than 1% of the gel volume in TERM applications (but is much higher for tissue sealants), and fluid–solid interactions that dictates the gel's response to external forces. Consequently, understanding how gel reconstitution conditions can impact the mechanical properties of the gel produced is important.

17.2.3 Controlling the fiber network structure

The microstructure that forms when fibrin is reconstituted (Figure 17.2, image A) is complex and dependent on a number of interdependent factors. Adjusting the concentration and ratio of fibrinogen and thrombin affects fiber size, network structure, and gelation time [22, 27, 35–38]. Fiber thickness and branching is also modulated by environmental conditions, such as pH, ionic strength, and temperature that affect the kinetics of lateral associations and axial growth between monomers and growing fibrils. For example, Carr *et al.* found that increasing the calcium concentration and the fibrinogen concentration, and decreasing the thrombin concentration and the ionic concentration

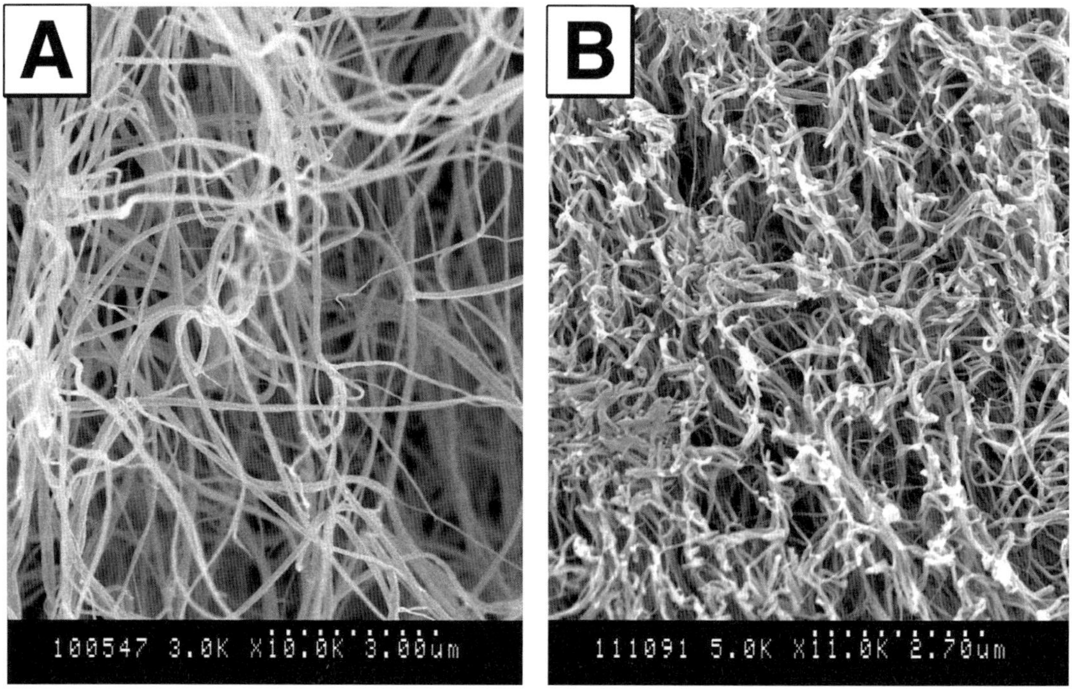

Figure 17.2 High-resolution scanning electron microscope (SEM) images showing the organization of bovine fibrin fibers in (A) an acellular 6-mg/ml fibrin gel and (B) a fibroblast-compacted 6-mg/ml fibrin gel after two weeks. Note the difference in magnification. For details on the reconstitution conditions see [56].

produces thicker fibers, and increasing the thrombin concentration accelerates gel formation [36]. Generally speaking, for gels with equal fibrin concentrations, those conditions that produce thick fibers will result in gels with larger pores (i.e. inter-fiber spacing) than in gels where the conditions produce thin fibers and smaller pores. Furthermore, gels with thicker fibers tend to have fewer branching junctions and thus longer fiber segments, whereas gels with thin fibers have many branching junctions and shorter segments [27]. These two types of gels are often referred to as "coarse" and "fine" clots, respectively [39].

Additional components in the blood are also known to affect fibrin structure. For example, plasma gels are known to assemble differently and form thicker fibers than gels made from purified fibrinogen [36]. In one study that examined clot morphology from different sources, a bimodal fiber distribution consisting of a fine meshwork of thin fibers overlapping thick fibers was observed in preparations using human platelet concentrate but not in fresh and lyophilized human-platelet-rich plasma [30]. Higher fibrinogen concentration, higher thrombin activity due to a higher initial concentration of platelets, and additional additives that reduce fibrinogen–platelet binding were all cited as potential contributors to the formation of the finer meshwork [30]. Many factors thus contribute to the kinetics of network and fiber formation and structure, which in turn controls the gel's mechanical properties, and should be considered carefully for the application at hand.

17.2.4 Mechanical properties

Fibrin gels are poroviscoelastic and exhibit a dependence on strain-rate and energy dissipation with loading

[40, 41]. The viscoelastic properties of fibrin gels have been studied extensively with dynamic shear tests, and these tests have revealed that behavior is directly tied to fibrin concentration, network microstructure, and the degree of crosslinking [22, 42–45]. These tests also indicate that, under small deformations and short time scales (10^{-3} to 6 seconds) the gels are elastic, and they exhibit little change in storage modulus or viscoelastic relaxation with frequency [40, 43].

The mechanical properties of individual fibrin fibers have also been assessed recently and shown to possess a rich spectrum of behavior [46–49]. The fibers are elastic and very extensible, capable of being stretched to more than six times their original length [46]. Fibers are also stiffer in tension than in flexion and increase in stiffness when crosslinked with factor XIIIa [48]. In one study that assessed properties using atomic force microscopy, fully crosslinked fibers had a higher elastic modulus (8.0 MPa versus 3.9 MPa), a lower maximum extensibility (147% versus 226%), and a lower elastic limit ($\leq$50% versus 120%) than did uncrosslinked fibers [47].

A distinguishing feature of fibrin gels is that they are highly extensible, much more so than collagen gels (Figure 17.3), and can easily be stretched to two or three times their initial length without rupturing [29, 40]. A typical loading curve for uniaxial extension begins with a linear increase in force that then transitions into a region with a steeper slope until failure occurs. This ability to accommodate such large strains comes from the network structure and the intrinsic properties of the fibrin molecule. Initially, fibers rotate and realign into the direction of applied force (unpublished data), a behavior shared with collagen gels [2, 50, 51]. Changes in fibrin molecular spacing, as assessed with small-angle X-ray scattering (SAXS), indicate that, once fibrin fibers are aligned in the direction of stretch, fibrinopeptides begin to unfold, most likely by their coiled-coil domains, to accommodate increasing strain [29]. Without the crosslinks introduced by factor XIIIa, protofibrils will instead slide past each other rather than unfold [29]. Once unfolding has been exhausted the fibers rapidly stiffen and more force is required to axially deform the fibers. The individual fibers then begin to fail by rupturing either at the connections between fibers or along the fiber in a manner dependent on the amount of crosslinking [52].

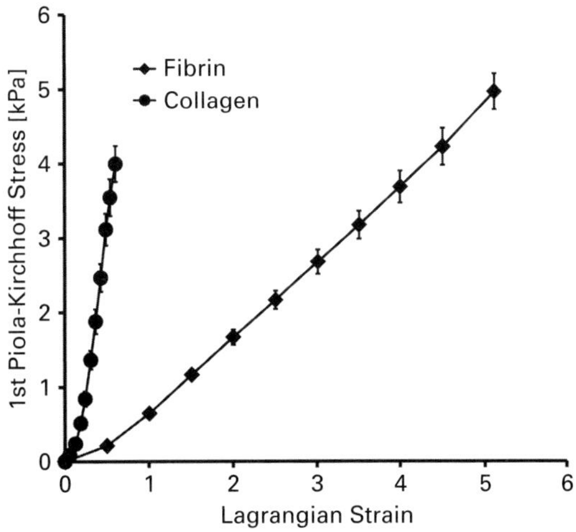

Figure 17.3 Load–displacement behavior of acellular 1.9-mg/ml fibrin gels ($n = 7$) and 2.1-mg/ml collagen gels ($n = 8$). The fibrin gel increases in stiffness after reaching ~50% strain, and it is significantly more compliant under uniaxial extension than the collagen gel, stretching to more than three times it original length (16.5 mm) before failure. Data provided courtesy of Victor Lai.

17.3 Cell entrapment

Once a fibrin gel forms from a fibrinogen–thrombin–Ca^{2+} solution containing tissue cells, cells quickly begin to interact with the network structure that has formed, as evidenced by cell elongation. Many cell types can compact and remodel the gel, as well as proliferating, such that the microstructure is reorganized and fibrin is degraded and replaced with other extracellular matrix (ECM) protein fibers. Fibrin interactions with several cell types have been investigated, including fibroblasts [53–56], myofibroblasts [57], smooth muscle cells [4, 31, 58–60], mesenchymal stem cells [61, 62], and endothelial cells [33, 63]. Each type of cell interacts with fibrin in a unique way, but common to most phenotypes is the tendency for cells to exert tractions on the matrix that compact the gel, which can lead to alignment of both cells and fibers.

17.3.1 Cell compaction

When cells are added to fibrin gels, they are generally mixed in with the solution of fibrinogen, thrombin, and $CaCl_2$ just prior to reconstitution in order to produce a homogeneous distribution of cells within the construct. Once gelation has occurred, tissue cells attach to the fibrin fibers and exert traction forces that pull the fibers inward, provided that these forces exceed the mechanical resistance of the fiber network. These cell tractions act collectively to significantly reduce gel volume and compact the gel through an increase in matrix density (Figure 17.2, image B) and a concomitant expulsion of interstitial fluid, a process sometimes referred to as syneresis [64]. As with cell-populated collagen gels, the rate and amount of gel compaction are dependent on a number of factors, including cell concentration, fibrin concentration, and other cell culture conditions. Furthermore, if the gels are prevented from fully compacting (i.e. the gels are mechanically constrained), then, instead of compacting into an isotropic and stress-free state (as is the case when they are unattached and free-floating) [53], tension is sustained in the network and fibrin fiber alignment develops [65]. Both the amount of tension and the degree of alignment in the gel appears to play an important role in fibroblast proliferation and ECM synthesis, and has implications for the trajectory that ECM remodeling will follow [56].

17.3.2 Controlling fiber alignment

A key advantage to using fibrin gels as a temporary scaffold is that the fiber alignment that results during cell compaction of the gel can serve as a template for the alignment of ECM fibers that are deposited as the fibrin degrades [65–67]. Creating fiber alignment from cell-induced compaction significantly improves the mechanical properties of the gel. The fibrin alignment that develops mirrors that observed in collagen gels of the same geometry (tubes [50, 68], valves [66, 69], and cruciform shapes [56, 70]) (Figure 17.4). In order to control fiber alignment, resistance to cell traction on the network is required. This resistance is provided by mechanical constraints on the gel that often take the form of adherent surfaces or embedded obstructions. These constraints, which change the boundary conditions of the gel, can be designed into the molds used to form the gel's initial geometry. For example, if one forms a rectangular gel where the two gel surfaces normal to the long axis are prevented from contracting inward, the gel will compact along directions perpendicular to the remaining four free surfaces, such that the gel contracts inward and axial fiber alignment forms between the two constraining surfaces. Alternatively, if one forms a tubular gel in a mold with non-adherent surfaces, the gel will compact radially and axially, and this process will generate circumferential alignment similar to that found in the arterial wall. We will see in a later section how these tubular constructs are used to form tissue-engineered blood vessels, and how mold design can be used to achieve more complicated geometries with prescribed fiber alignment patterns, and thus fibrin templates, that more closely resemble the structural heterogeneity of the ECM in other tissues and serve as templates for engineered heart valves.

17.3.3 Mechanical properties

As the cells compact and remodel a fibrin gel, the gel's mechanical properties begin to change considerably, with increases in stiffness and strength leading to tissue-like properties as cells proliferate and remodel the gel with newly synthesized collagen and other ECM proteins [56, 71, 72]. Once the compaction process begins, the gel stiffens rapidly along the direction of fiber alignment, primarily because of consolidation of and changes in fiber orientation [68, 73]. The stiffening process, as it develops over the long term, is dependent in part on the initial cell density [74]. It is also dependent on the initial configuration of the microstructure because, even though it quickly changes as the cells remodel the matrix, it provides constraints and cues that direct the subsequent remodeling events [56]. The biggest changes occur when the fibrin is replaced with collagen fibers and other ECM components [55, 56]. However, it is not just composition that is important. Collagen crosslinking with lysyl oxidase is critical to the development of

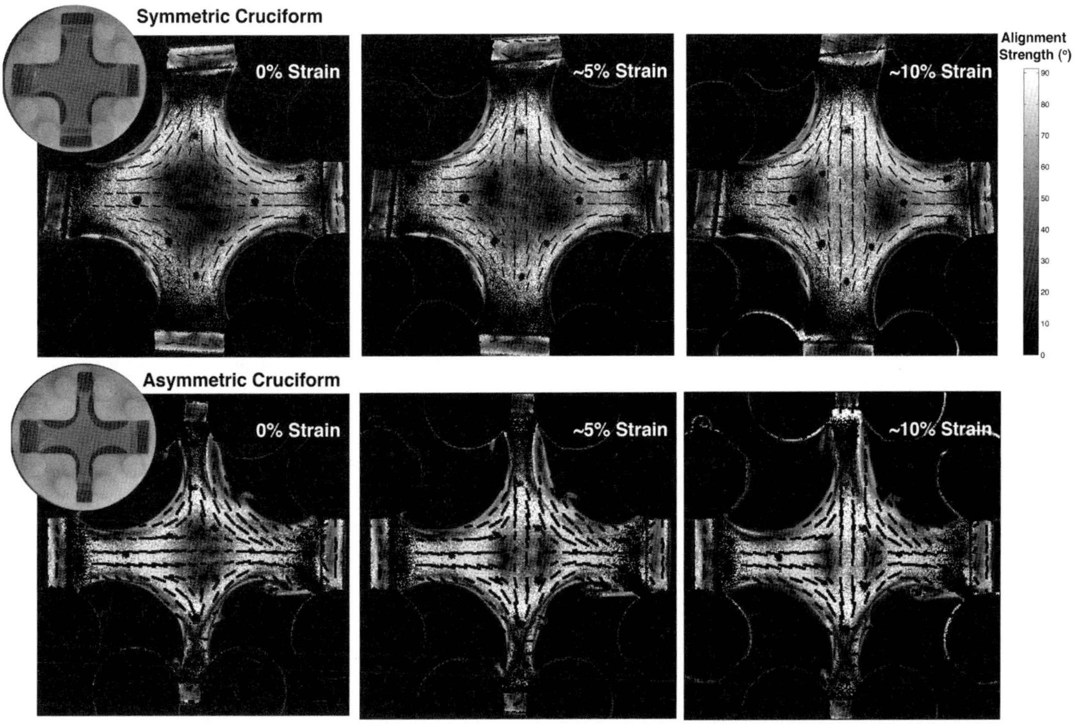

Figure 17.4 Alignment maps for cross-shaped fibrin gels seeded with neonatal human dermal fibroblasts and allowed to remodel for 10 weeks. The interplay among cell compaction of the gel, the gel geometry, and the mechanical constraints to compaction produces fiber alignment (black lines) in the fibrin gels. For the symmetric cruciform, there is strong alignment (assessed with polarized light) in the arms and little alignment in the center region at 0% strain. The asymmetric cruciform also has strong alignment in the arms at 0% strain, but in the center there is moderate horizontal alignment. During an off-axis hold test, where the vertical axis is displaced while the horizontal axis remains stationary, there is increasing fiber re-alignment toward the vertical axis. See [56] for more details.

tissue strength and integrity, as evidenced by the poor mechanical strength in gels where lysyl oxidase crosslinking was inhibited [55]. In fact, the authors of several studies have investigated methods to promote fibrin crosslinking in order to increase gel stiffness, including the use of ruthenium-catalyzed photocrosslinking [75, 76] and genipin [77]. Both of these crosslinking methods stiffen the tissues, thereby retarding compaction [76], without demonstrable changes in viability or cellularity, but it remains unclear how such crosslinks impact the long-term remodeling of the construct. The events involved in the remodeling process unfold in a complex and integrated manner that is application-specific, so we will reserve further discussion on cell-based changes in mechanical properties for later sections.

17.3.4 Advantages over collagen

Compositional changes and further cellular refinements to the ECM microstructure continue to enhance the mechanical functionality of remodeling fibrin-based constructs, bringing them closer to the properties of native tissues. A key benefit to using fibrin over collagen as the biopolymer scaffold is that there is a significant increase in the production of both collagen and total protein when tissue cells, such as fibroblasts [65, 78] and smooth muscle cells (SMCs) [65], are cultured in fibrin gels instead of collagen gels. For example, SMCs in fibrin gels produced more than triple the amount of collagen and detectable amounts of elastin produced by their counterparts in collagen gels [65]. Furthermore, even though there is less total collagen in a remodeled fibrin-based construct than in an analogous collagen-based construct, the fibrin-based constructs develop superior mechanical properties, including modulus and ultimate tensile strength, because the constructs contain cell-produced collagen that is properly assembled and crosslinked compared with reconstituted collagen. Fibrin also promotes cell proliferation for many cell phenotypes, such as fibroblasts [54], SMCs [60], and MSCs [38]. However, high initial concentrations of fibrinogen (17–50 mg/ml) have been shown to reduce fibroblast proliferation rates compared with rates obtained with lower concentrations (2–5 mg/ml), at least for fibroblasts maintained in vitro [38, 74]. Even in the physiological range of fibrin concentrations (1–6 mg/ml), cell-proliferation and collagen-synthesis rates were found to be inversely correlated with fibrin concentration [79], a result that may reflect reduced nutrient transport as a consequence of the formation of smaller pores at higher fibrin concentrations [38, 79]. Nevertheless, several attempts that employed fibrin sealant (>90 mg/ml) for in-vivo cell delivery have been successful (see Section 17.6.1), perhaps illustrating differences in cell type and between in-vitro and in-vivo conditions. Furthermore, there are a number of circulating proteins and growth factors that bind to fibrin and presumably enhance its biological activity compared with that of collagen [80, 81]. Finally, fibrinogen can be obtained from a patient's blood in sufficient amounts to produce an autologous graft, if necessary, thereby mitigating the risks of disease transmission or an immune/inflammatory response, something that is not possible with collagen.

17.4 Fibrinolysis

17.4.1 Mechanism

Fibrinolysis is the process by which fibrin is enzymatically degraded (see [82] for an extensive review). It is a two-step process that begins with the activation of plasminogen into the active form of the enzyme, plasmin, and continues with fibrin cleavage by plasmin into soluble fragments called fibrin degradation products (FDPs). Plasminogen is primarily activated by tissue plasminogen activator (tPA), which is secreted by vascular endothelial cells, but there are other plasminogen activators too, such as urokinase-type plasminogen activator (uPA) [82]. tPA binds first to the outside of a fibrin fiber and then activates bound plasminogen to plasmin. Fibrinolysis then proceeds by “transverse cutting” rather than by uniform and progressive cutting on the fiber surface, which means that thick fibers do not transition into thin fibers but instead progressively fragment [35, 83]. In addition, as fibers are digested, dissected fragments can associate laterally, such that fiber diameter and pore size both increase during fibrinolysis [82]. The rate of degradation is dependent on a number of factors besides plasmin concentration, including fibrin fiber diameter and network microstructure [35] and the degree and type of fibrin crosslinking [32]. Although thin fibers degrade faster than thick fibers [35], coarse gels containing thick fibers with large pores dissolve faster than fine gels with thin fibers and small pores, most likely because the fine gels have more fibers to cut through and a slower tPA binding front [82]. This finding thus illustrates the complex interplay between fiber and network architecture. Furthermore, the degradation rate is also influenced by the state of tension in the gel. Recent work has shown that fibrin networks under tension are more resistant to degradation than are unloaded networks [84]. Here, the rates of both plasminogen activation and fibrin lysis were reduced in stretched fibers.

17.4.2 Inhibiting fibrinolysis

One challenge in using fibrin as a scaffold for engineered tissues is that the fibrin matrix can degrade rapidly, depending on the cell type and culture conditions used. In the worst case, the construct disintegrates before enough ECM can be produced to maintain the stability of the construct. In such cases, it is beneficial to reduce the rate of fibrinolysis by adding chemical inhibitors to the culture medium in order to provide sufficient time for the replacement ECM to form. Several fibrinolysis inhibitors have been used successfully to reduce the rate of fibrin degradation, including aprotinin [53, 57, 85] and ε-amino caproic acid (ACA) [68, 86–88]. ACA inhibits plasmin [89], uPA [90], and tPA [91]. For SMCs entrapped in a fibrin gel, the amount and temporal profile of FDPs in the medium was dependent on the concentration of ACA in the medium [92]. At lower inhibitor concentrations (e.g. 3 mM), the level of FDP in the medium was substantially higher and peaked sooner than was the case for higher ACA concentrations (e.g. 12 mM). The use of a lower ACA concentration – which led to less inhibition of fibrin degradation – also resulted in greater deposition of collagen and elastin, greater cellularity, and better mechanical properties [92].

The necessity of including a fibrinolysis inhibitor is cell-type-dependent, and therefore application-specific. Ye *et al.* found that myofibroblasts completely degrade 3.5 mg/ml fibrin gel with 5 μg/ml or less aprotinin [57]. Some fibrinolysis was detected with 15 μg/ml aprotinin, but no visible fibrinolysis was observed with 20 μg/ml aprotinin. In another study, rat SMCs entrapped in 3.3 mg/ml fibrinogen completely degraded the fibrin gel within 24 hours without exogenous inhibitors [92]. On the other hand, fibrin degraded at a much slower rate and still persisted in constructs with neonatal human dermal fibroblasts after 10 weeks of culture without exogenous inhibitors [56]. The reduced rate of degradation observed for fibroblasts is a direct consequence of lower plasmin levels, but it could also be modulated by the internal tensions exerted by fibroblasts on the fibers, since degradation rates are lower for stretched fibers than for unstretched ones [84].

17.4.3 Fibrin degradation products

Fibrin degradation products (FDPs) are biologically active and are known to influence cell behavior and the remodeling process in a number of ways. Some examples are that FDPs can influence fibroblasts and neutrophil migration [93], SMC [31, 58] and hemopoietic cell [94] proliferation, collagen production in a chorioallantoic membrane model [95], and fibrinogen synthesis by rat hepatocytes [96]. In one study, the addition of 250 or 500 μg/ml of FDP to the medium of SMCs in either monolayer culture or in fibrin constructs for one week induced SMCs to produce significantly more collagen per cell than did untreated controls [92]. These results suggest that FDPs positively stimulate ECM synthesis. However, various growth factors are also sequestered in the ECM and can be activated by plasmin activity [97, 98], which makes it difficult to determine whether the FDPs themselves or the growth factors attached to them are directing cell activity. Regardless of the exact mechanism, the course of ECM remodeling is clearly affected by the intricate interplay and balance between degrading and replacing the provisional fibrin matrix with new ECM and maintaining the stability of the structure.

17.5 Fibrin remodeling and tissue growth

17.5.1 Biochemical stimulation

Growth factors, hormones, cytokines, and other biochemicals are important chemical messengers that are routinely included in culture medium to direct cell activity and improve ECM synthesis. TGF-β_1 is commonly added to the medium because it is known to improve ECM synthesis [99] and stimulate production of the collagen-crosslinking enzyme lysyl oxidase [100], activities that both increase tissue stiffness and strength. For example, Clark *et al.* found that including TGF-β_1 significantly improved collagen production by fibroblasts maintained on tissue culture plastic [101]. Enhanced synthetic activity in the presence of TGF-β_1 has also been observed for fibroblasts in fibrin gel, but in collagen gel the synthetic response is attenuated [3, 78]. In one study, when 100 pM TGF-β_1 was added to fibroblasts in fibrin gel, collagen and non-collagen synthesis increased 4.4- and 3.4-fold, respectively, compared with the case of gels without TGF-β_1 [3]. Insulin also has been shown to increase collagen synthesis and improve mechanical properties, but it is most effective when combined with TGF-β_1, in which case it acts synergistically to up-regulate latent TGF-β_1 synthesis [102]. In our own studies we have found that substantial improvements in ECM remodeling and mechanical properties occur when TGF-β_1 and insulin are combined [55, 60, 68, 103]. For example, after 51 days with 5 ng/ml TBF-β_1 and 2 μg/ml insulin added to the medium, fibrin constructs seeded with fibroblasts produced nearly 20 times more collagen than, and had a 10-fold increase in tensile strength compared with, those without the additives [55]. In another study, SMCs were stimulated with 5 ng/ml TBF-β_1 and 2 μg/ml insulin, and increased collagen production six-fold and UTS and tangent modulus 15–20-fold after three weeks of culture [68]. Furthermore, TBF-β_1 and insulin also increased elastic fiber production [60, 103]. We have also found recently that TGF-β_1 activity is influenced by the mechanical environment [73]. Fibrin-based constructs cyclically stretched for seven weeks and supplemented with TGF-β_1 had lower collagen content, UTS/modulus, and extracellular signal-regulated kinase (ERK) phosphorylation, but higher elastin content than did samples without TGF-β_1 supplementation, even though at two weeks no differences between the two groups were observed. The idea that chemical and mechanical stimulation are coupled is supported by earlier work that showed that TGF-β_1 activity was modulated by whether gels were allowed to retract or prevented from retracting [78]. Fibrin gels that were prevented from contracting produced significantly more collagen, suggesting that the state of tension in the fibrin network, and hence the mechanical environment, is important for directing the remodeling process.

17.5.2 Mechanical stimulation

It is well established that mechanical conditioning can provide important stimulatory cues during the remodeling process that increase the mechanical stiffness and strength of a tissue [104]. These signals can be delivered externally to the gel via a number of modalities, including compression, tension, bending, and shear, where the duration and magnitude are altered accordingly. For example, Balestrini *et al.* studied fibroblast response to dynamic equibiaxial stretch (16% stretch at 0.2 Hz) over eight days and found increased collagen deposition and crosslinking that was correlated with a significant increase in construct strength over that of static controls (although some of the improvements in strength were also attributed to increased fibrin compaction and other organizational changes that were also observed in acellular controls) [105]. When the stretch magnitude and duration (i.e. continuous (24 hours per day) versus intermittent (6 hours per day) stretch) were varied, the construct strength increased with the stretch magnitude, and the failure tension, stiffness, and collagen synthesis increased with intermittent stretch [72]. Why intermittent stretch produced better results than continuous stretch is unknown, but one possibility is that rest disrupted the adaptive response that the fibroblasts developed to continuous conditioning, such that the daily renewal of cyclic stretch following rest continued to activate cell signaling pathways necessary to stimulate collagen production. Syedain *et al.* also observed cellular adaptation to long-term continuous cyclic distention [67]. However, instead of implementing a rest period, the strain amplitude was periodically increased in step-wise fashion to the same final strain amplitude as for the continuously conditioned constructs. The change in mechanical environment with each strain step significantly improved collagen deposition and mechanical properties and correlated with an increase in ERK phosphorylation, which has been shown to be necessary for stretch-induced collagen transcription by cardiac fibroblasts [106]. From these studies, it is clear that, in order to provide positive mechanical stimulation for increased collagen deposition, the loading environment must change faster than the cells adapt to it. Furthermore, because the relationship between external loading and cell stimulation is a dynamic and evolving one, theoretical models are required to provide a full appreciation and understanding of these complex and interdependent relationships so that an optimized conditioning strategy for producing functional engineered tissues can be designed.

Another potentially significant and less appreciated source of mechanical stimulation is the endogenous gel tension that develops during the compaction process. In collagen gels, it has been clearly demonstrated that cell tension is an important stimulatory signal for fibroblasts that is reduced or absent in unconstrained, free-floating gels [107, 108]. Internal tension is also important in fibrin gels. As mentioned in the previous section, substantially more collagen was produced in constrained fibrin gels than in unconstrained free-floating fibrin gels [78]. In addition, gels that are constrained compared with their unconstrained counterparts have shown modulated responses to platelet-derived growth factor BB [109], decreased tPA levels and fibrinolysis rates [110], and improved organization and crimp of deposited collagen [111]. A recent study on the cell-induced compaction and fiber alignment process in cross-shaped fibrin gels found regional differences in ECM deposition that were correlated with regional differences in fiber alignment [56]. Simulations of the experiment suggest that the regional mechanical stress environment produced by internal cell tension influences collagen deposition, and that a high local mechanical stress produced via cell compaction and fiber alignment induces more collagen and, to a lesser extent, elastin synthesis than occurs in regions where this stress is less. These results illustrate clearly that complex relationships exist among external mechanical conditioning/stimulation, internal cell-generated tension, and ECM remodeling, and that the final outcomes reported are dependent on a number of experimental conditions. For this reason, we continue our discussion on mechanical stimulation as it applies to each application in the next section.

17.6 Tissue engineering applications

The use of fibrin to facilitate tissue regeneration has its origins in fibrin's usage as a sealant in surgery. Here, solutions of fibrinogen (at high concentrations – e.g. ARTISS by Baxter contains >90 mg/ml of fibrinogen) and thrombin are typically delivered via a dual-syringe system to the surgical site in order to stop bleeding (hemostasis), to seal tissues (i.e. contain fluids in their proper compartments), or to bond tissues together until they can heal [112–114]. In addition to serving as a biocompatible, biodegradable, and moldable adhesive, fibrin sealant also promotes wound healing, angiogenesis, and tissue growth. For these reasons, fibrin continues to be explored for its potential in many clinical applications, including in the field of tissue-engineering [115, 116]. Below we summarize the major areas where fibrin-based tissue engineering technologies are being developed.

17.6.1 Fibrin as a cell-delivery vehicle

Perhaps the most straightforward extension of using fibrin as a sealant is for the delivery of cells to a specific location in the body. For example, Bach *et al.* reconstructed a urethra by introducing a mixture of autologous urothelial cells and fibrin to a connective tissue capsule tube formed in vivo [117]. In a similar type of study, skeletal myoblasts encapsulated in fibrin were injected into rat infarcted left ventricles to replace necrotic cardiomyoctes [118]. The use of fibrin increased the rate of survival of transplanted cells, reduced the size of the infarcted region, and increased blood flow to the region compared with direct injection of cells in bovine serum albumin. Use of fibrin has also been explored as a potential method for delivering mesenchymal stem cells to sites of bone fracture [61], defects in tendons [62, 119], and cutaneous wounds [120, 121] to enhance healing. Other investigators have used fibrin as a carrier for seeding cells within other more rigid scaffolds. Mol *et al.* found that such an approach led to greater retention of cell-produced collagen and more mature ECM formation then was achieved without the fibrin gel [86]. In a somewhat different capacity, fibrin has also been used to bond engineered tissue to the surgical site, for example with skin grafts [122] or a composite neotrachea [123].

17.6.2 Skin tissue engineering and wound healing

In addition to its usage as an adhesive for skin grafts [122, 124], fibrin has also been studied for its potential to aid in wound healing and as a scaffold for engineered skin [122]. For skin tissue engineering applications, efforts with fibrin-based materials have focussed on either engineering a dermis in vitro that becomes populated with the host's keratinocytes after grafting

[125, 126], or recreating the epidermal–dermal structure of native skin [85, 127, 128] so that the grafts have better tissue integrity and function than cultured epithelium provides. One obstacle to using fibrin in the latter capacity is that the keratinocytes that make up the epidermal layer lack $\alpha v\beta_3$ integrins, and therefore cannot attach directly to fibrin, being able to attach only indirectly through bridges formed with other ECM proteins, such as fibronectin [129]. Nevertheless, after 15 days of culture, Meana *et al.* [85] were able to form a stratified epithelium with basement membrane (as indicated by the presence of type IV collagen) on a fibrin gel containing fibroblasts. They were likely successful because the fibrin used was obtained from human plasma, which is known to contain fibronectin and other biomolecules [130, 131]. Furthermore, the fibroblasts in the gel also provided essential support to the keratinocytes in forming a basement membrane, a finding that has long been observed with other engineered skin systems [132, 133]. More recent studies have also demonstrated successful bilayer formation when keratinocytes are combined with fibrin from plasma and fibroblasts [127, 128]. Another benefit of using fibrin as a scaffold is that it appears to induce greater VEGF production in keratinocytes than do collagen scaffolds, which could have important implications in improving graft vascularization and implantation success rates [134]. Remaining challenges for this technology include increasing construct mechanical strength in vitro to minimize damage during surgery, incorporating skin appendages, such as sweat glands and hair follicles, reducing scar formation, and improving the cosmetic appearance and composition of the constructs as they remodel on the patient so that the grafts are indistinguishable from native skin.

17.6.3 Cardiovascular tissue engineering

Regenerative technologies involving fibrin have also been explored in many cardiovascular applications, including the production of tissue-engineered blood vessels, heart valves, and myocardium. Tissue-engineered blood vessels (TEBVs) are perhaps the simplest of these to produce, and involve forming tubular-tissue constructs with entrapped cells from different sources. As discussed previously, by controlling the geometry and boundary conditions of the gel, one can control the fiber alignment pattern that develops as the cells compact the gel so that the circumferential alignment observed in native vessels develops. This strategy was first implemented with smooth muscle cells (SMCs) embedded in collagen gels [135, 136] and later extended to fibrin gels [60, 65, 68, 103] due to significant improvements in collagen deposition and mechanical properties with fibrin [65]. Early work on fibrin TEBVs with neonatal SMCs and cultured in vitro with 1 ng/ml TBF-β, 1 mg/ml ACA, and 2 μg/ml insulin found extensive remodeling and substantial improvements in mechanical properties after six weeks [68]. The modulus and UTS values (15.4 ± 5.3 MPa and 1.4 ± 6.1 MPa, respectively) were comparable to those of the rat abdominal aorta (8.4 ± 2.2 MPa and 2.1 ± 9.0 MPa, respectively), but the constructs were thin and the burst strength was still quite low, around 120–140 mm Hg [137] and well below the requirements of a replacement artery. Swartz *et al.* added ECs to SMC-seeded TEBVs after they had remodeled in vitro for two weeks. After 3–10 days, these constructs were grafted into the external jugular veins of lambs, and they were still patent 15 weeks after the operation. Furthermore, they contained significant amounts of collagen and elastin, as well as multiple layers of SMCs covered by a lumenal monolayer of endothelial cells [138, 139]. However, these TEBVs also lacked the burst strength needed for arterial implantation, which is the major clinical need.

Several bioreactors have been developed to provide environmental conditions that better mimic the in-vivo environment and further aid in construct development prior to implantation [67, 140–143]. Many of these systems provide pulsatile flow for mimicking in-vivo cyclic distension and/or shear-flow profiles. Others provide for cyclic distension alone by inflating an internal elastic tube that contacts the luminal surface [67, 140, 142]. Such configurations provide mechanical as well as chemical stimulation, which greatly enhances TEBV development over static culture conditions.

Since the loading conditions are often unchanged for the duration of the experiment (i.e. strain amplitude, loading wave form, flow rate, etc.), it was hypothesized that the initial stimulatory response can quickly fade as cells adapt to the environment. When periodic incremental increases in the cyclic strain amplitude from 5% to 15% circumferential strain were applied to TEBVs containing either porcine valve interstitial cells or human dermal fibroblasts, greater collagen deposition and significantly better mechanical properties were achieved than with a constant strain amplitude (~300% higher modulus and 50% higher UTS, respectively, compared with static controls) [67]. Furthermore, it appears that with each step in strain amplitude, the cells were stimulated by the change in the mechanical environment, consistent with an increase in ERK phosphorylation, and perhaps responded by remodeling the ECM in order to return to a baseline environment (i.e. an adaptive response), as hypothesized in "tensional homeostasis" [145]. This notion is supported by the finding that there was a better outcome when four 2.5% strain steps were taken from 5% to 15% strain over the three-week culture period rather than two equal 5% steps. To overcome nutrient limitations inside TEBVs, transmural flow through the vessel wall was also investigated [141] and incorporated into a new bioreactor system so that beneficial components of cyclic stretching and controlled luminal, abluminal, and transmural flow could be applied to the TEBV [146]. Superior results were obtained in this pulsed-flow-stretch bioreactor, with burst pressures in the range 1400–1600 mm Hg, with compliance comparable to that of native arteries being achieved, in comparison with values in the range 300–500 mm Hg using just static culture for a similar duration [140].

Prosthetic heart-valve replacements suffer from several problems that stem from their inability to mimic native valve mechanics or to grow and adapt throughout the patient's lifetime, an issue of particular importance to pediatric patients. Tissue-engineered heart valves (TEHVs) offer a potential solution by providing a living replacement valve [147, 148]. Current strategies to realize this potential using fibrin generally involve creating a valve-shaped fibrin gel that the entrapped tissue cells remodel (Figure 17.5). Jockenhoevel *et al.* first introduced molds to fabricate myofibroblast-encapsulated fibrin gels with the

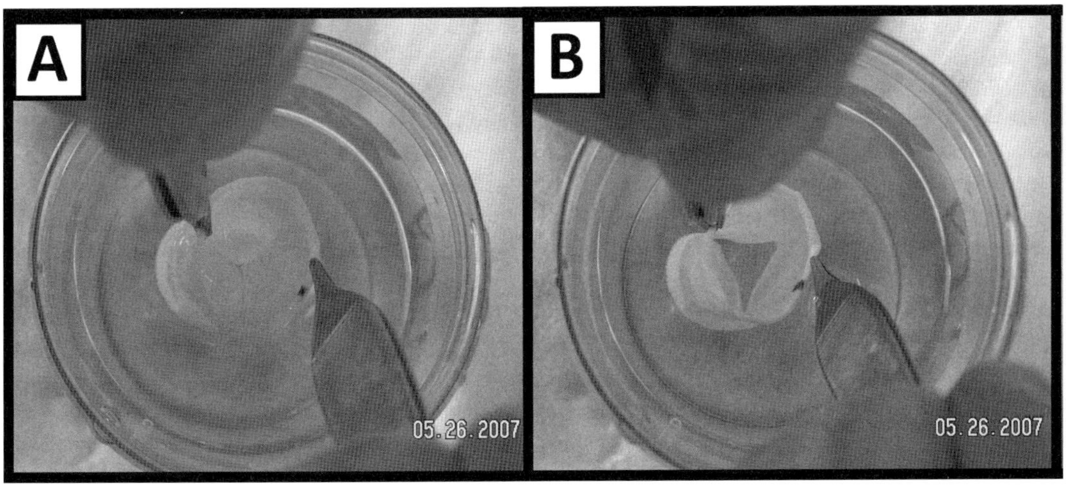

Figure 17.5 A fibrin-based engineered heart valve in the (A) closed and (B) open position. The process of constrained fibrin gel compaction in a casting mold was used to fabricate a tri-leaflet valve, with coaptation of the leaflets evident, as described previously [66, 144, 155]. The mold is designed so that fibrin and subsequent cell-produced collagen have the characteristic circumferential alignment in the root and commisural alignment in the leaflets.

complex 3D geometry of native heart valves [149, 150]. In order to prevent significant changes in valve geometry from cell-induced compaction ("gel shrinkage" was cited as a major problem), these constructs were fixed at the boundaries, either chemically with poly-L-lysine or mechanically with a polystyrene plate [149]. However, despite several weeks of culture and ECM remodeling, the valves were too weak for implantation. Rather than trying to prevent gel shrinkage, Neidert *et al.* [69] designed molds that take advantage of the cell compaction process to produce stronger constructs with alignment. By applying the same concepts as those used to fabricate arteries, molds were designed to produce collagen TEHVs [69] (as proof-of-concept work) and fibrin TEHVs [66] that possessed commissure-to-commissure alignment in the leaflets and circumferential alignment in the aortic root that resembles the gross fiber alignment patterns observed in the native valve. Although both TEHVs incorporated neonatal human dermal fibroblasts that compacted the gel to produce anisotropic fiber alignment and mechanical properties, the fibrin TEHVs had higher circumferential modulus and UTS values than did the collagen TEHVs (2343 kPa and 530 kPa versus 28 kPa and 320 kPa, respectively) when the TEHVs were cultured statically on the casting mold for the five-week duration [66]. Also, even though the fibrin TEHVs had an average circumferential modulus and UTS approximately 15% and 50% of native porcine valve values, the fibrin-based constructs did compare favorably with porcine aortic valves in many other respects, including fully opening and allowing flow at −10 mm Hg, sustaining a maximum back pressure of ~330 mm Hg when pressurized to failure at a rate of 100 mm Hg/s, and functioning within the estimated in-vivo range of maximum stress (500 kPa) and tension (175 kPa) in the aortic valve [66].

Despite these improvements, the compositional, microstructural, and mechanical properties of fibrin-based TEHVs fabricated under static culture conditions still differed substantially from those of native valves, particularly in terms of elastin content and viscoelastic behavior [151]. As discussed earlier, mechanical stimulation from dynamic culture conditions can provide important cues that direct tissue growth and improve mechanical properties. Bioreactors have been designed to deliver mechanical stimulation and improve nutrient transport for TEHVs [144, 146, 152–154]. These bioreactors generally involve incorporating a pulsatile-flow loop that opens and closes the valve leaflets, and mimics some aspect of in-vivo physiological conditions. Such a system provides dynamic stimulation in the form of shear stress, pressure gradients, and tissue deformation, and it also improves nutrient and waste transport. Common to each of these systems is the finding that the dynamic environment significantly improved the remodeling response compared with static controls. For fibrin TEHVs, Flanagan *et al.* observed increased cellularity and expression of α-smooth muscle actin and greater ECM deposition and organization with pulsatile flow and low pressure differences across the closed leaflets than for control TEHVs cultured under stirred conditions [153]. Syedain *et al.* incorporated both cyclic pressurization and stretching via a distensible latex tube placed around the TEHV [144, 146]. Incremental increases in the strain amplitude applied over a three-week culture period produced TEHVs with improved compositional and mechanical properties, including tensile stiffness and ability to accommodate cyclic pulmonary pressure comparable to that of sheep pulmonary valves [144].

Some groups have reached the stage where their TEHVs are stable enough for implantation into animals [155, 156]. Flanagan *et al.* [156] implanted TEHVs mechanically conditioned for 28 days and consisting of autologous aortic fibroblasts, smooth muscle cells, and endothelial cells into sheep. After three months in vivo, harvested TEHVs were found to have undergone substantial remodeling and development toward native valve structure. However, leaflet shrinkage did lead to valvular insufficiency problems, which led the authors to suggest that a biodegradable support material will need to be incorporated into the fibrin gel to mitigate tissue contraction. Syedain *et al.* implanted TEHVs that had been mechanically conditioned for 21 days consisting of human dermal fibroblasts into immunosuppressed and heparinized sheep [155]. In all sheep, echocardiography at implantation showed coapting leaflets, with minimal valve regurgitation and no turbulence. Orifice area and pressure gradients at systole attained the native pulmonary valve values. However, as in the study by Flanagan *et al.*, leaflet shrinkage occurred over eight weeks, leading to regurgitation. Immunocytochemistry indicated that this was due to sustained tissue contraction caused by the fibroblasts, not by the invading host cells, which included a subpopulation consistent with bone-marrow-derived cells. Nevertheless, these results are highly encouraging and suggest that the realization of TEHVs for clinical usage is within sight.

Other areas where fibrin is being incorporated into cardiovascular tissue engineering applications include the development of myocardium [157] and vascular supply via angiogenesis [158, 159].

17.6.4 Other applications

There are other TERM applications where fibrin has been explored for its potential as a scaffold, most notably for cartilage [77, 88, 160–162], but also for cornea [163], tendon [79], and neural tissue [164–167]. In many of these applications, fibrin is combined with a synthetic material to leverage the advantages of fibrin with the mechanical strength and other favorable properties of the other materials [71, 168–170]. In all these applications, the potential of fibrin or a fibrin-based engineered tissue has been demonstrated. However, many significant challenges for this technology yet remain, the most pressing and overarching being that these engineered constructs generally do not possess enough of the compositional and structural features of the native tissue, and therefore cannot provide the functional requirements of the tissues they are intended to replace.

17.7 Conclusion

Fibrin possesses a combination of properties that make it an attractive material for TERM applications. As a result, it has been investigated for use in producing a number of engineered tissues. Some studies have demonstrated the feasibility of using fibrin in certain applications. However, many complex and interdependent factors contribute to the formation, development, and maturation of the engineered tissue, and additional research is required in order to understand how these factors can be better controlled to achieve the functional requirements it must possess to be successful clinically.

REFERENCES

[1] Fratzl, P. 2008. *Collagen: Structure and Mechanics.* Berlin: Springer-Verlag.

[2] Sander, E., Barocas, V. and Fratzl, P. 2008. *Biomimetic Collagen Tissues: Collagenous Tissue Engineering and Other Applications.* New York: Springer.

[3] Clark, R., Nielsen, L. D., Welch, M. P. and McPherson, J. M. 1995. Collagen matrices attenuate the collagen-synthetic response of cultured fibroblasts to TGF-β. *J. Cell Sci.*, **108**(3), 1251.

[4] Thie, M., Schlumberger, W., Semich, R., Rauterberg, J. and Robenek H. 1991. Aortic smooth muscle cells in collagen lattice culture: effects on ultrastructure, proliferation and collagen synthesis. *Eur. J. Cell Biol.*, **55**(2), 295–304.

[5] Mosesson M. 2005. Fibrinogen and fibrin structure and functions. *J. Thrombosis Haemostasis*, **3**(8), 1894–904.

[6] Lord, S. T. 2011. Molecular mechanisms affecting fibrin structure and stability. *Arterioscler. Thromb. Vasc. Biol.*, **31**(3), 494–9.

[7] Weisel, J. W. 2005. Fibrinogen and fibrin. *Adv. Protein Chem.*, **70**, 247–99.

[8] Medved, L. and Weisel, J. 2009. Recommendations for nomenclature on fibrinogen and fibrin. *J. Thrombosis Haemostasis*, **7**(2), 355–9.

[9] Herrick, S., Blanc-Brude, O., Gray, A. and Laurent, G. 1999. Fibrinogen. *Int. J. Biochem. Cell Biol.*, **31**(7), 741–6.

[10] Henschen, A. and Mcdonagh, J. 1986. Fibrinogen, fibrin and factor XIII. *New Comprehensive Biochem.*, **13**, 171–241.

[11] Yee, V. C., Pratt, K. P., Côté, H. C. F. *et al.* 1997. Crystal structure of a 30 kDa C-terminal fragment from the γ chain of human fibrinogen. *Structure*, **5**(1), 125–38.

[12] Spraggon, G., Everse, S. J. and Doolittle, R. F. 1997. Crystal structures of fragment D from human fibrinogen and its crosslinked counterpart from fibrin. *Nature*, **389**(6650), 455–62.

[13] Lewis, S. D., Shields, P. and Shafer, J. 1985. Characterization of the kinetic pathway for liberation of

fibrinopeptides during assembly of fibrin. *J. Biol. Chem.*, **260**(18), 10192.

[14] Doolittle, R. F. 1984. Fibrinogen and fibrin. In *Encyclopedia of Life Sciences.* London: Nature Publishing Group.

[15] Laudano, A. P. and Doolittle, R. F. 1978. Synthetic peptide derivatives that bind to fibrinogen and prevent the polymerization of fibrin monomers. *Proc. Nat. Acad. Sci.*, **75**(7), 3085.

[16] Litvinov, R. I., Gorkun, O. V., Galanakis, D. K. *et al.* 2007. Polymerization of fibrin: direct observation and quantification of individual B: b knob-hole interactions. *Blood*, **109**(1), 130.

[17] Laudano, A. P. and Doolittle, R. F. 1980. Studies on synthetic peptides that bind to fibrinogen and prevent fibrin polymerization. Structural requirements, number of binding sites, and species differences. *Biochemistry*, **19**(5), 1013–19.

[18] Gorkun, O. V., Veklich, Y. I., Weisel, J. W. and Lord, S. T. 1997. The conversion of fibrinogen to fibrin: recombinant fibrinogen typifies plasma fibrinogen. *Blood*, **89**(12), 4407.

[19] Collet, J. P., Moen, J. L., Veklich, Y. I. *et al.* 2005. The αC domains of fibrinogen affect the structure of the fibrin clot, its physical properties, and its susceptibility to fibrinolysis. *Blood*, **106**(12), 3824.

[20] Ferry, J. D. 1952. The mechanism of polymerization of fibrinogen. *Proc. Natl. Acad. Sci. USA*, **38**(7), 566.

[21] Kaibara, M., Fukada, E. and Sakaoku, K. 1981. Rheological study on network structure of fibrin clots under various conditions. *Biorheology*, **18**(1), 23–35.

[22] Ryan, E. A., Mockros, L. F., Weisel, J. W. and Lorand, L. 1999. Structural origins of fibrin clot rheology. *Biophys. J.*, **77**(5), 2813–26.

[23] Muller, M. F., Ris, H. and Ferry, J. D. 1984. Electron microscopy of fine fibrin clots and fine and coarse fibrin films: observations of fibers in cross-section and in deformed states. *J. Molec. Biol.*, **174**(2), 369–84.

[24] Weisel, J. W., Nagaswami, C. and Makowski, L. 1987. Twisting of fibrin fibers limits their radial growth. *Proc. Nat. Acad. Sci.*, **84**(24), 89–91.

[25] Mosesson, M., DiOrio, J., Siebenlist, K., Wall, J. and Hainfeld, J. 1993. Evidence for a second type of fibril branch point in fibrin polymer networks, the trimolecular junction. *Blood*, **82**(5), 15–17.

[26] Mosesson, M. W., Siebenlist, K. R., Amrani, D. L. and DiOrio, J. P. 1989. Identification of covalently linked trimeric and tetrameric D domains in crosslinked fibrin. *Proc. Nat. Acad. Sci.*, **86**(4), 11–13.

[27] Baradet, T. C., Haselgrove, J. C. and Weisel, J. W. 1995. Three-dimensional reconstruction of fibrin clot networks from stereoscopic intermediate voltage electron microscope images and analysis of branching. *Biophys. J.*, **68**(4), 1551–60.

[28] Ariëns, R. A. S., Lai, T. S., Weisel, J. W., Greenberg, C. S. and Grant, P. J. 2002. Role of factor XIII in fibrin clot formation and effects of genetic polymorphisms. *Blood*, **100**(3), 743.

[29] Brown, A. E. X., Litvinov, R. I., Discher, D. E., Purohit, P. K. and Weisel, J. W. 2009. Multiscale mechanics of fibrin polymer: gel stretching with protein unfolding and loss of water. *Science*, **325**(5941), 741.

[30] Pretorius, E., Briedenhann, S., Marx, J. *et al.* 2007. Ultrastructural comparison of the morphology of three different platelet and fibrin fiber preparations. *Anatomical Record: Adv. Integrative Anatomy Evolutionary Biol.*, **290**(2), 188–98.

[31] Ishida, T. and Tanaka, K. 1982. Effects of fibrin and fibrinogen-degradation products on the growth of rabbit aortic smooth muscle cells in culture. *Atherosclerosis*, **44**(2), 161–74.

[32] Greenberg, C. S., Birckbichler, P. J. and Rice, R. H. 1991. Transglutaminases: multifunctional cross-linking enzymes that stabilize tissues. *FASEB J.*, **5**(15), 3071.

[33] Watanabe, K. and Tanaka, K. 1983. Influence of fibrin, fibrinogen and fibrinogen degradation products on cultured endothelial cells. *Atherosclerosis*, **48**(1), 57–70.

[34] Weaver, F. A., Lew, W., Granke, K. *et al.* 2008. A comparison of recombinant thrombin to bovine thrombin as a hemostatic ancillary in patients undergoing peripheral arterial bypass and arteriovenous graft procedures. *J. Vascular Surgery*, **47**(6), 1266–73.

[35] Collet, J., Park, D., Lesty, C. *et al.* 2000. Influence of fibrin network conformation and fibrin fiber diameter on fibrinolysis speed: dynamic and structural approaches by confocal microscopy. *Arterioscler. Thromb. Vasc. Biol.*, **20**(5), 1354–61.

[36] Carr, M. E. 1988. Fibrin formed in plasma is composed of fibers more massive than those formed from purified fibrinogen. *Thromb. Haemost.*, **59**(3), 535–9.

[37] Blomback, B., Carlsson, K., Hessel, B. *et al.* 1989. Native fibrin gel networks observed by 3D microscopy, permeation and turbidity. *Bioch. Biophys. Acta – Protein Structure Molec. Enzymol.*, **997**(1–2), 96–110.

[38] Ho, W., Tawil, B., Dunn, J. C. Y. and Wu, B M. 2006. The behavior of human mesenchymal stem cells in 3D fibrin

clots: dependence on fibrinogen concentration and clot structure. *Tissue Eng.*, **12**(6), 1587–95.

[39] Ferry, J. D. and Morrison, P. R. 1947. Preparation and properties of serum and plasma proteins. VIII. The conversion of human fibrinogen to fibrin under various conditions. *J. Am. Chem. Soc.*, **69**(2), 388–400.

[40] Weisel, J. W. 2004. The mechanical properties of fibrin for basic scientists and clinicians. *Biophys. Chem.*, **112**(2–3), 267–76.

[41] Janmey, P. A., Winer, J. P. and Weisel, J. W. 2009. Fibrin gels and their clinical and bioengineering applications. *J. Roy. Soc. Interface*, **6**(30), 1.

[42] Mockros, L., Roberts, W. and Lorand, L. 1974. Viscoelastic properties of ligation-inhibited fibrin clots. *Biophys. Chem.*, **2**(2), 164.

[43] Roberts, W. W., Lorand, L. and Mockros, L. 1973. Viscoelastic properties of fibrin clots. *Biorheology*, **10**(1), 29.

[44] Gerth, C., Roberts, W. W. and Ferry, J. D. 1974. Rheology of fibrin clots II: linear viscoelastic behavior in shear creep. *Biophys. Chem.*, **2**(3), 208–17.

[45] Nelb, G. W., Gerth, C., Ferry, J. D. and Lorand, L. 1976. Rheology of fibrin clots: III. Shear creep and creep recovery of fine ligated and coarse unligated clots. *Biophys. Chem.*, **5**(3), 377–87.

[46] Liu, W., Jawerth, L., Sparks, E. *et al.* 2006. Fibrin fibers have extraordinary extensibility and elasticity. *Science*, **313**(5787), 634.

[47] Liu, W., Carlisle, C., Sparks, E. and Guthold, M. 2010. The mechanical properties of single fibrin fibers. *J. Thromb. Haemost.*, **8**(5), 1030–6.

[48] Collet, J. P., Shuman, H., Ledger, R. E., Lee, S. and Weisel, J. W. 2005. The elasticity of an individual fibrin fiber in a clot. *Proc. Nat. Acad. Sci. USA*, **102**(26), 9133–7.

[49] Guthold, M., Liu, W., Stephens, B. *et al.* 2004. Visualization and mechanical manipulations of individual fibrin fibers suggest that fiber cross section has fractal dimension 1.3. *Biophys. J.*, **87**(6), 4226–36.

[50] Tower, T. T., Neidert, M. R. and Tranquillo, R. T. 2002. Fiber alignment imaging during mechanical testing of soft tissues. *Ann. Biomed. Eng.*, **30**(10), 1221–33.

[51] Sander, E. A., Stylianopoulos, T., Tranquillo, R. T. and Barocas, V. H. 2009. Image-based multiscale modeling predicts tissue-level and network-level fiber reorganization in stretched cell-compacted collagen gels. *Proc. Nat. Acad. Sci.*, **106**(42), 17675.

[52] Carlisle, C., Sparks, E., Der Loughian, C. and Guthold, M. 2010. Strength and failure of fibrin fiber branchpoints. *J. Thromb. Haemost.*, **8**(5), 1135–8.

[53] Tuan, T. L. and Grinnell, F. 1989. Fibronectin and fibrinolysis are not required for fibrin gel contraction by human skin fibroblasts. *J. Cell Physiol.*, **140**(3), 577–83.

[54] Tuan, T. L., Song, A., Chang, S., Younai, S. and Nimni, M. E. 1996. In vitro fibroplasia: matrix contraction, cell growth, and collagen production of fibroblasts cultured in fibrin gels. *Exp. Cell Res.*, **223**(1), 127–34.

[55] Neidert, M., Lee, E., Oegema, T. and Tranquillo, R. 2002. Enhanced fibrin remodeling in vitro with TGF-β_1, insulin and plasmin for improved tissue-equivalents. *Biomaterials*, **23**(17), 3717–31.

[56] Sander, E., Barocas, V. and Tranquillo, R. 2011. Initial fiber alignment pattern alters extracellular matrix synthesis in fibroblast-populated fibrin gel cruciforms and correlates with predicted tension. *Ann. Biomed. Eng.*, 1–16.

[57] Ye, Q., Zünd, G., Benedikt, P. *et al.* 2000. Fibrin gel as a three dimensional matrix in cardiovascular tissue engineering. *Eur. J. Cardio-Thoracic Surgery*, **17**(5), 587–91.

[58] Naito, M., Nomura, H. and Iguchi, A. 1996. Migration of cultured vascular smooth muscle cells into non-crosslinked fibrin gels. *Thromb. Res.*, **84**(2), 129–36.

[59] Weinbaum, J. S., Qi, J. and Tranquillo, R. T. 2009. Monitoring collagen transcription by vascular smooth muscle cells in fibrin-based tissue constructs. *Tissue Eng. Part C: Methods*, **16**(3), 459–67.

[60] Ross, J. and Tranquillo, R. 2003. ECM gene expression correlates with in vitro tissue growth and development in fibrin gel remodeled by neonatal smooth muscle cells. *Matrix Biol.*, **22**(6), 477–90.

[61] Bensaïd, W., Triffitt, J., Blanchat, C. *et al.* 2003. A biodegradable fibrin scaffold for mesenchymal stem cell transplantation. *Biomaterials*, **24**(14), 2497–502.

[62] Chong, A., Ang, A., Goh, J. *et al.* 2007. Bone marrow-derived mesenchymal stem cells influence early tendon-healing in a rabbit achilles tendon model. *J. Bone Joint Surgery Am. Volume*, **89**(1), 74.

[63] Nakatsu, M. N., Sainson, R. C. A., Aoto, J. N. *et al.* 2003. Angiogenic sprouting and capillary lumen formation modeled by human umbilical vein endothelial cells (HUVEC) in fibrin gels: the role of fibroblasts and angiopoietin-1. *Microvasc. Res.*, **66**(2), 102–12.

[64] Tranquillo, R. T. 1999. Self-organization of tissue-equivalents: the nature and role of contact guidance. *Biochem. Soc. Symp.*, **65**, 27–42.

[65] Grassl, E., Oegema, T. and Tranquillo, R. 2002. Fibrin as an alternative biopolymer to type-I collagen for the fabrication of a media equivalent. *J. Biomed. Mater. Res.*, **60**(4), 607–612.

[66] Robinson, P. S., Johnson, S. L., Evans, M. C., Barocas, V. H. and Tranquillo, R. T. 2008. Functional tissue-engineered valves from cell-remodeled fibrin with commissural alignment of cell-produced collagen. *Tissue Eng. Part A*, **14**(1), 83–95.

[67] Syedain, Z. H., Weinberg, J. S. and Tranquillo, R. T. 2008. Cyclic distension of fibrin-based tissue constructs: evidence of adaptation during growth of engineered connective tissue. *Proc. Nat. Acad. Sci.*, **105**(18), 6537.

[68] Grassl, E., Oegema, T. and Tranquillo, R. 2003. A fibrin-based arterial media equivalent. *J. Biomed. Mater. Res. Part A*, **66**(3), 550–61.

[69] Neidert, M. R. and Tranquillo, R. T. 2006. Tissue-engineered valves with commissural alignment. *Tissue Eng.*, **12**(4), 891–903.

[70] Jhun, C. S., Evans, M. C., Barocas, V. H. and Tranquillo, R. T. 2009 Planar biaxial mechanical behavior of bio-artificial tissues possessing prescribed fiber alignment. *J. Biomech. Eng.*, **131**, 081006.

[71] Cummings, C. L., Gawlitta, D., Nerem, R. M. and Stegemann, J. P. 2004. Properties of engineered vascular constructs made from collagen, fibrin, and collagen-fibrin mixtures. *Biomaterials*, **25**(17), 3699–706.

[72] Balestrini, J. L. and Billiar, K. L. 2009. Magnitude and duration of stretch modulate fibroblast remodeling. *J. Biomech. Eng.*, **131**, 051005.

[73] Syedain, Z. H. and Tranquillo, R. T. 2011. TGF-β_1 diminishes collagen production during long-term cyclic stretching of engineered connective tissue: implication of decreased ERK signaling. *J. Biomech.*, **44**(5), 848–55.

[74] Duong, H., Wu, B. and Tawil, B. 2009. Modulation of 3D fibrin matrix stiffness by intrinsic fibrinogen–thrombin compositions and by extrinsic cellular activity. *Tissue Eng. Part A*, **15**(7), 1865–76.

[75] Bjork, J. W., Johnson, S. L. and Tranquillo, R. T. 2011. Ruthenium-catalyzed photo cross-linking of fibrin-based engineered tissue. *Biomaterials*, **32**(10), 2479–88.

[76] Syedain, Z. H., Bjork, J., Sando, L. and Tranquillo, R. T. 2009. Controlled compaction with ruthenium-catalyzed photochemical cross-linking of fibrin-based engineered connective tissue. *Biomaterials*, **30**(35), 6695–701.

[77] Dare, E. V., Griffith, M., Poitras, P. *et al.* 2009. Genipin cross-linked fibrin hydrogels for in vitro human articular cartilage tissue-engineered regeneration. *Cells Tissues Organs (Print)*, **190**(6), 313–25.

[78] Coustry, F., Gillery, P., Maquart, F. X. and Borel, J. P. 1990. Effect of transforming growth factor β on fibroblasts in three-dimensional lattice cultures. *FEBS Lett.*, **262**(2), 339–41.

[79] Vavken, P., Joshi, S. M. and Murray, M. M. 2011. Fibrin concentration affects ACL fibroblast proliferation and collagen synthesis. *Knee*, **18**(1), 42–6.

[80] Sahni, A., Odrljin, T. and Francis, C. W. 1998. Binding of basic fibroblast growth factor to fibrinogen and fibrin. *J. Biol. Chem.*, **273**(13), 7554.

[81] Sahni, A. and Francis, C. W. 2000. Vascular endothelial growth factor binds to fibrinogen and fibrin and stimulates endothelial cell proliferation. *Blood*, **96**(12), 3772.

[82] Weisel, J. and Litvinov, R. 2008. The biochemical and physical process of fibrinolysis and effects of clot structure and stability on the lysis rate. *Cardiovasc. Hematol. Agents Med. Chem.*, **6**(3), 161–80.

[83] Veklich, Y., Francis, C. W., White, J. and Weisel, J. W. 1998. Structural studies of fibrinolysis by electron microscopy. *Blood*, **92**(12), 4721.

[84] Varjú, I., Sótonyi, P., Machovich, R. *et al.* 2011. Hindered dissolution of fibrin formed under mechanical stress. *J. Thromb. Haemost.*, **9**(5), 979–86.

[85] Meana, A., Iglesias, J., Del Rio, M. *et al.* 1998. Large surface of cultured human epithelium obtained on a dermal matrix based on live fibroblast-containing fibrin gels. *Burns*, **24**(7), 621–30.

[86] Mol, A., van Lieshout, M. I., Dam-de Veen, C. G. *et al.* 2005. Fibrin as a cell carrier in cardiovascular tissue engineering applications. *Biomaterials*, **26**(16), 3113–21.

[87] Rowe, S. L. and Lee, S. Y. and Stegemann, J. P. 2007. Influence of thrombin concentration on the mechanical and morphological properties of cell-seeded fibrin hydrogels. *Acta Biomater.*, **3**(1), 59–67.

[88] Kupcsik, L., Alini, M. and Stoddart, M. J. 2009. Epsilon-aminocaproic acid is a useful fibrin degradation inhibitor for cartilage tissue engineering. *Tissue Eng. Part A*, **15**(8), 2309–13.

[89] Anonick, P. K., Vasudevan, J. and Gonias, S L. 1992. Antifibrinolytic activities of α-N-acetyl-L-lysine methyl ester, ε-aminocaproic acid, and tranexamic acid. Importance of kringle interactions and active site inhibition. *Arterioscler. Thromb. Vasc. Biol.*, **12**(6), 708.

[90] Sun, Z., Chen, Y., Wang, P. *et al.* 2002. The blockage of the high-affinity lysine binding sites of plasminogen by EACA significantly inhibits prourokinase-induced plasminogen activation. *Biochim. Biophys. Acta – Protein Structure Molec. Enzymol.*, **1596**(2), 182–92.

[91] Bakker, A. H. F, Weening-Verhoeff, E. J. D. and Verheijen, J. H. 1995. The role of the lysyl binding site of tissue-type plasminogen activator in the interaction with a forming fibrin clot. *J. Biol. Chem.*, **270**(21), 12355.

[92] Ahmann, K. A., Weinbaum, J. S., Johnson, S. L. and Tranquillo, R. T. 2010. Fibrin degradation enhances vascular smooth muscle cell proliferation and matrix deposition in fibrin-based tissue constructs fabricated in vitro. *Tissue Eng. Part A*, **16**(10), 3261–70.

[93] Senior, R. M., Skogen, W. F., Griffin, G. L. and Wilner, G. D. 1986. Effects of fibrinogen derivatives upon the inflammatory response. Studies with human fibrinopeptide B. *J. Clin. Invest.*, **77**(3), 10–14.

[94] Hatzfeld, J. A., Hatzfeld, A. and Maigne, J. 1982. Fibrinogen and its fragment D stimulate proliferation of human hemopoietic cells in vitro. *Proc. Nat. Acad. Sci.*, **79**(20), 62–80.

[95] Thompson, W., Ervans, A. and Campbell, R. 1986. The control of fibrogenesis: stimulation and suppression of collagen synthesis in the chick chorioallantoic membrane with fibrin degradation products, wound extracts and proteases. *J. Pathol.*, **148**(3), 207–15.

[96] Qureshi, G. D., Guzelian, P. S., Vennart, R. M. and Evans, H. J. 1985. Stimulation of fibrinogen synthesis in cultured rat hepatocytes by fibrinogen fragment E. *Biochim. Biophys. Acta - Molec. Cell Res.*, **844**(3), 288–95.

[97] Campbell, P. G., Novak, J. F., Yanosick, T. and McMaster, J. 1992. Involvement of the plasmin system in dissociation of the insulin-like growth factor-binding protein complex. *Endocrinology*, **130**(3), 1401.

[98] George, S. J., Johnson, J. L., Smith, M. A., Angelini, G. D. and Jackson, C. L. 2005. Transforming growth factor-β is activated by plasmin and inhibits smooth muscle cell death in human saphenous vein. *J. Vasc. Res.*, **42**(3), 247–54.

[99] Roberts, A. B., Mccune, B. K. and Sporn, M. B. 1992. TGF-β: regulation of extracellular matrix. *Kidney Int.*, **41**, 557–9.

[100] Hong, H. H., Mehmet, I. U., Chunni, D., Sheff, M. C. and Trackman, P. C. 1999. Regulation of lysyl oxidase, collagen, and connective tissue growth factor by TGF-β_1 and detection in human gingiva. *Lab. Investigation*, **79**(12), 1655–67.

[101] Clark, R. A. F., McCoy, G. A., Folkvord, J. M. and McPherson, J. M. 1997. TGF-β_1 stimulates cultured human fibroblasts to proliferate and produce tissue-like fibroplasia: a fibronectin matrix-dependent event. *J. Cell Physiol.*, **170**(1), 69–80.

[102] Ghahary, A., Tredget, E. E., Mi, L. and Yang, L. 1999. Cellular response to latent TGF-β_1 is facilitated by insulin-like growth factor-II/mannose-6-phosphate receptors on MS-9 cells. *Exp. Cell. Res.*, **251**(1), 111–20.

[103] Long, J. L. and Tranquillo, R. T. 2003. Elastic fiber production in cardiovascular tissue-equivalents. *Matrix Biol.*, **22**(4), 339–50.

[104] Pedersen, J. A. and Swartz, M. A. 2005. Mechanobiology in the third dimension. *Ann. Biomed. Eng.*, **33**(11), 1469–90.

[105] Balestrini, J. L. and Billiar, K. L. 2006. Equibiaxial cyclic stretch stimulates fibroblasts to rapidly remodel fibrin. *J. Biomech.*, **39**(16), 2983–90.

[106] Papakrivopoulou, J., Lindahl, G. E., Bishop, J. E. and Laurent, G. J. 2004. Differential roles of extracellular signal-regulated kinase 1/2 and p38MAPK in mechanical load-induced procollagen α_1(I) gene expression in cardiac fibroblasts. *Cardiovasc. Res.*, **61**(4), 736–44.

[107] Grinnell, F., Zhu, M., Carlson, M. A. and Abrams, J. M. 1999. Release of mechanical tension triggers apoptosis of human fibroblasts in a model of regressing granulation tissue. *Exp. Cell Res.*, **248**(2), 608–19.

[108] Mochitate, K., Pawelek, P. and Grinnell, F. 1991. Stress relaxation of contracted collagen gels: disruption of actin filament bundles, release of cell surface fibronectin, and down-regulation of DNA and protein synthesis. *Exp. Cell Res.*, **193**(1), 198–207.

[109] Shreiber, D. I., Enever, P. A. J. and Tranquillo, R. T. 2001. Effects of PDGF-BB on rat dermal fibroblast behavior in mechanically stressed and unstressed collagen and fibrin gels. *Exp. Cell Res.*, **266**(1), 155–66.

[110] Lorimier, S., Bouthors, S., Droulle, C. *et al.* 1997. The rate of fibrinolysis is increased by free retraction of human gingival fibroblast populated fibrin lattices. *Int. J. Biochem. Cell Biol.*, **29**(1), 181–9.

[111] Kapacee, Z., Richardson, S. H., Lu, Y. *et al.* 2008. Tension is required for fibripositor formation. *Matrix Biol.*, **27**(4), 371–5.

[112] MacGillivray, T. E. 2003. Fibrin sealants and glues. *J. Card. Surg.*, **18**(6), 480–5.

[113] Radosevich, M., Goubran, H. and Burnouf, T. 1997. Fibrin sealant: scientific rationale, production methods, properties, and current clinical use. *Vox Sang.*, **72**(3), 133–43.

[114] Spotnitz, W. D. 2010. Fibrin sealant: past, present, and future: a brief review. *World J. Surg.*, **34**(4), 632–4.

[115] Eyrich, D., Göpferich, A. and Blunk, T. 2007. Fibrin in tissue engineering. *Tissue Eng.*, **13**(2), 379–92.

[116] Ahmed, T. A. E., Dare, E. V. and Hincke, M. 2008. Fibrin: a versatile scaffold for tissue engineering applications. *Tissue Eng. Part B: Rev.*, **14**(2), 199–215.

[117] Bach, A., Bannasch, H., Galla, T., Bittner, K. and Stark, G. 2001. Fibrin glue as matrix for cultured autologous urothelial cells in urethral reconstruction. *Tissue Eng.*, **7**(1), 45–53.

[118] Christman, K. L., Vardanian, A. J., Fang, Q. *et al.* 2004. Injectable fibrin scaffold improves cell transplant survival, reduces infarct expansion, and induces neovasculature formation in ischemic myocardium. *J. Am. Coll. Cardiol.*, **44**(3), 654–60.

[119] Hankemeier, S., van Griensven, M., Ezechieli, M. *et al.* 2007. Tissue engineering of tendons and ligaments by human bone marrow stromal cells in a liquid fibrin matrix in immunodeficient rats: results of a histologic study. *Arch. Orthop. Trauma Surg.*, **127**(9), 815–21.

[120] Falanga, V., Iwamoto, S., Chartier, M. *et al.* 2007. Autologous bone marrow-derived cultured mesenchymal stem cells delivered in a fibrin spray accelerate healing in murine and human cutaneous wounds. *Tissue Eng.*, **13**(6), 1299–312.

[121] Grant, I., Warwick, K., Marshall, J., Green, C. and Martin, R. 2002. The co-application of sprayed cultured autologous keratinocytes and autologous fibrin sealant in a porcine wound model. *Br. J. Plast. Surg.*, **55**(3), 219–27.

[122] Currie, L. J., Sharpe, J. R. and Martin, R. 2001. The use of fibrin glue in skin grafts and tissue-engineered skin replacements: a review. *Plast. Reconstr. Surg.*, **108**(6), 1713.

[123] Doolin, E. J., Strande, L. F., Sheng, X. and Hewitt, C. W. 2002. Engineering a composite neotrachea with surgical adhesives. *J. Pediatr. Surg.*, **37**(7), 1034–7.

[124] Auger, F. and Guignard, R. 1993. Role and innocuity of Tisseel®, a tissue glue, in the grafting process and in vivo evolution of human cultured epidermis. *Br. J. Plast. Surg.*, **46**(2), 136–42.

[125] Flasza, M., Kemp, P., Shering, D. *et al.* 2007. Development and manufacture of an investigational human living dermal equivalent (ICX-SKN). *Regen. Med.*, **2**(6), 903–18.

[126] Boyd, M., Flasza, M., Johnson, P. A., Roberts, J. S. C. and Kemp, P. 2007. Integration and persistence of an investigational human living skin equivalent (ICX-SKN) in human surgical wounds. *Regen. Med.*, **2**(4), 363–70.

[127] Llames, S. G., Del Rio, M., Larcher, F. *et al.* 2004. Human plasma as a dermal scaffold for the generation of a completely autologous bioengineered skin. *Transplantation*, **77**(3), 350.

[128] Mazlyzam, A., Aminuddin, B., Fuzina, N. *et al.* 2007. Reconstruction of living bilayer human skin equivalent utilizing human fibrin as a scaffold. *Burns*, **33**(3), 355–63.

[129] Kubo, M., Van De Water, L., Plantefaber, L. C. *et al.* 2001. Fibrinogen and fibrin are anti-adhesive for keratinocytes: a mechanism for fibrin eschar slough during wound repair. *J. Invest. Dermatol.*, **117**(6), 1369–81.

[130] Clark, R. A. F. 2003. Fibrin glue for wound repair: facts and fancy. *Thromb. Haemost.* **90**(6), 1003–6.

[131] Clark, R. A. F. 2003. Fibrin is a many splendored thing. *J. Invest. Dermatol.* **121**(5), xxi–xxii.

[132] Hansbrough, J. F., Boyce, S. T., Cooper, M. L. and Foreman, T. J. 1989. Burn wound closure with cultured autologous keratinocytes and fibroblasts attached to a collagen-glycosaminoglycan substrate. *JAMA: J. Am. Med. Assoc.*, **262**(15), 21–25.

[133] Boyce, S. T., Supp, A. P., Swope, V. B. and Warden, G. D. 2002. Vitamin C regulates keratinocyte viability, epidermal barrier, and basement membrane in vitro, and reduces wound contraction after grafting of cultured skin substitutes. *J. Invest. Dermatol.*, **118**(4), 565–72.

[134] Hojo, M., Inokuchi, S., Kidokoro, M. *et al.* 2003. Induction of vascular endothelial growth factor by fibrin as a dermal substrate for cultured skin substitute. *Plast. Reconstr. Surg.*, **111**(5), 1638.

[135] Barocas, V., Girton, T. and Tranquillo, R. 1998. Engineered alignment in media equivalents: magnetic prealignment and mandrel compaction. *J. Biomech. Eng.*, **120**, 660.

[136] Girton, T., Oegema, T. and Tranquillo, R. 1999. Exploiting glycation to stiffen and strengthen tissue equivalents for tissue engineering. *J. Biomed. Mater. Res.*, **46**(1), 87–92.

[137] Ma, P. X. and Elisseeff, J. H. 2005. *Scaffolding in Tissue Engineering.* Boca Raton, FL: CRC Press.

[138] Swartz, D. D., Russell, J. A. and Andreadis, S. T. 2005. Engineering of fibrin-based functional and implantable small-diameter blood vessels. *Am. J. Physiol. - Heart Circulatory Physiol.*, **288**(3), H1451.

[139] Solan, A., Mitchell, S., Moses, M. and Niklason, L. 2003. Effect of pulse rate on collagen deposition in the tissue-engineered blood vessel. *Tissue Eng.*, **9**(4), 579–86.

[140] Isenberg, B. C., Williams, C. and Tranquillo, R. T. 2006. Endothelialization and flow conditioning of fibrin-based media-equivalents. *Ann. Biomed. Eng.*, **34**(6), 971–85.

[141] Bjork, J. W. and Tranquillo, R. T. 2009. Transmural flow bioreactor for vascular tissue engineering. *Biotechnol. Bioeng.*, **104**(6), 1197–206.

[142] Seliktar, D., Black, R. A., Vito, R. P. and Nerem, R. M. 2000. Dynamic mechanical conditioning of collagen-gel blood vessel constructs induces remodeling in vitro. *Ann. Biomed. Eng.*, **28**(4), 351–62.

[143] Niklason, L., Gao, J., Abbott, W. *et al.* 1999. Functional arteries grown in vitro. *Science*, **284**(5413), 489.

[144] Syedain, Z. H. and Tranquillo, R. T. 2009. Controlled cyclic stretch bioreactor for tissue-engineered heart valves. *Biomaterials*, **30**(25), 4078–84.

[145] Brown, R., Prajapati, R., McGrouther, D., Yannas, I. and Eastwood, M. 1998. Tensional homeostasis in dermal fibroblasts: mechanical responses to mechanical loading in three-dimensional substrates. *J. Cell Physiol.*, **175**(3), 323–32.

[146] Syedain, Z. H., Meier, L. A., Bjork, J. W., Lee, A. and Tranquillo, R. T. 2011. Implantable arterial grafts from human fibroblasts and fibrin using a multi-graft pulsed flow-stretch bioreactor with noninvasive strength monitoring. *Biomaterials*, **32**(3), 714–22.

[147] Vesely, I. 2005. Heart valve tissue engineering. *Circ. Res.*, **97**(8), 743.

[148] Neuenschwander, S. 2004. Heart valve tissue engineering. *Transpl. Immunol.*, **12**(3–4), 359–65.

[149] Jockenhoevel, S., Zund, G., Hoerstrup, S. P. *et al.* 2001. Fibrin gel – advantages of a new scaffold in cardiovascular tissue engineering. *Eur. J. Cardio-thoracic Surg.*, **19**(4), 424–30.

[150] Jockenhoevel, S., Chalabi, K., Sachweh, J. *et al.* 2001. Tissue engineering: complete autologous valve conduit – a new moulding technique. *Thorac. Cardiovasc. Surg.*, **49**(5), 287–90.

[151] Robinson, P. S. and Tranquillo, R. T. 2009. Planar biaxial behavior of fibrin-based tissue-engineered heart valve leaflets. *Tissue Eng. Part A*, **15**(10), 2763–72.

[152] Mol, A., Driessen, N. J. B., Rutten, M. C. M. *et al.* 2005. Tissue engineering of human heart valve leaflets: a novel bioreactor for a strain-based conditioning approach. *Ann. Biomed. Eng.*, **33**(12), 1778–88.

[153] Flanagan, T. C., Cornelissen, C., Koch, S. *et al.* 2007. The in vitro development of autologous fibrin-based tissue-engineered heart valves through optimised dynamic conditioning. *Biomaterials*, **28**(23), 3388–97.

[154] Hoerstrup, S. P., Sodian, R., Sperling, J. S., Vacanti, J. P. and Mayer, J. E. Jr. 2006. New pulsatile bioreactor for in vitro formation of tissue engineered heart valves. *Tissue Eng.*, **6**(1), 75–9.

[155] Syedain, Z. H., Lahti, M. T., Johnson, S. L. *et al.* 2011. Implantation of a tissue-engineered heart valve from human fibroblasts exhibiting short term function in the sheep pulmonary artery. *Cardiovasc. Eng. Technol.*, **2**, 101–12.

[156] Flanagan, T. C., Sachweh, J. S., Frese, J. *et al.* 2009. In vivo remodeling and structural characterization of fibrin-based tissue-engineered heart valves in the adult sheep model. *Tissue Eng. Part A*, **15**(10), 2965–76.

[157] Black, L. D. III, Meyers, J. D., Weinbaum, J. S., Shvelidze, Y. A. and Tranquillo, R. T. 2009. Cell-induced alignment augments twitch force in fibrin gel-based engineered myocardium via gap junction modification. *Tissue Eng. Part A*, **15**(10), 3099–108.

[158] Morin, K. T. and Tranquillo, R. T. 2011. Guided sprouting from endothelial spheroids in fibrin gels aligned by magnetic fields and cell-induced gel compaction. *Biomaterials*, **32**(26), 6111–18.

[159] Chen, X., Aledia, A. S., Ghajar, C. M. *et al.* 2008. Prevascularization of a fibrin-based tissue construct accelerates the formation of functional anastomosis with host vasculature. *Tissue Eng. Part A*, **15**(6), 1363–71.

[160] Eyrich, D., Brandl, F., Appel, B. *et al.* 2007. Long-term stable fibrin gels for cartilage engineering. *Biomaterials*, **28**(1), 55–65.

[161] Pelaez, D. C., Huang, C. Y. and Cheung, H. S. 2009. Cyclic compression maintains viability and induces chondrogenesis of human mesenchymal stem cells in fibrin gel scaffolds. *Stem Cells Development*, **18**(1), 93–102.

[162] Hunter, C. J., Mouw, J. K. and Levenston, M. E. 2004. Dynamic compression of chondrocyte-seeded fibrin gels: effects on matrix accumulation and mechanical stiffness. *Osteoarthritis Cartilage*, **12**(2), 117–30.

[163] Han, B., Schwab, I. R., Madsen, T. K. and Isseroff, R. R. 2002. A fibrin-based bioengineered ocular surface with human corneal epithelial stem cells. *Cornea*, **21**(5), 505.

[164] Dubey, N., Letourneau, P. and Tranquillo, R. 2001. Neuronal contact guidance in magnetically aligned fibrin gels: effect of variation in gel mechano-structural properties. *Biomaterials*, **22**(10), 1065–75.

[165] Willerth, S. M., Arendas, K. J., Gottlieb, D. I. and Sakiyama-Elbert, S. E. 2006. Optimization of fibrin scaffolds for differentiation of murine embryonic stem cells into neural lineage cells. *Biomaterials*, **27**(36), 5990–6003.

[166] Johnson, P. J., Parker, S. R. and Sakiyama-Elbert, S. E. 2010. Fibrin-based tissue engineering scaffolds enhance neural fiber sprouting and delay the accumulation of

reactive astrocytes at the lesion in a subacute model of spinal cord injury. *J. Biomed. Mater. Res. Part A*, **92**(1), 152–63.

[167] Schense, J. C., Bloch, J., Aebischer, P. and Hubbell, J. A. 2000. Enzymatic incorporation of bioactive peptides into fibrin matrices enhances neurite extension. *Nature Biotechnol.*, **18**(4), 415–19.

[168] Osathanon, T., Linnes, M. L., Rajachar, R. M. *et al.* 2008. Microporous nanofibrous fibrin-based scaffolds for bone tissue engineering. *Biomaterials*, **29**(30), 4091–9.

[169] Zhang, G., Hu, Q., Braunlin, E. A., Suggs, L. J. and Zhang, J. 2006. Enhancing efficacy of cell transplantation in hearts with post-infarction LV remodeling by an injectable biomatrix. *Circulation*, **114**(18, Suppl. II), 239.

[170] Zhang, G., Drinnan, C. T., Geuss, L. R. and Suggs, L. J. 2010. Vascular differentiation of bone marrow stem cells is directed by a tunable three-dimensional matrix. *Acta Biomater.*, **6**(9), 3395–403.

18

Microfabricated gels for tissue engineering

Gulden Camci-Unal, Jesper Hjortnaes, Hojae Bae, Mehmet Remzi Dokmeci and Ali Khademhosseini

18.1 Introduction

Tissue engineering aims to develop biological substitutes that repair or replace damaged tissues or whole organs by combining technologies from engineering and medical sciences [1]. Although tissue engineering has enabled successful generation of various artificial tissue substitutes, such as skin [2], bladder [3], cartilage [4], bone [5], heart valves [6], and blood vessels [7], a number of challenges remain to be solved. It has been challenging to engineer large and vascularized organs such as the heart or liver. These tissues depend on adequate vascularization for the supply of nutrients and oxygen. In tissue engineering, this translates into not only creating the specific tissue but also making the highly organized vasculature. On the other hand, avascular tissues such as heart valves or cartilage depend on adequate diffusion for their supply of nutrients and oxygen. In terms of engineering, an avascular biomimetic construct cannot be too thick [8, 9], since this would lead to a limited supply of nutrients and oxygen [1]. Microfabrication strategies aim to overcome these limitations by controlling the size, geometry and features of three-dimensional (3D) in-vitro tissue-engineered constructs. Recent advances in biomaterials combined with developments in microengineering methods have enabled the development of vascular networks, prevascularized tissue constructs, and creation of well-ordered tissue constructs from microgel units with different cell types. [10].

Native tissues consist of cells that reside in a framework called the extracellular matrix (ECM). The ECM is composed of proteins (e.g. collagen), fibers (e.g. elastin), polysaccharides (e.g. hyaluronic acid), glycosaminoglycans (e.g. heparan sulfate), and growth factors (e.g. fibroblast growth factor). The ECM functions as a support system for cells to exert their biological function and can be viewed as the scaffolding environment for the tissues. Traditional tissue engineering uses synthetic scaffolds or biomaterials as molds to create tissue constructs. These scaffolds are typically porous, biocompatible, and degradable, and allow sufficient diffusion to occur [11]. Furthermore, such scaffolds enable cell adhesion, proliferation, and differentation, and tissue organization that are similar to those in their native counterparts [12]. Over time, the synthetic scaffold will degrade in vivo, while the cells deposit new natural scaffolding (ECM), thus leading to the formation of new tissue.

Some of the most common biomaterials used as 3D scaffolding materials in tissue engineering are hydrogels. Hydrogels are generated by crosslinking hydrophilic polymer precursors using a range of external stimuli, such as ultraviolet (UV) light, pH, or temperature. Hydrogels resemble native ECM [13] because they have high water content [12, 14], are sufficiently flexible, and can be fabricated using natural ECM components, such as collagen, hyaluronic acid (HA), chondroitin sulfate, heparin, and elastin. Hydrogels are used as 3D scaffolds or matrices to entrap cells [15] and provide a sufficiently hydrophilic environment for cell survival, growth, and new ECM production [12]. Hydrogels can also be used as building blocks to fabricate scaffolds [15], which provide structural support and regulate cellular function and signaling [12].

The chemical, biological, and mechanical features of hydrogels can be tailored to modulate cellular function. For example, various growth factors, adhesive peptides, proteins, fibers, and degradable peptides have been used to modify hydrogels for tissue engineering applications [12]. Additionally, modifications in degradation or mechanical properties of hydrogels induce modulation of cell response in the final engineered construct due to the resulting changes in the substrate properties. Such tunable hydrogels can potentially be useful for various engineering applications [12, 16], such as bone [17] or cartilage [14] tissue engineering.

Communication between cells is essential for them to function properly [18], and this is largely facilitated by integration and interaction of cells with the ECM [16]. In an ideal engineered tissue, cells are homogeneously distributed and sufficiently organized to allow the transport of oxygen, nutrients, and waste throughout the porous scaffold. In addition, such constructs should possess suitable mechanical properties to support the growing tissue. Cell–cell, cell–substrate, and cell–soluble-factor interactions can be controlled by creating cellular microenvironments with the aid of microfabrication techniques [19, 20]. For instance, the alignment of cells or behavior of co-cultures can be controlled by these strategies. Additionally, patterned substrates can be used to influence cellular behavior, such as adhesion, survival, spreading, migration, proliferation, elongation, biological function, and direction of stem cell fate.

In tissue engineering, selecting the proper biomaterial is crucial for directing interactions between cells and the surrounding microenvironment. Cell–biomaterial interactions on hydrogel surfaces play a significant role in influencing cellular behavior. For instance, photocured HA–gelatin methacrylate hydrogels have been synthesized to capture endothelial progenitor cells (EPCs) [21]. Similarly, HA–heparin-containing hydrogels were generated to promote adhesion and spreading of EPCs for endothelialization purposes [22]. Furthermore, cells or biological molecules have been patterned on surfaces to study cellular interactions in two dimensions (2D) by utilizing various microfabrication techniques [23–31]. However, 2D cultures are not suitable for simulating the natural environment of cells, because they lack the complexity and organization that are present in native tissues. To address this need, cells have been embedded in 3D hydrogels [32, 33].

Hydrogel microengineering strategies are potentially powerful tools to create 3D tissue models to mimic the natural environment of living tissues. The ability to engineer hydrogels laden with cells or other biological molecules has enabled the fabrication of in-vitro tissue constructs. Microengineered hydrogels can be produced by utilizing techniques such as bioprinting, micromolding, photopatterning, emulsification, and microfluidics. Cells are encapsulated in the hydrogel precursors with these techniques to create controlled architectures for different tissue engineering applications [34].

In this chapter, we will classify hydrogel microfabrication strategies and highlight tissue engineering applications by discussing top-down and bottom-up tissue engineering approaches.

18.2 Microfabrication techniques

Microfabrication strategies for the generation of hydrogels have emerged as powerful tools in tissue engineering and regenerative medicine to precisely control the cellular microenvironment. These fabrication techniques may yield complex features resembling highly organized architectures in native organs. For instance, micropatterned co-cultures can control homotypic and heterotypic cellular interactions in engineered tissue constructs [18]. The major microfabrication techniques to synthesize engineered hydrogels can be classified into the following groups: bioprinting, micromolding, photolithograpy, emulsification, and microfluidics.

18.2.1 Bioprinting

Bioprinting is a technique that uses printing technology to create tissue-like structures. In essence, this technology "prints" tissue. Cells or biological molecules can be embedded within hydrogels and used

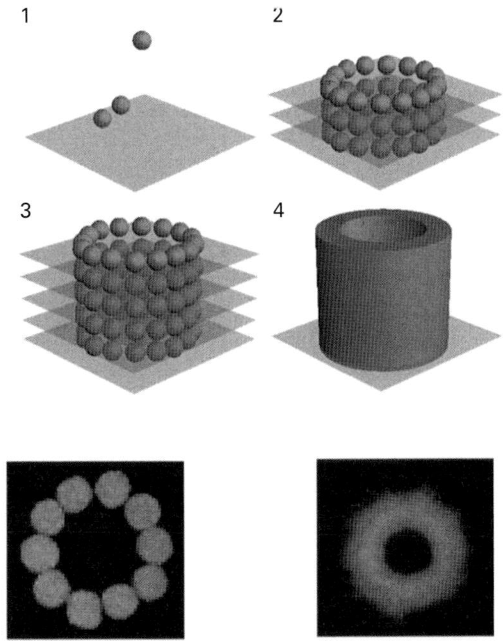

Figure 18.1 Bioprinting strategy to build tissues and organs by making use of hydrogel precursors [35]. Reproduced by permission of The Royal Society of Chemistry.

as "ink" to generate engineered constructs [12]. More specifically, gels with or without cells/biological factors are printed on predefined positions utilizing a layer-by-layer approach (Figure 18.1) [35]. This technique allows the creation of 3D tissue constructs, which could be used to repair damaged or diseased tissues [11, 12]. Using this technique, cells can be homogeneously distributed within a hydrogel matrix at predefined positions. To alter physical, chemical, or mechanical properties of printed gels, such as size, shape, or stiffness, one can change the nozzle diameter, cell density, fluid flow rate, liquid rheology, and printing temperature [13, 36, 37] in bioprinting systems.

The hydrogel precursors for bioprinting are chosen according to the target application. The following polymers are commonly used as hydrogel precursors in bioprinting studies: gelatin [38], chitosan [39], Matrigel [40–43], alginate [44–46], HA [47], starch [48], collagen [40, 49–51], fibrin [13], polyethylene glycol diacrylate (PEGDA) [52], and agarose [13]. Numerous cell types have been utilized in bioprinting techniques to build artificial tissue units. For example, endothelial cells [42], smooth muscle cells [40], and osteoblasts [45] have successfully been encapsulated in hydrogel-based matrices. Moreover, nerve, bone, and cartilage tissues have also been fabricated using bioprinting [11]. Although bioprinting enables creation of well-controlled 3D cell-laden structures such as lines, dots etc., such rapid prototyping techniques have some limitations. For instance, due to harsh printing conditions, such as shear stress, variation in pH or elevated temperatures, it may be challenging to maintain high cell viability during the printing process [53].

Printing strategies can also be used for cell-patterning or creating biological-molecule-loaded hydrogels [54]. In these approaches, cells or biological molecules, such as growth factors, are resuspended in the prepolymer solution and dispensed by a printing mechanism on predetermined positions on a solid surface. The resulting droplets are subsequently cross-linked to form individual building blocks and this process is repeated to form layers for the final tissue construct. This approach enables the deposition of multiple cell types or aggregates of cells encapsulated in hydrogels [53]. Ten to several hundreds of micrometers is typically the range for spatial resolution obtained by computer-assisted design (CAD) strategies [55].

Stereolithography, another bioprinting technique, is also used to generate cell-laden hydrogels and print tissue-engineered constructs. In stereolithography, selective polymerization of the hydrogel precursor is carried out by an ordered layer-by-layer procedure to obtain multilayered cell-embedded scaffolds [12] by utilizing photocrosslinking (see Section 2.3 for details of this technique) induced by exposure to UV light [11, 13, 56–58].

18.2.2 Micromolding

Creating highly organized complex tissue architectures is one of the main challenges in tissue engineering [16, 59–61], especially because the spatial distribution of cells modulates tissue function [62]. Micromolding

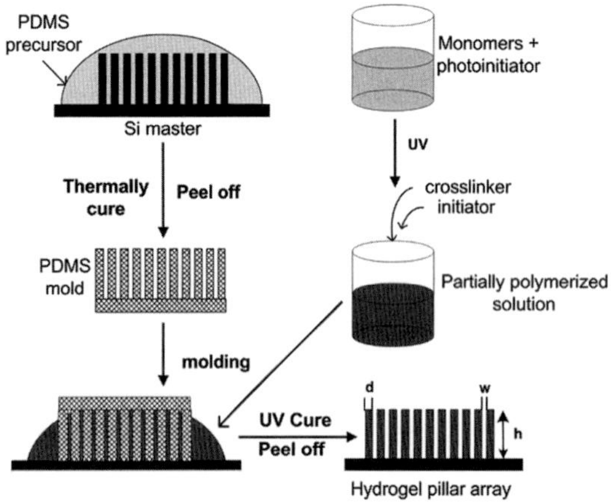

Figure 18.2 The soft lithographic fabrication process for PDMS molds [70]. Reproduced by permission of The Royal Society of Chemistry.

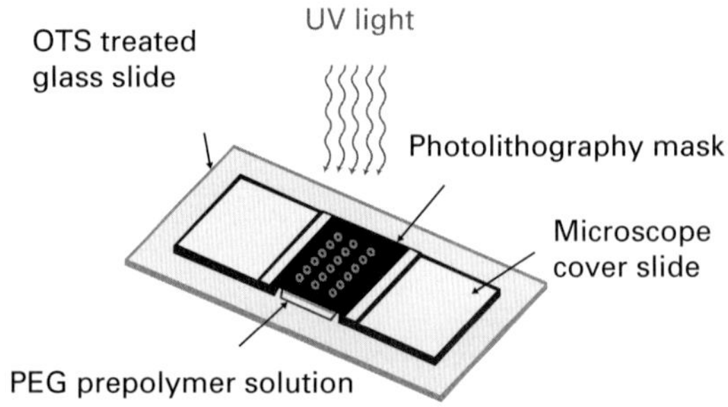

Figure 18.3 Photolithography utilizes photocurable hydrogel precursors with a photomask with desired shapes on it to generate microfabricated structures [78]. Reproduced by permission of John Wiley and Sons.

techniques are used to control the spatial distribution of cells in 3D tissue-like structures [23, 63, 64] by regulating the size and shape of microscale hydrogels [16, 19, 32]. This technique can produce hydrogel patterns with micron or nanometer resolutions [65]. Basically, this technology utilizes the shape of molds to create the desired features for different materials. More specifically, with micromolding, prepolymer solutions are crosslinked within patterns of elastomeric molds [16, 66] to regulate the dimensions, shapes, and sizes of the resulting hydrogels [67]. Micromolding is a simple and low-cost technique [67, 68], and has been used extensively to fabricate microengineered constructs [19, 23, 62, 64, 69–71]. However, the major limitation of micromolding is that it is challenging to use this technique for chemically crosslinked hydrogels [66].

The micromolds are typically made from polydimethoxysilane (PDMS), which is an elastomer that is widely used to transfer specific patterns from silicon wafers [67, 70, 72] (Figure 18.2). PDMS is a highly porous, transparent, and biocompatible material. In addition to PDMS, also polyimines and polyurethanes are used as molds in micromolding-based techniques. Additionally, fluoropolymers (e.g. perfluoropolyether) have been utilized as molding materials to obtain easily harvestable hydrogel units due to their unique non-adhesive properties [73]. Micromolding is used to create microscale gels from a variety of polymer precursors, such as chitosan [19], PEG [32, 70, 74], HA [23, 32], and agarose [75]. Micromolding has successfully been used to create 3D tissue-like structures [23, 63, 64, 76] by encapsulating cells within hydrogels. For example, the spatial distributions of NIH-3T3 fibroblast cells in PEG- and HA-based hydrogel patterns have been controlled by micromolding strategies [32]. In another study, microvasculature networks in hepatocyte-laden agarose-based hydrogel channels were created [77]. Additionally, alignment and differentiation of skeletal muscle cells were studied in fibrin–collagen gels by micromolding techniques [64].

18.2.3 Photolithography

Another strategy to fabricate hydrogels of controlled size and shape is photolithography [72]. In this process, photolabile hydrogel precursors are crosslinked via exposure to light. A photomask with predefined patterns is placed above the prepolymer mixture and crosslinked via radical polymerization by means of UV light [66, 78] (Figure 18.3). As a result, patterns from the photomask are transferred onto the prepolymer solution residing on the substrate. Once the polymerization has gone to completion, the unreacted polymer mixture is rinsed away. The resolution of photolithographic techniques varies from the sub-micron to the millimeter range [16]. Photolithography is a simple

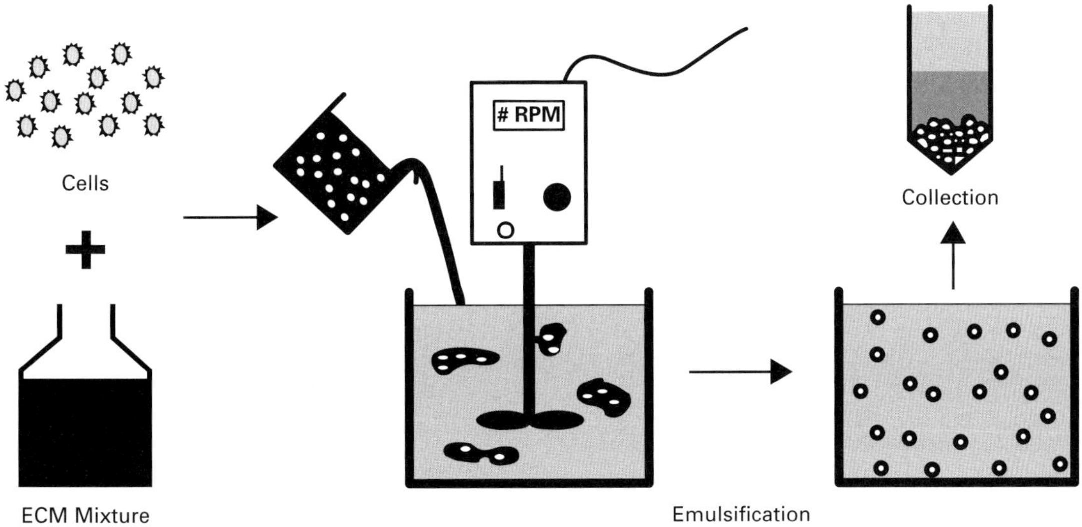

Figure 18.4 The process of emulsification yielding cell-loaded hydrogel particles [86]. Reproduced by permission of John Wiley and Sons.

technique enabling a high degree of spatial control [16]; however, the major drawback of photolithography is that it uses exposure to UV light to induce crosslinking, which can be cytotoxic [66].

There are various hydrogel precursors, which can be modified with photocrosslinkable functional groups. Photolithography is a simple procedure to fabricate micropatterns with varying size and shapes [72, 79, 80]. In addition, photolithographic approaches enable encapsulation of cells in patterned hydrogels with spatial control [16]. For instance, micropatterns of PEG-based hydrogels have been generated by encapsulating hepatocytes, fibroblasts, or macrophages [80, 81]. Similarly, NIH-3T3 fibroblasts have been encapsulated in microchannel patterns made of gelatin methacrylate hydrogel to study cell alignment [82].

Scanning or focussing light are other approaches to generate 3D hydrogel patterns [66]. For example, photocurable polymers have been crosslinked using scanning laser lithography [83–85]. In another study, a similar approach has been utilized to generate 3D hydrogel scaffolds with heterogeneous properties [52]. In this report, porous scaffolds in honeycomb or woodpile geometries were fabricated with protein-modied sites to study cell adhesion.

18.2.4 Other techniques

18.2.4.1 Emulsification

Emulsification is a technique used to produce microscale hydrogel structures [16]. In emulsification, two phase-separating liquids [72] are mixed by agitation [66] to generate droplets, which can subsequently be crosslinked (Figure 18.4) [86]. For example, water-in-oil emulsion systems are often used to obtain emulsified phases [67]. Mineral oil, hexane, and cyclohexane are commonly used as the hydrophobic phase to produce emulsions [67, 72]. In this process, the shape and size of the hydrogel particles can be controlled by manipulating a number of factors, such as the rotation speed, surface tension, and viscosity [16] of the liquid phases. The droplets which are formed as a result of mixing can then be crosslinked using different stimuli, such as temperature, pH, or UV exposure [16]. Although emulsification is a simple technique, the size distribution of hydrogel particles varies more than in the other microfabrication methods [16, 66]. Additionally, there is less control over the shapes of the gels produced by this technique.

Common hydrogel precursors used to generate droplets by emulsification-based techniques are agarose [16], alginate [16], collagen [16], HA [67, 87, 88], and gelatin [67, 89]. In addition to producing hydrogel beads, cells can easily be incorporated within hydrogels by means of emulsification [16, 67, 90, 91]. For instance, in one study, embryoid bodies were encapsulated in alginate-based hydrogels by emulsification, which promoted cardiomyogenic differentiation resulting in spontaneous beating areas in the hydrogel beads [92]. The authors of another study demonstrated successful encapsulation of human mesenchymal stem cells (hMSCs) in agarose–collagen-based hydrogel beads by emulsification [86].

18.2.4.2 Microfluidics

Microfluidics is another method used for the fabrication of microscale hydrogels. The most common microfluidic strategies to fabricate microgels are based on single-phase flows or two-phase immiscible liquid mixtures [16]. In single-phase systems, UV light is exposed to a particular area of the flowing prepolymer to form hydrogels. In multiphase systems, first the droplets are formed under continuous fluid flow and then these droplets are crosslinked using a variety of methods, such as UV irradiation or ionic stimuli [67]. The surface tension and viscosity [16] of the fluids and the reaction time [67] are the main parameters to control during the droplet fabrication process. Microfluidic channels are commonly produced from elastomeric PDMS molds. The flow rates of the fluids and the dimensions of the microfluidic channels also affect the final properties of the hydrogels [16]. This method enables precise generation of size and shape-controlled hydrogel particles [93]. The major limitation of microfluidic systems is that they usually use photolabile polymer precursors to form hydrogels [94].

Recently, new technologies to produce hydrogel units using microfluidic strategies have been reported. For example, stop-flow lithography combines microfluidics and photopatterning approaches [16]. This method can be used to create gels under continuous-flow conditions via exposure to UV light [95]. Optofluidic maskless lithography (OFML) is another microfluidic approach, which enables *in situ* formation of hydrogels in microfluidic channels under continuous flow [96]. In this technique, projection of UV light on the flowing photocrosslinkable resin is controlled by a computer. Hydrogel patterns are formed by selective crosslinking of photocurable resin induced by UV light exposure. In one study, OMFL has been utilized with a membrane to control the size of the hydrogels by manipulating the height of the channel (Figure 18.5) [97]. In addition to plain hydrogel units, cell-encapsulated hydrogels can be generated by microfluidic techniques [81, 98, 99]. For example, layer-by-layer fabrication of co-cultures using different polymers has been performed [100]. Similarly, HeLa cells were encapsulated within PEGDA hydrogels using an OMFL technique to study cellular interactions in co-cultures [97].

Microfluidics is also used to generate concentration gradients of soluble or growth factors inside the hydrogel channels. This has important implications for tissue engineering applications where production of a gradient is needed [72, 101]. For example, NIH-3T3 fibroblasts have been encapsulated in a gelatin–HA gradient within a microchannel demonstrating gradient-dependent cell spreading [102]. This result is observed due to the adhesive and non-adhesive nature of gelatin and HA hydrogels, respectively. Similarly, elasticity gradients have been generated using microfluidic systems to control cellular behavior, such as adhesion and spreading, by using substrate stiffness [103].

18.3 Tissue engineering applications

Owing to the complexity of interactions among cells, ECM, and soluble factors of the cellular niche, it has been challenging to mimic the 3D organization of native microenvironments. To address these issues, different approaches were developed to fabricate biomimetic tissue constructs in vitro. There are two main strategies to utilize microfabrication techniques in tissue engineering: top-down and bottom-up approaches.

18.3.1 Top-down approach

Traditionally in tissue engineering cells are seeded onto 3D scaffolds and stimulated to deposit their own

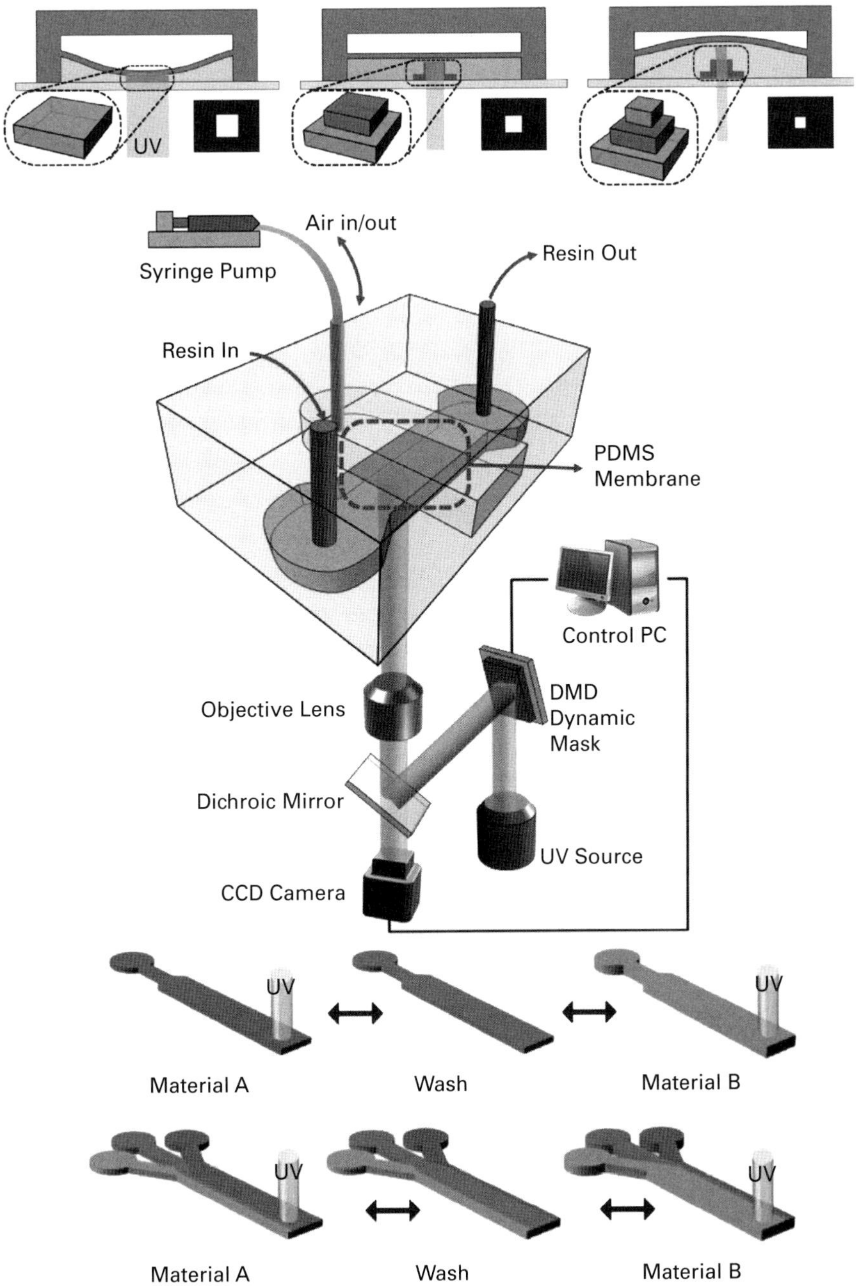

Figure 18.5 Fabrication of hydrogel units by a microfluidics method using optofluidic maskless lithography (OFML). Two-layered OFML is performed to control the thickness of the hydrogel [97]. Reproduced by permission of The Royal Society of Chemistry.

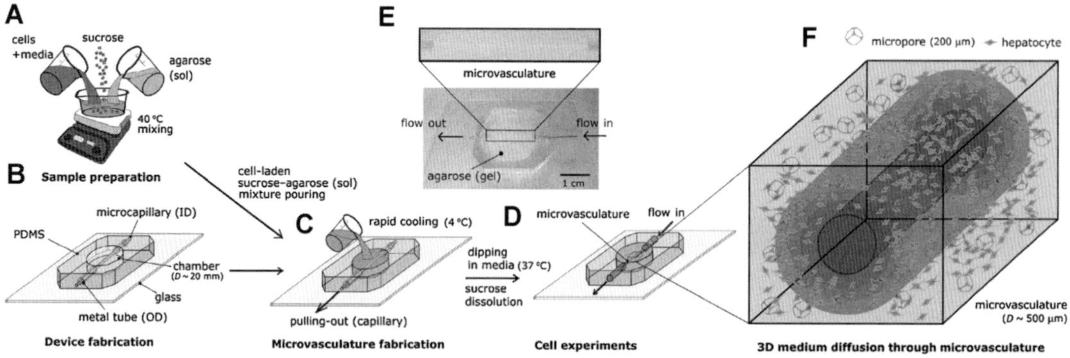

Figure 18.6 The production process used to obtain a microporous hydrogel construct with potential tissue engineering applications to mimic vasculatures. The cell-encapsulated hydrogel block was perfused with media to maintain high cell viability [77]. (Reproduced by permission of John Wiley and Sons.)

ECM structure while the scaffolds degrade. Theoretically, the resulting structure would have the shape of the scaffold [1]. However, it has been shown that this approach will not necessarily recreate all the complex tissue architecture that exists in native tissues. The most successful applications of tissue engineering using this approach are for relatively simple tissues such as cartilage and skin due to their relatively simple structures, their low requirements for oxygen and nutrients, and their ability to be supported by vascular structures in the host. Creating connective tissues such as the bladder and bone has also been successful over the past decades using this tissue engineering approach. In addition, several promising advances have been reported in heart valve and vascular tissue engineering [7, 58, 104–107].

Top-down microfabrication strategies aim to control and modify the properties of relatively large hydrogel units in microscale. To achieve this goal, researchers have engineered controlled features within macroscale scaffolds. In principle, the goal of this approach is to engineer a tissue's vasculature in vitro [61, 108]. For instance, microvasculature structures were engineered within tissue engineering scaffolds [108]. Similarly, microfluidic channels can be created to form vascular networks by generating size- and shape-controlled patterns [109–111]. Additionally, microtubular structures were generated in collagen gels, and endothelialization on the walls of the lumens was achieved [112].

A different approach to engineer microvascular structures was used to fabricate a HepG2-laden agarose hydrogel system containing micropores (Figure 18.6) that were created by dissolving sucrose crystals, which causes leaching [77]. These porous structures can improve oxygen and protein transport and nutrient diffusion, thus providing a synthetic environment that can mimic native tissue structures. In addition, this technique was able to control the microporosity of the scaffold. Similarly, AML-12 murine hepatocytes were encapsulated within hydrogel channels fabricated from agarose [110]. Medium was perfused through the channels to demonstrate the effect of oxygen and nutrient delivery on viability of cells. Creating microfluidic channels within macroscaffolds holds great potential for creating biomimetic synthetic vasculature [110].

Another top-down strategy has been demonstrated by using microengineering to yield 3D scaffolds with appropriate tissue architecture. For instance, layers of hydrogels, with or without cells, were fabricated by controlled porosity. Then the layers were combined to create 3D scaffolds, which resulted in specific architectures. By using a layer-by-layer microfluidic approach researchers have immobilized cell-loaded hydrogel units to build multilayered constructs. In this study, three different types of vascular cells were used to generate constructs that can mimic the arterial structure [100].

Researchers have also used lithography to pattern bioactive features into photolabile materials using an adaptation of established photolithographic techniques [84]. For example, single-photon absorption photolithography was used to generate biochemical and mechanical patterns in hydrogels in 3D, but this method results in limited pattern complexity. To overcome this limitation, complex 3D patterns and gradients in photoactive biomaterials have been created by using two-photon absorption lithography [84].

Top-down approaches in microengineering aim to control features of macroscale scaffolds. This has led to the fabrication of functional capillary networks on scaffold materials and also to controlling biochemical and mechanical features of existing scaffold materials. Although more research is warranted before translation from bench to bed, these techniques are a vital addition for engineering vascularized tissue constructs.

18.3.2 Bottom-up approach

Bottom-up approaches are used to engineer tissues by assembling microscale building blocks made solely of cells or cell-laden biomaterials [113]. This is an efficient strategy to create biomimetic structures, because some of the complex organs in the body, such as the pancreas, kidney, muscles, and liver, consist of repeating functional units. For example, hepatocytes have been encapsulated in hydrogels to mimic one lobule of liver [114]. Although bottom-up strategies provide unique opportunities to generate microengineered constructs, it is challenging to assemble the individual building blocks with sufficient mechanical strength. For example, the secondary crosslinking step to attach the individual building blocks should be optimized in such a way that the crosslink mechanically supports the entire tissue construct [115]. In addition, the feasibility and reproducibility of the assembly processes require improvements if one is to fabricate successfully functioning tissue constructs [116].

The geometrical architecture of the tissues in the body consists of small vascularized repeating functional units [115]. Tightly assembled tissue-like building blocks provide precisely organized elements, which may resemble actual tissues. To implement this principle, lock-and-key approaches have been developed to create highly organized engineered constructs, which could potentially yield clinically relevant tissue units [54]. Hydrogels with controlled sizes and shapes created by microfabrication techniques can be assembled using such lock-and-key approaches. For instance, different geometries, such as a solid ball, a casquet, or cylindrical tubes, can be formed by directed aggregation of small hydrogel units [117]. Once micron-size hydrogels had been fabricated by photolithography, a small amount of prepolymer was added to the gels and then they were transferred onto a PDMS mold with the desired final geometry. The excess prepolymer was removed, and then gels were allowed to assemble, and subsequently crosslinked to stabilize the shape. Then, PDMS mold was removed to create the final geometry of tightly packed building blocks. In this work, capillary forces were used as the major driving force of the assembly process. To demonstrate the applicability of this strategy in tissue engineering, cell-laden gels were fabricated and allowed to assemble for the desired geometries. Hepatocytes were encapsulated in 20% (wt/vol) PEG dimethacrylate (PEGDM) to form 500-μm-sized cubic units, and these gel units were assembled to form a cylindrical tube structure of inner diameter 5 mm. Moreover, the lock-and-key approach was utilized to assemble microgels with different shapes (e.g. rods and crosses) to obtain final geometries such as blocks and tubes. This is a useful technique to fabricate cell-encapsulated artificial tissue-like structures.

In another bottom-up approach, surface tension was used as a driving force to assemble individual cell-laden hyrogels [118]. Macroscale constructs were fabricated by assembling cuboidic hydrogels with dimensions ranging from 100 to 200 μm. Such scalable approaches could promote incorporation of multiple types of cells in different types of hydrogels to study co-cultures. Secondary UV crosslinking was used to stabilize the assembled hydrogel units. Similarly, directed assembly of PEGDM-based hydrogel units was achieved in a mineral oil/water system following a bottom-up strategy [119]. Once cell-laden microscale

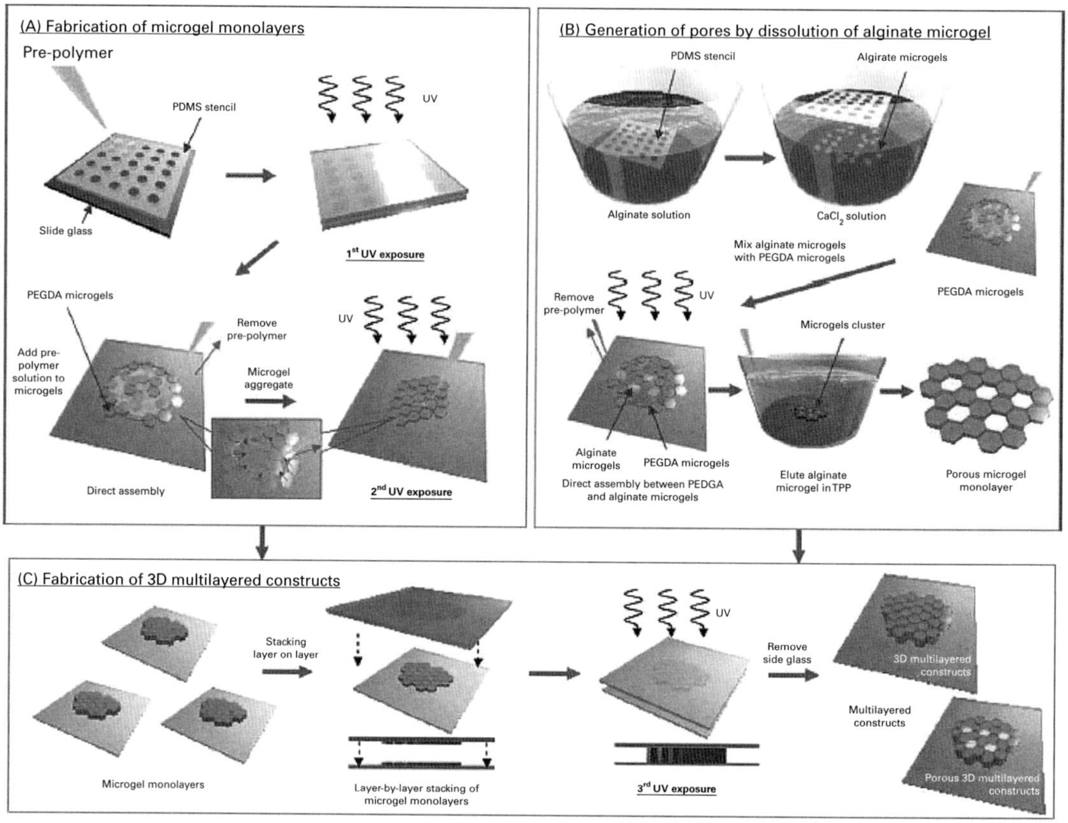

Figure 18.7 Fabrication and assembly of PEGDA-based hydrogel units. Photolithography was used to generate individual hydrogel building blocks. Then the gels were exposed to UV irradiation a second time to stabilize the assembled groups. Alginate was used as an additional component to generate pores throughout the construct. Then 3D layered constructs were prepared by stacking the monolayers on top of each other and crosslinking further to stabilize the entire construct [121]. (Reproduced by permission of John Wiley and Sons.)

hydrogels had been generated by UV light exposure, they were placed in a Petri dish with mineral oil. By agitation, directed assembly of microgels was promoted, and the gels were stabilized by a secondary UV light exposure. In this approach, hydrophilic/hydrophobic effects were considered to be dominant by virtue of their minimizing the surface energy. This method enables fabrication of co-cultured hydrogels by encapsulation of different cell types. Another scalable example of a bottom-up strategy was used to form fibroblast-loaded hydrogels with a size range of 200–1000 μm with 150 μm thickness [120].

Bottom-up strategies were also utilized to fabricate millimeter-size 3D tissue-like structures [121]. For example, directed assembly of cell-laden photocured PEGDA hydrogels was performed. Hexagon-shaped micron-size hydrogel patterns were created using PDMS stencils (Figure 18.7). Then, by addition of pre-polymer, hydrogel units were packed, followed by secondary crosslinking. In the last step, individual layers of hydrogels were stacked together by additional crosslinking via UV exposure. Furthermore, alginate was used as sacrificial element to create pores throughout the engineered unit.

In addition to assembling hydrogel units, bottom-up approaches can also be utilized to generate vascular tissue-engineered constructs. Vascularized structures were fabricated by packing collagen gels in a tube where blood or medium is passed through the gel units [33]. For instance, HepG2 cells were encapsulated in micron-size collagen rods, and were seeded with human umbilical vein endothelial cells (HUVECs) to obtain endothelialized constructs, taking advantage of their non-thrombogenic properties. Then endothelialized gels were packed in a tube and subsequently perfused with blood or medium. The resulting tissue units demonstrated high viability, offering opportunities toward the creation of functional tissue units with potential use for in-vivo studies.

In another attempt to create vasculature-like hydrogel structures, microgel units from 20% (wt/vol) PEGDA were assembled to obtain cylindrical tubes with connected lumens [78]. These hydrogels were assembled sequentially to mimic vasculature geometries. First, NIH-3T3 cells were encapsulated to optimize the viability in the engineered units. Then, endothelial cells and smooth muscle cells were encapsulated in PEGDA hydrogels to create a construct resembling a blood vessel. This strategy allowed fabrication of engineered structures with potential applications in vascular tissue engineering.

All in all, bottom-up tissue engineering strategies enable formation of multicellular tissue structures, which can improve the existing methods to generate medically relevant biomimetic constructs.

18.4 Conclusions

In this chapter, we described various microfabrication strategies to generate cell-laden microscale hydrogels and provided detailed examples related to their use in tissue engineering. We reviewed applications of bottom-up and top-down tissue engineering strategies for controlling cellular microenvironments, such as differentiation, vascularization, and cell guidance. The fabrication of complex engineered constructs is considered a challenge; however, this can be addressed by the use of elastomeric hydrogels with tunable properties and patterns to direct cellular behavior. For this reason, new biomaterial design strategies are needed for tissue engineering applications. The future success of engineering artificial organs will be closely associated with fabrication of biomimetic cell-loaded constructs. Controlled cell-laden hydrogel systems are expected to lead to significant developments for in-vitro tissue models, which could potentially be transformed into applications relevant to in-vivo systems.

ACKNOWLEDGEMENTS

This work was supported by the US Army Corps of Engineers, the Institute for Soldier Nanotechnologies, the National Science Foundation (DMR0847287) and the National Institutes of Health (AR057837, HL092836, EB008392, HL099073, and DE019024).

REFERENCES

[1] Langer, R. and Vacanti, J. P. 1993. Tissue engineering. *Science*, **260**, 920–6.

[2] Auger, F. A., Lacroix, D. and Germain, L. 2009. Skin substitutes and wound healing. *Skin Pharmacol. Physiology*, **22**, 94–102.

[3] Atala, A., Bauer, S. B., Soker, S., Yoo, J. J. and Retik, A. B. 2006. Tissue-engineered autologous bladders for patients needing cystoplasty. *Lancet*, **367**, 1241–6.

[4] Ashiku, S. K., Randolph, M. A. and Vacanti, C. A. 1997. Tissue engineered cartilage. *Porous Mater. Tissue Eng.*, **250**, 129–50.

[5] Petite, H., Viateau, V., Bensaid, W. *et al.* 2000. Tissue-engineered bone regeneration, *Nature Biotechnol.*, **18**, 959–63.

[6] Cebotari, S., Lichtenberg, A., Tudorache, I. *et al.* 2006. Clinical application of tissue engineered human heart valves using autologous progenitor cells. *Circulation*, **114**, I132–7.

[7] L'Heureux, N., Dusserre, N., Konig, G. *et al.* 2006. Human tissue-engineered blood vessels for adult arterial revascularization. *Nature Med.*, **12**, 361–5.

[8] Liu, B., Liu, Y., Lewis, A. K. and Shen, W. 2010. Modularly assembled porous cell-laden hydrogels. *Biomaterials*, **31**, 4918–25.

[9] Muschler, G. E., Nakamoto, C. and Griffith, L. G. 2004. Engineering principles of clinical cell-based tissue engineering. *J. Bone Joint Surg.*, **86A**, 1541–58.

[10] Nichol, J. W., Bae, H., Kachouie, N. *et al.* 2011. Microscale technologies for tissue engineering and stem cell differentiation. In *Stem Cell and Tissue Engineering*, ed. Li, S., L'Heureux, N., and Elisseeff, J., Singapore: World Scientific Publishing Company.

[11] Pescosolido, L., Schuurman, W., Malda, J. *et al.* 2011. Hyaluronic acid and dextran-based semi-IPN hydrogels as biomaterials for bioprinting. *Biomacromolecules*, **12**, 1831–8.

[12] Fedorovich, N. E., Alblas, J., de Wijn, J. R. *et al.* 2007. Hydrogels as extracellular matrices for skeletal tissue engineering: state-of-the-art and novel application in organ printing, *Tissue Eng.*, **13**, 1905–25.

[13] Landers, R., Hubner, U., Schmelzeisen, R. and Mulhaupt, R. 2002. Rapid prototyping of scaffolds derived from thermoreversible hydrogels and tailored for applications in tissue engineering. *Biomaterials*, **23**, 4437–47.

[14] DeKosky, B. J., Dormer, N. H., Ingavle, G. C. *et al.* 2010. Hierarchically designed agarose and poly(ethylene glycol) interpenetrating network hydrogels for cartilage tissue engineering. *Tissue Eng. Part C*, **16**, 1533–42.

[15] Lutolf, M. P. 2009. Spotlight on hydrogels. *Nature Mater.*, **8**, 451–3.

[16] Khademhosseini, A. and Langer, R. 2007. Microengineered hydrogels for tissue engineering. *Biomaterials*, **28**, 5087–92.

[17] Benoit, D. S. W., Durney, A. R. and Anseth, K. S. 2006. Manipulations in hydrogel degradation behavior enhance osteoblast function and mineralized tissue formation, *Tissue Eng.*, **12**, 1663–73.

[18] Kaji, H., Camci-Unal, G., Langer, R. and Khademhosseini, A. 2011. Engineering systems for the generation of patterned co-cultures for controlling cell–cell interactions. *Biochim. Biophys. Acta – General Subjects*, **1810**, 239–50.

[19] Fukuda, J., Khademhosseini, A., Yeo, Y. *et al.* 2006. Micromolding of photocrosslinkable chitosan hydrogel for spheroid microarray and co-cultures. *Biomaterials*, **27**, 5259–67.

[20] Wheeldon, I., Fernandez, J., Bae, H., Kaji, H. and Khademhosseini, A. 2011. Microscale biomaterials for regenerative medicine and engineered cellular microenvironments. In *Biomaterials for Tissue Engineering: A Review of the Past and Future Trends*, ed. Burdick, J. A., and Mauck, R. L., New York: Springer.

[21] Camci-Unal, G., Aubin, H., Ahari, A. F. *et al.* 2010. Surface-modified hyaluronic acid hydrogels to capture endothelial progenitor cells. *Soft Matter*, **6**, 5120–6.

[22] Camci-Unal, G., Nichol, J. W., Bae, H. *et al.* 2013. Hydrogel surfaces to promote attachment and spreading of endothelial progenitor cells. *J. Tissue Eng. Regen. Med.*, **7**(5), 337–47.

[23] Khademhosseini, A., Eng, G., Yeh, J. *et al.* 2006. Micromolding of photocrosslinkable hyaluronic acid for cell encapsulation and entrapment. *J. Biomed. Mater. Res. A*, **79**, 522–32.

[24] Chung, B. G., Kang, L. and Khademhosseini, A. 2007. Micro- and nanoscale technologies for tissue engineering and drug discovery applications. *Expert Opinion Drug Discovery*, **2**, 1653–68.

[25] Karp, J. M., Yeh, J., Eng, G. *et al.* 2007. Controlling size, shape and homogeneity of embryoid bodies using poly (ethylene glycol) microwells. *Lab Chip*, **7**, 786–94.

[26] Moeller, H. C., Mian, M. K., Shrivastava, S., Chung, B. G. and Khademhosseini, A. 2008. A microwell array system for stem cell culture. *Biomaterials*, **29**, 752–63.

[27] Yamazoe, H., Uemura, T. and Tanabe, T. 2008. Facile cell patterning on an albumin-coated surface. *Langmuir*, **24**, 8402–4.

[28] Wojciak-Stothard, B., Curtis, A., Monaghan, W., Macdonald, K. and Wilkinson, C. 1996. Guidance and activation of murine macrophages by nanometric scale topography. *Exp. Cell Res.*, **223**, 426–35.

[29] Meyle, J., Gultig, K., Wolburg, H. and Von Recum, A. F. 1993. Fibroblast anchorage to microtextured surfaces. *J. Biomed. Mater. Res. A*, **27**, 1553–7.

[30] Rajnicek, A. M., Britland, S. and McCaig, C. D. 1997. Contact guidance of CNS neurites on grooved quartz: influence of groove dimensions, neuronal age and cell type. *J. Cell Sci.*, **110**, 2905–13.

[31] Chen, C. S., Mrksich, M., Huang, S., Whitesides, G. M. and Ingber, D. E. 1997. Geometric control of cell life and death. *Science*, **276**, 1425–8.

[32] Yeh, J., Ling, Y., Karp, J. M. *et al.* 2006. Micromolding of shape-controlled, harvestable cell-laden hydrogels. *Biomaterials*, **27**, 5391–8.

[33] McGuigan, A. P. and Sefton, M. V. 2006. Vascularized organoid engineered by modular assembly enables blood perfusion. *Proc. Nat. Acad. Sci. USA*, **103**, 11461–6.

[34] Nguyen, K. T. and West, J. L. 2002. Photopolymerizable hydrogels for tissue engineering applications. *Biomaterials*, **23**, 4307–14.

[35] Mironov, V., Prestwich, G. and Forgacs, G. 2007. Bioprinting living structures. *J. Mater. Chem.*, **17**, 2054–60.

[36] Fedorovich, N. E., Swennen, I., Girones, J. *et al.* 2009. Evaluation of photocrosslinked lutrol hydrogel for tissue printing applications. *Biomacromolecules*, **10**, 1689–96.

[37] Seitz, H., Rieder, W., Irsen, S., Leukers, B. and Tille, C. 2005. Three-dimensional printing of porous ceramic scaffolds for bone tissue engineering. *J. Biomed. Mater. Res. Part B - Appl. Biomater.*, **74**, 782–8.

[38] Wang, X. H., Yan, Y. N., Pan, Y. Q. *et al.* 2006. Generation of three-dimensional hepatocyte/gelatin structures with rapid prototyping system. *Tissue Eng.*, **12**, 83–90.

[39] Ang, T. H., Sultana, F. S. A., Hutmacher, D. W. *et al.* 2002. Fabrication of 3D chitosan–hydroxyapatite scaffolds using a robotic dispensing system. *Mater. Sci. Eng. C - Biomimetic Supramolec. Systems*, **20**, 35–42.

[40] Wilson, W. C. Jr. and Boland, T. 2003. Cell and organ printing 1: protein and cell printers. *Anat. Rec. A Discov. Molec. Cell Evol. Biol.*, **272**, 491–6.

[41] Odde, D. J. and Renn, M. J. 2000. Laser-guided direct writing of living cells. *Biotechnol. Bioeng.*, **67**, 312–18.

[42] Barron, J. A., Wu, P., Ladouceur, H. D. and Ringeisen, B. R. 2004. Biological laser printing: a novel technique for creating heterogeneous 3-dimensional cell patterns. *Biomed. Microdevices*, **6**, 139–47.

[43] Ringeisen, B. R., Kim, H., Barron, J. A. *et al.* 2004. Laser printing of pluripotent embryonal carcinoma cells. *Tissue Eng.*, **10**, 483–91.

[44] Cohen, D. L., Malone, E., Lipson, H. and Bonassar, L. J. 2006. Direct freeform fabrication of seeded hydrogels in arbitrary geometries. *Tissue Eng.*, **12**, 1325–35.

[45] Varghese, D., Deshpande, M., Xu, T. *et al.* 2005. Advances in tissue engineering: cell printing. *J. Thorac. Cardiovasc. Surg.*, **129**, 470–2.

[46] Landers, R., Pfister, A., Hubner, U. *et al.* 2002. Fabrication of soft tissue engineering scaffolds by means of rapid prototyping techniques. *J. Mater. Sci.*, **37**, 3107–16.

[47] Skardal, A., Zhang, J. X. and Prestwich, G. D. 2010. Bioprinting vessel-like constructs using hyaluronan hydrogels crosslinked with tetrahedral polyethylene glycol tetracrylates. *Biomaterials*, **31**, 6173–81.

[48] Lam, C. X. F., Mo, X. M., Teoh, S. H. and Hutmacher, D. W. 2002. Scaffold development using 3D printing with a starch-based polymer. *Mater. Sci. Eng. C - Biomimetic Supramolec. Systems*, **20**, 49–56.

[49] Nahmias, Y., Schwartz, R. E., Verfaillie, C. M. and Odde, D. J. 2005. Laser-guided direct writing for three-dimensional tissue engineering. *Biotechnol. Bioeng.*, **92**, 129–36.

[50] Boland, T., Mironov, V., Gutowska, A., Roth, E. A. and Markwald, R. R. 2003. Cell and organ printing 2: fusion of cell aggregates in three-dimensional gels. *Anatomical Record Part A - Discoveries Molec. Cellular Evolutionary Biol.*, **272**, 497–502.

[51] Smith, C. M., Stone, A. L., Parkhill, R. L. *et al.* 2004. Three-dimensional bioassembly tool for generating viable tissue-engineered constructs. *Tissue Eng.*, **10**, 1566–76.

[52] Han, L. H., Suri, S., Schmidt, C. E. and Chen, S. C. 2010. Fabrication of three-dimensional scaffolds for heterogeneous tissue engineering. *Biomed. Microdevices*, **12**, 721–5.

[53] Chen, C. Y., Barron, J. A. and Ringeisen, B. R. 2006. Cell patterning without chemical surface modification: cell–cell interactions between printed bovine aortic endothelial cells (BAEC) on a homogeneous cell-adherent hydrogel. *Appl. Surf. Sci.*, **252**, 8641–5.

[54] Guillotin, B. and Guillemot, F., Cell patterning technologies for organotypic tissue fabrication. *Trends Biotechnol.*, **29**, 183–90.

[55] Ovsianikov, A., Gruene, M., Pflaum, M. *et al.* 2010. Laser printing of cells into 3D scaffolds. *Biofabrication*, **2**, 014104.

[56] Kikuchi, A. and Okano, T. 2005. Nanostructured designs of biomedical materials: applications of cell sheet engineering to functional regenerative tissues and organs. *J. Controll. Release*, **101**, 69–84.

[57] Shimizu, T., Sekine, H., Isoi, Y. *et al.* 2006. Long-term survival and growth of pulsatile myocardial tissue grafts engineered by the layering of cardiomyocyte sheets. *Tissue Eng.*, **12**, 499–507.

[58] L'Heureux, N., Paquet, S., Labbe, R., Germain, L. and Auger, F. A. 1998. A completely biological tissue-engineered human blood vessel. *FASEB J.*, **12**, 47–56.

[59] Mikos, A. G., Herring, S. W., Ochareon, P. *et al.* 2006. Engineering complex tissues. *Tissue Eng.*, **12**, 3307–39.

[60] Lee, K. Y. and Mooney, D. J. 2001. Hydrogels for tissue engineering. *Chem. Rev.*, **101**, 1869–79.

[61] Kaihara, S., Borenstein, J., Koka, R. *et al.* 2000. Silicon micromachining to tissue engineer branched vascular channels for liver fabrication. *Tissue Eng.*, **6**, 105–17.

[62] Stevens, M. M., Mayer, M., Anderson, D. G. *et al.* 2005. Direct patterning of mammalian cells onto porous tissue engineering substrates using agarose stamps. *Biomaterials*, **26**, 7636–41.

[63] Tekin, H., Ozaydin-Ince, G., Tsinman, T. *et al.* 2011. Responsive microgrooves for the formation of harvestable tissue constructs. *Langmuir*, **27**, 5671–9.

[64] Bian, W. N. and Bursac, N. 2009. Engineered skeletal muscle tissue networks with controllable architecture. *Biomaterials*, **30**, 1401–12.

[65] Xia, Y. N. and Whitesides, G. M. 1998. Soft lithography. *Ann. Rev. Mater. Sci.*, **28**, 153–84.

[66] Slaughter, B. V., Khurshid, S. S., Fisher, O. Z., Khademhosseini, A. and Peppas, N. A. 2009. Hydrogels in regenerative medicine. *Adv. Mater.*, **21**, 3307–29.

[67] Oh, J. K., Lee, D. I. and Park, J. M. 2009. Biopolymer-based microgels/nanogels for drug delivery applications. *Prog. Polymer Sci.*, **34**, 1261–82.

[68] Folch, A. and Toner, M. 2000. Microengineering of cellular interactions. *Ann. Rev. Biomed. Eng.*, **2**, 227–56.

[69] Suh, K. Y., Choi, S. J., Baek, S. J., Kim, T. W. and Langer, R. 2005. Observation of high-aspect-ratio nanostructures using capillary lithography. *Adv. Mater.*, **17**, 560–4.

[70] Chandra, D., Taylor, J. A. and Yang, S. 2008. Replica molding of high-aspect-ratio (sub-)micron hydrogel pillar arrays and their stability in air and solvents. *Soft Matter*, **4**, 979–84.

[71] Johann, R. M., Baiotto, C. and Renaud, P. 2007. Micropatterned surfaces of PDMS as growth templates for HEK 293 cells. *Biomed. Microdevices*, **9**, 475–85.

[72] Rivest, C., Morrison, D. W. G., Ni, B. *et al.* 2007. Microscale hydrogels for medicine and biology: synthesis, characteristics and applications. *J. Mechanics Mater. Structures*, **2**, 1103–19.

[73] Rolland, J. P., Maynor, B. W., Euliss, L. E. *et al.* 2005. Direct fabrication and harvesting of monodisperse, shape-specific nanobiomaterials. *J. Am. Chem. Soc.*, **127**, 10096–100.

[74] Khademhosseini, A., Yeh, J., Jon, S. *et al.* 2004. Molded polyethylene glycol microstructures for capturing cells within microfluidic channels. *Lab Chip*, **4**, 425–30.

[75] Tekin, H., Tsinman, T., Sanchez, J. G. *et al.* 2011. Responsive micromolds for sequential patterning of hydrogel microstructures. *J. Am. Chem. Soc.*, **133**, 12944–7.

[76] Khademhosseini, A., Ferreira, L., Blumling, J. III *et al.* 2006. Co-culture of human embryonic stem cells with murine embryonic fibroblasts on microwell-patterned substrates. *Biomaterials*, **27**, 5968–77.

[77] Park, J. H., Chung, B. G., Lee, W. G. *et al.* 2010. Microporous cell-laden hydrogels for engineered tissue constructs. *Biotechnol. Bioeng.*, **106**, 138–48.

[78] Du, Y., Ghodousi, M., Qi, H. *et al.* 2011. Sequential assembly of cell-laden hydrogel constructs to engineer vascular-like microchannels. *Biotechnol. Bioeng.*, **108**, 1693–703.

[79] Koh, W. G., Revzin, A. and Pishko, M. V. 2002. Poly(ethylene glycol) hydrogel microstructures encapsulating living cells. *Langmuir*, **18**, 2459–62.

[80] Liu, V. A. and Bhatia, S. N. 2002. Three-dimensional photopatterning of hydrogels containing living cells. *Biomed. Microdevices*, **4**, 257–66.

[81] Koh, W. G., Itle, L. J. and Pishko, M. V. 2003. Molding of hydrogel multiphenotype cell microstructures to create microarrays. *Anal. Chem.*, **75**, 5783–9.

[82] Aubin, H., Nichol, J. W., Hutson, C. B. *et al.* 2010. Directed 3D cell alignment and elongation in microengineered hydrogels. *Biomaterials*, **31**, 6941–51.

[83] Mapili, G., Lu, Y., Chen, S. C. and Roy, K. 2005. Laser-layered microfabrication of spatially patterned functionalized tissue-engineering scaffolds. *J. Biomed. Mater. Res. Part B - Appl. Biomater.* **75**, 414–24.

[84] Hahn, M. S., Miller, J. S. and West, J. L. 2006. Three-dimensional biochemical and biomechanical patterning of hydrogels for guiding cell behavior. *Adv. Mater.*, **18**, 2679–84.

[85] Fozdar, D. Y., Soman, P., Lee, J. W., Han, L. H. and Chen, S. C. 2011. Three-dimensional polymer constructs exhibiting a tunable negative Poisson's ratio. *Adv. Functional Mater.*, **21**, 2712–20.

[86] Batorsky, A., Liao, J. H., Lund, A. W., Plopper, G. E. and Stegemann, J. P. 2005. Encapsulation of adult human mesenchymal stem cells within collagen–agarose microenvironments. *Biotechnol. Bioeng.*, **92**, 492–500.

[87] Jia, X. Q., Yeo, Y., Clifton, R. J. *et al.* 2006. Hyaluronic acid-based microgels and microgel networks for vocal fold regeneration. *Biomacromolecules*, **7**, 3336–44.

[88] Laroui, H., Grossin, L., Leonard, M. *et al.* 2007. Hyaluronate-covered nanoparticles for the therapeutic targeting of cartilage. *Biomacromolecules*, **8**, 3879–85.

[89] Ethirajan, A., Ziener, U., Chuvilin, A. *et al.* 2008. Biomimetic hydroxyapatite crystallization in gelatin nanoparticles synthesized using a miniemulsion process. *Adv. Functional Mater.*, **18**, 2221–7.

[90] Dang, S. M., Kyba, M., Perlingeiro, R., Daley, G. Q. and Zandstra, P. W. 2002. Efficiency of embryoid body formation and hematopoietic development from embryonic stem cells in different culture systems. *Biotechnol. Bioeng.*, **78**, 442–53.

[91] Dang, S. and Zandstra, P. 2005. Scalable production of embryonic stem cell-derived cells. *Methods Molec. Biol.*, **290**, 353–64.

[92] Magyar, J. P., Nemir, M., Ehler, E. *et al.* 2001. Mass production of embryoid bodies in microbeads. *Ann. New York Acad. Sci.*, **944**, 135–43.

[93] Xu, S., Nie, Z., Seo, M. *et al.* 2005. Generation of monodisperse particles by using microfluidics: control over size, shape, and composition. *Angewandte Chem. Int. Edition Engl.*, **44**, 3799.

[94] Franzesi, G. T., Ni, B., Ling, Y. B. and Khademhosseini, A. 2006. A controlled-release strategy for the generation of

cross-linked hydrogel microstructures. *J. Am. Chem. Soc.*, **128**, 15064–5.

[95] Dendukuri, D., Pregibon, D. C., Collins, J., Hatton, T. A. and Doyle, P. S. 2006. Continuous-flow lithography for high-throughput microparticle synthesis. *Nature Mater.*, **5**, 365–9.

[96] Chung, S. E., Park, W., Park, H. *et al.* 2007. Optofluidic maskless lithography system for real-time synthesis of photopolymerized microstructures in microfluidic channels. *Appl. Phys. Lett.*, **91**, 041106.

[97] Lee, S. A., Chung, S. E., Park, W., Lee, S. H. and Kwon, S. 2009. Three-dimensional fabrication of heterogeneous microstructures using soft membrane deformation and optofluidic maskless lithography. *Lab Chip*, **9**, 1670–5.

[98] Panda, P., Ali, S., Lo, E. *et al.* 2008. Stop-flow lithography to generate cell-laden microgel particles. *Lab Chip*, **8**, 1056–61.

[99] Braschler, T., Johann, R., Heule, M., Metref, L. and Renaud, P. 2005. Gentle cell trapping and release on a microfluidic chip by *in situ* alginate hydrogel formation. *Lab Chip*, **5**, 553–9.

[100] Tan, W. and Desai, T. A. 2004. Layer-by-layer microfluidics for biomimetic three-dimensional structures. *Biomaterials*, **25**, 1355–64.

[101] Burdick, J. A., Khademhosseini, A. and Langer, R. 2004. Fabrication of gradient hydrogels using a microfluidics/photopolymerization process. *Langmuir*, **20**, 5153–6.

[102] Hancock, M. J., Piraino, F., Camci-Unal, G., Rasponi, M. and Khademhosseini, A. 2011. Anisotropic material synthesis by capillary flow in fluid stripes. *Biomaterials*, **32**, 6493–504.

[103] Zaari, N., Rajagopalan, P., Kim, S. K., Engler, A. J. and Wong, J. Y. 2004. Photopolymerization in microfluidic gradient generators: microscale control of substrate compliance to manipulate cell response. *Adv. Mater.*, **16**, 2133–7.

[104] Hoerstrup, S. P., Zund, G., Sodian, R. *et al.* 2001. Tissue engineering of small caliber vascular grafts. *Eur. J. Cardio-Thorac. Surg.*, **20**, 164–9.

[105] Shin'oka, T., Matsumura, G., Hibino, N. *et al.* 2005. Midterm clinical result of tissue-engineered vascular autografts seeded with autologous bone marrow cells. *J. Thorac. Cardiovasc. Surg.*, **129**, 1330–8.

[106] Hjortnaes, J., Gottlieb, D., Figueiredo, J. L. *et al.* 2010. Intravital molecular imaging of small-diameter tissue-engineered vascular grafts in mice: a feasibility study. *Tissue Eng. Part C – Methods*, **16**, 597–607.

[107] L'Heureux, N., Germain, L., Labbe, R. and Auger, F. A. 1993. In vitro construction of a human blood-vessel from cultured vascular cells – a morphologic study. *J. Vasc. Surg.*, **17**, 499–509.

[108] Borenstein, J. T., Terai, H., King, K. R. *et al.* 2002. Microfabrication technology for vascularized tissue engineering. *Biomed. Microdevices*, **4**, 167–75.

[109] Fidkowski, C., Kaazempur-Mofrad, M. R., Borenstein, J. *et al.* 2005. Endothelialized microvasculature based on a biodegradable elastomer. *Tissue Eng.*, **11**, 302–9.

[110] Ling, Y., Rubin, J., Deng, Y. *et al.* 2007. A cell-laden microfluidic hydrogel. *Lab Chip*, **7**, 756–62.

[111] Golden, A. P. and Tien, J. 2007. Fabrication of microfluidic hydrogels using molded gelatin as a sacrificial element. *Lab Chip*, **7**, 720–5.

[112] Chrobak, K. M., Potter, D. R. and Tien, J. 2006. Formation of perfused, functional microvascular tubes in vitro. *Microvasc. Res.*, **71**, 185–96.

[113] Nichol, J. W. and Khademhosseini, A. 2009. Modular tissue engineering: engineering biological tissues from the bottom up. *Soft Matter*, **5**, 1312–19.

[114] Tsang, V. L., Chen, A. A., Cho, L. M. *et al.* 2007. Fabrication of 3D hepatic tissues by additive photopatterning of cellular hydrogels. *FASEB J.*, **21**, 790–801.

[115] Wheeldon, I., Ahari, A. F. and Khademhosseini, A. 2010. Microengineering hydrogels for stem cell bioengineering and tissue regeneration. *J. Assoc. Lab. Automation*, **15**, 440–8.

[116] Peppas, N. A., Hilt, J. Z., Khademhosseini, A. and Langer, R. 2006. Hydrogels in biology and medicine: from molecular principles to bionanotechnology, *Adv. Mater.*, **18**, 1345–60.

[117] Fernandez, J. G. and Khademhosseini, A. 2010. Micromasonry: construction of 3D structures by microscale self-assembly. *Adv. Mater.*, **22**, 2538–41.

[118] Du, Y., Ghodousi, M., Lo, E. *et al.* 2010. Surface-directed assembly of cell-laden microgels. *Biotechnol. Bioeng.*, **105**, 655–62.

[119] Du, Y., Lo, E., Vidula, M. K., Khabiry, M. and Khademhosseini, A. 2008. Method of bottom-up directed assembly of cell-laden microgels. *Cellular Molec. Bioeng.*, **1**, 157–62.

[120] Du, Y., Lo, E., Ali, S. and Khademhosseini, A. 2008. Directed assembly of cell-laden microgels for fabrication of 3D tissue constructs. *Proc. Nat. Acad. Sci.*, **105**, 9522–7.

[121] Yanagawa, F., Kaji, H., Jang, Y. H. *et al.* 2011. Directed assembly of cell-laden microgels for building porous three-dimensional tissue constructs. *J. Biomed. Mater. Res. Part A*, **97**, 93–102.

19

Organ printing

Tao Xu, Daniel Reyna-Soriano, Jorge I. Rodríguez-Dévora, Mohammod Bhuyan and Thomas Boland

19.1 Introduction

Since the first successful organ transplantation with a kidney in 1954 [1], scientists have maintained the dream of being able to fabricate organs on request. Organogenesis – or the creation of organs from artificial manipulation of cells, materials, growth factors (GFs), and other organ elements – has been waiting for the appropriate technology to emerge. This futuristic technique should be capable of rebuilding the compositional and structural complexities of human tissues and organs. The recent development of bioprinting technologies (defined by their high resolution and high-speed construction) has revived interest in applying those emerging methods for organogenesis. The term "organ printing" has become standard since the 2000s [2–4]. It refers to the line of investigations related to the development of the technologies for the construction of three-dimensional (3D) structures based on the deposition of different cell lines and biochemical promoters.

Although individual tissue systems have been successfully engineered for various applications using the basic tissue engineering approach, the means for the building of complex tissues that consist of multiple cell and tissue components have not been established. This is due to various challenges encountered in the tissue building process. One of the challenges has been the inability to recreate the well-defined cellular configurations and functions of a native tissue. Living tissues contain multiple cell types and various extracellular materials arranged in specific patterns that are difficult to replicate in vitro. Thus, one important goal of tissue engineering and regenerative medicine is to develop a tissue fabrication method that allows specific control over the placement of various cells and matrices in three dimensions in order to mimic the complexity of native tissue architecture. Emerging "organ printing" or "bioprinting" methodologies are being investigated in order to create tissue-engineered constructs that initially have more defined spatial organization. The underlying hypothesis is that with these biomimetic patterns one can achieve improved therapeutic outcomes [5].

The following sections provide a brief and concise introduction of basic elements and current trends as they pertain to cell and organ printing, including bio-blueprints, bio-ink, bio-paper, and bio-printer and printing methods. Organ printing stands at the forefront of tissue engineering since recent studies have demonstrated the feasibility and benefits of implementing bioprinting of biomolecules and cells for tissue engineering and biological applications.

19.2 Bio-blueprint

The bio-blueprint for organ printing is known as a preprocessing step in the bioprinting process. In order to print an artificial organ, a detailed description and representation of morphology, anatomy, cell and tissue characteristics, and vascular systems at different organ levels is first needed. The computer model for this information is defined as a bio-blueprint for organ printing [5], which can generally be obtained from non-invasive medical imaging data of a natural organ [3]. The purposes of the bio-blueprint model are the following: (1) to set forth the anatomy, geometry, and extracellular matrix (ECM) of an organ, tissue heterogeneity, individual tissue geometry, and boundary distinction within the organ; (2) to define a vascular network in an organ; and (3) to provide a database on an organ's geometry, heterogeneity, and vascular network that can be used for printing-path generation of organ printing [6].

19.2.1 Current bio-blueprint modeling methods

Bio-blueprint organ modeling consists of two principal processes: non-invasive imaging data acquisition and 3D reconstruction. Often the anatomical data are obtained from an appropriate imaging process modality to construct a specific organ, which is referred to as image-based organ modeling. In this modeling, the imaging should be able to create 3D views of anatomy, differentiate heterogeneous cell tissue types, show the vascular architecture, and generate organ models for other downstream approaches, such as analysis and simulation. Figure 19.1 shows the process for obtaining a computer-assisted design (CAD) model from medical imaging data [6]. The three major approaches used for this process will be introduced below.

19.2.1.1 MedCAD interface

The MedCAD interface, which is normally available as a standard module of medical imaging processing software, is intended to bridge the gap between medical imaging and CAD design software. The MedCAD interface can export data from the imaging system to the CAD platform and vice versa in International Graphics Exchange Standard (IGES), Standard for Exchange of Product (STEP), or stereolithography (STL) format. The interface provides for the fitting of primitives, such as cylinders, planes, and spheres at the imaging two-dimensional (2D) segmentation slices. It also provides the limited ability to model a free-form surface (such as B-spline surfaces). The limitation of using MedCAD interface is the incapability to capture detail and complex tissue anatomical features, particularly for features with complex geometry [6].

19.2.1.2 Reverse-engineering interface

The reverse-engineering-interface approach uses a 3D voxel model created from the segmentation. The 3D voxel model is converted to point-data form and the points are loaded into reverse-engineering software. The points are then triangulated to form a faceted model. The faceted model is further refined and enhanced to reduce the file sizes and unwanted features. The free-form surfaces of Non-Uniform Rational B-Spline (NURBS) patches are used to fit across the outer shape of the model. Although the process has a comparatively longer processing time, the results obtained are significantly better than those achieved with the other two methods. The CAD model is much more aesthetically pleasing, stable in configuration, and associated with less error in data-transfer formats, particularly for an integrated CAD and finite-element analysis application [6].

19.2.1.3 STL: a triangulated model converting approach

The 3D voxel model can also be converted to an STL file, and this STL file can then be imported into reverse-engineering software for surface refinement and NURBS surface generation. The difference between this approach and the reverse-engineering approach is that this approach uses the STL triangulated surface as modeling input rather than the point clouds data. Although the processing time is shorter, this approach inherits all of the limitations of the STL format [6].

19.2.2 Data acquisition

There are non-invasive and tactile data acquisition methods. For bio-blueprint design it is preferable to use a non-invasive data acquisition method [6], often involving the application of light, sound, or magnetic fields. In each case an appropriate analysis must be performed to determine positions of points

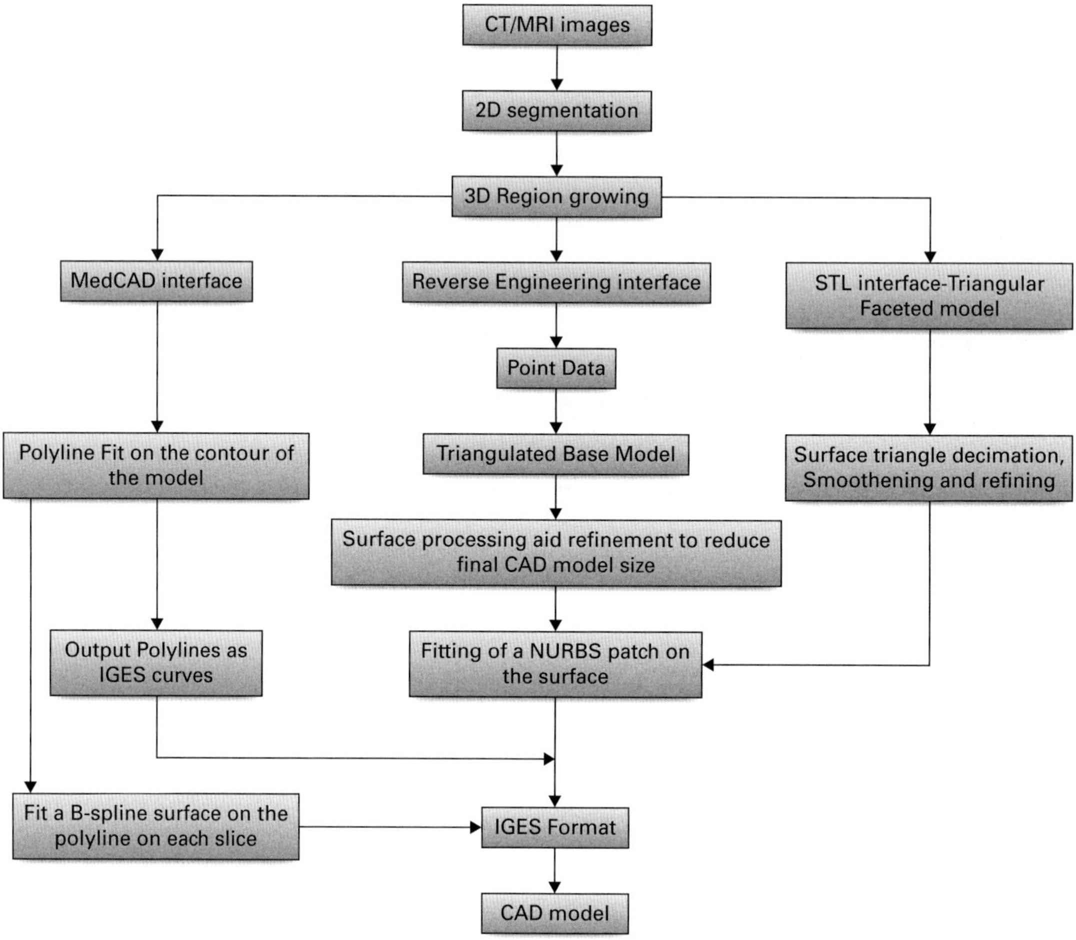

Figure 19.1 Process definition to arrive at a CAD model from CT/MRI data [7].

on the organ's surface from physical readings obtained. Each method has strengths and weaknesses, meaning that the data acquisition system must be carefully selected for the shape-capture functionality desired [8].

19.2.2.1 Non-invasive imaging data acquisition

The primary imaging modalities used in the tissue modeling are computed tomography (CT) scans, magnetic resonance imaging (MRI), and optical microscopy, each with its own advantages and limitations.

19.2.2.1.1 Organ data acquisition by CT scanning

With CT and μCT scans a sample is exposed to small quantities of ionizing radiation, the absorption of which is detected and imaged. This results in a series of 2D images displaying a density map of the sample. Stacking these images creates a 3D representation of the scanned area. The main advantage of CT and μCT as an imaging modality for tissue engineering purposes is the reasonably high resolution. The latest development of μCT technology has been successfully used to quantify the microstructure-function relationship of tissues and the designed tissue

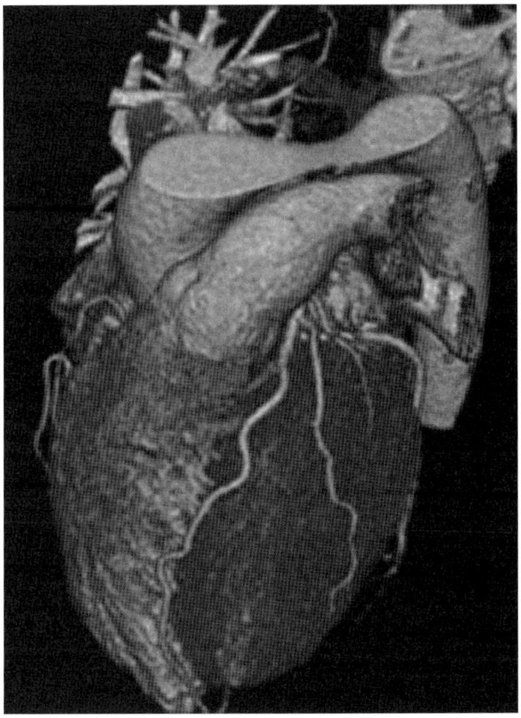

Figure 19.2 Heart imaging obtained by CT scan [18].

structures [9]. For example, recent reports have shown that a μCT system was capable of characterizing the micro-architectural and mechanical properties of tissue scaffolds [10], helping in the design and fabrication of tailored tissue microstructures [11, 12], quantifying the bone-tissue morphologies and internal stress–strain behavior [13–15], and non-destructively evaluating angiography. In addition, certain metals, metal salts, and metal particulates significantly increase contrast in CT. Owing to the toxicity and side effects of heavy metals in vivo, few of these metallic contrast agents are in widespread clinical use [16, 17]. The assembly of an organ blueprint model from a cadaveric sample allows one to avoid these deleterious side effects, and metal-bearing contrast agents may be useful [6]. Figure 19.2 shows a representative example of imaging obtained by CT scan.

19.2.2.1.2 Organ data acquisition by MRI

Compared with CT technology, MRI does not expose the sample to ionizing radiation, thus giving MRI a broader range of clinical applications. It images soft tissues as well as bone, and hence is vastly superior in differentiating soft-tissue types and recognizing border regions of tissues of similar densities. Much like CT, the output of MRI is a series of 2D images that may be stacked and segmented by signal intensity. Further segmentation may be achieved through region-growing selection of voxels of similar signal values that are contiguous. This can create models of regions of similar signal intensity that are part of an individual structure, e.g. selecting a single ligament rather than all the ligaments in the image [6]. Although the resolution of MRI is inferior to that of CT scans, it has been of great use in assembling anatomic atlases of increasingly fine resolution as the technology matures [6]. Figure 19.3 shows a representative example of imaging obtained by a MRI scan.

19.2.2.1.3 Organ data acquisition by optical methods

Without modeling software capable of reassembling dissected histology slices, optical-microscopic methods of developing 3D tissue modeling would not be possible. To examine a sample in high resolution using optical microscopy, it must be physically sectioned to a thickness of between 5 and 80 μm and placed onto slides, providing a square sample of dimensions perhaps 1 cm × 1 cm for fine resolution. The division into these slides is a labor-intensive process, and the resulting images of the target organ would be thousands of 2D images that must be both digitally stacked into 3D columns as in CT and MRI and arranged in correct *X* and *Y* positions. This is computationally cumbersome and memory-intensive, but within the capabilities of many computer-modeling programs [6].

With the understanding that the technique would be labor-intensive and require a great deal of computer time, optical microscopy also brings the benefit of a century of refinement. Pathologists have become skilled at identifying any individual cell in the body

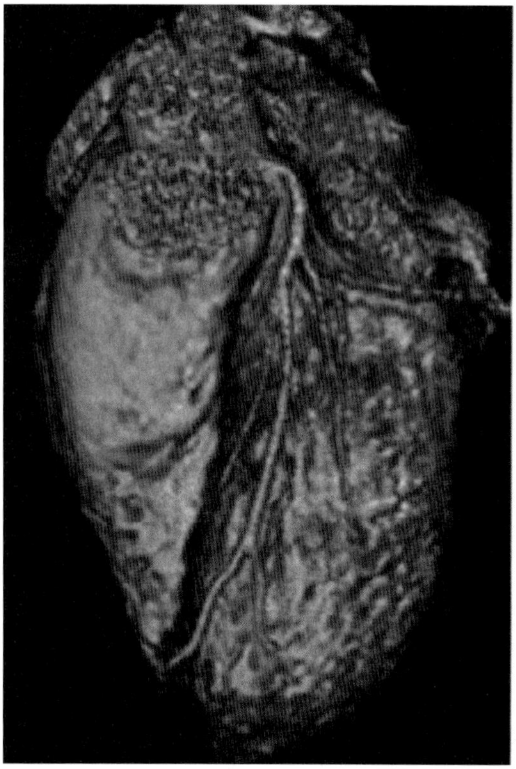

Figure 19.3 Heart imaging obtained by MRI scan [19].

visually, even in cases of diseased tissue, the origin of their name. Stains may be applied to individual slides or all slides. These stains may be as simple as dyes or as complex as fluorescing antibodies that bind only to a single type of cell. Differentiating every tissue type down to the level of the individual cell is possible for optical microscopy in ways far beyond what can be done with either CT or MRI, not by density or signal intensity, but by the features of the cells themselves. One particular example of optical microscopy used in tissue modeling was reported in regard to the imaging of lung tissue, detecting fluorescence from the lung parenchyma above 545 nm. The individual images taken were then stacked, and carefully re-aligned, for a 3D representation. While the alveoli were modeled at extremely high resolution, the main drawbacks of this method were made readily apparent. Specifically, both the sectioning and the imaging are time-consuming processes, and the sectioning can result in distortion of the individual slides. Also, from a practicality point of view, pathologists cannot be expected to examine thousands of individual slides of an entire organ and identify each and every cell in the image. Therefore, it will be a significant challenge to train computers to identify individual cells by their visual characteristics, even with the aid of complex staining [6].

19.2.2.2 Imaging-based 3D reconstruction

The basic 3D interpretation format of consecutive slice images is a volumetric model consisting of voxels. The volumetric model consists of brick-like components, each representing a set height, width, and depth. Like pixels, each voxel represents a yes/no value indicating its existence in the model and a grayscale or color value. Hence volumetric models tend to have rough surface textures with many right angles at the scale of the individual voxel, as shown in Figure 19.4 [6].

Although volumetric data from medical image data can be directly altered to STL format and printed on a rapid prototyping system, there are many advantages to further converting the images model into a CAD-based solid model. CAD-based solid modeling relies upon boundary representation by means of which a solid model is defined by the boundaries that enclose it. These bounding surfaces are mathematically described by polynomial functions such as NURBS functions. This method facilitates the construction of the model by minimizing the size of the files and ensuring the closure of bounding surfaces. Figure 19.5 illustrates the difference between volumetric and surface representations: (a) the left panel represents a series of slice images, with a single-pixel protuberance from a vertical flat surface; (b) the middle panel displays this single-pixel volumetric model as a voxel; and (c) the surface interpretation of these 2D pixels is different, however, and, when expressed as a NURBS surface, as in the right panel, the single offshoot pixel is expressed as the apex of a curve [6].

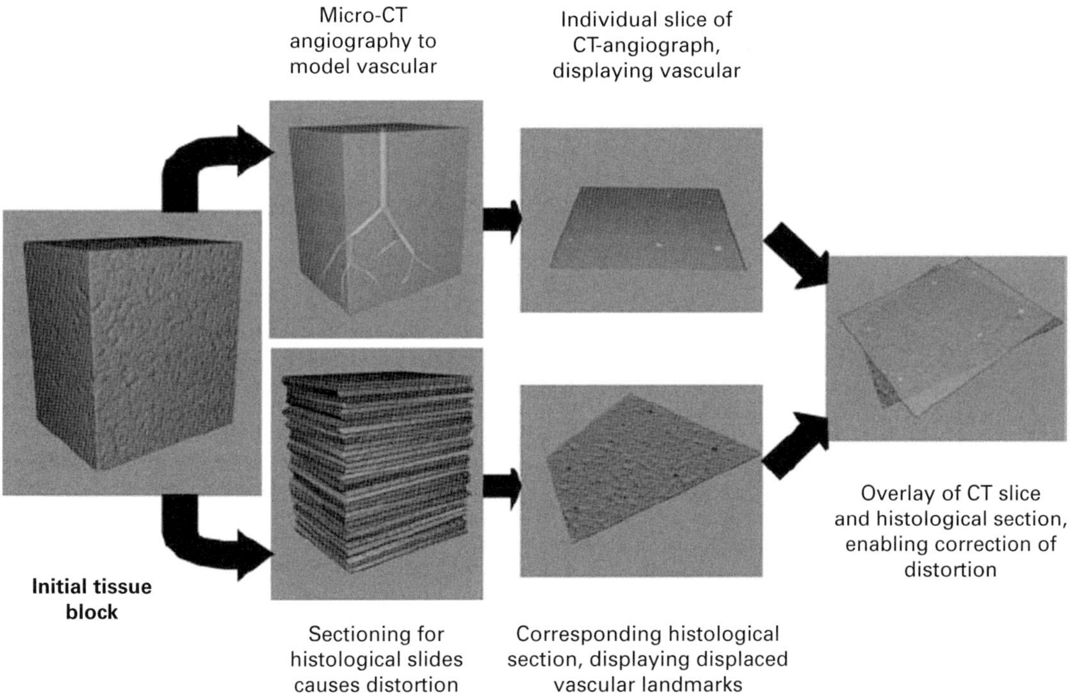

Figure 19.4 An illustration of the micro-CT/optical-microscopy hybrid model [6].

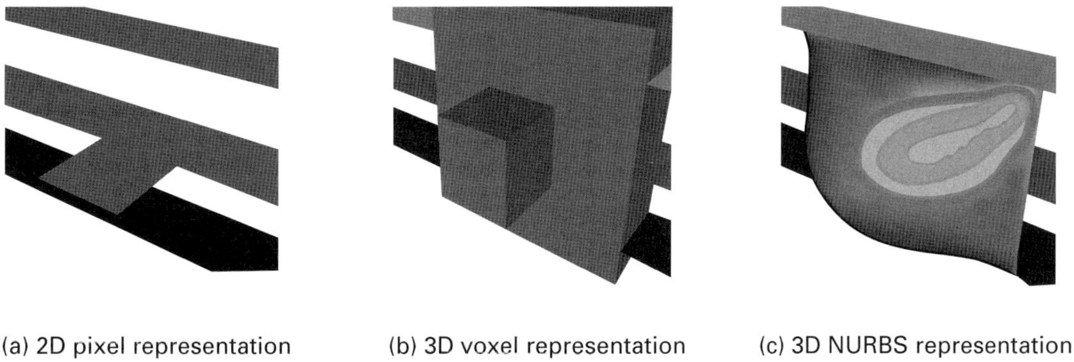

Figure 19.5 Image volumetric representation [6].

19.2.3 Blueprint development

The framework of development of a biomimetic model is outlined through the following major steps: (1) development of a computer modeling representation of a 3D organ, (2) development of a 3D vascularization network, and (3) development of a CAD-based organ bio-blueprint model.

The development of a bio-blueprint model starts from 3D reconstruction of organ anatomy (without the vascular system) from the given modalities

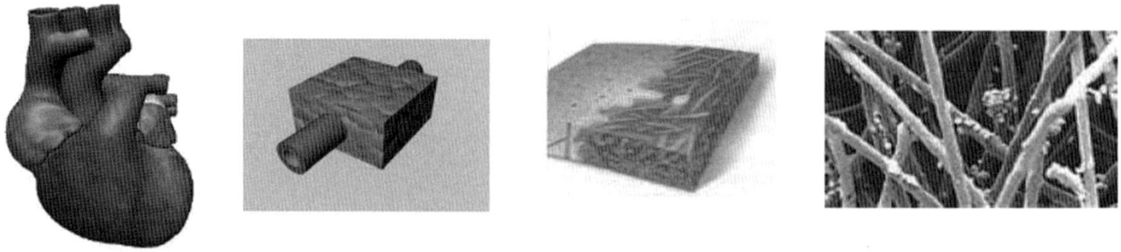

Figure 19.6 Hierarchical scales of organ structure [6].

(medical imaging data) and a CAD-based modeling representation that can be used to explicitly describe organ geometry, topology, and individual tissues. The model development involves using state-of-the-art 3D reconstruction, reverse engineering, CAD platforms, and in-house heterogeneous modeling algorithms [20, 21]. A bio-blueprint model is generated from non-invasive medical imaging for capturing and replicating organ anatomy including detailed internal and external morphology, geometry, vascularization, and tissue identification. Therefore, all of the following three hierarchical scales, as shown in Figure 19.6, need to be considered in the construction of the bio-blueprint model:

(1) the scale of the organ (to consider the organ's macrostructure tissue types, vasculature, ducting, and anatomical compatibility);
(2) the scale of the tissue, or sub-organ (to consider the heterogeneity of tissue with appropriate types of cells and their interaction);
(3) the scale at the cellular level (to consider the selection of ECM or scaffold materials and to divide the bio-blueprint model into small blocks to enable local definition of ECM/scaffold materials).

The bio-blueprint model is represented in a CAD format that adopts "boundary representation" by which an organ or tissue anatomy and topology can be explicitly described by the enclosed and adjacent boundaries through mathematically defined NURBS functions [6]. Reducing the memory usage of the bio-blueprint or of interpolating structures not visible in medical imaging can be done by reducing the combinations of feature primitives. This method also smoothes out irregularities in continuous features caused by noise in the imaging modality. For instance, a feature-primitive-based reconstruction method for vascular networks is used to generate a 3D biological vascular system for organ growth. In this primitive feature modeling approach, the basic vascular primitive characteristic parameters are determined from patient-specific CT/MRI images, and further use of Boolean operation algebra forms a high-level vessel assembly. The vascular feature primitives are represented as NURBS bases, and the parameters in the NURBS equations can be determined by measuring the spatial positions of the vascular CT/MRI images at different projections [6].

In summary, the bio-blueprint is a crucial step for the organ printing process because it provides a description and representation of details of organ anatomy, morphology, tissue heterogeneity, and vascular systems at different organizational scales. Reverse engineering plays an important role for the organ printing process, transforming a real organ into engineering models and concepts. The methods currently used to obtain the organ modeling data involve non-invasive data acquisition by CT scanning, MRI scanning, and optical methods. The bio-blueprint procedure is at an early stage and more research is required in order to decrease the current limitations. The future goal is to realize an "artificially intelligent" organ using reverse engineering to create an optimal bio-blueprint model not only to define the dimensions and parameters, but also to focus on simulating the functionality.

19.3 Bio-ink

As one of the key elements to effectively pursue organ printing, bio-inks and associated additives are being developed. The term bio-ink originates from the fact that inkjet technologies with the ultra-precise characteristics needed in order to achieve organogenesis have been developed. While inkjet technologies were initially used for printing applications (texts and pictures), the method has found its way toward more interesting uses such as the construction of electronic components and biomedical applications. Ink was developed for years [22–27] to optimize its characteristics in order to improve printing quality (precision and accuracy) and speed by creating a controlled flow of ink and preventing clogging and drying of ink at the print head; these outcomes are also key for the desired futuristic organ printing devices. Therefore, intensive research has been focussed on developing so-called bio-inks in order to advance toward organogenesis. Such research is reviewed in the present section.

Strategies based on the types of materials utilized have been pursued. All kinds of living cells, small proteins, and plasmids have been utilized in different techniques to create 3D structures in vitro. In general, the requirements for a viable suspension for a bio-ink are high biocompatibility, low sedimentation, high control of viscosity, the ability to be arranged three-dimensionally, and so forth, justifying the focus on improving one or more of these characteristics by different research groups worldwide. In the following paragraphs a description divided by suspension source is provided in order to illustrate contemporary strategies.

19.3.1 Cell suspensions

The human body is formed by many structures such as muscles, bones, nerves, vessels, skin, and so on. Each structure has its purpose within the system (body); therefore, as expected, each structure is formed from many different types of cell in such a way as to achieve its function. If the intention of organ printing consists of the fabrication of living structures to overcome the lack of organ donation, it is expected that all these types of cells will need to be tested to evaluate the engineering capabilities required for assembling viable 3D structures. To date, many of these cell types have been used for tissue engineering applications [28]. Within these experiments, we can identify two strategies. The first involves using differentiated cells such as epithelial, muscle, bone, and nerve cells, and so forth. However, therapeutic rejection of such cells is common, because the implanted cells have to perfectly match the ones contained within the patient's body. On the other hand, cell proliferation of a patient's biopsied cells can be approached as an alternative solution (autologous treatment). As a second strategy, the pluripotency of stem cells makes their use a promising approach for creating human-made organs. Even though there are still ethical concerns regarding the acquisition of stem cells, research using them has been initiated and continues to grow. Further details of specific usage of the cell lines are described below.

19.3.1.1 Differentiated cells

The term differentiated cells refers to those that have followed a maturation process either in a host environment or in vitro to provide specific functions within a tissue or organ. During the embryological developmental process, primary cell tissue layers (mesoderm, endoderm, and ectoderm) initiate their restricted roads toward their final fates. From the three primary tissue layers, more than 200 cell types are differentiated to form the human body. However, organs are not typically constructed by a single type of cell, being more likely to have many types that are highly crosslinked. The crosslinked nature of cells provides a challenge by itself; nevertheless, biologists have developed disassociation technologies that accurately isolate cells from donated tissue. Such technological advances have made available to biomedical engineering the resources with which to start trials with the ultimate goal of building an artificial organ.

Applications in tissue engineering leading toward organ fabrication had emerged by the late 1990s, when a direct writing system utilizing a laser was used to dispense arrays of embryonic-chick spinal-cord cells [29, 30]. Further progress has been made, allowing one to isolate cells from tissues, enabling a vast range of differentiated cells to be tried via printing systems. The types of cells which have been investigated include epithelial [23, 31], cardiac muscle [32], bone [33, 34], and nerve [26, 30, 35] cells. In all cases it has been demonstrated that organ printing precursor systems are able to create viable cell assemblies. However, development is still required in order to attain fully viable macro-scalable 3D structures.

19.3.1.2 Stem cells

Stem cells have been utilized for therapeutic purposes for quite a long time. Even though their working mechanisms have yet to be fully understood, their unique characteristics are envisioned as bearing great promise for clinical therapies and future organogenesis. The main two advantages of stem cells are their increased capability of renewal (high proliferation rate) and the fact that they act as a joker in the sense of being capable of differentiating into many types of specialized cells (as discussed previously) depending on specific conditions during their development. To date, the widely accepted classification of stem cell sources assigns them to the following categories:

(1) Adult stem cells. Adult bone marrow transplants were the first successful stem cell therapies, and since then (1968 [36]) they have been used widely, mainly in patients with ongoing chemotherapy. However, in the 1980s isolation of stem cells from circulating blood was achieved [37]. Some other sources are fat [38] and skin [39].

(2) Embryonic stem cells. Compared with adult stem cells, embryonic stem cells have a better proliferation rate and greater therapeutic potential. However, ever since they were first isolated (1998), there has been a great ethical controversy due to the embryo's destruction during the isolation process. This controversy has meant that, in the USA, the National Institutes of Health (NIH) have restricted stem cell research to 15 cell lines, despite complaints expressed by the scientific community to the effect that the therapeutic benefits of its usage are being jeopardized.

(3) Fetal and early born stem cells. Isolation from such sources as amniotic fluid [34], placenta [40], and umbilical cord [41, 42] has been done. Umbilical cord preservation is gaining popularity nowadays since a decent number of stem cells can be obtained from there. However, the properties of embryonic stem cells remain superior [36].

Biological research is a key factor to understanding prior to initiating the journey toward organ printing. Stem cells provide tremendous potential for research in comparison with differentiated cells. The seeding of stem cells opens the possibility in "organ engineering" to accurately arrange cell suspensions along with growth factors (GFs) (and so forth) in organ-like 3D structures, provide controlled incubation conditions, and let the nature of stem cells do the rest of the work toward organogenesis. With this objective in mind, research trying to create simple tissues, has been done and differentiation evaluation tests involving this strategy have been performed.

Recent studies have focussed on the construction of surrounding microenvironments (niches) to create biomedical replacements at such a scale. It has been found that there are many factors affecting success, such as materials, structural architectures, external signals, and intercellular interactions. Such factors have been widely investigated [28], with the aim of controlling them in such a manner that stem cells' fate can be predicted and manipulated. However, further research is required in order to get closer to the requirements of organ fabrication.

19.3.2 Growth factors/cytokines

Along with the utilization of differentiated and stem cells, other factors have been found helpful in the attempt to artificially create living tissues. The natural organization of living tissues is governed by environmental signals such as biochemical cues (i.e. GFs, cytokines). For instance, vascular endothelial growth factor (VEGF), a GF well known for its angiogenesis property, is a potential factor to improve the vascularization of printed organs, emphasizing the need for investigation of these cues to further advance toward organ printing in reality.

By employing different GFs, Campbell's group [43] has achieved recent progress in experiments eliciting musculoskeletal tissues using inkjet printing technologies to accurately dispense the GF-loaded bio-inks. Spatial patterns of GFs were built over oriented submicron fibers (mimicking musculoskeletal ECM), which were evaluated in vitro to demonstrate that control over cell fate had been achieved. In further studies [44] bone morphogenetic protein-2 was used to guide stem cells toward osteoblast differentiation by employing the same inkjet technology. This protein was patterned over 200-μm (on average)-thick scaffolds, which are promising for controlling cell differentiation in 3D structures. These results represent first steps toward fabrication of more complicated structures.

19.3.3 Other additives

Other materials have been used to modify the characteristics of bio-ink to improve its printability and assembly features. Printability is highly related to viscosity and surface tension, while assembly features require the contrary characteristics by means of quick solidification (i.e. via gelation) and structural properties to enable 3D organ-like structures. Very few studies have been focussed on the intrinsic characteristics of the bio-ink as an enhanced agent, which represents a potentially promising field for broad investigations. Among the first types of agent investigated for improving sedimentation and aggregation rates are surfactants. Surfactants decrease shear stress via diminishing surface tension. For instance, pluronic surfactant is known to decrease cell aggregation [45]. In a recent study, pluronic surfactant has been proven biocompatible, and more importantly decreases cell aggregation and sedimentation when dispensed by a piezoelectric inkjet printing system [46]. Another alternative for improving bio-ink printability characteristics has been polyethylene glycol (PEG). Studies have shown that 10% concentration in cell suspensions effectively improves the circulation time and biocompatibility of bio-ink [47, 48].

The ECM is crucial for cell homeostasis in vivo. The cell containing bio-ink should accordingly be composed of an ECM fraction. Consistently with the layer-by-layer 3D building strategy, the solidification of the bio-ink onto the substrate is necessary and should be controlled for at least three reasons: (1) to stabilize the printed 2D pattern, (2) to mechanically support the subsequent bio-ink layer, and (3) to mimic cell-type-specific ECM with the ability to regulate cell fate [49]. The solidification process of the bio-ink should not be harmful to the cells. In laser-based printing methods [50], cell suspensions have been supplemented with 1% (wt/vol) alginate hydrogel as a preliminary approach to mimicking the ECM. Cell adhesion proteins have been printed successfully since Klebe's pioneering work [51]. Fibrin is a versatile biopolymer, which presents potential for tissue engineering applications [52]. Cui and Boland recently printed a cellularized pattern reminiscent of microvasculature using an inkjet bioprinter to print cells in combination with fibrin hydrogel [53].

In summary, a key characteristic in organ printing is the selection of a mixture of cells, additives, cytokines, and GFs. These components will provide unique properties, with different effects on the final product.

19.3.4 Bio-paper

Efficacious organ printing requires appropriate substrates or scaffolds to use as bio-paper that are complemented with the organ constituents concerned, to contribute biological cues in order to elicit explicit cellular responses and direct new tissue formation [27, 54]. Bio-paper is usually used as a scaffolding material in organ printing, contributing a biological and structural support for cells to attach, proliferate, and differentiate in. Bio-papers are printed for the accommodation of cells, the supervision of cellular augmentation, and the revival of 3D tissues with proper support and functions. The most important task of a bio-paper is to guarantee a challengeable support to body structures to allow stress transfer over time to implanted sites, and promote tissue regeneration on the paper structure. Some general properties for biomaterials, including biocompatibility, and some special properties with which we should be concerned for the materials used for bio-printing applications, including viscosity, and mechanical and physical requirements, are the main criteria when choosing materials for organ printing applications. Bio-paper is chosen from biomaterials and the commonly available materials used for bio-printing can be classified into three major categories, namely natural polymers, synthetic polymers, and ceramics.

19.3.4.1 Natural polymers used as bio-paper

Natural polymers are commonly used as bio-paper due to their excellent properties, together with the ease of handling and shaping them under certain conditions. Natural biomaterials are enormously diverse and complex, and are obtained from proteins and carbohydrates. These proteins and carbohydrates have evolved to execute very specialized biological, mechanical, biochemical, and structural roles. Natural biodegradable polymers such as alginate, gelatin, collagen, silk fibroin, and chitosan show potential advantages over synthetic polymers because of their favourable properties, including splendid biocompatibility, biodegradability, and biorestorability.

19.3.4.1.1 Collagen

Collagen is a fibrous naturally occurring protein with a triple-helix configuration and has excellent biocompatibility, biodegradability, and synergic capability with bioactive components. Thus collagen has served as the primary scaffolding resource in tissue engineering. For organ printing applications, collagen gels are often used. These are thermally reversible, mechanically weak matrices that provide good cell adhesion and are degraded by cells. Since collagen is a mechanically weak substrate, it is easy to process, which facilitates laser-guided direct writing of cells, ink-jet printing of cells and cell aggregates [31, 55], and construction of layered anatomical shapes [56]. Collagen also has some limitations, including poor mechanical strength, complex handling, high cost, and being useless for the managing of an infected site. Its mechanical strength can be enhanced by introducing crosslinks by physical treatment, such as ultraviolet/gamma-ray irradiation and dehydrothermalization treatment [57, 58].

Collagen can form a gel by itself under post-processing conditions. "Bio-ink" such as a suspension of living cells and/or a combination of nutrients, GFs, therapeutic drugs, and other essential components can be printed on collagen solution without any reaction or adverse effect. Boland *et al.* have used a collagen solution as 2D paper for QCE-6 cell printing with the aid of a modified commercial Hewlett Packard (HP) Deskjet printer (model 550C) [59]. The collagen solution formed a gel after printing cells in an incubation process carried out at 37 °C, under an atmosphere of 5% CO_2, at a relative humidity of 99%. After printing, the printed cells maintain their viability and undergo proliferation on the collagen gel, rendering them satisfactory for further subculture or implantation.

Collagen can also easily form a hard 3D gel structure together with other molecules. Xu *et al.* have applied collagen gel for 3D constructs of bone graft entrapped with amniotic fluid stem cells (AFSCs) and primary bovine aortic endothelial cells with the aid of a model 550C HP DeskJet printer [60, 61]. Collagen gel was formed by mixing autoclaved ice-cold alginate solution (sodium alginate and guluronic) and neutralized ice-cold rat-tail collagen. During the printing process, alginate in the presence of $CaCl_2$ formed a biodegradable hydrogel scaffold. Bio-paper/cell constructs were fabricated by layer-by-layer printing of the endothelial cells or AFSCs onto the collagen/alginate composite gel they implanted in mice for in-vivo testing; the resulting collagen bio-paper proved to be hard, limiting the movement of water in the bone graft and providing adequate 3D vascularization for viability of cells in an osteogenic medium.

Bio-printing systems experience a loss of cell viability and clogging. Collagen can protect the bioactivity and prevent physical damage of cells by being encapsulated with cells and printed together with them rather than serving as a substrate for cell printing in 2D and 3D. Moon *et al.* have applied collagen gel as a carrier for delivery of smooth muscle cells (cell-laden hydrogel) to protect the cells during the printing process and immediate shaping of cell constructs upon printing [62]. By cell encapsulation, multiple layers of collagen with cells can be used to construct a designed organ without distortion or diffusion of geometry.

However, the use of collagen gels remains limited due to the lack of geometric consistency through shrinkage and qualitative variations of batch production. During the dry-freezing process, collagen shrinks by almost 40%, which leads to mismatching with the internal pore structure for vascularization as well as with implantation in the host body. Viscosity, a key parameter in organ printing, increases with collagen concentration [63]. As a result, a solution with a high concentration of collagen is simply unable to flow through the small nozzle of the bio-printer. Further investigation is under way to improve the properties of collagen bio-paper for organ printing applications.

19.3.4.1.2 Alginate

Alginate is a naturally occurring water-soluble linear polysaccharide, typically obtained from three species (*Laminaria hyperborean*, *Ascophyllum nodosum*, and *Macrocystis pyrifera*) of brown algae. Alternating blocks of 1–4-linked α-L-guluronic and β-D-mannuronic acid residues are the main constituents of alginate. Alginates are biocompatible, low-toxicity, pH-sensitive and less expensive natural polymers. Owing to its superior properties, alginate has been widely used as bio-paper for organ printing. Gel formation is the key phenomenon in jet technology to mechanically support the printed construct. Alginate forms a gel just after mixing with other solutions by an ionic bonding reaction. Alginate gel maintains the orthogonal morphological structural design of the substrate and the location of the living cells in the structures. Both 2D and 3D structures can be constructed using alginate by ink-jet or laser-jet technology with convenient additives.

Porosity is one of the prime characteristics of scaffolding, which facilitates delivery of nutrients and waste product elimination [64], and permits ingrowth of blood vessels [65]. Alginate hydrogel can be printed as a porous heterogeneous substrate using highly viscous alginate powder, which supports both osteogenic and chondrogenic differentiation. By a 3D fiber deposition (3DF) [96] method, Fedorovich *et al.* have used alginate to fabricate cell-laden, heterogeneous hydrogel constructs as osteochondral grafts for in-vitro use. They demonstrated that cell-laden heterogeneous grafts in vitro stayed in their original deposited position over the entire culture period.

The ionic crosslinking of alginate is well suited to *in situ* applications due to the formation of gel on site [66]. Cohen *et al.* have directly printed alginate (alginate solution and calcium sulfate) onto bone defects since this does not rely upon external cues for a phase change in vitro [67]. The hydrogel construct was printed directly into the bone hole *in situ* five times. The bone matrix formed by alginate had a similar surface texture and its geometry matched the intended geometry specified by the CT scan.

Although Cohen's 3D printing application described above seems to have potential, there are explicit challenges for alginate bio-paper, which is subject to high levels of variability and cytotoxicity, and poor cell viability, mechanical integrity, surface texture, and fidelity of geometry. Improperly mixed gels, with non-uniform calcium ion concentration, lead to localized pockets of under- and over-crosslinked gel, resulting in varying flow rates. The variable deposition rate militates against geometric fidelity of printing. To overcome these limitations, Cohen *et al.* have developed a novel quantitative method for characterizing hydrogel homogeneity by using a vortex spinner [68]. Boosted mixing of the alginate and crosslinker improved gel homogeneity by systematic recirculation of the ions; the extra mixing energy more evenly distributed the crosslink ions throughout the alginate solution. The increased mixing of alginate solution yielded very much higher reduction of mechanical noise, more accurate geometric fidelity, smoother surface texture, and higher viability of seeded cells.

It is generally considered that crosslinks mainly contribute to the mechanical properties of the network. However, crosslinked alginate hydrogels lose more than 60% of their initial mechanical strength within 15 hours of exposure to physiological buffers [69], due to an outbound flux of ions into the surrounding medium. Increasing the proportion of guluronic and monomers and covalent linkages improves the mechanical properties of alginate [70]. However, for a high density of crosslinking molecules, the moduli of the gels began to decrease irrespective of their high conversion. Another weak point of alginate is its non-biodegradability under normal physiological conditions; however, this can be improved by truncating chains using partial oxidation [71] and gamma-ray irradiation [72]. On top of that, alginate hydrogels are nanoporous structures that do not support cell attachment unless they are modified chemically, with ligands or other adhesion peptides [73].

19.3.4.1.3 Fibrin

Fibrin is a fibrous, insoluble, mechanically hard protein, available from animal sources. It is a fast-gelling biodegradable biopolymeric gel, which enables the fabrication of 3D structures. Since fibrin is a printable hydrogel, Xu *et al.* were able to use fibrin gel (fibrinogen and thrombin) to form NT2 neurons into specific patterns [26]. The 3D neural cell-based constructs with specific forms were fabricated by alternately printing fibrin gels and NT2 neurons into a 3D functional structure. In the printed cellular construct, the fibrin gel provided enough mechanical and biological support for attachment of cells.

Fibrin has been proven a good substrate for vasculature formation and angiogenesis. Lately, fibrin has been applied for tissue engineering purposes as a key scaffold material for engineered cardiovascular and neural tissues. Researchers have recently taken advantage of this important feature to print vascular endothelial cells for microvasculature formation. Cui and Boland have developed fibrinogen bio-paper polymerizations of a range of arrangements of fibrinogen, thrombin, and Ca^{2+} concentrations to print human microvascular endothelial cells [53]. A model 500 HP Deskjet thermal inkjet printer was used to instantaneously place those cells and fibrin into a well-aligned structure with the appropriate microvasculature. Simultaneous deposition of endothelial cells and fibrin gel using thermal inkjet printing skills for fabrication of living microvasculature could be a promising future technology for organ printing.

Fibrin has versatile characteristics for different applications. Besides being used as 2D or 3D substrate materials, fibrins are also used with a variety of native GFs to enhance cellular functions. Miller *et al.* have combined fibrin with fibroblast growth factor-2 (FGF-2) as a printing substrate for proliferation and migration of human osteosarcoma cell line MG63 cells [74]. They found that the surface concentration gradient of FGF-2 can control cell density and migration throughout the pattern. In recent in-vitro studies it was found that fibrin gels can also support matrix synthesis, apart from cell migration and proliferation [75]. With those novel properties of the fibrin gel, printed fibrin-based neural constructs have potential to offer appropriate cell or tissue sources with in-vivo affinity for medical healing of severe neural damage and degenerative diseases, such as Parkinson's disease and spinal cord injury.

19.3.4.1.4 Matrigel™

Matrigel™ is the trade name of reconstituted basement membrane matrix. It is similar to the composite extracellular environment available in many tissues. The main constituents of Matrigel™ are structural proteins such as laminin, entactin, and type IV collagen. It is preserved as a frozen solution, becomes liquid at 4 °C, and becomes a gel at room temperature (24–37 °C) within 30 minutes.

Owing to the ease with which it undergoes gel formation and the fact that it is rich in GFs, Matrigel™ has been widely used as substrate for cell seeding in laser-guided direct writing and biological laser printing. Matrigel™ also can form lumen to imitate the original branch and stem of the vascular system, which is a network of arteries or capillaries that extends throughout the volume of a tissue. Using GF-rich Matrigel™ hydrogel, Wu *et al.* have constructed branch–stem structures of human umbilical vein smooth muscle cells (HUVSMCs) and human umbilical vein endothelial cells (HUVECs) [76]. By means of biological laser printing (BioLP™), thin hydrogel layers were constructed instead of the thick layers, in order to obtain more nutrients through diffusion. The purpose of the construction is to investigate the viability of the vascular network as well as subsequent cell growth and development. After printing and culturing the development and differentiation of these structures were compared with either HUVECs or HUVSMCs alone. The research revealed that co-deposition of various cells, bearing the unique capability to manage cell–cell communications, occurred in 3D hydrogel scaffolds.

19.3.4.2 Synthetic polymers

Synthetic biopolymers are the combination of two or more materials, whether by design or by natural processes. Compared with natural polymers, synthetic bio-papers are more promising for organ printing applications, since their block structures, gelation dynamics, crosslinkings, pore structures, and mechanical properties can be manipulated and are reproducible in the laboratory.

19.3.4.2.1 Polylactic-co-glycolic acid (PLGA)

PLGA is an amorphous copolymer, produced by means of arbitrary ring-gap copolymerization of monomers of lactic acid and glycolic acid. It degrades by hydrolysis of its ester linkages in the presence of water. Owing to its low toxicity, and to its biodegradability, biocompatibility, and porous structure, PLGA has been widely used in organ printing as a bio-substrate. Apart from extensive use in organ printing, PLGA is also used in biomedical applications such as prosthetic devices, implants, sutures, and grafts.

With solid free-form fabrication processes, controllable interconnected pore size and porosity can be achieved with PLGA. Since PLGA provides enough osteogenic and vascular support, Kim *et al.* used PLGA to produce a novel bio-substrate to print mesenchymal stem cells (MC3T3-E1) [77]. Post-cell-deposition evaluation revealed that cell interaction, adhesion, proliferation, and viability were superior to what could be achieved with other synthetic hydrogels due to the hydrophilicity of the substrates.

Besides providing biological support, PLGA is an accepted option for biodegradability with no toxic effects in a cell culture environment. PLGA is biocompatible, and can be deployed using a natural hydrogel coating or a hydrogel filled with ECM. It is also mechanically firm enough to be manipulated with tweezers both in soaked and in dehydrated environments. Pirlo *et al.* have chosen PLG to develop 2D bio-papers to generate layered 3D constructs with well-defined pore sizes and shapes using BioLP™ [78]. They prepared the substrate by a solvent casting method and added collagen and Matrigel™ for better biocompatibility and microvascular network formation. HUVECs were deposited onto the bio-substrate with BioLP™. After the cell seeding, microscopy observations showed that mechanical stability and high cell permeation and endurance had been achieved throughout the extensive porous gel-loaded compound constructs. These results indicated that it was also feasible to use the 2D cell-printing technique to stack bio-paper to build 3D vascularized tissues.

19.3.4.2.2 Polycaprolacton (PCL)

PCL is biodegradable polyester with a low melting point of about 60 °C. In addition to excellent biocompatibility, PCL provides a shock-absorbing mattress for the printed cells and supports cell viability and proliferation. Given these advantageous features, PCL is considered an extensive bio-substrate suitable for deposition of soft material. An electrospun PCL membrane can serve as bio-paper from which to construct 3D living structures with a managed interior architecture of chronological layers of cells and scaffolds. Catros *et al.* have applied electrospun PCL membrane to serve as bio-paper to print human osteosarcoma cell line MG63 cells [79] by using the laser bio-printing method. The reliability of the printed patterns was preserved by the use of PCL bio-papers, which protected the viability of MG63 cells after processing. The printed structure also provided a suitable environment for cell nourishment and function. Because of the high proliferation and appropriate vascularization support rate, the layer-by-layer cells/PCL construct was used for an animal study using NOD-SCID mice. In-vivo studies revealed that PCL bio-paper has good biocompatibility and strong enough mechanical properties to support the cells/PCL sandwich structure. For the thinner structure, PCL provided enough nutrients and oxygen supply. However, it may be necessary to develop a vasculature system within the thicker material for the diffusion of nutrients and oxygen as well as the elimination of metabolic waste. To achieve clinical-size 3D cellularized constructs, proper pore size (300 μm is recommended) and post-processing of printed elements are mandatory in order to maintain cell position and viability.

19.3.4.2.3 Polyethylene glycol (PEG)

PEGs are conjugated amphiphilic synthetic polymers made of repeating ethylene oxide units. PEG polymers' chain lengths are easily controllable and tunable, allowing one to elicit cellular responses with varying reflex properties. PEG has been widely used as a building block material in biomedical applications due to its good mechanical and physical properties. Copolymers of PEG and Tetra are multi-armed regular dense porous structures and very suitable for forming multi-functional biomaterials for vessel-like construct. Skardal *et al.* have used PEG to build bio-artificial vessel-like grafts [80] with two four-armed PEG derivatives with varying PEG strings. This hydrogel encapsulated NIH3T3 fibroblast cells as macrofilaments, which were printed into tubular PEG tissue constructs by using a layer-by-layer deposition method. This study showed that the cells in this construct were viable for a defined period of time. The extruded encapsulated cells of macrofilaments maintained their geometry both during printing and after printing. The physical properties, rheology, and composition of cell structures indicated that cellularized hydrogels prepared using PEG may possibly be printed as healthy tubular assembles with outstanding cell viability.

19.3.5 Bio-printers and different printing methods

Bioprinting is an emerging field represented by various biologically applied deposition systems, which range from direct writing, micro-stamping, photolithography, laser writing, electro-printing, microfluidics, electrospraying, stereolithography, and extrusion to inkjet deposition. To date, much of the bioprinting work has focussed on 2D patterning for basic biological studies. However, the development of fabrication methods and their adaptation to 3D cellular or tissue constructs will be required for organogenesis. To date, those technologies inspired by rapid prototyping based on layer-by-layer fabrications for 3D structures are more attractive to researchers. Thus extrusion, inkjet (thermal and piezoelectric), and laser printing devices will be the main focus for bio-printers in this chapter, since much progress in creating biological structures has been made with these techniques.

The ideal organ bio-printer has specific system requirements that must be met in order to achieve its goal. These include high resolution, high throughput, the ability to dispense various materials simultaneously, biocompatibility, cell viability, process repeatability, and the ability to control dispensability of bio-inks by modification of properties such as viscosity, surface tension, and density. Resolution is a critical factor for reconstruction of the details of organ structures; for instance, layers of vessels are at most a few micrometers in thickness. The throughput or process speed is also important, since the main material used for organ biofabrication is living cells, and their viability can be compromised if the fabrication process is lengthy. However, an alternative solution can be the usage of a special bio-reactor that provides an environment in which one can maintain cells alive. Organs are naturally constituted by many diverse types of cells and structures, which encourages researchers to develop organ bio-printers to assemble different cells and materials. The organ bio-printer has to be safe in the sense of avoiding any potential cross-contamination by isolating material reservoirs. Furthermore, the organ bio-printer should dispense materials where intended, to ensure biocompatibility and cell viability within the system. As discussed in previous sections, manipulation of bio-ink properties is essential for the future organ bio-printer. This system is not allowed to accommodate clogging and/or changes in dispensing rates; therefore, bio-ink conditions have to be monitored and controlled to avoid these potential drawbacks. Another concern is the possibility that the printing process could adversely affect cellular phenotypes and genotypes, which calls for detection methods to assure cell integrity throughout the bioprinting process.

The great opportunity and potential financial interest which the organ printing technology can bring has motivated the biomedical industry to develop and start commercializing 3D bio-printer systems. Even though actual organs are far from being accomplished, the launching of these prototyping systems supports the technical investigation needed to move this emerging

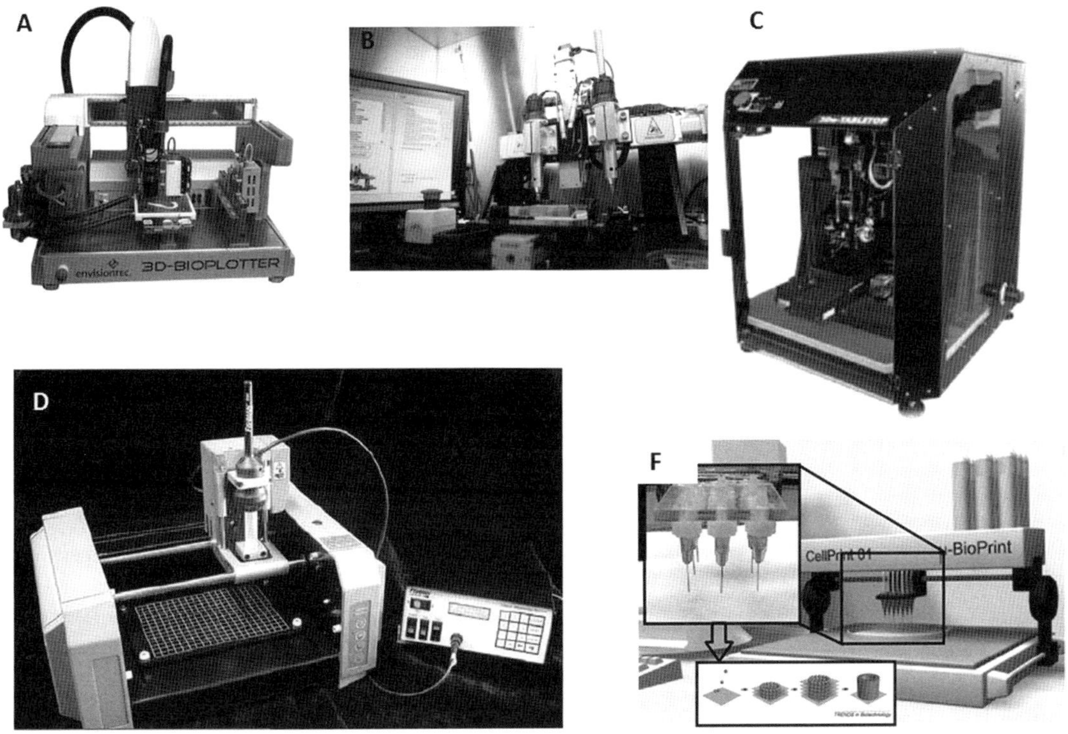

Figure 19.7 Examples of available bio-printers: (A) Envisiontech 3D bio-plotter, (B) NovoGen MMX Bioprinter™, (C) Sciperio-nScript bio-printer, (D) Neatco bio-printer, and (E) the bio-printer developed by Boland's group at Clemson University [81].

technology forward. Currently, the commercially available 3D bio-printers are produced by envisionTEC, Organovo, Tengion, Sciperio, and Neatco. In Figure 19.7, examples of their systems are shown. These systems have found major applications in drug discovery, biological assays, experimental biological depositions, stem cell experiments, and much more.

Various strategies can be followed in order to accomplish organ printing. For example, some groups have focussed on adopting high-resolution technologies (nanometer range) for use in biomedical applications. Moreover, strategies have been named after their methods for assembly of cells and materials [28]: (1) structural, organ structure is to be achieved by dispensing a mixture of cells and structural entities by the same bio-printing system (either via different heads or using a single head); (2) conformal, in this approach prefabricated scaffolds (i.e. hydrogel layers) are used as substrates for sites of deposition of cell suspension; and (3) aggregational, as its name implies, cells are expected to be aggregated (organized analogously to "bricks") in such a manner that "bricks" are utilized to biofabricate macroscaled biological structures. In this aggregational approach, genetic cell modification is expected to occur to maintain "brick" integrity. Alternatively, strategies based on the basic work mechanism can be elucidated. Here the most promising technologies investigated have been extrusion-, inkjet-, and laser-deposition-based systems. Since they have many key characteristics required by the ideal organ printer, it is worth reviewing them in this chapter.

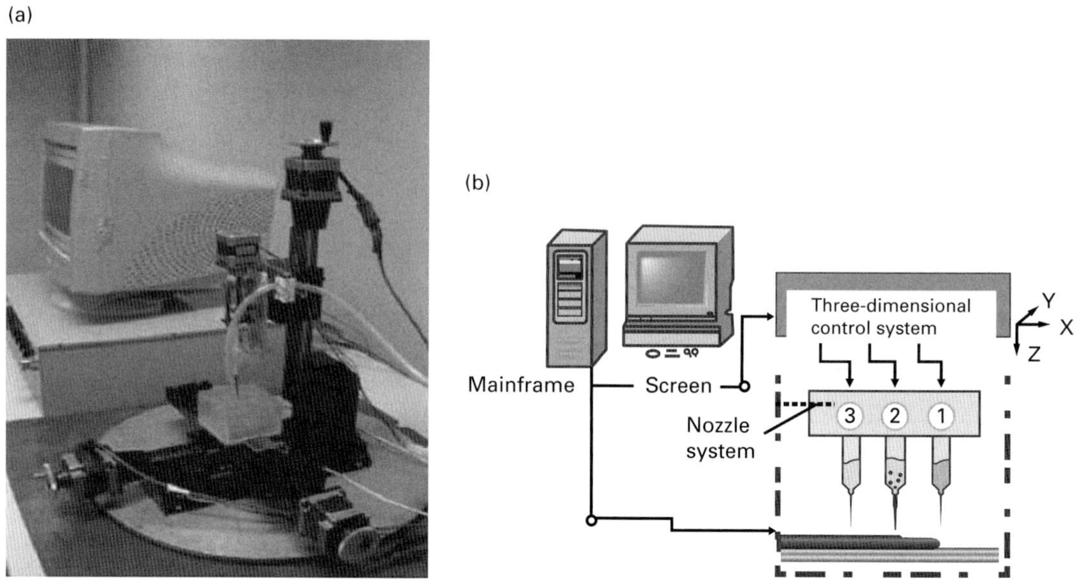

Figure 19.8 Tsinghua University group's cell-assembling machine [90]: (a) the actual machine and (b) a schematic diagram of the cell-assembling device.

19.3.5.1 Extrusion printing

The pressure- or extrusion-based method had historically been used for quite a long time, mainly for material transportation. The work mechanism is best explained by invoking the syringe mechanism, where the plunger exerts pressure on liquid enclosed in the barrel to dispense a controlled volume through the needle. When tissue engineering was introduced by Langer and Vacanti [82] last century, this technology also started to be investigated as a promising technique for creating living tissues [83–85]. Many researchers have worked on creating and adapting more complex systems that can accommodate tissue bio-construction [86–88]. The main advantage lies in its ability to deposit highly viscous materials; however, the major drawbacks are its low resolution and high droplet volume.

One of its widely researched applications is in the drug discovery industry, where it is being used as a high-throughput combinatorial system to evaluate different biochemical entities. As a result of this need, the development of robotic systems that improve system speed has been pursued, taking the system to throughputs above 200,000 assays/day [89]. More interestingly in the context of this chapter, an extrusion system to create living 3D structures was developed. Approximately 600-μm-tall hepatic tissue was built by Tsinghua University's group in China [90]. In this study, hepatocyte cells were entrapped in an artificial matrix (a mixture of gelatin and chitosan hydrogels), and were proven to remain viable and functional after 3D biofabrication. Their cell-assembling machine is illustrated in Figure 19.8. Moreover, the same cell-assembling system was applied to treat traumatic brain injury [91]. In this study porous scaffolds made of gelatin and a mixture of gelatin and hyaluronan hydrogels were fabricated. These scaffolds were implanted in a rat's brain and evaluated for their biocompatibility and biodegradation properties. The results indicate that the printed scaffolds improved tissue regeneration by infiltration. Even though brain construction is currently not within the scope of organ printing, it is important to work on characterization and fabrication methods for this type of tissue.

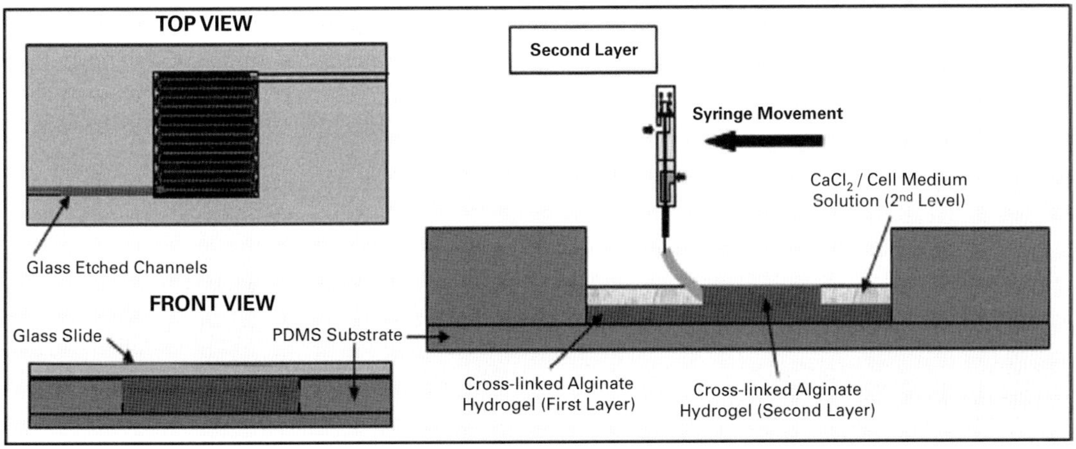

Figure 19.9 An overview of the DCW 3D microorgan approach, in a schematic representation [4].

Moreover, extrusion systems (i.e. direct cell writing (DCW)) have been combined with the use of microfluidic devices for the fabrication of a pharmacokinetic model [4]. The DCW process is integrated with a microfluidic device to fabricate 3D tissue/organ constructs/chambers, as opposed to producing 2D cell monolayers (Figure 19.9). Biological studies revealed the unstable cellular phenotype and reduced tissue-specific gene expression with conventional monolayer in-vitro culture techniques [83–85, 92]. A 3D tissue model will, in contrast, foster improved retention of cell-specific function. The study resulted in tissue structures that more closely resembled the corresponding in-vivo physiological state where cell–cell communication either from direct contact or by paracrine signaling is important for proper cellular behavior, differentiation, and proliferation, along with the concomitant ECM produced by the neighboring cells. Further, process parameters (nozzle pressure, motion-arm velocity, nozzle-tip size, etc.) and material parameters (biopolymer viscosity, crosslinking agent concentrations, etc.) were optimized to achieve high-fidelity 3D structures and seamless integration onto microfluidic tissue micro-organ chambers.

Modifications to classical extrusion systems have emerged in recent years. Sun's group at Drexel University has developed a temperature-controlled system that enables an expansion of an extrusion system's library of biomaterials [88]. As illustrated in Figure 19.10, the system consists of three main components: (1) material delivery system, (2) 3D motion device, and (3) a computer-aided modeling system. As shown in Figure 19.10(c), there are two heating elements that control the temperature along the material delivery chamber. The top heating element (heating element 1), located at the inlet of the chamber, is typically set at a higher temperature than the bottom heating element (heating element 2) located at the nozzle [5, 93]. The primary goal of heating element 1 is to heat the biopolymer until the polymer's phase changes from solid to liquid. The second heating element then maintains the biopolymer's viscosity through the chamber until it is extruded. Moreover, demand for a device that would fabricate scaffolds from high-melting-point biopolymers has increased. As a result, a cooling system has been integrated to control the temperature of filaments as they are extruded, enabling the system to use biomaterials with melting points as high as 250 °C (the prior limit was 100 °C). Some 3D structures made of high-melting-point biomaterials were fabricated with this method, demonstrating viability and proliferation of cells under different patterns of porosity.

The extrusion technique has been investigated in order to pursue the construction of skin-like tissue by Yoo's group. A 10-layered scaffold has been

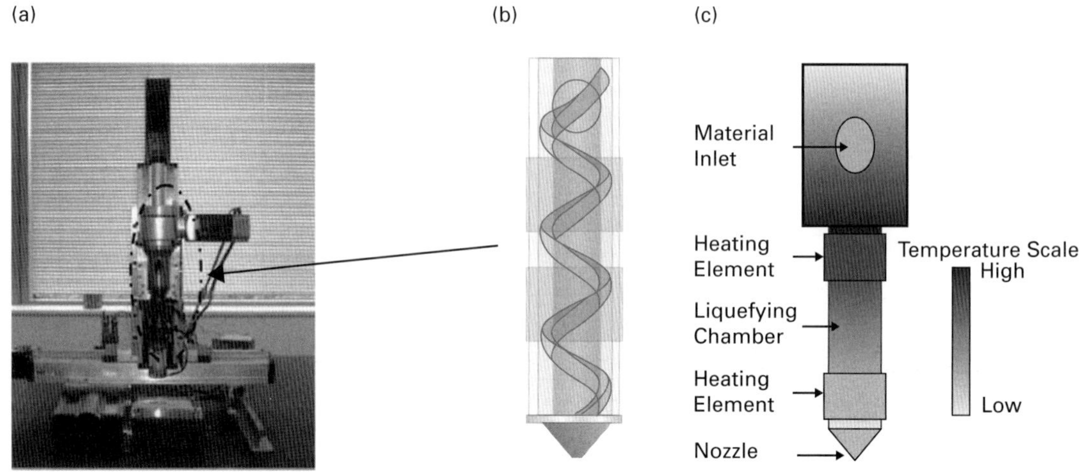

Figure 19.10 The extrusion system. (a) Front view of the precision extrusion deposition, (b) schematic view of the material delivery chamber, and (c) schematic illustration of the temperature gradient of the material delivery chamber where the top heating element has a higher working temperature than the lower heating element [88].

constructed with embedded human skin fibroblasts (FB) and keratinocytes (KC) at intermediate layers [94], imitating the skin's natural structure. As illustrated in Figure 19.11, the system utilized consists of four microvalves connected to reservoirs (disposable syringes dispensing 5–10 ml) with camera-based monitoring systems to assure printing quality. Moreover, one of the dispenser units and the vertical stage were temperature-controlled (with an operating temperature between 5 and 40 °C). In this system, more than 30 human and animal cell lines [95] have been dispensed with high survival rates (above 95%). These results suggest that this technique can be generally applied to most cell types and demonstrate the ability to print and culture multilayered cell–hydrogel composites on planar and non-planar surfaces.

19.3.5.2 Nozzle-based printing

The main types of printers at the forefront of this technology are inkjet, pipette, piezoelectric, and nozzle printers. Let it be understood though that the inkjet printers consist of nozzles and some inkjet printers are piezoelectric, but in terms of the technology of layered printing these need to be differentiated. One of the main reasons is because many of the new proprietary printers specifically use the piezoelectric aspect of the printer. They can also be piezoelectric without the inkjet technology. The nozzle printers typically used have little relation to inkjet printers; in fact, they resemble more closely the pipette printers. The pipette printers along with the nozzle printers are sometimes referred to as bioprinters, but that title is non-specific [96]. Each of these printers is interfaced with a computer, and software is used to design and control the printer output.

The inkjet printer is the most common [97], primarily because the parts are readily available and simple modifications and changes to the ink cartridge and printer itself make it ready to dispense biomaterials [97]. The piezoelectric printer is the next most common, since it too can be bought as an off-the-shelf item. This printer has many of the same benefits as the inkjet printer except that the technology is not advancing at such a rapid pace.

Pipette printers are essentially pipettes interfaced with a dispenser and a computer. The computer can interface not only with the dispenser but also with a one-, two-, or three-axis coordinate system that controls the spatial operation of the pipette. Thus the

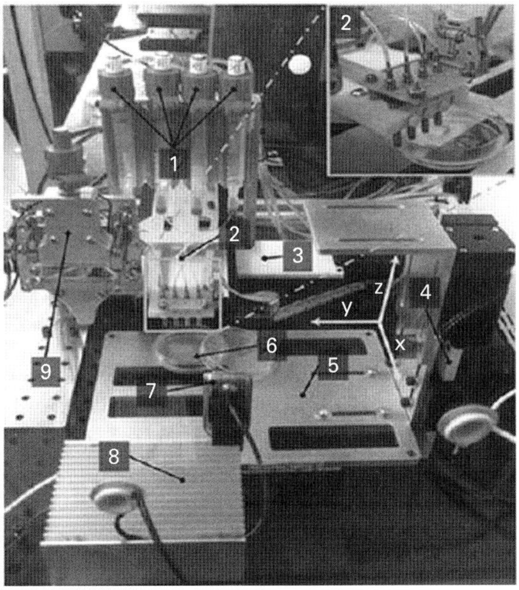

Figure 19.11 A picture of the modular tissue printing platform; (1) four syringes used as "cartridges" to load cell suspensions and hydrogel precursors; (2) an array of four-channel dispensers; (3) horizontal stage; (4) vertical stage; (5) target platform; (6) target substrate; (7) camera, (8) stage heater, vertical stage heater; and (9) independently heated/cooled dispenser [95].

computer software controls not only the amount pipetted but also the location. Typically this works by having either a pressure system or a syringe system that pushes the material through and out of the pipette. The nozzle printers are typically proprietary and are rare, but are primarily used for hydrogels. The dispensing volumes in these nozzles are typically controlled by a type of cutting mechanism. This method is similar to pipette printing except that, instead of a syringe system or a pressure system to extrude the material, gravity is sometimes the force extruding the material. An open-and-close mechanism or in some cases a cutting mechanism is the technology used to control the volume. The mechanism of control usually depends on the turgidity of the hydrogel or material.

Generally speaking, a crosslinker or binding agent is supplied in the cleaned and modified printer cartridge. If the printer does not contain a cartridge, then the binding agent or crosslinker is contained in the dispensing reservoir. The cartridge prints the binding agent onto a material in the design specified by the software, and then a one-dimensional, (1D), 2D, or 3D construct is formed. In some cases the material is printed onto a binding agent or crosslinker. All currently known suitable materials and their crosslinkers, binding agents, or substrates are listed in Table 19.1.

The nozzle of an inkjet printer is approximately the size of a typical cell (20 μm) and can rapidly deliver reagents over an area in the same way as a sheet of cells. Given a suitable gel acceptor layer, it would be possible to deliver a sequence of catalysts and reagents to build a layer of material as cells do. Thus a printing system with enough "colors" ought to be capable of forming materials with the various structures and properties associated with tissue matrices. Other printing processes could also be used, but non-contact, digital printing has many advantages.

19.3.5.2.1 Piezoelectric printers

Piezoelectric inkjet printers are most commonly used in industry because they can be driven at higher frequencies and can be tuned for optimum performance. In a piezoelectric inkjet printer a drop is ejected as the result of a pressure wave generated in the column of liquid above the nozzle. Rapidly alternating expansions and contractions of the ceramic material will cause the fluid to separate into droplets, which have a large amount of kinetic energy.

The inks used in piezoelectric printers have a fairly narrow range of surface tension and viscosity. However, once a fluid has been identified, one can optimize the voltage pulse to the ceramic elements in order to avoid satellite drops and the long-tails hallmark of this process. This can insure uniform drop speeds and sizes from adjacent nozzles for precise positioning. In addition to rheological properties, the possibility of chemical attack on the head by the ink must be considered. Water-based inks are often a concern because the moisture and salt may eventually short out the high voltages needed to drive the piezoelectric pulse. Particle-containing inks may abrade the nozzle and cause the drop size or firing direction to change.

Table 19.1 Biomaterials currently used with printing technology, their applications, and references

Material	Printer	Application	Notes	Reference
Alginate	Inkjet	Soft tissue	$CaCl_2$ crosslinker	[23]
	Nozzle	Hydrogel	$CaCl_2$ crosslinker	[98, 99]
	Pipette	Hydrogel		[54]
	Pipette	Bone	$CaCl_2$ crosslinker	[96]
Gelatin	Inkjet	Soft tissue	$CaCl_2$ crosslinker	[23]
Tricalcium phosphate	Inkjet	Bone	Chondroitin sulfate/succinate binding agents	[100]
Polyurethane	Inkjet	Scaffolds	Acetic acid or $CaCl_2$ binding agent	[101, 102]
Fibrinogen	Inkjet	Neurons	Thrombin binding agent	[26]
	Piezoelectric	Wound repair	FGF-2 substrate	[103]
Thrombin	Inkjet	Neurons		[26]
Polyaniline	Inkjet	Sensor		[104]
Collagen	Pipette	Soft tissue		[105]
PEO	Pipette	Hydrogel	PEO-PPO-PEO	[54]
Matrigel™	Pipette	Hydrogel		[54]
Agarose	Pipette	Hydrogel		[54]
Methylcellulose	Pipette	Hydrogel		[54]
Lectins	Piezoelectric	Biomarker identification		[106]

Modern piezoelectric printheads have hundreds or thousands of nozzles, and are therefore very expensive. They are generally intended to be used with one type of ink with a tightly controlled formulation. Often, the ink is supplied by the company that produces the printhead. Frequently they are sold as part of a complete system built for the customer by "integrators" and containing cameras to monitor the drops and sample, and the transport and alignment systems, and sophisticated software to convert images into nozzle firing sequences.

Commercial piezoelectric systems may have applications in laboratory settings for bioprinting applications. The chief drivers for commercial printer development are speed, resolution (which is determined by droplet size), precision of drop positioning, and the elimination of smaller satellite drops often produced in the firing process. These may also be important in some laboratory applications but are often not crucial. Laboratory printing can impose limitations that rarely occur commercially. Laboratory printing processes may involve solvents, or strong acids or bases, that should not harm the printing system. The system may need to be sterilized. Inks may contain particles or polymers that aggregate over time so that printheads may need to be disposable or readily cleanable. Inks used in bioprinting may have high viscosity, or low surface tension, interfering with normal droplet formation.

19.3.5.2.2 Thermal inkjet printers

Thermal printers operate by heating of a small air bubble that ejects a drop of ink from the nozzle as it expands. A typical heating pulse lasts a few microseconds and drops are fired at a rate of about 1 kHz. For the authors, home-built systems based on HP pens have proved an excellent combination of robustness and inexpensive replacement. However, they offer only a narrow window of nozzle voltages and fluid properties within which jetting can be achieved. Therefore ink formulations must fall within a relatively narrow range of viscosities and surface tensions. In addition, they have limited tolerance to solvents and strong acids. Customizing cartridges of thermal printers for biological inks is currently being investigated by manufacturers such as HP and Olivetti, thus in the future one may be able to use more viscous fluids and avoid the relatively large amount of "dead volume" that is found in current pen designs.

Although thermal inkjets operate at lower pressure with less ability to control the pulse and the head lifetime tends to be shorter, they can be seen as having advantages for bioprinting. Thermal printheads can be mass-produced and are therefore inexpensive and disposable, which makes ink development considerably less expensive. Most piezoelectric printheads can be cleaned ultrasonically, but irreversible damage is still common. Existing thermal inkjet heads are not very solvent-resistant and have limited resistance to acids and bases, but bioprinting solutions are mostly aqueous and neutral. While piezoelectric inkjet heads can be solvent- and acid-resistant, many commercial heads run at high voltages and can be vulnerable to slow degradation in water.

Thermal inkjets seem to be much more robust than piezoelectric inkjets in terms of the range of inks that can be printed, which is a valuable attribute for research systems. The ranges of viscosity and surface tension of inks printable by each technology are not well documented, since in many cases the printer makers are also the ink makers. In general, inks with viscosities up to 20 cP and surface tensions around 30–40 mN/m are printable. Thermal droplet ejection is a rugged process that is relatively insensitive to the ink properties, as long as some component of the ink can be vaporized. Rheological properties are less important in determining drop formation and jettability than for piezo-based printheads. Thus even high-molecular-weight polymers at higher concentrations may be jettable. There may still be some limitation for biopolymers due to refilling of the ink chamber at the appropriate time to allow subsequent nozzle firings. Ink formulation is discussed further below.

19.3.5.2.3 *Rapid prototyping and inkjet printing*

Since the development of stereolithography in 1986, many methods to build 3D structures from a CAD file have been developed [107]. Many of these techniques can be used to make 3D scaffolds for biofabrication, either by direct deposition of the material [108] or by forming a negative that is removed after the scaffold material has been molded around it [109]. Stereolithography has also been used to directly form hydrogel scaffolds with embedded cells [110, 111].

Some biofabrication methods do involve inkjet printing of one component. Binder can be printed into a powder bed [112], or low-molecular-weight polymers and waxes can be printed directly, but they do not offer the materials versatility needed for biological structures.

Biofabrication using extrusion methods whereby a bead of material is pushed out through a fine nozzle has been done successfully. Nozzle sizes down to about 100 μm can be used to extrude ceramics [113], polymers [108], hydrogels [114], composites [115, 116], and metals [117]. Biofabrication by extrusion is easier than inkjet printing, but inkjet printing offers some functions that extrusion cannot. The two could be regarded as complementary. In terms of resolution they are similar. Linewidths and features generated by inkjets are about 10–100 μm in the x–y plane. Typical free-form extrusion generates a linewidth of 100 μm, although both can give much finer lines in special cases [118, 119]. In both cases, the discontinuity between lines and drops makes it difficult to form pore-free films. For extrusion methods the vertical (z-axis) resolution is also about 100 μm, whereas an inkjet drop dried on a flat surface will form a pancake about 100 nm thick. Sun and co-workers have modeled the flow of encapsulated cells through various extrusion needles and compared the results with those from experimental studies. They concluded that the high pressures observed in needles smaller than 250 μm will cause high morbidity and cell death [120].

Biofabricated structures made from high-viscosity materials such as concentrated polymer solutions or particle suspensions can be realized using extrusion methods, provided that there is a rapid solidification process to hold the 3D shape. Final curing processes can occur slowly or after the part has been built. Biofabrication using inkjets is limited to inks of much lower viscosity, but the drops dry rapidly, allowing structures to be built. As a non-contact process, the inkjet procedure is also more suited to adding material to porous, curved, or uneven surfaces. Extrusion methods require that the nozzle height be maintained at about one linewidth above the surface. When the linewidth is below 100 μm, this is possible only with rigid surfaces and very careful alignment. Finally, using inkjets in the biofabrication process allows multiple inks to be mixed or reacted chemically, while extruded layers remain chemically distinct.

In the long term, industrial printing of diagnostic sensors or other disposable biological systems would require the fast, reproducible printing that both thermal and piezoelectric systems can offer. On the other hand, it may be that systems for use during surgery would be better delivered from sterile apparatus.

19.3.5.2.4 Applications

Typical inks used in bioprinting are composed of an aqueous solution containing salts and other small solutes, coiled-chain polymers, globular proteins, cells, and/or particles. The rheology of such mixtures is complex and non-Newtonian. Aggregation, settling, thermal denaturation, and other changes may occur during storage or printing. So far there are no clear rules or guidelines to help in designing inks for bioprinting, so it is up to the researcher to develop a proper ink formulation for the particular application.

The concentration and molecular-weight dependences of solution viscosities of linear polymers are well established [121]. For low molecular weights, the relationships are roughly linear. For larger molecular weights, when chain entanglement starts to influence flow behavior, the viscosity increases with molecular weight to the power 3.4 and concentration to the power 5. Higher-molecular-weight polymers behave differently under the high shear rates and extensional flow found in an inkjet printer from low-molecular-weight polymers. Recent work has addressed the role of viscoelastic effects in inkjet printing [121, 122]. These studies have mostly been carried out on solutions of synthetic polymers, for which samples with a wide range of well-characterized molecular weights are available. While concentrations of 10–50 ppm of 300-kD polymers will prevent satellite droplet formation, higher concentrations are often not printable. Hoath, Hutchings, and Martin have found that linear polymers are printable with piezoelectric devices if $cM < 100$, where c is the concentration of the polymer in %wt/wt and M is the molecular weight in kD [123]. Thus, for most biomedical linear polymers, such as polysaccharides, only dilute solutions are expected to be printable. Most soluble proteins have a globular conformation in solution and so will have a much smaller effect on viscosity. One possible solution for depositing high concentrations of polymers consists of printing monomers, precursers, or prepolymers and initiators followed by polymerization, typically with UV irradiation [124].

Biopolymers fall into two categories, coiled and globular. The former include the water-soluble polysaccharides such as alginates, chitosan, and various gums, soluble polypeptides such as polylysine and polyglutamate, and some forms of DNA. Since all biopolymers are susceptible to being charged, the viscosity will depend on the pH and ionic strength of the solution, which can be adjusted.

19.3.5.2.5 Coiled biopolymers

Alginates have long been used as matrix materials for tissue engineering [125]. They are normally produced from seaweed for a variety of thickening applications in food and pharmaceuticals. They can also be produced in medical grades by bacterial fermentation. These medical grades are free of bacterial endotoxins, which will cause illness in humans and will kill cells in culture. The attraction of alginates is that they are rapidly crosslinked by solutions of calcium ions, or other polyvalent cations. A drawback is that gelation is reversed if the calcium level falls below a level that depends on the chain structure of the polymer but is in the region of 10 mM [126].

Alginate gels can be inkjet printed by printing drops of calcium chloride solution into alginate solution or vice versa. Nakamura and co-workers have described printing a suspension of cells in low-concentration (<1% wt/vol) sodium alginate solution into an aqueous solution of calcium chloride and polyvinylalcohol [127]. Xu *et al* have described a system for printing 3D cellular constructs by printing calcium chloride and cells, or sodium alginate and cells, into a solution of alginate or calcium salt. As with stereolithography, a platform is submerged below the surface of the liquid and drops as each new layer of gel is added [128].

Other polysaccharides can be printed. Gellan and xanthan have been inkjet printed as dispersants and matrices for carbon nanotubes [129]. Structural proteins such as collagen are insoluble at high concentration and physiological pH. However, dilute solutions of silk and collagen can be printed [63] but do tend to precipitate and occlude nozzles so that the printing system will have to be cleaned periodically.

In principle, bioprinting is an excellent route to preparing biopolymer hydrogel matrices for tissue engineering, drug delivery, and other applications, given that self-assembly, pH shift, enzymatic modification, or other routes can be used to convert soluble polymers into gels. In practice, most potential biopolymer matrix materials are of high molecular weight, which makes the solutions too viscous at concentrations above 1%. In addition, most commercial materials are intended for industrial use and are poorly characterized and quite variable between batches.

19.3.5.2.6 Globular proteins

Most non-structural proteins have a globular, folded structure, which is succeptable to denaturation, especially in the presence of hydrophobic surfaces, under high shear or temperatures. As a result proteins would be expected to denature on the surfaces in an inkjet printer cartridge, at the air interface of the ejected drop, and at the surfaces of the delivered drop. Globular proteins have a compact structure and so do not greatly increase the viscosity of an inkjet ink. Hence the main concern relates to whether the printing process actually denatures the protein.

Experimental shear studies on denaturing of proteins have recently been reviewed [130]. Most proteins show denaturation when experiencing several hundreds s^{-1} shear in various flow configurations. In addition to shear, piezoelectric printers set up a fast pressure pulse to eject a drop. Nishioka *et al.* suggest that this pulse causes denaturation of enzymes (peroxidase), which increases as the compression rate increases [131]. The effect is reduced by addition of a sugar, such as trehalose. It is perhaps surprising that denaturation can occur within the very short time of a pressure pulse, and it is possible that some other effect related to drop velocity is the immediate cause of degradation. Likewise the addition of "sacrificial" protein such as serum albumin may help protect the protein of interest.

In thermal printers, the heating pulse raises the question of whether any damage is caused to biopolymers during the process. For small molecules it is possible that thermal degradation occurs, while polymers of very high molecular weight and cells may also be damaged by shear processes. This has been studied in the context of the possible use of inkjet printing for delivery of drugs in aerosol form. Proteins (insulin) were found to be unaffected by passage through a thermal inkjet printhead [132]. In our experience of printing lysozyme with a thermal printhead, its activity as measured by a bacterial assay was unchanged. Denaturation is a kinetic process and so will not necessarily occur.

In other studies, the ECM and the GFs have been co-jetted [133]; however, because gelled fibrin cannot be jetted, the authors used multiple printheads for independent and concurrent deposition of fibrinogen, thrombin, and GF bio-inks. Some 3D fibrin–hormone structures were built up, layer-by-layer, by jetted droplets mixing and gelling locally at the printed surface [134].

19.3.5.3 Printing cells

19.3.5.3.1 Cell-directing patterns

In order to build structured tissues, we can deposit combinations of cell-adhesive and cell-repulsive polymers in patterns, and then deposit cells over the patterns. In one of the first examples, collagen mixtures were printed on dried agarose-coated glass coverslips. Smooth muscle cells adhered to the patterns in less than one day and dorsal root ganglion neurons were seen to attach to the patterns and extend neuritis on the patterns [63]. Other variations of this approach included collagen being printed onto glass coverslips coated with polyethyleneglycol [135]. After 8 days in culture the neurons patterned on the adhesive regions. A variation of this approach is the spotting of cytokines on hydrogels. Campbell *et al.* have printed the bone growth factor BMP-2 and inhibitory factors Noggin and TGF-β onto the commercially available hydrogel DemaMatrix. When printed alone, the growth factor caused bone to form in broad diffused patterns; however, when combined with the inhibitory factors, bone grew along the patterned semicircles [44]. These technologies seem promising for directed growth of tissues.

19.3.5.3.2 Cellular inks

Most of the early cellular inks were a single cell type suspended in saline solution [136] at concentrations of typically 1–10 million cells/ml. Initially hypertonic solutions were used to reduce the cell volume; however, this has largely been abandoned [23]. Many types of ink contain additional nutrients such as glucose or amino acids; some contain serum-free media. Electromechanical printing systems will accept up to 10% or more serum being added; however, thermal inkjet systems will stop ejecting drops when serum proteins are added, presumably due to the proteins being adsorbed onto the heating elements and thereby "poisoning" the mechanism.

More recently, cellular ink has included other functional macromolecules, such as proteins and DNA. The authors of one study took advantage of the transient pores that develop in membranes of thermally printed cells to deliver DNA vectors into porcine aortic endothelial cells, and measured the effective transfer by detecting expression of green fluorescent protein in the cells [137]. Cui and Boland added thrombin and calcium ions to human capillary endothelial cells to build fibrin networks *in situ* [138]. Much of the progress in building functional tissues will depend on the judicious choice of ions, macromolecules, and cells to make up the ink of a delivery device, thus it is thought that the area of biological ink development will see much future growth.

Cell damage due to shear during drop ejection in inkjet printing is clearly a concern. Cell diameters are very dependent on cell type but are typically 20 μm or less. This corresponds to the size of a 1-picoliter nozzle, and nozzle diameters can thus range from less than a cell diameter to several cell diameters. Hence the degree of interaction between the cell and the fluid flow in the nozzle can be very variable. In most cases larger nozzles are used for cell printing. Shear damage to cells is an issue in many medical devices. For instance, Lee *et al.* reported on shear damage to red blood cells in a microchannel system [139]. Therefore the design of printheads for cell printers must be undertaken to minimize small channels and chambers. Future designs may insure that the nozzle orifice is the smallest constriction in the system.

19.3.5.3.3 Effect of piezo and thermal printers on cells

To date living cells have been printed successfully with two electromechanically driven systems, namely the static-electricity-actuated printhead manufactured by Seiko Epson [140] and a commercially available system using a piezoelectrically driven Microjet MJ-AB-01 printhead (Microfab Inc., Plano, TX) [141]. The authors of these studies used bovine endothelial cells and human fibroblast cells, and found 97% viability after ejection. As the driving voltage for droplet ejection was increased, droplet velocity and the forces generated during drop generation and impact increased. There was a small decrease in cell survival rate from about 98% at a pulse amplitude of 40 V to 94% at 80 V (compared with >98% for the unprinted control). However, more detailed investigations are required in order to distinguish between the influence of the forces experienced by the cells during droplet generation and that of droplet impact and develop sophisticated experiments to separate the influence of these processes.

Cell survival after extrusion through a nozzle [142], or electrostatic extraction through a nozzle, a process known as electrospraying, has been studied [143, 144]. However, these systems are limited by the resolution that can be achieved because of the cell morbidity experienced in needles of diameter <250 μm [142].

Thermally driven systems were used earlier and with more success than electromechanical systems to eject viable cells or clusters of cells. Several groups are using systems that employ the heat of a laser to eject cells embedded in a matrix. Early work examined bacteria [145], but the technique was later perfected to include rat Schwann and astroglial cells and pig lens epithelial cells [146]. More recently, the resolution of these systems has been improved to single-cell level and 97% viability of rat olfactory ensheathing cells [147]. Thermal inkjet printers have been used successfully to deliver cells into predescribed patterns. Earlier work examined the viability of Chinese hamster ovary (CHO) cells [136], but was later extended to neuronal cells [26]. This work showed that the growth rate of printed ganglial neurons was not statistically different from that of pipetted cells.

Moreover, since, presumably, the cell membrane may be the most vulnerable part of a cell exposed to shear forces, the electrophysiology of primary hippocampal and cortical neurons was examined after two weeks of culturing. No difference between printed and normal cultured cells was found in terms of their resting membrane potential, input resistance, membrane capacitance, and a host of other electrophysiological quantities [26]. The short-term integrity of the membrane of printed CHO cells was investigated more recently. It was found that the printing process caused pores of diameter 100 nm to develop, which close up after about 2 hours in culture. In this study it was also found that no over-expression of heat-shock proteins occurs due to the printing of those cells compared with that of normally cultured cells [148].

High-concentration cellular inks have also been used successfully. Spheroids of cell aggregates up to 300 μm thick can be prepared by gyratory shaking. These aggregates can be assembled into structures within a sacrificial hydrogel. A variation of this method is the extrusion of paletted cell suspensions through a capillary tube. Forgacs and co-workers have created vessels by horizontally laying the cell tubes onto agarose rods [149]. After removal of the rods and maturation in a bioreactor, a cell tube is obtained. Presumably the morbidity observed with other extrusion techniques is avoided here by using 300–500-μm extrusion pipettes. However, diffusion of oxygen through such thick cellular aggregates may be a problem if necrosis is not desired.

19.3.5.3.4 Cell attachment and growth

The is no simple way to identify a suitable material to support cell growth or to enable growth of embedded cells. The first consideration is whether the material releases cytotoxic compounds, either due to residual contamination or from a degradation process. Even if the cells are not killed outright, many cell types are attachment-dependent and will not grow on a surface unless they can attach. Cells embedded in a matrix will also be dependent on attachment sites if they are to multiply. Embedded cells also need nutrition and hence depend on diffusion through the matrix. The following brief summary is intended to act as a guide to the complexities of the current literature.

Cytotoxicity can readily be tested with cells grown on conventional tissue culture plates in the presence of solutions of extracts from the matrix material to be tested. The most common problem arises from residual solvents. If solvent is used in depositing solid polymer layers, some will be trapped and thereafter will slowly be released.

Most human cell types will not multiply without attachment to a surface. Those which do not attach will eventually undergo aptosis and die. Cells do not attach to most neutral and anionic gel surfaces, but attachment may be induced induced through chemical modification with recognition sequences for specific amino acids, such as RGD, or through the use of cationic surface groups [150, 151]. Chondrocytes and some types of tumor cells are exceptions and can multiply without attachment. A recent review of cell growth on polyelectrolyte gels formed by layer-by-layer deposition addresses these questions [152].

While neutral and anionic gel surfaces do not promote cell attachment, the equivalent solid surface may, and there is no clear distinction between a gel and a solid except a difference in elastic modulus. Since cells are normally cultured from plasma containing a complex mix of proteins, cell attachment is preceded by adsorption of proteins such as fibronectin that then promote cell attachment.

There is not much systematic understanding of the requirements for attachment of cells embedded in matrices. Fibrin gels can provide suitable attachment sites to promote differentiation of embedded mesenchymal stems cells [153, 154]. Cell growth in matrices must also depend on oxygen and nutrient supply. As a rule of thumb, these factors limit growth to a distance of about 100 μm below the matrix surface [155].

Stem cells are a special case in that they can survive without attachment but do not multiply until they attach and differentiate into a specific cell type. The differentiation is driven by chemical and mechanical signals that have not yet been fully identified.

19.3.5.4 Reactive inks

The use of crosslinking ions in alginate as a component of ink was investigated a few years ago using alginate as the gellable hydrogel material [156]. This type of ink reacts with the target substrate, solidifying it. Reactive ink is an attractive concept, because it will allow one to build 3D structures, while limiting the amount of reactive compounds used. The amounts can thus be targeted to react only locally, producing structures that closely mimic the printed patterns. To date this concept of reactive ink is only beginning to be studied. Some simple patterns such as hollow spheres and hollow tubes have been described [59, 128]. However, the technique holds promise for building vascular capillary structures, as was demonstrated recently [138].

In nature, in order to avoid premature precipitation, insoluble biopolymer structures are formed by various strategies involving a soluble precursor polymer followed by self-assembly [157, 158]. Synthetic polypeptides containing large fractions of cationic and anionic amino acids can be induced to self-assemble by a pH shift from strong acid or strong base whereby only the amines or acids are ionized to neutral pH, whereupon both are ionized and form an ionic bond [159, 160]. A similar strategy has been used to form structures from pairs of synthetic cationic polymers and anionic polymers by careful choice of the polymer ratios [119]. Capsules made of biopolymer gels can be formed by dropping a solution of cationic polymer, such as chitosan, into an anionic polymer such as alginate [161]. These self-assembled gels can also be formed as thin films using layer-by-layer dipping methods [162, 163].

Inkjet printing can be used to form similar self-assembled hydrogels from cationic and anionic polymers [164]. Alternately printing layers of the two polymers or simultaneous printing from two cartridges results in thin multilayer sandwiches of the two polymers, which can then diffuse and combine to form a gel. Inkjet printing is commonly used to print hot waxes that freeze on contact with the substrate, and this could be applied to thermally gelling biopolymers such as agarose or gelatin. Apart from the need to use a heated printed head, there would be severe limitations on molecular weight and concentration of the biopolymer.

Ultraviolet-curable inkjet inks are widely used, and this approach could be applied to printing hydrogels. Ultraviolet-cured gels with embedded cells have been formed by stereolithography [111]. The main barrier to inkjet printed gels or cell supports cured with blue or UV light would be inhibition of the curing reaction by oxygen. It might therefore prove difficult simultaneously to retain cell viability and monomer curability.

There is a real need for better gel matrix materials to support bioprinting of cells. Calcium-crosslinked alginate is widely used, but these gels are very weak and will solubilize in solutions that are low in calcium. The target support should mimic the ECM, for which the best model is Matrigel, a commercial protein mixture secreted by Engelbreth-Swarm (EHS) mouse sarcoma cells and marketed by BD Biosciences. The chief components of Matrigel are structural proteins such as laminin and collagen that present cultured cells with the adhesive peptide sequences they would encounter in their natural environment. Also present are growth factors that promote differentiation and proliferation of many cell types.

Functionalized polysaccharides can be crosslinked by the Michael-type addition reaction [165, 166] without damage to entrained cells. Long-wavelength UV [111] or blue light [167] can be used to crosslink cytocompatible PEG diacrylate solutions. It should also be possible to inkjet thermally gelling systems to print cold- or hot-gelling polymers over cells at room temperature. In addition to processability and mechanical strength, matrix gels will need well-defined transport properties for oxygen, nutrients, and other small and large molecules, stability of size in a range of solution environments, compatibility at implant sites,

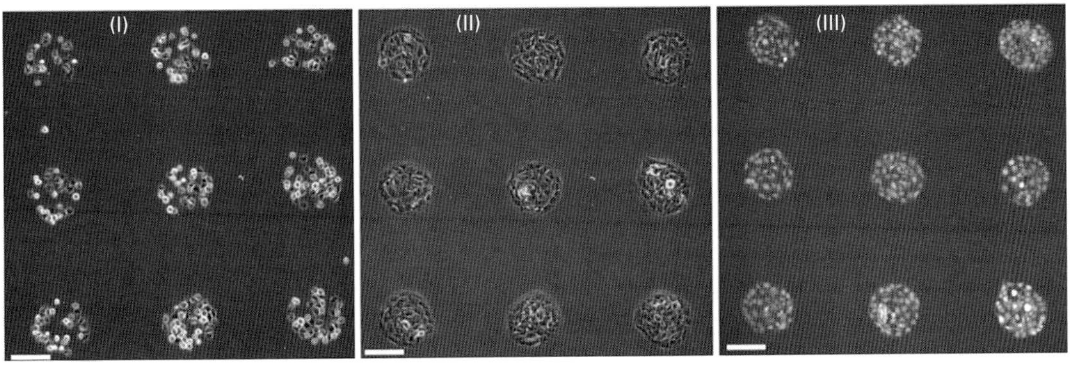

Figure 19.12 NIH3T3 fibroblast cells array formation on a collagen pattern printed from 0.9-mg/ml collagen solution at a cell seeding density of 2.5×10^5 cells/cm^2. Phase-contrast images of cells on the pattern after (I) 2 h incubation and (II) 24 h culture, and (III) the fluorescence image of cells from (II) after the calcein-AM assay. Most of the cells emit fluorescence, showing a high viability of the cells on the array. All of the scale bars are 150 μm. From [168].

anchoring surfaces for cell attachment, and probably more. The immediate need is to expand the range of available printable matrices which can be adapted for different systems.

19.3.5.5 Other inkjet systems

Different areas of improvements exist for current inkjet printing systems; for instance, inkjet printing has a lower resolution than photolithographic and microfluidic techniques. Moreover, this technique is restricted to low-viscosity fluids and low cell density to avoid clogging [63]. In addition, control of the particles dispensed is lost once the liquid has left the confinement of the ejection nozzle; consequently this method suffers from issues related to drying and spreading of the ink on the surface, and provides a relatively lower resolution (no smaller than 20–30 μm) [63]. A novel approach to resolve the last issue has emerged [168]. Droplets were printed at volume rates of 10 and 330 pl with a Dimatix® ©FUJIFILM Material Printer DMP-2800 and a Perkin–Elmer Piezoarray™ microarray spotter, respectively. The printing voltage was tuned to minimize satellite-droplet formation. The method involves a reliable silanization method to create an effective non-adhesive PEG layer on glass. The results demonstrate, for the first time, that micropatterned protein spots remained stable on the PEG surface even after extensive washing (as shown in Figure 19.12). A focus on the assemby and fixation properties of bio-inks is important if we are to advance toward organogenesis.

An alternative system intended to overcome limitations in inkjet printing has recently been developed by Demirci's group [62]. This system utilizes mechanical valves that enable higher-viscosity materials to be printed. They have demonstrated that this new printing system is able to create hydrogel structures characterized by (1) printing of multilayered 3D cell-laden hydrogel structures (16.2 μm thick per layer) with controlled spatial resolution (proximal axis 18.0 ± 7.0 μm and distal axis 0.5 ± 4.9 μm), (2) high-throughput droplet generation (1 s per layer, 160 droplets/s), (3) cell-seeding uniformity (26 ± 2 cells/mm^2 at 1 million cells/ml, 122 ± 20 cells/mm^2 at 5 million cells/ml, and 216 ± 38 cells/mm^2 at 10 million cells/ml), and (4) long-term viability in culture (>90% after 14 days). An illustration of the system is presented in Figure 19.13.

19.3.5.6 Laser printing

Laser printing has attracted interest since it was first introduced into the biomedical engineering field [31, 50, 169, 170] because of its major benefits, such as high resolution and throughput. As illustrated in

(a)

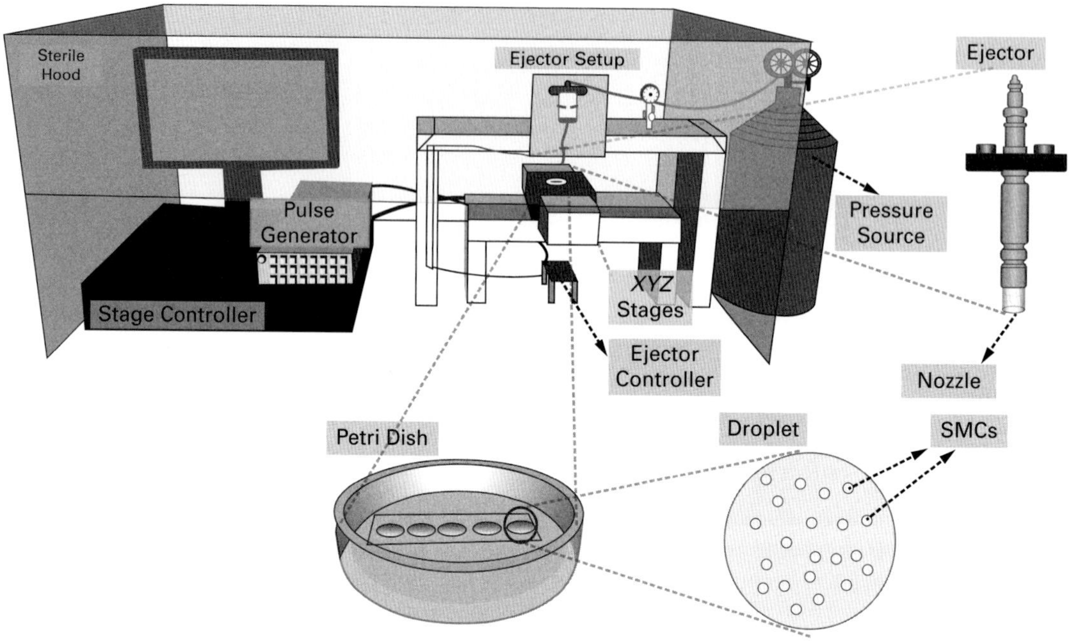

Figure 19.13 Illustration of cell-encapsulating droplet printing onto a substrate. The cell printing setup is enclosed in a sterile field (Cleanroom International, Grand Rapids, MI). Cells and collagen mixture flow into the valve, driven by constant air pressure. A mixture of cells and collagen solution is loaded into a 10-ml syringe reservoir. The *XYZ* stage is controlled by a controller that was synchronized with a pulse generator and a control PC. With programmed sequences to build a three-dimensional (3D) structure, the apparatus can control ejection conditions, that is, the stage speed, pressure, valve on/off frequency, and valve opening duration.

Figure 19.14, laser-based biological deposition is based on ejection of materials via a laser-powered beam. Different layers of materials are disposed of in such a manner that the first layer absorbs a great part of the beam energy, but letting through just enough of the energy to push adjacent layers (biological materials of interest) toward the desired substrate at a precise location. The laser beam is extremely small, which provides this method with great precision. Moreover, this laser can be computer-controlled to create complex patterns. The nozzle-free nature of the method enables the usage of high-viscosity materials, an advantage that makes it worth investigating, since inkjet and extrusion systems work only for materials of limited viscosity. The creation of stable gels will certainly increase the chances of constructing 3D organ-like structures on a layer-by-layer basis.

An important issue specific to laser direct writing (LDW) of biological solutions is their absorption properties with respect to the laser wavelength [171]. Most biomaterials are dissolved in water-based solvents, making these solutions transparent to a wide range of common laser wavelengths, for instance, the second and third harmonics of a Nd:YAG laser, preventing laser transfer. For wavelengths to be absorbed, one must be cautious not to denature the biomolecules due to thermal effects. Researchers have circumvented these difficulties by employing optical manipulation and laser-guided techniques to position cells [30], or by using a biocompatible, sacrificial absorbing layer [172] deposited on the donor substrate, prior to source fabrication for LDW printing. These techniques have a variety of names in the literature, such as BioLP™ [173] or absorbing-film-assisted laser-induced forward

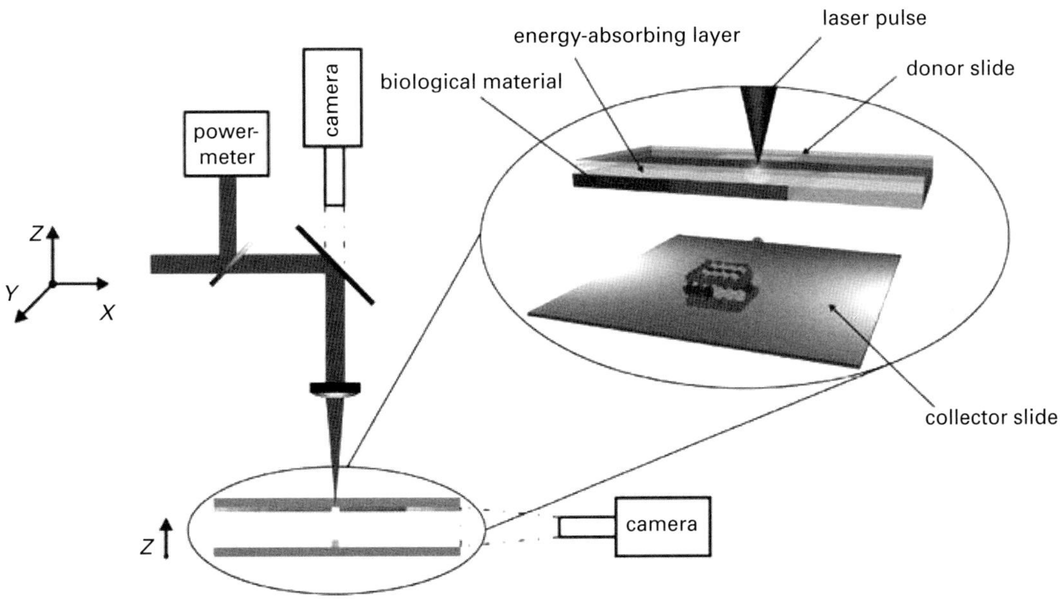

Figure 19.14 A schematic diagram of laser printing.

transfer (AFA-LIFT) [174], but, in general, they work on the same LDW principle. More recent work has employed polymer-based absorbing layers that decompose upon laser irradiation, thereby preventing contamination of the transferred solution [175].

LGDW is a unique cellular patterning technique able to deposit cells with micrometer accuracy on arbitrary matrices, including soft gels such as collagen and Matrigel™ [29–31, 176]. The unique ability of LGDW to micropattern cells on the basement membrane Matrigel™ allows researchers to use the intrinsic ability of endothelial cells to self-assemble into vascular structures [177, 178] for the assembly of liver tissue.

To avoid optical damage to cells, LGDW uses the near-infrared part of the electromagnetic spectrum (700–1000 nm), which is beyond the absorption spectra of most proteins and before the infrared absorption of water. Photons in this range of the spectrum lack the energy to create free radicals (as in the UV) and are not absorbed by DNA, suggesting that the laser has little chance of creating mutations or causing cell death, although precise wavelength optimization remains an issue [179, 180]. LGDW has been used to pattern living embryonic chick neurons [29, 30], multipotent adult progenitor cells [176], endothelial cells [31], and bacteria and other particles [30, 181, 182], with no apparent deleterious effect on cellular viability and function. The LGDW variant, optical trapping, has been commercially available for the past decade and has been used extensively in the field.

The LGDW system developed by Odde [183] represents a basic protocol to micropattern the formation of endothelial vascular structures on biological gels, such as Matrigel™. The actual system and set-up are shown in Figure 19.15. In addition, the protocol describes the formation of hepatic–endothelial organoids in both random and patterned formats. Minor alterations of this protocol might yield other important structures such as cardiac muscle [184] and pancreas [185]. The simplicity of the LGDW technique enables most laboratories to create small, arbitrary patterns of cells with little expertise in optics or microfabrication. However, several other techniques offer important improvements but need expertise. For example, a time-multiplexed array of optical tweezers can be formed using two diffractive elements to create 3D

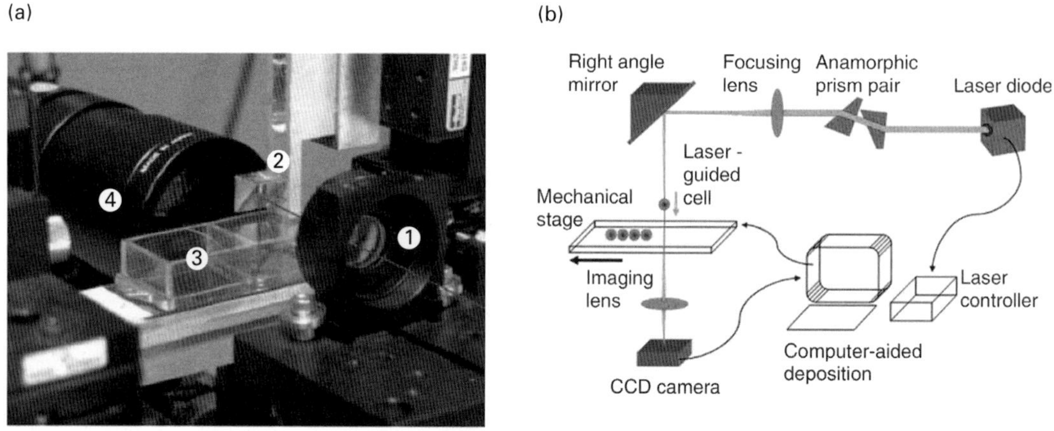

Figure 19.15 The LGDW system. (a) An image of the LGDW setup: (1) focusing lens (12 mm diameter), (2) right-angle mirror, (3) sealed glass chamber-slide, and (4) an optional side-on imaging lens for monitoring particle trajectory. (b) A schematic depiction of the LGDW setup [183].

patterns [186]. Alternatively, a microfabricated array of electrodes can be used to pattern thousands of cells in well-defined geometries using an enhanced field-induced dielectrophoresis trap [187].

Laser-induced forward transfer (LIFT), also referred to as laser printing, has been investigated as a means to transfer small amounts of various materials (including living cells) in preset 2D or 3D patterns. LIFT has been used for printing single cells to tens of cells simultaneously without any observable damage to phenotype and genotype [188]. Laser jet printing has successfully been used to generate cellular patterns either by printing cell-adhesive molecules for subsequent cell seeding or by directly depositing cells onto substrates with predesigned patterns. Koch *et al.* [189] have used this approach to transfer living cells in a 2D structure. Further, Barron *et al.* [173] and Othon *et al.* [147] transferred single cells, also in a 3D structure, by using a layer-by-layer technique. The cells survived the transfer procedure with rates of 98% ± 1% standard error of the mean (skin cells) and 90% ± 10% (human musculoskeletal cells). These results demonstrate that LIFT is a suitable technique for unharmed computer-controlled positioning of different cell types and a promising tool for future applications in the ex-vivo generation of tissue replacements [189].

As stated previously, nozzle-based cell printing has the limitation of the printer head clogging issues when the cell concentration of the bio-ink exceeds 10^7 cells/ml. In contrast, it has recently been demonstrated that laser-based printing (in particular the laser-assisted bioprinter (LAB) system [50]) can print a high cell fraction per droplet volume (i.e. cells with little surrounding bio-ink volume). Accordingly, the LAB can print cells one by one from a high-cell-concentration bio-ink (10^8 cells/ml) with high viscosity (above 100 mPa s) to fabricate a tissue-engineered product with comparable organization and cell density to those of living tissues, in which cells are in physical contact with each other. Further development may focus on the implementation of a cell- recognition scanning technology on the ribbon prior to printing, so that the laser beam could exactly aim a single cell per pulse. Moreover, previous studies have shown that the LAB can print mammalian cells undamaged in terms of cell viability, DNA integrity, and function [147, 174, 190–192]. However, current investigations are in progress to confirm the functional integrity of printed cell suspensions [50]. More information regarding the LAB system can be found in the previous report [193].

Understanding jet dynamics is crucial to developing laser printing toward organ printing. A condition

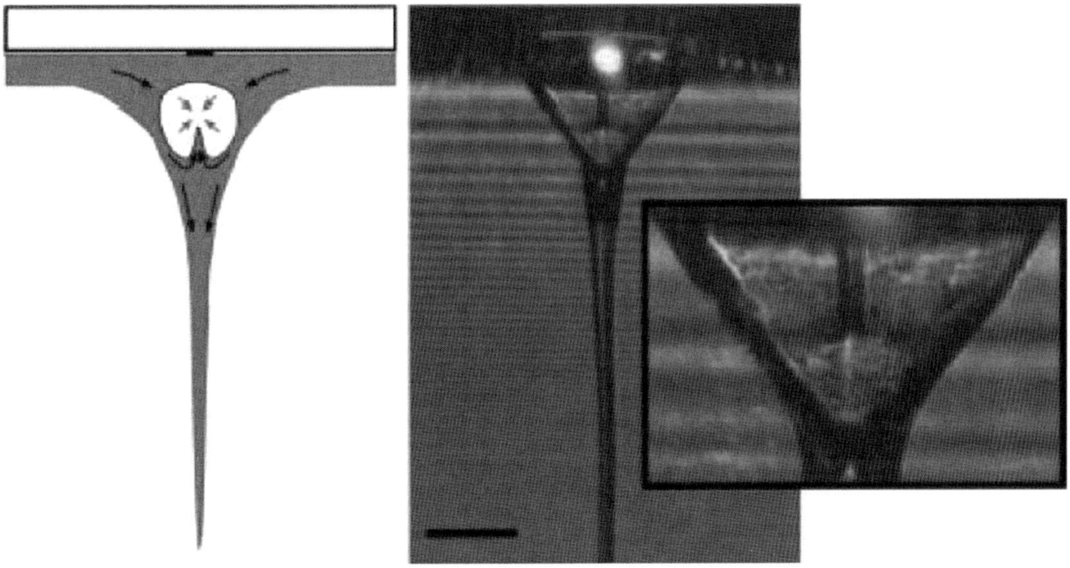

Figure 19.16 In the sketch, grey arrows indicate expansion or contraction of the vapor and black arrows mark the fluid flow inside the jet. For the time-resolved images hydrogel with viscosity $\eta = 0.1477$ Pa · s was coated as a 66-μm-thick layer onto the donor slide. The black scale bars correspond to 200 μm. The delay of the image was 100 μs. To visualize the small counterjet higher energy levels were necessary (60 μJ).

assumed to occur during laser printing was the so-called counterjet. Counterjet phenomena consist of microbubbles formed at the moment of ejecting liquids using this technique. This phenomenon was suspected during initial studies [194, 195]; however, it was not until recent studies [196] that such a phenomenon was confirmed. To enable the visualization of the counterjet, an increase in the laser energy was required. Figure 19.16 shows a clear image of the bubble formed, together with a sketch clarifying it. This finding corroborates the bubble-collapse theory of jet formation.

The need to understand the relation between the laser pulse energy and bio-ink properties has attracted interest. Characteristics such as hydrogel viscosity and layer height have been elicited in a recent study [196], revealing a linear relationship between the laser pulse energy and the droplet volume. On the other hand, the authors failed to relate the droplet viscosity to the printed hydrogel viscosity insofar as no systematic dependence was found. However, it was observed that a maximum droplet volume occurred at a specific viscosity; moreover, on varying the layer height a pronounced effect was observed. As a result, the following statements can be said to hold.

(1) For every layer thickness there exists a specific viscosity at which the printed droplet volume reaches its maximum.
(2) The specific viscosity at which the printed droplet volume reaches its maximum is lower for a lower thickness of the hydrogel layer.

Findings of this nature are important for managing the optimization of parameters for creating viable 3D structures.

Despite its advantages, the LAB also suffers from several drawbacks [197]. First, during the printing process, the metallic laser-absorbing layer is vaporized and metallic residues can be found in the final tissue engineering product. Recent and promising developments to avoid this limitation include the use of a polyimide membrane as the laser-absorbing layer, which is capable of dissipating shock energy through

Table 19.2 A comparison of different bioprinting methods

Technology	Resolution/ density	Cell viability	Load volume (ml)	Bio-ink viscosity	Throughput (print speed)	Advantages	Disadvantages
Needle-based							
Extrusion	2–500 μm [63]/ ~30,000 spots per mm^2 (hiScan by Illumina®)	>90 [67, 95]	0.2–5 [95]	Up to 200 Pa/s [95]	2×10^5 droplets/day [89] equivalent to 138.89 droplets/s	Controlled volume, validated technology for decades	Expensive, robotic, and infrastructure required
Nozzle-based							
Thermal	15–50 μm/64 spots per mm^2 [199]	Up to 97% [26, 27]	0.3–0.5 [200]	0.5–20 mPa/s [141]	1×10^4 drops/s [200]	Low investment, high throughput	Obstruction and blockage, drying and spreading of the ink, limited to low-viscosity materials
Piezoelectric		Up to 98% at 40-V pulse [141]		0.5–20 mPa/s [141]	1000 droplets/s [201] at 5×10^6 cells/ml [27]	Fair precision, picoliter scale volume control, additive operation	
Nozzle-free							
Laser-based	1–3 μm [202] /100 spots per mm^2 [203]	Modified LIFT 95–100 [200]	Modified LIFT $(0.5–20) \times 10^{-3}$, 10–70,000 pl [196], 12 fl [171]	1–300 mPa/s [197]	10^2 drops/s, 5000 droplets/s [50]	Printing of high-viscosity materials, ultra-high throughput, high resolution and density, additive operation	Laser source might have adverse effects on cellular genetic material

elastoplastic deformation [198], or the generation of the cavitation bubble without the use of a laser-absorbing layer [169]. Second, owing to the manner of spreading cell suspensions onto the ribbon, cell printing is still random. To address this issue, it has been shown that statistical cell printing can be optimized by using a ribbon with a confluent-like cell concentration [50]. An "aim and shoot" procedure could be helpful when driving the laser beam onto the ribbon to ensure that each printed droplet contains a predefined number of cells. Finally, the printing speed of the LAB could be enhanced by increasing the laser pulse rate (up to 100 MHz) and by mounting multiple laser beams in parallel.

19.4 Summary

Organ printing is the natural evolution of medicine, manufacturing, biology, and tissue engineering science. Recent research in this field is showing that gaining control of the 3D environment offers better results and much better reproducibility. Even though organ printing has not yet been achieved, estimations give a 15–20-year window before biomedical companies will start producing organs or organ parts ready for implantation. For wider in-vivo applications of bioprinting, it is necessary to develop new materials and methods to fabricate 3D layer-by-layer printed biopaper that will allow manipulation and implantation. The next step also includes the improvement of bioink formulations in order for the printed cells to be minimally damaged during printing and so that they maintain their specific genotype and phenotype.

Table 19.2 gives a comparison of bioprinting methods.

Computer-aided layer-by-layer assembly of biological tissues and organs is currently feasible, fast-evolving, and predicted to be a major technology in tissue engineering. Organ printing uses the principle of cellular self-assembly into tissues, similarly to the way embryonic-like tissues sort and fuse into functional forms dictated by the rules laid out in developmental biology. At present several groups around the world are actively working on improvement of organ inkjet printing technology. Inkjet bioprinting technology would benefit enormously from being more affordable. Moreover, in the long term, the existence of profitable and well-established inkjet printer technology with global companies such as HP, Lexmark, Cannon, and Xerox will represent an important advantage especially when the technology becomes mature enough for commercialization. Besides their obvious application for organ transplantation, 3D perfused, vascularized, printed human tissues (or structural-functional units of human organs) could become popular screening assays for drug discovery and testing and further biomedical research. It is safe to predict that, in the twenty-first century, cell and organ printers will be as broadly used as biomedical research tools as was the electron microscope in the twentieth century.

ACKNOWLEDGEMENTS

The authors would like to thank the NIH National Heart, Lung, and Blood Institute (NHLBI) (grant #1SC2HL107235-01), National Science Foundation (grant #CBET0936238), and Department of Education (grant #P116V090013) for funding this project. The authors would like to thank Randi Bossie for her assistance with editing.

REFERENCES

[1] Murray, J. E. 2005. The 50th anniversary of the first successful human organ transplant. *Rev. Invest. Clin.*, **57**(2), 118–19.

[2] Mironov, V. 2006. Toward human organ printing: Charleston Bioprinting Symposium. *ASAIO J.*, **52**(6), e27–30.

[3] Mironov, V., Boland, T., Trusk, T., Forgacs, G. and Markwald, R. R. 2003. Organ printing: computer-aided jet-based 3D tissue engineering. *Trends Biotechnol.*, **21**(4), 157–61.

[4] Chang, R., Nam, J. and Sun, W. 2008. Direct cell writing of 3D microorgan for in vitro pharmacokinetic model. *Tissue Eng. Part C Methods*, **14**(2), 157–66.

[5] Sun, W., Starly, B., Darling, A. and Gomez, C. 2004. Computer-aided tissue engineering: application to

biomimetic modelling and design of tissue scaffolds. *Biotechnol. Appl. Biochem.*, **39**(Part 1), 49–58.

[6] Sun, W., Darling, A., Starly, B. and Nam, J. 2004. Computer-aided tissue engineering: overview, scope and challenges. *Biotechnol. Appl. Biochem.*, **39**, 29–47.

[7] Sun, W., Starly, B., Nam, J. and Darling, A. 2005. Bio-CAD modeling and its applications in computer-aided tissue engineering. *Comput. Aided Design*, **37**(11), 1097–114.

[8] Varady, T., Martin, R. R. and Cox, J. 1997. Reverse engineering of geometric models – an introduction. *Comput. Aided Design*, **29**(4), 255–68.

[9] Sun, W. and Lal, P. 2002. Recent development on computer aided tissue engineering – a review. *Comput. Meth. Prog. Biol.*, **67**(2), 85–103.

[10] Lin, A. S. P., Barrows, T. H., Cartmell, S. H. and Guldberg, R. E. 2003. Microarchitectural and mechanical characterization of oriented porous polymer scaffolds. *Biomaterials*, **24**(3), 481–9.

[11] Folch, A. and Toner, M. 2000. Microengineering of cellular interactions. *Ann. Rev. Biomed. Eng.*, **2**, 227–56.

[12] Landers, R., Hubner, U., Schmelzeisen, R. and Mulhaupt, R. 2002. Rapid prototyping of scaffolds derived from thermoreversible hydrogels and tailored for applications in tissue engineering. *Biomaterials*, **23**(23), 4437–47.

[13] Muller, R. and Ruegsegger, P. 1997. Micro-tomographic imaging for the nondestructive evaluation of trabecular bone architecture. *Stud. Health Technol. Inform.*, **40**, 61–79.

[14] Ulrich, D., Hildebrand, T., Van Rietbergen, B., Muller, R. and Ruegsegger, P. 1997. The quality of trabecular bone evaluated with micro-computed tomography, FEA and mechanical testing. *Stud. Health Technol. Inform.*, **40**, 97–112.

[15] Van Rietbergen, B., Muller, R., Ulrich, D., Ruegsegger, P. and Huiskes, R. 1999. Tissue stresses and strain in trabeculae of a canine proximal femur can be quantified from computer reconstructions. *J. Biomech.*, **32**(4), 443–51.

[16] Krause, W., Handreke, K., Schuhmann-Giampieri, G. and Rupp, K. 2002. Efficacy of the iodine-free computed tomography liver contrast agent, Dy-EOB-DTPA, in comparison with a conventional iodinated agent in normal and in tumor-bearing rabbits. *Invest. Radiol.*, **37**(5), 241–7.

[17] Watanabe, M., Shin'oka, T., Tohyama, S. *et al.* 2001. Tissue-engineered vascular autograft: inferior vena cava replacement in a dog model. *Tissue Eng.*, **7**(4), 429–39.

[18] Micläuş, G. M.-V. B. and Clipicioiu, D. 2007. New perspectives in exploring cardiac patient imaging – cardiac CT. *Timişoara Med. J.* **57**, 162–6.

[19] Bandettini, W. P. and Arai, A. E. 2008. Advances in clinical applications of cardiovascular magnetic resonance imaging. *Heart*, **94**(11), 1485–95.

[20] Sun, W. 2000. Multi-volume CAD modeling for heterogeneous object design and fabrication. *J. Comput. Sci. Technol.*, **15**(1), 27–36.

[21] Sun, W. and Hu, X. 2002. Reasoning Boolean operation based modeling for heterogeneous objects. *Comput. Aided Design*, **34**(6), 481–8.

[22] Boland, T., Cui, X., Chaubey, A. *et al.* 2007. Precision printing of cells and biomaterials onto 3D matrices. *In Proceedings of the ASME International Conference on Manufacturing Science and Engineering*, pp. 77–81.

[23] Boland, T., Tao, X., Damon, B. J. *et al.* 2007. Drop-on-demand printing of cells and materials for designer tissue constructs. *Mater. Sci. Eng. C – Biol.*, **27**(3), 372–6.

[24] Cui, X. F. and Boland, T. 2008. Simultaneous deposition of human microvascular endothelial cells and biomaterials for human microvasculature fabrication using inkjet printing. In *Nip24/Digital Fabrication 2008: 24th International Conference on Digital Printing Technologies, Technical Program and Proceedings*, pp. 480–3.

[25] Kesari. P., Xu, T. and Boland, T. 2005. Layer-by-layer printing of cells and its application to tissue engineering. *Mater. Res. Soc. Symp. Proc.*, **845**:111–17.

[26] Xu, T., Gregory, C. A., Molnar, P. *et al.* 2006. Viability and electrophysiology of neural cell structures generated by the inkjet printing method. *Biomaterials*, **27**(19), 3580–8.

[27] Xu, T., Jin, J., Gregory, C. *et al.* 2005. Inkjet printing of viable mammalian cells. *Biomaterials*, **26**(1), 93–9.

[28] Narayan, R., Boland, T. and Lee, Y.-S. 2010. *Printed Biomaterials: Novel Processing and Modeling Techniques for Medicine and Surgery.* New York: Springer.

[29] Odde, D. J. and Renn, M. J. 1999. Laser-guided direct writing for applications in biotechnology. *Trends Biotechnol.*, **17**(10), 385–9.

[30] Odde, D. J. and Renn, M. J. 2000. Laser-guided direct writing of living cells. *Biotechnol. Bioeng.*, **67**(3), 312–18.

[31] Nahmias, Y., Schwartz, R. E., Verfaillie, C. M. and Odde, D. J. 2005. Laser-guided direct writing for three-dimensional tissue engineering. *Biotechnol. Bioeng.*, **92**(2), 129–36.

[32] Barron, J. A., Spargo, B. J. and Ringeisen, B. R. 2004. Biological laser printing of three dimensional cellular structures. *Appl. Phys. A – Mater.*, **79**(4–6), 1027–30.

[33] Saunders, R., Gough, J. and Derby, B. 2005. Ink jet printing of mammalian primary cells for tissue engineering applications. *Mater. Res. Soc. Symp. Proc.*, **845**, 57–62.

[34] De Coppi, P., Bartsch, G. Jr., Siddiqui, M. M. *et al.* 2007. Isolation of amniotic stem cell lines with potential for therapy. *Nature Biotechnol.*, **25**(1), 100–6.

[35] Eagles, P. A., Qureshi, A. N. and Jayasinghe, S. N. 2006. Electrohydrodynamic jetting of mouse neuronal cells. *Biochem. J.*, **394**(Part 2), 375–8.

[36] Printz, C. 2011. American Cancer Society reports progress in reducing cancer deaths. However, some groups still lag behind this trend. *Cancer – Am. Cancer Soc.*, **117**(20), 4573–4.

[37] Asahara, T., Murohara, T., Sullivan, A. *et al.* 1997. Isolation of putative progenitor endothelial cells for angiogenesis. *Science*, **275**(5302), 964–7.

[38] Gimble, J. M., Katz, A. J. and Bunnell, B. A. 2007. Adipose-derived stem cells for regenerative medicine. *Circ. Res.*, **100**(9), 1249–60.

[39] Bartsch, G., Yoo, J. J., De Coppi, P. *et al.* 2005. Propagation, expansion, and multilineage differentiation of human somatic stem cells from dermal progenitors. *Stem Cells Dev.*, **14**(3), 337–48.

[40] Delo, D. M., De Coppi, P., Bartsch, G. Jr. and Atala, A. 2006. Amniotic fluid and placental stem cells. *Methods Enzymol.*, **419**, 426–38.

[41] Cutler, C. and Ballen, K. 2009. Reduced-intensity conditioning and umbilical cord blood transplantation in adults. *Bone Marrow Transplant.*, **44**(10), 667–71.

[42] Delaney, C., Ratajczak, M. Z. and Laughlin, M. J. 2010. Strategies to enhance umbilical cord blood stem cell engraftment in adult patients. *Expert Rev. Hematol.*, **3**(3), 273–83.

[43] Ker, E. D. P., Nain, A. S., Weiss, L. E. *et al.* 2011. Bioprinting of growth factors onto aligned sub-micron fibrous scaffolds for simultaneous control of cell differentiation and alignment. *Biomaterials*, **32**(32), 8097–107.

[44] Cooper, G. M., Miller, E. D., DeCesare, G. E. *et al.* 2010. Inkjet-based biopatterning of bone morphogenetic protein-2 to spatially control calvarial bone formation. *Tissue Eng. Part A*, **16**(5), 1749 59.

[45] Ma, N. N., Chalmers, J. J., Aunins, J. G., Zhou, W. C. and Xie, L. Z. Quantitative studies of cell-bubble interactions and cell damage at different pluronic F-68 and cell concentrations. *Biotechnol. Progr.*, **20**(4), 1183–91.

[46] Parsa, S., Gupta, M., Loizeau, F. and Cheung, K. C. 2010. Effects of surfactant and gentle agitation on inkjet dispensing of living cells. *Biofabrication*, **2**(2), 025003.

[47] Holtsberg, F. W., Ensor, C. M., Steiner, M. R., Bomalaski, J. S. and Clark, M. A. 2002. Poly(ethylene glycol) (PEG) conjugated arginine deiminase: effects of PEG formulations on its pharmacological properties. *J. Control. Release*, **80**(1–3), 259–71.

[48] Bomalaski, J. S., Holtsberg, F. W., Ensor, C. M. and Clark, M. A. 2002. Uricase formulated with polyethylene glycol (uricase-PEG 20): biochemical rationale and preclinical studies. *J. Rheumatol.*, **29**(9), 1942–9.

[49] Engler, A. J., Sen, S., Sweeney, H. L. and Discher, D. E. 2006. Matrix elasticity directs stem cell lineage specification. *Cell*, **126**(4), 677–89.

[50] Guillotin, B., Souquet, A., Catros, S. *et al.* 2010. Laser assisted bioprinting of engineered tissue with high cell density and microscale organization. *Biomaterials*, **31** (28), 7250–6.

[51] Klebe, R. J. 1988. Cytoscribing: a method for micropositioning cells and the construction of two- and three-dimensional synthetic tissues. *Exp. Cell Res.*, **179**(2), 362–73.

[52] Ahmed, T. A., Dare, E. V. and Hincke, M. 2008. Fibrin: a versatile scaffold for tissue engineering applications. *Tissue Eng. Part B Rev.*, **14**(2), 199–215.

[53] Cui, X. F. and Boland, T. 2009. Human microvasculature fabrication using thermal inkjet printing technology. *Biomaterials*, **30**(31), 6221–7.

[54] Fedorovich, N. E., Alblas, J., de Wijn, J. R. *et al.* 2007. Hydrogels as extracellular matrices for skeletal tissue engineering: state-of-the-art and novel application in organ printing. *Tissue Eng.*, **13**(8), 1905–25.

[55] Wilson, W. C. Jr. and Boland, T. 2003. Cell and organ printing 1: protein and cell printers. *Anat. Rec. A Discov. Molec. Cell Evol. Biol.*, **272**(2), 491–6.

[56] Smith, C. M., Stone, A. L., Parkhill, R. L. *et al.* 2004. Three-dimensional bioassembly tool for generating viable tissue-engineered constructs. *Tissue Eng.*, **10**(9–10), 1566–76.

[57] Harkness, R. D. 1966. Collagen. *Sci. Prog.*, **54**(214), 257–74.

[58] Stenzel, K. H., Dunn, M. W., Rubin, A. L. and Miyata, T. 1969. Collagen gels: design for a vitreous replacement. *Science*, **164**(885), 1282–3.

[59] Boland, T., Xu, T., Damon, B. and Cui, X. 2006. Application of inkjet printing to tissue engineering. *Biotechnol. J.*, **1**(9), 910–17.

[60] Xu, T., Petridou, S., Lee, E. H. *et al.* 2004. Construction of high-density bacterial colony arrays and patterns by the ink-jet method. *Biotechnol. Bioeng.*, **85**(1), 29–33.

[61] Xu, T., Olson, J., Zhao, W. X. *et al.* 2008. Characterization of cell constructs generated with inkjet printing

technology using in vivo magnetic resonance imaging. *J. Manuf. Sci. Technol.*, **130**(2), 020601.

[62] Moon, S., Hasan, S. K., Song, Y. S. *et al.* 2010. Layer by layer three-dimensional tissue epitaxy by cell-laden hydrogel droplets. *Tissue Eng. Part C Methods*, **16**(1), 157–66.

[63] Roth, E. A., Xu, T., Das, M. *et al.* 2004. Inkjet printing for high-throughput cell patterning. *Biomaterials*, **25**(17), 3707–15.

[64] Malda, J., Woodfield, T. B., van der Vloodt, F. *et al.* 2004. The effect of PEGT/PBT scaffold architecture on oxygen gradients in tissue engineered cartilaginous constructs. *Biomaterials*, **25**(26), 5773–80.

[65] Karageorgiou, V. and Kaplan, D. 2005. Porosity of 3D biomaterial scaffolds and osteogenesis. *Biomaterials*, **26**(27), 5474–91.

[66] Cotterill, A. M., Camacho-Hübner, C., Woods, K. *et al.* 1994. The insulin-like growth factor I generation test in the investigation of short stature. *Acta Paediatr.*, **399**(Suppl.), 128–30.

[67] Cohen, D. L., Malone, E., Lipson, H. and Bonassar, L. J. 2006. Direct freeform fabrication of seeded hydrogels in arbitrary geometries. *Tissue Eng.*, **12**(5), 1325–35.

[68] Cohen, D. L., Lipton, J. I., Bonassar, L. J. and Lipson, H. 2010. Additive manufacturing for in situ repair of osteochondral defects. *Biofabrication*, **2**(3), 035004.

[69] LeRoux, M. A., Guilak, F. and Setton, L. A. 1999. Compressive and shear properties of alginate gel: effects of sodium ions and alginate concentration. *J. Biomed. Mater. Res.*, **47**(1), 46–53.

[70] Shoichet, M. S., Li, R. H., White, M. L. and Winn, S. R. 1996. Stability of hydrogels used in cell encapsulation: an in vitro comparison of alginate and agarose. *Biotechnol. Bioeng.*, **50**(4), 374–81.

[71] Bouhadir, K. H., Lee, K. Y., Alsberg, E. *et al.* 2001. Degradation of partially oxidized alginate and its potential application for tissue engineering. *Biotechnol. Prog.*, **17**(5), 945–50.

[72] Lee, W. J., Chia, W. J., Wang, J. *et al.* 2010. Role of surfaces and interfaces in controlling the mechanical properties of metallic alloys. *Langmuir*, **26**(21), 16254–60.

[73] Alsberg, E., Kong, H. J., Hirano, Y. *et al.* 2003. Regulating bone formation via controlled scaffold degradation. *J. Dent. Res.*, **82**(11), 903–8.

[74] Miller, E. D., Fisher, G. W., Weiss, L. E., Walker, L. M. and Campbell, P. G. 2006. Dose-dependent cell growth in response to concentration modulated patterns of FGF-2 printed on fibrin. *Biomaterials*, **27**(10), 2213–21.

[75] Fortier, L. A., Lust, G., Mohammed, H. O. and Nixon, A. J. 1999. Coordinate upregulation of cartilage matrix synthesis in fibrin cultures supplemented with exogenous insulin-like growth factor-I. *J. Orthop. Res.*, **17**(4), 467–74.

[76] Wu, P. K. and Ringeisen, B. R. 2010. Development of human umbilical vein endothelial cell (HUVEC) and human umbilical vein smooth muscle cell (HUVSMC) branch/stem structures on hydrogel layers via biological laser printing (BioLP). *Biofabrication*, **2**(1), 014111.

[77] Kim, J. Y., Park, E. K., Kim, S.-Y., Shin, J.-W. and Cho, D.-W. 2008. Fabrication of a SFF-based three-dimensional scaffold using a precision deposition system in tissue engineering. *J. Micromech. Microeng.*, **18**(5), 055027.

[78] Pirlo, R. K., Wu, P., Liu, J. and Ringeisen, B. 2012. PLGA/hydrogel biopapers as a stackable substrate for printing HUVEC networks via BioLP™. *Biotechnol. Bioeng.*, **109**(1), 262–73.

[79] Catros, S., Guillemot, F., Nandakumar, A. *et al.* 2011. Layer-by-layer tissue microfabrication supports cell proliferation in vitro and in vivo. *Tissue Eng. Part C Methods*, **18**(1), 62–70.

[80] Skardal, A., Zhang, J. and Prestwich, G. D. 2010. Bioprinting vessel-like constructs using hyaluronan hydrogels crosslinked with tetrahedral polyethylene glycol tetracrylates. *Biomaterials*, **31**(24), 6173–81.

[81] Mironov, V., Boland, T., Trusk, T., Forgacs, G. and Markwald, R. R. 2003. Organ printing: computer-aided jet-based 3D tissue engineering. *Trends Biotechnol.*, **21**(4), 157–61.

[82] Langer, R. and Vacanti, J. P. 1993. Tissue engineering. *Science*, **260**(5110), 920–6.

[83] Roskelley, C. D., Desprez, P. Y. and Bissell, M. J. 1994. Extracellular matrix-dependent tissue-specific gene expression in mammary epithelial cells requires both physical and biochemical signal transduction. *Proc. Nat. Acad. Sci. USA*, **91**(26), 12378–82.

[84] Mooney, D. J., Sano, K., Kaufmann, P. M. *et al.* 1997. Long-term engraftment of hepatocytes transplanted on biodegradable polymer sponges. *J. Biomed. Mater. Res.*, **37**(3), 413–20.

[85] Knight, B., Laukaitis, C., Akhtar, N. *et al.* 2000. Visualizing muscle cell migration *in situ*. *Curr. Biol.*, **10**(10), 576–85.

[86] Chang, R., Nam, J. and Sun, W. 2008. Effects of dispensing pressure and nozzle diameter on cell survival from solid freeform fabrication-based direct cell writing. *Tissue Eng. Part A*, **14**(1), 41–8.

[87] Lee, W., Pinckney, J., Lee, V. *et al.* 2009. Three-dimensional bioprinting of rat embryonic neural cells. *Neuroreport*, **20**(8), 798–803.

[88] Hamid, Q., Snyder, J., Wang, C. *et al.* 2011. Fabrication of three-dimensional scaffolds using precision extrusion deposition with an assisted cooling device. *Biofabrication*, **3**(3), 034109.

[89] Mayr, L. M. and Bojanic, D. 2009. Novel trends in high-throughput screening. *Curr. Opin. Pharmacol.*, **9**(5), 580–8.

[90] Yan, Y., Wang, X., Pan, Y. *et al.* 2005. Fabrication of viable tissue-engineered constructs with 3D cell-assembly technique. *Biomaterials*, **26**(29), 5864–71.

[91] Zhang, T., Yan, Y. N., Wang, X. H. *et al.* 2007. Three-dimensional gelatin and gelatin/hyaluronan hydrogel structures for traumatic brain injury. *J. Bioact. Compat. Pol.*, **22**(1), 19–29.

[92] Patz, T. M., Doraiswamy, A., Narayan, R. J. *et al.* 2006. Three-dimensional direct writing of B35 neuronal cells. *J. Biomed. Mater. Res. B Appl. Biomater.*, **78**(1), 124–30.

[93] Shor, L., Guceri, S., Wen, X. J., Gandhi, M. and Sun, W. 2007. Fabrication of three-dimensional polycaprolactone/hydroxyapatite tissue scaffolds and osteoblast-scaffold interactions in vitro. *Biomaterials*, **28**(35), 5291–7.

[94] Lee, W., Debasitis, J. C., Lee, V. K. *et al.* 2009. Multi-layered culture of human skin fibroblasts and keratinocytes through three-dimensional freeform fabrication. *Biomaterials*, **30**(8), 1587–95.

[95] Ringeisen, B. R., Spargo, B. J. and Wu, P. K. 2010. *Cell and Organ Printing*. New York: Springer.

[96] Fedorovich, N. E., Dewijn, J. R., Verbout, A. J., Alblas, J. and Dhert, W. J. A. 2008. Three-dimensional fiber deposition of cell-laden, viable, patterned constructs for bone tissue printing. *Tissue Eng. Part A*, **14**(1), 127–33.

[97] Hon, K. K. B., Li, L. and Hutchings, I. M. 2008. Direct writing technology – advances and developments. *CIRP Ann. – Manufacturing Technol.*, **57**(2), 601.

[98] Chang, R., Nam, J., Holtorf, H. *et al.* 2008. Direct cell writing of 3D tissue micro-organs for drug metabolism study. *J. Biotechnol.*, **136**(Suppl. 1), S144.

[99] Chang, R. and Sun, W. 2008. Effects of dispensing pressure and nozzle diameter on cell survival from solid freeform fabrication-based direct cell writing. *Tissue Eng. Part A*, **14**(1), 41–8.

[100] Igawa, K., Mochizuki, M., Sugimori, O. *et al.* 2006. Tailor-made tricalcium phosphate bone implant directly fabricated by a three-dimensional ink-jet printer. *J. Artificial Organs*, **9**(4), 234.

[101] Zhang, C., Zhao, K., Hu, T. *et al.* 2008. Loading dependent swelling and release properties of novel biodegradable, elastic and environmental stimuli-sensitive polyurethanes. *J. Controll. Release*, **131**(2), 128.

[102] Zhang, C., Wen, X., Vyavahare, N. R. and Boland, T. 2008. Synthesis and characterization of biodegradable elastomeric polyurethane scaffolds fabricated by the inkjet technique. *Biomaterials*, **29**(28), 3781.

[103] Miller, E. D., Fisher, G. W., Weiss, L. E., Walker, L. M. and Campbell, P. G. 2006. Dose-dependent cell growth in response to concentration modulated patterns of FGF-2 printed on fibrin. *Biomaterials*, **27**(10), 2213.

[104] Crowley, K., Morrin, A., Hernandez, A. *et al.* 2008. Fabrication of an ammonia gas sensor using inkjet-printed polyaniline nanoparticles. *Talanta*, **77**(2), 710.

[105] Jakab, K., Norotte, C., Damon, B. *et al.* 2008. Tissue engineering by self-assembly of cells printed into topologically defined structures. *Tissue Eng. Part A*, **14**(3), 413–21.

[106] Nagaraj, V. J., Eaton, S., Thirstrup, D. and Wiktor, P. 2008. Piezoelectric printing and probing of Lectin NanoProbeArrays for glycosylation analysis. *Biochem. Biophys. Res. Commun.*, **375**(4), 526.

[107] Calvert, P. and Crockett, R. 1997. Chemical solid freeform fabrication: making shapes without molds. *Chem. Mater.*, **9**, 650.

[108] Zein, I., Hutmacher, D. W., Tan, K. C. and Teoh, S. H. 2002. Fused deposition modeling of novel scaffold architectures for tissue engineering applications. *Biomaterials*, **23**(4), 1169–85.

[109] Liu, C., Sachlos, E., Wahl, D., Han, Z. and Czernuszka, J. 2007. On the manufacturability of scaffold mould using a 3D printing technology. *Rapid Prototyping J.*, **13**, 163.

[110] Dhariwala, B., Hunt, E. and Boland, T. 2004. Rapid prototyping of tissue-engineering constructs, using photopolymerizable hydrogels and stereolithography. *Tissue Eng.*, **10**(9–10), 1316–22.

[111] Arcaute, K., Mann, B. K. and Wicker, R. B. 2006. Stereolithography of three-dimensional bioactive poly(ethylene glycol) constructs with encapsulated cells. *Ann. Biomed. Eng.*, **34**(9), 1429–41.

[112] Dimitrov, D., Schreve, K. and De Beer, N. 2006. Advances in three dimensional printing: state of the art and future perspectives. *Rapid Prototyping J.*, **12**(3), 136–47.

[113] Morissette, S. L., Lewis, J. A., Cesarano, J., Dimos, D. B. and Baer, T. 2000. Solid freeform fabrication of aqueous

alumina-poly(vinyl alcohol) gelcasting suspensions. *J. Am. Ceram. Soc.*, **83**, 2409.

[114] Cohen, D. L., Malone, E., Lipson, H. and Bonassar, L. J. 2006. Direct freeform fabrication of seeded hydrogels in arbitrary geometries. *Tissue Eng.*, **12**(5), 1325–35.

[115] Liu, Z. S., Erhan, S. Z., Xu, J. and Calvert, P. D. 2002. Development of soybean oil-based composites by solid freeform fabrication method: epoxidized soybean oil with bis or polyalkyleneamine curing agents system. *J. Appl. Polymer Sci.*, **85**, 2100.

[116] Peng, J., Lin, T. L. and Calvert, P. 1999. Orientation effects in freeformed short-fiber composites. *Composites A*, **30**, 133.

[117] Sercombe, T. B., Schaffer, G. B. and Calvert, P. 1999. Freeform fabrication of functional aluminium prototypes using powder metallurgy. *J. Mater. Sci.*, **34**, 4245.

[118] Sirringhaus, H., Kawase, T., Friend, R. H. *et al.* 2000. High-resolution inkjet printing of all-polymer transistor circuits. *Science*, **290**(5499), 2123–6.

[119] Gratson, G. M., Xu, M. and Lewis, J. A. 2004. Microperiodic structures: direct writing of three-dimensional webs. *Nature*, **428**(6981), 386.

[120] Yan, K. C., Nair, K. and Sun, W. 2010. Three dimensional multi-scale modelling and analysis of cell damage in cell-encapsulated alginate constructs. *J. Biomech.*, **43**(6), 1031–8.

[121] van Krevelen, D. W. 1990. *Properties of Polymers*. Amsterdam: Elsevier.

[122] Alamry, K. A., Nixon, K., Hindley, R., Odell, J. A. and Yeates, S. G. 2010. Flow-induced polymer degradation during ink-jet printing. In *Nip 26: Digital Fabrication*, p. 284.

[123] Hoath, S., Hutchings, I., Martin, G. *et al.* 2009. Links between ink rheology, drop-on-demand jet formation, and printability. *J. Imaging Sci. Technol.*, **53**(4), 041208–041210.

[124] Hancock, A. and Lin, L. 2004. Challenges of UV curable inkjet printing inks – a formulator's perspective. *Pigment Resin Technol.*, **33**, 280.

[125] Rowley, J. A., Madlambayan, G. and Mooney, D. J. 1999. Alginate hydrogels as synthetic extracellular matrix materials. *Biomaterials*, **20**(1), 45–53.

[126] Jorgensen, T. E., Sletmoen, M., Draget, K. I. and Stokke, B. T. 2007. Influence of oligoguluronates on alginate gelation, kinetics, and polymer organization. *Biomacromolecules*, **8**(8), 2388–97.

[127] Nishiyama, Y., Nakamura, M., Henmi, C. *et al.* 2009. Development of a three-dimensional bioprinter: construction of cell supporting structures using hydrogel and state-of-the-art inkjet technology. *J. Biomech. Eng.*, **131**(3), 035001.

[128] Xu, T., Baicu, C., Aho, M., Zile, M. and Boland, T. 2009. Fabrication and characterization of bio-engineered cardiac pseudo tissues. *Biofabrication*, **1**(3), 035001.

[129] in het Panhuis, M., Heurtematte, A., Small, W. R., and Paunov, V. N. 2007. Inkjet printed water sensitive transparent films from natural gum–carbon nanotube composites. *Soft Matter*, **3**, 840–3.

[130] Bekard, I. B., Asimakis, P., Bertolini, J. and Dunstan, D. E. 2011. The effects of shear flow on protein structure and function. *Biopolymers*, **95**(11), 733–45.

[131] Nishioka, G. M., Markey, A. A. and Holloway, C. K. 2004. Protein damage in drop-on-demand printers. *J. Am. Chem. Soc.*, **126**(50), 16320–1.

[132] Goodall, S., Chew, N., Chan, K., Auriac, D. and Waters, M. J. Aerosolization of protein solutions using thermal inkjet technology. *J. Aerosol. Med.*, **15**(3), 351–7.

[133] Campbell, P. G. and Weiss, L. E. 2007. Tissue engineering with the aid of inkjet printers. *Expert Opin. Biol. Ther.*, **7**(8), 1123–7.

[134] Weiss, L. E., Amon, C. H., Finger, S. *et al.* 2005. Bayesian computer-aided experimental design of heterogeneous scaffolds for tissue engineering. *Comput. Aided Design*, **37**(11), 1127–39.

[135] Sanjana, N. E. and Fuller, S. B. 2004. A fast flexible inkjet printing method for patterning dissociated neurons in culture. *J. Neurosci. Methods*, **136**(2), 151–63.

[136] Xu, T., Jin, J., Gregory, C., Hickman, J. J. and Boland, T. Inkjet printing of viable mammalian cells. *Biomaterials*, **26**(1), 93–9.

[137] Xu, T., Rohozinski, J., Zhao, W. *et al.* 2009. Inkjet-mediated gene transfection into living cells combined with targeted delivery. *Tissue Eng. Part A*, **15**(1), 95–101.

[138] Cui, X. and Boland, T. 2009. Human microvasculature fabrication using thermal inkjet printing technology. *Biomaterials*, **30**(31), 6221–7.

[139] Lee, S. S., Yim, Y., Ahn, K. H. and Lee, S. J. 2009. Extensional flow-based assessment of red blood cell deformability using hyperbolic converging microchannel. *Biomed. Microdevices*, **11**(5), 1021–7.

[140] Nakamura, M., Kobayashi, A., Takagi, F. *et al.* 2005. Biocompatible inkjet printing technique for designed seeding of individual living cells. *Tissue Eng.*, **11**(11–12), 1658–66.

[141] Saunders, R. E., Gough, J. E. and Derby, B. 2008. Delivery of human fibroblast cells by piezoelectric drop-on-demand inkjet printing. *Biomaterials*, **29**(2), 193–203.

[142] Nair, K., Gandhi, M., Khalil, S. *et al.* 2009. Characterization of cell viability during bioprinting processes. *Biotechnol. J.*, **4**(8), 1168–77.

[143] Joly, P., Chavda, N., Eddaoudi, A. and Jayasinghe, S. N. 2010. Bio-electrospraying and aerodynamically assisted bio-jetting whole human blood: interrogating cell surface marker integrity. *Biomicrofluidics*, **4**(1), 11101.

[144] Mongkoldhumrongkul, N., Flanagan, J. M. and Jayasinghe, S. N. 2009. Direct jetting approaches for handling stem cells. *Biomed. Mater.*, **4**(1), 015018.

[145] Ringeisen, B. R., Chrisey, D. B., Pique, A. *et al.* 2002. Generation of mesoscopic patterns of viable *Escherichia coli* by ambient laser transfer. *Biomaterials*, **23**(1), 161–6.

[146] Hopp, B., Smausz, T., Kresz, N. *et al.* 2005. Survival and proliferative ability of various living cell types after laser-induced forward transfer. *Tissue Eng.*, **11**(11–12), 1817–23.

[147] Othon, C. M., Wu, X., Anders, J. J. and Ringeisen, B. R. 2008. Single-cell printing to form three-dimensional lines of olfactory ensheathing cells. *Biomed. Mater.*, **3**(3), 034101.

[148] Cui, X., Dean, D., Ruggeri, Z. M. and Boland, T. 2010. Cell damage evaluation of thermal inkjet printed Chinese hamster ovary cells. *Biotechnol. Bioeng.*, **106**(6), 963–9.

[149] Norotte, C., Marga, F. S., Niklason, L. E. and Forgacs, G. 2009. Scaffold-free vascular tissue engineering using bioprinting. *Biomaterials*, **30**(30), 5910–17.

[150] De Rosa, M., Carteni, M., Petillo, O. *et al.* 2004. Cationic polyelectrolyte hydrogel fosters fibroblast spreading, proliferation, and extracellular matrix production: implications for tissue engineering. *J. Cell Physiol.*, **198**(1), 133–43.

[151] La Gatta, A., Schiraldi, C., Esposito, A., D'Agostino, A. and De Rosa, A. 2009. Novel poly(HEMA-co-METAC)/alginate semi-interpenetrating hydrogels for biomedical applications: synthesis and characterization. *J. Biomed. Mater. Res. A*, **90**(1), 292–302.

[152] Detzel, C. J., Larkin, A. L. and Rajagopalan, P. 2011. Polyelectrolyte multilayers in tissue engineering. *Tissue Eng. Part B Rev.*, **17**(2), 101–13.

[153] Ho, S. T., Cool, S. M., Hui, J. H. and Hutmacher, D. W. 2010. The influence of fibrin based hydrogels on the chondrogenic differentiation of human bone marrow stromal cells. *Biomaterials*, **31**(1), 38–47.

[154] Huang, N. F. and Li, S. 2011. Regulation of the matrix microenvironment for stem cell engineering and regenerative medicine. *Ann. Biomed. Eng.*, **39**(4), 1201–14.

[155] Bhatia, S. R., Khattak, S. F. and Roberts, S. C. 2005. Polyelectrolytes for cell encapsulation. *Curr. Opin. Colloid Interf. Sci.*, **10**, 45.

[156] Varghese, D., Deshpande, M., Xu, T. *et al.* 2005. Advances in tissue engineering: cell printing. *J. Thorac. Cardiovasc. Surg.*, **129**(2), 470–72.

[157] Silver, F. H., Freeman, J. W. and Seehra, G. P. 2003. Collagen self-assembly and the development of tendon mechanical properties. *J. Biomech.*, **36**(10), 1529–53.

[158] Huang, J., Foo, C. W. P. and Kaplan, D. L. 2007. Biosynthesis and applications of silk-like and collagen-like proteins. *Polym. Rev.*, **47**, 29–62.

[159] Zhao, X. and Zhang, S. 2007. Designer self-assembling peptide materials. *Macromolec. Biosci.*, **7**(1), 13–22.

[160] Zhang, S. 2002. Emerging biological materials through molecular self-assembly. *Biotechnol. Adv.*, **20**(5–6), 321–39.

[161] Simsek-Ege, F. A., Bond, G. M. and Stringer, J. 2002. Matrix molecular weight cut-off for encapsulation of carbonic anhydrase in polyelectrolyte beads. *J. Biomater. Sci. Polym. Edition*, **13**(11), 1175–87.

[162] Decher, G., Hong, J. D. and Schmitt, J. 1992. Buildup of ultrathin multilayer films by a self-assembly process: III. Consecutively alternating adsorption of anionic and cationic polyelectrolytes on charged surfaces. *Thin Solid Films*, **210/211**, 831.

[163] Bertrand, P., Jonas, A., Laschewsky, A. and Legras, R. 2000. Ultrathin polymer coatings by complexation of polyelectrolytes at interfaces: suitable materials, structure and properties. *Macromolec. Rapid Commun.*, **21**, 319.

[164] Limem, S., Li, D. P., Iyengar, S. and Calvert, P. 2009. Multi-material inkjet printing of self-assembling and reacting coatings. *J. Macromolec. Sci. Part A – Pure Appl. Chem.*, **46**, 1205.

[165] Cellesi, F., Tirelli, N. and Hubbell, J. A. 2004. Towards a fully-synthetic substitute of alginate: development of a new process using thermal gelation and chemical crosslinking. *Biomaterials*, **25**(21), 5115–24.

[166] Vernon, B., Tirelli, N., Bachi, T., Haldimann, D. and Hubbell, J. A. 2003. Water-borne, in situ crosslinked biomaterials from phase-segregated precursors. *J. Biomed. Mater. Res. A*, **64**(3), 447–56.

[167] Biase, M. D., Saunders, R. E., Tirelli, N. and Derby, B. 2011. Inkjet printing and cell seeding thermoreversible photocurable gel structures. *Soft Matter*, **7**, 2639.

[168] Zarowna-Dabrowska, A., McKenna, E. O., Schutte, M. E. *et al.* 2012. Generation of primary hepatocyte microarrays by piezoelectric printing. *Colloids Surf. B Biointerfaces*, **89**, 126–32.

[169] Duocastella, M., Fernandez-Pradas, J. M., Morenza, J. L., Zafra, D. and Serra, P. 2010. Novel laser printing technique for miniaturized biosensors preparation. *Sensors Actuat. B - Chem.*, **145**(1), 596–600.

[170] Kattamis, N., Brown, M. and Arnold, C. B. 2010. Incident beam shape effects on thick-film laser induced forward transfer. In *2010 Conference on Lasers and Electro-Optics (CLEO) and Quantum Electronics and Laser Science Conference (QELS) 2010.*

[171] Arnold, C. B., Serra, P. and Pique, A. 2007. Laser direct-write techniques for printing of complex materials. *Mater. Res. Soc. Bull.*, **32**(1), 23–31.

[172] Tolbert, W. A., Lee, I. Y. S., Wen, X. N. *et al.* 1993. Laser-ablation transfer imaging using picosecond optical pulses - ultra-high-speed, lower threshold and high-resolution. *J. Imaging Sci. Technol.*, **37**(5), 485–9.

[173] Barron, J. A., Wu, P., Ladouceur, H. D. and Ringeisen, B. R. 2004. Biological laser printing: a novel technique for creating heterogeneous 3-dimensional cell patterns. *Biomed. Microdevices*, **6**(2), 139–47.

[174] Hopp, B., Smausz, T., Kresz, N. *et al.* 2005. Survival and proliferative ability of various living cell types after laser-induced forward transfer. *Tissue Eng.*, **11**(11–12), 1817–23.

[175] Doraiswamy, A., Narayan, R. J., Lippert, T. *et al.* 2006. Excimer laser forward transfer of mammalian cells using a novel triazene absorbing layer. *Appl. Surf. Sci.*, **252**(13), 4743–7.

[176] Nahmias, Y. K., Gao, B. Z. and Odde, D. J. 2004. Dimensionless parameters for the design of optical traps and laser guidance systems. *Appl. Opt.*, **43**(20), 3999–4006.

[177] Kubota, Y., Kleinman, H. K., Martin, G. R. and Lawley, T. J. 1988. Role of laminin and basement membrane in the morphological differentiation of human endothelial cells into capillary-like structures. *J. Cell Biol.*, **107**(4), 1589–98.

[178] Vernon, R. B., Angello, J. C., Iruela-Arispe, M. L., Lane, T. F. and Sage, E. H. 1992. Reorganization of basement membrane matrices by cellular traction promotes the formation of cellular networks in vitro. *Lab. Invest.*, **66**(5), 536–47.

[179] Neuman, K. C., Chadd, E. H., Liou, G. F., Bergman, K. and Block, S. M. 1999. Characterization of photodamage to *Escherichia coli* in optical traps. *Biophys. J.*, **77**(5), 2856–63.

[180] Liang, H., Vu, K. T., Krishnan, P. *et al.* 1996. Wavelength dependence of cell cloning efficiency after optical trapping. *Biophys. J.*, **70**(3), 1529–33.

[181] Renn, M. J., Montgomery, D., Vdovin, O. *et al.* 1995. Laser-guided atoms in hollow-core optical fibers. *Phys. Rev. Lett.*, **75**(18), 3253–6.

[182] Renn, M. J. and Pastel, R. 1998. Particle manipulation and surface patterning by laser guidance. *J. Vac. Sci. Technol. B*, **16**(6), 3859–63.

[183] Nahmias, Y. and Odde, D. J. 2006. Micropatterning of living cells by laser-guided direct writing: application to fabrication of hepatic-endothelial sinusoid-like structures. *Nature Protoc.* **1**(5), 2288–96.

[184] Narmoneva, D. A., Vukmirovic, R., Davis, M. E., Kamm, R. D. and Lee, R. T. 2004. Endothelial cells promote cardiac myocyte survival and spatial reorganization: implications for cardiac regeneration. *Circulation*, **110**(8), 962–8.

[185] Lammert, E., Cleaver, O. and Melton, D. 2001. Induction of pancreatic differentiation by signals from blood vessels. *Science*, **294**(5542), 564–7.

[186] Akselrod, G. M., Timp, W., Mirsaidov, U. *et al.* 2006. Laser-guided assembly of heterotypic three-dimensional living cell microarrays. *Biophys. J.*, **91**(9), 3465–73.

[187] Ho, C. T., Lin, R. Z., Chang, W. Y., Chang, H. Y. and Liu, C. H. 2006. Rapid heterogeneous liver-cell on-chip patterning via the enhanced field-induced dielectrophoresis trap. *Lab Chip*, **6**(6), 724–34.

[188] Gruene, M., Deiwick, A., Koch, L. *et al.* 2014. Laser printing of stem cells for biofabrication of scaffold-free autologous grafts. *Tissue Eng. Part C Methods*, to be published.

[189] Koch, L., Kuhn, S., Sorg, H. *et al.* 2010. Laser printing of skin cells and human stem cells. *Tissue Eng. Part C Methods*, **16**(5), 847–54.

[190] Chen, C. Y., Barron, J. A., Ringeisen, B. R. 2006. Cell patterning without chemical surface modification: cell–cell interactions between printed bovine aortic endothelial cells (BAEC) on a homogeneous cell-adherent hydrogel. *Appl. Surf. Sci.*, **252**(24), 8641–5.

[191] Barron, J. A., Ringeisen, B. R., Kim, H. S., Spargo, B. J. and Chrisey, D. B. 2004. Application of laser printing to mammalian cells. *Thin Solid Films*, **453**, 383–7.

[192] Ringeisen, B. R., Kim, H., Barron, J. A. *et al.* 2004. Laser printing of pluripotent embryonal carcinoma cells. *Tissue Eng.*, **10**(3–4), 483–91.

[193] Guillemot, F., Souquet, A., Catros, S. *et al.* 2010. High-throughput laser printing of cells and biomaterials for tissue engineering. *Acta Biomater.*, **6**(7), 2494–500.

[194] Duocastella, M., Fernandez-Pradas, J. M., Morenza, J. L. and Serra, P. 2009. Time-resolved imaging of the laser forward transfer of liquids. *J. Appl. Phys.*, **15**, 106 (8 pp.).

[195] Unger, C., Gruene, M., Koch, L., Koch, J. and Chichkov, B. N. 2011. Time-resolved imaging of hydrogel printing via laser-induced forward transfer. *Appl. Phys. A - Mater.*, **103**(2), 271–7.

[196] Gruene, M., Unger, C., Koch, L., Deiwick, A. and Chichkov, B. 2011. Dispensing pico to nanolitre of a natural hydrogel by laser-assisted bioprinting. *Biomed. Eng.*, doi:10.1186/1475-925X-10-19.

[197] Guillotin, B. and Guillemot, F. 2011. Cell patterning technologies for organotypic tissue fabrication. *Trends Biotechnol.*, **29**(4), 183–90.

[198] Kattamis, N. T., Purnick, P. E., Weiss, R. and Arnold, C. B. 2007. Thick film laser induced forward transfer for deposition of thermally and mechanically sensitive materials. *Appl. Phys. Lett.*, **91**, 171120.

[199] Arrabito, G. and Pignataro, B. 2010. Inkjet printing methodologies for drug screening. *Anal. Chem.*, **82**(8), 3104–7.

[200] Ringeisen, B. R., Othon, C. M., Barron, J. A., Young, D. and Spargo, B. J. 2006. Jet-based methods to print living cells. *Biotechnol. J.*, **1**(9), 930–48.

[201] Nakamura, M., Kobayashi, A., Takagi, F. *et al.* 2005. Biocompatible inkjet printing technique for designed seeding of individual living cells. *Tissue Eng.*, **11**(11–12), 1658–66.

[202] Schiele, N. R., Corr, D. T., Huang, Y. *et al.* 2010. Laser-based direct-write techniques for cell printing. *Biofabrication*, **2**(3), 032001.

[203] Duocastella, M., Colina, M., Fernandez-Pradas, J. M. *et al.* 2007. Study of the laser-induced forward transfer of liquids for laser bioprinting. *Appl. Surf. Sci.*, **253**(19), 7855–9.

PART IV

Biological factor delivery

20

Growth factor delivery on scaffolds

Kai Feng, Jiang Hu, Zubad Newaz and Peter X. Ma

20.1 Introduction

Traditionally tissue engineering entails the seeding and culturing of differentiated somatic cells onto biodegradable scaffolds, with subsequent implantation of the cell–scaffold constructs into the defective or damaged sites to regenerate tissues [1]. In this approach, the scaffold acts as a three-dimensional (3D) framework to provide physical support and accommodate cell growth and deposition of extracellular matrices, and its biodegradability allows the scaffold material to be resorbed in pace with new tissue formation. Despite some encouraging successes in clinical trials [2, 3], two key limitations with this approach include the limited source of exogenous donor cells and the lack of adequate vascularity to maintain vitality of the newly regenerated tissues. To address these limitations, current advanced tissue engineering techniques gear toward harnessing a biomimetic scaffold that provides a synthetic regenerative microenvironment to support natural tissue regeneration and angiogenesis [4]. In addition to providing physical support, the ideal biomimetic scaffold would preferably also deliver bioactive factors, which instruct endogenous stem cell recruitment and differentiation three-dimensionally and in a controlled manner [5] (Figure 20.1). Various bioactive factors, including growth factors [6–8], nucleic acids [9], and integrin-binding ligands [10], have successfully been delivered or presented on biodegradable scaffolds. Among these, growth factors are the most important soluble signals in the natural regenerative microenvironment, being actively involved in stem cell recruitment, proliferation, and differentiation, angiogenesis, and tissue morphogenesis. Although they are potent, growth factors are expensive and have short half-lives in vivo. Therefore, scaffolds with controlled-release capacity are desired in order to preserve growth factor bioactivity and to prolong their function at therapeutic levels over an extended time period. However, there remain significant challenges in delivering growth factors effectively from scaffolds, including the need to preserve the bioactivity of growth factors during the possibly harsh incorporation process, the control of their release over an extended period during tissue regeneration, and the need for release to be restricted locally so as to avoid toxic or unwanted systemic side effects. Additionally, each individual delivery strategy is related, and sometimes restricted, to the type of scaffold utilized.

This chapter will review current advances in strategies and technologies to incorporate growth factor controlled-release systems into several major types of biodegradable tissue engineering scaffold, including hydrogel and porous polymer foams, and the newly developed nanofibrous polymer scaffolds. Considering the vast variety of growth factors and their multiple functions, we will limit our examples to the effects of delivered growth factors promoting angiogenesis and bone formation in the applications of these growth factor delivery scaffolds.

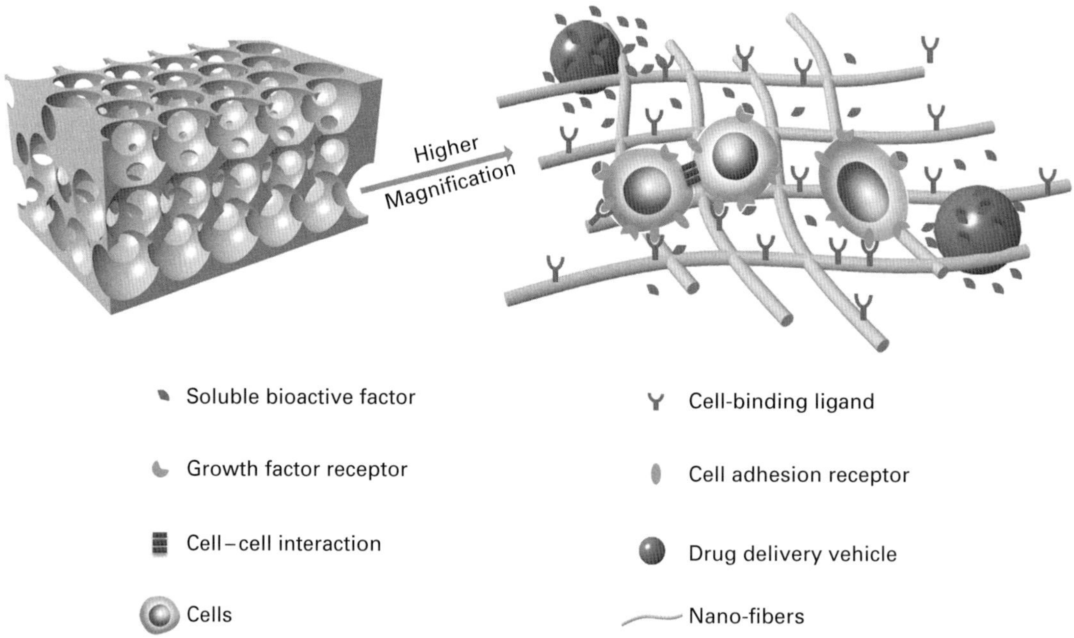

Figure 20.1 A schematic illustration of a biomimetic scaffold with an integrated synthetic regenerative microenvironment. The scaffold can not only provide a physical structure that accommodates cell growth and tissue formation, but also serve as extracellular matrix-mimicking matrices to enhance cell-scaffold interactions and deliver bioactive factors in a temporally and spatially controlled manner. (Reprinted from [5] *Advanced Drug Delivery Reviews*, **64**, Zhang, Z., Hu, J., and Ma, P.X., Nanofiber-based delivery of bioactive agents and stem cells to bone sites, 1129–41, Copyright (2012), with permission from Elsevier.)

20.2 Selected examples of growth factors used for mineralized tissue regeneration and angiogenesis

Recent progress in understanding the role of growth factors in tissue repair and regeneration has been a prime asset in the development of novel regenerative technologies. The molecular form of biologically active growth factors is a protein structure, which allows modulation of cellular activity via induction of conformational changes on cellular transmembrane receptors. Several consequences of cell-growth-factor interactions include chemotaxis, cell proliferation, differentiation, and angiogenesis – all instrumental in the formation of regenerated tissues. An essential consideration of growth factor molecular structure with respect to tissue engineering is the preservation of bioactivity, since the growth factors are susceptible to conformational changes or inactivation of functional groups if not protected in their interactions with scaffold material in the various incorporation processes.

The growth factors utilized particularly in the regeneration of highly mineralized tissues, such as bone or dentin, are bone morphogenetic proteins (BMPs). Among the 20 known BMPs, BMP-2, BMP-4, and BMP-7 are commonly used for bone and tooth tissue engineering. BMP-2 and BMP-7 induce osteoblast differentiation [11, 12], and play important roles in the development of bone and cartilage alike [13]. BMP-4 plays a role in bone mineralization, and is additionally known to be expressed throughout the stages of embryonic tooth development [14]. Angiogenic growth factors, such as basic fibroblast growth factor (bFGF) [15], platelet-derived growth factor (PDGF) [16], and

Table 20.1 Biological activity of a few select growth factors related to mineralized tissue regeneration and angiogenesis

Growth factor	Biological function	Reference
Bone morphogenetic protein-2	Induce osteoblast differentiation, stimulate bone and cartilage development	[12, 13]
Bone morphogenetic protein-4	Bone mineralization, embryonic tooth development	[14]
Bone morphogenetic protein-7	Induce osteoblast differentiation, stimulate bone and cartilage development	[11, 13]
Basic fibroblast growth factor	Potent inducer of endothelial cell proliferation	[15]
Platelet-derived growth factor	Differentiation of mesenchymal stem cells, recruitment of smooth muscle cells, angiogenesis, wound healing	[16]
Vascular endothelial growth factor	Stimulate endothelial cell mitogenesis and migration	[17]

vascular endothelial growth factor (VEGF) [17], have been used to promote vascularized tissue regeneration, including formation of mineralized tissue. As a few examples, the biological functions of some growth factors frequently used for mineralized tissue regeneration and angiogenesis are listed in Table 20.1.

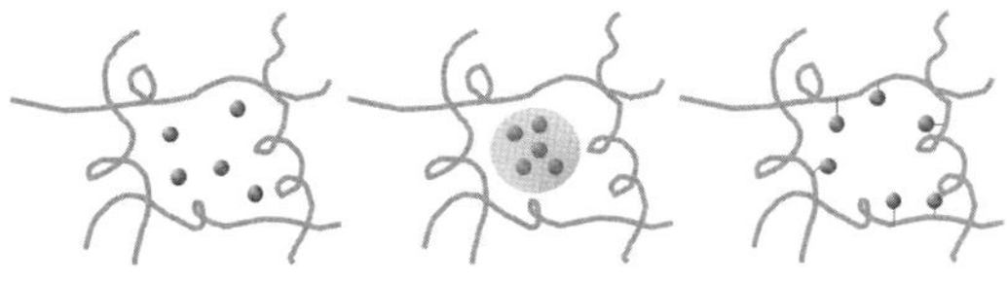

Figure 20.2 Schematic illustrations of growth factor delivery strategies on hydrogel scaffolds: (a) direct incorporation; (b) microparticle encapsulation; and (c) covalent immobilization.

20.3 Growth factor delivery from hydrogel scaffolds

Hydrogel scaffolds are frequently used to engineer highly metabolic soft tissues, for which the load-bearing capacity is less demanding but high permeabilities of oxygen and nutrients are desirable [18, 19]. Three major techniques have been applied to deliver growth factors from hydrogel scaffolds: direct incorporation, microparticle encapsulation, and covalent immobilization (Figure 20.2).

The typical release profile of directly incorporated growth factors from hydrogels (Figure 20.2(a)) consists of a rapid burst release during the initial swelling phase, followed by an extended release of protein retarded by the crosslink network of the hydrogel polymer. Since a hydrogel contains more than 90% water by weight, the diffusion of incorporated growth factors is mainly determined by the size of the growth factor relative to the density of chemical or physical crosslinks between polymer chains [20]. Several attempts have been made to adjust the crosslink density to tune the release profiles [21, 22]. A slower release rate can be achieved by introducing charged polymers such as gelatin to interact with the incorporated growth factors via oppositely charged functional groups [23]. Although the methodology itself is straightforward, concerns with this approach include the denaturation of growth factors due to chemical crosslinking if they are loaded into a hydrogel before crosslinking or the uneven distribution of the growth factors if they are loaded into a hydrogel after the crosslinking.

Microparticle-encapsulation systems made from hydrophobic non-swelling polymers [24], solid lipids [25] or hydrophilic polymers [26] can be incorporated into a hydrogel system (Figure 20.2(b)) to further alter the release profile. The growth factor release profile depends on the degradation of the microparticles, which allows several growth factors to be released at different release rates by using different types of microparticles [27].

The process of growth factor incorporation into hydrogel by chemical covalent immobilization (Figure 20.2(c)) entails the bonding of the functional groups of the growth factor to certain sites of the hydrogel polymer [28], and in some cases with an enzymatically cleavable tether [29]. These designed hydrogels with attached growth factors are useful in some tissue engineering applications, although concerns about the stability of the attached growth factors remain.

20.4 Growth factor delivery from porous foam scaffolds

Several techniques have been applied to incorporate and deliver growth factors from 3D porous foam scaffolds, including passive adsorption, covalent immobilization, polymer emulsion surface coating, and direct encapsulation (Figure 20.3).

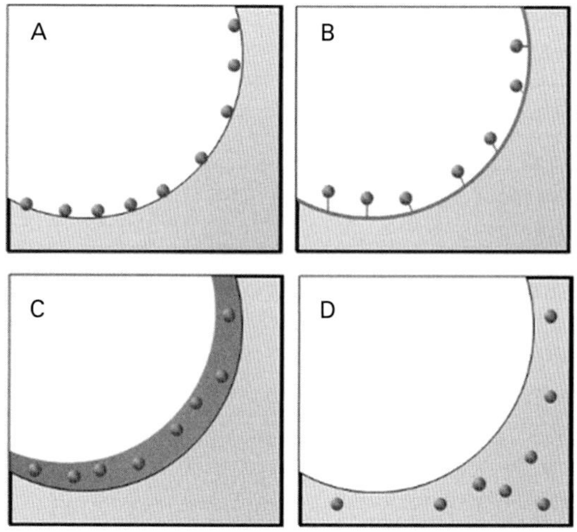

Figure 20.3 Schematic illustrations of growth factor delivery strategies on porous foam scaffolds: (a) passive absorption; (b) surface functionalization and covalent immobilization; (c) polymer emulsion surface coating; and (d) direct encapsulation.

Prefabricated porous scaffolds can be immersed in a protein solution to passively adsorb the proteins on the surface of scaffolds (Figure 20.3(a)). The adsorption process involves electrostatic interactions, hydrogen bonding, and hydrophobic interactions between the proteins and hydrophobic foam scaffolds, leading to potential protein conformational change and loss of bioactivity. The release profile of growth factors adsorbed on a scaffold is not controlled, resulting in a very short release period. Meanwhile, the growth factors are not protected, resulting in their denaturation and failure to achieve the desired biological effects over an extended period [30].

Covalent immobilization involves using chemical bonds to immobilize growth factors on the scaffold pore wall surface (Figure 20.3(b)). In many cases, the biodegradable scaffolds are fabricated from commercial polymers that lack functional groups to enable the conjugation reactions. Therefore the pore surface may need to be activated first in order to present functional groups, which are subsequently employed to conjugate with growth factors through appropriate reactions. There are various ways to activate the scaffold pore surface after scaffold fabrication. For example, plasma treatment and ultraviolet irradiation have been used to alter the polymer surface chemistry [31, 32]. Plasma treatment can create diverse functional groups, including amine and carboxyl groups, if the plasma source is properly configured. These functional groups or free radicals can be utilized to initiate surface graft polymerization in order to introduce the desired chemistry. It should be noted that these methods could be applied only to two-dimensional (2D) films or very thin 3D scaffolds due to the limited plasma penetration depth. Chemical etching is another method for surface modification [33, 34]. For the widely used biodegradable polyesters, the exposed ester bonds in the polymer backbone partially degrade under acidic or basic conditions, resulting in carboxyl and hydroxyl groups on the surface. However, strong reaction conditions should be avoided in order to maintain the integrity of the scaffold. Various conjugation techniques for protein immobilization have been developed. While most conjugation methods involve non-selective reactions between the functional groups of a protein and those on a biomaterial, there are more complicated techniques to achieve selective conjugation, which involve site-specific labeling of proteins and peptide tags [35]. Primary amine and carboxyl groups are the most frequently utilized reaction sites in growth factors for conjugation. The reaction rate between amine and carboxyl groups could be accelerated by using the 1-ethyl-3-(3-dimethylaminopropyl) carbodiimide (EDC)–N-hydroxysuccinimide (NHS) chemistry [36]. Recently, click chemistry has been attracting much attention and shows great potential in growth factor conjugation, because the reactions are irreversible, quantitative, and mild [37]. However, some widely used click reactions, such as the azide–alkyne Huisgen cycloaddition [38], employ metal catalysts with potential toxic effects on cells. Catalyst-free click reactions are more attractive for scaffold functionalization [39]. In addition, a stimuli-responsive release profile can be achieved when stimuli-responsive linkers are employed in the conjugation reaction [40]. A common concern with covalent immobilization is the inactivation of the growth factors during chemical reaction, especially when the active site of the growth factor is involved in the conjugation reaction.

Polymer emulsion surface coating is another method used to physically load growth factors on the surface of prefabricated porous foam scaffolds (Figure 20.3(c)). The bioactivity of growth factors can be protected, and the release time period is extended by the introduction of a protective polymer layer. However, the porous structure of the scaffold may be significantly altered by the coating process [41].

Alternatively, growth factors can be mixed with polymer emulsion and directly physically encapsulated inside porous scaffold walls during an emulsion freeze-drying scaffold fabrication process (Figure 20.3(d)). BMP-2 released from a scaffold prepared in such manner enhanced ectopic bone formation in rats [42]. While this method combines the scaffold fabrication and growth factor incorporation into a single step, the structure and mechanical properties of scaffolds are subject to inadvertent alteration. An additional limitation is that the growth factor release rate simply depends on the scaffold bulk degradation rate, leaving little room to tune the release profile to match regeneration rates of various tissues.

20.5 Growth factor delivery from nanofibrous scaffolds

The surface architecture of the scaffold can be engineered to more closely mimic an intrinsic extracellular microenvironment and thereby enhance the desired cell–scaffold interactions for tissue regeneration. Collagen is the major organic component of the extracellular matrices of many tissues, being present in the form of a fibrous network with fiber diameters ranging from 50 to 500 nm [43]. Numerous studies have shown that collagen fibers promote osteogenesis as well as the regeneration of other collagenous tissues [44, 45]. Scaffolds with nanofibrous architecture were developed on this premise to mimic the structural features and functional properties of collagenous extracellular matrices. For convenience of discussion, fibers with diameters ranging from a few nanometers to a few micrometers, intended for tissue engineering applications, are collectively referred to as "nanofibers." In many cases, higher amounts of growth factors can be loaded on nanofibrous scaffolds due to their larger surface-to-volume ratio. The delivery of growth factors from two commonly used techniques to fabricate nanofibrous structure, namely electrospinning and thermally induced phase separation, will be discussed.

20.5.1 Growth factor delivery on electrospun nanofibrous scaffolds

Owing to the wide variety of material choices and simplicity of fabrication, electrospun scaffolds have been applied in multiple types of tissue regeneration [46–48]. In general, four major techniques have been used to incorporate growth factors into electrospun scaffolds, namely physical adsorption, covalent immobilization, blend/emulsion electrospinning, and coaxial electrospinning.

Physical adsorption and covalent immobilization processes are similar to the above-mentioned modification techniques used for conventional porous foam scaffolds. Among the growth-factor-loading techniques, physical adsorption is the simplest method to incorporate growth factors into an electrospun scaffold, since the electrospun scaffold is simply dipped into an aqueous solution containing growth factors. The major disadvantages of this approach are the denaturation, uncontrolled release profile, and very short duration of release. Covalent immobilization utilizes the ability of functional groups both on the growth factors and on the electrospun scaffold surface to form a covalent bond, just as for conventional porous foam scaffolds.

The blend electrospinning approach mixes growth factors within the polymer solution and electrospins the mixed solution into a hybrid scaffold with growth factors localized within the fibers of the scaffold. This approach is also called "emulsion electrospinning" when growth factors are emulsified into polymer solution by ultrasonication or homogenization [49]. Compared with physical adsorption, blend electrospinning usually results in a more sustained growth factor release profile, which can last over several weeks. A typical growth factor release profile from blend electrospun scaffolds consists of an initial burst release followed by a sustained release. The major disadvantage of this approach is the loss of bioactivity of the incorporated growth factors due to their conformational changes in the organic solution environment or under harsh mixing conditions. Several strategies have been applied to address this issue, including the addition of hydrophilic polymers such as poly(ethylene glycol) (PEG) in the aqueous growth factor solution to improve protein stability [50], as well as the addition of hydrophilic hydroxyapatite (HAP) to adsorb growth factors [51], reducing the damage caused by the harsh electrospinning process.

Coaxial electrospinning is a specific electrospinning technique to produce growth factors containing composite nanofibers with a core–shell structure by coaxially and simultaneously electrospinning a growth factor solution and a polymer solution through different feeding capillary channels in one needle (Figure 20.4). The bioactivity of the growth factors in the core can be preserved because of its minimal contact with the organic solvent used in the shell. The growth factor release profile from a coaxial electrospun scaffold also consists of two stages. However, the burst release is significantly reduced and the release duration is prolonged [52], compared with the release profile from a blend electrospun scaffold. This is because the growth factors are mainly incorporated and distributed in the core part. The polymer shell provides a barrier membrane, which controls the protein diffusion rate. Introduction of porogens in the polymer shell is able to further tune the growth factor release profile [53]. One concern of co-axial electrospinning is the potential compromise of scaffold fiber morphology and mechanical properties.

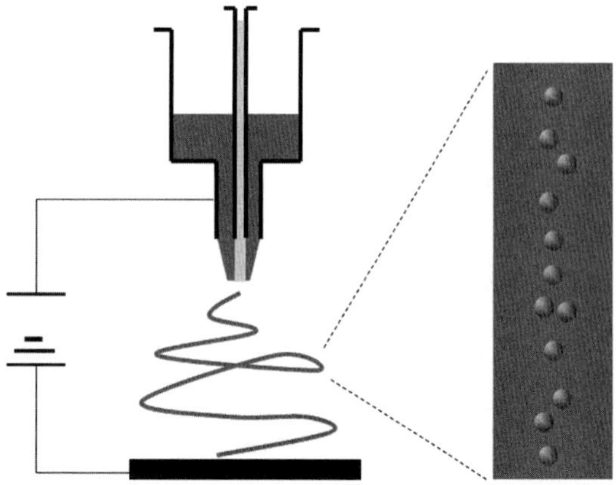

Figure 20.4 A schematic illustration of growth factor delivery via co-axial electrospinning.

As discussed above, electrospinning has been a very useful technique to generate nanofibrous scaffolds and to incorporate growth factors. However, the electrospinning technique remains a difficult modality for creating a macropore network and complex 3D shapes for large-scale tissue regeneration.

20.5.2 Growth factor delivery on phase-separated nanofibrous scaffolds

Three-dimensional nanofibrous scaffolds have been developed using thermally induced phase-separation (TIPS) techniques [54, 55]. The overall 3D shape of the scaffolds can be designed to simulate a specific human anatomical part or defect by a reverse solid free-form fabrication technique [56, 57]. Their interconnected spherical macropore network promotes cell penetration. Their nanofibrous architecture mimics intrinsic

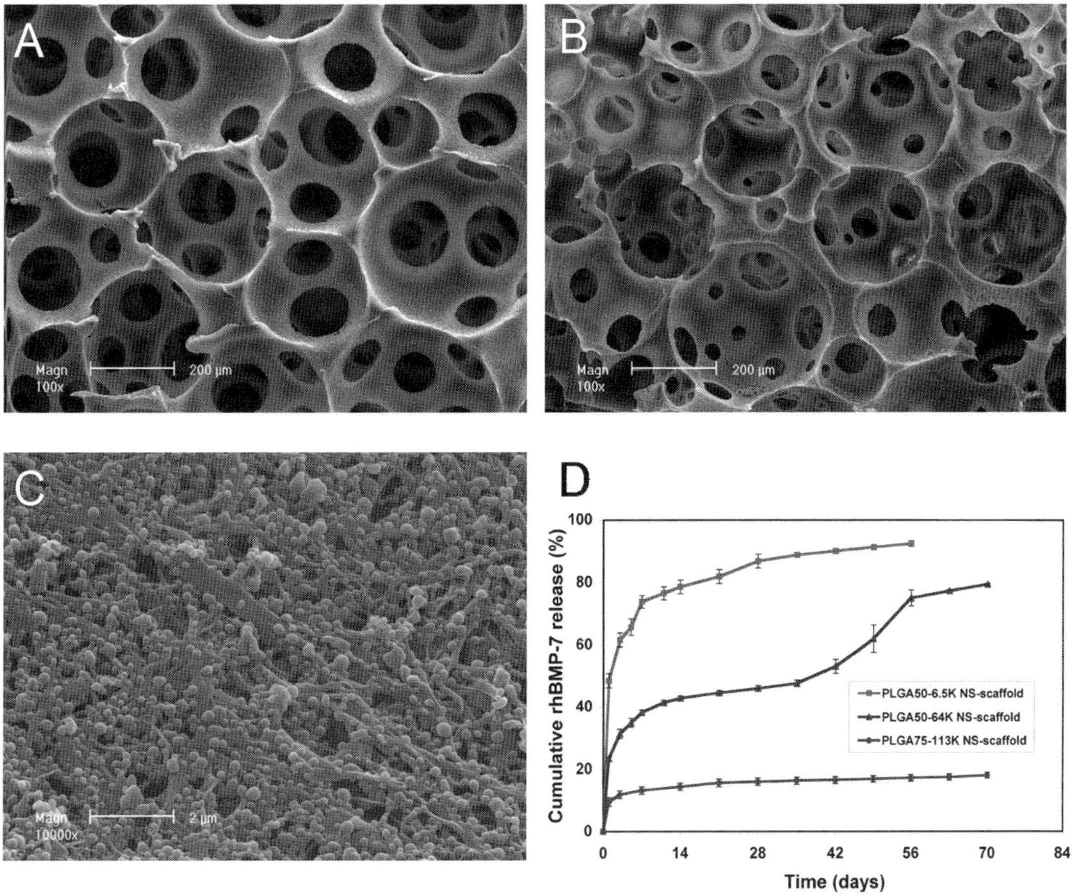

Figure 20.5 Growth factor delivery via microsphere (MS)/nanosphere (NS) encapsulation and immobilization on nanofibrous (NF) scaffolds. (A) Scanning electron micrographs of the macropore structure of poly(L-lactic acid) (PLLA) NF scaffolds before NS immobilization and (B) after NS immobilization. (C) NS immobilized on the NF wall matrices. (D) In-vitro release kinetics of bone morphogenetic protein-7 (BMP-7) from NS immobilized on NF scaffolds. Three distinct BMP-7 release profiles were achieved with NS composed of different poly(lactic-*co*-glycolic acid) (PLGA) formulations (PLGA50-6.5K, LA/GA ratio 50/50, molecular weight (MW) 6.5 kDa; PLGA50-64K, LA/GA ratio 50/50, MW 64 kDa; PLGA75-113K, LA/GA ratio 75/25, MW 113 kDa). (Reprinted from [64] *Biomaterials*, **28**, Wei, G., Jin, Q., Giannobile, W. V., and Ma, P. X., The enhancement of osteogenesis by nano-fibrous scaffolds incorporating rhBMP-7 nanospheres, 2087–96, Copyright (2007), with permission from Elsevier.)

extracellular matrices to promote cell attachment, proliferation, and differentiation. With these beneficial features, these 3D porous scaffolds have found applications in the regeneration of a variety of tissues [58, 59].

In order to overcome the shortcomings associated with the above-discussed growth-factor-incorporation methods for conventional porous foam scaffolds, a novel technique was developed. Growth factors are first encapsulated into polymer microspheres (MSs) or nanospheres (NSs), and then such spheres are immobilized onto the nanofibrous pore wall surface of prefabricated scaffolds via tight attachment of spheres to nanofibrous matrices [60] (Figure 20.5). Polymeric MSs and NSs have been widely applied to encapsulate a variety of bioactive factors, and their ability to protect the encapsulated bioactive factors from denaturation and degradation has been demonstrated in many reports [61, 62]. In a typical procedure, an aqueous growth factor solution is mixed with a poly (lactic-co-glycolic acid) (PLGA) polymer solution to encapsulate the growth factor into PLGA spheres using a water-in-oil-in-water double-emulsion process [63]. The sphere size ranges from nanometers to micrometers, depending on the emulsion parameters such as surfactant concentration and emulsion strength applied. Subsequently, these obtained growth-factor-containing PLGA MSs/NSs are immobilized onto the inner nanofibrous pore surface of a prefabricated scaffold via a post-seeding method. This MS/NS encapsulation and loading method offers several advantages over conventional direct encapsulation techniques. First, scaffold fabrication is separated from growth factor incorporation. The macroporous architecture and the mechanical and degradation properties of the scaffolds are not altered after growth factor incorporation. Therefore the growth factor release and the scaffold degradation can be individually rationally optimized. Second, the temporally differentiated release of different sets of growth factors from the same scaffold can be easily achieved, by employing the chemical and degradation properties of the MS/NS polymer formulation. The release of the encapsulated proteins occurs in two phases, with the early phase mainly controlled by diffusion and the late phase mainly controlled by polymer degradation. Release durations from several days to months can be easily achieved by adjusting polymer formulations such as the PLGA copolymer LA/GA ratio and/or the molecular weight (more formally, relative molecular mass) of the copolymer. Thirdly, the immobilization of MSs/NSs on porous nanofibrous scaffolds can reduce the burst release of growth factors and prolong the release duration [64].

20.6 Applications of growth factor delivery scaffolds in tissue regeneration

Examples of applications demonstrating the ability of growth factor delivery from scaffolds to promote angiogenesis and osteogenesis will be discussed in this section. The effect of controlled release of growth factors in instructing stem cell recruitment and differentiation, and recent advances in constructing a beneficial stem cell niche, will be stressed, since the stem cells are the key target of delivered growth factors.

Since most tissues are highly vascularized, the induction of rapid ingrowth of a vascular network can potentially accelerate tissue regeneration. In one study, PDGF, an angiogenic factor that has been demonstrated to promote wound healing [16], was encapsulated into nanofibrous poly(L-lactic acid) (PLLA) scaffolds using the above-described MS/NS encapsulation and loading method [60], and then the scaffolds were subcutaneously implanted into rats (Figure 20.6). After implantation, MS scaffolds promoted tissue penetration and angiogenesis within the scaffolds. The biological effects of released PDGF depended both on the release dosage and on the release profile, with scaffolds releasing PDGF at higher dosage and with an extended time course resulting in enhanced angiogenesis. How the delivered growth factors induce stem cell recruitment and participation in the construction and maintenance of new vasculature remains open for further investigation. A recent study showed that the gene expression profiles of several chemokines that have been found to play an import role in stem cell recruitment were related to the PDGF release profile [65].

In another study of applying growth factor delivery scaffolds to regenerate bone tissues, BMP-7 was encapsulated and loaded on nanofibrous PLLA scaffolds using the same method, and then the scaffolds were subcutaneously implanted into rats [64] (Figure 20.7). BMP-7 has been shown to promote new bone formation in animal models both at ectopic and at orthotopic sites [66, 67]. After implantation, NS scaffolds promoted ectopic new bone formation inside the scaffolds, while neither the control scaffolds without BMP-7 loading nor the scaffolds with passive adsorption of the same amount of BMP-7 could induce bone formation. The failure with the passive-adsorption scaffolds was probably due to the loss of bioactivity during adsorption, and the

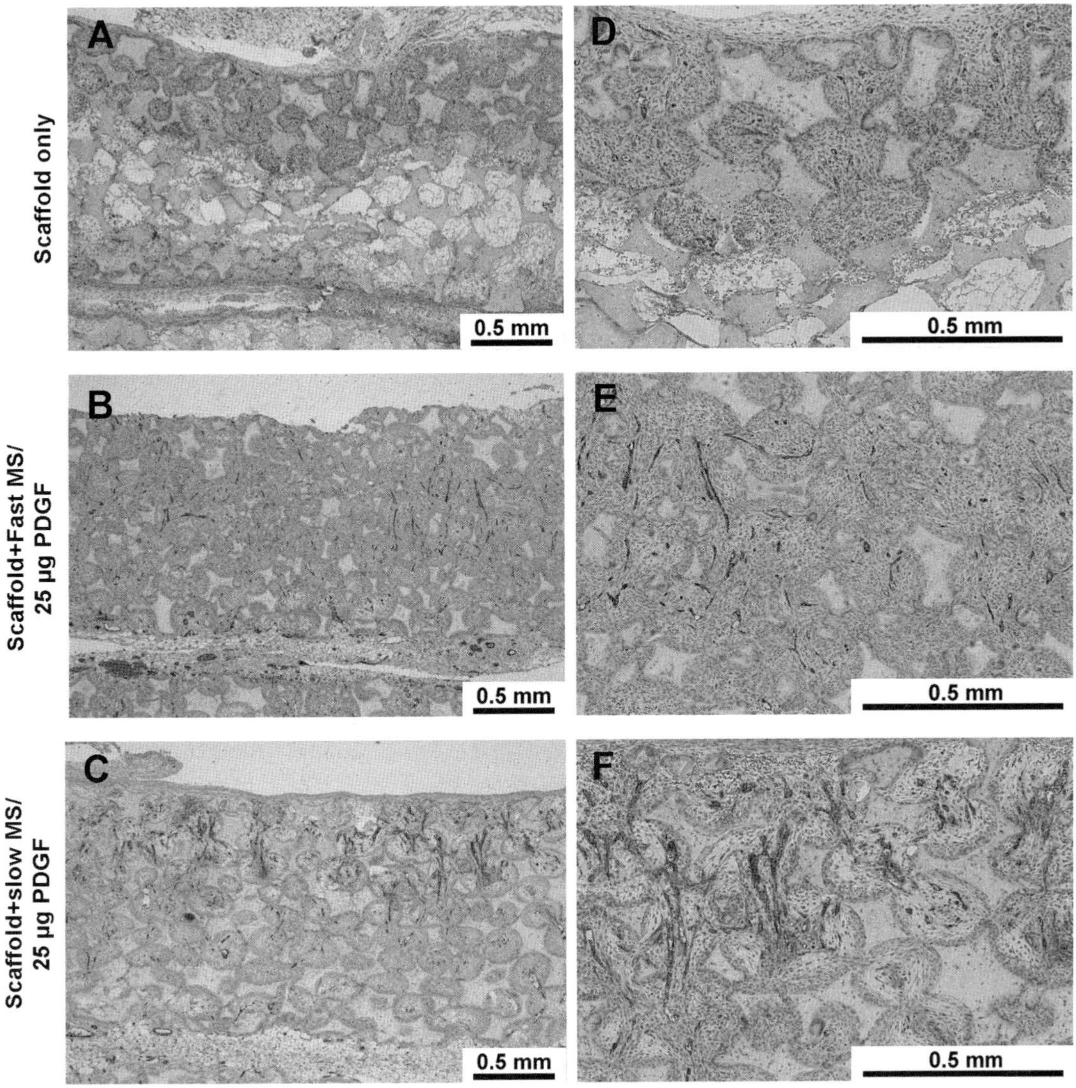

Figure 20.6 Nanofibrous scaffolds with platelet-derived growth factor (PDGF) microspheres (MS) promote angiogenesis in vivo after one week of subcutaneous implantation: left panels, low magnification; right panels, high magnification; (A) and (D) scaffold only; (B) and (E) MS scaffold with fast-releasing 25 µg of PDGF per scaffold; (C) and (F) MS scaffold with slow-releasing 25 µg of PDGF per scaffold. (Reprinted from [65] *PLoS One*, **3**, Jin, Q., Wei, G., Lin, Z., Sugai, J. V., Lynch, S. E., Ma, P. X., and Giannobile, W. V., Nanofibrous scaffolds incorporating PDGF-BB microspheres induce chemokine expression and tissue neogenesis in vivo, e1729, (2008).)

insufficient duration of release upon implantation. The ectopic bone formation occurs by an endochondral ossification process, with consequent events of mesenchymal stem cell (MSC) recruitment, stem cell differentiation into a cartilaginous template, vascular infiltration, and ossification, which is initiated and orchestrated principally by the controlled release of BMPs from the scaffolds.

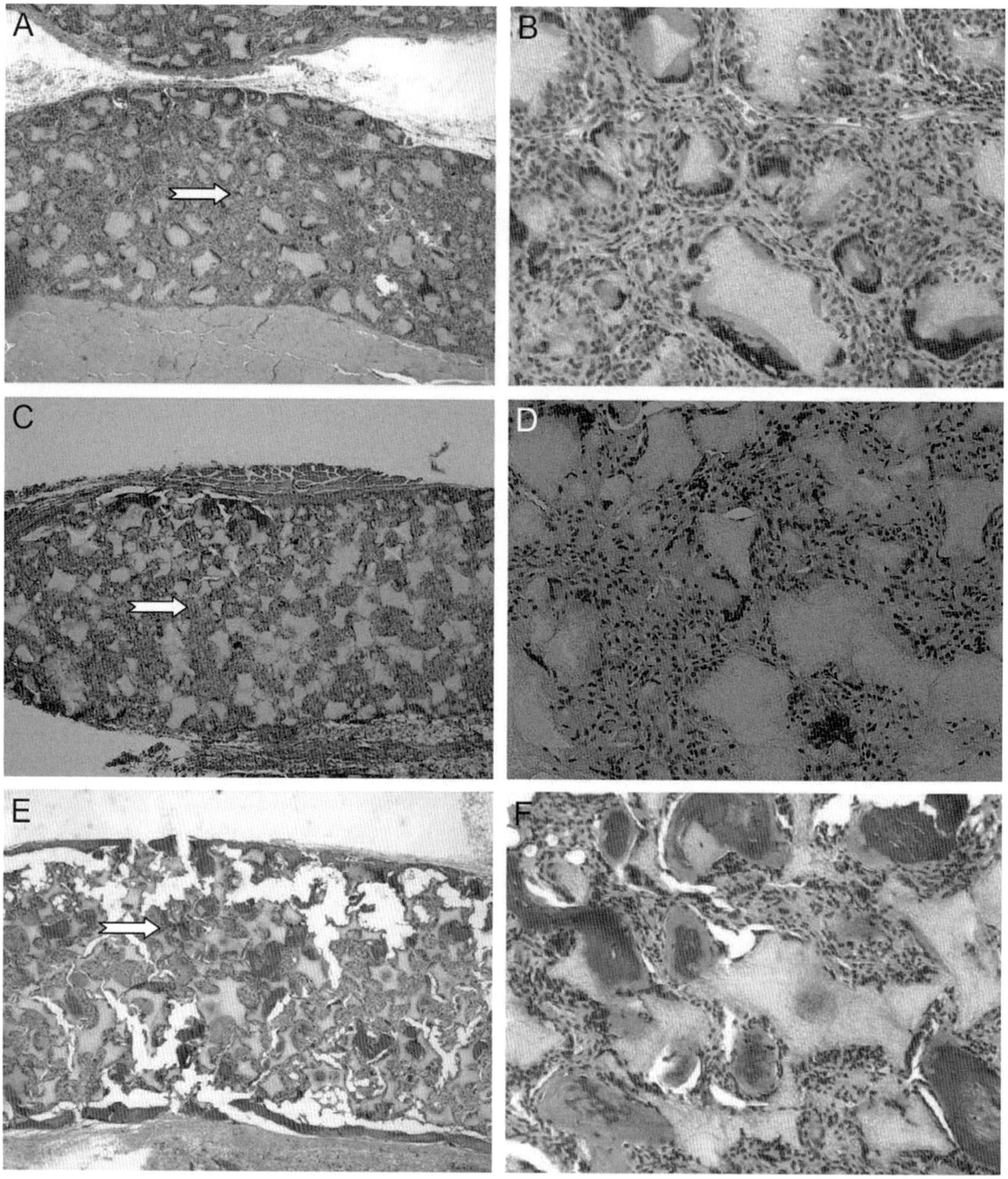

Figure 20.7 Nanofibrous scaffolds with bone morphogenetic protein-7 (BMP-7) nanospheres (NS) promote osteogenesis in vivo after six weeks of subcutaneous implantation: (A) and (B) scaffold only; (C) and (D) 5 μg of BMP-7 adsorbed to scaffold; (E) and (F) 5 μg BMP-7 incorporated in NS scaffold. Original magnifications: (A), (C), and (E) full cross-sections; and (B), (D), and (F) high-magnification views (arrows indicate the selected areas in (A), (C), and (E). (Reprinted from [64] *Biomaterials*, **28**, Wei, G., Jin, Q., Giannobile, W. V., and Ma, P. X., The enhancement of osteogenesis by nano-fibrous scaffolds incorporating rhBMP-7 nanospheres, 2087–96, Copyright (2007), with permission from Elsevier.)

The specialized microenvironment determining stem cell fate and modulating stem cell function, i.e. the stem cell niche, can also be the target of tissue regeneration technologies. Bone marrow niche is among the most studied of such niche microenvironments [68]. By delivering MSCs on scaffolds to construct bone tissues and organize bone marrow niche, host hematopoietic stem cells can migrate inward to eventually constitute functional bone marrow tissues [69], providing a potential live cell source for stem cell therapies. The delivery of BMPs on scaffolds, either alone or in combination with other kinds of growth factor, can provide an alternative on-shelf solution to instruct bone marrow niche development and construct functional bone marrow tissues, without the inherent immunocompatibility issues of the cell-delivery approach.

20.7 Conclusion

Since the emergence of tissue engineering technology late in the twentieth century, interest from scientists, engineers, and healthcare professionals has been generated globally. Tissue engineering has experienced tremendous growth in recent years with the advent of novel biomimetic scaffolds to serve both as functional structural support for cell growth and as temporally and spatially controlled delivery vehicles for growth factors to regulate stem cell behavior and tissue regeneration at multiple levels. This chapter summarizes the current approaches used in growth factor delivery on several major types of biodegradable scaffolds. Despite the significant progress in delivering growth factors from biomimetic scaffolds, noteworthy challenges and questions remain. The parameters of biomimetic scaffolds, including mechanical properties, growth factor release profile, and architectural features allowing them to accommodate or interact with stem cells, are all highly dependent on the fabrication technologies. While significant progress has been made in nanofiber technologies and their applications in tissue regeneration, there remains inadequate mechanistic understanding, limiting the pace of advancement of the field. More systematic and quantitative studies are needed in order to establish the relationships among nanostructural features, growth factor delivery, stem cell recruitment and differentiation, and tissue regeneration. Interdisciplinary and multidisciplinary approaches and collaborations are necessary to tackle these challenges. Moreover, while encouraging results show the potential of these biomimetic scaffolds in the laboratory, more translational studies are required before they can be widely applied clinically as therapeutic modalities.

ACKNOWLEDGEMENTS

The authors would like to acknowledge the financial support from the National Institutes of Health (NIDCR DE015384, DE017689 and DE022327: PXM), DOD (W81XWH-12-2-0008: PXM) and NSF (DMR-1206575: PXM). Z.N. was partially supported by an AADR Student Research Fellowship.

REFERENCES

[1] Langer, R. and Vacanti, J. P. 1993. Tissue engineering. *Science*, **260**(5110), 920–6.

[2] Shin'oka, T., Imai, Y. and Ikada, Y. 2001. Transplantation of a tissue-engineered pulmonary artery. *New Engl. J. Med.*, **344**(7), 532–3.

[3] Raya-Rivera, A., Esquiliano, D. R., Yoo, J. J. *et al.* 2011. Tissue-engineered autologous urethras for patients who need reconstruction: an observational study. *Lancet*, **377**(9772), 1175–82.

[4] Ma, P. X. 2008. Biomimetic materials for tissue engineering. *Adv. Drug Delivery Rev.*, **60**(2), 184–98.

[5] Zhang, Z., Hu, J. and Ma, P. X. 2012. Nanofiber-based delivery of bioactive agents and stem cells to bone sites. *Adv. Drug Delivery Rev.*, **64**(22), 1129–41.

[6] Whang, K., Tsai, D. C., Nam, E. K. *et al.* 1998. Ectopic bone formation via rhBMP-2 delivery from porous bioabsorbable polymer scaffolds. *J. Biomed. Mater. Res.*, **42**(4), 491–9.

[7] Oldham, J. B., Lu, L., Zhu, X. *et al.* 2000. Biological activity of rhBMP-2 released from PLGA microspheres. *J. Biomech. Eng. Trans. ASME*, **122**(3), 289–92.

[8] Peter, S. J., Lu, L., Kim, D. J. *et al.* 2000. Effects of transforming growth factor beta 1 released from biodegradable polymer microparticles on marrow stromal osteoblasts cultured on poly(propylene fumarate) substrates. *J. Biomed. Mater. Res.*, **50**(3), 452–62.

[9] Shea, L. D., Smiley, E., Bonadio, J. and Mooney, D. J. 1999. DNA delivery from polymer matrices for tissue engineering. *Nature Biotechnol.*, **17**(6), 551–4.

[10] Hern, D. L. and Hubbell, J. A. 1998. Incorporation of adhesion peptides into nonadhesive hydrogels useful for tissue resurfacing. *J. Biomed. Mater. Res.*, **39**(2), 266–76.

[11] Asahina, I., Sampath, T. K., Nishimura, I. and Hauschka, P. V. 1993. Human osteogenic protein-1 induces both chondroblastic and osteoblastic differentiation of osteoprogenitor cells derived from newborn rat calvaria. *J. Cell Biol.*, **123**(4), 921–33.

[12] Torii, Y., Hitomi, K. and Tsukagoshi, N. 1996. Synergistic effect of BMP-2 and ascorbate on the phenotypic expression of osteoblastic MC3T3-E1 cells. *Molec. Cellular Biochem.*, **165**(1), 25–9.

[13] Wozney, J. M. and Rosen, V. 1998. Bone morphogenetic protein and bone morphogenetic protein gene family in bone formation and repair. *Clin. Orthopaedics Related Res.*, **346**, 26–37.

[14] Neubuser, A., Peters, H., Balling, R. and Martin, G. R. 1997 Antagonistic interactions between FGF and BMP signaling pathways: a mechanism for positioning the sites of tooth formation. *Cell*, **90**(2), 247–55.

[15] Servold, S. A. 1991. Growth factor impact on wound healing. *Clinics Podiatric Med. Surg.*, **8**(4), 937–53.

[16] Robson, M. C., Mustoe, T. A. and Hunt, T. K. 1998. The future of recombinant growth factors in wound healing. *Am. J. Surg.*, **176**(Suppl. 2A), 80–2.

[17] Gerwins, P., Skoldenberg, E. and Claesson-Welsh, L. 2000. Function of fibroblast growth factors and vascular endothelial growth factors and their receptors in angiogenesis. *Crit. Rev. Oncol. Hematol.*, **34**(3), 185–94.

[18] Lee, K. Y. and Mooney, D. J. 2001. Hydrogels for tissue engineering. *Chem. Rev.*, **101**(7), 1869–79.

[19] Nguyen, K. T. and West, J. L. 2002. Photopolymerizable hydrogels for tissue engineering applications. *Biomaterials*, **23**(22), 4307–14.

[20] Siepmann, J. and Peppas, N. A. 2001. Mathematical modeling of controlled drug delivery. *Adv. Drug Delivery Rev.*, **48**(2–3), 137–8.

[21] Mellott, M. B., Searcy, K. and Pishko, M. V. 2001. Release of protein from highly cross-linked hydrogels of poly (ethylene glycol) diacrylate fabricated by UV polymerization. *Biomaterials*, **22**(9), 929–41.

[22] Cadee, J. A., de Groot, C. J., Jiskoot, W., den Otter, W. and Hennink, W. E. 2002. Release of recombinant human interleukin-2 from dextran-based hydrogels. *J. Controll. Release*, **78**(1–3), 1–13.

[23] Tabata, Y., Ishii, T., Muniruzzaman, M., Hirano, Y. and Ikada, Y. 2000. Influence of gelatin complexation on cell proliferation activity and proteolytic resistance of basic fibroblast growth factor. *J. Biomater. Sci. – Polymer Edition*, **11**(6), 571–82.

[24] Ungaro, F., Biondi, M., d'Angelo, I. *et al.* 2006. Microsphere-integrated collagen scaffolds for tissue engineering: effect of microsphere formulation and scaffold properties on protein release kinetics. *J. Controll. Release*, **113**(2), 128–36.

[25] Maschke, A., Becker, C., Eyrich, D. *et al.* 2007. Development of a spray congealing process for the preparation of insulin-loaded lipid microparticles and characterization thereof. *Eur. J. Pharmaceutics Biopharmaceutics*, **65**(2), 175–87.

[26] Holland, T. A., Tabata, Y. and Mikos, A. G. 2003. In vitro release of transforming growth factor-β_1 from gelatin microparticles encapsulated in biodegradable, injectable oligo(poly(ethylene glycol) fumarate) hydrogels. *J. Controll. Release*, **91**(3), 299–313.

[27] Holland, T. A., Tabata, Y. and Mikos, A. G. 2005. Dual growth factor delivery from degradable oligo(poly(ethylene glycol) fumarate) hydrogel scaffolds for cartilage tissue engineering. *J. Controll. Release*, **101**(1–3), 111–25.

[28] DeLong, S. A., Moon, J. J. and West, J. L. 2005. Covalently immobilized gradients of bFGF on hydrogel scaffolds for directed cell migration. *Biomaterials*, **26**(16), 3227–34.

[29] Rizzi, S. C., Ehrbar, M., Halstenberg, S. *et al.* 2006. Recombinant protein-co-PEG networks as cell-adhesive and proteolytically degradable hydrogel matrixes. Part II: biofunctional characteristics. *Biomacromolecules*, **7**(11), 3019–29.

[30] Park, K. E., Kang, H. K., Lee, S. J., Min, B. M. and Park, W. H. 2006. Biomimetic nanofibrous scaffolds: preparation and characterization of PGA/chitin blend nanofibers. *Biomacromolecules*, **7**(2), 635–43.

[31] Nitschke, M., Schmack, G., Janke, A. *et al.* 2002. Low pressure plasma treatment of poly(3-hydroxybutyrate): toward tailored polymer surfaces for tissue engineering scaffolds. *J. Biomed. Mater. Res.*, **59**(4), 632–8.

[32] Wan, Y. Q., Yang, J., Yang, J. L., Bei, J. Z. and Wang, S. G. 2003. Cell adhesion on gaseous plasma modified

poly-(L-lactide) surface under shear stress field. *Biomaterials*, **24**(21), 3757–64.

[33] Gao, J. M., Niklason, L. and Langer, R. 1998. Surface hydrolysis of poly(glycolic acid) meshes increases the seeding density of vascular smooth muscle cells. *J. Biomed. Mater. Res.*, **42**(3), 417–24.

[34] Park, G. E., Pattison, M. A., Park, K. and Webster, T. J. 2005. Accelerated chondrocyte functions on NaOH-treated PLGA scaffolds. *Biomaterials*, **26**(16), 3075–82.

[35] Duckworth, B. P., Xu, J. H., Taton, T. A., Guo, A. and Distefano, M. D. 2006. Site-specific, covalent attachment of proteins to a solid surface. *Bioconjugate Chem.*, **17**(4), 967–74.

[36] Kim, T. G. and Park, T. G. 2006. Surface functionalized electrospun biodegradable nanofibers for immobilization of bioactive molecules. *Biotechnol. Prog.*, **22**(4), 1108–13.

[37] Shi, Q., Chen, X. S., Lu, T. C. and Jing, X. B. 2008. The immobilization of proteins on biodegradable polymer fibers via click chemistry. *Biomaterials*, **29**(8), 1118–26.

[38] Fu, G. D., Xu, L. Q., Yao, F., Li, G. L. and Kang, E. T. 2009. Smart nanofibers with a photoresponsive surface for controlled release. *ACS Appl. Mater. Interfaces*, **1**(11), 2424–7.

[39] Killops, K. L., Campos, L. M. and Hawker, C. J. 2008. Robust, efficient, and orthogonal synthesis of dendrimers via thiol-ene "click" chemistry. *J. Am. Chem. Soc.*, **130**(15), 5062–4.

[40] Ehrbar, M., Rizzi, S. C., Hlushchuk, R. *et al.* 2007. Enzymatic formation of modular cell-instructive fibrin analogs for tissue engineering. *Biomaterials*, **28**(26), 3856–66.

[41] Sohier, J., Haan, R. E., de Groot, K. and Bezemer, J. M. 2003. A novel method to obtain protein release from porous polymer scaffolds: emulsion coating. *J. Controll. Release*, **87**(1–3), 57–68.

[42] Whang, K., Goldstick, T. K. and Healy, K. E. 2000. A biodegradable polymer scaffold for delivery of osteotropic factors. *Biomaterials*, **21**(24), 2545–51.

[43] Elsdale, T. and Bard, J. 1972. Collagen substrata for studies on cell behavior. *J. Cell Biol.*, **54**(3), 626–37.

[44] Franceschi, R. T. 1999. The developmental control of osteoblast-specific gene expression: role of specific transcription factors and the extracellular matrix environment. *Crit. Rev. Oral Biol. Med.*, **10**(1), 40–57.

[45] Xiao, G. Z., Gopalakrishnan, R., Jiang, D. *et al.* 2002. Bone morphogenetic proteins, extracellular matrix, and mitogen-activated protein kinase signaling pathways are required for osteoblast-specific gene expression and differentiation in MC3T3-E1 cells. *J. Bone Mineral Res.*, **17**(1), 101–10.

[46] Li, W. J., Laurencin, C. T., Caterson, E. J., Tuan, R. S. and Ko, F. K. 2002. Electrospun nanofibrous structure: a novel scaffold for tissue engineering. *J. Biomed. Mater. Res.*, **60**(4), 613–21.

[47] Matthews, J. A., Wnek, G. E., Simpson, D. G. and Bowlin, G. L. 2002. Electrospinning of collagen nanofibers. *Biomacromolecules*, **3**(2), 232–8.

[48] Yoshimoto, H., Shin, Y. M., Terai, H. and Vacanti, J. P. 2003. A biodegradable nanofiber scaffold by electrospinning and its potential for bone tissue engineering. *Biomaterials*, **24**(12), 2077–82.

[49] Li, C. M., Vepari, C., Jin, H. J., Kim, H. J. and Kaplan, D. L. 2006. Electrospun silk-BMP-2 scaffolds for bone tissue engineering. *Biomaterials*, **27**(16), 3115–24.

[50] Casper, C. L., Yamaguchi, N., Kiick, K. L. and Rabolt, J. F. 2005. Functionalizing electrospun fibers with biologically relevant macromolecules. *Biomacromolecules*, **6**(4), 1998–2007.

[51] Nie, H., Soh, B. W., Fu, Y. C. and Wang, C. H. 2008. Three-dimensional fibrous PLGA/HAp composite scaffold for BMP-2 delivery. *Biotechnol. Bioeng.*, **99**(1), 223–34.

[52] Zhang, Y. Z., Wang, X., Feng, Y. *et al.* 2006. Coaxial electrospinning of (fluorescein isothiocyanate-conjugated bovine serum albumin)-encapsulated poly(ε-caprolactone) nanofibers for sustained release. *Biomacromolecules*, **7**(4), 1049–57.

[53] Jiang, H. L., Hu, Y. Q., Zhao, P. C., Li, Y. and Zhu, K. J. 2006. Modulation of protein release from biodegradable core–shell structured fibers prepared by coaxial electrospinning. *J. Biomed. Mater. Res. Part B – Appl. Biomater.*, **79**(1), 50–7.

[54] Chen, V. J. and Ma, P. X. 2004. Nano-fibrous poly(L-lactic acid) scaffolds with interconnected spherical macropores. *Biomaterials*, **25**(11), 2065–73.

[55] Wei, G. B. and Ma, P. X. 2006. Macroporous and nanofibrous polymer scaffolds and polymer/bone-like apatite composite scaffolds generated by sugar spheres. *J. Biomed. Mater. Res. Part A*, **78**(2), 306–15.

[56] Chen, V. J., Smith, L. A. and Ma, P. X. 2006. Bone regeneration on computer-designed nano-fibrous scaffolds. *Biomaterials*, **27**(21), 3973–9.

[57] Wang, P., Hu, J. and Ma, P. X. 2009. The engineering of patient-specific, anatomically shaped, digits. *Biomaterials*, **30**(14), 2735–40.

[58] Woo, K. M., Jun, J. H., Chen, V. J. *et al.* 2007. Nanofibrous scaffolding promotes osteoblast differentiation and biomineralization. *Biomaterials*, **28**(2), 335–43.

[59] Hu, J. A., Sun, X. A., Ma, H. Y. *et al.* 2010. Porous nanofibrous PLLA scaffolds for vascular tissue engineering. *Biomaterials*, **31**(31), 7971–7.

[60] Wei, G. B., Jin, Q. M., Giannobile, W. V. and Ma, P. X. 2006. Nano-fibrous scaffold for controlled delivery of recombinant human PDGF-BB. *J. Controll. Release*, **112**(1), 103–10.

[61] Langer, R. 1990. New methods of drug delivery. *Science*, **249**(4976), 1527–33.

[62] Woodrow, K. A., Cu, Y., Booth, C. J. *et al.* 2009. Intravaginal gene silencing using biodegradable polymer nanoparticles densely loaded with small-interfering RNA. *Nature Mater.*, **8**(6), 526–33.

[63] Wei, G. B., Pettway, G. J., McCauley, L. K. and Ma, P. X. 2004. The release profiles and bioactivity of parathyroid hormone from poly(lactic-*co*-glycolic acid) microspheres. *Biomaterials*, **25**(2), 345–52.

[64] Wei, G. B., Jin, Q. M., Giannobile, W. V. and Ma, P. X. 2007. The enhancement of osteogenesis by nano-fibrous scaffolds incorporating rhBMP-7 nanospheres. *Biomaterials*, **28**(12), 2087–96.

[65] Jin, Q. M., Wei, G. B., Lin, Z. *et al.* 2008. Nanofibrous scaffolds incorporating PDGF-BB microspheres induce chemokine expression and tissue neogenesis in vivo. *PLOS One*, **3**(3), e1729.

[66] Ripamonti, U., VandenHeever, B., Sampath, T. K. *et al.* 1996. Complete regeneration of bone in the baboon by recombinant human osteogenic protein-1 (hOP-1, bone morphogenetic protein-7). *Growth Factors*, **13**(3–4), 273–89.

[67] Cook, S. D. 1999. Preclinical and clinical evaluation of osteogenic protein-1 (BMP-7) in bony sites. *Orthopedics*, **22**(7), 669–71.

[68] Xie, Y. C., Yin, T., Wiegraebe, W. *et al.* 2009. Detection of functional haematopoietic stem cell niche using real-time imaging. *Nature*, **457**(7225), U97–102.

[69] Miura, Y., Gao, Z. G., Miura, M. *et al.* 2006. Mesenchymal stem cell-organized bone marrow elements: an alternative hematopoietic progenitor resource. *Stem Cells*, **24**(11), 2428–36.

21

Gene delivery for periodontal regeneration

Andrei D. Taut and William V. Giannobile

21.1 Gene therapy for regenerative medicine

Gene therapy refers to the delivery of genetic material that will activate, hinder, or modify the expression of specific genes to facilitate the natural cellular production of a therapeutic agent to treat disease [1, 2]. The concept has emerged as an effective method to control the course of a disease/disorder, modulate the host-response triggered by pathogen, or regenerate compromised biological tissues [2]. As such, the use of gene delivery technologies offers a novel approach for delivery of putative regenerative molecules to sites in the oral cavity and craniofacial complex [2]. Gene therapy is more advantageous than the traditional therapeutic delivery of compounds and proteins. A greater sustainability in comparison with a single dosage or several of a protein or compound is one of the primary advantages of therapeutic gene delivery. Although the half-lives of conventional pharmaceutical compounds or recombinant proteins range from hours to a few days, viral vector-gene delivery of the corresponding genes can lead to in-vivo expression lasting from weeks to years. Gene therapy also alleviates technical challenges that arise with protein expression and purification. Furthermore, gene delivery of an entire group of regenerative factors combined with existing tissue regeneration therapies could potentially replicate natural biological healing processes and allow engineering of complex three-dimensional (3D), multitissue structures (Figure 21.1) [2]. Therapeutic gene delivery for tissue regeneration is achieved through the use of both viral and non-viral vectors (Table 21.1).

21.1.1 Therapeutic non-viral gene delivery

Non-viral genetic therapy strategies include disruption of the translation process in the cytoplasm to inhibit a defective gene or exogenous delivery of genetic material to compensate for a protein deficiency (Figure 21.2) [3, 4]. The requirements for creating a successful gene delivery system include safety, resistance to degradation, immune evasion, ability to enter a cellular compartment using target-site-specificity signals, and ability to modulate or express a protein of choice [3]. Furthermore, the ability to modulate/express the desired therapeutic protein to direct regenerative processes is largely dependent on discrete intracellular events following internalization of the genetic material (Figure 21.3). In general, non-viral gene delivery methods are safer than the viral alternatives; however, they are considered less effective due to the reduced and transient exogenous gene expression due to the low transfection efficiency [3].

21.1.1.1 Nucleic acid delivery

Plasmid DNA must be transported into cell nuclei, where transcription and translation result in protein synthesis independently of chromosomal DNA. In plasmid-mediated gene delivery, the expression of desired genes is controlled by the promoter and enhancer sequences within the plasmid [5].

Antisense oligonucleotides (AONs) are single-stranded nucleic acids complementary to a target mRNA. AONs down-regulate gene expression, and thus can be used to treat disorders characterized by

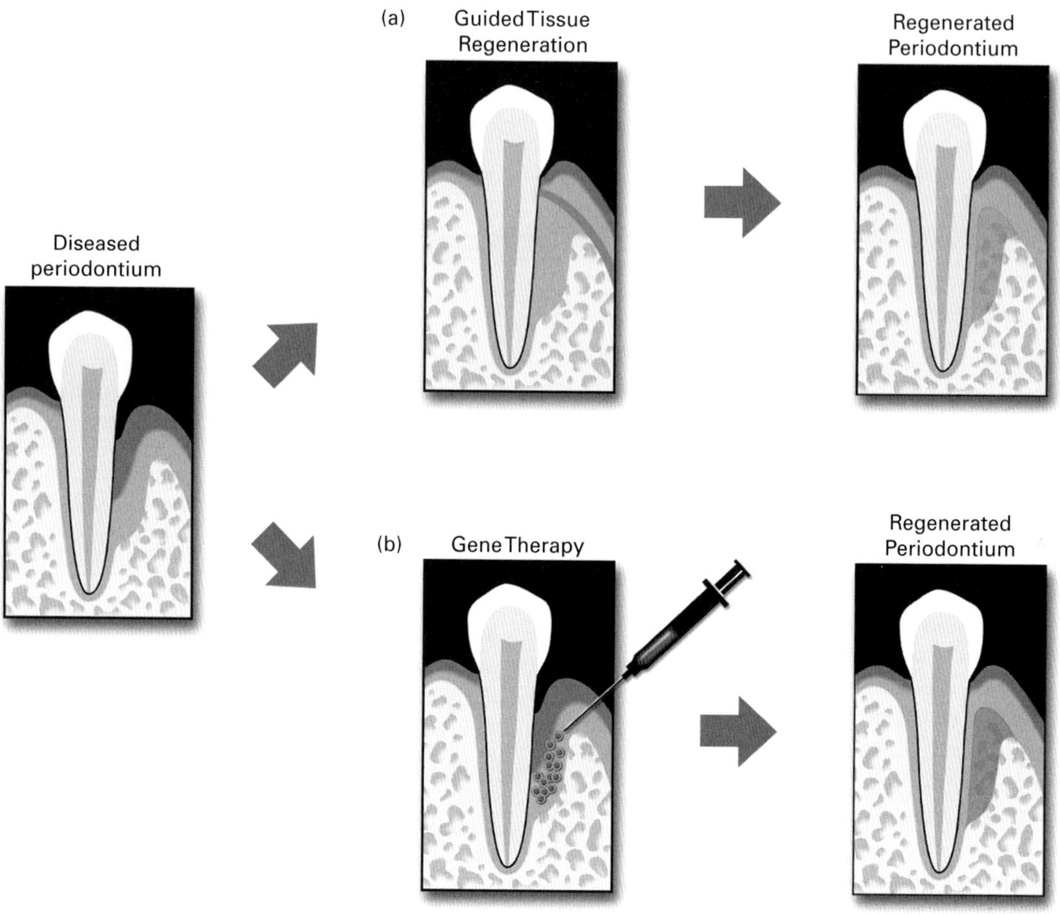

Figure 21.1 Traditional and gene delivery-based therapeutics for tissue regeneration in the periodontium. (a) Occlusive barrier membranes used in guided tissue regeneration promote healing and restoration of bone and gingival tissues. (b) Delivery of growth-factor-encoding vectors into periodontal defects can facilitate hard- and soft-tissue regenerative processes in the periodontium. (Reproduced with Permission from Ramseier *et al.* (2006) [29].)

excessive production of a protein product, but cannot be used to express a gene of interest [3]. Inhibition of target mRNA is accomplished via (1) induction of RNaseH endonuclease activity, resulting in degradation of target mRNA; (2) translational arrest and subsequent steric hindrance of ribosomes; and (3) interference with alternative splicing in the nucleus [6, 7]. In general, the nucleotide sequence and the insertion of chemically modified nucleotides into AONs can impact the success and mechanism of action of gene modulation [3, 8, 9].

21.1.1.2 Nucleic acid delivery for RNA interference

Small interfering RNAs (siRNAs) are short, double-stranded RNA segments that hinder protein expression by binding mRNA in the cytoplasm. The siRNAs involve central RNA interference (RNAi), a cellular regulatory system for gene expression, and mediate degradation of target mRNA via activation of the large protein assemblies called the RNA-induced silencing complex (RISC) [10].

Table 21.1 Viral and non-viral vectors utilized in tissue engineering [2]

Vector	Type	Advantages	Disadvantages
Retrovirus	Viral	Non-immunogenic Sustained gene expression	Risk of insertional mutagenesis Transduction limited to dividing cells
Lentivirus	Viral	Transduces dividing and non-dividing cells Low immunogenicity Sustained gene expression	Risk of insertional mutagenesis Potential pathogenicity High-titer production is difficult
Adenovirus	Viral	Transduces dividing and non-dividing cells Decreased risk of insertional mutagenesis	Potentially highly immunogenic Transient gene expression
Adeno-associated virus	Viral	Transduces dividing and non-dividing cells Low immunogenicity Non-pathogenic	Small transgenes High-titer production is difficult
Plasmid	Non-viral	Non-immunogenic Non-pathogenic	Low transfection efficiency
DNA/RNA polymer complexes	Non-viral	Transfects dividing and non-dividing cells Nuclear and cell-specific targeting	Low transfection efficiency Potential for cytotoxicity
Transposon	Non-viral	Sustained gene expression Relatively large transgenes Non-immunogenic	Risk of insertional mutagenesis Low transfection efficiency

Similarly, small hairpin RNAs (shRNAs) also induce gene silencing via RNA interference through activation of the RISC [11]. However, shRNA vectors can be engineered to generate more pronounced and effective gene silencing via initiation of both RNA interference and translational arrest [12].

Mature micro-RNAs (miRNA) also represent an emerging class of endogenous molecules for therapeutic targeting. The miRNA naturally binds to partially complementary sites on the target mRNA to down-regulate mRNA post-transcriptionally and inhibit uncontrolled gene expression [3, 13]. Furthermore, it has been demonstrated that some miRNAs can target hundreds of different mRNAs

Transposon systems, such as the *Sleeping Beauty* (*SB*) transposon, are discrete DNA sequences that randomly integrate into the host cell genome using the transposase enzyme. In recent research, the *SB* transposon has been found to engage in efficient and stable gene transfer and sustained gene expression in primary cell types including human hematopoietic progenitors, mesenchymal stem cells, and myoblasts when delivered using a plasmid vector [14]. Transposon systems are non-disease-causing entities, but can result in reversible insertional mutagenesis [15].

21.1.1.3 Nucleic acid carriers for non-viral gene therapy

Introduction of naked nucleic acids into biological environments generally leads to their rapid degradation by protective enzymes prior to the genetic material reaching target tissues and cells. The hydrophilic properties of nucleic acids also restrict their cellular uptake, limiting their intracellular bioavailability [3]. Thus, delivery vectors or carriers protect complexed nucleic acids from degradation and increase their cellular uptake. Additionally, properties of carriers must complement those of the lipophilic, negatively charged plasma membrane for improved cellular uptake and possible delivery to the nucleus [16]. Finally, nucleic acid carriers must augment immune responses triggered against exogenous DNA and RNA [3]. Several types of carriers, including cationic lipids and peptides, have been demonstrated to improve protection and delivery of nucleic acids used in non-viral gene delivery.

Cationic lipids, such as liposomes and solid lipid nanoparticles, have a high capacity for packing genetic material, low immunogenicity, and potential

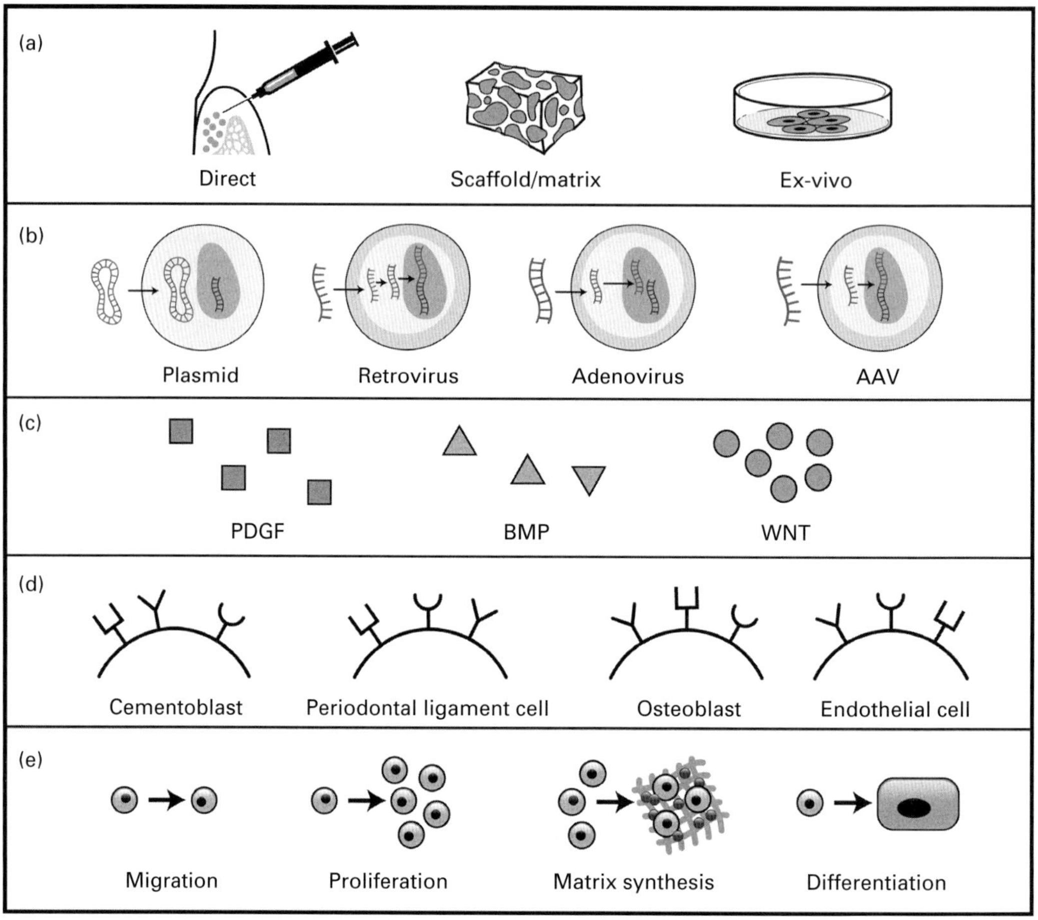

Figure 21.2 Various components of the current model of gene delivery for periodontal regeneration. The delivery method (a), vector type (b), tissue growth factor (c), target cell and cellular receptors (d), and local effect (e) can be customized to complement the wound site characteristics and achieve desired therapeutic outcome. (Adapted from Ramseier *et al.* (2006) [29].)

for mass production, but exhibit low transfection potential because of their rapid deactivation in serum [3, 17].

Polymers, including polyethylenimine (PEI) and poly(amido amine) (PAA), significantly increase cellular uptake and are highly stable under physiological conditions. Furthermore, polymers are generally quickly degraded following cellular internalization, allowing endosomal release of genetic material. However, the polymer's molecular weight (more formally, relative molecular mass) influences nucleic acid transfection efficiency and cytotoxicity, which has been a topic of extensive investigation in the polymer research field [18–20].

21.1.1.4 Targeting of nucleic acid carriers

Peptides, including CL22 and rPOA, are highly stable in extracellular spaces and also rapidly reduced within cells, facilitating endosomal escape following

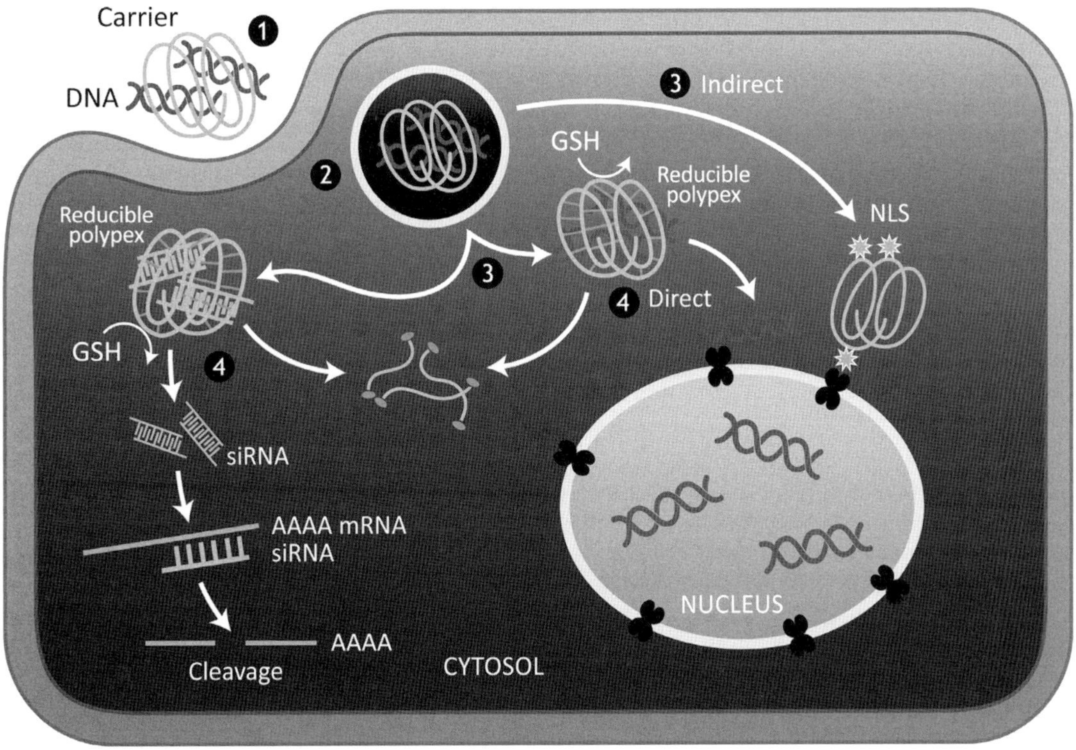

Figure 21.3 Biomechanistic depiction of non-viral gene delivery and subsequent cytoplasmic events influencing gene expression at the subcellular level. Targeted delivery and internalization of genetic material (plasmid DNA, siRNA, etc.) can be improved using appropriate carrier (cationic lipids, polymers, etc.). Following translocation and successful endosomal escape into the cytosol, the nucleic acid–carrier complex can follow one of several pathways in order to alter expression of the target gene(s). In the nuclear delivery pathway, nuclear localization signals embedded in the carrier material facilitate importin-mediated active transport of the exogene across the nuclear membrane. In the absence of nuclear localization signals, cytosolic glutathione (GSH) can direct the reduction/breakdown of polymer carriers to release of nucleic acid into the cytoplasm for nuclear DNA delivery (via passive diffusion through nuclear pore complex) and RNA interference/gene silencing. (Adapted from Won *et al.* (2011) [75].)

uptake by endocytosis to release genetic material into the cytoplasm [3]. Peptides allow active targeting of genetic material and can potentially be combined with other carriers to form hybrid carriers that exhibit improved targeting efficiency and protection against the degradation of nucleic acids [3]. Targeting can also be achieved by conjugating of non-viral vectors to other targeting entities, including antibodies, aptamers, vitamins, and sugar moieties [21–24].

21.1.1.5 Physical methods of gene delivery

Electroporation, or the use of an electric field to penetrate physical biological barriers for transfer of genetic material into cells, has been shown to improve delivery of plasmids into dental tissues following injection. Electroporation also enhances transfection of alveolar bone and surrounding dental tissues to aid in regulating tooth eruption [16, 25].

Ultrasound therapy is generally used in combination with (lipid or protein) microbubbles to create plasma membrane pores that allow for improved internalization of nucleic acid complexes [26]. In a recent study, plasmid DNA and lipid microbubbles, used in conjunction with ultrasound therapy, improved transfection in muscle cells of gingival tissues [27]. Furthermore, ultrasound-mediated therapy also improved transfection of dentin sialoprotein gene in dental pulp tissue to stimulate reparative dentin formation in canine teeth [28].

21.1.2 Therapeutic viral gene delivery

The use of viral gene therapy is one of the most common forms of gene targeting in vivo and includes many different vector constructs such as adenovirus, retrovirus, lentivirus, and other viridiae for clinical application. Viral gene therapy prolongs expression (ranging from a few weeks to years) of genes of interest, but exhibits immunogenic and mutagenic properties. Retroviral vectors are single-stranded RNA viruses utilizing reverse transcriptase to synthesize viral DNA and incorporate themselves into the host genome [29]. The cellular lineages then retain viral DNA material for sustained and efficient transgene expression. However, the potential for insertional mutagenesis and subsequent carcinogenesis does exist [30].

Lentiviruses are a subclass of retroviruses with an identical transfection mechanism to that of retroviruses, but with more restricted sites of insertion and longer incubation periods. The risk of mutagenesis persists with the use of lentiviral vectors, and there is potential for the formation of competent viruses (of HIV origin) through recombination events [31].

Adenoviral vectors are double-stranded DNA viruses, exhibiting higher stability than that of RNA viruses, but high immunogenicity. They are associated with mild disease and can transduce both dividing and non-dividing cells. Their non-integrating genome results in a decreased risk of insertional mutagenesis, but also leads to ineffective genetic manipulation of dividing cells. The generational loss of transgene leads to short-term gene expression. In non-dividing cells, adenoviruses can persist for years without immune responses against the virus or transgene protein products [32]. These vectors are some of the most common gene therapy vehicles.

Adeno-associated viruses (AAVs) are single-stranded DNA viruses with low immunogenicity, but exhibit some risk of mutagenesis. The AAVs integrate genetic material at a specific site on chromosome 19. Additionally, AAV vectors can carry only minute amounts of genetic material [32, 33].

21.2 Gene therapy for periodontal disease

Periodontal diseases affect more than 80% of adults worldwide and nearly 15% display severe forms of infection concomitant with early tooth loss [34]. The detrimental changes that the tooth-supporting tissues undergo are primarily the result of specific microbial challenges [35]. These alterations disrupt the functional and structural integrity of the tooth-supporting apparatus and may progress to modulate a number of systemic conditions [36]. Therefore, the periodontium represents an important entry that can be overcome by invasive oral microrganisms, triggering local and systemic inflammatory responses that characterize local infection. As such, the reconstruction of periodontal wounds represents an important form of therapy that could benefit by gene delivery of regenerative molecules (Figure 21.4).

21.2.1 Growth factors in periodontal regenerative medicine

Platelet-derived growth factor (PDGF) is a platelet-derived, multifunctional polypeptide growth factor originally found to trigger mitogenesis in cells of mesenchymal origin. PDGF exerts its biological effects to increase cell proliferation, migration, and extracellular matrix synthesis [37–39]. Furthermore, it has also been shown to exhibit anti-apoptotic properties, which, together with its additional biological functions, make it a critical initiator of tissue repair pathways in periodontal tissues, including bone, cementum, and the periodontal ligament [40, 41].

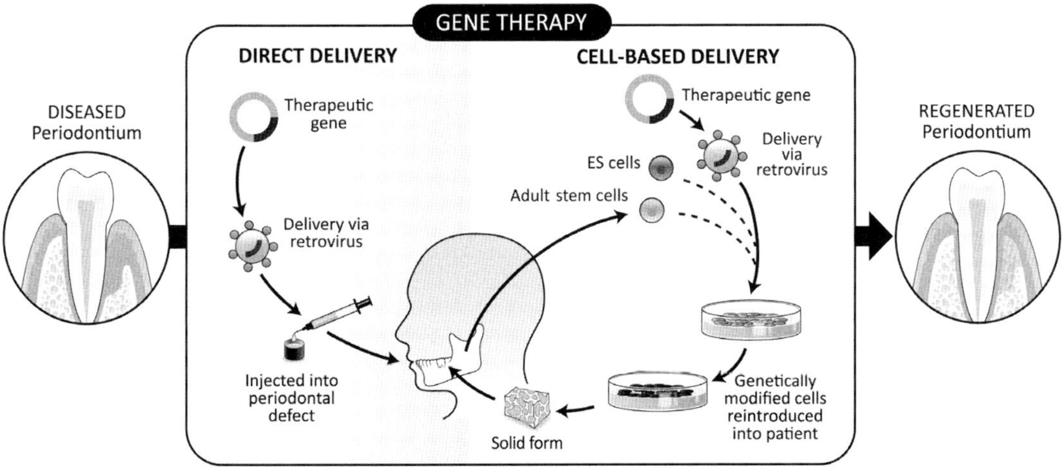

Figure 21.4 The direct and cell-based delivery of a therapeutic gene has been demonstrated to increase tissue regeneration and bioavailability of essential growth factors. The therapeutic gene(s) of interest can either be injected directly into the periodontal defect using viral or non-viral vectors or incorporated into embryonic/adult stem cells that are subsequently expanded and reintroduced into the periodontal defect. (Adapted from Rios *et al.* (2011) [2].)

Early research has shown evidence that adenoviral vectors encoding for PDGF successfully transduce periodontal tissue cells, including periodontal ligament cells, gingival fibroblasts, cementoblasts, and osteoblasts, leading to increased proliferation in all cell types [42, 43]. Additionally, adenoviral PDGF (Ad-PDGF) delivery has been shown to increase the duration of PDGF signaling, as well as continuous and localized PDGF gene expression, for up to 35 days following delivery in periodontal defects [44–46]. Analysis of the systemic distribution of the vector revealed minimal viral presence in the blood, lungs, spleen, and other major organs, indicating that Ad-PDGF seeded in a collagen matrix exhibits an adequate biosafety profile for potential human clinical studies [2, 46].

Several studies have demonstrated the therapeutic and regenerative potential of PDGF gene therapy for periodontal disease. Jin *et al.* delivered Ad-PDGF-B in collagen carrier to large periodontal lesions, giving a significant increase in defect bone fill, nearly a fourfold increase in bridging bone, and a six-fold increase in cementum regeneration compared with the use of adenoviral loss-of-function mutant PDGF [47]. Further analysis revealed that Ad-PDGF-B transduction of cells promotes the migration and proliferation of human gingival fibroblasts into the defect region, revealing one potential factor contributing to increased alveolar bone regeneration [2]. Although PDGF has been shown to be a stimulator of alveolar bone regeneration, prolonged delivery of PDGF-A can have inhibitory effects on cementogenesis. Continuous exogenous delivery of PDGF-A for at least 3 weeks postpones mineral deposition by cementoblasts [48].

Bone morphogenetic proteins (BMPs) are a diverse group of soluble polypeptide molecules capable of initiating bone matrix deposition and morphogeneis [49]. Furthermore, BMPs are potent regulators of cartilage and bone formation, and have also shown increased expression during alveolar bone healing in the periodontium [49–51]. Clinically, BMPs are most relevant for the ability to stimulate alveolar bone formation.

Ex-vivo methods of BMP gene delivery have been studied as treatment modalities for periodontal disease. Transduction of both rat syngeneic dermal fibroblasts and human periodontal ligament cells with adenoviral BMP-7, and subsequent implantation into oral osseous lesions, has shown predictable regeneration of alveolar bone (bone volume and density), cementum, and periodontal ligament fibers [52, 53]. Interestingly, Ad-BMP-7-driven bone formation has been shown to occur via a cartilage intermediate, which then rapidly matures into a multitissue periodontal attachment complex [2, 52]. Thus, BMP-7 ex-vivo gene therapy has been shown to give rise to potentially more functional tissue structures that closely resemble the natural, healthy periodontium.

Wnts, including sclerostin and leucine-responsive regulatory protein 5 (Lrp5), are secreted glycoproteins that have been shown to play a crucial part in embryonic craniofacial morphogenesis, bone maintenance, and tooth morphogenesis through regulation of cell migration, proliferation, differentiation, and apoptosis [54, 55]. Research has shown that Wnts target a variety of cells, including periodontal fibroblasts, cementoblasts, osteoblasts, and osteocytes, indicating a potential role of Wnts in mediating bone and soft tissue homeostasis within periodontal structures [56, 57]. More specifically, Wnt pathway-linked sclerostin and Lrp5 have been identified as potential therapeutic targets for osteopathias and, more specifically, periodontal disease [58].

Although the roles of Wnt pathway proteins are not completely understood within the realms of periodontal homeostasis and regeneration, several studies have revealed the therapeutic potential of regulating the Wnt pathway using gene delivery. Chang *et al.* demonstrated that human periodontal ligament MSCs modified to express *Wnt-4* (using a retroviral vector) promoted healing and bone regeneration in an experimental periodontal defect model. Furthermore, no significant inflammatory response was evident against the retroviral vector-transduced cells. *Wnt-4*-engineered MSCs also promoted an increase in blood vessel formation within the defect, resulting in higher quantities of bone than in natural healing [59].

21.2.2 Transcription factors in periodontal regenerative medicine

Transcription factors and regulators have also recently emerged as potential targets for periodontal gene therapy and, more specifically, alveolar bone augmentation. Although the research on transcription regulators is extensive, *Runx2*, Osterix (*Osx*), and LMP show promise in periodontal tissue engineering.

Runx2, a major transcription activator of osteoblast differentiation, has been shown to direct both bone marrow stromal cells and dermal fibroblasts to differentiate into osteoblasts following gene delivery using adenoviral and retroviral vectors, respectively [60, 61]. Additionally, *Runx2* gene delivery induces osteogenic gene expression for up to 3 weeks following delivery, resulting in the formation of mineralized tissue and enhanced healing of craniofacial bone defects [60].

Osx is a zinc-finger-containing transcription factor functioning downstream of *Runx2* and is essential in osteoblast differentiation and bone formation. Its importance is revealed in *Osx* gene knockout experiments. Preosteoblastic cells in the periosteum and skeleton fail to differentiate into osteoblasts, and *Osx*-null mice exhibit absence of bone formation [62]. Consequently, *Osx* over-expression in bone marrow stromal cells using a retroviral vector has been shown to enhance bone healing of critical-sized craniofacial defects [62].

LIM domain mineralization proteins (LMPs) are non-secreted, intracellular proteins that have been found to be highly up-regulated during early stages of osteoblast differentiation. In recent studies, LMP-3 gene delivery to preosteoblastic and fibroblastic cells has been shown to increase expression of bone-specific genes, as well as to induce bone mineralization in a dose-dependent manner [63]. More so, autologous dermal fibroblasts transduced with Ad-LMP-3 aided in the successful regeneration of bone within mandibular lesions [64].

21.2.3 Modulation of host responses to periodontal disease

Another strategy for using gene delivery to provide long-term, stable treatment to patients with periodontal disease involves modulation of host immune responses in order to control disease progression and prevent destruction of the periodontal structures [65]. In fact, combinatorial gene delivery of tissue regenerative growth factors, with host modulatory genes or antimicrobials, may emerge as an effective treatment modality for patients with severe periodontal disease [2]. Current understanding of the progression of periodontitis indicates that the host immune response against the bacterial load is a major contributor to periodontal tissue destruction. As a result, several modulatory molecules, including MMPs, cathepsins, and other osteoclast-derived mediators of bone resorption, have been identified as potential targets for regulating the host immune response using viral and non-viral gene delivery [2, 65].

One approach focusses on delivery of genes to prolong expression of therapeutic host modulatory molecules. Cirelli *et al.* used AAV vectors to deliver TNF receptor-immunoglobulin Fc (TNFR:Fc) fusion gene locally in periodontia to combat experimental *P. gingivalis (Pg)*-LPS-mediated experimental periodontitis. TNFR:Fc gene delivery was used to hinder the pro-inflammatory functions of TNF-α in the periodontium and prevent subsequent destruction of periodontal tissues. Results demonstrated the prolonged expression, for at least 2 months, of serum TNFR:Fc following a single administration, as well as inhibition of local inflammatory cell infiltration and suppression of bone resorptive cytokine expression. Additionally, AAV TNFR:Fc administration also preserves the linear height, volume, and density of tooth-supporting alveolar bone during experimental periodontitis [66].

Tristetraprolin (TTP), a cytokine-regulating RNA-binding protein, has been shown to down-regulate expression of pro-inflammatory cytokines by initiating the degradation of corresponding mRNA transcripts. Consequently, over-expression of TTP via adenoviral vector hinders the in-vitro expression of interleukin-6, TNF-α, and prostaglandin E_2, and inhibits local inflammatory cell infiltration to protect against inflammation-mediated bone loss in an experimental periodontitis model [2, 67]. Similarly, adenoviral delivery of mitogen-activated protein kinase (MAPK) phosphatase 1 (MKP-1) has also been shown to dampen immune responses and prevent inflammation-mediated alveolar bone loss [68].

The success of growth and transcription factor gene delivery in directing an individual's own cells to produce the desired therapeutic outcome can be dependent on their incorporation and delivery using a variety of matrix delivery systems. Naturally derived materials include, but are not limited to, porcine collagen membranes and mineralized allografts and xenografts. Synthetic materials encompass scaffolds made from various polymers, such as polylactic acid, and matrices composed of naturally occurring hydroxyapatite. Scaffolding matrices can control the spatial and temporal release of growth, transcription, and modulatory factor gene therapy, and enhance effectiveness in treating periodontal disease [69].

21.3 Gene therapy for oral implant osseointegration

21.3.1 Gene expression during peri-implant healing as a model for gene therapy

Dental implants restore functionality in the oral cavity following tooth loss. Thus, both enhancement of alveolar bone formation for dental implant placement and implant osseointegration have been a major focus of recent oral implant research. Understanding the molecular events that occur during oral implant osseointegration can lead to the development of improved treatments for more successful implant outcomes [70]. Lin and colleagues classified gene expression during dental implant osseointegration into three healing phases. During early healing stages, pro-inflammatory cytokines such as IL-1β and Cxcl2 exhibit increased gene expression that eventually decreases. The expression of extracellular matrix proteins and osteogenic factors such as osteopontin (*Opn*), periostin (*Postn*), and osteocalcin (*Ocn*) dominates late-stage osseointegration events, while other genes, such as scleraxis, are constitutively expressed throughout implant osseointegration [70]. Characterization of molecular events during implant osseointegration brings to light possible pathways that can be further explored or utilized for osseointegration acceleration strategies [70].

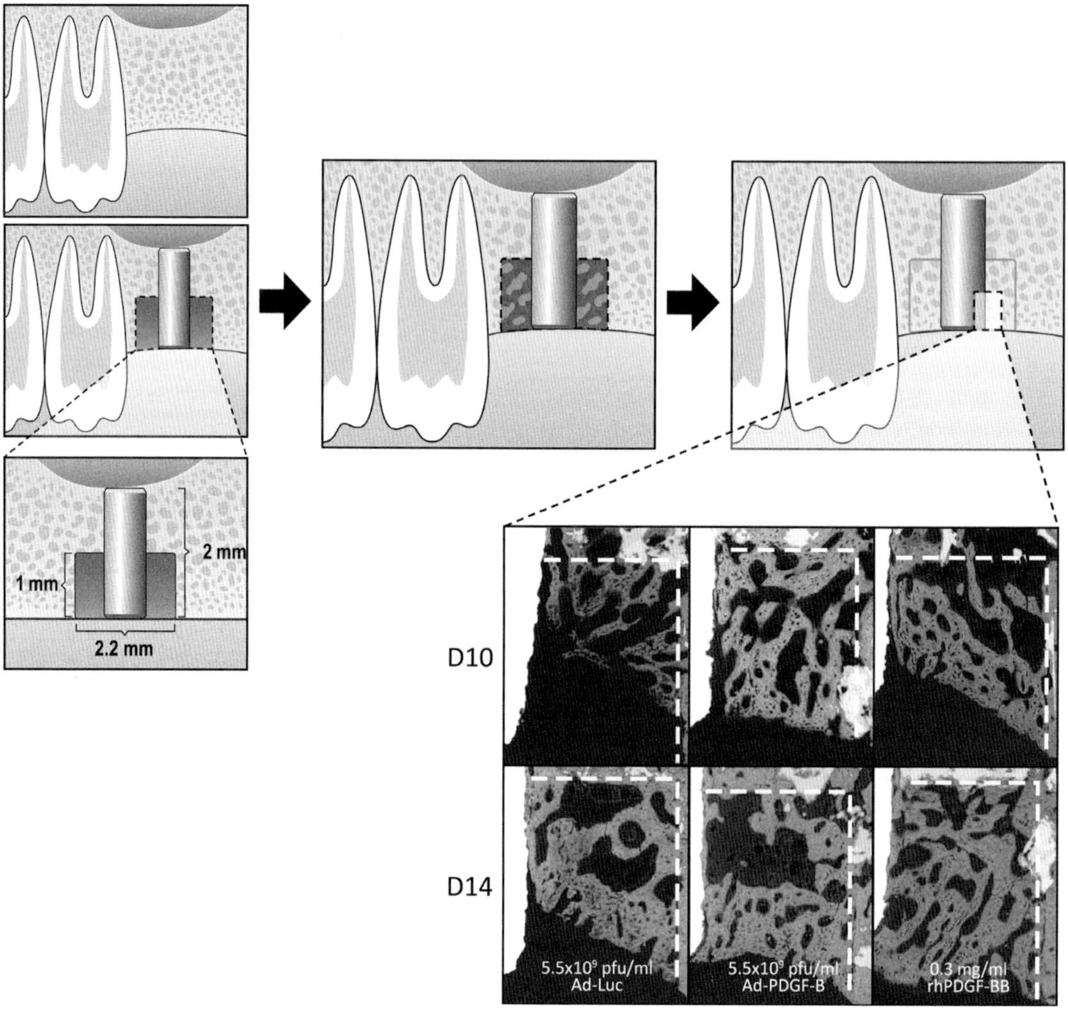

Figure 21.5 Dental implant placement as well as generation of a standardized peri-implant defect in a peri-implant healing model using gene therapy. Consequently, the model allows one to evaluate both alveolar bone healing and osseointegration of titanium implant within the created defect (the dashed line denotes the borders of the osseous defect and the white region represents the location of the titanium implant). The effects of PDGF protein (rhPDGF-BB) and adenovirus-mediated PDGF-B (Ad-PDGF-B) gene delivery were evaluated and compared with those of adenovirus-encoding luciferase negative control (Ad-Luc). Backscattered SEM (BS-SEM) cross-sections of defect region show increased mineralized tissue formation after 10 days (D10) with Ad-PDGF-B compared to Ad-Luc. Additionally, advanced bone formation against the oral implant surface is also present 14 days (D14) after PDGF treatment. (Adapted from Rios *et al.* (2011) and Chang *et al.* (2010) [2, 71].)

21.3.2 Gene therapy for improving oral implant osseointegration

PDGF, which is important to healing in the periodontium, has shown promise for both treatment of periodontal disease and enhancement of bone formation around dental implants. In a study by Chang *et al.* adenoviral vectors encoding for PDGF-B accelerated bone repair in an experimental dental implant model (Figure 21.5). Additionally, Ad-PDGF-B delivered in collagen matrix showed regenerative capabilities for bone tissue engineering and osseointegration in alveolar bone defects comparable with those of recombinant human PDGF-BB protein delivery in vivo, as measured by several methods of analysis, including biomechanical assessments (Figure 21.5) [71, 72].

Additionally, direct gene delivery of Ad-BMP-7 vectors seeded in a collagen scaffold significantly enhanced alveolar bone defect fill, new bone formation, and bone-to-implant contact compared with control in an experimental dental implant model – notably, targeted transgene expression persisted in osteotomy defects for up to 10 days following delivery [73]. In a related study, Ad-BMP-7 and human periodontal ligament cells seeded into a porous chitosan/collagen scaffold increased bone formation around dental implants. Further analysis revealed higher levels of ALP activity, as well as increased expression of osteopontin and bone sialoprotein in BMP-7-transduced experimental groups [74].

21.4 Future perspectives: targeted gene therapy in vivo

Significant progress has been made in the reconstruction of tooth-supporting periodontal defects and oral/craniofacial deficiencies using a variety of approaches including gene delivery. Gene transfer approaches to improve periodontal repair have now been under development for nearly a decade; however, many challenges remain. Both viral and non-viral approaches to target regenerative molecules to tooth, implant, and jaw bone defects have demonstrated success in preclinical models. Many aspects will need to be worked out from a regulatory standpoint through the FDA and EMEA to gain approval to embark on proof-of-concept early-stage human studies. We are optimistic that the next decade will see the application of these technologies to reconstruct oral defects due to disease, injury, or congenital malformations.

ACKNOWLEDGEMENTS

The authors thank Mr. Chris Jung for his help with the figures. These studies were supported by NIH/NIDCR grant RO1-DE13397, the ITI Foundation, and a grant from the AO Foundation to W.V.G.

REFERENCES

[1] Ditto, A. J., Shah, P. N. and Yun, Y. H. 2009. Non-viral gene delivery using nanoparticles. *Expert Opin. Drug Deliv.*, **6**(11), 1149–60.

[2] Rios, H. F., Lin, Z., Oh, B., Park, C. H. and Giannobile, W. V. 2011. Cell- and gene-based therapeutic strategies for periodontal regenerative medicine. *J. Periodontol.*, **82** (9), 1223–37.

[3] Elsabahy, M., Nazarali, A. and Foldvari, M. 2011. Non-viral nucleic acid delivery: key challenges and future directions. *Curr. Drug Deliv.*, **8**(3), 235–44.

[4] Watanabe, T., Umehara, T. and Kohara, M. 2007. Therapeutic application of RNA interference for hepatitis C virus. *Adv. Drug Deliv. Rev.*, **59**(12), 1263–76.

[5] Williams, J. A., Carnes, A. E. and Hodgson, C. P. 2009. Plasmid DNA vaccine vector design: impact on efficacy, safety and upstream production. *Biotechnol. Adv.*, **27**(4), 353–70.

[6] Liang, W. W., Shi, X., Deshpande, D., Malanga, C. J. and Rajanasakul, Y. 1996. Oligonucleotide targeting to alveolar macrophages by mannose receptor-mediated endocytosis. *Biochim. Biophys. Acta*, **1279**(2), 227–34.

[7] Chan, J. H., Lim, S. and Wong, W. S. 2006. Antisense oligonucleotides: from design to therapeutic application. *Clin. Exp. Pharmacol. Physiol.*, **33**(5–6), 533–40.

[8] Sazani, P. and Kole, R. 2003. Therapeutic potential of antisense oligonucleotides as modulators of alternative splicing. *J. Clin. Invest.*, **112**(4), 481–6.

[9] Hogrefe, R. I. 1999. An antisense oligonucleotide primer. *Antisense Nucleic Acid Drug Dev.*, **9**(4), 351–7.

[10] Preall, J. B. and Sontheimer, E. J. 2005. RNAi: RISC gets loaded. *Cell*, **123**(4), 543–5.

[11] Karikó, K., Bhuyan, P., Capodici, P. *et al.* 2004. Small interfering RNAs mediate sequence-independent gene suppression and induce immune activation by signaling through toll-like receptor 3. *J. Immunol.*, **172**(11), 6545–9.

[12] Rao, D. D., Vorhies, J. S., Senzer, N. and Nemunaitis, J. 2009. siRNA vs. shRNA: similarities and differences. *Adv. Drug Deliv. Rev.*, **61**(9), 746–59.

[13] Lee, Y., Jeon, K., Lee, J. T., Kim, S. and Kim, V. N. 2002. MicroRNA maturation: stepwise processing and subcellular localization. *EMBO J.*, **21**(17), 4663–70.

[14] Ivics, Z. and Izsvak, Z. 2011. Nonviral gene delivery with the sleeping beauty transposon system. *Hum. Gene Ther.*, **22**(9), 1043–51.

[15] Carlson, C. M. and Largaespada, D. A. 2005. Insertional mutagenesis in mice: new perspectives and tools. *Nature Rev. Genet.*, **6**(7), 568–80.

[16] Gao, X., Kim, K. S. and Liu, D. 2007. Nonviral gene delivery: what we know and what is next. *AAPS J.*, **9**(1), E92–104.

[17] Li, P., Liu, D., Sun, X. *et al.* 2011. A novel cationic liposome formulation for efficient gene delivery via a pulmonary route. *Nanotechnology*, **22**(24), 245104.

[18] Pi, Y., Zhang, X., Shi, J. *et al.* 2011. Targeted delivery of non-viral vectors to cartilage in vivo using a chondrocyte-homing peptide identified by phage display. *Biomaterials*, **32**(26), 6324–32.

[19] McLachlan, G., Davidson, H., Holder, E. *et al.* 2011. Pre-clinical evaluation of three non-viral gene transfer agents for cystic fibrosis after aerosol delivery to the ovine lung. *Gene Ther.*, **18**(10), 996–1005.

[20] Arote, R. B., Jiang, H. L., Kim, Y. K. *et al.* 2011. Degradable poly(amido amine)s as gene delivery carriers. *Expert Opin. Drug Deliv.*, **8**(9), 1237–46.

[21] Farokhzad, O. C., Karp, J. M. and Langer, R. 2006. Targeted nanoparticle–aptamer bioconjugates for cancer chemotherapy in vivo. *Proc. Nat. Acad. Sci. USA*, **103**(16), 6315–20.

[22] Kim, S. H., Jeong, J. H., Mok, H. *et al.* 2007. Folate receptor targeted delivery of polyelectrolyte complex micelles prepared from ODN–PEG–folate conjugate and cationic lipids. *Biotechnol. Prog.*, **23**(1), 232–7.

[23] Oishi, M., Kataoka, K. and Nagasaki, Y. 2006. pH-responsive three-layered PEGylated polyplex micelle based on a lactosylated ABC triblock copolymer as a targetable and endosome-disruptive nonviral gene vector. *Bioconjug. Chem.*, **17**(3), 677–88.

[24] Rozema, D. B., Lewis, D. L., Wakefield, D. H. *et al.* 2007. Dynamic PolyConjugates for targeted in vivo delivery of siRNA to hepatocytes. *Proc. Nat. Acad. Sci. USA*, **104**(32), 12982–7.

[25] Yao, S., Gutierrez, D. L., Ring, S., Liu, D. and Wise, G. E. 2010. Electroporation to deliver plasmid DNA into rat dental tissues. *J. Gene Med.*, **12**(12), 981–9.

[26] Song, S., Shen, Z., Chen, L., Brayman, A. A. and Miao, C. H. 2011. Explorations of high-intensity therapeutic ultrasound and microbubble-mediated gene delivery in mouse liver. *Gene Ther.*, **18**(10), 1006–14.

[27] Chen, R., Chiba, M., Mori, S., Fukumoto, M. and Kodama, T. 2009. Periodontal gene transfer by ultrasound and nano/microbubbles. *J. Dent. Res.*, **88**(11), 1008–13.

[28] Nakashima, M., Tachibana, K., Iohara, K. *et al.* 2003. Induction of reparative dentin formation by ultrasound-mediated gene delivery of growth/differentiation factor 11. *Hum. Gene Ther.*, **14**(6), 591–7.

[29] Ramseier, C. A., Abramson, Z. R., Jin, Q., Giannobile, W. V. 2006. Gene therapeutics for periodontal regenerative medicine. *Dent. Clin. North Am.*, **50**(2), 245–63 and ix.

[30] Waheed, A. A. and Freed, E. O. 2010. The role of lipids in retrovirus replication. *Viruses*, **2**(5), 1146–80.

[31] Telenti, A. and McLaren, P. 2010. Genomic approaches to the study of HIV-1 acquisition. *J. Infect. Dis.*, **202** (Suppl. 3), S382–6.

[32] Phillips, J. E., Gersbach, C. A. and Garcia, A. J. 2007. Virus-based gene therapy strategies for bone regeneration. *Biomaterials*, **28**(2), 211–29.

[33] Surosky, R. T., Urabe, M., Godwin, S. G. *et al.* 1997. Adeno-associated virus Rep proteins target DNA sequences to a unique locus in the human genome. *J. Virol.*, **71**(10), 7951–9.

[34] Pihlstrom, B. L., Michalowicz, B. S. and Johnson, N. W. 2005. Periodontal diseases. *Lancet*, **366**(9499), 1809–20.

[35] Socransky, S. S., Haffajee, A. D., Cugini, M. A., Smith, C. and Kent, R. L. Jr. 1998. Microbial complexes in subgingival plaque. *J. Clin. Periodontol.*, **25**(2), 134–44.

[36] Tobita, M. and Mizuno, H. 2010. Periodontal disease and periodontal tissue regeneration. *Curr. Stem Cell Res. Ther.*, **5**(2), 168–74.

[37] Heldin, P., Laurent, T. C. and Heldin, C. H. 1989. Effect of growth factors on hyaluronan synthesis in cultured human fibroblasts. *Biochem. J.*, **258**(3), 919–22.

[38] Kaplan, D. R., Chao, F. C., Stiles, C. D., Antoniades, H. N. and Scher, C. D. 1979. Platelet alpha granules contain a growth factor for fibroblasts. *Blood*, **53**(6), 1043–52.

[39] Seppä, H., Grotendorst, G., Seppä, S., Schiffmann, E. and Martin, G. R. 1982. Platelet-derived growth factor is chemotactic for fibroblasts. *J. Cell Biol.*, **92**(2), 584–8.

[40] Kaigler, D., Avila, G., Wisner-Lynch, L. *et al.* 2011. Platelet-derived growth factor applications in periodontal and peri-implant bone regeneration. *Expert Opin. Biol. Ther.*, **11**(3), 375–85.

[41] Rosenkranz, S. and Kazlauskas, A. 1999. Evidence for distinct signaling properties and biological responses induced by the PDGF receptor α and β subtypes. *Growth Factors*, **16**(3): p. 201–16.

[42] Zhu, Z., Lee, C. S., Tejeda, K. M. and Giannobile, W. V. 2001. Gene transfer and expression of platelet-derived growth factors modulate periodontal cellular activity. *J. Dent. Res.*, **80**(3), 892–7.

[43] Giannobile, W. V., Lee, C. S., Tomala, M. P. *et al.* 2001. Platelet-derived growth factor (PDGF) gene delivery for application in periodontal tissue engineering. *J. Periodontol.*, **72**(6), 815–23.

[44] Lin, Z., Sugai, J. V., Jin, Q., Chandler, L. A. and Giannobile, W. V. 2008. Platelet-derived growth factor-B gene delivery sustains gingival fibroblast signal transduction. *J. Periodontal Res.*, **43**(4), 440–9.

[45] Chen, Q. P. and Giannobile, W. V. 2002. Adenoviral gene transfer of PDGF downregulates gas gene product PDGFαR and prolongs ERK and Akt/PKB activation. *Am. J. Physiol. Cell Physiol.*, **282**(3), C538–44.

[46] Chang, P. C., Cirelli, J. A., Jin, Q. *et al.* 2009. Adenovirus encoding human platelet-derived growth factor-B delivered to alveolar bone defects exhibits safety and biodistribution profiles favorable for clinical use. *Hum. Gene Ther.*, **20**(5), 486–96.

[47] Jin, Q., Anusaksathien, O., Webb, S. A., Printz, M. A. and Giannobile, W. V. 2004. Engineering of tooth-supporting structures by delivery of PDGF gene therapy vectors. *Molec. Ther.*, **9**(4), 519–26.

[48] Anusaksathien, O., Jin, Q., Zhao, M., Somerman, M. J. and Giannobile, W. V. 2004. Effect of sustained gene delivery of platelet-derived growth factor or its antagonist (PDGF-1308) on tissue-engineered cementum. *J. Periodontol.*, **75**(3), 429–40.

[49] Urist, M. R. 1965. Bone: formation by autoinduction. *Science*, **150**(3698), 893–9.

[50] Reddi, A. H. 2001. Bone morphogenetic proteins: from basic science to clinical applications. *J. Bone Joint Surg. Am.*, **83A** (Suppl. 1, Part 1), S1–6.

[51] Amar, S., Chung, K. M., Nam, S. H. *et al.* 1997. Markers of bone and cementum formation accumulate in tissues regenerated in periodontal defects treated with expanded polytetrafluoroethylene membranes. *J. Periodontal Res.*, **32**(1, Part 2), 148–58.

[52] Jin, Q. M., Anusaksathien, O., Webb, S. A., Rutherford, W. B. and Giannobile, W. V. 2003. Gene therapy of bone morphogenetic protein for periodontal tissue engineering. *J. Periodontol.*, **74**(2), 202–13.

[53] Park, C. H., Rios, H. F., Taut, A. D. *et al.* 2011. Tissue engineering bone-ligament complexes using fiber-guiding scaffolds. *Biomaterials*, **33**(1), 137–45.

[54] Brugmann, S. A., Goodnough, L. H., Gregorieff, A. *et al.* 2007. Wnt signaling mediates regional specification in the vertebrate face. *Development*, **134**(18), 3283–95.

[55] van Amerongen, R. and Nusse, R. 2009. Towards an integrated view of Wnt signaling in development. *Development*, **136**(19), 3205–14.

[56] Fleming, H. E., Janzen, V., Lo Celso, C. *et al.* 2008. Wnt signaling in the niche enforces hematopoietic stem cell quiescence and is necessary to preserve self-renewal in vivo. *Cell Stem Cell*, **2**(3), 274–83.

[57] Galli, C., Passeri, G. and Macaluso, G. M. 2010. Osteocytes and WNT: the mechanical control of bone formation. *J. Dent. Res.*, **89**(4), 331–43.

[58] Krishnan, V., Bryant, H. U. and Macdougald, O. A. 2006. Regulation of bone mass by Wnt signaling. *J. Clin. Invest.*, **116**(5), 1202–9.

[59] Chang, J., Sonoyama, W., Wang, Z. *et al.* 2007. Noncanonical Wnt-4 signaling enhances bone regeneration of mesenchymal stem cells in craniofacial defects through activation of p38 MAPK. *J. Biol. Chem.*, **282**(42), 30938–48.

[60] Zhao, Z., Wang, Z., Ge, C., Krebsbach, P. and Franceschi, R. T. 2007. Healing cranial defects with AdRunx2-transduced marrow stromal cells. *J. Dent. Res.*, **86**(12), 1207–11.

[61] Phillips, J. E., Guldberg, R. E. and Garcia, A. J. 2007. Dermal fibroblasts genetically modified to express Runx2/Cbfa1 as a mineralizing cell source for bone tissue engineering. *Tissue Eng.*, **13**(8), 2029–40.

[62] Tu, Q., Valverde, P., Li, S. *et al.* 2007. Osterix overexpression in mesenchymal stem cells stimulates healing of critical-sized defects in murine calvarial bone. *Tissue Eng.*, **13**(10), 2431–40.

[63] Pola, E., Gao, W., Zhou, Y. *et al.* 2004. Efficient bone formation by gene transfer of human LIM mineralization protein-3. *Gene Ther.*, **11**(8), 683–93.

[64] Lattanzi, W., Parrilla, C., Fetoni, A. *et al.* 2008. Ex vivo-transduced autologous skin fibroblasts expressing human Lim mineralization protein-3 efficiently form new bone in animal models. *Gene Ther.*, **15**(19), 1330–43.

[65] Giannobile, W. V. 2008. Host-response therapeutics for periodontal diseases. *J. Periodontol.*, **79**(8, Suppl.), 1592–600.

[66] Cirelli, J. A., Park, C. H., MacKool, K. *et al.* 2009. AAV2/1-TNFR:Fc gene delivery prevents periodontal disease progression. *Gene Ther.*, **16**(3), 426–36.

[67] Patil, C. S., Liu, M., Zhao, W. *et al.* 2008. Targeting mRNA stability arrests inflammatory bone loss. *Molec. Ther.*, **16**(10), 1657–64.

[68] Yu, H., Li, Q., Herbert, B. *et al.* 2011. Anti-inflammatory effect of MAPK phosphatase-1 local gene transfer in inflammatory bone loss. *Gene Ther.*, **18**(4), 344–53.

[69] Hughes, F. J., Ghuman, M. and Talal, A. 2010. Periodontal regeneration: a challenge for the tissue engineer? *Proc. Inst. Mech. Eng. H*, **224**(12), 1345–58.

[70] Lin, Z., Rios, H. F., Volk, S. L. *et al.* 2011. Gene expression dynamics during bone healing and osseointegration. *J. Periodontol.*, **82**(7), 1007–17.

[71] Chang, P. C., Seol, Y. G., Cirelli, J. A. *et al.* 2010. PDGF-B gene therapy accelerates bone engineering and oral implant osseointegration. *Gene Ther.*, **17**(1), 95–104.

[72] Chang, P. C., Lang, N. P. and Giannobile, W. V. 2010. Evaluation of functional dynamics during osseointegration and regeneration associated with oral implants. *Clin. Oral Implants Res.*, **21**(1), 1–12.

[73] Dunn, C. A., Jin, Q., Taba, M. Jr. *et al.* 2005. BMP gene delivery for alveolar bone engineering at dental implant defects. *Molec. Ther.*, **11**(2), 294–9.

[74] Zhang, Y., Song, J., Shi, B. *et al.* 2007. Combination of scaffold and adenovirus vectors expressing bone morphogenetic protein-7 for alveolar bone regeneration at dental implant defects. *Biomaterials*, **28**(31), 4635–42.

[75] Won, Y. W., Lim, K. S. and Kim, Y. H. 2011. Intracellular organelle-targeted non-viral gene delivery systems. *J. Controlled Release*, **152**(1), 99–109.

22

Endogenous stem/progenitor cell recruitment for tissue regeneration

Mildred Embree, Chang Hun Lee, Ziming Dong, Mo Chen, Kimi Kong, Hemin Nie, Avital Mendelson, Bhranti Shah, Shoko Cho, Takahiro Suzuki, Rujing Yang, Nan Jiang and Jeremy J. Mao

22.1 Introduction: stem/progenitor cell recruitment vs. transplantation

The utilization of transplanted stem cells in regenerative medicine has been studied extensively as a potential therapy to repair or replace tissues that are lost due to trauma, congenital deformities, tumor resections, or infectious diseases [1–3]. The current cell transplantation model in regenerative medicine is founded on the principle that the application of transplanted stem cells could repopulate and regenerate damaged or diseased tissues, with restored tissue functions and homeostasis. However, cell transplantation is faced with a multitude of clinical and cell culture complications including the complexity of the multistep surgical procedures, donor-site trauma, immune rejection for allogeneic and xenogeneic cells, cell phenotypic variations due to in-vitro culture techniques, potential tumorigenesis associated with long-term cell expansion, failure of exogenous cell engraftment, and uncertainties and difficulties in the regulatory approval process [4–8]. The difficulties in the clinical application of stem cell transplantation are in strong contrast to the results of multiple experimental studies that demonstrate different levels of efficacy of cell delivery in a number of disease models such as Parkinson's disease [9, 10], blood cancers and diseases [11, 12], and muscle and spinal disorders/injuries [13, 14].

For a number of regenerative medicine applications, the use of stem cell transplantation might not be competitive with the cost-effectiveness of current clinical treatment modalities in the dental and musculoskeletal fields, including titanium joint replacements, dental implants, and operative dental procedures [15–17]. Alternatively, the concept of endogenous stem/progenitor cell recruitment in regenerative medicine is based on the idea that native stem/progenitor cells that already reside within mature tissue can be stimulated and functionally enhanced to repopulate, repair, and/or regenerate damaged tissues [18]. Relative to stem cell transplantation, the application of endogenous stem cell recruitment in regenerative medicine is still in its infancy. The combination of the use of biological factors, release technology, biomaterials, and bioengineered scaffolds to enhance endogenous stem cell recruitment seems very promising for potential use in translational regenerative medicine. However, further scientific experimentation is warranted, since many scientific questions concerning the mechanistic details remain unresolved and it will be necessary to validate the efficacy of this approach for clinical application.

22.2 Stem/progenitor cell sources and niche

Stem cells are unspecialized cells that are critical for organogenesis and tissue repair. Stem cells also play vital roles in tissue homeostasis and replenish more specialized cells undergoing apoptosis. In comparison with specialized cells, stem cells have unique properties of self-renewal, clonogenicity, and the ability to differentiate into multiple mature cell types [19, 20]. There are three main types of stem cells: embryonic stem cells (ESCs), adult stem/progenitor cells, and induced pluripotent stem cells (iPSs). The ESCs are derived from the inner mass of the blastocyst of early-stage embryos [20]. They have the ability to divide indefinitely, are pluripotent, and can differentiate into all three germ layers: the ectoderm, endoderm, and mesoderm [20]. However, the use of human embryos in research has raised ethical concerns [21]. To avoid the ethical dilemmas, adult or somatic cells have been reprogrammed as iPSs that possess many of the properties of ESCs, such as self-renewal and pluripotency [22]. Unlike with ESCs, an important feature of IPs is the ability to develop patient-specific stem-cell-based therapy [22, 23].

Resident adult stem/progenitor cells are the critical cell sources which are utilized for endogenous stem/progenitor cell recruitment therapy. Adult stem/progenitor cells have been identified in multiple tissues, including prostate [24], heart [25, 26], brain [27], bone marrow [28, 29], blood [30], orofacial [31], tendon [32], cartilage [33], skeletal muscle [34], and hair follicles [35]. The primary roles of adult stem/progenitor cells are to maintain tissue homeostasis and also to repair tissue in the event of injury or disease. In comparison with ESCs and iPSs, adult stem/progenitor cells can divide only a limited number of times, and are also limited in terms of the number of differentiated cell types they can produce [36]. Adult stem/progenitor cells generally exist in relatively low numbers within adult tissue, and remain in a quiescent or non-dividing state unless they are activated to maintain tissue homeostasis or by disease or tissue injury [26, 37]. Adult stem/progenitor cells reside within a specialized niche or a microenvironment that regulates how it contributes to tissue generation, homeostasis, and repair [38, 39]. The stem/progenitor cell niche is critical for modulating the signals that mediate the balanced response of stem cells to the requirements of the tissue homeostasis, and ultimately determines a balanced proportion of quiescent and activated stem cells [38].

22.3 Lessons learned from native stem/progenitor cell homing mechanisms

Homing is the process whereby stem cells migrate and engraft into tissue. Homing is involved both during embryological development and in adult tissue homeostasis or repair [40, 67]. During development stem cell homing is critical for organogenesis and morphogenesis [40]. The migration of neural crest cells is a fine example of stem cell homing [40]. In adult tissues, resident stem/progenitor cells receive biological cues that induce their migration from their corresponding cell niche to the targeted tissue destination in order to either maintain tissue homeostasis or repair tissue that has been damaged by disease/injury [41, 67]. Stem/progenitor cells are homed from a specific cell niche, such as the bone marrow, and enter into circulation in the blood stream. The circulating stem cells can then exit blood vessels and enter the target tissue to repopulate mature effector adult cells or home from the blood stream to sites of injury to exert local effects to repair the tissue [41]. In either case, homed stem/progenitor cells ultimately restore tissue function and maintain cellular balance. The mechanisms underlying stem/progenitor cell homing are poorly understood, but likely involve multiple, complex steps that are both tissue- and cell-specific [41].

One of the most well-characterized stem cell homing processes in adults involves homing of hematopoietic stem cells (HSCs) from the bone marrow niche into the bloodstream, across the endothelium to target organs, and finally back to the bone marrow niche [41]. This HSC homing entails a coordinated set of multifaceted events and molecular players, including growth factors, chemokines, and adhesion factors, which orchestrate the migration of circulating HSCs to specific tissue targets. In this process, chemoattractant cytokines or chemokines mobilize HSCs from the bone marrow niche. Stromal cell-derived factor 1 (SDF-α_1) is one example of a powerful chemokine that has been implicated in the migration, proliferation, differentiation, and survival of human and murine HSCs [42]. SDF-α_1 is produced in the bone marrow by immature osteoblasts in the endosteum region adjacent to stem cell niches [43], and is also highly expressed by human and murine bone marrow endothelium [43, 44]. CXCR4 (or CD184) is a transmembrane G-protein-coupled receptor of SDF-α_1 that is widely expressed by hematopoietic, endothelial, stromal, and neuronal cells [45]. More specifically, studies using both SDF-α_1- and CXCR4-null mice have demonstrated that interactions between SDF-α_1 and CXCR4 are critical for HSC localization in the bone marrow niche, since disruption of this interaction results in rapid mobilization of HSCs from their niches [42, 46]. Furthermore, ischemia within peripheral tissue causes increased SDF-α_1 expression on endothelial cells, which, in turn, mediates the recruitment of HSCs to the sites of vascular injury [47–49]. Given the critical role of the SDF-α_1–CXCR4 axis in the mobilization and homing of stem cells to target tissues, it is not surprising that augmentation of SDF-α_1 signals to induce stem cell homing has been studied as a potential therapy to repair injured tissues such as heart, kidney, and bone [50–52].

To migrate, HSCs must break away from their niche, which requires the activation of proteolytic enzymes, such as matrix metalloproteinase (MMP)-9, cysteine protease cathepsin K, and osteoclasts [53, 54]. Subsequently, HSCs enter the bloodstream, and must home to target sites by attaching to microvascular endothelial cells through adhesion molecules located on HSC and endothelial cell surfaces. Primary adhesion molecules, such as selectins and integrins, mediate the rolling and tethering of HSCs to the blood vessel wall and implement fast binding with high tensile strength but short bond lifetime [40, 41]. Subsequently, chemotactic activating stimuli are provided by chemokines to promote target specificity. Finally, more stable binding is mediated by secondary adhesion molecules, mostly integrins (a2 or a4) that interact with endothelial ligands of the immunoglobulin superfamily [41]. Finally, HSCs must return to the bone marrow niche to replenish the bone marrow cell population. The HSCs exit from the peripheral tissue back into circulation through the lymphatic system, which is tightly regulated by Sphingosine-1-phosphage (S1P) [55]. The a4b1 integrin (VLA-4) is expressed by most HSCs and interacts with vascular cell adhesion molecule (VCAM)-1 on stromal cells and endothelium of the bone marrow, which is critical for HSC engraftment to the bone marrow niche [56, 57].

Another stem cell population within the bone marrow niche consists of one of the most widely studied types of stem cell in tissue engineering, namely mesenchymal stem cells (MSCs). The MSCs exist within the blood circulation in relatively low numbers [58]. The mobilization of MSCs from the bone marrow niche to the bloodstream and peripheral tissues, and their return to the bone marrow niche, is a dynamic process. The migration of native MSCs from local tissue niches or from the bone marrow niche can be induced by injured tissue, whereby MSCs migrate toward the target site to solicit a repair response [59, 60]. More MSCs are seen in peripheral blood of injured subjects than in that of non-injured controls [60]. Furthermore, MSC mobilization to sites of injury correlates with significantly increased concentrations of cytokines, including VEGF and G-CSF [59, 60], emphasizing the roles of cytokines in MSC mobilization [60]. The cellular mechanisms regulating the homing of MSCs to sites of injury are similar to HSC homing mechanisms [61]. Circulating MSCs first engage in rolling, whereby MSCs establish low-affinity binding interactions with vascular endothelial cells. This process then leads to subsequent arrest of other fast-flowing MSC subpopulations within the circulation via chemokine-mediated integrin adhesion, followed by more stable adhesive binding. Finally, endothelial transmigration occurs, with subsequent chemotaxis to injured tissue. The engraftment of homed MSC into the injured tissue is largely dependent upon multiple factors, including chemotactic gradients established by the injured tissue, adhesive molecules, ECM digestion, and MSC cytoskeletal arrangement [61]. Given the role of native MSCs in repair of injured tissue, it is not surprising that the infusion of exogenous MSCs within the bloodstream has been tested as a potential therapy for musculoskeletal tissue [62, 63]. However, the complexity of guiding exogenous MSCs in sufficient numbers to the site of injury has hindered this methodology. A complete, in-depth understanding of the mechanistic details underlying the homing of native MSC to injured or diseased tissues could potentially enable bioengineers to develop improved endogenous stem/progenitor cell recruitment strategies to enhance and precisely control the regenerative process.

22.4 Activation of endogenous stem cells for tissue engineering and regeneration

The concept of endogenous stem/progenitor cell recruitment in tissue engineering is based on the concept that cytotactic cues such as growth factors (GFs) stimulate the endogenous stem/progenitor cells to migrate and repair the damaged tissues [67]. In a report in *The Lancet*, Lee *et al.* showed in 2010 that cells recruited into the microchannels of anatomically correct scaffolds regenerated a synovial joint defect [67]. In this approach, TGF-β_3 is integrated into biomaterial scaffolds mimicking native host extracellular matrices and the biomaterial/GF delivery vehicle can then be transplanted to the target host tissue defect (Figure 22.1(a)). Subsequently, GFs within biomaterial scaffold delivery system can act as biological cues to induce the recruitment of stem/progenitor cells from a local tissue cell niche and/or from the blood stream to the targeted tissue defect (Figure 22.1(b)). The recruited stem/progenitor cells can then orchestrate the regenerative process and repair/regenerate new tissue.

The GFs act as powerful and critical signaling molecules that direct and instruct cells during

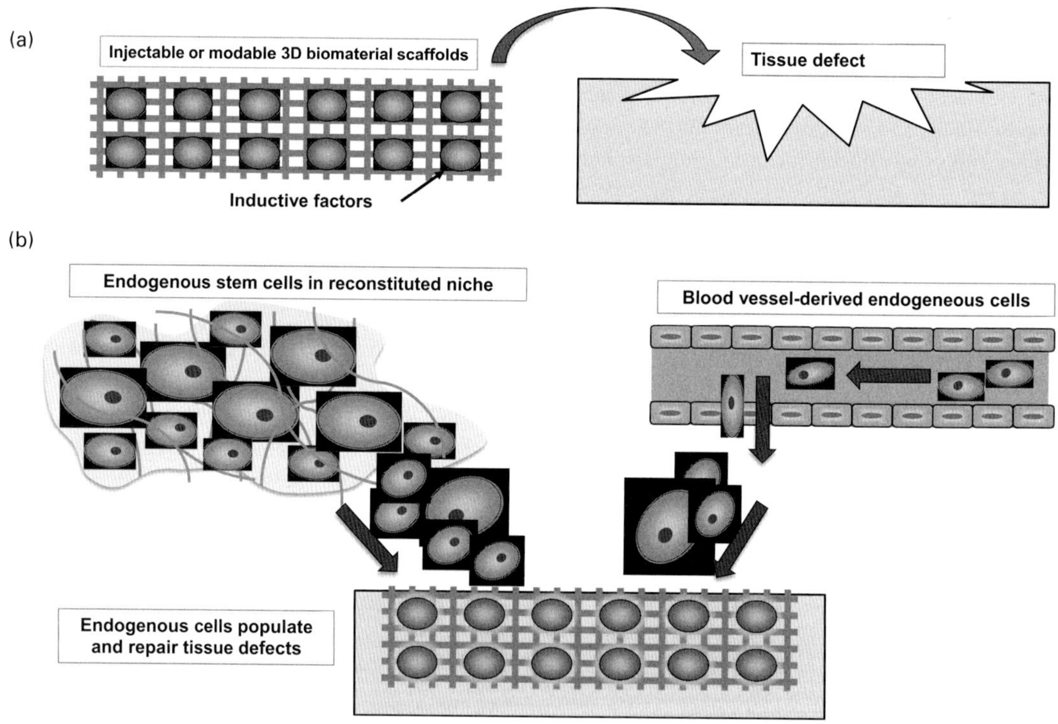

Figure 22.1 A schematic illustration showing the use of growth factors (GFs) embedded in a biomaterial scaffold for recruitment of endogenous stem/progenitor cells to a tissue defect site for regeneration. (a) Scaffolds composed of selected biomaterials specifically designed for the host tissue defect serve as GF delivery systems. Biomaterial scaffolds can consist of a prefabricated external shape and an internal porous architecture integrated with the appropriate GFs. The biomaterial/GF delivery vehicle can be transplanted to target the host tissue defect. (b) GFs within a biomaterial scaffold delivery system can act to induce the recruitment of stem/progenitor cells from local tissue extracellular matrix niche and/or from the blood stream.

development, in maintenance of tissue homeostasis, and in response to injury [64]. Generally, GFs have the ability to promote either one or a combination of the following cellular activities: recruitment, proliferation, and differentiation. Bioengineers have seized inspiration from native tissue design, and use a combination of carefully designed biomaterials to precisely apply and control exogenous GFs in a local area for the potential to initiate and/or augment the tissue regeneration. By harnessing therapeutic induction of tissue repair by GFs and/or GFs' ability to maintain functional tissue homeostasis, bioengineers aim to recapitulate the spatial and temporal microenvironments formed by native extracellular matrices. With an improved understanding of the critical pathways involved in the development of the targeted tissue of interest, the role of GFs in repair and regeneration, and the enhancement of GF biological activity through recombinant technologies, the use of GFs is an increasingly important strategy to repair or regenerate damaged tissue.

22.5 Growth factor delivery strategies and systems

The goals of GF delivery systems are to improve GF bioavailability and activity, provide a compatible three-dimensional (3D) framework for native cells, reduce side effects of GFs on the patient, and facilitate administration [18]. Current GF delivery systems usually utilize scaffolding biomaterials specifically designed for the host tissue defect. Such scaffolds consist of a prefabricated external shape and an internal porous architecture integrated with the appropriate GFs [65]. For different tissue defects the specific GF and its concentration and release rate are optimized to promote the restoration of tissue integrity and function. Bioscaffolds can be defined as scaffolds that are composed of biomaterials and house the selected GF used in tissue engineering. Bioscaffolds afford the required mechanical properties, and are designed to emulate the native ECM tissue architecture to provide an optimal and instructive microenvironment in which native cells can attach, grow, and differentiate into new tissue.

Several barriers may negatively impact on GF efficacy, including short half-life and the cellular/tissue toxicity caused by administration of multiple doses or high concentrations. Furthermore, in therapies that involve direct GF delivery locally to the tissue defect via injected solutions, GFs have the tendency to diffuse away from the site and undergo enzymatic degradation [70–72]. Consequently, controlled-release technology was developed to maximize the biological effect of GFs and minimize negative side effects on native tissue and cells [66–69]. Advanced controlled-release technology provides controlled, predictable, and sustained delivery of GFs to drive stem/progenitor cell recruitment.

Controlled-release technology involves the encapsulation of GFs into bioscaffolds, nanoparticles, and/or microspheres with predictable degradation rates and allows precise control of GF release [73, 74]. Moreover, most biomaterials are not readily internalized by the cells and are retained in the tissue, providing prolonged GF release [75]. Additionally, encapsulated GFs generally remain at the site of implantation and are too large to diffuse out of the target tissue to other sites. Therefore, encapsulated GFs typically have only local tissue/cell effects. For example, encapsulation of GFs such as granulocyte colony-stimulating factor in scaffolds with sustained release kinetics or scaffolds that permit expression of GFs by gene transfer has been shown to improve cardiac function after disease initiation [76]. Additionally, bioengineered ECMs with release technology have been demonstrated to provide control of spatiotemporal delivery of single or even multiple GFs [69, 77]. It has been demonstrated that, by crosslinking chemically modified hyaluronan hydrogels loaded with the two GFs VEGF and angiopoietin-1, localized microvessel regrowth rates could be controlled [78]. In this regard, the combined use and controlled release of multiple GFs should have the potential to provide additive and potentially synergistic effects, thus offering an advantage for the bioengineer who wants to carefully orchestrate and control the regenerative process.

In general, biomaterial vehicles for GF encapsulation and delivery should ideally (1) possess the ability to conform and/or adhere to the host damaged tissue; (2) provide the necessary biomechanical support to maintain structural integrity of native tissue and sustain the host's movements; (3) provide the optimal microenvironment for recruitment, proliferation, differentiation, and attachment of native cells, and new tissue formation; (4) maintain the biological activity and concentration of GFs over the desired time course; (5) cause no toxicity or immunogenic response to the host; and (6) not interfere with the regenerative process and be absorbed over time [69]. The selection of the biomaterial vehicle and design to encapsulate a GF for delivery for regenerative purposes is largely dependent upon the host target tissue, the nature of the damaged tissue, and the desired GF release and therapeutic effect.

Currently there are multiple choices of biomaterials for encapsulation for delivery of a GF that is either injected or surgically transplanted. Synthetic polymers afford several advantages, including physical adaptability to tissue defects, their availability in different sizes and shapes to suite the specific host, controllable mechanical and degradation properties, and the fact that GFs can be easily incorporated by adding functional groups and side chains [79]. Polymer properties such as the scaffold pore size, surface physiochemical properties, and substrate stiffness can also be modified to achieve the desired regenerative and GF therapeutic effect [80, 81]. The most commonly used synthetic polymers in tissue engineering for scaffold/GF delivery are polyglycolic acid (PGA), polylactic acid (PLA), and also copolymers such as poly(lactic-*co*-glycolic acid) (PLGA) and polycaprolactone (PCL) [80]. On the other hand, natural polymers that can be used in tissue engineering include collagen, alginate, agarose, chitosan, fibrin, and hyaluronic acid [74]. In comparison with synthetic polymers, natural polymers generally undergo adsorption readily and have only very minor side effects on the host [74]. However, natural polymers offer little structural integrity, and their biomechanical and chemical properties cannot be as easily modified as can those of synthetic polymers [74]. While the addition of crosslinking agents to natural polymers can aid in maintaining GF bioactivity, another common critical disadvantage in comparison with synthetic polymers is the loss of the GF's bioactivity [64]. A composite material is generally a combination of two or more materials that differ in composition that is intended to result in specific chemical, physical, and mechanical properties [82–84]. The advantage of using a composite material is that the resulting material may possess a combination of the best properties of its constituents for the desired regenerative effect. For example, a blend of PLG and poly(3-hydroxybutyrate-*co*-3-hydroxyvalerate) (PHBV) microspheres improves retention in the biomaterial during scaffold fabrication and produced a better encapsulating material than either PLG or PHBV alone [84].

The selection of the GF delivery rate is mainly contingent on the specific GF and targeted tissue. Usually the delivery rate can be controlled by the degree of encapsulation, irrespective of whether the GF is designed to have hydrophobic or hydrophilic interactions with the selected biomaterial, variations in biomaterial physical and chemical properties, the distribution of the GF within the biomaterial, and the porosity of the biomaterial [64]. For example, the size of nanospheres and microparticles encapsulating one or more GFs determines the delivery rate as a surface-area-to-GF-volume ratio [85]. For quick-burst and high-dose release, GFs can be administered via a bolus injection or released by being directly adsorbed onto biomaterial scaffold surfaces or in collagen sponges. In this regard, mainly natural polymers or readily degradable synthetic polymers are utilized for GF encapsulation [86–88]. To achieve a more sustained release, GFs may be non-covalently encapsulated into microspheres or nanoparticles that are not highly crosslinked [85]. A delayed release can be achieved by encapsulating GF non-convalently in highly crosslinked microspheres and/or in microspheres with an outer core shell [89]. A pulse-like release can be achieved using a combination of GF non-covalently adsorbed onto scaffolds incorporated into highly crosslinked microspheres with core shells [69]. By chemically covalently attaching GFs to biomaterial scaffolds or by designing core shells with high porosity to allow GF diffusion, a continuous and high-dose release can be achieved [90–92]. For example, VEGF-loaded core-shell fibrous membranes prepared by co-axial electrospinning with dextran (DEX) as the core component and PLGA as the shell polymer resulted in GF release being sustained for more than 28 days [92]. Finally, environment-sensitive materials can be utilized to generate pulsatile and on/off release in response to local and external changes in pH, temperature, or protease activity [93–96]. Taken together, GF delivery systems hold great promise as smart technology for precise controlled release of GFs that can be tailored for tissue- and patient-specific clinical applications. The appropriate choice of GF, encapsulating biomaterial, and biscaffold design may enable fast and precise cellular responses during tissue regeneration.

22.6 Cellular reponses to exogenously delivered growth factors

The regenerative effects of delivered growth factors that have so far been demonstrated in tissue regeneration have been both tissue- and GF-specific. Various GFs have been used as biological cues to induce stem cell recruitment in tissue engineering to mediate the regeneration of several tissues, such as bone [97–106], cartilage [67], tendon-to-bone insertion [107, 108], skeletal muscle [109], nerve [110–113], heart [114–116], dentin and pulp [117–121], dental periodontium [122–127], and temporomandibular joint [128–131]. A summary of selected experimental examples of tissue regeneration by GF recruitment of endogenous stem/progenitor cells is outlined in Table 22.1.

Several GFs have been used to promote bone regeneration; however, the role of bone morphogenetic proteins (BMPs) has perhaps been studied the most extensively [97–101, 132]. More specifically, one member, BMP-2, is critical for the chemotractant migration of human osteogenic precursor cells [70, 133]. However, extremely high doses of BMP-2 are typically required for achieving a substantial healing response due to disadvantages such as the short protein half-life [132, 134]. High doses of BMP-2 in bone have resulted in complications such as diffusion of protein to other tissues, and the treatment cost is high [135, 136]. In this regard, numerous sustained BMP delivery vehicles were developed to improve the protein pharmacokinetics in vivo, including a biodegradable hydrogel allowing controlled release of BMP-2 in a rabbit defect model [98]. Furthermore, synthetic poly(ethylene glycol) (PEG)-based hydrogels used as cell-ingrowth matrices containing a combination of crosslinking MMP substrates and pendant adhesion sites allowed controlled release of BMP-2, recruitment of osteogenic precursor cells, and new bone formation in critically sized cranial defects in rats [103]. Bone functional recovery has also been demonstrated, whereby a hybrid alginate–nanofiber mesh BMP-2 delivery system not only allowed a significant increase in bone mineral density, but also improved biomechanical function in a rat femoral segmental defect model [99].

Attempts to regenerate new bone often face the challenge of minimal vascularization [137], which can impede bone regeneration. Consequently, vascular endothelial factor (VEGF), which is a pro-angiogenic GF, is often utilized in combination with BMP-2 in biomaterial scaffolds to promote the endothelial cell recruitment and regeneration of new vascular supply [102, 104–106]. For example, dual delivery of VEGF and BMP-2 encapsulated in gelatin microparticles, which were incorporated onto a poly(propylene fumarate) scaffold, resulted in increased vascularity and increased bony bridging and bone formation when the microparticles were transplanted onto calvarial defects in rats [104]. Furthermore, enhanced neovascularization can also improve bone turnover,

The regeneration of an entire articular surface of rabbit synovial joint was also demonstrated by recruitment of endogenous stem/progenitor cells. A composite biomaterial consisting of PCL and hydroxyapatite was fabricated into an anatomically shaped humeral condyle in rabbits. In this case, the bioscaffolds were spatially infused with TGF-β_3 in hydrogels to induce stem/progenitor cell recruitment and differentiation into synovial joint [67]. Follow-up in-vitro studies demonstrated that delivery of TGF-β_3 and SDF-1β in a collagen sponge cube resulted in increases in numbers of recruited adipose, mesenchymal, and

Table 22.1 Selected examples of GF delivery for endogenous stem/progenitor cell recruitment and tissue regeneration

Tissue	Growth factor	Delivery vehicle	Animal species	References
Bone	BMP-2	Collagen sponges; biodegradable hydrogel; nanofibrous mesh-alginate hybrid system; PGA and β-TCP; PEG-based hydrogel	Goat, rabbit, rat	[97–100, 103]
	BMP-7	PLGA nanospheres on prefabricated nano-fibrous PLLA scaffolds	Rat	[101]
	VEGF and BMP-2	Gelatin microparticles on poly(propylene fumarate); alginate hydrogel and $P_{DL}LA$; poly(lactic-*co*-glycolic acid) microspheres embedded in a poly(propylene) scaffold surrounded by a gelatin hydrogel	Rat, mouse	[104–106]
Cartilage	TGF-β_3	Hydrogels spatially infused into PCL-HA	Rabbit	[67]
Skeletal muscle	IGF	EH and EH-PEG	Human	[109]
Tendon-to-bone insertion (fibrocartilage)	TGF-β_3	Heparin/fibrin; injectable calcium phosphate matrix	Rat	[107, 108]
Nerve	NGF	PCL; PLGA	Rat	[110, 111]
	GDNF	PLGA/PCL	Rat	[112]
	SHH	Peptide amphiphile nanofibers	Rat	[113]
Cardiac	IGF-1	Self-assembling peptide nanofibers	Rat	[114]
	HGF and IGF-1	Alginate	Rat	[115]
	SDF-1	Self-assembling peptide nanofibers	Rat	[116]
Dentin and pulp	TGF-β_1, TGF-β_2, TGF-β_3	Agarose beads	Rat	[117]
	TGF-β_1	Alginate beads	Human	[118]
	BMP-7	Agarose beads	Rat	[119]
	BMP-2,4	Collagen sponge	Human	[120]
	bFGF, VEGF, PDGF	Collagen gel	Mouse	[121]
Dental periodontium	FGF-2	Gelatinous carrier, collagen membrane	Canine	[122]
	IGF-1	Dextran-*co*-gelatin hydrogel microspheres	Human	[123]
	BMP-12	Collagen sponge	Canine	[124]
	BMP-2	Dissolving collagen membrane	Rat	[125]
	PDGF-BB	bTCP	Human	[126]
	BMP-7, SDF-1	PCL-HA composite	Rat	[127]
Temporo man-dibular joint (TMJ)	BMP-2	Collagen and PLA/PGA copolymer–gelatin sponge	Rabbit	[128, 129]
	TGF-β_1	Oligo(poly(ethylene glycol) fumarate) OPF	Rabbit	[130]
	TGF-β_3	Thermoreversible hydrogel/hyaluronic acid	Rabbit	[131]

synovial stem/progenitor cells, and also an increase in the expression of chondrogenic markers [68]. Taken together, the use of GFs incorporated within biomaterials as biological cues to recruit cells to targeted tissue sites has been demonstrated. The therapeutic effects are dependent upon the GF, GF release, selection of biomaterial design, and targeted cells/tissue.

22.7 Clinical translation: barriers and opportunities

Experimental studies, especially in-vivo findings, have demonstrated that certain GFs acting as bioactive cues immobilize endogenous stem/progenitor cells in order for them to participate in tissue regeneration. The selection of bioactive cues, including GFs, for endogenous regeneration remains a challenging task for active investigations, given the diversity of tissues to be regenerated, cell types, and molecular players involved in the regenerative process, and the structural complexity of the tissues to be regenerated. For example, selected GFs may specifically recruit undifferentiated stem/progenitor cells and/or more mature cells. Endogenous cell sources involved in the regenerative process also include mature, differentiated cells and inflammatory cells that must be kept under control. These questions are further confounded by the experimental limitations imposed by current scientific resources, whereby methods for tracking endogenous cell recruitment in vivo are restricted. Additionally, the long-term prognosis, the functional capabilities of the regenerated tissues, and the use of this approach in disease and complex wound models still warrant further investigations. Future advances in endogenous regeneration will likely rely on the selectivity of bioactive cues that specify multiple cellular processes including migration, ending of stemness, lineage specification, differentiation and regeneration/remodeling.

ACKNOWLEDGEMENTS

We thank Qiongfen Guo and Jacqueline Melendez for their administrative assistance. The work for this chapter was supported by NIH grants R01DE018248, R01EB009663, and RC2DE020767 (to J.J.M.)

REFERENCES

[1] Passier, R., van Laake, L. W. and Mummery, C. L. 2008. Stem-cell-based therapy and lessons from the heart. *Nature*, **453**(7193), 322–9.

[2] Lindvall, O. and Kokaia, Z. 2006. Stem cells for the treatment of neurological disorders. *Nature*, **441**(7097), 1094–6.

[3] Rafii, S. and Lyden, D. 2003. Therapeutic stem and progenitor cell transplantation for organ vascularization and regeneration. *Nature Med.*, **9**(6), 702–12.

[4] Burt, R. K., Shah, S. J., Diu, K. *et al.* 2011. Autologous non-myeloablative haemopoietic stem-cell transplantation compared with pulse cyclophosphamide once per month for systemic sclerosis (ASSIST): an open-label, randomised phase 2 trial. *Lancet*, **378**(9790), 498–506.

[5] Bongso, A., Fong, C. Y. and Gauthaman, K. 2008. Taking stem cells to the clinic: major challenges. *J. Cell Biochem.*, **105**(6), 1352–60.

[6] Condic, M. L. and Rao, M. 2008. Regulatory issues for personalized pluripotent cells. *Stem Cells*, **26**(11), 2753–8.

[7] Fujikawa, T., Oh, S. H., Pi, L. *et al.* 2005. Teratoma formation leads to failure of treatment for type I diabetes using embryonic stem cell-derived insulin-producing cells. *Am. J. Pathol.*, **166**(6), 1781–91.

[8] Nussbaum, J., Minami, E., Laflamme, M. A. *et al.* 2007. Transplantation of undifferentiated murine embryonic stem cells in the heart: teratoma formation and immune response. *FASEB J.*, **21**(7), 1345–57.

[9] Ben-Hur, T., Idelson, M., Khaner, H. *et al.* 2004. Transplantation of human embryonic stem cell-derived neural progenitors improves behavioral deficit in Parkinsonian rats. *Stem Cells*, **22**(7), 1246–55.

[10] Yang, D., Zhang, Z.-J., Oldenburg, M., Ayala, M. and Zhang, S.-C. 2008. Human embryonic stem cell-derived dopaminergic neurons reverse functional deficit in Parkinsonian rats. *Stem Cells*, **26**(1), 55–63.

[11] Andersson, B. S. 2010. Advances in CML: the role of allogeneic hematopoietic stem cell transplantation. *Clin. Adv. Hematol. Oncol.*, **8**(11), 746–8.

[12] Dreger, P., Döhner, H., Ritgen, M. *et al.* 2010. Allogeneic stem cell transplantation provides durable disease control in poor-risk chronic lymphocytic leukemia: long-term clinical and MRD results of the German CLL Study Group CLL3X trial. *Blood*, **116**(14), 2438–47.

[13] Ferrari, G., Cusella-De Angelis, G., Coletta, M. *et al.* 1998. Muscle regeneration by bone marrow-derived myogenic progenitors. *Science,* **279**(5356), 1528–30.

[14] Sahni, V. and Kessler, J. A. 2010. Stem cell therapies for spinal cord injury. *Nature Rev. Neurol.,* **6**(7), 363–72.

[15] Lindahl, A., Brittberg, M. and Peterson, L. 2003. Cartilage repair with chondrocytes: clinical and cellular aspects. *Novartis Found. Symp.,* **249**, p. 175–86; discussion 186–9, 234–8 and 239–41.

[16] Iacono, V. J. 2000. Dental implants in periodontal therapy. *J. Periodontol.,* **71**(12), 1934–42.

[17] Clar, C., Cummins, E., McIntyre, L. *et al.* 2005. Clinical and cost-effectiveness of autologous chondrocyte implantation for cartilage defects in knee joints: systematic review and economic evaluation. *Health Technol. Assess.,* **9**(47), iii–iv, ix–x, and 1–82.

[18] Chen, F. M., Wu, L. A., Zhang, M., Zhang, R. and Sun, H. H. 2011. Homing of endogenous stem/progenitor cells for in situ tissue regeneration: Promises, strategies, and translational perspectives. *Biomaterials,* **32**(12), 3189–209.

[19] Grossman, Z. 1986. The stem cell concept revisited: self-renewal capacity is a dynamic property of hemopoietic cells. *Leuk. Res.,* **10**(8), 937–50.

[20] Thomson, J. A., Itskovitz-Eldor, J., Shapiro, S. S. *et al.* 1998. Embryonic stem cell lines derived from human blastocysts. *Science,* **282**(5391), 1145–7.

[21] Volarević, V., Ljujić, B., Stojković, P. *et al.* 2011. Human stem cell research and regenerative medicine – present and future. *Br. Med. Bull.,* **99**, 155–68.

[22] Takahashi, K. and Yamanaka, S. 2006. Induction of pluripotent stem cells from mouse embryonic and adult fibroblast cultures by defined factors. *Cell,* **126** (4), 663–76.

[23] Yu, J., Hu, K., Smuga-Otto, K. *et al.* 2009. Human induced pluripotent stem cells free of vector and transgene sequences. *Science,* **324**(5928), 797–801.

[24] Leong, K. G., Wang, B. E., Johnson, L. and Gao, W. Q. 2008. Generation of a prostate from a single adult stem cell. *Nature,* **456**(7223), 804–8.

[25] Beltrami, A. P., Barlucchi, L., Torella, D. *et al.* 2003. Adult cardiac stem cells are multipotent and support myocardial regeneration. *Cell,* **114**(6), 763–76.

[26] Mishra, R., Vijayan, K., Colletti, E. J. *et al.* 2011. Characterization and functionality of cardiac progenitor cells in congenital heart patients. *Circulation,* **123**(4), 364–73.

[27] McKay, R. D. 1999. Brain stem cells change their identity. *Nature Med.,* **5**(3), 261–2.

[28] Liechty, K. W., MacKenzie, T. C., Shaaban, A. F. *et al.* 2000. Human mesenchymal stem cells engraft and demonstrate site-specific differentiation after in utero transplantation in sheep. *Nature Med.,* **6**(11), 1282–6.

[29] Gerson, S. L. 1999. Mesenchymal stem cells: no longer second class marrow citizens. *Nature Med.,* **5**(3), 262–4.

[30] Orkin, S. H. and Zon, L. I. 2008. Hematopoiesis: an evolving paradigm for stem cell biology. *Cell,* **132**(4), 631–44.

[31] Huang, G. T., Gronthos, S. and Shi, S. 2009. Mesenchymal stem cells derived from dental tissues vs. those from other sources: their biology and role in regenerative medicine. *J. Dent. Res.,* **88**(9), 792–806.

[32] Bi, Y., Ehirchiou, D., Kilts, T. M. *et al.* 2007. Identification of tendon stem/progenitor cells and the role of the extracellular matrix in their niche. *Nature Med.,* **13**(10), 1219–27.

[33] Koelling, S., Kruegel, J., Irmer, M. *et al.* 2009. Migratory chondrogenic progenitor cells from repair tissue during the later stages of human osteoarthritis. *Cell Stem Cell,* **4**(4), 324–35.

[34] Mitchell, K. J., Pannérec, A., Cadot, B. *et al.* 2010. Identification and characterization of a non-satellite cell muscle resident progenitor during postnatal development. *Nature Cell Biol.,* **12**(3), 257–66.

[35] Blanpain, C., Lowry, W. E., Geoghegan, A. *et al.* 2004. Self-renewal, multipotency, and the existence of two cell populations within an epithelial stem cell niche. *Cell,* **118**(5), 635–48.

[36] Bongso, A. and Richards, M. 2004. History and perspective of stem cell research. *Best Pract. Res. Clin. Obstet. Gynaecol.,* **18**(6), 827–42.

[37] Encinas, J. M., Michurina, T. V., Peunova, N. *et al.* 2011. Division-coupled astrocytic differentiation and age-related depletion of neural stem cells in the adult hippocampus. *Cell Stem Cell,* **8**(5), 566–79.

[38] Scadden, D. T. 2006. The stem-cell niche as an entity of action. *Nature,* **441**(7097), 1075–9.

[39] Voog, J. and Jones, D. L. 2010. Stem cells and the niche: a dynamic duo. *Cell Stem Cell,* **6**(2), 103–15.

[40] Laird, D. J., von Andrian, U. H. and Wagers, A. J. 2008. Stem cell trafficking in tissue development, growth, and disease. *Cell,* **132**(4), 612–30.

[41] Lapidot, T., Dar, A. and Kollet, O. 2005. How do stem cells find their way home? *Blood,* **106**(6), 1901–10.

[42] Lapidot, T. and Kollet, O. 2002. The essential roles of the chemokine SDF-1 and its receptor CXCR4 in human stem cell homing and repopulation of transplanted

immune-deficient NOD/SCID and NOD/SCID/B2m (null) mice. *Leukemia*, **16**(10), 1992–2003.

[43] Ponomaryov, T., Peled, A., Petit, I. *et al.* 2000. Induction of the chemokine stromal-derived factor-1 following DNA damage improves human stem cell function. *J. Clin. Invest.*, **106**(11), 1331–9.

[44] Imai, K., Kobayashi, M., Wang, J. *et al.* 1999. Selective secretion of chemoattractants for haemopoietic progenitor cells by bone marrow endothelial cells: a possible role in homing of haemopoietic progenitor cells to bone marrow. *Br. J. Haematol.*, **106**(4), 905–11.

[45] Loetscher, M., Geiser, T., O'Reilly, T. *et al.* 1994. Cloning of a human seven-transmembrane domain receptor, LESTR, that is highly expressed in leukocytes. *J. Biol. Chem.*, **269**(1), 232–7.

[46] Kawabata, K., Ujikawa, M., Egawa, T. *et al.* 1999. A cell-autonomous requirement for CXCR4 in long-term lymphoid and myeloid reconstitution. *Proc. Nat. Acad. Sci. USA*, **96**(10), 5663–7.

[47] Tachibana, K., Hirota, S., Iizasa, H. *et al.* 1998. The chemokine receptor CXCR4 is essential for vascularization of the gastrointestinal tract. *Nature*, **393**(6685), 591–4.

[48] Ceradini, D. J., Kulkarni, A. R., Callaghan, M. J. *et al.* 2004. Progenitor cell trafficking is regulated by hypoxic gradients through HIF-1 induction of SDF-1. *Nature Med.*, **10**(8), 858–64.

[49] Avecilla, S. T., Hattori, K., Heissig, B. *et al.* 2004. Chemokine-mediated interaction of hematopoietic progenitors with the bone marrow vascular niche is required for thrombopoiesis. *Nature Med.*, **10**(1), 64–71.

[50] Zaruba, M. M. and Franz, W. M. 2010. Role of the SDF-1–CXCR4 axis in stem cell-based therapies for ischemic cardiomyopathy. *Expert Opin. Biol. Ther.*, **10**(3), 321–35.

[51] Togel, F., Isaac, J., Hu, Z., Weiss, K. and Westenfelder, C. 2005. Renal SDF-1 signals mobilization and homing of CXCR4-positive cells to the kidney after ischemic injury. *Kidney Int.*, **67**(5), 1772–84.

[52] Ratanavaraporn, J., Furuya, H., Kohara, H. and Tabata, Y. 2011. Synergistic effects of the dual release of stromal cell-derived factor-1 and bone morphogenetic protein-2 from hydrogels on bone regeneration. *Biomaterials*, **32**(11), 2797–811.

[53] Heissig, B., Hattori, K., Dias, S. *et al.* 2002. Recruitment of stem and progenitor cells from the bone marrow niche requires MMP-9 mediated release of kit-ligand. *Cell*, **109**(5), 625–37.

[54] Kollet, O., Dar, A., Shirtiel, S. *et al.* 2006. Osteoclasts degrade endosteal components and promote mobilization of hematopoietic progenitor cells. *Nature Med.*, **12**(6), 657–64.

[55] Pappu, R., Schwab, S. R., Cornelissen, I. *et al.* 2007. Promotion of lymphocyte egress into blood and lymph by distinct sources of sphingosine-1-phosphate. *Science*, **316**(5822), 295–8.

[56] Lévesque, J. P., Takamatsu, Y., Nilsson, S. K., Haylock, D. N. and Simmons, P. J. 2001. Vascular cell adhesion molecule-1 (CD106) is cleaved by neutrophil proteases in the bone marrow following hematopoietic progenitor cell mobilization by granulocyte colony-stimulating factor. *Blood*, **98**(5), 1289–97.

[57] Papayannopoulou, T., Craddock, C., Nakamoto, B., Priestley, G. V. and Wolf, N. S. 1995. The VLA4/VCAM-1 adhesion pathway defines contrasting mechanisms of lodgement of transplanted murine hemopoietic progenitors between bone marrow and spleen. *Proc. Nat. Acad. Sci. USA*, **92**(21), 9647–51.

[58] Kuznetsov, S. A., Mankani, M. H., Gronthos, S. *et al.* 2001. Circulating skeletal stem cells. *J. Cell. Biol.*, **153**(5), 1133–40.

[59] Mauney, J., Olsen, B. R. and Volloch, V. 2010. Matrix remodeling as stem cell recruitment event: a novel in vitro model for homing of human bone marrow stromal cells to the site of injury shows crucial role of extracellular collagen matrix. *Matrix Biol.*, **29**(8), 657–63.

[60] Wang, J. A., He, A., Hu, X. *et al.* 2009. Anoxic preconditioning: a way to enhance the cardioprotection of mesenchymal stem cells. *Int. J. Cardiol.*, **133**(3), 410–12.

[61] Karp, J. M. and Leng Teo, G. S. 2009. Mesenchymal stem cell homing: the devil is in the details. *Cell Stem Cell*, **4**(3), 206–16.

[62] Lee, P. H., Kim, J. W., Bang, O. Y. *et al.* 2008. Autologous mesenchymal stem cell therapy delays the progression of neurological deficits in patients with multiple system atrophy. *Clin. Pharmacol. Ther.*, **83**(5), 723–30.

[63] Sackstein, R., Merzaban, J. S., Cain, D. W. *et al.* 2008. *Ex vivo* glycan engineering of CD44 programs human multipotent mesenchymal stromal cell trafficking to bone. *Nature Med.*, **14**(2), 181–7.

[64] Lee, K., Silva, E. A. and Mooney, D. J. 2011. Growth factor delivery-based tissue engineering: general approaches and a review of recent developments. *J. R. Soc. Interface*, **8**(55), 153–70.

[65] Moioli, E. K., Clark, P. A., Xin, X., Lal, S. and Mao, J. J. 2007. Matrices and scaffolds for drug delivery in dental, oral and craniofacial tissue engineering. *Adv. Drug Deliv. Rev.*, **59**(4–5), 308–24.

[66] Moioli, E. K. and Mao, J. J. 2006. Chondrogenesis of mesenchymal stem cells by controlled delivery of transforming growth factor-β_3. In *Conference Proceedings of the IEEE Engineering in Medicine and Biology Society*, pp. 2647–50.

[67] Lee, C. H., Cock, J. L., Mendelson, A. *et al.* 2010. Regeneration of the articular surface of the rabbit synovial joint by cell homing: a proof of concept study. *Lancet*, **376**(9739), 440–8.

[68] Mendelson, A., Frank, E., Allred, C. *et al.* 2011. Chondrogenesis by chemotactic homing of synovium, bone marrow, and adipose stem cells in vitro. *FASEB J.*, **25**(10), 3496–504.

[69] Chen, F. M., Zhang, M. and Wu, Z. F. 2010. Toward delivery of multiple growth factors in tissue engineering. *Biomaterials*, **31**(24), 6279–308.

[70] Kimura, Y., Miyazaki, N., Hayashi, N. *et al.* 2010. Controlled release of bone morphogenetic protein-2 enhances recruitment of osteogenic progenitor cells for de novo generation of bone tissue. *Tissue Eng. Part A*, **16**(4), 1263–70.

[71] Chen, F. M., Shelton, R. M., Jin, Y. and Chapple, I. L. 2009. Localized delivery of growth factors for periodontal tissue regeneration: role, strategies, and perspectives. *Med. Res. Rev.*, **29**(3), 472–513.

[72] Vasita, R. and Katti, D. S. 2006. Growth factor-delivery systems for tissue engineering: a materials perspective. *Expert Rev. Med. Devices*, **3**(1), 29–47.

[73] Zhang, S. and Uludag, H. 2009. Nanoparticulate systems for growth factor delivery. *Pharm. Res.*, **26**(7), 1561–80.

[74] Uebersax, L., Merkle, H. P. and Meinel, L. 2009. Biopolymer-based growth factor delivery for tissue repair: from natural concepts to engineered systems. *Tissue Eng. Part B Rev.*, **15**(3), 263–89.

[75] Robinson, R., Viviano, S. R., Criscione, J. M. *et al.* 2011. Nanospheres delivering the EGFR TKI AG1478 promote optic nerve regeneration: the role of size for intraocular drug delivery. *ACS Nano*, **5**(6), 4392–400.

[76] Askari, A. T., Unzek, S., Popovic, Z. B. *et al.* 2003. Effect of stromal-cell-derived factor 1 on stem-cell homing and tissue regeneration in ischaemic cardiomyopathy. *Lancet*, **362**(9385), 697–703.

[77] Guldberg, R. E. 2009. Spatiotemporal delivery strategies for promoting musculoskeletal tissue regeneration. *J. Bone Miner. Res.*, **24**(9), 1507–11.

[78] Riley, C. M., Fuegy, P. W., Firpo, M. A. *et al.* 2006. Stimulation of in vivo angiogenesis using dual growth factor-loaded crosslinked glycosaminoglycan hydrogels. *Biomaterials*, **27**(35), 5935–43.

[79] Ulery, B. D., Nair, L. S. and Laurencin, C. T. 2011. Biomedical applications of biodegradable polymers. *J. Polym. Sci. B Polym. Phys.*, **49**(12), 832–64.

[80] Place, E. S., George, J. H., Williams, C. K. and Stevens, M. M. 2009. Synthetic polymer scaffolds for tissue engineering. *Chem. Soc. Rev.*, **38**(4), 1139–51.

[81] Sokolsky-Papkov, M., Agashi, K., Olaye, A., Shakesheff, K. and Domb, A. J. 2007. Polymer carriers for drug delivery in tissue engineering. *Adv. Drug Deliv. Rev.*, **59**(4–5), 187–206.

[82] Godier-Furnémont, A. F., Marten, T. P., Koeckert, M. S. *et al.* 2011. Composite scaffold provides a cell delivery platform for cardiovascular repair. *Proc. Nat. Acad. Sci. USA*, **108**(19), 7974–9.

[83] Briganti, E., Spiller, D., Mirtelli, C. *et al.* 2010. A composite fibrin-based scaffold for controlled delivery of bioactive pro-angiogenetic growth factors. *J. Control. Release*, **142**(1), 14–21.

[84] Zhu, X. H., Wang, C. H. and Tong, Y. W. 2009. In vitro characterization of hepatocyte growth factor release from PHBV/PLGA microsphere scaffold. *J. Biomed. Mater. Res. A*, **89**(2), 411–23.

[85] Panyam, J. and Labhasetwar, V. 2003. Biodegradable nanoparticles for drug and gene delivery to cells and tissue. *Adv. Drug Deliv. Rev.*, **55**(3), 329–47.

[86] Lee, K. Y. and Mooney, D. J. 2001. Hydrogels for tissue engineering. *Chem. Rev.*, **101**(7), 1869–79.

[87] Santo, V. E., Frias, A. M., Carida, M. *et al.* 2009. Carrageenan-based hydrogels for the controlled delivery of PDGF-BB in bone tissue engineering applications. *Biomacromolecules*, **10**(6), 1392–401.

[88] Zisch, A. H., Lutolf, M. P., Ehrbar, M. *et al.* 2003. Cell-demanded release of VEGF from synthetic, biointeractive cell ingrowth matrices for vascularized tissue growth. *FASEB J.*, **17**(15), 2260–2.

[89] Siepmann, F., Siepmann, J., Walther, M., MacRae, R. J. and Bodmeier, R. 2008. Polymer blends for controlled release coatings. *J. Control. Release*, **125**(1), 1–15.

[90] Srouji, S., Ben-David, D., Lotan, R. *et al.* 2011. Slow-release human recombinant bone morphogenetic protein-2 embedded within electrospun scaffolds for regeneration of bone defect: in vitro and in vivo evaluation. *Tissue Eng. Part A*, **17**(3–4), 269–77.

[91] Liao, I. C., Chew, S. Y. and Leong, K. W. 2006. Aligned core–shell nanofibers delivering bioactive proteins. *Nanomedicine (Lond.)*, **1**(4), 465–71.

[92] Jia, X., Zhao, C., Li, P. *et al.* 2011. Sustained release of VEGF by coaxial electrospun dextran/PLGA fibrous membranes in vascular tissue engineering. *J. Biomater. Sci. Polym. Edn.*, **22**(13), 1811–27.

[93] Fu, K., Pack, D. W., Klibanov, A. M. and Langer, R. 2000. Visual evidence of acidic environment within degrading poly(lactic-*co*-glycolic acid) (PLGA) microspheres. *Pharm. Res.*, **17**(1), 100–6.

[94] Kim, H. K., Shim, W. S., Kim, S. E. *et al.* 2009. Injectable *in situ*-forming pH/thermo-sensitive hydrogel for bone tissue engineering. *Tissue Eng. Part A*, **15**(4), 923–33.

[95] Ehrick, J. D., Deo, S. K., Browning, T. W. *et al.* 2005. Genetically engineered protein in hydrogels tailors stimuli-responsive characteristics. *Nature Mater.*, **4**(4), 298–302.

[96] Klouda, L. and Mikos, A. G. 2008. Thermoresponsive hydrogels in biomedical applications. *Eur. J. Pharm. Biopharm.*, **68**(1), 34–45.

[97] Geiger, M., Li, R. H. and Friess, W. 2003. Collagen sponges for bone regeneration with rhBMP-2. *Adv. Drug Deliv. Rev.*, **55**(12), 1613–29.

[98] Yamamoto, M., Takahashi, Y. and Tabata, Y. 2006. Enhanced bone regeneration at a segmental bone defect by controlled release of bone morphogenetic protein-2 from a biodegradable hydrogel. *Tissue Eng.*, **12**(5), 1305–11.

[99] Kolambkar, Y. M., Boerckel, J. D., Dupont, K. M. *et al.* 2011. Spatiotemporal delivery of bone morphogenetic protein enhances functional repair of segmental bone defects. *Bone*, **49**(3), 485–92.

[100] Cao, H. and Kuboyama, N. 2010. A biodegradable porous composite scaffold of PGA/beta-TCP for bone tissue engineering. *Bone*, **46**(2), 386–95.

[101] Wei, G., Jin, Q., Giannobile, W. V. and Pa, P. X. 2007. The enhancement of osteogenesis by nano-fibrous scaffolds incorporating rhBMP-7 nanospheres. *Biomaterials*, **28**(12), 2087–96.

[102] Street, J., Bao, M., deGuzman, L. *et al.* 2002. Vascular endothelial growth factor stimulates bone repair by promoting angiogenesis and bone turnover. *Proc. Nat. Acad. Sci. USA*, **99**(15), 9656–61.

[103] Lutolf, M. P., Weber, F. E., Schmoekel, H. G. *et al.* 2003. Repair of bone defects using synthetic mimetics of collagenous extracellular matrices. *Nature Biotechnol.*, **21**(5), 513–8.

[104] Patel, Z. S., Young, S., Tabata, Y. *et al.* 2008. Dual delivery of an angiogenic and an osteogenic growth factor for bone regeneration in a critical size defect model. *Bone*, **43**(5), 931–40.

[105] Kanczler, J. M., Ginty, P. J., White, L. *et al.* 2010. The effect of the delivery of vascular endothelial growth factor and bone morphogenic protein-2 to osteoprogenitor cell populations on bone formation. *Biomaterials*, **31**(6), 1242–50.

[106] Kempen, D. H., Lu, L., Heijink, A. *et al.* 2009. Effect of local sequential VEGF and BMP-2 delivery on ectopic and orthotopic bone regeneration. *Biomaterials*, **30**(14), 2816–25.

[107] Manning, C. N., Kim, H. M., Sakiyama-Elbert, S. *et al.* 2011. Sustained delivery of transforming growth factor beta three enhances tendon-to-bone healing in a rat model. *J. Orthop. Res.*, **29**(7), 1099–105.

[108] Kovacevic, D., Fox, A. J., Bedi, A. *et al.* 2011. Calcium-phosphate matrix with or without TGF-β_3 improves tendon-bone healing after rotator cuff repair. *Am. J. Sports Med.*, **39**(4), 811–19.

[109] Falco, E. E., Wang, M. O., Thompson, J. A. *et al.* 2011. Porous EH and EH-PEG scaffolds as gene delivery vehicles to skeletal muscle. *Pharm. Res.*, **28**(6), 1306–16.

[110] Liu, J. J., Wang, C. Y., Wang, J. G., Ruan, H. J. and Fan, C. Y. 2011. Peripheral nerve regeneration using composite poly(lactic acid-caprolactone)/nerve growth factor conduits prepared by coaxial electrospinning. *J. Biomed. Mater. Res. A*, **96**(1), 13–20.

[111] de Boer, R., Knight, A. M., Borntraeger, A. *et al.* 2011. Rat sciatic nerve repair with a poly-lactic-*co*-glycolic acid scaffold and nerve growth factor releasing microspheres. *Microsurgery*, **31**(4), 293–302.

[112] Kokai, L. E., Bourbeau, D., Weber, D., McAtee, J. and Marra, K. G. 2011. Sustained growth factor delivery promotes axonal regeneration in long gap peripheral nerve repair. *Tissue Eng. Part A*, **17**(9–10), 1263–75.

[113] Angeloni, N. L., Bond, C. W., Tang, Y. *et al.* 2011. Regeneration of the cavernous nerve by Sonic hedgehog using aligned peptide amphiphile nanofibers. *Biomaterials*, **32**(4), 1091–101.

[114] Davis, M. E., Hsieh, P. C., Takahashi, T. *et al.* 2006. Local myocardial insulin-like growth factor 1 (IGF-1) delivery with biotinylated peptide nanofibers improves cell therapy for myocardial infarction. *Proc. Nat. Acad. Sci. USA*, **103**(21), 8155–60.

[115] Ruvinov, E., Leor, J. and Cohen, S. 2011. The promotion of myocardial repair by the sequential delivery of IGF-1 and HGF from an injectable alginate biomaterial in a model of acute myocardial infarction. *Biomaterials*, **32**(2), 565–78.

[116] Segers, V. F., Tokunou, T., Higgins, L. J. *et al.* 2007. Local delivery of protease-resistant stromal cell derived factor-1 for stem cell recruitment after myocardial infarction. *Circulation*, **116**(15), 1683–92.

[117] Sloan, A. J. and Smith, A. J. 1999. Stimulation of the dentine-pulp complex of rat incisor teeth by transforming growth factor-β isoforms 1–3 in vitro. *Arch. Oral Biol.*, **44**(2), 149–56.

[118] Dobie, K., Smith, G., Sloan, A. J. and Smith, A. J. 2002. Effects of alginate hydrogels and TGF-β_1 on human dental pulp repair in vitro. *Connect. Tissue Res.*, **43**(2–3), 387–90.

[119] Sloan, A. J., Rutherford, R. B. and Smith, A. J. 2000. Stimulation of the rat dentine-pulp complex by bone morphogenetic protein-7 in vitro. *Arch. Oral Biol.*, **45**(2), 173–7.

[120] Nakashima, M. 1994. Induction of dentin formation on canine amputated pulp by recombinant human bone morphogenetic proteins (BMP)-2 and -4. *J. Dent. Res.*, **73**(9), 1515–22.

[121] Kim, J. Y., Xin, X., Moioli, E. K. *et al.* 2010. Regeneration of dental-pulp-like tissue by chemotaxis-induced cell homing. *Tissue Eng. Part A*, **16**(10), 3023–31.

[122] Murakami, S., Takayama, S., Kitamura, M. *et al.* 2003. Recombinant human basic fibroblast growth factor (bFGF) stimulates periodontal regeneration in class II furcation defects created in beagle dogs. *J. Periodontal Res.*, **38**(1), 97–103.

[123] Takayama, S., Yoshida, J., Hirano, H. *et al.* 2002. Effects of basic fibroblast growth factor on human gingival epithelial cells. *J. Periodontol.*, **73**(12), 1467–73.

[124] Wikesjö, U. M., Lim, W. H., Thomson, R. C. *et al.* 2004. Periodontal repair in dogs: effect of recombinant human bone morphogenetic protein-12 (rhBMP-12) on regeneration of alveolar bone and periodontal attachment. *J. Clin. Periodontol.*, **31**(8), 662–70.

[125] King, G. N., King, N. and Hughes, F. J. 1998. Effect of two delivery systems for recombinant human bone morphogenetic protein-2 on periodontal regeneration in vivo. *J. Periodontal Res.*, **33**(4), 226–36.

[126] Cooke, J. W., Sarment, D. P., Whitesman, L. A. *et al.* 2006. Effect of rhPDGF-BB delivery on mediators of periodontal wound repair. *Tissue Eng.*, **12**(6), 1441–50.

[127] Kim, K., Lee, C. H., Kim, B. K. and Mao, J. J. 2010. Anatomically shaped tooth and periodontal regeneration by cell homing. *J. Dent. Res.*, **89**(8), 842–7.

[128] Suzuki, T., Bessho, K., Fujimura, K. *et al.* 2002. Regeneration of defects in the articular cartilage in rabbit temporomandibular joints by bone morphogenetic protein-2. *Br. J. Oral Maxillofac. Surg.*, **40**(3), 201–6.

[129] Ueki, K., Takazakura, D., Marukawa, K. *et al.* 2003. The use of polylactic acid/polyglycolic acid copolymer and gelatin sponge complex containing human recombinant bone morphogenetic protein-2 following condylectomy in rabbits. *J. Craniomaxillofac. Surg.*, **31**(2), 107–14.

[130] Holland, T. A., Bodde, E. W., Baggett, L. S. *et al.* 2005. Osteochondral repair in the rabbit model utilizing bilayered, degradable oligo(poly(ethylene glycol) fumarate) hydrogel scaffolds. *J. Biomed. Mater. Res. A*, **75**(1), 156–67.

[131] Na, K., Kim, S., Woo, D. G. *et al.* 2007. Synergistic effect of TGFβ-3 on chondrogenic differentiation of rabbit chondrocytes in thermo-reversible hydrogel constructs blended with hyaluronic acid by in vivo test. *J. Biotechnol.*, **128**(2), 412–22.

[132] Reddi, A. H. 1998. Role of morphogenetic proteins in skeletal tissue engineering and regeneration. *Nature Biotechnol.*, **16**(3), 247–52.

[133] Lind, M., Eriksen, E. F. and Bunger, C. 1996. Bone morphogenetic protein-2 but not bone morphogenetic protein-4 and -6 stimulates chemotactic migration of human osteoblasts, human marrow osteoblasts, and U2-OS cells. *Bone*, **18**(1), 53–7.

[134] Takaoka, K., Koezuka, M. and Nakahara, H. 1991. Telopeptide-depleted bovine skin collagen as a carrier for bone morphogenetic protein. *J. Orthop. Res.*, **9**(6), 902–7.

[135] Shields, L. B., Raque, G. H., Glassman, S. D. *et al.* 2006. Adverse effects associated with high-dose recombinant human bone morphogenetic protein-2 use in anterior cervical spine fusion. *Spine*, **31**(5), 542–7.

[136] Garrison, K. R., Donell, S., Ryder, J. *et al.* 2007. Clinical effectiveness and cost-effectiveness of bone morphogenetic proteins in the non-healing of fractures and spinal fusion: a systematic review. *Health Technol. Assess.*, **11**(30), 1–150 and iii–iv.

[137] Carano, R. A. and Filvaroff, E. H. 2003. Angiogenesis and bone repair. *Drug Discov. Today*, **8**(21), 980–9.

23

Affinity-based delivery systems

Jeffrey Mark Halpern and Horst A. von Recum

23.1 Scope

This chapter will focus on the basic and fundamental ideas of how to design an affinity-based drug delivery system. First, the various types of delivery mechanisms and the mathematics that govern these mechanisms will be discussed to reveal how affinity-based mechanisms are unique. Next, the most common affinity mechanisms will be described, with biological examples. Finally, the appropriate design of an affinity-based drug delivery system for specific applications will be expounded in detail. Literature examples will be used to explain general approaches to affinity mechanisms.

23.2 Description of polymer-based drug delivery mechanisms

As new materials and delivery systems are developed, polymer-delivery-based applications are becoming attractive because of their versatility in adapting the delivery system for specific applications [1–10]. These polymer systems can be designed with various release mechanisms: (1) a diffusion-controlled mechanism, in which the release of the drug into the body is achieved by means of a concentration gradient; (2) an erosion-controlled mechanism, in which the release of the drug is achieved by means of the polymer degrading in the body; and (3) an affinity-controlled mechanism, in which the release of the drug is achieved by means of an equilibrium relationship between the drug and polymer. See Figure 23.1 for a visual qualitative representation of these three drug delivery systems.

All three systems can be explained by the law of continuity of mass, which identifies the changes in concentration, α, of the drug, $\mathrm{\alpha}$, over time equal to the diffusion of the drug plus the generation of the drug [6, 8, 9, 11]:

$$\rho \frac{\mathrm{D}\alpha}{\mathrm{D}t} = \rho \, \nabla D_{\mathrm{\alpha,p}} \, \nabla \alpha + R_{\mathrm{\alpha}} \tag{23.1}$$

23.2.1 Diffusion-controlled delivery

The most common delivery method is diffusion-controlled delivery, in which a drug is loaded into a swelled polymer. The release is entirely dependent on how well the drug migrates through the polymer, represented by a diffusion coefficient ($D_{\mathrm{\alpha,p}}$) [5, 9, 12, 13], so the final delivery rate can be easily predicted and varied [2, 5]. The diffusion coefficient can be varied by changing the crosslinked density (density of the polymer), altering the ability of the drug to migrate through the polymer [2].

Equation (23.1) can be simplified because no reactions are occurring in the polymer and the diffusion coefficient is a constant. The result describes the situation in which the release is completely governed by a concentration gradient [8, 9, 11]:

$$\frac{\partial \alpha}{\partial t} = D_{\mathrm{\alpha,p}} \, \nabla^2 \alpha \tag{23.2}$$

23.2.2 Degradation-controlled delivery

After the drug has been released in a purely diffusion-controlled mechanism, the polymer remains in the body and does not degrade. Leaving a foreign object in the body can cause additional long-term problems.

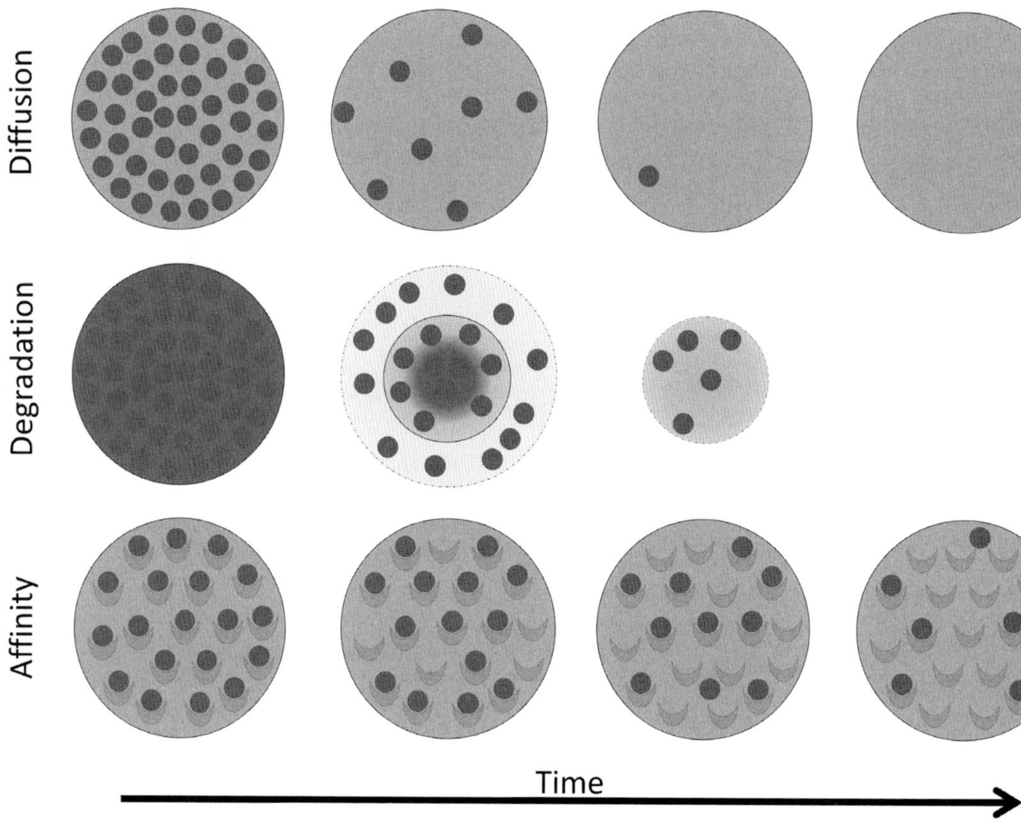

Figure 23.1 A qualitative visual representation of the three drug delivery mechanisms. The diffusion-controlled mechanism releases the drug the quickest, such that little to no drug remains to be released after a relatively short time. The degradation-controlled mechanism releases the drug slower, in such a way that the polymer degredation rate alters the speed at which the drug can be released. In regions of undegraded polymer (darker shading), the drug remains trapped in the polymer matrix. Over time, the polymer fully degrades (lighter shading) until no polymer remains and the drug is released. In an affinity-based mechanism the drug has an equilibrium relationship with the affinity molecules (represented by pockets). Once the drug has been released from the pocket, the drug travels through the polymer by diffusion. The equilibrium, affinity relationship causes the release to be slowed so that drug remains in the polymer for some time.

In degredation-controlled systems, the polymer degrades into biocompatible materials that can be broken down and removed by the body [4, 14, 15].

The release of the drug, entrapped in the polymer, is thus dependent on the rate at which the polymer system degrades. The polymer system degrading does not generate or remove drug through a reaction mechanism, so the reaction term in Equation (23.1) is zero. Because the polymer is degrading, the diffusion coefficient is no longer constant radially [8, 9, 14, 16, 17]. Equation (23.1) is reduced to

$$\frac{\partial \alpha}{\partial t} = \nabla D_{\alpha,\mathrm{p}} \nabla \alpha \tag{23.3}$$

23.2.3 Affinity-based delivery

Affinity-based systems are created when a guest molecule binds to a host system through van der

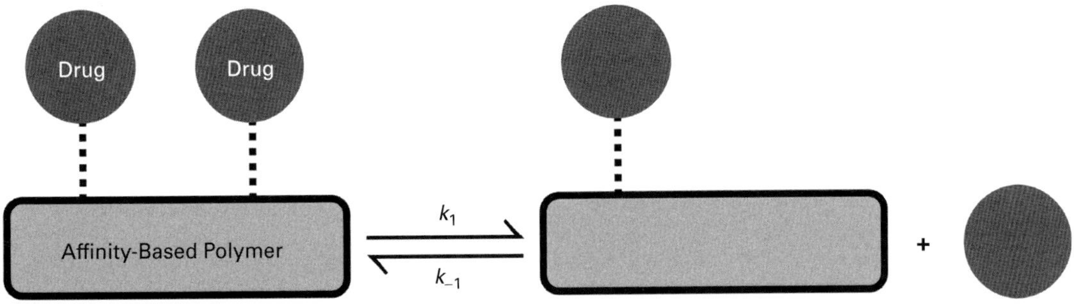

Figure 23.2 A reaction of an affinity-based polymer system with two drugs bound to the polymer with a 1:1 ratio. A single bond is released from the polymer, creating one free drug molecule. The chemical reaction is shown in Equation (23.4).

Waals interactions, electrostatic interactions, hydrogen bonding, or hydrophobic interactions [10]. The bound drug can be complexed; occasionally, there can be one drug for multiple affinity molecules within the polymer or vice versa [6]. The simplest affinity system, a 1:1 ratio (one drug molecule, DM, to one affinity molecule, AM), Figure 23.2, Equation (23.4), is often used as a first approximation:

$$\mathrm{DM{-}AM} \underset{k_{-1}}{\overset{k_1}{\rightleftharpoons}} \mathrm{DM} + \mathrm{AM} \tag{23.4}$$

Mathematically, the affinity interaction between the polymer and drug cannot be explained by a revaluation of the diffusivity term, because the molecules still diffuse according to a concentration gradient when unbound from the polymer. Instead, bound vs. unbound molecules are evaluated by the reaction term of Equation (23.1). The result is

$$\frac{\partial \alpha}{\partial t} = D_{\alpha,\mathrm{p}} \nabla^2 \alpha + k_1[\alpha\mathrm{{-}CD}] - k_{-1}[\alpha][\mathrm{CD}] \tag{23.5}$$

where CD is cyclodextrin. Equations (23.4) and (23.5) can be used only if the system is determined to have a 1:1 binding relationship; the R_α term will need to be redefined for affinity-based systems with a higher-order complexation than 1:1 [18]. Also, specific intermolecular forces for each affinity system can be defined and investigated [18, 19].

23.3 Affinity-based mechanisms that naturally occur in biological systems

Affinity interactions differ from chemical covalent and ionic bonds, which have a stoichiometry of atoms, are short range (~0.1 nm), and are directional in space. Affinity interactions, in contrast, involve well-separated molecules and lack directionality; they are strong intermolecular forces. One requires less energy to break apart the participating molecules than would be required to break a covalent or ionic bond [19]. Because of the properties of affinity interactions, various adhesive forces can occur without committing the participating molecules to long-term bonding (covalent or ionic), which increases the number of interactions between different molecules.

Affinity-based interactions are not novel to engineered polymer or drug delivery systems; they occur regularly in nature and are utilized in many different biological systems. Although there are many different types of affinity-based interaction, the four most commonly discussed are van der Waals forces, electrostatic interactions, hydrogen bonding, and hydrophobic interactions [19].

23.3.1 Van der Waals forces

The term van der Waals forces describes all (both permanent and temporary) dipole interactions involving molecular, atomic, and magnetic dipoles [19]. These forces can be powerful, resulting in strong molecular interactions, yet they can often be overcome with minimum energy by a shear force. Van der Waals forces are analogous to the forces holding a sticky note to a piece of paper. The note is stable until a shear force is applied by pulling it up and removing it. Another example of van der Waals forces is found in the hairs of a gecko's foot, which are bound to the surface with which the foot is in contact by van der Waals forces, allowing the gecko to climb up walls [20, 21]. This interaction can be overcome by a shear force, which gives the gecko the ability to control both the binding and the release of its foot.

23.3.2 Electrostatic interactions

Electrostatic interactions occur when unbound charges or dipoles interact, resulting in molecular attraction. One such example is the membrane potential that occurs because of the different concentrations on the two sides of the lipid membrane [22, 23]. These charges can migrate across the membrane when an ion channel opens fully, allowing the rush of charged ions across the membrane in an effort to equilibrate the potential [22]. Electrostatic interactions are also the cause of the pH-dependent properties of proteins [22, 24].

23.3.3 Hydrogen bonding

Hydrogen bonding is prevalent in biology; this interaction orients water molecules in a crystal-like form. Water has a natural dipole with oxygen, a negative dipole (π-acceptor), and hydrogen, a positive dipole (π-donor), and the water molecules orient themselves to match the two opposite dipoles [25, 26]. This structure aids in the dissolving and diffusion of ions through the water media.

Hydrogen can also interact with other negative dipoles to form a strong attraction. For example, N—H · · · O is a common hydrogen-bond donor-acceptor pair between nucleic acids, increasing interaction between two nucleic acid sequences [25, 26]. DNA base pairs have a specific complement related to hydrogen bonding [27]. This interaction is the basis for the double strand that exists in DNA [27, 28]. Hydrogen bonding is also present in polysaccharides, which have many carboxylic acid groups, leading to an O—H · · · O bond or a C=O · · · H bond [25, 26]. Finally, hydrogen bonding is also responsible for hydration shells that can occur around various types of molecules or membranes [25, 26].

23.3.4 Hydrophobic interactions

Unlike hydrogen or dipole interactions, where opposites attract, hydrophobic interactions encourage similar molecules to be attracted to each other. Hydrophobic molecules typically exhibit little or no dipole moment [29]. An example of hydrophobic interactions is the coalescence of hydrophobic molecules suspended in water.

There are multiple examples of hydrophobic interactions that occur naturally in biological systems. Hydrophobic interactions encourage protein folding by causing the protein to fold onto itself in order to avoid the water [29–33]. Another example is the lipid bilayer, which consists of hydrophobic and hydrophilic components, creating an effective separation barrier for the transport both of hydrophilic (molecules that like water) and hydrophobic molecules [22].

23.3.5 Conclusions on affinity-based examples

Simple examples of van der Waals forces, electrostatic interactions, hydrogen bonding, and hydrophobic interactions have been briefly described, yet the interactions are usually more complicated, consisting of multiple affinity interactions [19]. For example, protein folding is not entirely attributable to hydrophobic interactions but also consists of hydrogen bonding and electrostatic interactions [33]. Also, the DNA double-helix structure is attributable to van der Waals forces and electrostatic forces, as well as hydrogen bonding [28]. This basic understanding gives us a starting place for fabricating an affinity-based drug delivery system.

23.4 Current state of affinity-based delivery systems

The previous examples give a strong indication of what types of affinities are possible. On observing how these affinity systems occur in nature, it is possible to develop systems to release drugs by utilizing the same interactions. Ideally, the affinity attraction within these systems could be adjusted to optimize the delivery rate.

The most common affinity-based drug delivery systems use sulfated glycosaminoglycans, cyclodextrins, or molecularly imprinted polymers. These three systems have multiple applications and have been used with a wide range of drugs. This section will describe how these systems work, what drugs can be used within each system, and how to build/design each system.

23.4.1 Sulfated glycosaminoglycan affinity systems

Sulfated glycosaminoglycan (GAG) affinity systems utilize sulfate groups to bind drugs through electrostatic interactions or hydrogen bonding. The GAG affinity systems are most commonly used with growth factors and other proteins because of their natural mutual affinity, Figure 23.3. Although some of the earliest work was done with chondroitin sulfate [34], heparin and heparan sulfate derivatives are the most commonly used GAG molecules in drug delivery because they contain the greatest number of sulfate groups [35–37].

Heparin's inherent anticoagulant activity alludes to how heparin interacts with the delivery of growth factors. The sulfate group on heparin attracts antithrombin (AT) to the specific sulfate-binding sections of heparin. Upon binding, a protein conformation change occurs, which increases the rate of AT-mediated inhibition of thrombin [35, 38]. Specific sulfate groups have been identified as the active binding section for AT, which consists of only about a third of available heparin [37, 39]. The binding of heparin to growth factors is similar to the binding of heparin–AT,

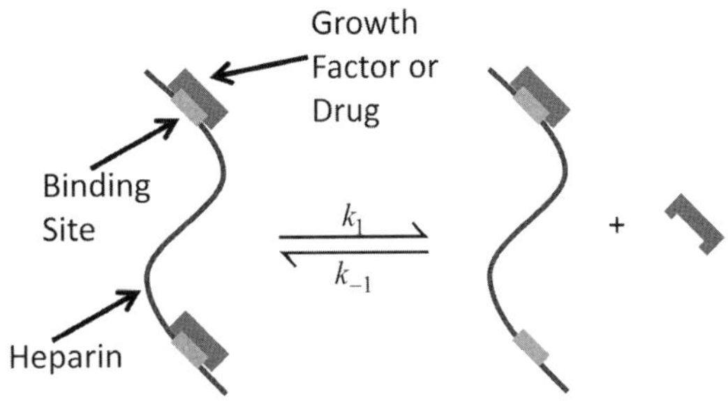

Figure 23.3 A graphical representation of a growth factor or drug binding to heparin at a specific binding site. Locally, these binding sites have multiple affinity interactions, making it favorable for the drug to stay bound to the heparin. Once all the affinity interactions have been released, the drug is free to travel away from the heparin into the surrounding medium.

where growth factors are also attracted to the specific active sulfate groups. The most prevalent use of heparin is in the affinity-based delivery of basic fibroblast growth factor, followed by vascular endothelial growth factor, with other growth factors (e.g. transforming growth factor-β, bone morphogenic protein 2, platelet-derived growth factor) being far less commonly used [10]. Our research group has recently been interested in the delivery of proteins that serve both as a growth factor and as a homing molecule [43]. A recent family of molecules investigated for this purpose consists of the chemokine (C–X–C motif and C–C motif) ligands (including stromal-derived factor 1, or CXCL12; macrophage inflammatory protein-1α, or CCL3; macrophage inflammatory protein-1β, or CCL4; monocyte chemotactic protein 3, or CCL7; and RANTES, or CCL5). As an example, the chemokine RANTES (Regulated upon Activation, Normal T-cell Expressed, and Secreted) has specific heparin-binding domains in its sequence, which have been mapped by various groups [40–42]. These binding sites on RANTES have been found to be very positive regions of the molecule (5 Lys, 5 Arg, 1 Asp, and 4 Glu with a net charge of +5 at neutral pH), with hydrogen dipoles [40, 41], and have been shown to be capable of being used for controlled release [43].

There are two possible primary affinity interactions between certain growth factors and heparin:

electrostatic interactions and hydrogen bonding, although both most likely occur. As described in Section 23.3, electrostatic interactions unite growth factors and heparin by virtue of the overall charge attraction between them, and hydrogen bonding will need direct negative dipole counterparts in order for a strong interaction to occur. The binding site of heparin has been identified as active sulfate groups (sulfate groups with the appropriate orientation and charge) [36, 40]. The positively charged sections of the growth factor or other cytokine become oriented to bind to the negatively charged sulfate sections of heparin [37, 40, 42]. Locally, multiple affinity interactions, either hydrogen bonding or electrostatic interactions, strengthen the interaction between the growth factor and heparin, making conditions more favorable for the growth factor to be bound to heparin than unbound.

Since chemokines bind specifically to the sulfate groups of GAGs, the binding affinity should be dependent on the concentration of active sulfate groups on the surface. This has been both tested and modeled by examining the chemokine protein binding to various sulfated GAG molecules, from largest to smallest number of active sulfate groups, heparin > heparan sulfate = chondroitin sulfate C > dermatan sulfate > chondroitin sulfate A [40]. In addition, the release of these proteins from immobilized heparin gels correlates with the concentration of active sulfate groups as well; thus, the release can be tailored for specific applications by choosing the appropriate sulfated GAG molecule [43].

There are various methods of immobilizing sulfated GAGs for an affinity-based delivery system. A method was developed by covalently incorporating a bi-domain peptide into a fibrin matrix using factor XIIIa [44, 45]. Heparin and a heparin-binding growth factor (such as VEGF or bFGF) are bound to the matrix through affinity interactions with the bi-domain peptide [4, 45, 46]. All components are mixed together *in situ*, immobilizing heparin and growth factors after the fibrin gel has formed [4, 45]. Another method was developed by reacting heparin (with an N-terminated cysteine) with vinyl sulfone-modified star PEG to create a PEG:heparin four-arm star copolymer [47, 48]. Various growth factors including VEGF have been released from this heparin star copolymer [47, 48]. Another method to immobilize heparin is by crosslinking it with bovine serum albumin using 1-ethyl-3-(3-dimethylpropyl)-carbodiimide (EDC) [43, 49]. While other methods of immobilizing heparin exist; the above are used as examples of the wide range of methods available [4, 10].

23.4.2 Heparin-like affinity models

Various hydrophilic drugs or growth factors do not have a strong affinity interaction with heparin, but the methods described previously can still be applied to release these drugs, with a minor alteration: an extra bi-domain peptide that has an affinity to both heparin and the non-heparin-binding growth factor can be synthesized [50, 51]. Willerth *et al.* demonstrated that two different peptides bind either directly to growth factors or indirectly, by first binding heparin [2, 18, 52]. These peptides can be immobilized within fibrin maxtrix, as described previously with factor XIIIa, with a bi-functional relationship: (1) the peptide binds to a fibrin matrix; and (2) a second domain binds either directly to the growth factor or indirectly by first binding heparin [4, 45, 50, 52, 53]. Although these multiple affinity interactions create complicated calculations to predict and model the release of the growth factor, this method has been shown to release growth factors by a slow, affinity-based mechanism [53].

23.4.3 Cyclodextrin affinity systems

Cyclodextrin (CD) is made up of six to eight glucose monomers, linked together, and shaped into a ring structure; see Figure 23.4 [54–56]. It has a three-dimensional (3D) toroid or ring shape that, due to the nature of the assembly, retains a relatively hydrophobic interior and can either partially or fully entrap a hydrophobic molecule within the interior of the ring (Figure 23.4). In larger-molecule drugs a hydrophobic portion will bind to the inside of the CD, while the remainder of the drug will remain outside the toroid [57–59]. Cyclodextrin can be incorporated into drug delivery systems by crosslinking or conjugating to polymers to create an affinity-based system.

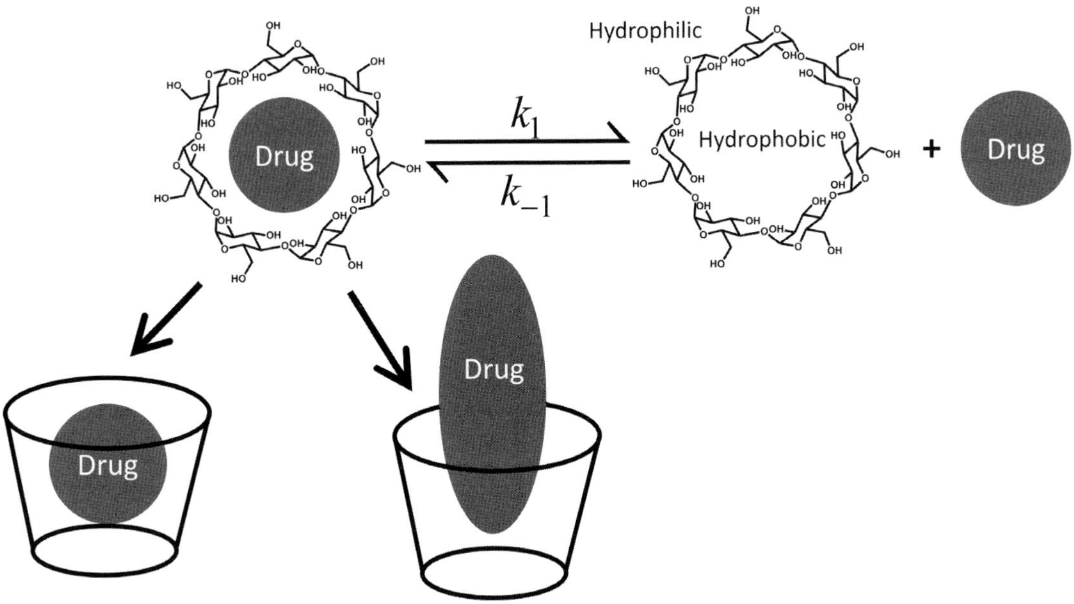

Figure 23.4 A graphical representation of a drug inside a cyclodextrin molecule. Left, the top view shows the drug inside the ring structure, yet a three-dimensional view shows that the entire drug may not sit in the ring. It is possible to have an affinity interaction even if some or most of the drug is outside the ring.

Owing to the hydrophobic core and hydrophilic exterior, drugs are released according to the probability that the hydrophobic portion will cross the hydrophobic/hydrophilic barrier of the CD (Figure 23.4) [54, 58, 59]. A hydrophobic drug is more likely to sit in the ring and not be released into the hydrophilic region; a hydrophilic drug may not even form an inclusion complex because it would not be attracted by the hydrophobic interior [54, 59, 60].

Many researchers have investigated the various natural forms of CD available (α-CD, β-CD, and γ-CD) as well as modifications to the CD molecule (e.g. HPCD). The forms α-CD, β-CD, and γ-CD (made from six, seven, or eight glucose monomers, respectively) have different-sized hydrophobic interiors, of diameters 0.57, 0.78, and 0.95 nm, respectively [54, 55]. Larger CD rings are available, but the rings of CDs larger than eight glucose monomers collapse in hydrophilic media and are not as useful [55]. The size of the CD ring can be chosen depending on the size of the drug that will be included in the affinity system. The hydrophobic exterior portion of the CD molecule can be modified to make the CD more soluble or easier to crosslink. For example, hydroxypropyl-β-CD (HP-β-CD) adds hydroxypropyl functional groups on the exterior hydroxyl molecules, making the β-CD more soluble [57, 60, 61]. Adding the hydroxypropyl functional groups can change the inclusion equilibrium by altering the hydrophobic/hydrophilic barrier without changing the size of the hydrophobic core [54, 57, 58, 60, 61].

There are various techniques to polymerize (or crosslink) CD to immobilize it for an appropriate affinity delivery system [10, 62]. Isocyanate and ethylene glycol diglycidyl ether crosslinkers were used to create a CD gel structure for the delivery of small-molecule drugs, in this case antibiotics [62–68]. In another system hydroxypropyl-β-CD was crosslinked with citric acid to release hydrophobic antibiotics [69–71]. Cyclodextrin copolymers have also been created by reacting the CD gel with NH_2—PEG—NH_2 to create a CD:PEG copolymer to release drugs [72].

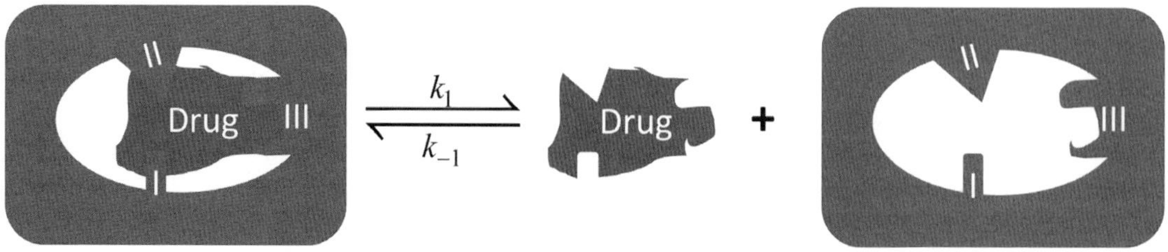

Figure 23.5 A graphical representation of a drug trapped within a molecularly imprinted polymer, bound with three affinity zones, I, II, and III. These zones can either be the same affinity groups or different ones to maximize the interaction between the drug and the polymer. All three affinity groups must release the drug in order for the drug to become free.

Although the primary affinity-based application using CD in the literature is for delivery of antibiotics, other small-molecule drugs have also been investigated. A β-CD polymer was fabricated by condensation of a CD monomer A with a diimidate comonomer B to form an AABBAABB block copolymer. This β-CD polymer has been shown to be successful for gene delivery and DNA release in vivo [73–77]. The affinity between anti-inflammatory steroid compounds and non-polymerized cyclodextrins has also been explored [78, 79]. Finally, β-CD has been used to increase the solubility and bioavailability of various hormones such as ovine growth hormone, testosterone, and interleukin-2 (glycoprotein) [80–82].

23.4.4 Molecularly imprinted polymers

Molecularly imprinted polymers (MIPs) are designed to release specific drugs at a particular rate. Originally created for the detection of trace species, they have been utilized by the drug delivery community for slow release of drugs [83]. MIPs have one or multiple affinity zones specifically designed for the drug of interest, Figure 23.5. The design of these systems is difficult and sensitive since all the affinity zones must be cross-linked together in a specific pattern around the drug but must not covalently attach the drug to the cross-linked network because that would mean that the drug would not be released. The swelling dynamics of the MIPs must also be taken into account, since swelling can greatly affect the orientation of the affinity zones, affecting the release of the drug. It has been recommended that one should create the polymer within the medium that the drug will be released in, or in a similar medium [84–86].

Figure 23.5 shows an example of the microstructure of a drug trapped and released by a MIP. Three zones of inhibition (I, II, and III) are shown in Figure 23.5; each of these zones can involve the same or different affinity groups, as described in Section 23.3 [87]. Each affinity zone has its own equilibrium relationship; the drug is not released until the affinity interactions from all zones have been released. This relationship, if the MIP is designed properly, creates a very specific, slow release of the drug.

There are many examples of MIPs in drug delivery. One common use is the release of ketotifen fumarate from therapeutic contact lenses. The MIP for contact lenses is fabricated using a free-radical UV photopolymerization with 2-hydroxyethylmethacrylate (HEMA) as the primary functional monomer [88, 89]. There has also been recent work to develop MIPs for protein delivery utilizing many different chemistries, yet they are typically based on methacrylate chemistries [90, 91].

23.5 Conclusions and future directions of affinity-based delivery systems

When designing an affinity-based drug delivery system, it is imperative to start with an investigation of the molecule being delivered to determine what inherent affinity mechanisms exist within the molecule. If the drug is hydrophobic, CD will work well because it creates an inherent separation between hydrophobic and hydrophilic molecules. If the drug is hydrophilic, it may have an affinity to sulfated GAG-family molecules such as heparin through hydrogen bonding or electrostatic forces. Other affinities that are being investigated exploit other biological interactions, such as exploiting the chaperone function of albumin as an affinity domain [92], or DNA molecular aptamers for drug delivery [93]. Finally, if neither CD nor heparin works sufficiently well, MIPs can be designed from broad categories of amphiphilic polymers to create more specific affinity interactions for a specific type of release profile.

Efforts are already being made to advance this field by combining the different types of affinity interactions and by combining affinity-based delivery with stimulus-controlled or degradation-controlled mechanisms [87, 94, 95]. The integration of the different types of affinity-based delivery systems will allow optimal delivery of large, complex molecules.

ACKNOWLEDGEMENTS

The authors were supported by grants from the National Institutes of Health (NIH T32 AR007505) (JMH) and NSF CAREER Award CBET-0954489 (HvR).

REFERENCES

[1] Pavlukhina, S. and Sukhishvili, S. 2011. Polymer assemblies for controlled delivery of bioactive molecules from surfaces. *Adv. Drug Delivery Rev.*, **63**, 822–36.

[2] Willerth, S. M. and Sakiyama-Elbert, S. E. 2007. Approaches to neural tissue engineering using scaffolds for drug delivery. *Adv. Drug Delivery Rev.*, **59**, 325–38.

[3] Stuart, M. A. C., Huck, W. T. S., Genzer, J. *et al.* 2010. Emerging applications of stimuli-responsive polymer materials. *Nature Mater.*, **9**, 101–13.

[4] Sakiyama-Elbert, S. E. and Hubbell, J. A. 2001. Functional biomaterials: design of novel biomaterials. *Ann. Rev. Mater. Res.*, **31**, 183–201.

[5] Naderi, H., Matin, M. M. and Bahrami, A. R. 2011. Critical issues in tissue engineering: biomaterials, cell sources, angiogenesis, and drug delivery systems. *J. Biomater. Appl.*, **26**(4), 383–417.

[6] Liechty, W. B., Kryscio, D. R., Slaughter, B. V. and Peppas, N. A. 2010. Polymers of drug delivery systems. *Ann. Rev. Chem. Biomed. Eng.*, **1**, 149–73.

[7] Liechty, W. B. and Peppas, N. A. 2012. Responsive polymer nanoparticles in cancer therapy. *Eur. J. Pharmaceutics Biopharmaceutics*, **80**(2), 241–6.

[8] Grassi, M. and Grassi, G. 2005. Mathematical modelling and controlled drug delivery: matrix systems. *Current Drug Delivery*, **2**, 97–116.

[9] Siepmann, J. and Siepmann, F. 2008. Mathematical modeling of drug delivery. *Int. J. Pharmaceutics*, **364**, 328–43.

[10] Wang, N. X. and von Recum, H. A. 2011. Affinity-based drug delivery. *Macromolec. Biosci.*, **11**, 321–32.

[11] Bird, R. B., Stewart, W. E. and Lightfoot, E. N. 2002. *Transport Phenomena*, 2nd edn. New York: John Wiley & Sons, Inc.

[12] Siepmann, J. and Peppas, N. A. 2001. Modeling of drug release from delivery systems based on hydroxypropyl methylcellulose (HPMC). *Adv. Drug Delivery Rev.*, **48**, 139–57.

[13] Lee, K., Silva, E. A. and Mooney, D. J. 2011. Growth factor delivery-based tissue engineering: general approaches and a review of recent developments. *J. R. Soc. Interface*, **8**, 153–70.

[14] Sackett, C. K. and Narasimhan, B. 2011. Mathematical modeling of polymer erosion: consequences for drug delivery. *Int. J. Pharmaceutics*, **418**, 104–14.

[15] Soppimath, K. S., Aminabhavi, T. M., Kulkarni, A. R. and Rudzinski, W. E. 2001. Biodegradable polymeric nanoparticles as drug delivery devices. *J. Controll. Release*, **70**, 1–20.

[16] Siepmann, J. and Gopferich, A. 2001. Mathematical modeling of bioerodible, polymeric drug delivery systems. *Adv. Drug Delivery Rev.*, **48**, 229–47.

[17] Edwards, D. A. and Cohen, D. S. 1995. A mathematical model for a dissolving polymer. *AIChE J.*, **41**, 2345–55.

[18] Willerth, S. M., Johnson, P. J., Maxwel, D. J. *et al.* 2007. Rationally designed peptides for controlled release of nerve growth factor from fibrin matrices. *J. Biomed. Mater. Res.*, **80A**, 13–23.

[19] Leckband, D. and Israelachvili, J. 2001. Intermolecular forces in biology. *Q. Rev. Biophys.*, **34**, 105–267.

[20] Autumn, K., Liang, Y. A., Hsieh, S. T. *et al.* 2000. Adhesive force of a single gecko foot-hair. *Nature*, **405**, 681–5.

[21] Autumn, K., Sitti, M., Liang, Y. A. *et al.* 2002. Evidence for van der Waals adhesion in gecko setae. *Proc. Nat. Acad. Sci. USA*, **99**, 12252–6.

[22] Honig, B. and Nicholls, A. 1995. Classical electrostatics in biology and chemistry. *Science*, **268**, 1144–9.

[23] Bostrom, M., Williams, D. R. M. and Ninham, B. W. 2001. Specific ion effects: why DLVO theory fails for biology and colloid systems. *Phys. Rev. Lett.*. **87**, 168103 (4 pp.).
[24] Fogolari, F., Brigo, A. and Molinari, H. 2002. The Poisson–Boltzmann equation for biomolecular electrostatics: a tool for structural biology. *J. Molec. Recognition*, **15**, 377–92.
[25] Desiraju, G. R. and Steiner, T. 1999. *The Weak Hydrogen Bond in Structural Chemistry and Biology*. New York: Oxford University Press.
[26] Jeffrey, G. A. and Saenger, W. 1991. *Hydrogen Bonding in Biological Structures*. Berlin: Springer-Verlag.
[27] Zimmer, C., Luck, G., Birch-Hirschfeld, E. *et al.* 1983. Chain length-dependent association of distamycin-type oligopeptides with A–T and G–C pairs in polydeoxynucleotide duplexes. *Biochim. Biophys. Acta*, **741**, 15–22.
[28] Dervan, P. B. 1986. Design of sequence-specific DNA-binding molecules. *Science*, **232**, 464–71.
[29] Langmuir, I. 1938. The role of attractive and repulsive forces in the formation of tactoids, thixotropic gels, protein crystals and cacervates. *J. Chem. Phys.*, **6**, 873–96.
[30] Dobson, C. M. 2003. Protein folding and misfolding. *Nature*, **426**, 884–90.
[31] Shea, J.-E. and Brooks, C. L. III 2001. From folding theories to folding proteins: a review and assessment of simulation studies of protein folding and unfolding. *Ann. Rev. Phys. Chem.*, **52**, 499–535.
[32] Kim, P. S. and Baldwin, R. L. 1982. Specific intermediates in the folding reactions of small proteins and the mechanism of protein folding. *Ann. Rev. Biochem.*, **51**, 459–89.
[33] Fersht, A. 1999. *Structure and Mechanism in Protein Science: A Guide to Enzyme Catalysis and Protein Folding*. New York: W. H. Freeman & Company.
[34] von Recum, H. A., Kikuchi, A., Yamato, M. *et al.* 1999. Growth factor and matrix molecules preserve cell function on thermally responsive culture surfaces. *Tissue Eng.*, **5**, 251–65.
[35] Conrad, H. E. 1998. *Heparin-Binding Proteins*. San Diego, CA: Academic Press.
[36] Rek, A., Brandner, B., Geretti, E. and Kungl, A. J. 2009. A biophysical insight into the RANTES–glycosaminoglycan interaction. *Biochim. Biophys. Acta*, **1794**, 577–82.
[37] Vives, R. R., Crublet, E., Andrieu, J.-P. *et al.* 2004. A novel strategy for defining critical amino acid residues involved in protein/glycosaminoglycan interactions. *J. Biol. Chem.*, **279**, 54327–33.
[38] Casu, B. 1994. Heparin and heparin-like polysaccharides. In *Polymeric Biomaterials*, ed. Dumintriu, S., New York: Marcel Dekker, Inc., pp. 159–78.
[39] Lau, E. K., Paavola, C. D., Johnson, Z. *et al.* 2004. Indentification of the glycosaminoglycan binding site of the CC chemokine, MCP-1. *J. Biol. Chem.*, **279**, 22294–305.
[40] Martin, L., Blanpain, C., Garnier, P. *et al.* 2001. Structural and functional analysis of the RANTES–glycosaminoglycans interactions. *Biochemistry*, **40**, 6303–18.
[41] Chung, C.-W., Cooker, R. M., Proudfoot, A. E. I. and Wells, T. N. C. 1995. The three-dimensional solution structure of RANTES. *Biochemistry*, **34**, 9307–14.
[42] Lortat-Jacob, H., Grosdidier, A. and Imberty, A. 2002. Structural diversity of heparan sulfate binding domains in chemokines. *Proc. Nat. Acad. Sci. USA*, **99**, 1229–34.
[43] Wang, N. X., Sieg, S. F., Lederman, M. *et al.* 2013. Using glycosaminoglycan/chemokine interactions for the affinity-based delivery of 5P12-RANTES for HIV prevention. *Molec. Pharmacol.*, **10**(10), 3564–73.
[44] Schense, J. C. and Hubbell, J. A. 1999. Cross-linking exogenous bifunctional peptides into fibrin gels with factor XIIIa. *Bioconjugate Chem.*, **10**, 75–81.
[45] Sakiyama-Elbert, S. E. and Hubbell, J. A. 2000. Development of fibrin derivatives for controlled release of heparin-binding growth factors. *J. Controll. Release*, **65**, 389–402.
[46] Naimy, H., Buczek-Thomas, J. A., Nugent, M. A., Leymarie, N. and Zaia, J. 2011. Highly sulfated nonreducing end-derived heparan sulfate domains bind fibroblast growth factor-2 with high affinity and are enriched in biologically active fractions. *J. Biol. Chem.*, **286**, 19311–19.
[47] Yamaguchi, N., Chae, B.-S., Zhang, L., Kiick, K. L. and Furst, E. M. 2005. Rheological characterization of polysaccharide–poly(ethylene glycol) star copolymer hydrogels. *Biomacromolecules*, **6**, 1931–40.
[48] Yamaguchi, N. and Kiick, K. L. 2005. Polysaccharide–poly(ethylene glycol) star copolymer as a scaffold for the production of bioactive hydrogels. *Biomacromolecules*, **6**, 1921–30.
[49] Hermanson, G. T. 1996. *Bioconjugate Techniques*. San Diego, CA: Academic Press.
[50] Maxwell, D. J., Hicks, B. C., Parsons, S. and Sakiyama-Elbert, S. E. 2005. Development of rationally designed affinity-based drug delivery systems. *Acta Biomater.*, **1**, 101–13.
[51] Felder, C. E., Prilusky, J., Silman, I. and Sussman, J. L. 2007. A server and database for dipole moments of proteins. *Nucl. Acids Res.*, **35**, W512–21.

[52] Sakiyama-Elbert, S. E. and Hubbell, J. A. 2000. Controlled release of nerve growth factor from heparin-containing fibrin-based cell ingrowth matrix. *J. Controll. Release*, **69**, 149–58.

[53] Wood, M. D. and Sakiyama-Elbert, S. E. 2008. Release rate controls biological activity of nerve growth factor released from firbin matrices containing affinty-based delivery systems. *J. Biomed. Mater. Res.*, **84A**, 300–12.

[54] Szejtli, J. 1998. Introduction and general overview of cyclodextrin chemistry. *Chem. Rev.*, **98**, 1743–53.

[55] Szejtli, J. 1988. *Cyclodextrin Technology*. Dordrecht: Kluwer Academic Publishers.

[56] Bender, M. L. and Komiyama, M. 1978. *Cyclodextrin Chemistry*. Berlin: Springer-Verlag.

[57] Szejtli, J. 1982. *Cyclodextrins and Their Inclusion Complexes*. Budapest: Akadémiai Kiadó.

[58] Challa, R., Ahuja, A., Ali, J. and Khar, R. K. 2005. Cyclodextrins in drug delivery: an updated review. *AAPS PharmSciTech*, **6**, E329–57.

[59] Kanjickal, D., Lopina, S., Evancho-Chapman, M. M., Schmidt, S. and Donovan, D. 2005. Improving delivery of hydrophobic drugs from hydrogels through cyclodextrins. *J. Biomed. Mater. Res.*, **74A**, 454–60.

[60] Uekama, K., Hirayama, F. and Irie, T. 1998. Cyclodextrin drug carrier systems. *Chem. Rev.*, **98**, 2045–76.

[61] Hirayama, F. and Uekama, K. 1999. Cyclodextrin-based controlled drug release system. *Adv. Drug Delivery Rev.*, **36**, 125–41.

[62] Alvarez-Lorenzo, C., Moya-Ortega, M. D., Loftsson, T., Concheiro, A., and Torres-Labandeira, J. J. 2011. Cyclodextrin-based hydrogels. In *Cyclodextrins in Pharmaceutics, Cosmetics, and Biomedicine*, ed. Bilensoy, E., Hoboken, NJ: John Wiley & Sons.

[63] Rodriguez-Tenreiro, C., Alvarez-Lorenzo, C., Rodriguez-Perez, A., Concheiro, A. and Torres-Labandeira, J. J. 2007. Estradiol sustained release from high affinity cyclodextrin hydrogels. *Eur. J. Pharm. Biopharm.*, 55–62.

[64] Rodriguez-Tenreiro, C., Alvarez-Lorenzo, C., Rodriguez-Perez, A., Concheiro, A. and Torres-Labandeira, J. J. 2006. New cyclodextrin hydrogels cross-linked with diglycidylethers with a high drug loading and controlled release ability. *Pharmaceutical Res.*, **23**, 121–30.

[65] Cesteros, L. C., Ramirez, C. A., Pecina, A. and Katime, I. 2006. Poly(ethylene glycol-β-cyclodextrin) gels: syntehsis and properties. *J. Appl. Polymer Sci.*, **102**, 1162–6.

[66] Wilson, L. D., Mohamed, M. H. and Headley, J. V. 2011. Surface area and pore structure properties of urethane-based copolymers containing β-cyclodextrin. *J. Colloid Interface Sci.*, **357**, 215–22.

[67] Thatiparti, T. R., Shoffstall, A. J. and von Recum, H. A. 2010. Cyclodextrin-based device coatings for affinity-based release of antibiotics. *Biomaterials*, **31**, 2335–47.

[68] Thatiparti, T. R. and von Recum, H. A. 2010. Cyclodextrin complexation for affinity-based antibiotic delivery. *Macromolec. Biosci.*, **10**, 82–90.

[69] Martel, B., Morcellet, M., Ruffin, D., Ducoroy, L. and Weltrowski, M. 2002. Finishing of polyester fabrics with cyclodextrins and polycarboxylic acids as crosslinking agents. *J. Inclusion Phenomena Macrocyclic Chem.*, **44**, 443–6.

[70] Blanchemain, N., Haulon, S., Boschin, F. *et al.* 2007. Vascular prostheses with controlled release of antibiotics part 1: surface modification with cyclodextrins of PET prostheses. *Biomolec. Eng.*, **24**, 149–53.

[71] Blanchemain, N., Haulon, S., Martel, B. *et al.* 2005. Vascular PET prostheses surface modification with cyclodextrin coating: development of new drug delivery system. *Eur. J. Vasc. Endovasc. Surg.*, **29**, 628–32.

[72] Salmaso, S., Semenzato, A., Bersani, S. *et al.* 2007. Cyclodextrin/PEG based hydrogels for multi-drug delivery. *Int. J. Pharmacol.*, **345**, 42–50.

[73] Park, I. K., von Recum, H. A., Jiang, S. and Pun, S. H. 2006. Supramolecular assembly of cyclodextrin-based nanoparticles on solid surfaces for gene delivery. *Langmuir*, **22**, 8478–84.

[74] Gonzalez, H., Hwang, S. J. and Davis, M. E. 1999. New class of polymers for the delivery of macromolecular therapeutics. *Bioconjugate Chem.*, **10**, 1068–1074.

[75] Hwang, S. J., Bellocq, C. N. and Davis, M. E. 2001. Effects of structure of β-cyclodextrin-containing polymers on gene delivery. *Bioconjugate Chem.*, **12**, 280–90.

[76] Park, T. G., Jeong, J. H. and Kim, S. W. 2006. Current status of polymeric gene delivery systems. *Adv. Drug Delivery Rev.*, **58**, 467–86.

[77] Pun, S. H., Bellocq, C. N., Liu, A. *et al.* 2004. Cyclodextrin-modified polyethylenimine polymers for gene delivery. *Bioconjugate Chem.*, **15**, 831–40.

[78] Cameron, K. S. and Fielding, L. 2002. NMR diffusion coefficient study of steroid-cyclodextrin inclusion complexes. *Magn. Reson. Chem.*, **40**, S106–9.

[79] Lin, S.-Z., Kohyama, N. and Tsuruta, H. 1996. Characterization of steroid/cyclodextrin inclusion compounds by X-ray powder diffractometry and thermal analysis. *Industrial Health*, **34**, 143–8.

[80] Lahiani-Skiba, M., Barbot, C., Bounoure, F., Joudieh, S. and Skiba, M. 2006. Solubility and dissolution rate of progesterone-cyclodextrin-polymer systems. *Drug Development Industrial Pharmacy*, **32**, 1043–58.

[81] Hedges, A. R. 1998. Industrial applications of cyclodextrins. *Chem. Rev.*, **98**, 2035–44.

[82] Brewster, M. E., Hora, M. S., Simpkins, J. W. and Bodor, N. 1991. Use of 2-hydroxypropyl-β-cyclodextrin as a solubilizing and stabilizing excipient for protein drugs. *Pharmaceutical Res.*, **8**, 792–5.

[83] Andersson, H. S., and Nicholls, I. A. 2001. A historical perspective of the development of molecular imprinting. In *Molecularly Imprinted Polymers: Man-Made Mimics of Antibodies and Their Applications in Analytical Chemistry*, ed. Sellergren, B., Amsterdam: Elsevier.

[84] Ekberg, B. and Mosbach, K. 1989. Molecular imprinting: a technique for producing specific separation materials. *TIBTECH*, **7**, 92–6.

[85] Sellergren, B., and Hall, A. J. 2001. Fundamental aspects on the synthesis and characterisation of imprinted network polymers. In *Molecularly Imprinted Polymers: Man-Made Mimics of Antibodies and Their Applications in Analytical Chemistry*, ed. Sellergren, B., Amsterdam: Elsevier.

[86] Wulff, G. 1995. Molecular imprinting in cross-linked materials with the aid of molecular templates – A way towards artificial antibodies. *Angew. Chem. Int. Edition Engl.*, **34**, 1812–32.

[87] Alvarez-Lorenzo, C. and Concheiro, A. 2004. Molecularly imprinted polymers for drug delivery. *J. Chromatography B*, **804**, 231–45.

[88] Ali, M., Horikawa, S., Venkatesh, S. *et al.* 2007. Zero-order therapeutic release from imprinted hydrogel contact lenses within in vitro physiological ocular tear flow. *J. Controll. Release*, **124**, 154–62.

[89] White, C. J. and Byrne, M. E. 2010. Molecularly imprinted therapeutic contact lenses. *Expert Opin. Drug Deliv.*, **7**, 765–80.

[90] Turner, N. W., Jeans, C. W., Brain, K. R. *et al.* 2006. From 3D to 2D: a review of the molecular imprinting of proteins. *Biotechnol. Prog.*, **22**, 1474–89.

[91] Ge, Y. and Turner, A. P. F. 2008. Too large to fit? Recent developments in molecular imprinting. *Trends Biotechnol.*, **26**, 218–23.

[92] Oss-Ronen, L. and Seliktar, D. 2011. Polymer-conjugated albumin and fibrinogen composite hydrogels as cell scaffolds designed for affinity-based drug delivery. *Acta Biomater.*, **7**, 163–70.

[93] Tan, W., Wang, H., Chen, Y. *et al.* 2011. Molecular aptamers for drug delivery. *Trends Biotechnol.* **29**(12), 634–40.

[94] Kryscio, D. R. and Peppas, N. A. 2008. Mimicking biological delivery through feedback-controlled drug release systems based on molecular imprinting. *AIChE J.*, **55**, 1311–24.

[95] Asanuma, H., Akiyama, T., Kajiya, K., Hishiya, T. and Komiyama, M. 2001. Molecular imprinting of cyclodextrin in water for the recognition of nonmeter-scaled guests. *Anal. Chim. Acta.* **435**, 25–33.

24

DNA delivery for regeneration

Stephanie K. Seidlits, Kelan Hlavaty and Lonnie D. Shea

24.1 Introduction

The delivery of nucleic acids is a powerful technique to regulate cellular processes that has profound implications for regenerative medicine. Nucleic acid delivery is most widely thought of as delivery of a gene to induce expression of a specific factor. This approach is highly versatile, insofar as it can readily target secreted factors (e.g. growth factors), membranous proteins (e.g. receptors), or intracellular proteins (e.g. transcription factors). Expression can potentially be modulated through the promoter, with control provided by soluble, inductive factors, or be restricted to specific cell populations. The alternative to delivering nucleic acids to induce expression of target genes is to reduce or block expression. The discovery of RNA interference (RNAi) has identified a powerful mechanism for nucleic acid delivery to catalyze the degradation of target mRNA. Similarly, oligonucleotides can bind to a complementary strand of mRNA (antisense) to terminate translation or act as decoys that bind to transcription factors and limit their ability to influence transcription. The delivery of nucleic acids has the potential to either promote or inhibit virtually any cell process; however, a major challenge to capitalizing on this potential lies in the need for effective delivery systems.

Delivery vehicles for nucleic acids can be categorized into viral and non-viral approaches. Non-viral approaches include direct delivery of naked plasmids or oligonucleotides, and the complexation of these nucleic acids with cationic polymers or lipids. Limiting factors in delivering naked plasmids or oligonucleotides include degradation, insufficient internalization, and intracellular trafficking (e.g. endosomal escape, nuclear entry) [1]. Complexation of these nucleic acids with cationic lipids or polymers via the negatively charged phosphate backbone forms lipoplexes and polyplexes, respectively, which can protect the nucleic acids from degradation, facilitate entry across the cell membrane, and promote intracellular trafficking [2]. While complexation can enhance the efficiency of delivery, the stability of the complexes and effective delivery systems beyond injection remain challenging [1, 3]. In contrast, viral delivery of nucleic acids is more efficient than non-viral systems [3, 4]. These viral vectors are derived from viral pathogens, from which the harmful sequences have been removed and into which therapeutic sequences can be inserted. Viruses have evolved mechanisms to efficiently infect cells, with some viruses integrating their genome with the host and others remaining episomal [5, 6]. Several viral vectors are currently being tested in clinical trials for various therapies, including retroviruses, lentiviruses, adenoviruses, and adeno-associated viruses. Several viral vectors are currently being tested in clinical trials for various therapies, including retroviruses, lentiviruses, adenoviruses, and adeno-associated viruses [7–12].

In the field of tissue engineering, gene delivery has enormous potential to promote tissue formation and regeneration. Gene delivery is typically targeted to the site for regeneration, and delivery from a tissue engineering scaffold provides the opportunity to localize gene expression, avoid toxicity associated with systemic dosing, and potentially reduce the immune response to the delivery vector [3, 13]. This chapter describes the biomaterial platforms that have been developed for delivery of nucleic acids. In addition to technologies, we discuss developments in understanding the relationship between the transgene expression profile and resultant tissue formation, namely the realization that improved delivery and greater expression do not necessarily improve regeneration. Although progress has been made, technologies that provide greater control over transgene expression are needed for the effective translation of gene delivery to regenerative medicine. Specific opportunities that will be discussed in this chapter include new attempts to better control the extent and duration of transgene expression, expression by targeted cell types, and integration of the scaffold with the native microenvironment.

24.2 Biomaterial platforms

Biomaterial-based delivery of gene therapy vectors, relative to bolus injection, can enhance the extent and duration of transgene expression at an implantation site [14–17]. Importantly, transgene expression can be designed to enhance or synergize with the intrinsic bioactivity of the scaffold and thereby create an environment that promotes tissue formation. The biomaterial provides a support for cell adhesion and an architecture that can serve to organize cells, and transgene expression can target cellular processes (e.g. proliferation and differentiation) that complement the structural functions provided by the biomaterial [18–20]. Interactions between the gene therapy vectors and the biomaterial scaffold can be tuned to modulate the release rate of vector, target specific internalization pathways, and potentially enhance intracellular trafficking [1]. Scaffolds can maintain elevated transgene expression on time scales ranging from weeks to months, with this duration of expression depending upon multiple factors such as the biomaterial, implantation site, and vector. For example, transgene expression after subcutaneous, intraperitoneal, or intramuscular delivery can persist for several months [21–26], whereas delivery into the spinal cord provides transgene expression on time scales of 4–8 weeks in vivo [17] (Figure 24.1). Multiple types of scaffolds have been employed, but they can be generally categorized as microporous scaffolds and hydrogels. The following paragraphs describe how the physical and chemical properties of the biomaterial scaffold and the mode of nucleic acid incorporation into the scaffold can be modified to control delivery of genetic material and the physiological response of surrounding cells or tissue.

Hydrogels are formed by the crosslinking or self-assembly of hydrophilic polymers. The hydrophilic polymers can be obtained from naturally occurring materials (e.g. fibrin, chitosan, and hyaluronan) or synthetic materials (e.g. polyethylene glycol (PEG) and polyvinyl alcohol (PVA)). The use of natural materials can be advantageous because of their biocompatibility and their inherent interactions with cells that effect cell attachment, migration, and differentiation. Alternatively, synthetic polymers offer the potential to create hydrogels with more precise control over the physical properties (e.g. mechanics and degradation) which directly affect both tissue formation and gene delivery. The mechanical properties of hydrogel scaffolds can be tuned to match those of native tissues [27–30], and has been implicated in differentiation [31] and gene delivery [32]. In addition, short, bioactive peptides derived from the extracellular matrix (ECM) (e.g. RGD) can be incorporated into scaffolds with precise control over the density of adhesive sites, which affects not only the overall strength of adhesion to the material, but also the type of receptor binding. Together with the density of adhesion sites, the degradation rate of the matrix modulates cell migration through the material, which influences integration with the host tissue. Importantly, the gelation conditions must be mild in order to preserve the viability of the encapsulated cells or the activity of entrapped vectors [33–36].

Alternatively, microporous scaffolds are formed from hydrophobic polymers, which are derived from either synthetic polymers (e.g. poly[lactide-*co*-glycolide] (PLG) or polycaprolactone (PCL)) or modified natural polymers (e.g. hydroxyapatite). The materials frequently used for scaffold fabrication have been utilized extensively for drug and gene delivery, and are

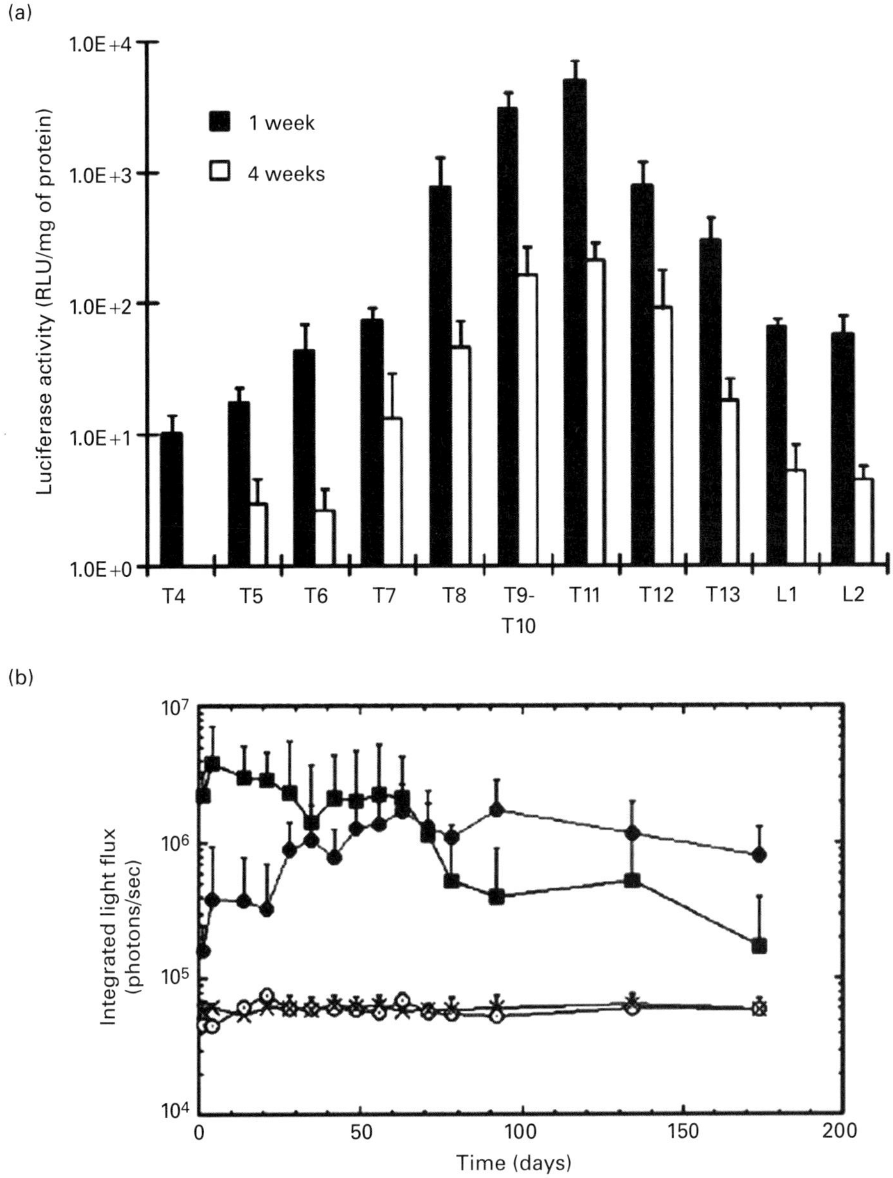

Figure 24.1 Localized transgene expression at multiple implant sites. (a) Expression of luciferase 1 and 4 weeks after implantation in the spinal cord of PLG scaffolds with immobilized lentivirus encoding for luciferase. (Reprinted from *Biomaterials*, Vol. 31(15), S. Shin, H.M. Tuinstra, D.M. Salvay and L.D. Shea, Phosphatidylserine immobilization of lentivirus for localized gene transfer, pp. 4353–9. Copyright 2010, with permission from Elsevier.) (b) Expression of luciferase up to 200 days after delivery of plasmid-encoding luciferase either as a bolus injection (closed squares) or encapsulation within PLG microspheres (closed circles) at an intramuscular site. The controls performed were microspheres without plasmid (×) and background light emission (open circles). (Reprinted from *J. Controlled Release*, Vol. 112(1), J. H. Jang and L. D. Shea, Intramuscular delivery of DNA releasing microspheres: microsphere properties and transgene expression, pp. 120–8. Copyright 2006, with permission from Elsevier.)

generally considered biocompatible. Porous scaffolds fabricated from materials such as PLG provide a three-dimensional (3D) structure that provides mechanical support following transplantation, and the porosity enables cell migration from the surrounding tissue into the scaffold [37, 38]. These scaffolds have been used extensively for cell transplantation [39–41], and as a delivery system for tissue inductive proteins that can regulate tissue development [42, 43]. More detailed reviews of scaffolds used for tissue engineering [44–48] and gene delivery [1, 3, 15, 49] are available.

24.3 Delivery strategies

The strategies for delivering gene therapy vectors from biomaterials have been broadly categorized as immobilization (i.e. association with the material) or physical entrapment in scaffolds. Many delivery systems for small molecules and proteins are developed with the objective of obtaining a controlled release. For gene delivery from scaffolds for tissue regeneration, an additional criterion is the amount of vector retained within the scaffold. The retention of vectors within the scaffold can facilitate gene transfer to infiltrating cells and promote transgene expression within the material, which contrasts with released vector that may target cells outside the scaffold. The method of scaffold fabrication and the material properties influence the extent to which vectors can be retained. Vector release from the hydrogel or microporous substrates typically occurs by diffusion, with the rate of release influenced by non-covalent vector–substrate interactions and the degradation rate of the scaffolds [14, 15, 34]. Scaffold design parameters such as porosity, tortuosity, hydrophobicity, and hydrophilicity, the rate and mechanism of degradation, and physical properties directly affect the host response (e.g. cell infiltration) and the vector (e.g. release rate), which combine to determine the overall efficiency of gene delivery.

24.3.1 Entrapment

The entrapment of vectors within the biomaterial scaffolds is typically employed to provide a sustained release that will maintain elevated concentrations of the vectors locally, which can extend the opportunities for cellular internalization and enhance gene delivery. Additional advantages of vector entrapment include increased stability through protection from extracellular degradative enzymes and recognition by the immune system [13, 50, 51]. Several natural and synthetic hydrogels have been used to entrap gene therapy vectors since these hydrogels undergo mild gelation that does not significantly impact the vector activity [34–36, 52]. Hydrogels with a mesh size larger than the vector diameter typically exhibit a rapid release, and hydrogels with a mesh size less than the vector diameter still exhibit some diffusive release, yet have release rates that are more dependent upon the degradation rate of the hydrogel. Protease-sensitive crosslinkers have served as a mode for vector release as infiltrating cells migrate through the hydrogel [34].

The encapsulation of vectors within hydrophobic materials can be more challenging than with hydrogels, since the processing conditions have the potential to significantly reduce the activity of the entrapped vectors. Nanospheres and microspheres with encapsulated vectors have been formed with PLG using an emulsion process, which is challenging because it involves organic solvents and lyophilization that can decrease activity [17, 50, 53, 54]. Despite the challenges, entrapped vectors retained activity, and encapsulation prevented recognition by the immune response. These particles can be injected locally to provide the localized release of a vector, yet do not provide a substrate for tissue growth. Alternatively, these particles could be seeded into microporous scaffolds or entrapped within a hydrogel to create a defined environment that stabilizes the implant site and delivers the vectors [35]. The vectors have also been directly encapsulated within micorporous scaffolds using a gas foaming process [14, 17, 53, 54]. The processes have been adapted to provide high encapsulation efficiencies (>75%) and released vectors have been able to induce extended transgene expression for times ranging from weeks to months, depending upon the implantation site [14, 19, 25].

24.3.2 Immobilization

The immobilization of vectors to materials can address several of the challenges associated with the entrapment approaches. For microporous scaffolds, immobilization would typically be applied after scaffold fabrication, thus the vectors would not be exposed to harsh processing conditions. The materials or vectors have been modified to provide for interactions with the vector. Nonspecific interactions between vectors and material surfaces (e.g. charged or protein-coated surfaces) have enabled vector retention on surfaces and have enhanced gene transfer [20, 21, 24, 25, 55]. Furthermore, this immobilization may function to co-localize the vectors with the cells and thus overcome mass-transport limitations. An alternative to simple adsorption of the vector has involved layer-by-layer deposition of cationic polymers and plasmid, which provides the opportunity for temporally controlled release as the plasmid on the outer surface is released first and that on the interior is released later [56]. Specific interactions, such as modification of viral and non-viral vectors with biotin to mediate interactions with avidin-modified materials [57], and the immobilization of antibodies that bind to the vector [58], have been used to better control vector immobilization and release. More recently, microporous and hydrogel scaffolds have been modified to specifically mediate interactions with VSV-G on lentivirus [17, 59]. For hydrogels, vectors are still encapsulated prior to gelation, unlike the microporous scaffolds. However, hydrophilic polymers can be modified prior to gelation to provide specific interactions with the vector. An initial strategy for this approach was the cationization of gelatin to provide binding sites for negatively charged plasmids [60, 61]. More recently, PEG hydrogels have been modified with affinity peptides to interact with entrapped lipoplexes and thereby retain the vectors. Importantly, the strength of interactions between scaffolds and vectors is critical, since excessive binding of the vector to the material can limit cell association and internalization [36].

24.4 Transgene expression profiles

Certain biomaterial systems have been demonstrated to have the ability to locally deliver DNA and obtain a localized transgene expression; however, the basic design parameters to maximize gene transfer remain to be fully identified. An aspect that has been the focus of many biomaterial-based delivery systems is achieving a sustained release of the vector. While sustained release has been consistently shown to enhance gene transfer in vitro [3, 33, 49], the role of sustained release in gene delivery in vivo is less clear. The potential for sustained release to promote gene transfer has been demonstrated with the intramuscular delivery of PLG microspheres, which exhibited increasing levels of gene expression over time [54]. This increasing expression over time contrasted with the bolus injection, for which transgene expression decreased with time. However, in a more recent study in which PLG scaffolds were modified with polydopamine (PD) to provide a sustained release of plasmid this did not significantly influence the profile of transgene expression relative to that with scaffolds that provided a rapid release (Figure 24.2) [20]. Interestingly, long-term transgene expression could be obtained only from a rapid release of the vector. The differences in results between sustained release and transgene expression likely reflect effects of the implantation site and variations in the host response, suggesting that a more thorough characterization of the number and type of cells expressing the transgene is needed.

The host response to the implant is expected to be a key factor influencing the extent and duration of transgene expression. The implantation of any biomaterial initiates a foreign-body response. Inflammatory cells such as neutrophils and macrophages are among the first responders which would be exposed to the released vectors (Figure 24.3(a)) [19, 26, 62]. Inflammatory cells are highly migratory and proliferative, which increases the probability that they will be transduced or transfected over cell types that arrive at scaffolds after the acute inflammatory response. Cell infiltration into scaffolds is thus a major determinant of transgene expression [26, 34, 35, 63]. A consideration

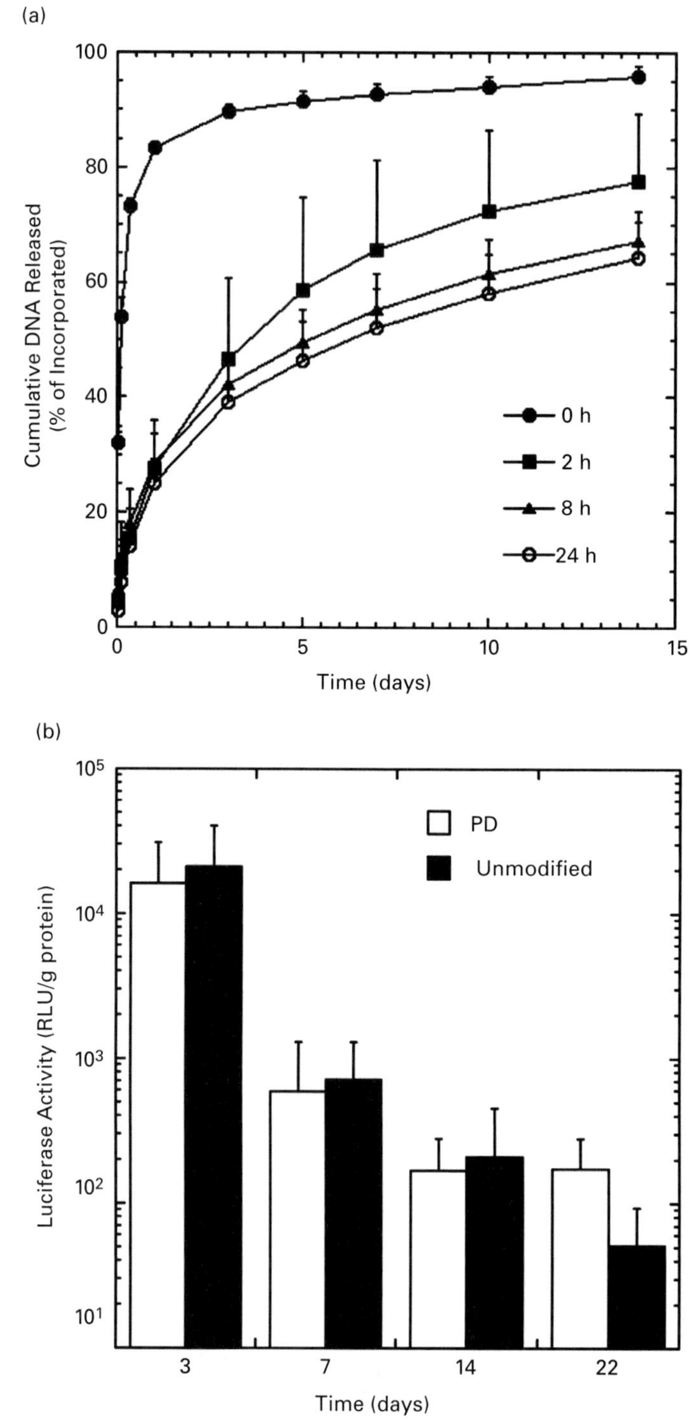

Figure 24.2 The relationship between DNA vector release and transgene expression profile in vivo. (a) PLG scaffolds were modified with PD for increasing amounts of time (0, 2, 8, or 24 h). Increased exposure of scaffolds to PD resulted in varying profiles

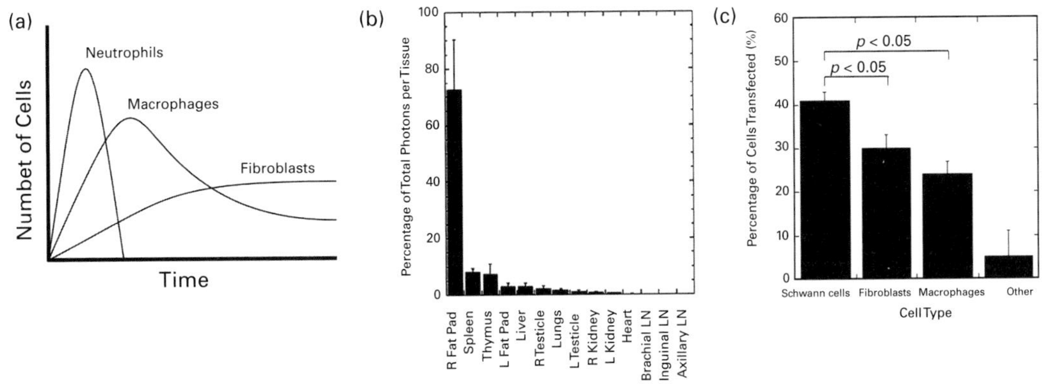

Figure 24.3 Transgene expression is typically dominated by immune cells. (a) The time course of cell infiltration into biomaterial scaffolds after implantation. (b) The percentage of total transgene expression in different organs in a mouse model three days after implantation of PLG scaffolds with immobilized lentivirus encoding luciferase. (With kind permission from Springer Informa HealthCare: *Drug Delivery Translational Research*, Hydrogels to modulate lentivirus delivery in vivo from microporous tissue engineering scaffolds, 1(1) 2011, 91–101, M. O. Avilés and L. D. Shea, Fig. 5C.) (c) Identification of transfected cell types after implantation in the spinal cord of PLG scaffolds loaded with plasmid encoding green fluorescent protein. (Reprinted by permission from Macmillan Publishers Ltd: *Molecular Therapy* 17(2):318–26, Plasmid releasing multiple channel bridges for transgene expression after spinal cord injury, L. De Laporte, Y. Yang, M. L. Zelivyanskaya, B. J. Cummings, A. J. Anderson and L. D. Shea, 2008.)

with delivery to these immune cells is their potential migration from the transplant site. Immune cells can exit through the lymphatic system and ultimately travel through the blood to the spleen and thymus. Localized delivery of viral vectors has produced transgene expression by immune cells in the spleen (Figure 24.3(b)) [26]. Within the implant, the immune cells are highly active and proliferative, which may contribute to the enhancement of gene transfer [63]. Immune cell types are consistently among the cells that express the transgene, along with a range of other cell types that are dependent upon the implantation site (Figure 24.3(c)) [17, 26, 41, 64].

Vector type and design are also determinants of transgene expression. Plasmids generally provide transient expression, which is most easily observed with in-vitro transfection [65]. The transient nature of expression with plasmids is attributed to a gradual decline in the number of plasmids per cell that occurs with cell division. Vectors that integrate the gene into the chromosome (e.g. retroviruses) have the potential for permanent expression in vitro. The in-vivo translation of these observations is more complex, in that non-viral vectors have induced transgene expression for months in some sites [24, 54], and expression with viral vectors may be transient, resulting from elimination of infected cells by the immune system [35]. Both for viral and for non-viral vectors, a factor limiting expression is silencing of the promoter. For example, in the peritoneal fat pad of mice, silencing of the

Caption for Figure 24.2 (*cont.*) of sustained release of loaded plasmid. (b) Despite the different DNA release profiles, subcutaneous implantation of PD-modified and unmodified PLG scaffolds with immobilized plasmid encoding for luciferase resulted in identical transgene expression profiles. (Reprinted from *Biomaterials*, Vol. 31(6), M. O. Avilés, C. H. Lin, M. Zelivyanskaya, J. G. Graham, R. M. Boehler, P. B. Messersmith and L. D. Shea, The contribution of plasmid design and release to in vivo gene expression following delivery from cationic polymer modified scaffolds, pp. 1140–7. Copyright 2010, with permission from Elsevier.)

cytomegalovirus (CMV) promoter resulted in significant loss of transgene expression over the course of 2 weeks, while transgene expression from the ubiquitin C (UqC) promoter was sustained at high levels for months [20]. Taken together, multiple aspects of the vector must be considered during the design of the system in order to achieve a specific expression profile.

The cell types transduced, and the extent and duration of expression, can be influenced by the microenvironment created by the biomaterial. The scaffolds typically present a combination of signals intended to promote tissue growth, and signals are presented in forms such as adhesion, mechanical properties, and the delivery of growth factors. Proteins or peptides that are conjugated to, or presented on, the scaffold can influence vector retention, yet may also influence cellular interactions with the material. The modification of scaffolds with ECM proteins has been extensively employed to influence cell adhesion and migration [66–68]. The identity of the ECM can also influence the internalization pathway and subsequent intracellular trafficking of viral and non-viral vectors, which can influence the extent of transgene expression [25, 41, 69, 70]. In addition to the ECM identity, the number of binding sites and their nanoscale spacing affects the level of trangene expression [71]. Specifically, the number of sites and nanoscale spacing influence receptor clustering, altering the intracellular response, including the cells' ability to endocytose non-viral vectors. Similarly, the mechanical strength of the material affects cytoskeletal organization and active signaling pathways within a cell. More rigid substrates are generally correlated with greater levels of transfection [32]. Since this study was performed with osteoblasts, which normally reside in a rigid environment (bone), it would be interesting to determine whether cells normally found in soft tissues would exhibit greater transfection efficiencies on soft substrates. Finally, the delivery of growth factors can enhance cell infiltration and/or cell proliferation, both of which may enhance gene transfer [63]. Taken together, the design of the microenvironment within the scaffold may influence the identity of infiltrating cells and also their phenotypic responses, which can influence the extent and duration of transgene expression.

Strategies that combine multiple material platforms may be able to target multiple barriers to efficient gene transfer, while creating an environment that supports tissue growth. Gene therapy vectors have increasingly been designed with multiple functional groups to enhance transport to the target tissue, promote binding to the target cell, and facilitate intracellular trafficking [72]. Biomaterial scaffolds can similarly be designed with these multiple functional components. Nanoparticles that bind the gene therapy vectors can be incorporated within hydrogels that provide a support for gene therapy vectors [35]. Microporous scaffolds that provide structural support have been filled with ECM-containing hydrogels that regulate cell adhesion and migration, and genes could be delivered either from the microporous scaffold or the hydrogel [26]. This multifaceted approach modulates cell adhesion and migration into the scaffold while simultaneously increasing vector bioavailability and delivery to cells.

24.5 Gene expression and tissue formation

While previous sections have addressed the design of biomaterials for gene delivery, the ultimate objective is to apply these gene delivery systems to promote the repair of injured tissues. Vector-loaded scaffolds have been applied to numerous applications, such as the repair of bone [73–76], angiogenesis [14, 77–79], and nerve regeneration [62, 65, 80, 81]. In addition to promoting tissue formation in vivo, scaffold-mediated gene delivery has also been investigated to model tissue formation in vitro. The design of these systems will need to focus not only on efficient delivery, but also on actually controlling the number and distribution of cells expressing the transgene, and the level and duration of expression. Vector-loaded scaffolds are a promising platform for artificially recapitulating the patterns of gene expression that may be observed during tissue development and tissue repair.

The number of cells expressing a transgene and the level of this expression can independently affect tissue formation [82, 83]. The impact of these parameters has been demonstrated in vitro using neurite outgrowth as

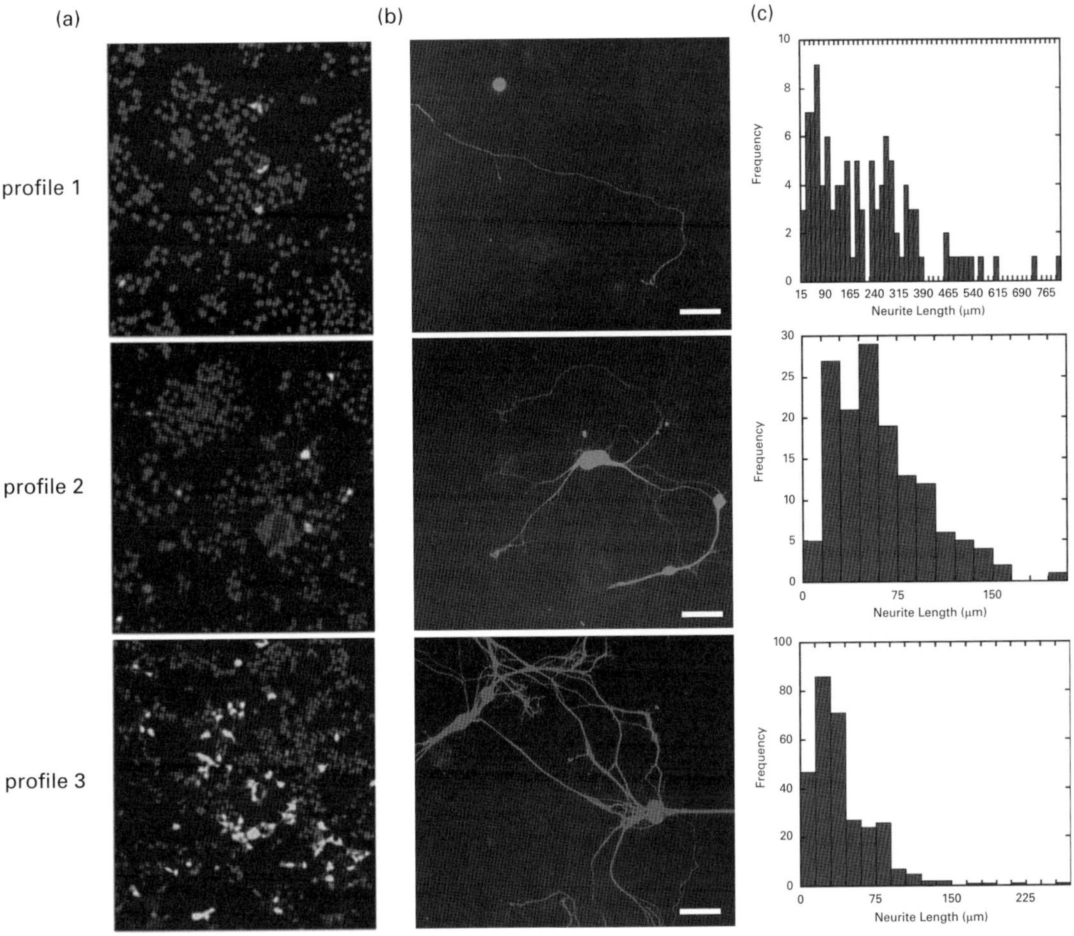

Figure 24.4 Dependence of physiological response on transgene expression profiles. Neurons were co-cultured with HEK293T cells expressing NGF in three distinct profiles. (a) Profiles were visualized by transfection of HEK293T cells with plasmid encoding green fluorescent protein. (b) Neurite outgrowth and branching in response to different expression profiles. Scale bars = 50 μm. (c) Quantification of neurite length and frequency. Profiles in (a) correspond to neurite images (b) and quantification (c) along each row. (From T. Houchin-Ray, M. Zelivyanskaya, A. Huang, and L. D. Shea. Non-viral gene delivery transfection profiles influence neuronal architecture in an in vitro co-culture model, *Biotechnology & Bioengineering*, 103(5), 1023–33, Copyright 2009. Reprinted by permission of John Wiley & Sons, Inc.)

a model [82]. Primary neurons were co-cultured with accessory cells, which were transfected with plasmid encoding for nerve growth factor (NGF) in three separate groups to obtain transfection profiles that were described as (i) high expression, with large numbers of transfected cells; (ii) high expression, with a low number of transfected cells; and (iii) low expression, with a low number of transfected cells. Specifically, profiles with low levels of NGF expression resulted in extension of longer, more unidirectional neurites, while high levels of NGF expression resulted in extension of shorter and more branched, multipolar neurites (Figure 24.4). Long neurites with less branching are suggestive of more directed axon growth, and the local concentration gradients generated around the fewer cells transfected were hypothesized to contribute to directional growth. This impact of cell number and expression level has similarly been observed to impact angiogenesis in vivo [83]. The in-vivo transplantation of myoblasts expressing vascular endothelial growth factor (VEGF) demonstrated that the number of cells determined the area over which a phenotypic response was observed. Importantly, only cells that expressed relatively low levels of VEGF were able to achieve the formation of normal, mature blood vessels, whereas cells expressing high levels of VEGF formed abnormal and immature vessels. Even when the total levels of VEGF production were equivalent (i.e. a small number of high VEGF expressers vs. a large number of low VEGF expressers), only the low expressers were able to elicit stable vessel formation. An improved understanding of the impact of these local concentration gradients on the phenotypic response will be essential for the application of gene delivery to tissue regeneration.

The micro-architecture of the material can synergize with the transgene expression to modulate tissue formation. This phenomenon has been demonstrated by the co-culture of neurons and accessory cells on topographically patterned PLG substrates [84]. Gene delivery to the accessory cells was achieved by immobilization to the PLG surface, which resulted in transfection efficiency and transgene expression that was dependent upon the channel width and DNA loading. The longest primary neurites were observed on surfaces with the smallest channels, and increasing the channel width gradually decreased the primary neurite length. Flat surfaces had the lowest extent of primary neurite growth. Interestingly, gene delivery was least efficient in the smallest channels as well. Taken together, these results indicate that there is a relationship between transgene expression and scaffold architecture that impacts the organization of the resulting tissue.

Spatial patterns of transgene expression have been employed to provide directional orientation to cellular processes or to create a tissue interface. The spatial patterning of gene therapy vectors on biomaterial scaffolds has been achieved using antibodies, biotin–avidin binding, and non-specific interactions, and researchers have been able to spatially control gene delivery both in vitro and in vivo [57, 64, 82, 85]. The patterned expression of soluble factors results in localized gradients, which may mimic those observed during developmental and repair processes, as previously demonstrated by observation of neurite extension, which occurs along high concentrations or towards high concentrations of neurotrophic factors [82]. In this study, the immobilization of vectors to narrow lines (100 μm) by microfluidics resulted in neuron survival and neurite outgrowth within the pattern. The patterning of vectors into larger features (500 μm) resulted in the directed growth of axons toward the vectors from distances up to 1.5 mm outside of the pattern.

An alternative to the expression of soluble factors to create gradients is the expression of transcription factors to direct differentiation and create an interface within a developing tissue. Biomaterials were modified with a retrovirus encoding for RunX2, which has been implicated in directing the differentiation of mesenchymal stem cells to an osteogenic phenotype [86]. Thus, a single cell type cultured on this surface was hypothesized to develop down an osteoblastic lineage or a fibroblastic lineage depending on which transgene was expressed. The gradient resulted in zonal organization of osteoblastic and fibroblastic phenotypes in vitro, and following subcutaneous implantation in vivo. This approach was able to generate a graded bone/soft tissue interface from a single cell type.

24.6 Emerging opportunities

Biomaterial-based systems for efficient, localized gene transfer are currently being developed to present controlled microenvironments that promote wound healing or tissue regeneration. Although much progress has been made in this area, numerous opportunities exist to improve the delivery systems to elicit the desired therapeutic result. While some of the design parameters dominating the tissue response to controlled gene delivery have been identified, further study will be required in order to develop a complete model relating gene transfer and the biomaterial design parameters. Recent studies have demonstrated that the phenotypic response to gene delivery depends on the number of cells that express a transgene and their level of expression. The efficiency of DNA uptake is highly dependent on the ability of cells to interact with, and migrate through, scaffolds. Scaffolds can be designed to regulate cell adhesion and migration by incorporating factors (e.g. ECM-derived peptides) that mimic the native tissue microenvironment. Similarly, biomaterial scaffolds can be designed to simultaneously promote gene formation and support tissue formation. Truly biomimetic materials would likely respond to the local environmental cues so that scaffold degradation, transgene expression, and tissue formation are timed with physiological events (inflammation, regeneration, etc.) and cell events (differentiation, migration, etc.) [87]. Future developments of biomaterial-mediated gene delivery should include better targeting of specific cell types, spatial control, and temporally dynamic gene delivery.

Development of more efficient cell- and tissue-specific delivery systems is critical to full realization of the potential of genetic therapies. The majority of genetic therapies have focussed on the delivery of genes encoding for secreted factors that can impact a broad area (e.g. NGF and VEGF), as described above. However, genetic vectors encoding for proteins involved in upstream intracellular signaling, such as transcription factors, may be necessary in order to effect drastic changes in cell differentiation and genotype. RNAi and other oligonucleotide therapies also work intracellularly, which amplifies the importance of targeting vector delivery to a specific cell population and delivering nucleic acid into sufficient numbers of cells for therapeutic efficacy. Tissue-specific therapies require consideration of the local cell population at an implant site, delivery of multiple genes in conjugation with soluble factors, presentation of adhesive ligands, and tissue mechanics. Few researchers have investigated tissue- or cell-specific promoters in regenerative medicine, while inducible promoters are improving and may provide additional control over expression.

With the development of improved delivery systems, spatial patterning of vectors on length scales of tens to hundreds of microns in vivo is expected to have great utility for promoting tissue regeneration. Gene expression is precisely localized during tissue development and in mature tissues, with spatial patterns in expression regulating the differentiation of multipotent progenitor cells into functional tissues. Recent studies have revealed strategies with the potential to spatially regulate gene transfer [64], and their extension to length scales of tens or hundreds of microns could be applied to recreate gene expression profiles observed during tissue and stem cell development. Delivery of genetic vectors from scaffolds provides a unique opportunity to capitalize on the potential synergy between the biomaterial design for cell processes and gene delivery. Co-patterning of cell adhesion, gene expression, and production of soluble factors can be combined in a single scaffold to create in-vitro models of tissue formation that mimic the complex microenvironments present during in-vivo tissue development. An ideal model of tissue development might entail culturing a single, multipotent stem cell type onto a scaffold presenting patterned gene transfer in a manner that promotes differentiation of the cells into various phenotypes depending on spatial location. In addition to spatial control, temporal control over gene expression is vital to differentiation of stem cells into mature phenotypes and wound healing (e.g. angiogenesis). For tissue engineers to recreate this process, temporally controlled delivery of multiple transgene vectors and soluble factors from scaffolds over periods of weeks or months will likely be required. For example, since viral vectors result in long-term expression at lower levels than do non-viral vectors, simultaneous delivery of multiple transgenes via different vectors could be used to gain temporal control.

A complementary aspect to creating a permissive microenvironment for cell infiltration is to enhance the number of progenitor cells available in vivo. The gene delivery systems described herein could potentially be employed for *in situ* cell programming. A greater understanding of transdifferentiation and induced pluripotent stem cells is emerging from fundamental biology studies, and may identify factors that could be delivered locally to safely create tissue-specific progenitor cells in vivo with greater potential for promoting regeneration than that of the endogenous progenitors recruited to an injury. This process of *in situ* programming is exemplified through targeting immune cells that infiltrate a scaffold to promote an immune response. Bacterially derived oligonucleotides (CpG) have been immobilized to PLG scaffolds using polyethylene imine (PEI) polyplexes and delivered in vivo to tumor sites in mice [88]. When this was done in conjunction with delivery of granulocyte macrophage-colony stimulating factor (GM-CSF), which stimulates migration, proliferation, phagocytosis, and differentiation of dendritic cells, mice developed a specific immunity to the cancerous tumor.

Biomaterial-mediated gene delivery systems have demonstrated enormous potential as effective therapies for tissue regeneration and organ replacement. While progress has been made in enhancing the efficiency of gene transfer of these systems, technological advancements must keep pace with the improved understanding of the underlying biology. Advanced tissue regeneration in vivo and tissue development in vitro could benefit tremendously from the creation of scaffolds that present an appropriate microenvironment for cell growth and mediate efficient spatially and temporally localized gene expression.

REFERENCES

[1] Jang, J. H., Houchin, T. L. and Shea, L. D. 2004. Gene delivery from polymer scaffolds for tissue engineering. *Expert Rev. Med. Dev.*, **1**(1), 127–38.

[2] Nishikawa, M. and Huang, L. 2001. Nonviral vectors in the new millennium: delivery barriers in gene transfer. *Human Gene Ther.*, **12**(8), 861–70.

[3] Pannier, A. K. and Shea, L. D. 2004. Controlled release systems for DNA delivery. *Molec. Ther.*, **10**(1), 19–26.

[4] Loser, P., Huser, A., Hillgenberg, M. *et al.* 2002. Advances in the development of non-human viral DNA-vectors for gene delivery. *Curr. Gene Ther.*, **2**(2), 161–71.

[5] Dull, T., Zufferey, R., Kelly, M. *et al.* 1998. A third-generation lentivirus vector with a conditional packaging system. *J. Virol.*, **72**(11), 8463–71.

[6] Kootstra, N. A. and Verma, I. M. 2003. Gene therapy with viral vectors. *Ann. Rev. Pharm. Toxicol.*, **43**, 413–39.

[7] Kay, M. A., Manno, C. S., Ragni, M. V. *et al.* 2000. Evidence for gene transfer and expression of factor IX in haemophilia B patients treated with an AAV vector. *Nature Genetics*, **24**(3), 257–61.

[8] Kaplitt, M. G., Feigin, A., Tang, C. *et al.* 2007. Safety and tolerability of gene therapy with an adeno-associated virus (AAV) borne GAD gene for Parkinson's disease: an open label, phase I trial. *Lancet*, **369**(9579), 2097–105.

[9] Maguire, A. M., Simonelli, F., Pierce, E. A. *et al.* 2008. Safety and efficacy of gene transfer for Leber's congenital amaurosis. *New Engl. J. Med.*, **358**(21), 2240–8.

[10] Cartier, N., Hacein-Bey-Abina, S., Bartholomae, C. C. *et al.* 2009. Hematopoietic stem cell gene therapy with a lentiviral vector in X-linked adrenoleukodystrophy. *Science*, **326**(5954), 818–23.

[11] Maguire, A. M., High, K. A., Auricchio, A. *et al.* 2009. Age-dependent effects of RPE65 gene therapy for Leber's congenital amaurosis: a phase 1 dose-escalation trial. *Lancet*, **374**(9701), 1597–605.

[12] Muramatsu, S., Fujimoto, K., Kato, S. *et al.* 2010. A phase I study of aromatic L-amino acid decarboxylase gene therapy for Parkinson's disease. *Molec. Ther.*, **18**(9), 1731–5.

[13] Sailaja, G., HogenEsch, H., North, A., Hays, J. and Mittal, S. K. 2002. Encapsulation of recombinant adenovirus into alginate microspheres circumvents vector-specific immune response. *Gene Ther.*, **9**(24), 1722–9.

[14] Shea, L. D., Smiley, E., Bonadio, J. and Mooney, D. J. 1999. DNA delivery from polymer matrices for tissue engineering. *Nature Biotechnol.*, **17**(6), 551–4.

[15] De Laporte, L. and Shea, L. D. 2007. Matrices and scaffolds for DNA delivery in tissue engineering. *Adv. Drug Del. Rev.*, **59**(4–5), 292–307.

[16] Huang, R., Liu, S., Shao, K. *et al.* 2010. Evaluation and mechanism studies of PEGylated dendrigraft poly-L-lysines as novel gene delivery vectors. *Nanotechnology*, **21**, 265101.

[17] Shin, S., Tuinstra, H. M., Salvay, D. M. and Shea, L. D. 2010. Phosphatidylserine immobilization of lentivirus for localized gene transfer. *Biomaterials*, **31**(15), 4353–9.

[18] Langer, R. 1998. Drug delivery and targeting. *Nature*, **392**(6679 Suppl.), 5–10.

[19] Rives, C. B., des Rieux, A., Zelivyanskaya, M. *et al.* 2009. Layered PLG scaffolds for in vivo plasmid delivery. *Biomaterials*, **30**(3), 394–401.

[20] Aviles, M. O., Lin, C. H., Zelivyanskaya, M. *et al.* 2010. The contribution of plasmid design and release to in vivo gene expression following delivery from cationic polymer modified scaffolds. *Biomaterials*, **31**(6), 1140–7.

[21] Huang, Y. C., Riddle, K., Rice, K. G. and Mooney, D. J. 2005. Long-term in vivo gene expression via delivery of PEI–DNA condensates from porous polymer scaffolds. *Human Gene Ther.*, **16**(5), 609–17.

[22] Jang, J. H. and Shea, L. D. 2006. Intramuscular delivery of DNA releasing microspheres: microsphere properties and transgene expression. *J. Controll. Rel.*, **112**(1), 120–8.

[23] Saul, J. M., Linnes, M. P., Ratner, B. D., Giachelli, C. M. and Pun, S. H. 2007. Delivery of non-viral gene carriers from sphere-templated fibrin scaffolds for sustained transgene expression. *Biomaterials*, **28**(31), 4705–16.

[24] Salvay, D. M., Zelivyanskaya, M. and Shea, L. D. 2010. Gene delivery by surface immobilization of plasmid to tissue-engineering scaffolds. *Gene Ther.*, **17**(9), 1134–41.

[25] Shin, S., Salvay, D. M. and Shea, L. D. 2010. Lentivirus delivery by adsorption to tissue engineering scaffolds. *J. Biomed. Mater. Res. A*, **93**(4), 1252–9.

[26] Aviles, M. O. and Shea, L. D. 2011. Hydrogels to modulate lentivirus delivery in vivo from microporous tissue engineering scaffolds. *Drug Del. Transl. Res.*, **1**(1), 91–101.

[27] Bryant, S. J. and Anseth, K. S. 2002. Hydrogel properties influence ECM production by chondrocytes photoencapsulated in poly(ethylene glycol) hydrogels. *J. Biomed. Mater. Res.*, **59**(1), 63–72.

[28] Burdick, J. A., Chung, C., Jia, X., Randolph, M. A. and Langer, R. 2005. Controlled degradation and mechanical behavior of photopolymerized hyaluronic acid networks. *Biomacromolecules*, **6**(1), 386–91.

[29] Banerjee, A., Arha, M., Choudhary, S. *et al.* 2009. The influence of hydrogel modulus on the proliferation and differentiation of encapsulated neural stem cells. *Biomaterials*, **30**(27), 4695–9.

[30] Seidlits, S. K., Khaing, Z. Z., Petersen, R. R. *et al.* 2010. The effects of hyaluronic acid hydrogels with tunable mechanical properties on neural progenitor cell differentiation. *Biomaterials*, **31**(14), 3930–40.

[31] Engler, A. J., Sen, S., Sweeney, H. L. and Discher, D. E. 2006. Matrix elasticity directs stem cell lineage specification. *Cell*, **126**(4), 677–89.

[32] Kong, H. J., Liu, J., Riddle, K. *et al.* 2005. Non-viral gene delivery regulated by stiffness of cell adhesion substrates. *Nature Mater.*, **4**(6), 460–4.

[33] Scherer, F., Schillinger, U., Putz, U., Stemberger, A. and Plank, C. 2002. Nonviral vector loaded collagen sponges for sustained gene delivery in vitro and in vivo. *J. Gene Med.*, **4**(6), 634–43.

[34] Shepard, J. A., Huang, A., Shikanov, A. and Shea, L. D. 2010. Balancing cell migration with matrix degradation enhances gene delivery to cells cultured three-dimensionally within hydrogels. *J. Controll. Rel.*, **146**(1), 128–35.

[35] Shin, S. and Shea, L. D. 2010. Lentivirus immobilization to nanoparticles for enhanced and localized delivery from hydrogels. *Molec. Ther.*, **18**(4), 700–6.

[36] Shepard, J. A., Wesson, P. J., Wang, C. E. *et al.* 2011. Gene therapy vectors with enhanced transfection based on hydrogels modified with affinity peptides. *Biomaterials*, **32**(22), 5092–9.

[37] Putnam, A. J. and Mooney, D. J. 1996. Tissue engineering using synthetic extracellular matrices. *Nature Med.*, **2**(7), 824–6.

[38] Kim, B. S. and Mooney, D. J. 1998. Development of biocompatible synthetic extracellular matrices for tissue engineering. *Trends Biotechnol.*, **16**(5), 224–30.

[39] Hill, E., Boontheekul, T. and Mooney, D. J. 2006. Regulating activation of transplanted cells controls tissue regeneration. *Proc. Nat. Acad. Sci. USA*, **103**(8), 2494–9.

[40] Smith, M. K., Riddle, K. W. and Mooney, D. J. 2006. Delivery of hepatotrophic factors fails to enhance longer-term survival of subcutaneously transplanted hepatocytes. *Tissue Eng.*, **12**(2), 235–44.

[41] Salvay, D. M., Rives, C. B., Zhang, X. *et al.* 2008. Extracellular matrix protein-coated scaffolds promote the reversal of diabetes after extrahepatic islet transplantation. *Transplantation*, **85**(10), 1456–64.

[42] Richardson, T. P., Peters, M. C., Ennett, A. B. and Mooney, D. J. 2001. Polymeric system for dual growth factor delivery. *Nature Biotechnol.*, **19**(11), 1029–34.

[43] Salvay, D. M. and Shea, L. D. 2005. Inductive tissue engineering with protein and DNA-releasing scaffolds. *Molec. BioSyst.*, **2**(1), 36–48.

[44] Ma, P. X. 2004. Scaffolds for tissue fabrication. *Mater. Today*, **7**(5), 30–40.

[45] Annabi, N., Nichol, J. W., Zhong, X. *et al.* 2010. Controlling the porosity and microarchitecture of hydrogels for tissue engineering. *Tissue Eng. B*, **16**(4), 371–83.

[46] Bhatia, S. K. 2010. Tissue engineering for clinical applications. *Biotech. J.*, **5**(12), 1309–23.

[47] Owen, S. C. and Shoichet, M. S. 2010. Design of three dimensional biomimetic scaffolds. *J. Biomed. Mater. Res. A*, **94**(4), 1321–31.

[48] Huang, N. F. and Li, S. 2011. Regulation of the matrix microenvironment for stem cell engineering and regenerative medicine. *Ann. Biomed. Eng.*, **39**(4), 1201–14.

[49] Mallapragada, S. K. and Agarwal, A. 2008. Synthetic sustained gene delivery systems. *Curr. Top. Med. Chem.*, **8**(4), 311–30.

[50] Mok, H., Park, J. W. and Park, T. G. 2007. Microencapsulation of PEGylated adenovirus within PLGA microspheres for enhanced stability and gene transfection efficiency. *Pharm. Res.*, **24**(12), 2263–9.

[51] Gary, D. J., Lee, H., Sharma, R. *et al.* 2011. Influence of nano-carrier architecture on in vitro siRNA delivery performance and in vivo biodistribution: polyplexes vs micelleplexes. *ACS Nano*, **5**(5), 3493–505.

[52] des Rieux, A., Shikanov, A. and Shea, L. D. 2009. Fibrin hydrogels for non-viral vector delivery in vitro. *J. Controll. Rel.*, **136**(2), 148–54.

[53] Jang, J. H. and Shea, L. D. 2003. Controllable delivery of non-viral DNA from porous scaffolds. *J. Controll. Rel.*, **86**(1), 157–68.

[54] Jang, J. H., Rives, C. B. and Shea, L. D. 2005. Plasmid delivery in vivo from porous tissue-engineering scaffolds: transgene expression and cellular transfection. *Molec. Ther.*, **12**(3), 475–83.

[55] Choi, S. and Murphy, W. L. 2010. Sustained plasmid DNA release from dissolving mineral coatings. *Acta Biomater.*, **6**(9), 3426–35.

[56] Shmueli, R. B., Anderson, D. G. and Green, J. J. 2010. Electrostatic surface modifications to improve gene delivery. *Expert Opin. Drug Del.*, **7**(4), 535–50.

[57] Segura, T., Anderson, B. C., Chung, P. H. *et al.* 2005. Crosslinked hyaluronic acid hydrogels: a strategy to functionalize and pattern. *Biomaterials*, **26**(4), 359–71.

[58] Zhang, L. H., Luo, T., Zhang, C. *et al.* 2011. Anti-DNA antibody modified coronary stent for plasmid gene delivery: results obtained from a porcine coronary stent model. *J. Gene Med.*, **13**(1), 37–45.

[59] Padmashali, R. M. and Andreadis, S. T. 2011. Engineering fibrinogen-binding VSV-G envelope for spatially- and cell-controlled lentivirus delivery through fibrin hydrogels. *Biomaterials*, **32**(12), 3330–9.

[60] Young, S., Wong, M., Tabata, Y. and Mikos, A. G. 2005. Gelatin as a delivery vehicle for the controlled release of bioactive molecules. *J. Controll. Rel.*, **109**(1–3), 256–74.

[61] Kasper, F. K., Kushibiki, T., Kimura, Y., Mikos, A. G. and Tabata, Y. 2005. In vivo release of plasmid DNA from composites of oligo(poly(ethylene glycol) fumarate) and cationized gelatin microspheres. *J. Controll. Rel.*, **107**(3), 547–61.

[62] Yang, Y., Laporte, L. D., Zelivyanskaya, M. L. *et al.* 2009. Multiple channel bridges for spinal cord injury: cellular characterization of host response. *Tissue Eng. A*, **15**(11), 3283–95.

[63] Riddle, K. W., Kong, H. J., Leach, J. K. *et al.* 2007. Modifying the proliferative state of target cells to control DNA expression and identifying cell types transfected in vivo. *Molec. Ther.*, **15**(2), 361–8.

[64] de Laporte, L, Huang, A., Ducommun, M. M. *et al.* 2010. Patterned transgene expression in multiple-channel bridges after spinal cord injury. *Acta Biomater.*, **6**(8), 2889–97.

[65] De Laporte, L., Yang, Y., Zelivyanskaya, M. L. *et al.* 2008. Plasmid releasing multiple channel bridges for transgene expression after spinal cord injury. *Molec. Ther.*, **17**(2), 318–26.

[66] Carson, A. E. and Barker, T. H. 2009. Emerging concepts in engineering extracellular matrix variants for directing cell phenotype. *Regen. Med.*, **4**(4), 593–600.

[67] Dutta, R. C. and Dutta, A. K. 2010. Comprehension of ECM-cell dynamics: a prerequisite for tissue regeneration. *Biotechnol. Adv.*, **28**(6), 764–9.

[68] Pradhan, S. and Farach-Carson, M. C. 2010. Mining the extracellular matrix for tissue engineering applications. *Regen. Med.*, **5**(6), 961–70.

[69] Bengali, Z., Rea, J. C. and Shea, L. D. 2007. Gene expression and internalization following vector adsorption to immobilized proteins: dependence on protein identity and density. *J. Gene Med.*, **9**(8), 668–78.

[70] Chang, K. L., Higuchi, Y., Kawakami, S., Yamashita, F. and Hashida, M. 2010. Efficient gene transfection by histidine-modified chitosan through enhancement of endosomal escape. *Bioconj. Chem.*, **21**(6), 1087–95.

[71] Kong, H. J., Hsiong, S. and Mooney, D. J. 2007. Nanoscale cell adhesion ligand presentation regulates nonviral gene delivery and expression. *Nano Lett.*, **7**(1), 161–6.

[72] Kay, M. A. 2011. State-of-the-art gene-based therapies: the road ahead. *Nature Rev. Genetics*, **12**(5), 316–28.

[73] Partridge, K., Yang, X., Clarke, N. M. P. *et al.* 2002. Adenoviral BMP-2 gene transfer in mesenchymal stem cells: in vitro and in vivo bone formation on biodegradable polymer scaffolds. *Biochem. Biophys. Res. Commun.*, **292**(1), 144–52.

[74] Kasper, F. K., Seidlits, S. K., Tang, A. *et al.* 2005. In vitro release of plasmid DNA from oligo(poly(ethylene glycol) fumarate) hydrogels. *J. Controll. Rel.*, **104**(3), 521–39.

[75] Jabbarzadeh, E., Starnes, T., Khan, Y. M. *et al.* 2008. Induction of angiogenesis in tissue-engineered scaffolds designed for bone repair: a combined gene therapy in cell transplantation approach. *Proc. Nat. Acad. Sci. USA*, **105**(32), 11099–104.

[76] Zhang, Y., Shi, B., Li, C. *et al.* 2009. The synergetic bone-forming effects of combinations of growth factors expressed by adenovirus vectors on chitosan/collagen scaffolds. *J. Controll. Rel.*, **136**(3), 172–8.

[77] Kyriakides, T. R., Hartzel, T., Huynh, G. and Bornstein, P. 2001. Regulation of angiogenesis and matrix remodeling by localized, matrix-mediated antisense gene delivery. *Molec. Ther.*, **3**(6), 842–9.

[78] Kasahara, H., Tanaka, E., Fukuyama, N. *et al.* 2003. Biodegradable gelatin hydrogel potentiates the angiogenic effect of fibroblast growth factor 4 plasmid in rabbit hind-limb ischemia. *J. Am. Coll. Cardiol.*, **41**(6), 1056–62.

[79] Mao, Z., Shi, H., Guo, R. *et al.* 2009. Enhanced angiogenesis of porous collagen scaffolds by incorporation of TMC/DNA complexes encoding vascular endothelial growth factor. *Acta Biomater.*, **5**(8), 2983–94.

[80] Berry, M., Gonzalez, A. M., Clarke, W. *et al.* 2001. Sustained effects of gene-activated matrices after CNS injury. *Molec. Cell Neurosci.*, **17**(4), 706–16.

[81] De Laporte, L., Yang, L. A. and Shea, L. D. 2009. Local gene delivery from ECM-coated poly(lactide-*co*-glycolide) multiple channel bridges after spinal cord injury. *Biomaterials*, **30**(12), 2361–8.

[82] Houchin-Ray, T., Zelivyanskaya, M., Huang, A. and Shea, L. D. 2009. Non-viral gene delivery transfection profiles influence neuronal architecture in an in vitro co-culture model. *Biotechnol. Bioeng.*, **103**(5), 1023–33.

[83] Ozawa, C. R., Banfi, A., Glazer, N. L. *et al.* 2004. Microenvironmental VEGF concentration, not total dose, determines a threshold between normal and aberrant angiogenesis. *J. Clin. Invest.*, **113**(4), 516–27.

[84] Houchin-Ray, T., Swift, L. A., Jang, J. H. and Shea, L. D. 2007. Patterned PLG substrates for localized DNA delivery and directed neurite extension. *Biomaterials*, **28**(16), 2603–11.

[85] Houchin-Ray, T., Huang, A., West, E. R., Zelivyanskaya, M. and Shea, L. D. 2009. Spatially patterned gene expression for guided neurite extension. *J. Neurosci. Res.*, **87**(4), 844–56.

[86] Zhao, Z., Zhao, M., Xiao, G. and Franceschi, R. T. 2005. Gene transfer of the Runx2 transcription factor enhances osteogenic activity of bone marrow stromal cells in vitro and in vivo. *Molec. Ther.*, **12**(2), 247–53.

[87] Jo, J. and Tabata, Y. 2008. Non-viral gene transfection technologies for genetic engineering of stem cells. *Eur. J. Pharmaceutics Biopharmaceutics*, **68**(1), 90–104.

[88] Ali, O. A., Huebsch, N., Cao, L., Dranoff, G. and Mooney, D. J. 2009. Infection-mimicking materials to program dendritic cells *in situ*. *Nature Mater.*, **8**(2), 151–8.

PART V

Animal models and clinical applications

25

Bone regeneration

Eric W. Hsu, Pedro Alvarez, Lyndsey Shutte, Amy Donovan, Shiguang Liu, Arun R. Shivats and Jeffrey O. Hollinger

25.1 Bone biology

Bone is a complex tissue-organ system integrating multiple components in hierarchical layers of molecular cues, cellular communities, and networking highways. Bone moves through space and time in a dynamic manner modulated by homeostatic mechanisms nuanced through a coordinated intercalation of biological and biomechanical rhythms. The price we vertebrate species pay for maintaining this magnificently orchestrated tissue-organ is daunting.

Bone is the most metabolically expensive tissue in the human body. For every ounce of bone, a pound of soft tissue is required for maintenance [1]. Moreover, the human skeletal system must be rugged in order to handle years of cyclic loading at high forces on the order of kilonewtons, and highly sensitive to the calibrated kinetics of calcium and phosphate release in order to maintain meticulously modulated ion levels [2]. Consequently, the intrinsic design of bone and the dynamics that sustain it are an instructional core for regenerative bone therapeutics.

In this chapter we will introduce the profoundly compelling biodynamic structural marvel that gives shape to the amorphous mass in which it is wrapped and provides the fulcrums and pulleys that propel our anatomy along the avenues and boulevards of our towns. We will probe the blueprint of bone as a defining mold that guides and mentors attempts in the laboratory to design and develop compositions to repair and regenerate this structural tour de force.

25.1.1 The cells and extracellular matrix of bone

There are three main bone cell phenotypes: the osteoblasts, the osteocytes, and the osteoclasts.

25.1.1.1 Osteoblasts

The osteoblasts are mononucleate cells that produce bone – or, more specifically, the organic osteoid and the proteins that facilitate its mineralization. Osteoblasts are derived from the mesenchymal stem cell line, either on the endosteal and periosteal surfaces of bone or from the marrow's stromal cells. These osteoprogenitors can be induced to differentiate by growth factors such as transforming growth factor-β (TGF-β) [3], platelet-derived growth factor (PDGF) [4, 5], fibroblast growth factor (FGF) [6–8], and certain bone morphogenetic proteins (BMPs) [9–12]. Once activated and situated on the surface of bone, osteoblasts will build up a surface layer of osteoid and mineralizing enzymes, such as alkaline phosphatase, that will cause hydroxyapatite crystals to form along the predominantly type I collagen strands of the osteoid. The osteoid is normally formed at a rate of roughly 1–2 μm/day and will mineralize afterwards at approximately 1 μm/day [13–15].

Osteoblasts may experience reduced activity and assume a quiescent state and fusiform morphology contiguous to the periosteal and endosteal envelopes. These are termed *bone-lining cells*. The bone-lining cells are also referred to as "resting osteoblasts," though this term has been used for cells that may be too small ($\lesssim$10–15 μm in diameter) to be active osteoblasts but are associated with a bone surface [16].

25.1.1.2 Osteocytes

Active osteoblasts that become entrapped within the mineralizing matrix front are called *osteocytes*. The *osteocytes* reside in the *lacunae* and elaborate filamentous-appearing protoplasmic extensions that form an intricate network of intercellular communication channels via gap junctions at the connecting termini. The *syncytium* formed enables a *mechanoreceptor* function for osteocytes that senses loading and directs modeling and remodeling, and thereby shapes and maintains the form and function of bone [17].

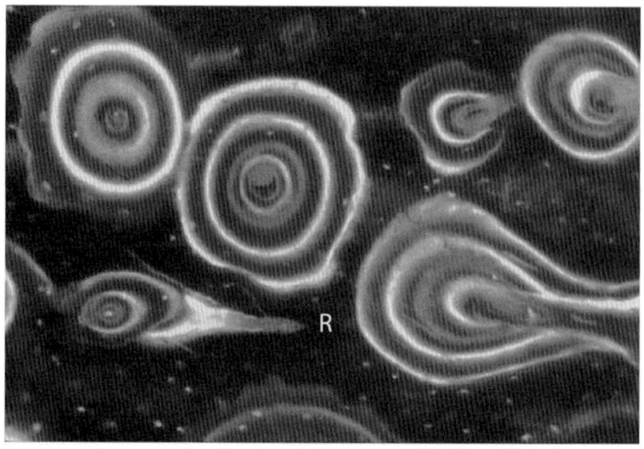

Figure 25.1 Multiple fluorochrome labels were administered at two-week intervals in a young dog. The concentric lines highlight the shape of the osteons. The osteocytes' lacunae can also be seen in this micrograph [22].

25.1.1.3 Osteoclasts

Osteoclasts are multinucleated giant cells ($\geq$100 μm in size with 3–10 nuclei) that resorb bone through a complex process of matrix dissolution [18, 19]. Cathepsin K and matrix metalloproteinase expressed by osteoclasts degrade the organic matrix while local acidification of the extracellular phagolysosomal compartment under the ruffled border of each osteoclast is responsible for the solubilization of the mineral components [20]. The outcome from this osteoclast-mediated process is the formation of resorptive pits, referred to as Howship's lacunae. Osteoclast lineage is derived from the hematopoietic monocyte–macrophage cell line – an entirely different family of stem cells from the osteoblastic line.

25.1.1.4 Extracellular matrix

These three cell phenotypes (osteoblasts, osteocytes, and osteoclasts) create and maintain the mineralized and organic extracellular matrices of bone. The matrix has multiple components arranged *anisotropically* (i.e. according to a defined spatial organization) to support the direction of primary load in each area of bone. *Osteoid* is secreted from the osteoblasts as organic molecules and fibrils. Ninety percent of this osteoid is type I collagen laid out in fibers parallel to the resorption surface; there are also proteoglycans and glycoproteins crucial to the elastic properties of the bone matrix. Other proteins incorporated in the bone include, but are not limited to, alkaline phosphatase (which appears to increase inorganic phosphate levels and decrease levels of pyrophosphate) [21], osteocalcin, osteopontin, osteonectin, bone sialoprotein, TGF-β, thrombospondin, insulin-like growth factor 1 (IGF-1), and FGF. While some of these proteins are immediately active in generating the mechanical properties of bone, others become functionally active only when released from the mineralized matrix by osteoclasts. See Figure 25.1.

The matrix is also different in areas that form the temporal and spatial markers between iterations of bone deposition. There are *resting lines or cement lines* dividing the bone into lamellar rings or encircling osteons (i.e. the bull's-eye-shaped areas where cortical bone has been remodeled). The *cement lines* are composed of higher levels of elastic fibrils that can prevent microfractures from propagating straight through the mineralized matrix. Macroscopically, cement lines are dark bands that can highlight the shape and orientation of the tissue – providing insight into the age of the bone, the orientation of the collagen fibers, and the direction of primary load.

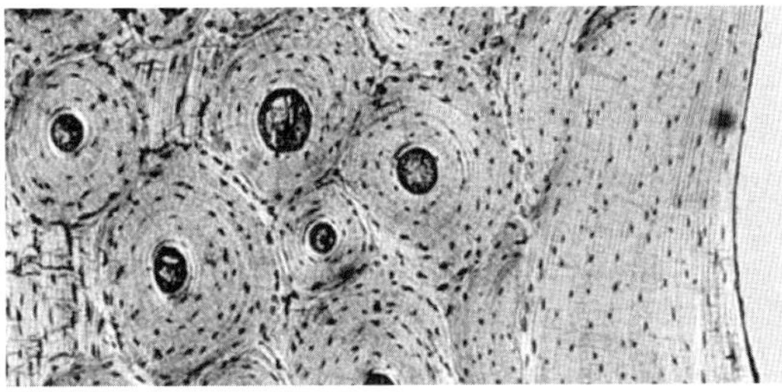

Figure 25.2 The bone to the right is composed of sheets of primary bone and the bone to the left, with the circular shape, is composed of osteons. The Haversian canals run through the center of the osteons. The black structures seen in this figure are the osteocyte lacunae [23].

25.1.2 Tissue-level structures of bone

At the macroscopic level, bone has two *distinctive morphologies*: cortical and trabecular. The *cortical* morphology is compact with an inner substructural microscopic component referred to as Haversian bone. Each *Haversian system* is composed of a blood vessel surrounded by concentric rings of lamellar bone, which is called an osteon. The cortical bone comprises the dense envelope of bone that supports the physiological mechanical loads. Rapidly forming bone in rabbits and mice, the cortical bone will be *primary bone*, that is, composed of either plexiform bone or primary osteons. Mature bone in adult vertebrates will remodel to include secondary osteons, which are identified by their 1–5-μm cement line border in the center of the cortical regions. See Figure 25.2.

The *trabecular* morphology (also known as cancellous) appears macroscopically as a spongy-looking network of thin rods and plates, which are microscopically referred to as *trabeculae*. The trabeculae are roughly 100–125 μm in length and 25–30 μm in width. The trabecular bone is key for homeostasis of calcium and phosphorus [24]. Moreover, the modeling and remodeling of bone predominantly involves the *turnover* of the trabecular compartment.

It is noteworthy that bone is a dynamic organ, responding to biomechanical and physiological cues. The processes involved, which include modeling, which forms and enlarges the skeleton, and remodeling, in which the skeleton is not changing shape but is still undergoing constant renewal, are directed both by mechanical and by endocrine needs. Consequently, bone, especially *trabecular bone*, is continually being replaced and renewed by remodeling over an average span of *seven years*.

Another morphological appearance of bone is *woven* bone, which is characterized by *isotropically* oriented trabeculae (i.e. random patterns of organization). Woven bone is found in fetal bones, heterotopic ossification, and the fracture-healing callus. For example, in fracture healing, woven bone forms internally (i.e. along the *endosteal envelope*) as well as along the *periosteal envelope*, that is, externally. The woven bone may be deposited at a rate of up to 50–100 μm/day in response to the phenomenon termed the rapid acceleratory phenomenon (RAP) by Frost [25]. This non-templated, accelerated process of bone formation produces a buttressing *callus* of woven bone to stabilize the fracture ends.

25.1.3 Bone remodeling

The remodeling of bone has two main forms, both carried out by a basic multicellular unit or bone remodeling unit (BMU), where the osteoclasts will lead the way by resorbing old bone and the osteoblasts will continue behind them, filling the resorption space back up with mineralizing osteoid. In the case of surface remodeling – of the trabeculae, or of the endosteal or the periosteal surfaces – the osteoclasts can resorb a pit called a Howship lacuna, which is usually 3–4 μm deep at the deepest part [26], which the osteoblasts fill back up (Figure 25.3). There is a new theory that this restoration of matrix occurs within a bone remodeling compartment under a tent of osteoblastic "bone canopy" cells that combine traits of angiogenic stem cells and osteoblastic stem cells, but more evidence for and against this theory remains to be collected.

Cortical bone also requires remodeling and renewal, but is too thick and dense to be repaired with Howship lacunae. In the case of cortical bone, the osteoclasts form a cone that resorbs a hollow cylinder out of the bone, almost always in the direction of primary load. A series of rings of osteoblasts and a new blood vessel follow closely behind this cone of osteoclasts, and each

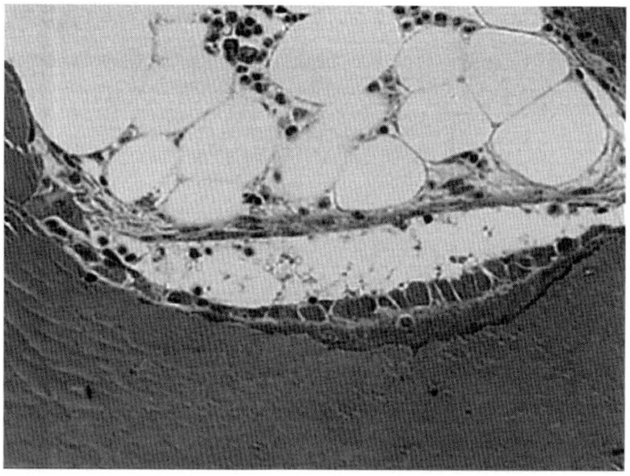

Figure 25.3 The resorption pit is filled with a row of osteoblasts producing new osteoid. Forming a layer between the remodeling surface and the marrow are the bone canopy cells [27].

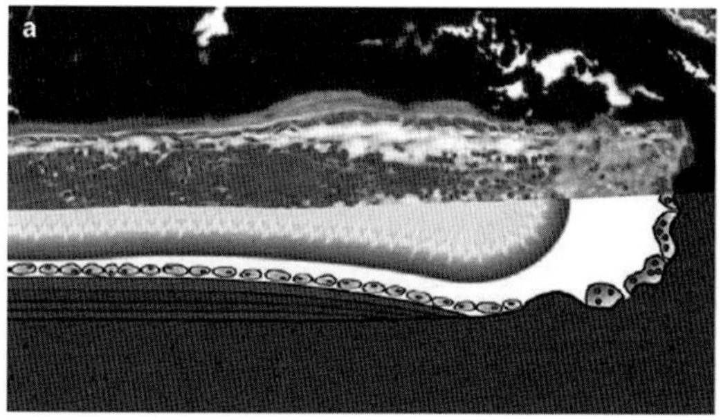

Figure 25.4 The structure of the cutting cone as seen through histology (top) and a diagram (bottom). Resorbing through old bone, the osteoclasts at the tip of the cutting cone will open a cylindrical void. The osteoclasts are followed by concentric circles of osteoblasts laying down mineralizing osteoid and forming a reversed closing cone that will refill the tunnel made by the osteoclasts [23]. The end result of the cutting cone is new matrix within the dense cortical bone that, when cut perpendicular to the direction of the cutting cone, is in the shape of an osteon.

centric ring will follow behind the previous one - depositing a new layer of osteoid and the occasional osteocyte. In this way, the osteoclasts and the osteoblasts form two cones oriented base to base that will move through the cortical bone, leaving behind a cylinder of new bone that, if cut through transversely, will show the canonical bull's-eye appearance of an osteon. This BMU, which creates the osteons and remodels the cortical bone, is called the cutting cone (see Figure 25.4).

25.1.4 Fracture healing

Bone has the remarkable property of being able to regenerate - to restore form and function indistinguishable from those of the pre-fractured state and without the formation of a scar. Fracture healing is the prototypical physiological process of bone regeneration.

When bone fractures, localized blood products, platelets, fibrin, and soluble signaling molecules (e.g. PDGF, FGF, and TGF-β) form a *hematoma*. The hematoma remodels into a vascularized clot including fibroblasts that produce collagen; this mass will undergo morphogenesis through a cartilaginous analog, mineralization, and subsequent bone formation. The quantity of cartilage in the fracture repair is commensurate to the stability of the fracture ends. Without stable fracture fixation, movement occurs; the more movement the more cartilage formed [28].

25.1.5 Mechanical properties of bones

Different bones within the anatomical skeleton have unique mechanical properties. Bones have been classified as either *load-bearing* or *non-load-bearing* bones. In fact, *non-load-bearing* bone is really *partially load-bearing*, for example the cranial vault. All bones are used in mechanical support of some kind, and this dynamic function must be considered in any scaffold design.

The precise mechanical properties of bone can defy simple definition. Variability is high among the 208 bones found in *Homo sapiens*, and each bone may yield different biomechanical values for different regions, orientations, and loading rates. Furthermore, much of the early work on bone mechanics was done ex vivo on dry or drying bones, which were later shown to have different mechanical properties from those of bones in vivo.

Table 25.1 Classification of osteoblasts by cell morphology

Type I	Pre-osteoblast: cytoplasm rarely seen; the presence of these cells apparently adjacent to the osteoid seam is probably an artifact
Type II	Active osteoblast: cuboidal or columnar shape with adjacent nuclear clear zone
Type III	Active osteoblast: cuboidal or columnar shape without adjacent nuclear clear zone; usually smaller than type II cells
Type IV	Lining osteoblast: flat nucleus and extremely thin cytoplasm
Type V	Apoptotic osteoblast: cuboidal or columnar shape with evident nuclear chromatin concentration

One study using bone-bonded strain gauges found that the peak microstrains for a variety of animals during normal activities were 2000–3500 microstrains (μE), where 1 E equaled a 1% deformation [29].

25.1.6 Identification of bone features in histology and pathology

The main cell types of bone have very diverse morphologies. The osteocytes are small and trapped within the lacunae, which are of diameter 10–20 μm. The osteoblasts, typically found in multiples in resorption pits or on the surfaces of seams of osteoid, are of diameter 20–30 μm. The osteoblastic cells also have been classified into types by Villanueva *et al.*, dependent on morphology (Table 25.1), with type I being the preosteoblasts, type II being young and very active osteoblasts, and type IV being the now more quiescent resting osteoblasts or bone-lining cells (Figure 25.5) [30]. The bone-lining cells may be so thinly stretched across the surface of bone that nothing but the soma will be viewable in light microscopy; however, viewed in SEM, they appear as 20–30-μm oval or polygonal cells on inactive bone surfaces [31].

A newly identified class of osteoblastic cell is the *canopy cell*. It is found closely associated with the marrow and forming a tent-like bone remodeling compartment over the active remodeling sites of trabecular

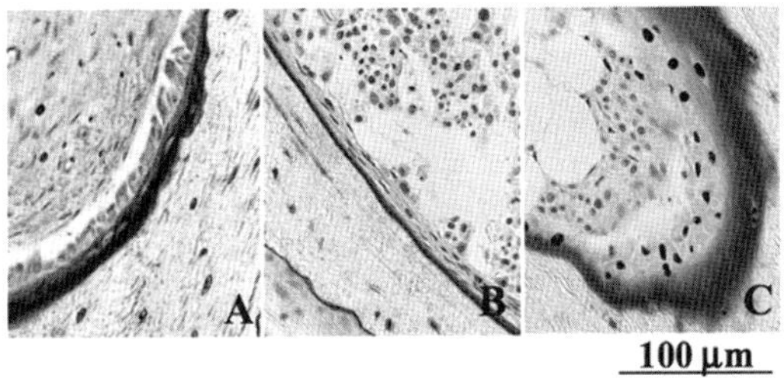

Figure 25.5 Typical appearance of (A) the type II osteoblasts (active osteoblasts), (B) the type IV osteoblasts (lining osteoblasts), and (C) the type V osteoblasts (apoptotic osteoblasts) [30].

bone (see Figure 25.3). These cells are typically flat, similar to bone-lining cells, but are not metabolically quiescent; rather they are likely associated with the signaling pathways occurring between cells in the Howship lacunae, the vasculature, and the marrow.

Many of the osteoblastic cells appear similar in light microscopy, even with appropriate histological stains. For more precise identification of osteoblasts, immunohistochemistry is an important tool. Active osteoblasts and canopy cells will immunostain for alkaline phosphatase, osteocalcin, and osteonectin. Bone-lining cells will not stain strongly for any of these molecules, especially alkaline phosphatase, since they are not metabolically active in producing bone. Barring the trapped osteocytes, the active osteoclasts are the easiest cells to identify. They have a distinct ruffled border, foamy cytoplasm, multiple nuclei, large size – sometimes 50 or hundreds of microns, and a possible resorption pit below them on the mineral surface. In a study of prehatched chicks, the mean number of nuclei was 6.92, only 4.5% had 5 or fewer nuclei, and only 11% had more than 10 nuclei [18]. The authors of this study also found a correlation between the number of nuclei and the volume of each osteoclast's resorption pit, though this relationship did not increase linearly. Using immunohistochemistry, active osteoclasts can be identified by the presence of tartrate-resistant acid phosphatase (TRAP).

Identification of new bone deposition can be done with the use of a toluidine blue stain or a Masson's trichrome stain that will visually separate the new osteoid from the older mineralized matrix. Another stain commonly used is Sanderson's Rapid Bone Stain, which is commonly used concurrently with Van Gieson's picrofuchsin to clearly differentiate non-mineralized tissue from mineralized bone (Figure 25.6). The amount of new bone deposition can be estimated using histology stains by determining the size of the osteoid seams or more precisely extrapolated by labeling the bone surface, at specific time intervals, with fluorescent markers that bind to calcium or phosphate, such as tetracycline. The *mineral apposition rate* (MAR) is calculated as the area of new bone (the length of the tetracycline label times the distance between two or more tetracycline labels) divided by the time between the administrations of the tetracycline doses.

Particular features to look for in a test of a new bone scaffold, drug, or therapeutic technique include

(1) a seamless interface, without a fibrotic capsule, between the recipient bone and implanted material, sometimes referred to as *osseointegration*;
(2) the ingrowth of host bone from the recipient site into the implanted structure (referred to as *osteoconduction*); and
(3) the transient appearance of leukocytic phenotypes associated with acute (e.g. neutrophils) or chronic (e.g. monocytes) inflammation, and signs of apoptotic and necrotic cellular debris.

Moreover, since bone is highly cellular and vascular, zones of acellularity and avascularity portend a poor survival outcome. Further, cartilage and fibrous tissues in a healing bone site are indicative of an environment where the bone-promoting implant failed to inspire the progression of osteoblast lineage differentiation, or where the bone implant degraded before new bone formation occurred. Thus, soft-tissue prolapse may have occurred.

25.2 Animal models

The goal of tissue engineering and regenerative medicine is to *restore the form and function* of damaged organs to their original state. To achieve this, a dynamic system of spatial and temporal interactions among specific concentrations of cell signaling molecules, progenitor stem cells, and extracellular matrix scaffolds must be fully understood.

The key to achieving restoration in bone (which includes repair, augmentation, replacement, and regeneration) lies in the formation of new bone tissue via osteogenic cells. These cells can be recruited in a variety of ways, including targeting local stem cells, transplanting stem cells from another site, and homing in stem cells from the systemic circulation. Biological signaling molecules then initiate the differentiation of these osteoprogenitors to osteogenic cells through the up-regulation of certain genes and proteins. Consequently, this highly complex process means that many variables are involved, and thus an accurate model is difficult to obtain.

Animal models (in-vivo models) must be utilized; in-vitro models will not capture with sufficient fidelity the intricacies of the human body. However, each animal model has unique attributes that affect its responses to biological stimuli. Therefore, a rational design must be incorporated when choosing the clinically relevant animal model for biomaterial testing. Researchers must understand the physiological limitations of each model, and select the model most similar to what is encountered in a clinical setting.

The use of animal models covers three domains in the tissue engineering field [32]:

(1) fundamental discovery,
(2) feasibility and bioactivity testing, and
(3) clinical modeling and efficacy prediction.

Fundamental discovery experiments may elucidate biological mechanisms. Animal models exploited for fundamental discuovery must satisfy several criteria, such as a *short* life cycle (days to months) so that one can assess biological outcomes. With results from fundamental discoveries one can proceed to feasibility experiments, where mechanisms are modulated to determine the impact on potential therapeutic targets. This can be accomplished through either local or systemic applications of a therapeutic modality (drug or biomaterial) to inhibit disease advancement or encourage tissue repair. Feasibility tests are normally performed on small mammals such as inbred mice and rats. However, larger animals such as dogs, sheep,

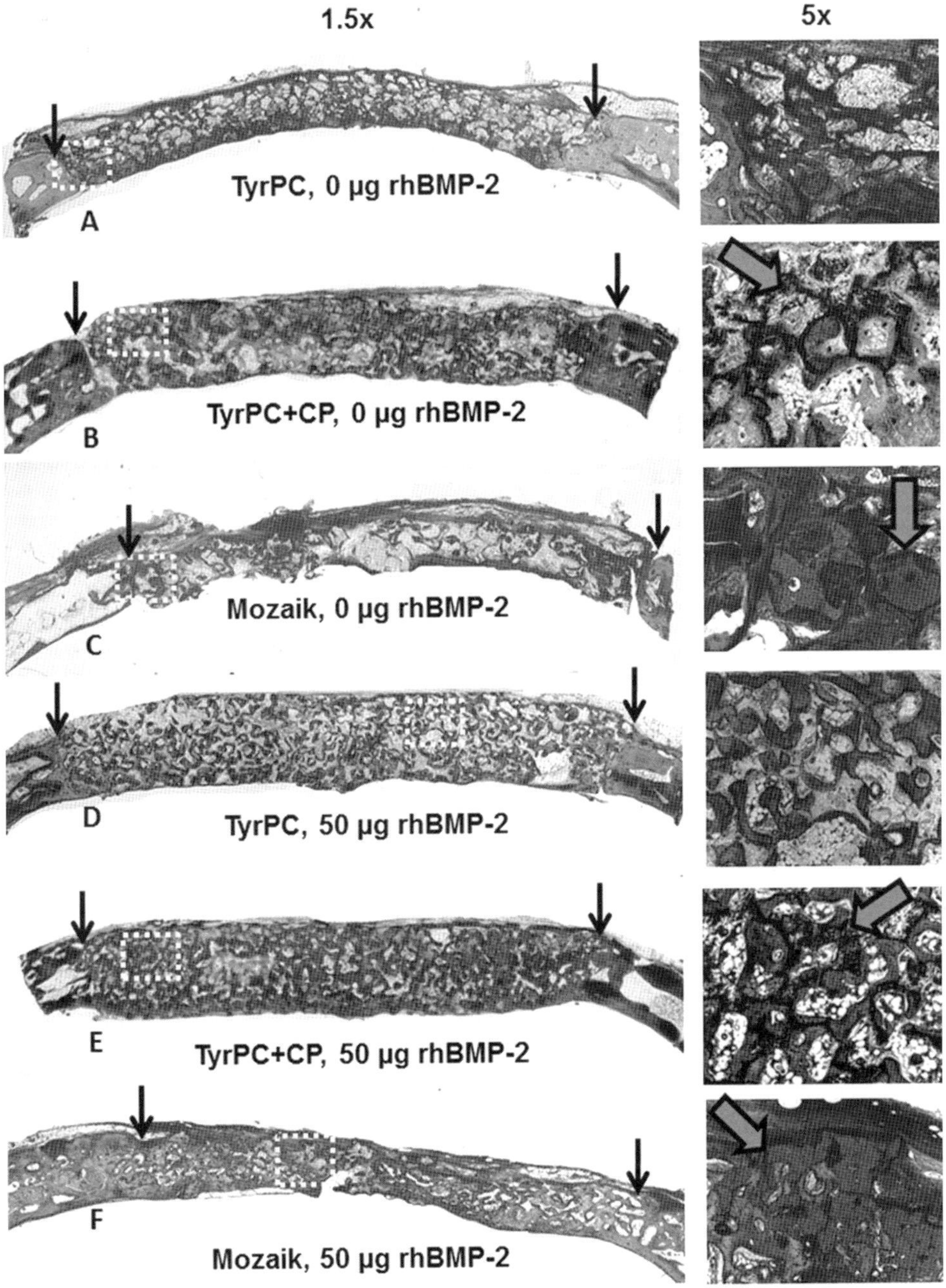

Figure 25.6 Bone healing in rabbit calvaria using scaffolds, 6 weeks after implantation. New bone formation was assessed by histology. The coronal plane of the histological section, stained with Sanderson's Rapid Bone Stain and counterstained with van Gieson's picrofuchsin, indicated soft tissue staining and bone staining. Panels on the left are at 1.5× magnification; the insert on the right is at 5× magnification. Black arrows identify the defect site. Mozaik (Integra LifeSciences Corporation, Plainsboro, NJ) is an FDA-approved composite bone void filler comprised of β-beta tricalcium phosphate and type I bovine collagen. Tyrosine polycarbonates (TyrPC) are a class of polymeric biomaterials being developed as an alternative to bone void fillers.

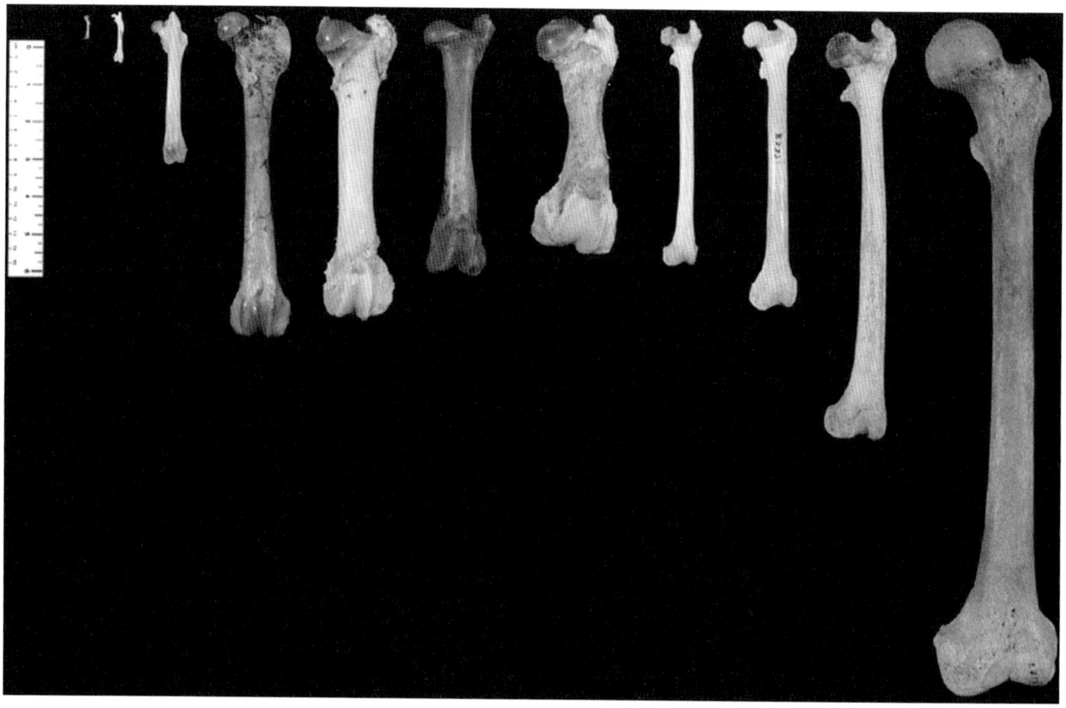

Figure 25.7 Comparison of femoral size and anatomy among animal species commonly used for bone regeneration research. Anterior view of left femurs of adult animals, from left to right: mouse, rat, rabbit, dog, goat, sheep, pig, South African monkey, rhesus, baboon, and human [32].

and goats may also be used. Small vertebrate animals have several limitations, including the following.

1. Surgery involving the spine and rotator cuff repair may be technically difficult to perform and reproduce.
2. It may be physically impossible to embed certain implants and devices in them.
3. It might not be possible to replicate clinically relevant void volumes and diffusion distances.

The specifics of these circumstances will be discussed later on in the chapter. The disparity in size among different species is readily apparent in Figure 25.7.

Clinical modeling and efficacy prediction studies are where the therapy's performance criteria are optimized. These studies must be accomplished in a manner that is clinically relevant. Hence the animal model used should have a physiological response similar to that of humans. In addition, the surgical technique, instruments, and site should mimic as closely as possible those used in a "human" clinical setting [32].

Therapeutic modalities for bone tissue engineering should be assessed depending on how they perform in the six domains of bone tissue activity [33]:

(1) *osteogenesis*, the process of synthesizing new bone tissue via osteoblasts;
(2) *osteoconduction*, the ingrowth of bone into a scaffold;
(3) *osteoinduction*, the process of stimulating osteoprogenitors to differentiate into osteoblasts;
(4) mass transport (fluxes of chemical entities);
(5) biophysical effects (mechanical, electric, and magnetic forces); and
(6) anatomical locale (the site of bone regeneration).

These *performance criteria* will dictate the animal model that should be used. The ideal animal model for a particular study should be one that limits variation among the different samples, increases the sensitivity of experimental outcome, and for which there exist clinically relevant testing environments and conditions [32]. In addition to being biologically analogous, the animal model must also be recognizable as an appropriate challenge to human physiology, and the defect introduced into the bone must fail to heal unless it is treated with the tissue engineering strategy under study [34]. This second criterion implies a *critical-sized defect* (CSD), which by definition, is "the smallest-size intraosseous wound in a particular bone and species of animal that will not heal spontaneously during the lifetime of the animal" [35]. The critical size is 2–2.5 times the diameter of the affected bone in most animal models, and 3 times the diameter of the corresponding diaphysis for sheep [35]. The four main types of defects are calvarial, segmental (long bone or mandible), partial cortical (cortical window, wedge defect, or transcortical drill hole), and cancellous bone defects. These defects and their use in specific animal models will be discussed further in the sections that follow.

An important aspect of the bone in which the defect is made is its loading characteristics. If a therapeutic modality is designed to aid in the regeneration of load-bearing bone (femur, tibia, fibula, vertebrae, pelvis) in humans, it must be tested in a load-bearing bone defect in an animal model. Modalities for non-load-bearing bone applications (such as craniofacial reconstruction) need be tested only in a non-load-bearing bone defect in an animal model (such as the rabbit calvaria model).

25.2.1 Small mammals

The three species of small mammals most commonly used are the mouse (*Mus musculus*), rat (*Rattus norvegicus*), and rabbit (*Oryctolagus cuniculus*). The first two belong to the rodent family, and have short longevities that allow experimental outcomes to be determined in a matter of weeks at most. Rodents and rabbits are most useful for fundamental discovery and initial feasibility-testing experiments. In particular, they are suitable for biocompatibility, degradation, and osteoconduction studies involving biomaterials up to 5 mm in length. Small mammals have been used in fracture repair studies, though this usually involves either no gaps or non-critical-sized gap defects together with external fixation [36]. In addition, they are widely used for osteoprogenitor cell homing [37] and cell transplantation studies [38].

25.2.1.1 Mouse and rat

The short development cycle and life span of the mouse (*Mus musculus*) and rat (*Rattus norvegicus*) have led to their inclusion in "fundamental discovery research" for discovering and characterizing biological mechanisms and "feasibility and biocompatibility testing" to assess biocompatibility and toxicity, to screen for adverse reactions, and to evaluate the delivery capability of a device or agent [32]. Rodents are not commonly used in "pre-clinical animal testing" because the anatomy and composition of autogenous bone and marrow in these species are not comparable to those of the human. The physiological composition of rodent bone marrow is significantly different from that of human bone marrow; only 10%–20% of the rodent marrow consists of osteogenic colony-forming units [39], whereas in human marrow up to 90% does [40]. Rodents also undergo continual bone growth and remodeling, processes that are not lifelong in humans, and results from mice and rat model studies can be difficult to correlate to human skeletal conditions.

Investigations involving rat cancellous bone defects are useful and cost-effective if the goal of the study is to evaluate the level of osteoconduction and bone ingrowth in a bony environment. A cancellous bone defect is generated by preparing a hole through cortical bone extending into the cancellous bone (e.g. the proximal femur of a rat) [34].

25.2.1.2 Rabbit

The New Zealand white rabbit (*Oryctolagus cuniculus*) is a popular animal model for testing bone implant materials [41]. This model permits the biocompatibility, osteogenesis, osteoconduction, mass transport ability, and biophysical effects of an implant to be determined antecedent to large-animal pre-clinical trials. Although the anatomical differences between rabbit and human bone are obvious, many attributes of the rabbit model make it a preferable choice for initial in-vivo musculoskeletal research studies. These attributes include the relatively low cost, availability, ease of housing, tolerance to captivity, low-maintenance care, ease of handling, inter-animal uniformity, tolerance of surgery, availability of adequate facilities and support staff, relatively short lifespan, and well-understood species-specific bone characteristics, and the existence of a database of biological information for the species [32].

The rabbit is often the lowest phylogenic model acceptable for bone regeneration studies. While international standards limit the size and maximum number of implants recommended per rabbit, the amount of rabbits used per study is often greater than the amount of larger animals that would be tested because of the low cost, ease of handling, size, and relatively short lifespan of these small mammals. For the same reasons, rabbit models are often used to test engineered bone products before trials with larger animals (such as goats or sheep) are performed. The results from the rabbit model can be used to fine-tune the bone regeneration therapy for the next level of pre-clinical animal trials, in a larger animal with anatomy more similar to that of humans [32].

Rabbits have a primary vascular longitudinal tissue structure composed of vascular canals of osteons running parallel with the long axis of the bone, surrounding the medullary canal and the periosteal surface. The bone between these layers is dense Haversian bone. There are similarities in the bone mineral density and fracture toughness of mid-diaphyseal bones in rabbits and humans [32]. Skeletal change and bone turnover occur at a faster rate in rabbits than in humans.

Three popular rabbit CSD models are the calvarial, radial, and femoral plug models for testing implant materials. In these models, a CSD is introduced surgically and filled with an implant material. After a designated time period, the implant and surrounding tissues are removed and analyzed via micro-computed tomography (micro-CT), histology, and other methods.

The rabbit calvarial model, as mentioned previously, can be used to test therapies for regenerating bone in craniofacial defects. A rabbit calvaria CSD is 15 mm in diameter. The rabbit calvaria defect model has been thoroughly used and studied, and is popular for many reasons. The rabbit calvaria model is reproducible since the coronal and sagittal sutures define a landmark for centering the defect in each animal, as can be seen in Figures 25.8(a) and (c). The calvaria is easy to access and sufficiently large, allowing surgical access and specimen handling. Moreover, no fixation is required with a calvarial defect. The orthopedic skeleton, for example, will require some form of fixation apparatus to stabilize and "fixate" bone fragments distal and proximal to a bone gap (i.e. ostectomy). The rabbit is a relatively small, easily maintained animal; the rabbit calvaria defect model is an economical alternative to larger animal models [34].

Moreover, the rabbit may be advantageous for orthopedic bone segmental defects; the radius and ulna models are commonly used, as shown in Figures 25.8(b) and (d). For example, an ostectomy 15 mm in length is considered a CSD in the rabbit radius. Further, the tubular anatomical form of the bone is convenient for radiographical and histological tests. A mid-diaphyseal ostectomy either in the radius or in the ulna may be prepared without the need for supplemental fixation. The mid-diaphyseal ostectomy, with an intact radius or ulna, is splinted proximally and distally by a robust synchondrosis, thus providing a "natural" method of stably fixing the osteotomized bone. This model should not exploit a bilateral procedure; it is too biomechanically challenging post-operatively for the rabbits and militates against the ability to favor the osteotomized limb for the first 24–36 hours after the operation [34].

25.2.2 Large animals

The large mammals most commonly utilized for in-vivo studies include dogs (*Canis familiaris*), goats (*Capra hircus*), sheep (*Ovis aries*), and pigs (*Sus scrofa*). These animals are mainly utilized for pre-clinical translational testing. An animal model should possess physiological similarities to humans. Their

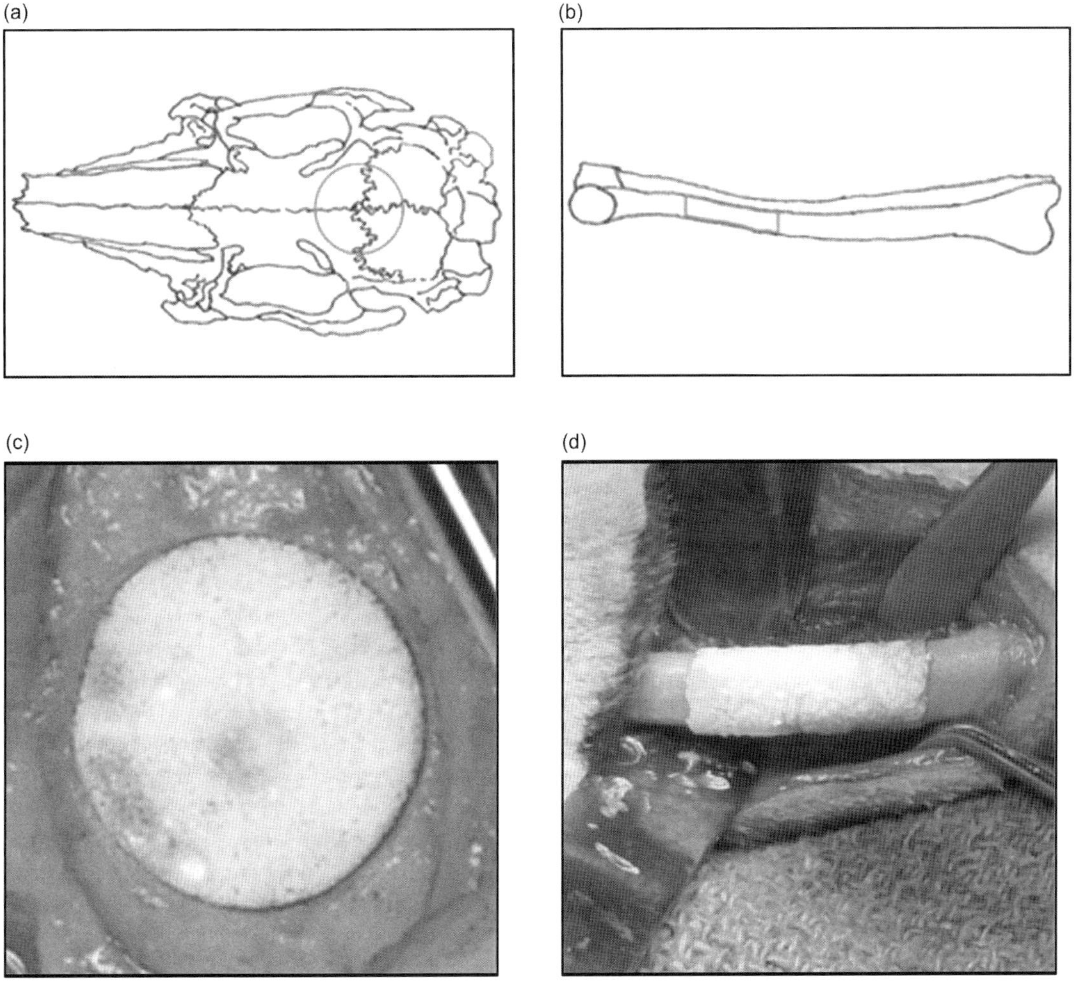

Figure 25.8 Two popular critically sized defects used in the rabbit model. (a) The intersection of the sagittal and coronal sutures provides a landmark for centering a 15-mm-diameter calvarial defect. (b) The ulna runs perpendicular to the radius, and provides support for a 15-mm-long radial defect. (c) A 15-mm-diameter bone substitute implant fits securely in the calvarial defect. (d) A 15-mm-long cylindrical bone substitute implant fills the ostectomy gap in the radial radius.

comparable size makes large animals suitable for the development of bone regeneration therapeutics. Although the most commonly used large-animal models (dog, sheep, goat, and pig) are more similar in size to humans than rabbits and smaller mammals, they share the same quadrupedal gait, which results in discrepancies between bone loading in humans and that in animal models [41].

25.2.2.1 Dog

While the canine model provides bone composition more similar to human bone than the other models discussed, it is no longer used as often as other large-animal models for bone regeneration studies. Dogs are companion animals (i.e. *pets*) in the USA, and their use as *research* animal models raises ethical issues.

Despite social concerns, the abundance of literature characterizing canine models supports their continued use as animal models for bone regeneration modality research.

Dogs are purpose-bred in both relatively large (e.g. coon hound) and small (e.g. beagle) breeds for musculoskeletal animal models. As with any other animal species, differences among breeds can add unnecessary variability to an experiment, so the use of a specific breed, rather than mongrel dogs of questionable background, is often preferred [32].

One desirable aspect of the canine model is the availability of specialized canine surgical equipment and implants. Dogs are also very tractable, and can be trained to take an active role in the recuperation process [41].

Unlike the secondary osteonal structure of human bone, canine bone has a mixed microstructure of predominantly secondary osteonal bone, but with areas of plexiform or laminar bone interspersed. This plexiform bone is mechanically stronger than woven, secondary osteonal tissue, which leads to mechanical differences between human and canine bone. These mechanical differences are apparent in failure tests, which indicate that canine trabecular bone is able to withstand higher compressive strains before failure than can human bone. While canine bone has been found to have a slightly higher mineral density than human bone, it has a very similar organic composition and bone density. In terms of bone composition, the canine model represents the characteristics of human bone more closely than does any other large-animal model discussed in this chapter [41].

A canine model that has been reported is the canine femoral multidefect model (CFMD). This defect model provides four 10-mm-diameter and 15-mm-long defects per animal, instead of a single graft site per animal, which is usually the case for large-animal models. A common argument against the CFMD model is the placement of multiple defects contiguous to one another and in a relatively confined area. Thus, there is a strong and logical concern about the impact of interactions among closely placed defects with multiple treatments within the same limb and within the same experimental animal. Consequently, the experimentalist should strongly consider the value of more independent test recipients versus *over-testing* of too many materials or therapies in a limited number of recipients, such as in the CFMD, where data overlap will obscure outcome differences.

25.2.2.2 Sheep

Sheep are most often used for orthopedic research involving fractures, osteoporosis, bone-lengthening, and osteoarthritis. Unlike rabbits and small breeds of dogs, adult sheep are large enough for the implantation of human implants and prostheses. Sheep bones closely resemble human bones on the macroscopic level, but histological analyses show vast differences on the microscopic level. Sheep have a predominantly primary bone structure, and secondary remodeling becomes more prevalent with age. Sheep bone, like canine bone, is also denser, and consequently stronger, than human bone. The trabecular bone density of a sheep femur is 1.5–2 times greater than that of a human femur. However, sheep and humans do show similar patterns of bone ingrowth into porous implants over time. Sheep tend to have slightly more ingrowth, but this difference could be attributed to the greater amount of cancellous bone in the distal femur of sheep, where ingrowth was observed. Aged sheep are suitable models for studies into human osteopenic and osteoporotic bone. The mechanical and physical properties of sheep bone change greatly with age; therefore, a consistent age must be established within a study and among different studies in order for proper comparisons to be made [41].

25.2.2.3 Goat

Adult goats have a body weight comparable to that of humans. Goats (and sheep) are food-producing animals, which contributes to there being less moral aversion to their use in research than there is for companion animals (such as dogs).

Goats can be more challenging than sheep to confine for long studies, but their relatively large size allows the use of human implants and prostheses, and multiple implants per animal. In goats, Haversian systems are non-uniformly distributed throughout the bones and are primarily located in the cranial, craniolateral, and medial sectors of the tibial diaphysis. The caudal sector is mainly comprised of lamellar bone. Goats are considered to have a metabolic rate and bone remodeling rate similar to that of humans. Moreover, their bone healing capacity and tibial blood supply are also comparable to those of humans. Goats are especially useful for studying the incorporation of bone grafts because the sequence of events during bone graft incorporation in goats is similar to that in humans. The main difference lies in the rate of revascularization and conversion into trabecular bone, which occurs in 3 months for goats but 8 months for humans [41].

25.2.2.4 Pig

Pigs are most often used in studies of osteonecrosis of the femoral head, bone and cartilage fractures, bone ingrowth, and dental implant design evaluations. Pigs can be difficult to handle because they are noisy and aggressive. Commercial pigs are also undesirable as an animal model for human bone regeneration because of their accelerated growth rates and excessive final body weights, in relation to humans. In order to overcome these drawbacks to the use of pigs as animal models, miniature pigs and micropigs have been developed and bred for research purposes. While miniature pigs weigh around 30 kg when fully mature, they are typically used once sexual maturity has been reached (aged ~3 months), and weigh approximately 7–8 kg [42].

The macrostructure of porcine bone is close to that of human bone, but pig bone tends to have a denser trabecular network. When compared with human and other large-animal bones, pig bones are anatomically short and thick. The pig also has a lamellar bone structure similar to that of humans. An aspect of pigs that make them particularly suited as an animal model for human bone regeneration studies is a rate of bone regeneration more similar to that of humans than the bone regeneration rate of dogs. Porcine bones are also remodeled in processes similar to those of human bones, namely trabecular and intracortical BMU-based remodeling.

25.2.3 Non-human primates

The rationale for utilizing non-human primates (NHPs) is their genetic similarities to humans, which should correlate to similar kinetics in terms of immunological and biological responses. The NHPs that have been used for in-vivo studies include the South African monkey (*Cercopithecus mona*), the rhesus monkey (*Macaca nemestrina*), and the baboon (*Papio hamdryas*). Spinal fusion studies have been performed on NHPs, but only for evaluating the lumbar spine.

Most NHPs used for animal studies, such as rhesus monkeys, are physiologically smaller than humans, thus prohibiting their use in certain experiments for the same reasons as apply to small mammals. Furthermore, biological responses may also deviate significantly from those of a human. For example, baboons have been shown to be hypersensitive to BMPs. Thus, while the genetic background of NHPs may resemble that of humans, specific biological and immunological responses should also be taken into consideration in order to mimic the clinical setting [32].

25.2.4 Testing and evaluation

Using animal models requires standard operating procedures in performing surgeries to create fracture repair or bone defects that are relevant to the clinical setting. Organizations such as the American Society for Testing Materials (ASTM) and the International Standards Organization (ISO) have standardized procedures that are related to bone tissue engineering (see Tables 25.2 and 25.3) [32].

Equally important are standardizing techniques used to quantify and evaluate the experimental outcomes. The majority of in-vivo bone tissue engineering studies involve quantifying the extent of mineralized bone matrix through an array of imaging techniques, such as radiographs and micro-CT. Micro-CT is particularly useful in that three-dimensional (3D) distributions of bone can be quantified (Figures 25.9 and 25.10). Histological techniques can be used to determine the amounts of other components present in bone, such as fat, fibrous tissue, and all cells involved in bone remodeling.

Table 25.2 ASTM standards for bone tissue engineering (TEMPs stands for tissue-engineered medical products)

ASTM standards	Description
F04.04	Division IV - TEMPs
F04.05	Computer-assisted orthopedic surgical systems
F04.11	Polymeric materials
F04.12	Metallurgical materials
F04.13	Ceramic materials
F04.15	Material test methods
F04.16	Biocompatibility test methods
F04.21	Osteosynthesis
F04.22	Arthroplasty
F04.25	Spinal devices
F04.33	Medical/surgical instruments
F04.41	Classification and terminology for TEMPs
F04.42	Biomaterials and biomolecules for TEMPs
F04.43	Cells and tissue-engineered constructs for TEMPs
F04.44	Assessment for TEMPs
F04.46	Cell signaling

Light microscopy is commonly used to observe and analyze histological slides of recovered bone and implants from in-vivo studies. In brief, the surgical defect/implant and surrounding tissue are harvested during necropsy and stored in a fixative, usually formalin. The specimen is then processed using hard- or soft-tissue histology processes. Bone specimens can be fixed and subsequently embedded in soft paraffin or resin, usually polymethyl methacrylate (PMMA), for sectioning. Paraffin-embedded bone specimens are usually decalcified so that they can be sliced into thin (5–7-μm) sections, via a microtome, and mounted onto slides. PMMA-embedded specimens can be cut into thin sections (5–10 μm) using a sliding-sledge microtome, or cut and ground down to thin sections (25–30 μm) that are affixed to PMMA slides. A variety of stains can be employed to highlight specific structures and components within the specimen, as dictated by the aim of the study. Some popular traditional stains used for bone specimens, the components that are stained, and a reference for each stain are listed in Table 25.4.

Table 25.3 ISO standards for bone tissue engineering

Name	Description
ISO 10993-1:2003	Evaluation and testing
ISO 10993-2:2006	Animal welfare requirements
ISO 10993-3:2003	Tests for genotoxicity, carcinogenicity, and reproductive toxicity
ISO 10993-4:2002	Selection of tests for interactions with blood
ISO 10993-5:1999	Tests for in-vitro cytotoxicity
ISO 10993-6:2007	Tests for local effects after implantation
ISO 10993-7:1995	Ethylene oxide sterilization residuals
ISO 10993-8:	Selection of reference materials
ISO 10993-9:1999	Framework for identification and quantification of potential degradation products
ISO 10993-10:2002	Tests for irritation and delayed-type hypersensitivity
ISO 10993-11:2006	Tests for systemic toxicity
ISO 10993-12:2007	Sample preparation and reference materials (available in English only)
ISO 10993-13:1998	Identification and quantification of degradation products from polymeric medical devices
ISO 10993-14:2001	Identification and quantification of degradation products from ceramics
ISO 10993-15:2000	Identification and quantification of degradation products from metals and alloys
ISO 10993-16:1997	Toxicokinetic study design for degradation products and leachables
ISO 10993-17:2002	Establishment of allowable limits for leachable substances
ISO 10993-18:2005	Chemical characterization of materials
ISO/TS 10993-19:2006	Physicochemical, morphological, and topographical characterization of materials
ISO/TS 10993-20:2006	Principles and methods for immunotoxicology testing of medical devices

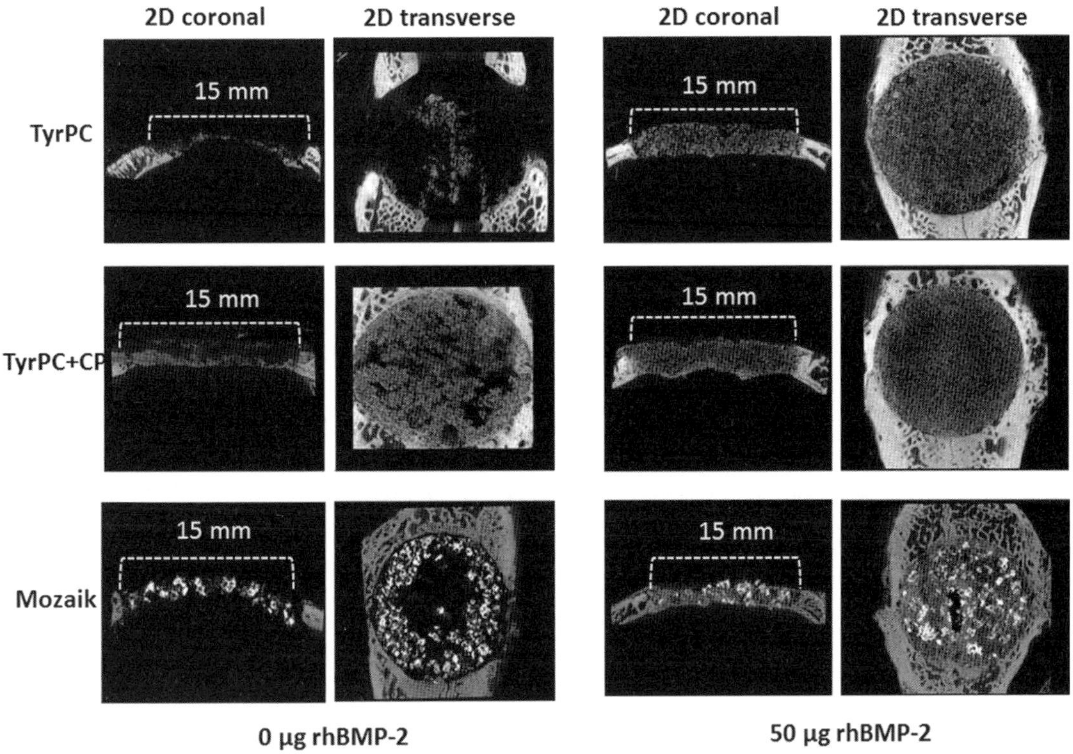

Figure 25.9 Micro-CT images of rabbit calvarial bone regeneration. Two-dimensional (2D) sections (coronal and transverse) of micro-CT calvarial specimens of each treatment showed that, without rhBMP-2, Mozaik and Tyr-PC scaffolds barely induced new bone formation, whereas rhBMP-2-treated scaffolds (50 μg/scaffold) appeared to have induced substantial bone regeneration after 6 weeks. Mozaik (Integra LifeSciences Corporation, Plainsboro, NJ) is a predicate composite bone void filler composed of β-tricalcium phosphate and type I bovine collagen. Tyrosine polycarbonates (TyrPC) are a class of polymeric biomaterials undergoing testing as an alternative to bone void fillers.

25.2.5 Conclusion

The selection of the correct animal models that duplicate a specific clinical indication will provide compelling opportunities to interrogate bone regenerative therapeutics for tissue engineering. Animal models must be clinically relevant. Moreover, researchers who use research animal models must comply with all of the stringent and highly appropriate laws governing the ethical use of animals for research promulgated by federal, state, and university institutions. Further, adherence to sound experimental design must satisfy power-analysis models in order to ensure that the quantity of experimental animals used is the smallest number that will provide data needed to make decisions on the safety and efficacy of tissue-engineered therapies. Moreover, whenever possible, outcome analyses must provide unambiguous quantitative data, and data must be tested using proper statistical analyses. In addition, animal models that are standardized and widely accepted among researchers must be emphasized [32]. Experimental research animal models used for scientific investigation must have a commonality among laboratories to ensure their reproducibility and validation among laboratories. Consequently, consensus must be achieved among bone tissue engineering groups

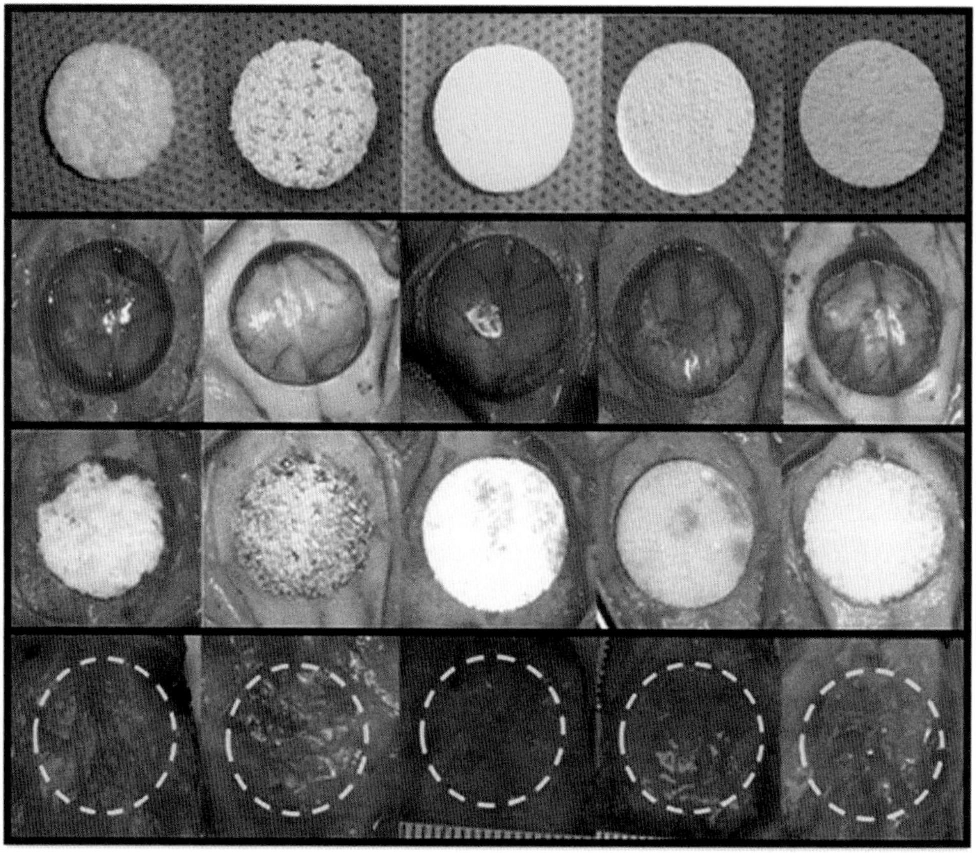

Figure 25.10 Implant images before and after surgical placement in a critical-size (15 mm) rabbit calvarial defect of a collection of biomaterials used for bone regeneration. Mozaik and ChronOS are both FDA-approved composite biomaterials. Non-coated tyrosine polycarbonates (TyrPC) and TyrPC coated with calcium phosphate (CP) and bone mineral matrix (bmm) were tested in comparison with the predicate materials. There were no adverse tissue observations at necropsy (the dotted circles show each implant site).

regarding the selection of animal models and testing paradigms that are standardized, uniform, quantitative in outcome, and properly statistically powered.

25.3 Bone regenerative materials

The goal of the use of regenerative materials is to promote the regeneration of functional tissue and to increase bioactivity, while minimizing the immune response. Biomaterials can be synthetic, naturally derived, or semi-synthetic (hybrids). Bone tissue engineering materials need to be resorbable, biointeractive, and integrative materials that will fully restore the form and function of bone [50].

25.3.1 Bone grafts

Bone grafts are classified as autografts, allografts, and xenografts. In the traditional nomenclature, the root term *graft* signifies *viable cells*.

Table 25.4 Common histological stains used for bone samples

Stain	Application	Details	References
Alizarin red	Mineralization	Mineralized bone (calcium) is stained red upon forming chelate complexes with alizarins.	[43, 44]
Hematoxylin and eosin (H&E)	Cellular detail; for decalcified bone	Hematoxylin stains nucleic acids and calcium blue. Eosin stains connective tissue (collagen fibers, elastic fibers, reticular fibers) pink and red blood cells (RBCs) orange.	[43, 45]
Goldner's modified trichrome	Differentiation of both mineralized and non-mineralized bone	Goldner's modified trichrome stains mineralized bone green, osteoid orange-red, nuclei blue-gray, and cartilage purple.	[43, 46]
Masson's trichrome	Highlight cell nuclei from surrounding connective tissue	Nuclei are stained dark brown or black, while the cytoplasm is stained red. Collagen fibers and osteoid are stained blue-green. RBCs and elastic fibrils stain pink.	[43]
Movat's pentachrome	Distinguish different types of connective tissue	Nuclei and elastic fibers are stained black. Collagen is stained yellow. Fibrin and muscle are stained bright red and red, respectively. Ground substances, such as mucin, are stained blue.	[43]
Sanderson's Rapid Bone	Allows differentiation between bone and soft tissue	Usually used with a counterstain (e.g. van Gieson). When used in conjunction with van Gieson's counterstain, mineralized bone appears red and soft tissue and cellular constituents of bone stain blue.	[43, 47, 48]
Toluidine blue	Highlights structural details	Bone and soft tissue are stained subtly different shades of blue.	[28]
von Kossa	Mineralization	Silver ions react with phosphate, which causes mineralized bone (calcium phosphate) to be stained black.	[49]

Autografts are harvested from a patient's body and are acknowledged as the "gold standard" in bone regeneration. However, since donor surgery has to be performed to obtain the graft, there can be complications such as donor-site morbidity, infection, hemorrhage, and cosmetic deformation. There are also limitations to how much bone can be recovered.

Allografts are frequent alternatives to autografts, and are grafts from a genetically matched, same-species donor (e.g. human to human). Through jargon, the usage of *allograft* has evolved to mean bone-bank-prepared allogeneic bone (i.e. cadaver bone). Bone-bank allografts are usually acellular; the logic is that this allows the removal of antigenic components, that is, cell-surface antigens. Allografts may be equivalent or superior to autografts in some respects. Allografts may carry the risk of immunogenicity, viral transmission, and different physiological properties. Contemporary bone banking by reputable tissue banks has markedly reduced these concerns.

The limited supply of autografts and allografts opens the opportunity for other candidate materials. Xenografts are from non-human species. However, the risk of cross-species disease transmission, as well as ethical factors, will prevent them from being compelling choices as synthetic materials. However, anorganic xenogenic bone matrix and xenogeneic organic matrix products are used in contemporary operating rooms to treat human patients. Examples include the organic Synthes XCM Biologic™ and the inorganic Geistlich Bio-Oss® matrix, which are porcine- and bovine-derived, respectively.

25.3.2 Ceramic scaffolds

Absorbable inorganic materials have been investigated as scaffolds for bone tissue regeneration. The most commonly used are calcium phosphate ceramics like hydroxyapatite, tricalcium phosphate, and the newer tetracalcium phosphate [51, 52]. Calcium phosphates are biocompatible, free of proteins, and have minimal immunological and systemic toxicity [51, 52]. While bone ceramics do not have inherent osteoinductive properties, they can be osteoconductive. However, bone growth behavior varies depending on the different ceramic material used. This is partly due to the morphological properties of the scaffold [53]. The granule size can affect the particle packing characteristics, affecting bone ingrowth, by altering the interstices [53]. The porosity of the ceramic has been demonstrated to affect the osteogenic platform for osteoprogenitor cells, while surface chemistry modifications have an impact on the cells' response to the material [53–56]. Surfaces can be modified by treating them with laminin or fibronectin, enhancing cell attachment [53, 57].

25.3.3 Polymeric scaffolds

Polymeric bone scaffolds are typically biocompatible and biodegradable materials that will support tissue growth, while simultaneously minimizing a host response. Polymeric constructs are of significant importance for bone tissue engineering due to their abundance and tunability. Variables that can be modified according to the application include the mechanical properties, surface chemistry, degradation rate and process, and pore size. These variables are influenced by the morphology, composition, ratio of components, chemical structure, and polydispersity [58]. Physical characteristics, such as chemistry and structure, impact cells' ability to attach, proliferate, migrate, or differentiate. While not all polymers promote all these characteristics, optimizing the previously discussed variables will ultimately affect cell–material interactions. The objective is that these biomaterials will be resorbed, while new bone is forming, eventually replacing the material for trabecular bone [53]. Polymers replace bone by serving as a carrier for cells and proteins, including growth factors, allowing the local introduction of osteogenic signaling cues to the site of injury, while providing a framework for ingrowth of trabecular bone [53, 59–65]. Biological polymers are excellent candidates, with much success in the clinic. Among the most widely used biological scaffolds for bone regeneration are those made from type I collagen. However, collagen's relatively weaker mechanical properties compared with those of bone have made scientists look for more tunable alternatives. Synthetic polymers like poly(lactic-*co*-glycolic acid) (PLGA), polyfumarates, poly(lactic acid) (PLA), poly(glycolic acid) (PGA), and polycaprolactone (PCL) have shown great versatility, in that their resorption time and mechanical durability can be adjusted to suit the needs of the patient [66] (Table 25.5).

25.3.3.1 Biodegradable poly(α-hydroxy acids)

Poly(α-hydroxy acids) have been extensively studied for bone tissue engineering. These synthetic constructs are thermoplastic and can be customized into desired shapes via solvent processing, extrusion, and molding [81]. Glycolic and lactic acid-based polymers are among the most commonly used polyesters for implantation due to their extensive safety record and controllable degradation rates [82]. PGA, also known as polyglycolide, has a low solubility in organic solvents, as well as a high tensile strength and a higher stiffness (modulus of 12.5 GPa) than other degradable polymeric constructs [81, 83]. In contrast to PGA, which is a highly crystalline polymer, PLA, or polylactide, tends to have a lower crystallinity, while retaining strong mechanical properties. PLA's high tensile strength and modulus (4.8 GPa), as well as its slow degradation, make it an ideal material for load-bearing applications [81]. PLGA, or poly(lactide-*co*-glycolide), is made by copolymerizing PLAs and PGAs. The LA/GA ratio of the PLGA polymers can be varied to obtain the optimal degradation rates for specific applications, making it a very successful material for drug delivery systems and tissue engineering [84].

25.3.3.2 Hydrogels

Hydrogels differ from other commonly used materials (which have a hydrophobic nature) in that their hydrophilic properties give them the potential to viably incorporate cells and growth factors. The polymeric

Table 25.5 A comparison of biomaterials commonly used for bone regeneration

Material	Advantages	Disadvantages	Reference
Chitosan sponge	Biodegradable; N-acetylglucosamine residues accelerate wound healing and bone formation; hemostatic	Weak mechanical properties	[67]
Bone mineral matrix	Well-documented success and minimal host response	Transmission of disease, weak mechanical properties, limited supply	[68]
Hydroxyapatite	Well-documented success; rapid integration; low immune response; bond to bone, undistinguishable unions	Difficulty in placing and keeping the material in the defect, length of time needed full bony restoration is achieved	[69]
Collagen sponge	High biocompatibility and weak antigenicity; biodegradable	Weak mechanical properties	[70]
Collagen–ceramic composite	High biocompatibility, biodegradable, higher stiffness compared to collagen alone	Weak mechanical properties	[71, 72]
Poly(lactic-*co*-glycolic acid)	Resorbable, biodegradable	Acidic degradation products; high levels of acid in the core can damage drug delivery; loss of mechanical properties early in degradation	[73, 74]
Hyaluronic acid	Low immunogenicity; injectable; serves as a delivery system	Poor mechanical properties; doesn't support cell attachment on its own; difficult to sterilize	[75]
Polyurethane	Biocompatibility; tailored for broad range of mechanical properties	Toxicity of degradation products with certain types	[74]
Polyphosphazenes	Biodegradable; injectable; supports cell attachment	Acidic degradation	[74]
Alginate	Biodegradable; controlled degradation; used as a delivery system	Weak mechanical properties	[76, 77]
Polycaprolactone	Degrades slowly, lasts longer in the body; used as a drug delivery system	Hydrophobic (bulk degradation)	[78, 79]
Tyrosine-derived polycarbonates	Biodegradable, low immunogenicity, used as delivery system	Weak mechanical properties	[80]

chains of hydrogels, either of synthetic or of natural origin, provide biodegradability, together with mechanical (modulus of 250–5000 Pa) and structural properties similar to those of many tissues and ECM [85, 86]. Hydrogels have many functions in tissue engineering, but, due to their mechanical weakness, are usually applied for non-load-bearing applications in bone. They serve as delivery systems for growth factors while simultaneously acting as space-filling agents for critical defects. Hydrogel scaffolds are particularly appealing for cell delivery because of their potential to encourage cells to adhere, proliferate, and differentiate. Most commonly used naturally derived hydrogels are alginate, chitosan, agarose, gelation, collagen, fibrin, and hyaluronic acid (Table 25.6).

25.3.4 Current advances in biomaterials

Biomaterials may be used as bone regenerative therapies to deliver cell modulating factors in register with the wound-healing cascade. Medtronic's Infuse® (bovine type I collagen sponge carrier with rhBMP-2), which was originally approved by the Food and Drug Administration (FDA) for spinal fusion procedures,

Table 25.6 Biomaterials and their use in bone regeneration

Materials	Use	Reference
Poly(lactic acid)	Bone screws, bone void filler	[87–89]
Poly(glycolic acid)	Bone void filler	[88]
Poly(lactic-*co*-glycolic acid)	Fracture fixation, microparticle delivery system, bone void filler	[90, 91]
PLGA/composite	Osteochondral defects	[92]
Polypropopylene fumarate	Bone defects (tibia), mandibular reconstruction	[93, 94]
Collagen sponge	Bone void filler, spine fusion, osteochondral defects	[95–97]
Collagen–ceramic sponge	Bone void filler, spine fusion	[71, 72]
Calcium phosphates	Bone void fillers, coatings for orthopedics	[91, 98]
Polymer/calcium phosphate	Bone void filler	[99]
Hyaluronic acid	Intra-articular (osteoarthritis)	[100]
Tyrosine-derived polycarbonate	Craniofacial reconstruction, bone void filler	[80]

and Gem 21S® (β-tricalcium phosphate with rhPDGF-BB), FDA-approved for periodontal bone defects, are currently the only medical devices incorporating recombinant human growth factor for bone regeneration. It is noteworthy that the doses of rhBMP-2 and rh-PDGF-BB delivered are greater than intrinsic physiological levels. Improvements in biomaterials as delivery vehicles for these wound healing molecules will enable lower dosing levels for therapeutic effectiveness.

Nanotechnology may offer options to overcome limitations associated with current therapies. Nanotechnology could enable the design of innovative materials that will provide for cell chemotaxis, cell proliferation, and osteogenic differentiation with a physiologically ineffective dose recapitulating *natural* pharmacokinetics [101]. Currently, nanoparticle research has focussed on the generation of nanoparticle composites to improve the mechanical properties of materials. Moreover, the fabrication of nanofiber biomaterials may improve cell attachment and expand overall regenerative capabilities [101].

25.3.4.1 Nanodelivery systems

Research is in progress on transfecting siRNA and DNA plasmids, as well as incorporating growth factors into 6–50-nm-sized particles [102], which can in turn be incorporated into another material [103]. The purpose is to fine-tune the release of signaling molecules in bone in register with the wound-healing cascade, in order to improve the expected outcome. Osteogenic gene transfer experiments that promote osteoblast-lineage progression may be an alternative to the high cost of rhBMP-2 and -7 [104–106].

25.3.5 Future of polymers in bone regeneration

The constant design and innovation of polymeric materials makes bone tissue regeneration a continuously dynamic field. The use of signaling molecules, such as growth factors, cytokines and hormones, as well as stem cells within various polymeric structures, makes it promising [107].

25.4 Clinical applications of bone regeneration

The skeletal integrity of the body can be compromised as a consequence of a myriad of factors that may be of traumatic origin, or may arise from developmental malformation, degenerative processes, and neoplastic disorders. Current understanding of the dynamics of bone biology and morphogenesis has accelerated the development of a comprehensive tool kit of treatment options to address many of these issues. However, there is a tremendous need to boost the quality and quantity of the tool kit.

The goal for a therapeutic modality associated with bone regeneration is restoration of *form and function* completely indistinguishable from those of the original state. At this time, bone grafting remains the major procedure for bone regeneration. However, in recent years gene and stem-cell-based bone tissue engineering, as well as the delivery of growth factors using biocompatible carriers, have emerged as potential means to regenerate bone [108–111]. For most regenerative applications, autogenous cancellous and, to a lesser degree, cortical bone are the gold standards in bone grafting. Other options include allogeneic bone (bone tissue obtained from another member of the same species), xenogeneic bone (bone tissue obtained from a different species altogether), and synthetic bone substitute materials.

25.4.1 Bone regeneration in dental medicine

In dental medicine, bone regeneration can be a useful therapeutic modality for orofacial disorders. These include

(1) periodontal defects,
(2) defects following cyst or tumor resection,
(3) post-extraction defects,
(4) peri-implant defects,
(5) resorbed or atrophic alveolar ridges,
(6) developmental abnormalities, and
(7) defects in the tooth root apex.

The recurring issue with all the above is the loss of specialized tissue (specifically, the gingival epithelium, the cementum of the tooth root, periodontal ligament, and the alveolar bone) to secure the teeth to the alveolar bone. To regenerate these important architectures, periodontal ligament and bone cells must be provided with an environment suitable for proliferation. This necessitates the use of a scaffold to provide support and anchorage for cells to initiate osteogenesis, osteoinduction, and osteoconduction, which will eventually lead to bone regeneration.

Common materials and techniques used for bone regeneration in dental medicine include autogenous bone grafts (usually obtained from the mandibular symphysis or ascending ramus, and from the iliac crest), alloplast, allogeneic, and xenogeneic bone, and growth factors [112].

25.4.2 Bone regeneration in craniofacial repair

Birth defects and genetic disorders are one category of craniofacial pathology that may require bone regeneration procedures. It is estimated that up to 7% of children born annually are affected by defects in the craniofacial area. These can include cleft palate, Down syndrome, Treacher Collins syndrome, and Apert and Crouzon syndromes [113]. Cleft palate has an incidence of 1 in 700 children, and occurs when the two plates that form the hard palate, namely the palatine process of the maxilla and the horizontal plate of palatine bone, do not develop properly and fail to join together. The result is a cleft, or fissure, that can potentially lead to the nasal cavity. Cleft palate can be debilitating by causing not only feeding and speech impediments, but also hearing impairments and ear infections. Therefore, bone regeneration and surgical intervention are required in order to fully establish these necessary functions. Down syndrome patients can have delayed closure of the large fontanelles and patent metopic sutures, which can decrease protection of the brain. Treacher Collins patients can have small jaws that obstruct airflow and breathing. Apert and Crouzon syndromes are usually associated with craniosynostosis, which is the premature fusion of calvarial sutures via ossification. This event would severely impact normal brain development and growth, so surgical treatment is required in order to remove the fused suture and correct the skull to a normal morphology. A combination of stem cell and growth factor therapies can be applied to minimize surgical trauma [114].

Craniofacial fractures may arise from both blunt and sharp trauma. In real-world situations, this is mostly the result of automobile accidents, assaults, and domestic violence. Common areas of fracture include the nasal and cranial bones, as well as the mandible, zygoma, and orbital bones. The level of treatment required will depend on the severity of the condition, which is usually diagnosed through imaging techniques such as X-ray scans and micro-CT. Tumor destruction can also be responsible for the need for craniofacial repair that requires bone regeneration. The cancers concerned include cancers of the skin of the face, the esophagus, the larynx, the mouth, and the nasal passages. Tumor resection localized in the head or neck may remove significant amounts of healthy tissue, which would necessitate the need for bone grafts as well as skin flaps.

Current therapies for craniofacial reconstruction include bone grafting with autografts or allogeneic banked bones, distraction osteogenesis, autogenous tissue implantation, and surgical palatoplasty. Fractures can be plated with either metallic or biodegradable miniplates. The FDA has also approved certain bone grafting substitutes including synthetic polymers, such as polymethylmethacrylate (PMMA), polytetrafluoroethylene (PTFE), and polyhydroxyethylmethacrylate (PHEMA). Organic scaffolds such as collagen, demineralized bone materials, and hydroxyapatites can also be used. Novel tissue engineering strategies are currently being developed by combining the expertise of clinical experts, developmental biologists, cell and molecular biologists, and polymer chemists [115].

25.4.3 Bone regeneration in the treatment for delayed union and non-union

The time required for bone to heal will vary depending on the gender, age, anatomical locus, and extent of injury. The term delayed union refers to a fracture that requires a longer than average period of time before bone union occurs. The term bone non-union describes a complete failure of bone healing. Many risk factors have been identified, such as open fracture, infection, and impaired blood supply [116]. The most frequent method of treatment for non-union is local augmentation through bone grafting, using autologous bone grafts, allograft bone, or synthetic bone substitutes. Results from animal studies and human trials have demonstrated the effectiveness of the growth factor bone morphogenetic protein (BMP) in treating fractures due to its mitogenic and osteoinductive characteristics. By harnessing recombinant DNA technology, recombinant human (rh) BMP-2 and BMP-7 (rhBMP-2 and rhBMP-7) been generated. These have attained FDA approval, and have been widely used to improve healing of patients with non-union, open fractures, and CSDs [117]. Additional growth factors, including TGF-β, insulin-like growth factor-1 (IGF-1), vascular endothelial growth factor (VEGF), and fibroblast growth factor (FGF), have chemotactic and angiogenic properties that are currently being analyzed for bone regeneration [118, 119]. Gene therapy is an alternative to growth factor delivery, in which exogenous genetic material is transfected into cells to induce regeneration. For clinical applications, this can be accomplished either in vivo (with genetic material directly introduced to the site of injury on the host), or ex vivo (tissue is harvested and undergoes genetic modification in vitro before implantation back into the host) [119].

25.4.4 Bone regeneration for spinal fusion

Spinal fusion is a surgical procedure in which two or more of the vertebrae undergo arthrodesis. In essence, an autologous bone graft or allograft is placed between the vertebrae, and fusion occurs as a result of ossification. Fixation using metal screws and plates is usually required in order to immobilize the spine while the bone graft ossifies. The most common reasons for fusing the vertebrae include treatment for fracture, correction of a deformity, treatment of certain cervical disk herniation, and elimination of pain from motion. Non-union is the most common complication after spinal fusion [120].

25.4.5 Bone regeneration in the treatment for osteonecrosis

Osteonecrosis is a disease where cellular death of bone occurs as a result of reduced local blood supply or avascularity. The risk factors are long-term steroidal treatment, alcohol abuse, trauma, bisphosphonates, and certain diseases such as infections and cancer. The most common treatment for femoral head osteonecrosis is total hip replacement. Alternative options

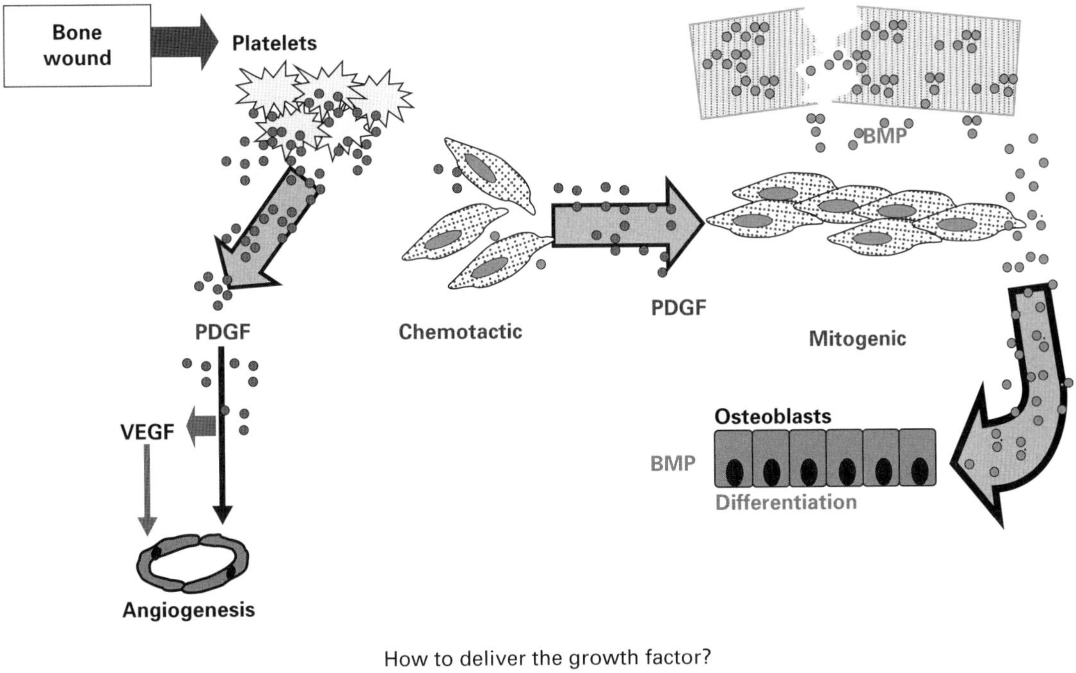

Figure 25.11 The PDGF-BB mechanism of action and bone regeneration. (Reprinted with permission from Hollinger, J. O., Hart, C., Gruber, R., and Doll, B. Protein therapeutics and bone healing. In Lynch, S. E., Wisner-Lynch, L. A., Nevins, M., and Marx, R. E., editors. *Tissue Engineering: Applications in Oral and Maxillofacial Surgery and Periodontics*. 2nd edn. Chicago: Quitessence; 2008, p. 5.)

include vascularized fibular grafts, in which a portion of the fibula and its associated blood supply are removed and transplanted into the femoral head [121]. Jaw (i.e. maxilla and mandible) necrosis may require surgical resection to excise necrotic bone followed by bone grafting [122]. Angiogenic factors such as vascular endothelial growth factor (VEGF), rhPDGF-BB, and rhBMP-2 may provide compelling ancillary options with bone grafting for treating the osteonecrosis. See Figure 25.11.

25.4.6 Bone regeneration in the treatment for osteoporosis

Osteoporosis is a chronic disease characterized by a decrease in bone mineral density (BMD), which can severely compromise mechanical properties of bone and its ability to withstand tensile and compressive forces. The World Health Organization has defined osteoporosis as having a BMD that is at least 2.5 standard deviations below the normal mean of an adult female. Unlike the previous examples, osteoporosis is a systemic condition that can affect the entire skeletal system. The mechanism is believed to be largely caused by hormonal imbalances that either decrease the activity of osteoblasts for bone formation, or increase bone resorption via osteoclasts, thereby upsetting homeostasis.

Owing to the systemic nature of the disease, a different approach has to be used to treat osteoporosis. The recruitment of mesenchymal stem cells (MSCs) by anabolic parathyroid hormone (PTH) [123] or transplantation with MSCs [124] exhibit the most promise in terms of increasing bone formation and decreasing the chance of bone fracture in a person with osteoporosis. Of these, two PTH analogs, PTH 1–34 and PTH 1–84, are currently undergoing clinical trials to treat osteoporosis [125].

25.4.7 Conclusion

Through developing a comprehensive understanding of normal bone formation and rigorously testing on animal models, therapeutics to augment or regenerate bone in a variety of local and systemic bone deficiencies have been developed. However, there still exist gaps in our knowledge of bone regeneration. There is still much debate over which types of stem cells are actually involved in fracture healing, as well as the timing and concentration of cytokines and growth factors. Harnessing this knowledge will inspire the design and development of new and improved therapies.

Current therapeutics have shortcomings and must be refined. For example, it seems that the collagen scaffold used in Medtronic's Infuse® encourages a burst release of rhBMP-2, which has been linked to inflammation, ectopic ossification, osteolysis, cancer, and even death [126]. This shows the need for scaffolds that can calibrate the release of growth factors at kinetic rates that match the wound-healing cascade. Furthermore, gene therapy modalities in humans still remain largely unsuccessful.

The development of new biomaterials to address current challenges must continue to undergo rigorous testing to ensure safety and efficacy. Currently, the best way to predict success in clinical trials is through using clinically relevant animal models and testing methods to screen new biomaterials. The path forward is to exploit quantifiable outcome measures in all modes of in-vivo testing and to insist on using accepted standard animal models. By furthering our knowledge of the normal bone-formation cascade and refining current technologies, we can continue to construct and improve biomimetic strategies to achieve bone regeneration.

REFERENCES

[1] Martin, R. B. 2007. The importance of mechanical loading in bone biology and medicine. *J. Musculoskelet. Neuronal Interact.*, **7**(1), 48–53.

[2] Kaplan, F. S., Hayes, W. C., Keaveny, T. M. *et al.* 1994. Form and function of bone. In Simon, S. P., editor. *Orthopaedic Basic Science.* Columbus, OH: American Academy of Orthopaedic Surgeons, pp. 127–85.

[3] Wergedal, J. E., Matsuyama, T. and Strong, D. D. 1992. Differentiation of normal human bone cells by transforming growth factor-beta and 1,25(OH)2 vitamin D3. *Metabolism: Clin. Exp.*, **41**(1), 42–8.

[4] Hollinger, J. O., Hart, C. E., Hirsch, S. N., Lynch, S. and Friedlaender, G. E. 2008. Recombinant human platelet-derived growth factor: biology and clinical applications. *J. Bone Joint Surg. Am. Vol.*, **90**(Suppl 1), 48–54.

[5] Pountos, I., Georgouli, T., Henshaw, K. *et al.* 2010. The effect of bone morphogenetic protein-2, bone morphogenetic protein-7, parathyroid hormone, and platelet-derived growth factor on the proliferation and osteogenic differentiation of mesenchymal stem cells derived from osteoporotic bone. *J. Orthopaedic Trauma*, **24**(9), 552–6.

[6] Minamide, A., Yoshida, M., Kawakami, M. *et al.* 2007. The effects of bone morphogenetic protein and basic fibroblast growth factor on cultured mesenchymal stem cells for spine fusion. *Spine*, **32**(10), 1067–71.

[7] Kubota, K., Iseki, S., Kuroda, S. *et al.* 2002. Synergistic effect of fibroblast growth factor-4 in ectopic bone formation induced by bone morphogenetic protein-2. *Bone*, **31**(4), 465–71.

[8] Visser, R., Arrabal, P. M., Santos-Ruiz, L., Becerra, J. and Cifuentes, M. 2012. Basic fibroblast growth factor enhances the osteogenic differentiation induced by bone morphogenetic protein-6 in vitro and in vivo. *Cytokine*, **58**(1), 27–33.

[9] Kim, J. and Hollinger, J. O. 2012. Recombinant human bone morphogenetic protein-2 released from polyurethane-based scaffolds promotes early osteogenic differentiation of human mesenchymal stem cells. *Biomed. Mater.*, **7**(4), 045008.

[10] Yang, X., Han, G., Pang, X. and Fan, M. 2012. Chitosan/collagen scaffold containing bone morphogenetic protein-7 DNA supports dental pulp stem cell differentiation in vitro and in vivo. *J. Biomed. Mater. Res. Part A*, doi:10.1002/jbm.a.34064.

[11] Sammons, J., Ahmed, N., El-Sheemy, M. and Hassan, H. T. 2004. The role of BMP-6, IL-6, and BMP-4 in mesenchymal stem cell-dependent bone development: effects on osteoblastic differentiation induced by parathyroid hormone and vitamin D(3). *Stem Cells Development*, **13**(3), 273–80.

[12] Yuan, S., Pan, Q., Liu, W. *et al.* 2011. Recombinant, B.M.P 4/7 fusion protein induces differentiation of bone marrow stem cells. *J. Cellular Biochem.*, **112**(10), 3054–60.

[13] Frost, H. M. 1964. Dynamics of bone remodeling. In Frost, H. M., editor. *Bone Biodynamics*. Boston, MA: Little, Brown and Company, pp. 315–33.

[14] Parfitt, A. M., Qiu, S. J. and Rao, D. S. 2004. The mineralization index – A new approach to the histomorphometric appraisal of osteomalacia. *Bone*, **35**(1), 320–5.

[15] Schen, S., Villanue, A. R. and Frost, H. M. 1965. Number of osteoblasts per unit area of osteoid seam in human cortical bone. *Can. J. Physiol. Pharm.*, **43**(2), 319–25.

[16] Deldar, A., Lewis, H. and Weiss, L. 1985. Bone lining cells and hematopoiesis – An electron-microscopic study of canine bone-marrow. *Anat. Rec.*, **213**(2), 187–201.

[17] Frost, H. M. 1987. The mechanostat: a proposed pathogenic mechanism of osteoporoses and the bone mass effects of mechanical and nonmechanical agents. *Bone Miner.*, **2**(2), 73–85.

[18] Piper, K., Boyde, A. and Jones, S. J. 1992. The relationship between the number of nuclei of an osteoclast and its resorptive capability in vitro. *Anatomy Embryol.*, **186**(4), 291–9.

[19] Jaworski, Z. F. G., Duck, B. and Sekaly, G. 1981. Kinetics of osteoclasts and their nuclei in evolving secondary Haversian systems. *J. Anat.*, **133**(Oct), 397–405.

[20] Delaisse, J. M., Andersen, T. L., Engsig, M. T. *et al.* 2003. Matrix metalloproteinases (MMP) and cathepsin K contribute differently to osteoclastic activities. *Microsc. Res. Technol.*, **61**(6), 504–13.

[21] Golub, E. E. and Boesze-Battaglia, K. 2007. The role of alkaline phosphatase in mineralization. *Curr. Opin. Orthop.*, **18**, 444–8.

[22] Roberts, W. E., Roberts, J. A., Epker, B. N., Burr, D. B. and Harsfield, J. K. 2006. Remodeling of mineralized tissues, part 1: the Frost legacy. *Seminars Orthodontics*, **12**(4), 216–37.

[23] Robling, A. G., Castillo, A. B. and Turner, C. H. 2006. Biomechanical and molecular regulation of bone remodeling. *Ann. Rev. Biomed. Eng.*, **8**, 455–98.

[24] Swartz, S. M., Parker, A. and Huo, C. 1998. Theoretical and empirical scaling patterns and topological homology in bone trabeculae. *J. Exp. Biol.*, **201**(4), 573–90.

[25] Frost, H. M. 1983. The regional acceleratory phenomenon: a review. *Henry Ford Hosp. Med. J.*, **31**(1), 3–9.

[26] Soe, K. and Delaisse, J. M. 2010. Glucocorticoids maintain human osteoclasts in the active mode of their resorption cycle. *J. Bone Miner. Res.*, **25**(10), 2184–92.

[27] Hauge, E. M., Qvesel, D., Eriksen, E. F., Mosekilde, L. and Melsen, F. 2001. Cancellous bone remodeling occurs in specialized compartments lined by cells expressing osteoblastic markers. *J. Bone Miner. Res.*, **16**(9), 1575–82.

[28] Hollinger, J. and Wong, M. E. 1996. The integrated processes of hard tissue regeneration with special emphasis on fracture healing. *Oral Surg. Oral Med. Oral Pathol. Oral Radiol. Endod.*, **82**(6), 594–606.

[29] Rubin, C. T. and Lanyon, L. E. 1984. Dynamic strain similarity in vertebrates; an alternative to allometric limb bone scaling. *J. Theor. Biol.*, **107**(2), 321–7.

[30] Villanueva, A. R., Mathews, C. H. and Parfitt, A. M. 1997. Relationship between the size and shape of osteoblasts and the width of osteoid seams in bone. In Takahashi, H., editor. *Handbook of Bone Morphometry*. Niigata: Nishimura, pp. 45–55.

[31] Yamazaki, K. and Eyden, B. P. 1995. A study of intercellular relationships between trabecular bone and marrow stromal cells in the murine femoral metaphysis. *Anat. Embryol. (Berlin)*, **192**(1), 9–20.

[32] Muschler, G. F., Raut, V. P., Patterson, T. E., Wenke, J. C. and Hollinger, J. O. 2010. The design and use of animal models for translational research in bone tissue engineering and regenerative medicine. *Tissue Eng. Part B*, **16**(1), 123–45.

[33] Muschler, G. E., Nakamoto, C. and Griffith, L. G. 2004. Engineering principles of clinical cell-based tissue engineering. *J. Bone Joint Surgery Am. Vol.*, **86A**(7), 1541–58.

[34] Salgado, A. J., Coutinho, O. P. and Reis, R. L. 2004. Bone tissue engineering: state of the art and future trends. *Macromolec. Biosci.*, **4**(8), 743–65.

[35] Hutmacher, D. W., Reichert, J. C., Saifzadeh, S. *et al.* 2009. The challenge of establishing preclinical models for segmental bone defect research. *Biomaterials*, **30**(12), 2149–63.

[36] O'Loughlin, P. F., Morr, S., Bogunovic, L. *et al.* 2008. Selection and development of preclinical models in fracture-healing research. *J. Bone Joint Surg. Am.*, **90**(Suppl. 1), 79–84.

[37] Kumagai, K., Vasanji, A., Drazba, J. A., Butler, R. S. and Muschler, G. F. 2008. Circulating cells with osteogenic potential are physiologically mobilized into the fracture healing site in the parabiotic mice model. *J. Orthop. Res.*, **26**(2), 165–75.

[38] Stevenson, S. 1999. Biology of bone grafts. *Orthop. Clin. N. Am.*, **30**(4), 543–52.

[39] Malaval, L., Modrowski, D., Gupta, A. K. and Aubin, J. E. 1994. Cellular expression of bone-related proteins during in vitro osteogenesis in rat bone marrow stromal cell cultures. *J. Cell. Physiol.*, **158**(3), 555–72.

[40] Majors, A. K., Boehm, C. A., Nitto, H., Midura, R. J. and Muschler, G. F. 1997. Characterization of human bone marrow stromal cells with respect to osteoblastic differentiation. *J. Orthop. Res.*, **15**(4), 546–57.

[41] Pearce, A. I., Richards, R. G., Milz, S., Schneider, E. and Pearce, S. G. 2007. Animal models for implant biomaterial research in bone: a review. *Eur. Cell Mater.*, **13**, 1–10.

[42] Bode, G., Clausing, P., Gervais, F. *et al.* 2010. The utility of the minipig as an animal model in regulatory toxicology. *J. Pharmacol. Toxicol. Methods*, **62**(3), 196–220.

[43] Bancroft, J. D. and Stevens, A. 1990. *Theory and Practice of Histological Techniques*, 3rd edn. Edinburgh: Churchill Livingstone.

[44] Dahl, L. K. 1952. A simple and sensitive histochemical method for calcium. *Proc. Soc. Exp. Biol. Med.*, **80**(3), 474–9.

[45] Harris, H. F. 1900. On the rapid conversion of hematoxylin into haematein in staining reactions. *J. Appl. Microsc. Lab. Methods*, **3**, 777.

[46] Goldner, J. 1937. A modification of the Masson trichrome technique for routine laboratory purposes. *Am. J. Clin. Pathol.*, **20**, 237–43.

[47] Wojtowicz, A. M., Shekaran, A., Oest, M. E. *et al.* 2010. Coating of biomaterial scaffolds with the collagen-mimetic peptide GFOGER for bone defect repair. *Biomaterials*, **31**(9), 2574–82.

[48] Van Gieson, I. 1889. Laboratory notes of technical methods for the nervous system. *NY Med. J.*, **50**, 57–60.

[49] von Kossa, J. 1901. Nachweis von Kalk. *Beiträge pathol. Anatomie allgem. Pathol.*, **29**, 163.

[50] Rabkin, E. and Schoen, F. J. 2002. Cardiovascular tissue engineering. *Cardiovasc. Pathol.*, **11**(6), 305–17.

[51] Hollinger, J. O. and Battistone, G. C. 1986. Biodegradable bone repair materials. Synthetic polymers and ceramics. *Clin. Orthop. Rel. Res.*, **207**, 290–305.

[52] Burg, K. J., Porter, S. and Kellam, J. F. 2000. Biomaterial developments for bone tissue engineering. *Biomaterials*, **21**(23), 2347–59.

[53] Laurencin, C. T. 2003. *Bone Graft Substitutes*. W. Conshohocken, PA: ASTM International.

[54] Goshima, J., Goldberg, V. M. and Caplan, A. I. 1991. Osteogenic potential of culture-expanded rat marrow cells as assayed in vivo with porous calcium phosphate ceramic. *Biomaterials*, **12**(2), 253–8.

[55] Ohgushi, H., Goldberg, V. M. and Caplan, A. I. 1989. Repair of bone defects with marrow cells and porous ceramic. Experiments in rats. *Acta Orthop. Scand.*, **60**(3), 334–9.

[56] Zreiqat, H., Evans, P. and Howlett, C. R. 1999. Effect of surface chemical modification of bioceramic on phenotype of human bone-derived cells. *J. Biomed. Mater. Res.*, **44**(4), 389–96.

[57] Dennis, J. E. and Caplan, A. I. 1993. Porous ceramic vehicles for rat-marrow-derived (*Rattus norvegicus*) osteogenic cell delivery: effects of pre-treatment with fibronectin or laminin. *J. Oral Implantol*, **19**(2), 106–15; discussion 36–7.

[58] Miller-Chou, B. A. and Koenig, J. L. 2003. A review of polymer dissolution. *Prog. Polymer Sci.*, **28**(8), 1223–70.

[59] Athanasiou, K. A., Singhal, A. R., Agrawal, C. M. and Boyan, B. D. 1995. In vitro degradation and release characteristics of biodegradable implants containing trypsin inhibitor. *Clin. Orthop. Relat. Res.*, **315**, 272–81.

[60] Lu, L., Stamatas, G. N. and Mikos, A. G. 2000. Controlled release of transforming growth factor beta1 from biodegradable polymer microparticles. *J. Biomed. Mater. Res.*, **50**(3), 440–51.

[61] Oldham, J. B., Lu, L., Zhu, X. *et al.* 2000. Biological activity of rhBMP-2 released from PLGA microspheres. *J. Biomech. Eng.*, **122**(3), 289–92.

[62] Heckman, J. D., Ehler, W., Brooks, B. P. *et al.* 1999. Bone morphogenetic protein but not transforming growth factor-beta enhances bone formation in canine diaphyseal nonunions implanted with a biodegradable composite polymer. *J. Bone Joint Surgery Am. Vol.*, **81**(12), 1717–29.

[63] Agrawal, C. M., Best, J., Heckman, J. D. and Boyan, B. D. 1995. Protein release kinetics of a biodegradable implant for fracture non-unions. *Biomaterials*, **16**(16), 1255–60.

[64] Whang, K., Tsai, D. C., Nam, E. K. *et al.* 1998. Ectopic bone formation via rhBMP-2 delivery from porous bioabsorbable polymer scaffolds. *J. Biomed. Mater. Res.*, **42**(4), 491–9.

[65] Boyan, B. D., Lohmann, C. H., Somers, A. *et al.* 1999. Potential of porous poly-D,L-lactide-*co*-glycolide particles as a carrier for recombinant human bone morphogenetic protein-2 during osteoinduction in vivo. *J. Biomed. Mater. Res.*, **46**(1), 51–9.

[66] Asikainen, A. J., Noponen, J., Lindqvist, C. *et al.* 2006. Tyrosine-derived polycarbonate membrane in treating mandibular bone defects. An experimental study. *J. R. Soc. Interface*, **3**(10), 629–35.

[67] Park, Y. J., Lee, Y. M., Park, S. N. *et al.* 2000. Platelet derived growth factor releasing chitosan sponge for periodontal bone regeneration. *Biomaterials*, **21**(2), 153–9.

[68] Acarturk, T. O. and Hollinger, J. O. 2006. Commercially available demineralized bone matrix compositions to regenerate calvarial critical-sized bone defects. *Plast. Reconstr. Surg.*, **118**(4), 862–73.

[69] Oonishi, H., Kushitani, S., Yasukawa, E. *et al.* 1997. Particulate bioglass compared with hydroxyapatite as a bone graft substitute. *Clin. Orthop. Relat. Res.*, **334**, 316–25.

[70] Vigier, S., Helary, C., Fromigue, O., Marie, P. and Giraud-Guille, M. M. 2010. Collagen supramolecular and suprafibrillar organizations on osteoblasts long-term behavior: benefits for bone healing materials. *J. Biomed. Mater. Res. A*, **94**(2), 556–67.

[71] Kraiwattanapong, C., Boden, S. D., Louis-Ugbo, J. *et al.* 2005. Comparison of Healos/bone marrow to INFUSE (rhBMP-2/ACS) with a collagen–ceramic sponge bulking agent as graft substitutes for lumbar spine fusion. *Spine*, **30**(9), 1001–7; discussion 7.

[72] Lyons, F. G., Al-Munajjed, A. A., Kieran, S. M. *et al.* 2010. The healing of bony defects by cell-free collagen-based scaffolds compared to stem cell-seeded tissue engineered constructs. *Biomaterials*, **31**(35), 9232–43.

[73] Karp, J. M., Shoichet, M. S. and Davies, J. E. 2003. Bone formation on two-dimensional poly(DL-lactide-*co*-glycolide) (PLGA) films and three-dimensional PLGA tissue engineering scaffolds in vitro. *J. Biomed. Mater. Res. A*, **64**(2), 388–96.

[74] Gunatillake, P. A. and Adhikari, R. 2003. Biodegradable synthetic polymers for tissue engineering. *Eur. Cell Mater.*, **5**, 1–16.

[75] Aslan, M., Simsek, G. and Dayi, E. 2006. The effect of hyaluronic acid-supplemented bone graft in bone healing: experimental study in rabbits. *J. Biomater. Appl.*, **20**(3), 209–20.

[76] Suzuki, Y., Tanihara, M., Suzuki, K. *et al.* 2000. Alginate hydrogel linked with synthetic oligopeptide derived from BMP-2 allows ectopic osteoinduction in vivo. *J. Biomed. Mater. Res.*, **50**(3), 405–9.

[77] Chueh, B. H., Zheng, Y., Torisawa, Y. S. *et al.* 2010. Patterning alginate hydrogels using light-directed release of caged calcium in a microfluidic device. *Biomed. Microdevices*, **12**(1), 145–51.

[78] Yeo, A., Wong, W. J., Khoo, H. H. and Teoh, S. H. 2010. Surface modification of PCL–TCP scaffolds improve interfacial mechanical interlock and enhance early bone formation: an in vitro and in vivo characterization. *J. Biomed. Mater. Res. A*, **92**(1), 311–21.

[79] Duling, R. R., Dupaix, R. B., Katsube, N. and Lannutti, J. 2008. Mechanical characterization of electrospun polycaprolactone (PCL): a potential scaffold for tissue engineering. *J. Biomech. Eng.*, **130**(1), 011006.

[80] Kim, J., Magno, M. H., Alvarez, P. *et al.* 2011. Osteogenic differentiation of pre-osteoblasts on biomimetic tyrosine-derived polycarbonate scaffolds. *Biomacromolecules*, **12**(10), 3520–7.

[81] Buring, K. 1975. On the origin of cells in heterotopic bone formation. *Clin. Orthop. Relat. Res.*, **110**, 293–301.

[82] Okie, S. 2005. Traumatic brain injury in the war zone. *N. Engl. J. Med.*, **352**(20), 2043–7.

[83] Garland, D. E., Blum, C. E. and Waters, R. L. 1980. Periarticular heterotopic ossification in head-injured adults. Incidence and location. *J. Bone Joint Surg. Am.*, **62**(7), 1143–6.

[84] Nair, L. S. and Laurencin, C. T. 2007. Biodegradable polymers as biomaterials. *Prog. Polymer Sci.*, **32**(8–9), 762–98.

[85] Drury, J. L. and Mooney, D. J. 2003. Hydrogels for tissue engineering: scaffold design variables and applications. *Biomaterials*, **24**(24), 4337–51.

[86] Sangaj, N. and Varghese, S. 2010. Controlling stem cells with biomaterials. In Burdick J. A. and Mauck, R. L., editors. *Biomaterials for Tissue Engineering Applications: A Review of the Past and Future Trends.* Berlin: Springer, p. 564.

[87] Anselme, K., Flautre, B., Hardouin, P. *et al.* 1993. Fate of bioresorbable poly(lactic acid) microbeads implanted in artificial bone defects for cortical bone augmentation in dog mandible. *Biomaterials*, **14**(1), 44–50.

[88] Tschon, M., Fini, M., Giavaresi, G. *et al.* 2007. In vitro and in vivo behaviour of biodegradable and injectable PLA/PGA copolymers related to different matrices. *Int. J. Artif. Organs*, **30**(4), 352–62.

[89] De Jong, W. H., Eelco Bergsma, J., Robinson, J. E. and Bos, R. R. 2005. Tissue response to partially in vitro predegraded poly-L-lactide implants. *Biomaterials*, **26**(14), 1781–91.

[90] Liu, H., Slamovich, E. B. and Webster, T. J. 2006. Less harmful acidic degradation of poly(lactic-*co*-glycolic acid) bone tissue engineering scaffolds through titania nanoparticle addition. *Int. J. Nanomedicine*, **1**(4), 541–5.

[91] Félix Lanao, R. P., Leeuwenburgh, S. C., Wolke, J. G. and Jansen, J. A. 2011. Bone response to fast-degrading, injectable calcium phosphate cements containing PLGA microparticles. *Biomaterials*, **32**(34), 8839–47.

[92] Zhu, S., Zhang, B., Man, C., Ma, Y. and Hu, J. 2011. NEL-like molecule-1-modified bone marrow mesenchymal stem cells/poly lactic-*co*-glycolic acid composite improves repair of large osteochondral defects in mandibular condyle. *Osteoarthritis Cartilage*, **19**(6), 743–50.

[93] Cai, Z., Zhang, T., Di, L. *et al.* 2011. Morphological and histological analysis on the in vivo degradation of poly(propylene fumarate)/(calcium sulfate/β-tricalcium phosphate). *Biomed. Microdevices,* **13**(4), 623–31.

[94] Trantolo, D. J., Sonis, S. T., Thompson, B. M. *et al.* 2003. Evaluation of a porous, biodegradable biopolymer scaffold for mandibular reconstruction. *Int. J. Oral Maxillofac. Implants,* **18**(2), 182–8.

[95] Burkus, J. K., Gornet, M. F., Glassman, S. D. *et al.* 2011. Blood serum antibody analysis and long-term follow-up of patients treated with recombinant human bone morphogenetic protein-2 in the lumbar spine. *Spine,* **36**(25), 2158–67.

[96] Kawaguchi, Y., Kondo, E., Kitamura, N. *et al.* 2011. In vivo effects of isolated implantation of salmon-derived crosslinked atelocollagen sponge into an osteochondral defect. *J. Mater. Sci. Mater. Med.,* **22**(2), 397–404.

[97] Kinsella, C. R. Jr., Bykowski, M. R., Lin, A. Y. *et al.* 2011. BMP-2-mediated regeneration of large-scale cranial defects in the canine: an examination of different carriers. *Plast. Reconstr. Surg.,* **127**(5), 1865–73.

[98] Kim, S. G., Hahn, B. D., Park, D. S. *et al.* 2011. Aerosol deposition of hydroxyapatite and 4-hexylresorcinol coatings on titanium alloys for dental implants. *J. Oral Maxillofac. Surg.,* **69**(11), e354–63.

[99] Sun, F., Zhou, H. and Lee, J. 2011. Various preparation methods of highly porous hydroxyapatite/polymer nanoscale biocomposites for bone regeneration. *Acta Biomater.,* **7**(11), 3813–28.

[100] McNeil, J. D. 2011. Intra-articular hyaluronic acid preparations for use in the treatment of osteoarthritis. *Int. J. Evid. Based Healthcare,* **9**(3), 261–4.

[101] Kim, K. and Fisher, J. P. 2007. Nanoparticle technology in bone tissue engineering. *J. Drug Target.* **15**(4), 241–52.

[102] Hu, Q., Ji, H., Liu, Y. *et al.* 2010. Preparing nano-calcium phosphate particles via a biologically friendly pathway. *Biomed. Mater.,* **5**(4), 041001.

[103] Endo, M., Kuroda, S., Kondo, H. *et al.* 2006. Bone regeneration by modified gene-activated matrix: effectiveness in segmental tibial defects in rats. *Tissue Eng.,* **12**(3), 489–97.

[104] Park, J., Ries, J., Gelse, K. *et al.* 2003. Bone regeneration in critical size defects by cell-mediated BMP-2 gene transfer: a comparison of adenoviral vectors and liposomes. *Gene Ther.,* **10**(13), 1089–98.

[105] Itaka, K., Ohba, S., Miyata, K. *et al.* 2007. Bone regeneration by regulated in vivo gene transfer using biocompatible polyplex nanomicelles. *Molec. Ther.,* **15**(9), 1655–62.

[106] Luo, J., Sun, M. H., Kang, Q. *et al.* 2005. Gene therapy for bone regeneration. *Curr. Gene Ther.,* **5**(2), 167–79.

[107] Marra, K. G. 2004. Biodegradable poylmers and microspheres in tissue engineering. In Hollinger, J. O., Einhorn, T. A., Doll, B. A. and Sfeir, C, editors. *Bone Tissue Engineering.* Boca Raton, FL: CRC Press.

[108] Winn, S. R., Hu, Y., Sfeir, C. and Hollinger, J. O. 2000. Gene therapy approaches for modulating bone regeneration. *Adv. Drug. Deliv. Rev.,* **42**(1–2), 121–38.

[109] Santos, J. L., Pandita, D., Rodrigues, J. *et al.* 2011. Non-viral gene delivery to mesenchymal stem cells: methods, strategies and application in bone tissue engineering and regeneration. *Curr. Gene Ther.,* **11**(1), 46–57.

[110] Betz, V. M., Betz, O. B., Harris, M. B., Vrahas, M. S. and Evans, C. H. 2008. Bone tissue engineering and repair by gene therapy. *Front. Biosci.,* **13**, 833–41.

[111] Griffin, M., Iqbal, S. A. and Bayat, A. 2011. Exploring the application of mesenchymal stem cells in bone repair and regeneration. *J. Bone Joint Surg. Br.,* **93**(4), 427–34.

[112] Lynch, S. E. 2005. Bone regeneration techniques in the orofacial region. In Lieberman, J. R. and Friedlaender, G. E., editors. *Bone Regeneration and Repair: Biology and Clinical Applications.* Totowa: Humana Press.

[113] *Craniofacial Reconstruction. 2007–2011,* available from http://www.surgeryencyclopedia.com/Ce-Fi/Craniofacial-Reconstruction.html.

[114] Moioli, E. K., Clark, P. A., Sumner, D. R. and Mao, J. J. 2008. Autologous stem cell regeneration in craniosynostosis. *Bone,* **42**(2), 332–40.

[115] Doll, B. A., Sfeir, C., Azari, K., Holland, S. and Hollinger, J. O. 2005. Craniofacial repair. In Lieberman, J. R. and Friedlaender, G. E., editors. *Bone Regeneration and Repair: Biology and Clinical Applications.* Totowa: Humana Press, p. 337.

[116] Boyd, H. B., Lipinski, S. W., Wiley, J. H. 1961. Observations on non-union of the shaft of the long bones, with a statistical analysis of 842 patients. *J. Bone Joint Surg. Am.,* **43**(2), 159–68.

[117] Giannoudis, P. V. and Einhorn, T. A. 2009. Bone morphogenetic proteins in musculoskeletal medicine. *Injury,* **40** (Suppl. 3), S1–3.

[118] Dimitriou, R., Tsiridis, E. and Giannoudis, P. V. 2005. Current concepts of molecular aspects of bone healing. *Injury,* **36**(12), 1392–404.

[119] Dimitriou, R., Jones, E., McGonagle, D. and Giannoudis, P. V. 2011. Bone regeneration: current concepts and future directions. *BMC Medicine*, **9**, 66.

[120] Pneumaticos, S. G., Triantafyllopoulos, G. K., Chatziioannou, S., Basdra, E. K. and Papavassiliou, A. G. 2011. Biomolecular strategies of bone augmentation in spinal surgery. *Trends Molec. Med.*, **17**(4), 215–22.

[121] Judet, H. and Gilbert, A. 2001. Long-term results of free vascularized fibular grafting for femoral head necrosis. *Clin. Orthop. Relat. Res.*, **386**, 114–9.

[122] Seth, R., Futran, N. D., Alam, D. S. and Knott, P. D. 2010. Outcomes of vascularized bone graft reconstruction of the mandible in bisphosphonate-related osteonecrosis of the jaws. *Laryngoscope*, **120**(11), 2165–71.

[123] Clines, G. A. 2010. Prospects for osteoprogenitor stem cells in fracture repair and osteoporosis. *Curr. Opin. Organ Transplant.*, **15**(1), 73–8.

[124] Ikehara, S. 2005. Intra-bone marrow-bone marrow transplantation: a new strategy for treatment of stem cell disorders. *Ann. NY Acad. Sci.*, **1051**, 626–34.

[125] Verhaar, H. J. and Lems, W. F. 2010. PTH analogues and osteoporotic fractures. *Expert Opin. Biol. Ther.*, **10**(9), 1387–94.

[126] Carragee, E. J., Hurwitz, E. L. and Weiner, B. K. 2011. A critical review of recombinant human bone morphogenetic protein-2 trials in spinal surgery: emerging safety concerns and lessons learned. *Spine J.*, **11**(6), 471–91.

26

Biomaterials for engineered tendon regeneration

Wei Liu and Yilin Cao

26.1 Tendon introduction

Tendon is one of the important components of the musculoskeletal system, which links muscles to bones, so that the tensile force created by muscles can be transmitted to bone for body movement. Tendon injury and defects are common diseases of the musculoskeletal system. Nevertheless, the treatment of tendon defects remains a major challenge to reconstructive surgery, partly because there is limited availability of autologous tendon grafts.

Regenerative medicine represents the future direction for tendon repair and functional recovery, in which stem cell therapy, tissue engineering, and regenerative materials will play important roles in tendon regeneration. Actually, engineered tendon repair might be the major contributor to tendon regeneration, because it can also integrate stem cells and biomaterials into tendon regeneration, although we are a long way from its ultimate translation to clinical therapy.

26.2 Scaffold materials

26.2.1 General requirements on tendon scaffold materials

As the major contributor to tissue regeneration, biomaterial plays a key role in engineered tendon regeneration, because it provides an essential scaffold for extracellular matrix (ECM) production and tissue formation. The main tendon extracellular matrix is type I collagen, which is highly organized in a hierarchy of bundles that are aligned in a parallel fashion. In addition, there are small amounts of other collagens and proteoglycans, such as collagens type III, V, XII, and XIV, decorin, and tenascin. In particular, the small linking proteins play important roles in enabling the structural integrity of tendon and affording it mechanical strength. This unique structure provides the unique biomechanical properties of tendon tissues. Therefore, the parallel alignment structure and mechanical strength should be considered for tendon scaffold design. It was proposed that an ideal tendon scaffold should fulfill the following requirements [1]:

(1) biodegradability with adjustable degradation rate;
(2) biocompatibility before, during, and after degradation;
(3) superior mechanical properties and maintenance of mechanical strength during the tissue regeneration process;
(4) biofunctionality (the ability to support cell proliferation and differentiation, ECM secretion, and tissue formation); and
(5) processability, to form desired constructs of complicated structures and shapes, such as woven or knitted scaffolds etc.

26.2.2 Categories of tendon scaffold

As reported in the literature, the major categories of scaffold materials for tendon engineering include poly(α-hydroxy) acids, collagen derivatives, acelluar tendon, xenogenic acellular extracelluar matrix, silk derivatives, and polysaccharides.

26.2.3 Synthetic materials for tendon engineering

Polyglycolic acid (PGA) fibers were the first scaffold biomaterials reported for tendon engineering. In 1994, Cao *et al.* reported their pioneering research into neo-tendon engineering using parallel aligned unwoven PGA fibers and seeded calf tenocytes in a nude mouse model. The results showed that tendon-like tissue could be regenerated after 12 weeks of in-vivo implantation, which produced longitudinally aligned collagen fibers [2].

Afterwards, a PGA scaffold was also employed in tendon engineering in a hen claw model as a test in an immunocompetent animal. In that study, autologous tenocytes were isolated and seeded on unwoven PGA fibers, and the cell–scaffold construct was implanted in vivo after one week of in-vitro culture to repair a 3-cm-long defect of the flexor digitorum profundus tendon. After 14 weeks, mature tendon tissue was formed when observed grossly (Figure 26.1, top panel). Histology revealed longitudinally aligned collagen fibers and tenocytes with a curving pattern representing a characteristic histology of tendon tissue (Figure 1, bottom panel). The regenerated tendon also reached 83% of the native tendon's tensile strength [3].

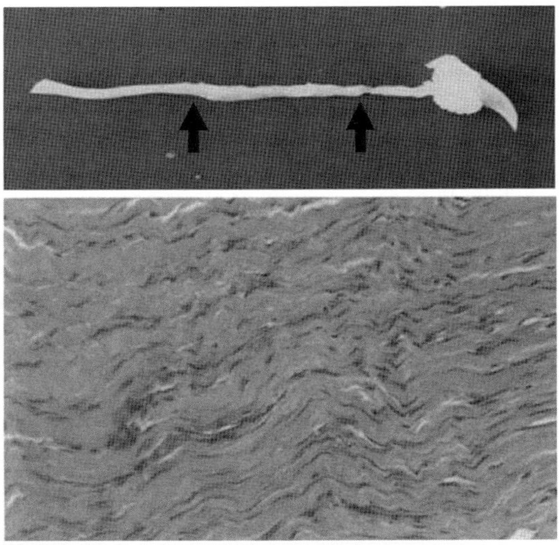

Figure 26.1 Tissue-engineered tendon 14 weeks after in-vivo implantation (modified from [3]). Top panel: gross view of engineered tendon (between arrows); bottom panel: H&E staining of engineered tendon.

A similar approach has also been applied to engineered tendon regeneration in a large-animal model, in which cells were seeded on unwoven PGA fibers and subjected to in-vitro culture for one week, and then the cell–scaffold constructs were implanted in vivo to repair a 3-cm-long defect created on the flexor digitorum superficialis tendon in a porcine model. After 26 weeks of in-vivo implantation, mature tendon tissue was formed grossly, and histology showed that the tissue structure was similar to that of native tendon, with good mechanical strength, indicating the possibility of engineered tendon regeneration in pre-clinical studies (Figure 26.2) [4].

Nevertheless, an obvious disadvantage of unwoven fibers is the lack of proper mechanical support during tendogenesis, therefore an acellular small intestinal submucosa membrane was needed to wrap around the cell-loaded PGA fibers in order to enhance the mechanical property of the cell–scaffold constructs [3, 4]. Compared with PGA, PLGA, the copolymer of PGA and polylactic acid (PLA), can retain good cell compatibility while degrading much slower, and thus can better maintain the mechanical strength during tendogenesis. In addition, the change of physical form of the polymer will also help to further enhance the mechanical strength of the scaffold to be used.

Ouyang *et al.* reported using knitted PLGA and allogeneic bome marrow stromal cells (BMSCs) for in-vivo tendon engineering and the repair of rabbit Achilles tendon. In the study, the tendon defect was repaired with either a BMSC-loaded PLGA scaffold or a PLGA scaffold alone as a control. The results showed that Achilles tendon could be better regenerated with the BMSC-seeded scaffold, demonstrating that PLGA could also serve as a scaffold for in-vivo tendon engineering and repair [5]. Similarly, Cooper *et al.* employed three-dimensional (3D) braiding technology to fabricate PLGA (10:90 ratio) polymer fibers for ACL ligament replacement and the resulting microporous scaffold exhibited optimal pore diameter with a range of 175–233 μm. Additionally, the initial mechanical strength of the construct reached a level similar to that of native ligament [6].

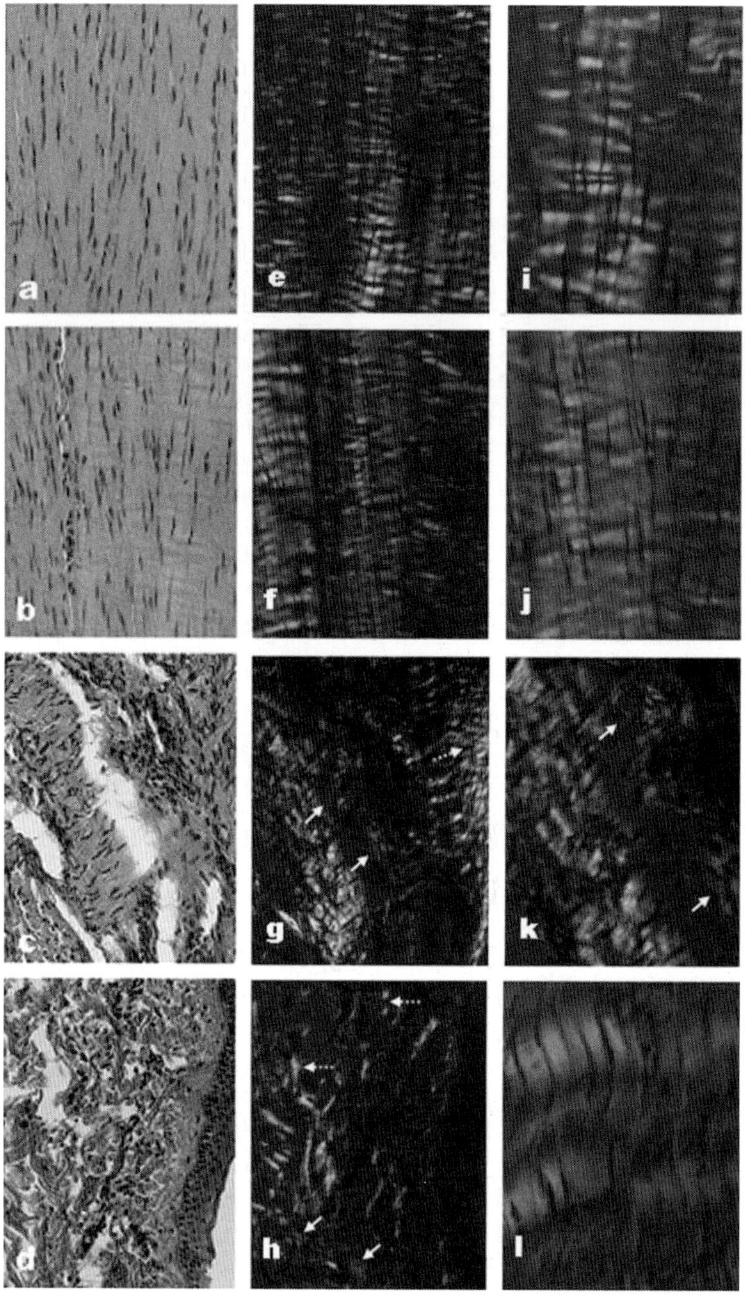

Figure 26.2 Histological finding of tissue formed after 26 weeks. H&E staining shows histological structures of fibroblast (a), tenocyte (b) engineered tendons, a control tissue in control group 2 (c) and normal pig skin (d). Collagen type III (delicate collagen fibers with a light-green color) is detected only in the polarized images of control tissues (g and k) and in normal pig skin (h), as indicated by white full arrows. In addition, collagen I (indicated by white dotted arrows) is also detected in these tissues. In the polarized images of fibroblast (e and i) and tenocyte (f and j) engineered tendons and natural tendons (l), collagen type I is the predominant collagen type. Original magnification ×400 for i–k; ×200, all others. (Reprinted from [4].)

To further improve cell attachment and cell proliferation on knitted PLGA scaffolds, Sahoo *et al.* reported creating hybrid polyester scaffolds by coating the knitted scaffolds with a thin film of poly(ε-caprolactone) or poly(D,L-lactide-*co*-glycolide) nanofibers or type 1 collagen. The study showed that the coating of knitted PLGA could modulate the mechanical properties and facilitate cell attachment and proliferation in the hybrid scaffold, and thus could be applied in tendons/ligament engineering [7].

Although PGA, PLA and PLGA all belong to the group of poly-α-hydroxy acids or poly-α-hydroxyesters, they vary greatly individually in terms of their degradation rate and their cell compatibility. Generally, the degradation rate increases in the order PLA, PLGA, and PGA. For example, unwoven PGA fibers had usually completely degraded 8–12 weeks after in-vivo implantation [2–4], whereas PLA fibers will not be completely degraded before 12 months have elapsed according to our recent study. The degradation rate of PLGA falls between those of PGA and PLA, and depends on the percentage of PLA in the copolymer. On the other hand, PGA exhibited the best cell compatibility, whereas PLA revealed the worst compatibility, relatively speaking. Similarly, the cell compatibility for PLGA is between those of PGA and PLA, depending on the percentage of PLA in the copolymer. It is often observed that PGA exhibits hydrophilic behavior, whereas PLA usually has a hydrophobic character, leading to poor compatibility of PLA to cells. The other factor that might affect cell compatibility is the acidic degradation product, which can disturb the cell survival environment. This is a common problem with all poly-α-hydroxyester polymers. In particular, the accumulated degradation product of lactic acid derived from PLA polymer is harmful to seeded cells, which may explain why PGA and PGLA are often used as tissue engineering scaffolds, whereas PLA is usually used as a medical suture or for orthopedic devices that need good biocompatibility, but not necessarily good cell compatibility because their primary use is not for tissue regeneration. Furthermore, the acidic degradation products also induce a strong host inflammatory reaction, which causes further deterioration of the in-vivo environment for tissue regeneration. This explains why unwoven PGA fibers behave differently in in-vivo environments for tissue formation depending on whether one is using immnodeficient or immunocompetent animal models [8].

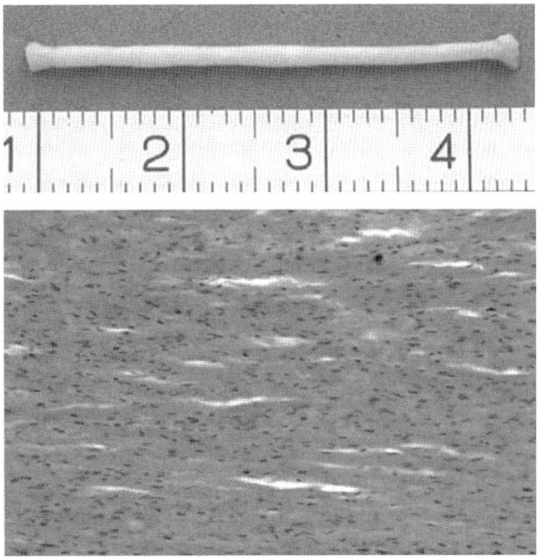

Figure 26.3 Gross view (top) and histology (bottom) of in-vitro engineered tendon using hen tenocytes and unwoven PGA fibers after 10 weeks of in-vitro culture. Note, PGA fibers were completely degraded. (Modified from [9].)

The challenge of using a poly-α-hydroxy acid as a scaffold is how to take the advantage of its good cell compatibility and meanwhile avoid the accumulation of undesired degradation products during tendogenesis. One approach is to develop techniques to engineer tendon grafting in vitro for in-vivo implantation. Cao *et al.* reported a preliminary study on tendon engineering in vitro using hen tenocytes and unwoven PGA fibers [9], which showed that a neo-tendon could be generated in a culture dish when examined grossly (Figure 26.3, top panel) after 6–10 weeks of in-vitro culture. Histologically, collagen fibers with longitudinal alignment were observed in the tissue section. Interestingly, PGA fibers were mostly degraded by in-vitro culture (Figure 3, bottom panel). Apparently, in-vivo implantation of neo-tendon tissue instead of cell-seeded polymer may avoid the formation of acidic degradation products that will adversely affect tissue formation. Importantly, when a properly designed bioreactor is used for in-vitro tendon engineering, the system can provide perfusion of culture medium to efficiently remove the acidic degradation products, which might further improve the tissue quality of engineered tendon. In another study performed in our center, unwoven PGA fibers and human dermal fibroblasts were similarly used to generate human neo-tendon tissue after in-vitro culture for 14 weeks on a U-spring (Figure 26.4) [10]. No matter what kinds of cells were used, the neo-tendon formed exhibited very weak mechanical strength (usually less than 5 N), probably due to the lack of proper mechanical loading that is applied to tendon tissue in daily life.

In a recent study performed in our center, we developed a bioreactor to provide dynamic mechanical loading to the in-vitro-engineered tendon at a certain frequency, and the tissue quality as well as the mechanical strength of loaded engineered tendon were significantly improved after 10–12 weeks of in-vitro culture. It is, however, worth noting that in-vitro-engineered tendon tissue remains weaker in mechanical strength than native tendon tissue.

To determine the optimal conditions for tissue-engineering-mediated tendogenesis [11], one more study was performed in our center. In this study, long PGA fibers and human fetal extensor tenoctyes (isolated from a 3-month-old aborted fetus donated by the parents for research only) were used to engineer extensor tendon equivalent. The long PGA fibers were arranged to mimic the extensor-tendon-complex-like structure (Figure 26.5) followed by cell seeding onto the scaffold. After in-vitro culture for 6 weeks, the cell-scaffold constructs were further divided into three groups: (1) in-vitro culture with mechanical loading; (2) in-vivo implantation without mechanical loading;

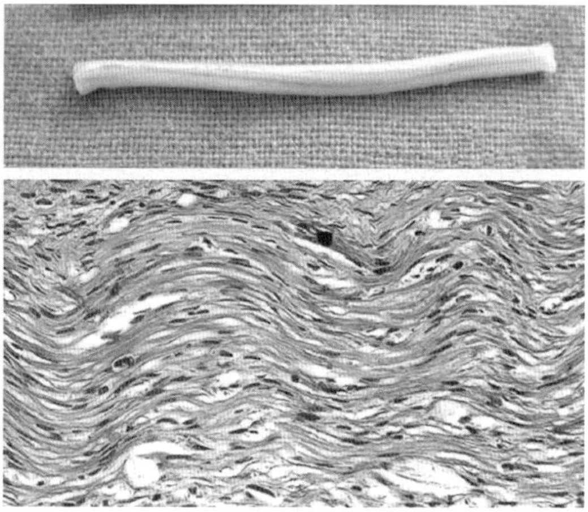

Figure 26.4 Gross view (top) and histology (bottom) of in-vitro engineered tendon using human dermal fibroblasts and unwoven PGA fibers after 14 weeks of in-vitro culture. (Reprinted from [10].)

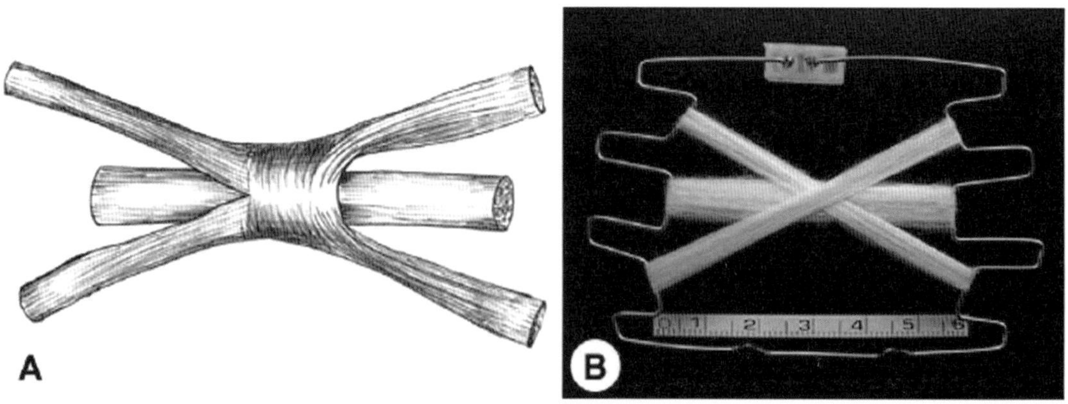

Figure 26.5 Design of extensor tendon complex scaffold. (A) A schematic chart showing the central slip and two lateral bands. (B) A PGA scaffold secured on a custom-made spring to mimic the complex structure. (Reprinted from [11].)

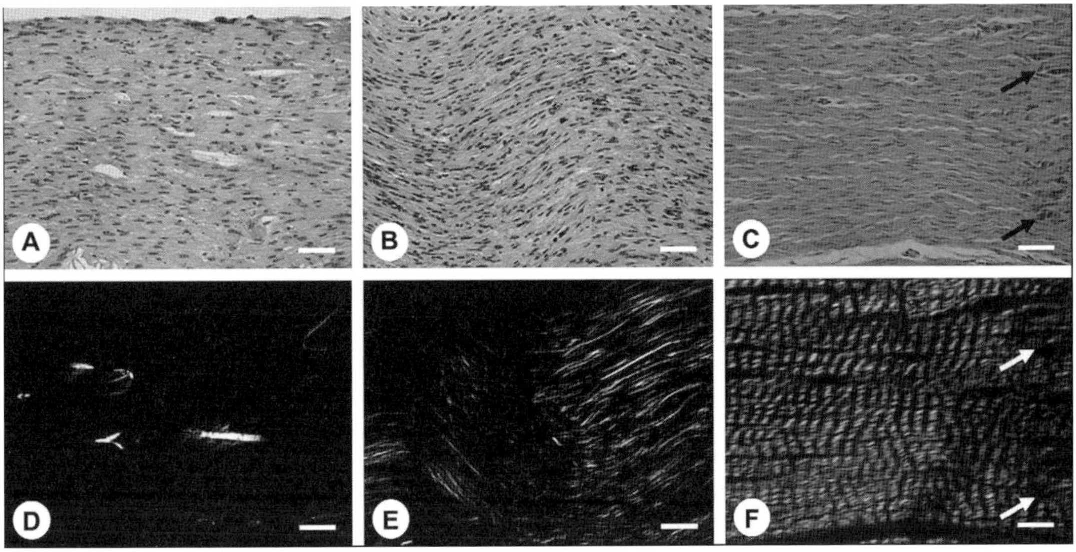

Figure 26.6 H&E staining (A–C) and polarized microscopic views (D–F) of in-vitro engineered tendon after total 12 weeks (A and D) and of in-vivo implanted tendons for 14 weeks without (B and E) and with (C and F) loading. Original magnifications: ×200; the bar represents 50 mm for all. (Reprinted from [11].)

and (3) in-vivo implantation with mechanical loading by suturing the construct to fascia, and thus mouse movement could provide a natural dynamic loading. The results showed that human fetal cells could form an extensor tendon complex structure in vitro, and could be made to become further matured in vivo by mechanical stimulation. In contrast to in-vitro loaded and in-vivo non-loaded tendons, in-vivo loaded tendons exhibited bigger tissue volume, better aligned collagen fibers, more mature collagen fibril structure with D-band periodicity, and stronger mechanical properties (Figure 26.6). These results indicate that in-vivo mechanical loading via an ex-vivo approach might be an optimal approach for engineering functional tendon tissue. Therefore, a reasonable strategy for engineered functional repair of tendon defects might be to generate a neo-tendon tissue first in vitro and then implant it in vivo for its further maturation while carrying out its functions. In our recent studies, use of a long-fiber braided scaffold for in-vitro tendon engineering could actually generate neo-tendon graft in vitro in a bioreactor, which was strong enough for in-vivo implantation for functional tendon repair.

26.2.3.1 Collagen materials for tendon engineering

In addition to poly-α-hydroxy acids, collagen derivatives have also been intensively investigated for application in tendon tissue engineering. This is because tendon tissues are mainly composed of type I collagen, and the collagen derivatives would be highly biocompatible to seeded cells and would support cell adhesion, proliferation, and matrix production, thus being highly biomimetic. Gel is a common form for collagen scaffolds. Collagen gels are usually employed for studying the effect of mechanical loading on neo-tendon formation in an in-vitro culture system. For example, Garvin *et al.* used a bioreactor to stretch a collagen gel construct containing avian flexor tenocytes, and they found that mechanical loading could significantly enhance the tensile strength of mechanically loaded constructs within a short time period [12]. However, collagen gel is apparently not suitable for practical application due to its shortcomings of quick degradation and lack of sufficient mechanical strength. Therefore, it was suggested that one could combine collagen gel itself with other materials for tendon engineering or repair. For example, Awad *et al.* applied the gel together with polyglyconate suture for patellar tendon repair [13]. Or collagen gel could be combined with collagen fibers or sponges to further enhance the mechanical strength [14]. Crosslinking with chemical agents may also enhance the mechanical strength of collagen-based scaffolds.

26.2.3.2 Acellular tissue for tendon engineering

The other approach to employing collagen matrix as a scaffold for tendon engineering is to use acellular collagen matrix. Tischer *et al.* reported the preparation of acellular tendon scaffold for cruciate ligament reconstructions [15]. They used sodium dodecyl sulfate (SDS) as the main ingredient to decellularize cell components from the tendon tissue. After acellularization, dermal fibroblasts were injected into the tendon and cultured for different time periods at 37 °C in 5% CO_2. The results showed that acellularized tendon exhibited similar mechanical properties for processed and native tendons, including the maximum load to failure, stiffness, and elongation. Additionally, a cell-seeded graft was able to produce pro-collagen I, as was revealed by immunohistochemistry. However, it was reported that tenocytes usually failed to penetrate into the decellularized scaffold, although the cells were able to attach to the processed tendon tissues.

Ingram *et al.* reported the use of ultrasonication to assist recellularization of acellular tissue scaffolds for potential reconstruction of anterior cruciate ligament [16]. They showed that ultrasonication plus a standard acellularization process could significantly enhance the cell penetration, which allowed extrinsic cells to migrate into the center of the acellular scaffold. This was because the sonification process could produce a microscopically more open porous matrix, but would not damage the overall architecture of the scaffold, and the essential biomechanical characteristics of the native tissue's biochemical constituents (collagen, glycosaminoglycans) could be well retained. However, the viability of the cells in the center of the scaffold was compromised. Therefore, how to promote cell survival might remain a challenge to the use of acellular dense connective tissue like acellularized tendon grafts.

In contrast, Badylak *et al.* reported the application of acellularized small intestinal submucosa (SIS) membrane for tendon regeneration [17]. Porcine SIS membrane was generated and then used to repair a 1.5-cm segmental defect of the Achilles tendon created in dogs. The animals were killed at different times after repair, and the neotendons were evaluated. The results showed that implanted SIS could be penetrated by host cells and the implanted materials could be gradually remodeled into neotendons. More importantly, the remodeled neotendon could achieve good mechanical strength, indicating that a functional repair of the tendon had been achieved. Their result suggests that the implanted SIS biomaterial probably underwent slow degradation within the first several weeks and served as a temporary scaffold around which the host could deposit appropriate and organized connective tissue. This cell-free approach may also become a promising approach for tendon tissue regeneration and defect repair.

26.2.3.3 Silk materials for tendon repair

In addition to the aforementioned scaffolds, silk fibers have also been used as the scaffold materials for tissue engineering because of their unique mechanical properties and the possibility of modifying them with growth factors and adhesion molecules on the side chains of the fibers. In particular, silk fibers will be a good candidate for scaffold materials if sericin (glue-like protein), a potential antigenic protein, can be completely removed [18]. Fan *et al.* reported the use of knitted silk mesh incorporating microporous silk sponges as a scaffold to investigate the regeneration of anterior cruciate ligament by using mesenchymal stem cells (MSCs) as the cell source [19]. In addition, knitted silk fiber scaffold was also impregnated with gelatin [20] or collagen matrix [21] for ligament regeneration experiments. It was noted that silk fibers elicited little inflammatory reaction and degraded slowly, and thus could provide mechanical support for ligament regeneration and repair [21]. This approach is likely to be applied to tendon engineering and repair as well. However, these reports also revealed that silk fibers were usually very slowly degraded, and no apparent mass loss could be observed even one year after repair [21]. This may cause a challenge to tendon engineering because the long-term presence of the scaffold materials may cause a foreign-body reaction and further fibrosis, and prevent implanted scaffold from bringing about tissue regeneration by occupying the space where tissue is intended to regenerate. It is expected that further refinement of the processing technique might allow one to modify silk fibers into scaffold materials with an appropriate degradation rate and high mechanical strength [18].

26.2.3.4 Polysaccharides for tendon engineering

Polysaccharides might also be a potential material category for tendon engineering. The polysaccharides include chitin, chitosan, alginate, and agarose. Bagnaninchi *et al.* reported that porous chitosan scaffolds with microchannels could be designed to engineer tendon tissues [22]. However, hybridization of chitosan with other polysaccharides seems to be a more practical approach for its application. For example, a hybridized chitosan–hyaloronan scaffold exhibited not only enhanced mechanical strength, but also better bioreactivity, with enhanced cell attachment and matrix production [23]. More detailed studies regarding their cell compatibility as well as their performance in tendon regeneration in vivo might provide valuable information to guide their application.

26.3 Cell sources for tendon engineering

The other key component of engineered tendon regeneration is the cell source. Several types of cell source have been employed in engineered tendon regeneration. Tenocytes were the first cell source that was investigated for engineered tendon regeneration both in vivo and in vitro [2, 3, 9]. Despite the success in animal studies, this is not a practical cell source due to the lack of tendon donors for cell extraction, particularly in the case of severe trauma. In contrast, dermal fibroblasts, which are similar to tenocytes in cell morphology and function have been used for tendon engineering either in vitro or in vivo in large-animal models [4, 10], indicating their potential in translating pre-clinical work to clinical therapy.

The other important source is adult mesenchymal stem cells. As mentioned above, BMSCs have been applied widely and successfully in engineered repair and regeneration of tendon or ligament in rabbit and porcine models [5, 13, 14, 19–22]. In addition to the engineered tissue approach, MSC-based cell therapy has also revealed its great potential in tendon/ligament regeneration [24, 25].

One of the disadvantages of using BMSCs is the need to sacrifice hematopoietic stem cells and immune system cells, which in the long run may to a certain extent adversely affect the health of the patient. In contrast, adipose-derived stem cells (ASCs) are a cell source that will not have any influence on health once the adipose tissue has been removed from the body [26]. Currently, ASCs have already been widely applied in musculoskeletal tissue regeneration [27], and there have been rare reports of their application to tendon regeneration.

One of the advantages of using MSCs is the possibility of their serving as an allogeneic cell source for tissue regeneration. It has been shown that ASCs are only slightly immunogenic and are able to modulate the immune reaction [28]. More importantly, ASCs have been employed for allogeneic cell-based tissue regeneration [29]. It is expected that the application of adult mesenchymal stem cells, particularly ASCs as a cell source, may lead to a new revolution of tendon repair in a regenerative way [30]. Recent research has isolated tendon stem/progenitor cells (TSCs) in human, mice, and rabbit tendon tissues, which play a critical role in maintaining tendon homeostasis and repair. Therefore this type of cell may also become an important cell source for engineered tendon regeneration [31, 32].

26.4 Conclusion

Overall, the progress in biomaterial research in the past few decades has contributed greatly to the development of regenerative medicine, including engineered tendon regeneration. In the future, advances in the design and manufacture of intelligent scaffold materials that are able to induce tenogenic differentiation of seeded adult MSCs will be an important area of biomaterial-mediated tendon regeneration. Additionally, determining how to prevent the adhesion of engineered tendon to surrounding tissue would also be a key aspect of future research, particularly for engineered repair of flexor tendon defects. Our recent study of engineered tendon sheath in a hen model may become an important step toward the achievement of functional recovery [33].

REFERENCES

[1] Liu, Y., Ramanath, H. S. and Wang, D. A., 2008. Tendon tissue engineering using scaffold enhancing strategies. *Trends Biotechnol.*, **26**, 201–9.

[2] Cao, Y., Vacanti, J. P., Ma, X., *et al.* 1994. Generation of neo-tendon using synthetic polymers seeded with tenocytes. *Transplant Proc.*, **26**, 3390–2.

[3] Cao, Y., Liu, Y., Liu, W. *et al.* 2002. Bridging tendon defects using autologous tenocyte engineered tendon in a hen model. *Plast. Reconstr. Surg.*, **110**, 1280–9.

[4] Liu, W., Chen, B., Deng, D. *et al.* 2006. Repair of tendon defect with dermal fibroblast engineered tendon in a porcine model. *Tissue Eng.*, **12**, 775–88.

[5] Ouyang, H. W., Goh, J. C., Thambyah, A., Teoh, S. H. and Lee, E. H. 2003. Knitted poly-lactide-*co*-glycolide scaffold loaded with bone marrow stromal cells in repair and regeneration of rabbit Achilles tendon. *Tissue Eng.*, **9**, 431–9.

[6] Cooper, J. A., Lu, H. H., Ko, F. K., Freeman, J. W. and Laurencin, C. T. 2005. Fiber-based tissue-engineered scaffold for ligament replacement: design considerations and in vitro evaluation. *Biomaterials*, **26**, 1523–32.

[7] Sahoo, S., Cho-Hong, J. G. and Siew-Lok, T. 2007. Development of hybrid polymer scaffolds for potential applications in ligament and tendon tissue engineering. *Biomed Mater*, **2**, 169–73.

[8] Liu, W. and Cao, Y. 2007. Application of scaffold materials in tissue reconstruction in immunocompetent mammals: our experience and future requirements. *Biomaterials*, **28**, 5078–86.

[9] Cao, D., Liu, W., Wei, X. *et al.* 2006. In vitro tendon engineering with avain tenocytes and polyglycolic acids: a preliminary report. *Tissue Eng.*, **12**, 1369–77.

[10] Deng, D., Liu, W., Xu, F. *et al.* 2009. Engineering human neo-tendon tissue in vitro with human dermal fibroblasts under static mechanical strain. *Biomaterials.*, **30**(35), 6724–30.

[11] Wang, B., Liu, W., Zhang, Y. *et al.* 2008. Engineering of extensor tendon complex by an ex vivo approach. *Biomaterials*, **29**, 2954–61.

[12] Garvin, J., Qi, J., Maloney, M. and Banes, A. J., 2003. Novel system for engineering bioartificial tendons and application of mechanical load. *Tissue Eng.*, **9**, 967–79.

[13] Awad, H. A., Boivin, G. P., Dressler, M. R. *et al.* 2003. Repair of patellar tendon injuries using a cell–collagen composite. *J. Orthop. Res.*, **21**, 420–31.

[14] Juncosa-Melvin, N., Boivin, G. P., Gooch, C. *et al.* 2006. The effect of autologous mesenchymal stem cells on the biomechanics and histology of gel–collagen sponge constructs used for rabbit patellar tendon repair. *Tissue Eng.*, **12**, 369–79.

[15] Tischer, T., Vogt, S., Aryee, S. *et al.* 2007. Tissue engineering of the anterior cruciate ligament: a new method using acellularized tendon allografts and autologous fibroblasts. *Arch. Orthop. Trauma Surg.*, **127**, 735–41.

[16] Ingram, J. H., Korossis, S., Howling, G., Fisher, J. and Ingham, E. 2007. The use of ultrasonication to aid recellularization of acellular natural tissue scaffolds for use in anterior cruciate ligament reconstruction. *Tissue Eng.*, **13**, 1561–72.

[17] Badylak, S. F., Tullius, R., Kokini, K. *et al.* 1995. The use of xenogeneic small intestinal submucosa as a biomaterial for Achilles tendon repair in a dog model. *J. Biomed. Mater. Res.*, **29**, 977–85.

[18] Altman, G. H., Diaz, F., Jakuba, C. *et al.* 2003. Silk-based biomaterials. *Biomaterials*, **24**, 401–16.

[19] Fan, H., Liu, H., Wong, E. J., Toh, S. L. and Goh, J. C. 2008. In vivo study of anterior cruciate ligament regeneration using mesenchymal stem cells and silk scaffold. *Biomaterials*, **29**, 3324–37.

[20] Fan, H., Liu, H., Toh, S. L. and Goh, J. C. 2008. Enhanced differentiation of mesenchymal stem cells co-cultured with ligament fibroblasts on gelatin/silk fibroin hybrid scaffold. *Biomaterials*, **29**, 1017–27.

[21] Chen, X., Qi, Y. Y., Wang, L. L. *et al.* 2008. Ligament regeneration using a knitted silk scaffold combined with collagen matrix. *Biomaterials*, **29**, 3683–92.

[22] Bagnaninchi, P. O., Yang, Y., Zghoul, N. *et al.* 2007. Chitosan microchannel scaffolds for tendon tissue engineering characterized using optical coherence tomography. *Tissue Eng.*, **13**, 323–31.

[23] Funakoshi, T., Majima, T., Iwasaki, N. *et al.* 2005. Novel chitosan-based hyaluronan hybrid polymer fibers as a

scaffold in ligament tissue engineering. *J. Biomed. Mater. Res. A*, **74**, 338–46.

[24] Okamoto, N., Kushida, T., Oe, K. *et al.* 2010. Treating Achilles tendon rupture in rats with bone-marrow-cell transplantation therapy. *J. Bone Joint Surg. Am.*, **92**, 2776–84.

[25] Gulotta, L. V., Kovacevic, D., Packer, J. D., Deng, X. H. and Rodeo, S. A. 2011. Bone marrow-derived mesenchymal stem cells transduced with scleraxis improve rotator cuff healing in a rat model. *Am. J. Sports Med.*, **39**, 1282–9.

[26] Zuk, P. A., Zhu, M., Mizuno, H. *et al.* 2001. Multilineage cells from human adipose tissue: implications for cell-based therapies. *Tissue Eng.*, **7**, 211–28.

[27] Gimble, J. M., Katz, A. J. and Bunnell, B. A. 2007. Adipose-derived stem cells for regenerative medicine *Circ Res.*, **100**, 1249–60.

[28] Kang, J. W., Kang, K. S., Koo, H. C. *et al.* 2008. Soluble factors-mediated immunomodulatory effects of canine adipose tissue-derived mesenchymal stem cells. *Stem Cells Dev.*, **17**, 681–93.

[29] Ryu, H. H., Lim, J. H., Byeon, Y. E. *et al.* 2009. Functional recovery and neural differentiation after transplantation of allogenic adipose-derived stem cells in a canine model of acute spinal cord injury. *J. Vet. Sci.*, **10**(4), 273–84.

[30] Zhang, Z. Y., Teoh, S. H., Hui, J. H. *et al.* 2012. The potential of human fetal mesenchymal stem cells for off-the-shelf bone tissue engineering application. *Biomaterials*, **33**, 2656–72.

[31] Bi, Y., Ehirchiou, D., Kilts, T. M. *et al.* 2007. Identification of tendon stem/progenitor cells and the role of the extracellular matrix in their niche. *Nature Med.*, **13**, 1219–27.

[32] Zhang, J., Keenan, C. and Wang, J. H. 2012. The effects of dexamethasone on human patellar tendon stem cells: implications for dexamethasone treatment of tendon injury. *J. Orthop. Res.*, **31**(1), 105–10.

[33] Xu, L., Cao, D., Liu, W. *et al.* 2010. In vivo engineering of a functional tendon sheath in a hen model. *Biomaterials*, **31**, 3894–902.

27

Advancing articular cartilage repair through tissue engineering: from materials and cells to clinical translation

Megan J. Farrell and Robert L. Mauck

27.1 Introduction

Owing to the inability of cartilage to heal even minor defects, as well as the prevalence of osteoarthritis, the biological repair of this tissue has been the primary focus of decades of basic science and pre-clinical research. This research focussed on cartilage repair has witnessed marked advances via developments in biomaterials science as well as in tissue engineering methodologies. In this chapter, we review select topics in cartilage tissue engineering, describe current clinical cartilage repair procedures, and discuss ongoing considerations relating to the realization of these advances through pre-clinical animal models.

27.2 Cartilage

Cartilage is a collagenous, proteoglycan-rich, and water-saturated flexible soft connective tissue. A single cell type, the chondrocyte, is responsible for cartilage tissue maintenance and homeostasis. The tissue is aneural and avascular in the adult and relies on diffusion for nutrient and waste exchange (Brodin, 1955; Strangeways, 1920). The structure and function of cartilage categorizes these soft connective tissues into three broad groupings: elastic cartilage, fibrocartilage, and hyaline cartilage (Gray and Goss, 1973).

Elastic cartilage is a flexible type of cartilage with elastin as a main component of the extracellular matrix. Elastic cartilage can be found in the Eustachian tube, the epiglottis, and portions of the larynx, as well as in auricular cartilage. In the broadest terms, fibrocartilages contain both type I and type II collagen. Some fibrocartilages, such as the meniscus or annulus fibrosus of the intervertebral disk, have highly organized hierarchical designs that lend themselves to specific load transmission and load dispersion. However, when referring to cartilage repair, particularly insofar as it relates to articular cartilage repair (hyaline cartilage), the term "fibrocartilage" often refers to a fibrous, disorganized, scar tissue with inappropriate matrix constituents and inadequate mechanical properties. Hyaline cartilage includes articular cartilage, costal cartilage, and cartilage found in the trachea and some portions of the larynx. It is the most common type of cartilage found within the body, and is referenced as having a glistening white or bluish tint (Gray and Goss, 1973). A range of biomaterials has been used for the repair of the various cartilaginous tissues mentioned, including the trachea (Macchiarini *et al.*, 2008), meniscus (Ionescu *et al.*, 2012; Kon *et al.*, 2012; Mandal *et al.*, 2011), and intervertebral disk (Bowles *et al.*, 2011; Nerurkar *et al.*, 2010; Park *et al.*, 2012); however, repair of articular cartilage will be the focus of the sections to follow.

27.2.1 Structure and function of articular cartilage

27.2.1.1 Articular cartilage structure

Articular cartilage lines the joint surfaces of bones, transmits load across the joint, and provides a low-friction surface that is critical for joint motion. Articular cartilage is comprised primarily of water

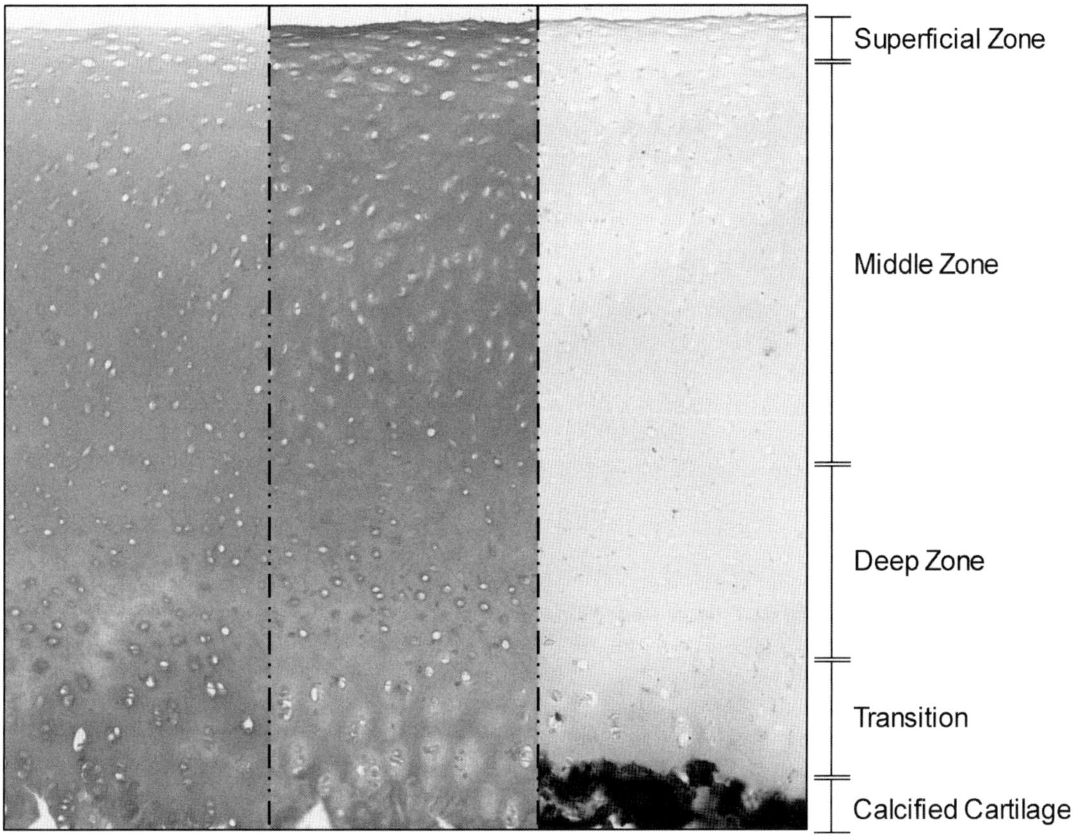

Figure 27.1 Depth-dependent histological staining of adult bovine cartilage from the femoral condyle. Alcian Blue (proteoglycans, left), Picrosirius Red (collagens, center), and Alizarin Red (calcium deposits, right) staining.

(60%–85%), type II collagen (15%–22%), and the proteoglycan aggrecan (4%–7%), although additional ground matrix, including minor collagens and proteoglycans, plays a significant role in its structure and function (Mow and Huiskes, 2005). Articular cartilage (Figure 27.1) has a graded distribution of matrix, organization (Figure 27.2), and mechanical properties through its depth (Freeman, 1979; Huang *et al.*, 2005; Schinagl *et al.*, 1997), and is segregated into the following zones: the superficial zone, the middle zone, the deep zone, and calcified cartilage (Figure 27.1). Although cartilage has one primary cell type, the chondrocyte, phenotype changes through the tissue depth to play specific roles in each of these regions (Klein *et al.*, 2007; Youn *et al.*, 2006).

Within the superficial (tangential) zone, the collagen content is high and fibers are oriented tangentially to the articulating surface, while the proteoglycan content is lower than in the deeper zones. In this most superficial zone, the chondrocytes are ellipsoidal in morphology and synthesize molecules such as proteoglycan 4 (Schumacher *et al.*, 1994), previously referred to as lubricin or superficial zone protein, that help to maintain a low friction coefficient between the two articulating surfaces (Swann *et al.*, 1985).

Progressing further through the depth to the middle (transitional) zone, the collagen content decreases and the proteoglycan content increases compared with the levels in the superficial zone. In this zone, which comprises the majority of the cartilage thickness, the

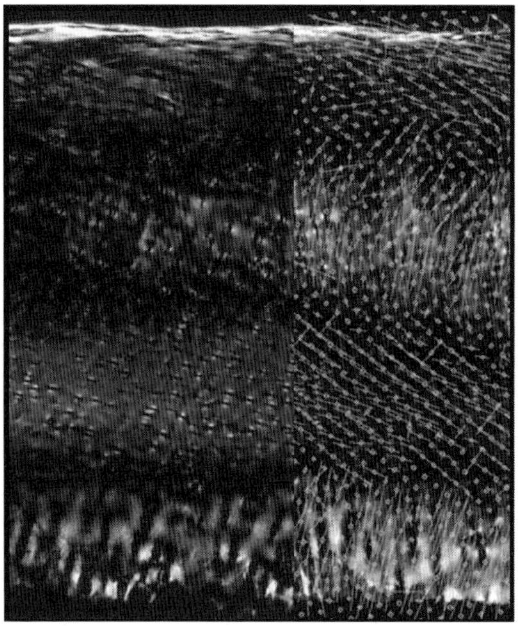

Figure 27.2 Cartilage organization as a function of depth. Left: polarized light imaging of adult bovine cartilage from the femoral condyle. Right: an alignment map generated from quantitative polarized light microscopy analysis (extinction angles with 5° rotation increments of polarizer) as in Thomopoulos *et al.* (2003).

collagen fibrils have a less dense, random orientation, and the chondrocytes adopt a more rounded morphology.

The deep zone is marked by a shift in collagen fiber orientation, with larger bundles that run perpendicular to the articular surface. The chondrocytes within this zone appear in columnar arrangements. The deep zone is separated from the underlying calcified cartilage by a tidemark. This calcified cartilage, the result of hypertrophic differentiation of chondrocytes, contains matrix-specific markers such as type X collagen, and forms a transition between the cartilage and subchondral bone.

27.2.1.2 Mechanical function

Cartilage exhibits anisotropic, viscoelastic, and depth-dependent mechanical properties (Huang *et al.*, 2005; Schinagl *et al.*, 1997). The mechanical properties can vary with species, age, tissue location, and tissue health (Armstrong and Mow, 1982; Athanasiou *et al.*, 1991; Treppo *et al.*, 2000; Williamson *et al.*, 2001). For example, bovine articular cartilage has an aggregate compressive modulus of 0.079 MPa in the superficial zone, 1.14 MPa in the middle zone, and 2.10 MPa in the deepest zone, with a full-thickness modulus of 0.38 MPa (Schinagl *et al.*, 1997). Insofar as it relates to location, the equilibrium aggregate modulus of bovine cartilage is on the order of 0.89 MPa in the lateral condyle and 0.47 MPa in the patellar grove (Athanasiou *et al.*, 1991). Cartilage withstands high physiological compressive loads, and therefore it is most commonly tested in compression. However, due to the tension placed on the collagen network by osmotic swelling, a significant contributor to the mechanical role of cartilage, an understanding of the tensile mechanical behavior of the tissue is also important. Furthermore, the tissue is subjected to both torsional and shear strains during normal physiological activities, so properties under these loading configurations must be considered when developing cartilage replacements.

27.2.2 The knee – A synovial joint

The knee is a diarthrodial joint enclosed in a synovial membrane and bathed in synovial fluid, an ultrafiltrate of blood plasma (Ropes *et al.*, 1939), that supports the nutritional demands of cartilage and lowers friction in the joint (Ogston and Stanier, 1953; Reimann, 1976; Swann *et al.*, 1985). Owing to the lack of blood supply in the adult, cells within articular cartilage experience low oxygen tension (Zhou *et al.*, 2004). Ligaments and menisci stabilize the knee (Figure 27.3) (Flandry and Hommel, 2011), with the menisci playing an additional role in load transmission and distribution (Jones *et al.*, 1996). Articular cartilage covers the joint surfaces of the femur, tibia, and patella, transferring load at three articulating surfaces: two femoral condyles contacting menisci and adjacent tibial surfaces and the patella contacting the trochlear grove of the femur (Gray and Goss, 1973).

27.2.3 Articular cartilage disease and clinical approaches to replacement and repair

Osteoarthritis is the chronic, progressive degeneration of articular cartilage, affecting upwards of 30 million adults in the USA (Lawrence *et al.*, 2008). This disease is associated with extensive pain, which is due not to the direct degeneration of the cartilage itself (Figure 27.4) (cartilage lacks a nerve supply), but rather to exposure and contact of highly innervated bone, osteophyte formation, and activation of nociceptors in the synovial capsule by inflammatory molecules (Mease *et al.*, 2011). Since cartilage in the adult lacks a blood supply, it has a limited intrinsic healing capacity. Surgical intervention is therefore necessary for the treatment of osteoarthritis. While osteoarthritis poses the most difficulty for clinical cartilage repair, there are other conditions that must be addressed. For example, trauma-induced focal defects can be painful and impact quality of life (Heir *et al.*, 2010), and, if left untreated, can alter tissue strains and ultimately progress to joint-wide osteoarthritis.

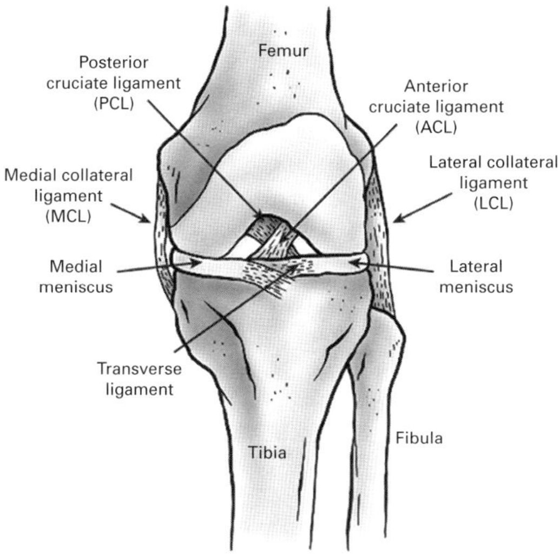

Figure 27.3 A schematic diagram of basic knee anatomy adapted with permission from Makris *et al.* (2011).

Severe joint damage caused by chronic osteoarthritis cannot be treated with conservative methods and requires joint arthroplasty (Figure 27.4) or joint resurfacing to alleviate pain. Arthroplasty is most commonly performed in the hip or knee joints. This technique is highly invasive and involves the surgical removal of the diseased cartilage and the underlying bone, followed by the implantation of a prosthetic articular surface with a stem that is cemented or press fit into the intermedulary canal of the primary bones of the affected joint. Implants can be comprised of ceramics, metals, and ultra-high-molecular-weight polymers with the primary goal of providing a stable, low-friction surface with good wear properties that will maintain joint stability and restore some aspects of normal joint motion (Wong *et al.*, 2011). While joint arthroplasty is one of the more successful long-term osteoarthritis treatments, the extreme invasiveness leaves little room for additional surgical repair if implant failure occurs. Joint arthoplasty is a particularly unattractive option

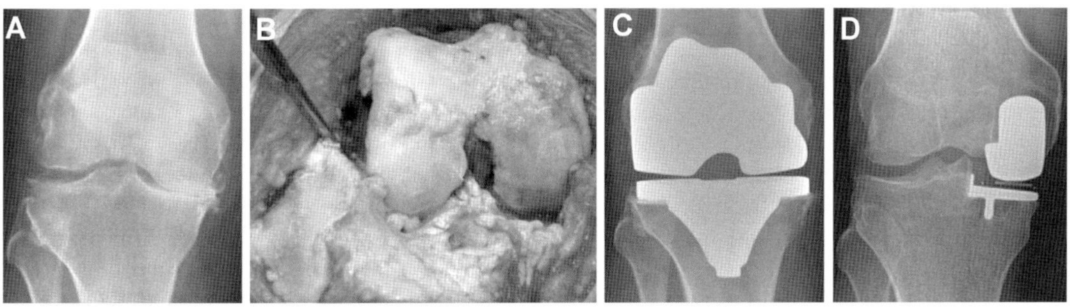

Figure 27.4 Clinical signs and current treatment of osteoarthritis. (A) A radiograph showing joint space narrowing of an osteoarthritic knee. (B) Gross appearance of osteoarthritic cartilage. (C) A radiograph of total knee arthroplasty. (D) A radiograph of partial knee arthroplasty. Images adapted from Carr *et al.* (2012) with permission.

for younger individuals (Li *et al.*, 2012), since implant failure can occur during the lifespan of the patient (Mulhall *et al.*, 2006). To allow the performance of additional future joint arthroplasty surgery if necessary, less invasive, yet similar repair techniques have been used as a first line of treatment, including partial joint replacement (i.e. unicompartmental knee replacement) and joint resurfacing.

In instances where damage or osteoarthritic tissue is localized to smaller lesion sites, biologically based cartilage repair techniques are clinically available. One such treatment, microfracture, induces de-novo tissue formation from a bone marrow clot in the lesion site (Gomoll, 2012; Gomoll and Minas, 2011). Microfracture is a marrow-stimulation technique that involves debridement of the lesion followed by the perforation of the subchondral bone using an awl (Figure 27.5). The microfracture perforations allow flooding of the lesion site by blood and bone marrow, which in turn results in the formation of a clot and the development of tissue by cells within the bone marrow. The limitations of this procedure include long recovery periods, inadequate tissue development (the tissue which forms is often fibrocartilagenous and disorganized (Figure 27.6)), and short-term efficacy (LaPrade *et al.*, 2008; Mithoefer *et al.*, 2009).

Alternatively, living osteochondral tissue can be grafted into a defect site. This procedure is referred to as osteochondral allografting (Gomoll and Minas, 2011) when donor tissue is used, or osteochondral autograft transfer (OAT) when the patient's own tissue is used. When numerous osteochondral plugs are used to fill a single, large defect, the procedures is termed mosaicplasty, given the resemblance of the repair site to a mosaic (Figure 27.5). To conduct OAT procedures, osteochondral plugs are harvested from non-load-bearing sites of the joint, such as the trochlear ridge or the interchondylar notch, using a sharp harvesting tool. This tissue is then typically press fit into the defect site. The limitations associated with such techniques can be tissue availability, chondrocyte viability at the plug-harvest interface (Huntley *et al.*, 2005), decreased cell viability or tissue degeneration during storage (Fening *et al.*, 2011; Pallante *et al.*, 2009), donor-site morbidity (Matricali *et al.*, 2010), poor lateral tissue integration, and donor-to-patient disease transmission in the case of allografts.

Finally, autologous chondrocyte implantation (ACI) (Minas, 2001), is a cell-based therapy for cartilage repair that uses transplanted chondrocytes to form de-novo cartilage development within the defect site. ACI, also referred to as autologous chondrocyte transplantation (ACT) is a two-stage surgical procedure, which first involves the harvesting of cartilage from a non-load-bearing donor site of the patient (Figure 27.5). This harvested cartilage is then shipped to a laboratory and digested to isolate the chondrocytes within, which are subsequently expanded in a tissue culture facility to obtain a sufficient number for re-implantation. The cells are returned to the surgeon and injected under a covering (typically a periosteal or collagen-based flap) fixed over the cartilage defect with sutures and fibrin glue. The primary indication for use of ACI, as suggested by Genzyme©, provider of Carticel® autologous cultured chondrocytes, is for cartilage lesions that have been treated unsuccessfully with other methods, and the use of ACI is not suggested for the treatment of generalized osteoarthritis. A high rate of subsequent surgical procedures is amongst the limitations associated with this procedure. Additionally, there remains a vigorous debate in the field as to whether the cartilage formed is true hyaline cartilage rather than being fibrous (Figure 27.6), as well as ongoing considerations as to the cost/benefit ratio relative to simpler microfracture procedures (Nehrer *et al.*, 1999; Van Assche *et al.*, 2010).

27.3 Cartilage regeneration and tissue engineering

Limitations associated with clinical cartilage repair, the inability of cartilage to heal a critically sized lesion, and the progressive nature of general osteoarthritis have all resulted in an increased focus on methods to regenerate or tissue engineer articular cartilage. The sections to follow will discuss some of the more prevalent cell types, growth factors, and materials that have been used to address these challenges.

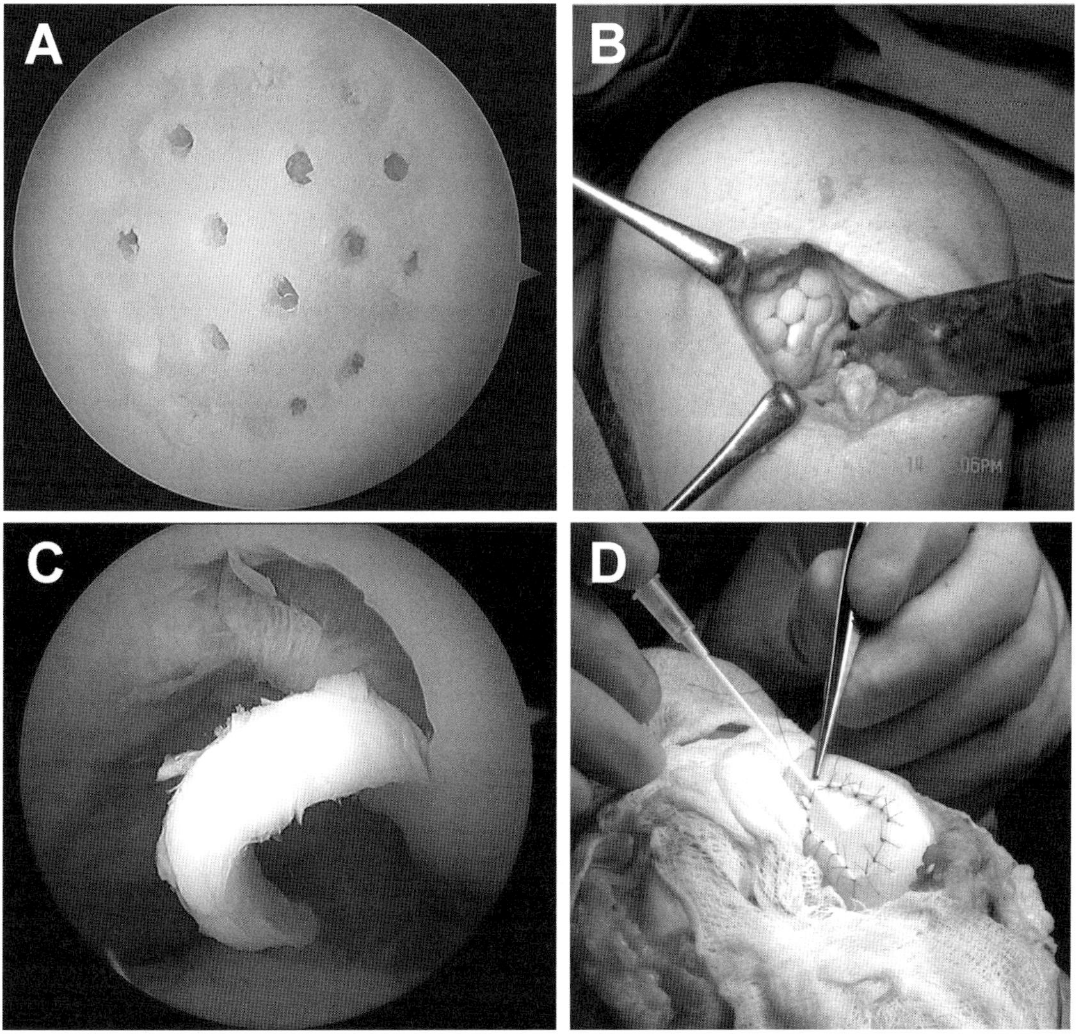

Figure 27.5 Current methods for biological articular cartilage repair. (A) Microfracture holes are created with an awl, after which tourniquet is released and blood floods the defect site. (B) Mosaicplasty of the medial femoral chondyle. (C) ACI: a cartilage biopsy is removed from a non-load-bearing donor site of the intercondyle notch from which chondrocytes are isolated. (D) ACI: a chondrocyte suspension is injected under a flap fixed over the defect site. Images adapted with permission from Gomoll *et al.* (2010) and Hangody *et al.* (2008).

27.3.1 Cells

Chondrocytes are the sole cell type in cartilage, and are therefore the primary cells of interest for cartilage regeneration and engineering. Chondrocytes isolated from articular cartilage produce tissue rich in proteoglycans (aggrecan, biglycan, decorin) and type II collagen. Important considerations for the use of chondrocytes for tissue engineering purposes include cell health and matrix-producing capacity as a function of zonal location (Hu and Athanasiou, 2006; Kim *et al.*, 2003; Ng *et al.*, 2009), patient age (Skaalure *et al.*, 2012;

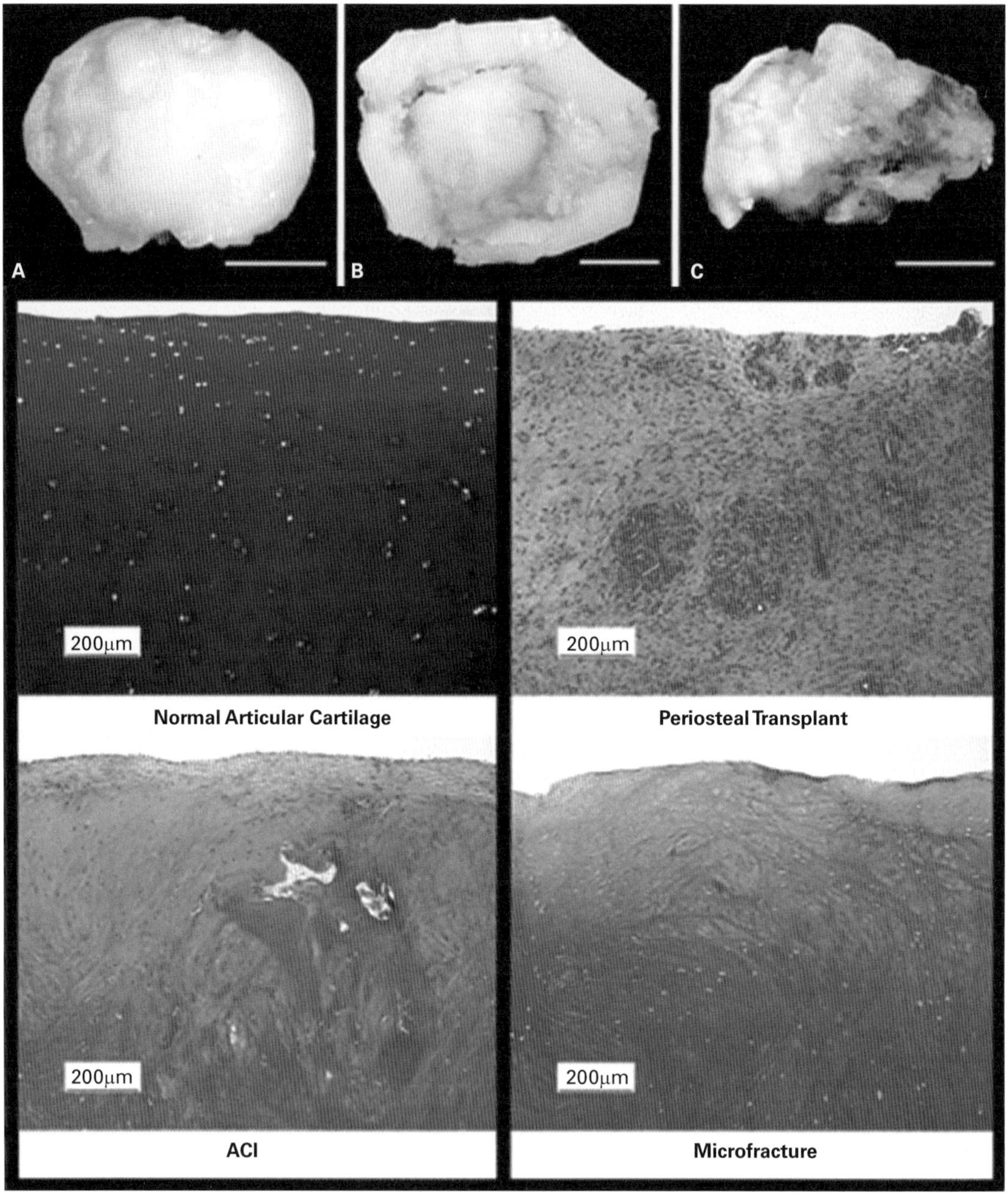

Figure 27.6 Top: gross appearance of human repair tissue from ACI (left), microfracture (center), and periosteal transplant (right). Bottom: toluidine blue staining of repair tissue from various repair techniques shows a decrease in staining intensity and increased levels of fibrous tissue ("200um" denotes 200 μm). Adapted from LaPrade *et al.* (2008) with permission.

Tran-Khanh *et al.*, 2005), disease state of the isolated tissue (Dorotka *et al.*, 2005a; Hsieh-Bonassera *et al.*, 2009), and phenotypic and metabolic changes as a result of expansion conditions (Benya and Shaffer, 1982; Heywood and Lee, 2010; Schiltz *et al.*, 1973).

One alternative to chondrocytes for cartilage tissue engineering applications is the use of chondrocyte progenitor cells such as embryonic stem cells (Toh *et al.*, 2011), adipose-derived stem cells (Estes *et al.*, 2010), synovium-derived stem cells (Jones and Pei, 2012), or bone-marrow-derived mesenchymal stem cells (Johnstone *et al.*, 1998; Mauck *et al.*, 2006; Pittenger *et al.*, 1999) (MSCs). The differentiation capacity of stem cells is impacted by factors including the tissue source (El Tamer and Reis, 2009), growth factor supplementation (Freyria and Mallein-Gerin, 2012), and oxygen tension (Adesida *et al.*, 2012; Malda *et al.*, 2003). Although chondrogenic stem cells hold promise for cartilage regeneration and tissue engineering applications, in-vivo hypertrophic terminal differentiation, marked by cell enlargement, production of types I and X collagen, increased alkaline phosphatase activity, cell apoptosis, and tissue mineralization (Pelttari *et al.*, 2006) remain significant challenges to be overcome before these cell types can find clinical application.

27.3.2 Growth factors

In essence, the role of growth factors in cartilage regeneration and tissue engineering is to enhance matrix production and promote chondrogenesis, reduce inflammatory responses and catabolic matrix degradation, and prevent hypertrophic differentiation. To accomplish this, media cocktails including one or more of the following growth factors have been used.

27.3.2.1 TGF-β superfamily

Members of the transforming growth factor-β (TGF-β) superfamily include TGF-β itself and bone morphogenetic proteins (BMPs). These factors are morphogens that activate SMAD signaling pathways and ultimately alter expression of cartilage-related genes (Watanabe *et al.*, 2001). TGF-β has been shown to initiate the expression of chondrogenic markers including SRY (sex-determining region Y)-box 9 (SOX9), cartilage oligomeric matrix protein (COMP), aggrecan, and type II collagen (Denker *et al.*, 1995; Johnstone *et al.*, 1998; Mauck *et al.*, 2006). The most frequently used isoforms for chondrogenic differentiation are TGF-β_1 (Cals *et al.*, 2012; Estes *et al.*; Johnstone *et al.*, 1998) and TGF-β_3 (Buckley *et al.*, 2012; Cals *et al.*, 2012; Huang *et al.*, 2010), although TGF-β_2 (Barry *et al.*, 2001; Cals *et al.*, 2012; Kim and Im, 2009) has also been used. BMPs can induce chondrogenic and osteogenic differentiation, depending on the context in which they are applied. BMPs used for cartilage tissue engineering include BMP-2,-4,-6, and-7 (Weiss *et al.*, 2010).

27.3.2.2 FGF, PTH-rP, IGF, dexamethasone

Other commonly used growth factors and steroids for cartilage regeneration and tissue engineering include the following.

(1) Fibroblast growth factor (FGF), which is categorized as a mitogen. The FGF isoforms which have been used to enhance proliferation, chondrogenesis, and osteogenesis include FGF-18 (Davidson *et al.*, 2005) and FGF-2 (Hellingman *et al.*, 2010; Hsieh-Bonassera *et al.*, 2009) (also referred to as basic fibroblast growth factor (bFGF)).
(2) Parathyroid hormone-related protein (PTH-rP), which is a protein that is used to promote chondrocyte proliferation and suppress terminal hypertrophic differentiation (Harrington *et al.*, 2004; Weiss *et al.*, 2010).
(3) Insulin-like growth factor (IGF), which is a chondrogenic anabolic factor that has been used to reduce chondrocyte apoptosis and increase matrix synthesis, particularly of proteoglycans (Guenther *et al.*, 1982; Starkman *et al.*, 2005).
(4) Dexamethasone, which is an anti-inflammatory steroidal hormone that is commonly used in culture in chemically defined media of tissue-engineered cartilage (Johnstone *et al.*, 1998; Mauck *et al.*, 2006; Ng *et al.*, 2009). Although dexamethasone has been shown to enhance chondrogenesis, it has also been linked to increased alkaline phosphatase activity (Johnstone *et al.*, 1998).

27.3.3 Materials

Biomaterials are instrumental for cartilage tissue engineering and regeneration. Their roles include providing immediate mechanical function in the cartilage lesion, serving as three-dimensional (3D) scaffolds to guide or enhance cell matrix deposition, and acting as delivery vehicles for controlled drug release. In the section to follow, examples of natural and synthetic materials used for cartilage regeneration and tissue engineering will be provided.

27.3.3.1 Classifications of materials and examples in cartilage regeneration and tissue engineering

27.3.3.1.1 Scaffold-free materials

Cartilage formation during development occurs via condensation of cells of the mesenchyme into high-density masses in the limb bud. Scaffold-free, or self-assembling, tissue replacements attempt to emulate this developmental process by aggregating cells into micromasses or high-density monolayer-type aggregates, supporting the chondrogenic phenotype and the production of de-novo cartilaginous matrix in vitro (Kim *et al.*, 2011; Natoli *et al.*, 2009; Solorio *et al.*, 2012). The result is the development of a dense, cartilaginous tissue. This method has been used both with chondrocytes and with MSCs, and is similar to clinical cell-based cartilage repair techniques such as ACI and microfracture, though in this formulation the initial tissue formation and condensation would be carried out prior to implantation.

27.3.3.1.2 Scaffold materials

Although it has been done less commonly, *metals* have been implanted in vivo into chondral defects in animal models. Such metals include oxidized zirconium (Custers *et al.*, 2010), cobalt-chromium (Custers *et al.*, 2009, 2010), porous tantalum (Mardones *et al.*, 2005; Mrosek *et al.*, 2010), and titanium (Karagianes *et al.*, 1975). While some success has been achieved in using metal implants to enhance bone integration as part of an osteochondral repair with cartilage overgrowth, the implantation of metals into cartilage lesion defects to prevent osteoarthritis progression has not been successful.

The primary use of *ceramics* in cartilage tissue engineering applications is within composite osteochondral grafts, where bone integration may contribute to implant success. Some examples include bioactive glasses (Jiang *et al.*, 2010), hydroxyapatite (Schek *et al.*, 2004; Tampieri *et al.*, 2008), and calcium phosphate (Guo *et al.*, 2004; Kandel *et al.*, 2006; Tanaka *et al.*, 2005).

Polymers are the most widely used materials for cartilage tissue engineering and regeneration. The versatility of polymers, such as their tunable mechanical and degradative properties, the possibility of hierarchical structure, and their controllable geometry, is instrumental for recreating the complex structure and function of cartilage.

Hydrogels are hydrophilic polymer networks that, depending on the polymer, may be formed through physical or chemical crosslinks. Hydrogels are porous and water-retentive, which is an important factor when one is attempting to regenerate or engineer a viscoelastic tissue with a high water content such as cartilage. Hydrogels used for cartilage tissue engineering include combinations of synthetic polymers created from polyethylene-glycol (PEG) and polyethylene-glycol diacrylate (PEG-DA) (Hwang *et al.*, 2011; Johnstone *et al.*, 1998; Nguyen *et al.*, 2012), polyglycolic acid (PGA) (Shahin and Doran, 2011; Terada *et al.*, 2005), and poly(lactic-*co*-glycolic acid) (PLGA) (Chang *et al.*, 2012; Spiller *et al.*, 2009, 2011). Naturally occurring polymers include those derived from mammalian species (type I collagen (Schulz *et al.*, 2008; Yuan *et al.*, 2010), type II collagen (Jurgens *et al.*, 2012), and hyaluronic acid (Chung *et al.*, 2008; Erickson *et al.*, 2012; Toh *et al.*, 2012)), polymers derived from other plants and fungi (e.g. agarose (Buckley *et al.*, 2012; Farrell *et al.*, 2012; Lima *et al.*, 2007), alginate (Coates *et al.*, 2012; Degala *et al.*, 2012; Estes *et al.*, 2010), and chitosan (Bhardwaj *et al.*, 2011; Lahiji *et al.*, 2000; Sechriest *et al.*, 2000)), and commercially available engineered proteins and composites (e.g. Puramatrix (Dickhut *et al.*, 2008; Erickson *et al.*, 2009; Maher *et al.*, 2010) and Matrigel (Basic *et al.*, 1996; Bradham *et al.*, 1995; Dickhut *et al.*, 2008)). Hydrogels are particularly

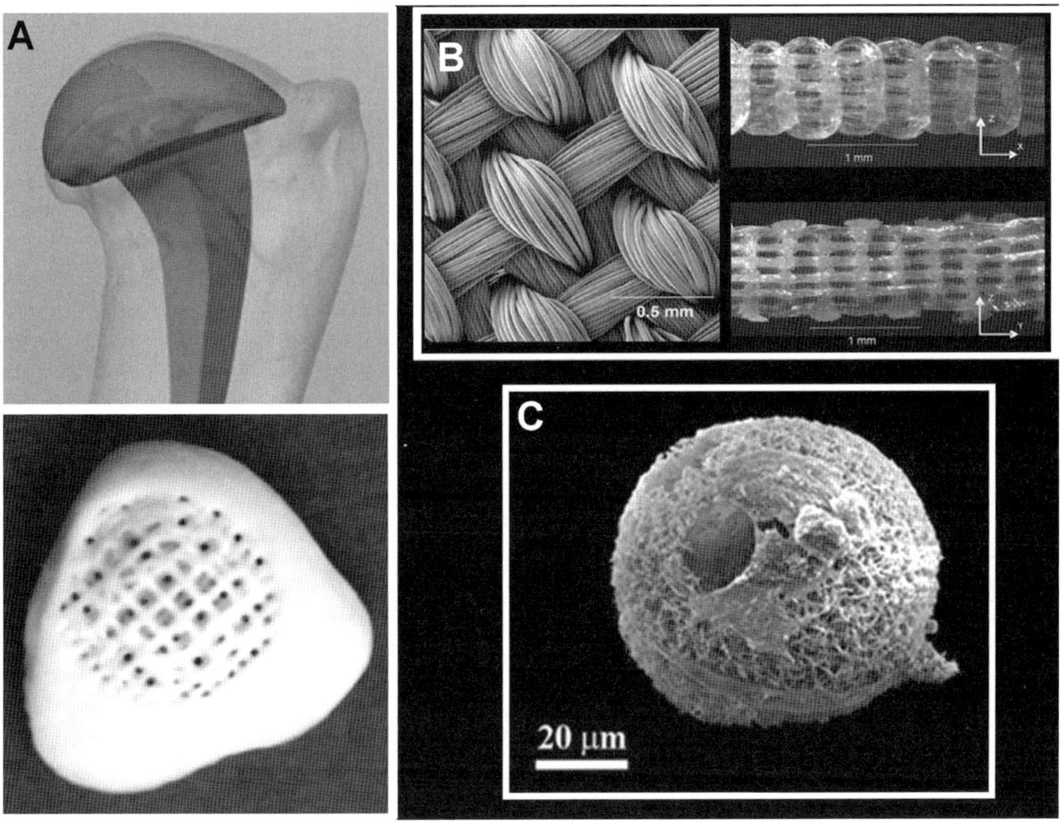

Figure 27.7 (A) An anatomically correct porous osteo- and chondro-inductive implant fabricated via computer-aided design and bioprinting. (B) A fibrous three-dimensional woven scaffold with anisotropic properties. (C) Nanofibrous hollow microspheres that support the chondrogenic phenotype and foster tissue repair in vivo. Images adapted from Lee *et al.* (2010), Moutos and Guilak (2010), and Liu *et al.* (2011), with permission.

beneficial for cartilage tissue engineering in that polymerization processes are often conducive to cell encapsulation.

Advances in fabrication techniques such as *textile* creation or controlled scaffold design via electrospinning, weaving, or microprinting have generated cartilage replacements with more advanced geometric shapes and hierarchical structures (Figure 27.7). These structures have the potential to provide immediate mechanical support to mimic the mechanical role of cartilage, or may function to allow cell infiltration and tissue integration. Examples of such scaffold designs used for cartilage repair are fibrous woven scaffolds with high tensile strength created using poly (ε-caprolactone) (PCL) (Moutos and Guilak, 2010) and anatomic 3D porous grafts created from PCL and hydroxyapatite composites (Lee *et al.*, 2010).

As noted above, growth factors can play a significant role in development and regeneration of cartilage. The porosity and degradability of polymers and the ability to functionalize, or attach moieties, to the polymers can provide spatial and temporal control of growth factor presentation. Examples of controlled growth factor release or presentation in cartilage tissue engineering and regeneration applications include growth factor incorporation into acellular constructs to enhance cell homing (Huang *et al.*, 2002), spatial release of growth factors (such as TGF-β and BMP) to control matrix development of biphasic osteochondral tissues (Re'em *et al.*, 2012), and temporal and sustained release of growth factors such as TGF-β_3 and PTH-rP from microspheres in vivo for the enhancement of chondrogenesis and prevention of terminal hypertrophic differentiation (Bian *et al.*, 2011), respectively.

Another polymer that is used for a variety of cartilage repair strategies is fibrin. Fibrin is a naturally occurring polymer that is active in the clotting cascade. Fibrin glue can be prepared from autologous plasma, or may be purchased from commercial sources. Owing to fibrin's ability to provide hemostasis, it has been used to reduce blood loss during total joint arthroplasty (Ahmed *et al.*, 2008; Thoms and Marwin, 2009). While fibrin glue has been used to attach loose cartilage fragments and to secure graft materials to defect sites (Kaplonyi *et al.*, 1988; McCormick *et al.*, 2008), it is more commonly used to aid in securing the periosteal or collagen-based flap for cell-based therapies such as ACI (Minas, 2001). However, the use of chondrocyte-seeded fibrin materials for cartilage repair has been reported (Deponti *et al.*, 2012; Hendrickson *et al.*, 1994; Sage *et al.*, 2009).

Composite scaffolds increase the potential for the formation of more complex tissue-engineered cartilage replacements. Osteochondral implants can be created from a mixture of different classes of materials, such as metals or ceramics spatially composited with a polymer to form a layered implant. However, where composites may be most beneficial is in their ability to overcome deficits of the primary structural component. Two such examples of constructs that benefit from polymer-polymer composites are the use of a hydrogel material as a cell delivery vehicle integrated into a mechanically supportive woven tissue-engineered construct where cell infiltration may be limited (Moutos *et al.*, 2007; Schatti *et al.*, 2011), and the use of secondary polymer networks that are swelled into a primary polymer hydrogel, forming a double network to synergistically increase the mechanical response of the gel (Yokota *et al.*, 2011). Fabrication techniques used for the development of polymer composites can be adopted to control porosity (Baker *et al.*, 2008) and/or create a more complex hierarchical design (Moutos *et al.*, 2007).

27.4 Animal models

Articular cartilage is exposed to a unique mechanical and nutritional environment in vivo. Although subcutaneous implantations in small-animal models (e.g. murine, lapine) serve well as screening tools for biocompatibility and proof-of-concept evaluation, larger-animal models provide the platform needed to test the long-term efficacy of tissue development and remodeling, integration, and mechanical performance. It is very difficult to accomplish work of this level of complexity in vitro, even with the most sophisticated bioreactors. In the sections to follow, various considerations relating to, and examples of, animal models used to study articular cartilage regeneration in the knee will be discussed.

27.4.1 Considerations for choice of animal model

The choice of animal model for cartilage regeneration strategies is dependent on a balance of cost, feasibility, and the nature of the research question being asked (Ahern *et al.*, 2009; ASTM, 2010; Chu *et al.*, 2010; Hurtig *et al.*, 2011; Reinholz *et al.*, 2004). The commonly used animal models for cartilage repair include mouse, rat, rabbit, dog, pig, sheep, goat, horse, and non-human primate (Ahern *et al.*, 2009; ASTM, 2010; Chu *et al.*, 2010; Hurtig *et al.*, 2011; Reinholz *et al.*, 2004). Below we will address some of the considerations that will influence model choice.

1. *Defect size/width.* A critically sized defect is necessary for the investigation of cartilage repair. In other repair situations (i.e. bone defects), the "critical size" is defined as the minimum defect size that is incapable of spontaneous regeneration and healing (Figure 27.8), and will vary from species to species. Since cartilage is incapable of healing a defect of almost any size once skeletal maturity has been reached, the definition of critical size in terms of cartilage repair more commonly refers to defect fill,

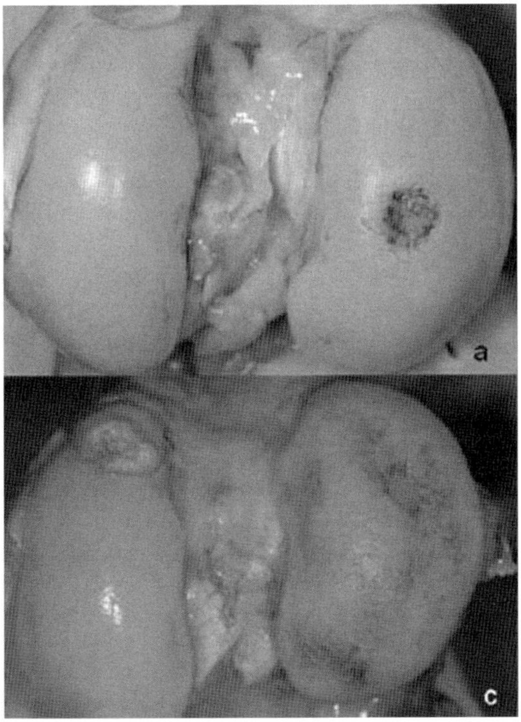

Figure 27.8 A critically sized defect (non-healing; 7 mm in ovine model) can cause progressive osteoarthritis after 6 (top) and 12 weeks (bottom). Fissures and defects are stained with India ink. Images adapted from Schinhan *et al.* (2012) with permission.

not the quality of the tissue forming within the defect. Above a certain threshold in size, defects of a "critical size" will remain void of any material.

2. *Cartilage thickness.* Cartilage thickness varies greatly with species, age, and location. Thin cartilage may result in difficulty in creating appropriate defects as well as difficulty in interpreting healing responses and repair efficacy.
3. *Defect thickness.* Defects can be created as partial or full-thickness defects or osteochondral defects. Although osteochondral defects are easier to execute and appear to be preferentially used in large-animal models, injury to the subchondral bone may result in undesirable tissue response and bone resorption. Furthermore, most clinical models of cartilage repair (i.e. ACI) protect the subchondral bone.
4. *Defect location.* Defect locations for cartilage repair include the femoral condyle, trochlear groove, tibial plateau, patella, and radial carpal. Femoral condyle defect sites are most commonly used. The loads experienced, cartilage thickness, and joint articulation can all vary with respect to location.
5. *Acute and chronic defects.* Osteoarthritis is a progressive catabolic disease that can be induced with the formation of a focal defect in an animal model. The timing of defect creation with respect to the timing of repair may therefore impact the repair potential. Although creation and repair of a fresh defect within a single session of surgery is more straightforward, it might not represent the clinical scenario. The creation of chronic defects and generation of an osteoarthritic pathology may therefore be necessary.
6. *Age.* The architecture, content, thickness, and healing response of cartilage vary with age. An animal that has reached cartilage maturity, as marked by zonal organization and decreased spontaneous healing capacity, is recommended. Cartilage maturity need not directly coincide with skeletal maturity, which is marked by the fusing of the epiphyseal plates.
7. *Cost and duration of study.* In addition to animal purchase costs, housing costs must be considered. Less costly small-animal models (murine and lapine) are adequate for proof-of-concept studies of repair and biocompatibility with study periods of 6–8 weeks. For assessment of the efficacy of cartilage repair, large-animal models with studies spanning at least 6–12 months are recommended; however, shorter periods of 8–12 weeks can serve to assess biocompatibility and the cellular response.
8. *Gait, weight, and anatomy.* Cartilage is a mechanically responsive tissue with mechanical function. Gait, weight, and anatomy (Figure 27.9) will have implications for joint kinematics and biomechanics, cartilage function, and cartilage repair.
9. *Postoperative care.* The activity level of the animal, its metabolic rate, and joint mobilization/immobilization all have the potential to impact the success

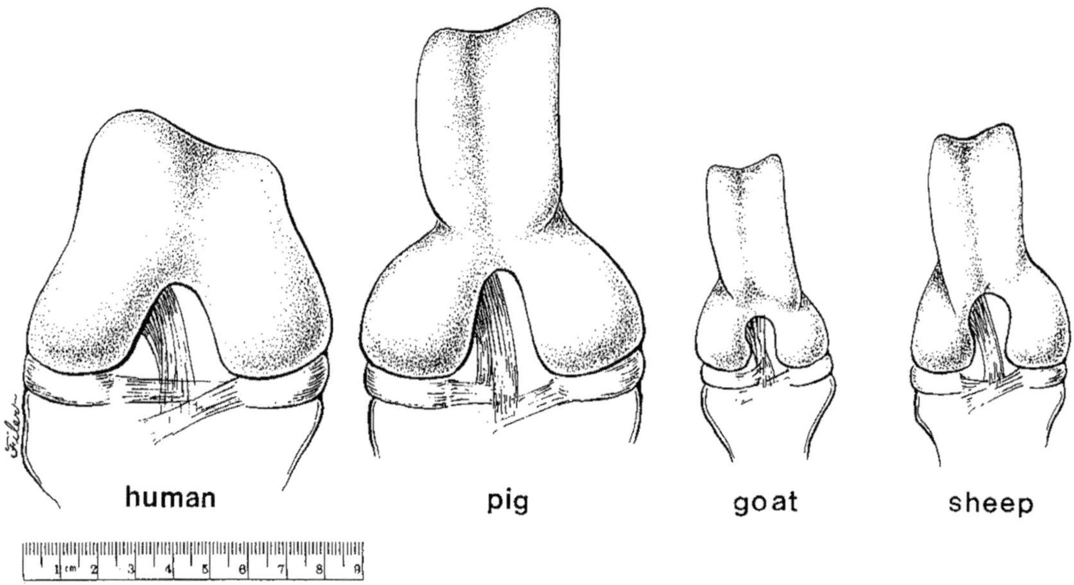

Figure 27.9 Artistic renderings of human, pig, goat, and sheep knees showing relative size and anatomy. Note: many of the porcine models for cartilage repair are minipig models, and therefore the joint size is smaller. Adapted from Xerogeanes *et al.* (1998) with permission.

of the implant and repair of the cartilage. These should at least be considered in the choice of animal, as should the design of the repair strategy, with the overall goal being to best approximate the expected therapeutic post-cartilage-repair procedures applied to humans (which generally consist of a period of non-weight-bearing activity).

27.4.2 Species

With the aforementioned considerations for choice of animal model in mind, Table 27.1 outlines some of the characteristics of each candidate species, with examples of biomaterials that have been implanted in the large-animal models outlined in Table 27.2. Below, some of the advantages and disadvantages of each species are highlighted.

1. *Murine.* Mouse and rat models are valuable for safety and biocompatibility studies. Availability and low cost are advantages of these models. Furthermore, genetic manipulations provide the opportunity to examine disease models and the role of specific pathways in cartilage repair. However, the disadvantages are that these animals have small joints with thin cartilage and purely chondral defects of a critical size are difficult to create.
2. *Lapine.* The advantages and disadvantages of lapine models are similar to those of murine ones in that the animals are easily obtained at low cost; however, they have small joints and thin cartilage. Furthermore, the high metabolic rate of rabbits can affect drug metabolism, in addition to resulting in accelerated healing responses. As a result, defects in lapine cartilage can heal spontaneously.
3. *Canine.* The advantages of canine models include arthroscopic accessibility of the knee joint. Veterinary experience, extensive knowledge of GI physiology, and easy postoperative management are also advantages. Thin cartilage as well as public

Table 27.1 Characteristics of species used for cartilage repair models

	Murine	Lapine	Canine	Porcine	Ovine	Caprine	Equine
Age of adult equivalency		9 months	>1–2 years	10 months to 1 year	2–3 years	2–3 years	2–4 years
Cartilage thickness (mm)	0.1	0.25–0.75	0.95–1.3	1.5	1.7	1.1–2	2–3
Critical-size defect (mm)	3 (in xiphoid process of rat)	3	4[a]	6.3	7	6	9

[a] No study pinpointing the canine critical-size defect was found, but defects 2 mm in size did not heal spontaneously (Shortkroff *et al.*, 1996). According to Ahern *et al.* (2009), 4 mm is a common size.

The data are from Ahern *et al.* (2009), ASTM (2010), Frisbie *et al.* (2006), Gotterbarm *et al.* (2008), Jackson *et al.* (2001), and Shortkroff *et al.* (1996).

disapproval of the use of these animals in a research setting are among the disadvantages.

4. *Porcine.* Larger joint size and the lower level of ethical concern of the public make these animals a feasible alternative when large-animal housing facilities are limited. Thin cartilage, large size, aggressiveness, and difficult handling are disadvantages; however, the use of miniature pig strains can alleviate some of these limitations.
5. *Ovine.* As a large-animal model, sheep are less expensive than equine models, and they have similar knee anatomy to humans, and thicker cartilage than porcine models. However, the difficulty of postoperative care, relatively high likelihood of disease, and variability of animal quality and cartilage are disadvantages with the use of sheep.
6. *Caprine.* Caprine models are popular for cartilage repair given their larger joint size and relatively thick cartilage compared with smaller-animal models. Cost makes caprine models a more feasible option for large-animal studies than equine models. The difficulty of postoperative care and weight-bearing control in addition to difficulties with arthroscopic accessibility are disadvantages.
7. *Equine.* Equine models are advantageous in that there is a market for cartilage repair in horses, horses have thicker cartilage, larger and more clinically relevant sized defects can be created, and the joint can be arthroscopically examined. Cost and availability, in addition to size, safety, compartmentalized joints, and postoperative care are disadvantages of equine models.
8. *Non-human primates.* Although midsized-to-large non-human primates may have the most anatomically relevant joints for pre-clinical assessment of cartilage repair, their use in cartilage repair studies has been limited due to cost, availability, and public opposition. However, a few studies have been conducted in smaller non-human primate models (Gill *et al.*, 2005; Girdler, 1997; Robinson, 1993).

27.4.3 Study outcomes

The *ASTM Standard Guide for in vivo Assessment of Implantable Devices Intended to Repair or Regenerate Articular Cartilage* suggests that outcome measures for cartilage repair studies include histology, biochemical content, and mechanical testing of repair tissue (ASTM, 2010; Hoemann *et al.*, 2011). Histological assessment allows spatial characterization of repair response, cell presence, and the characterization of the type of repair tissue elaborated. The histological stains suggested in these guidelines include Weigerts, hemotoxylin and eosin, and modified trichrome (used with or without the combination of analine blue for the staining of collagens) for overall tissue integrity, and Safranin-O and toluidine blue for detection of proteoglycans. Scoring systems such as the ICRS-II system

Table 27.2 Examples of biomaterials used in large-animal models

Biomaterial	Species	Defect type/location	Cells seeded	Study duration	Reference
Fibrin	Horse	Full thickness/trochlea	Chondrocytes	8 months	Hendrickson *et al.* (1994)
Type I collagen hydrogel	Horse	Osteochondral/trochlea	Chondrocytes	8 months	Sams and Nixon (1995)
Polyglactin/polydioxanone	Horse	Full thickness/tubular condyle	Chondrocytes	12 months	Barnewitz *et al.* (2006)
Layered collagen fibrils/hydroxyapatite nanoparticles	Horse	Osteochondral/metacarpal bone epiphysis	None	6 months	Kon *et al.* (2010)
Poly(D,L)lactide-*co*-glycolide + PGA fibers, bioglass, or calcium sulfate	Goat	Osteochondral/medial femoral condyle and patellar grove	Chondrocytes	16 weeks	Niederauer *et al.* (2000)
Crosslinkable elastin-like polypeptide	Goat	Osteochondral/medial femoral condyle	Acellular	6 months	Nettles *et al.* (2008)
Porous methoxypolyethyleneglycol/ poly(lactic-*co*-glycolic) scaffold + fibrin hydrogel	Goat	Osteochondral/femoral condyle	Chondrocytes	4 months	Lind *et al.* (2008)
Hyaluronic acid (HYAFF-11)	Goat	Osteochondral/trochlea	Chondrocytes	8 months	Miot *et al.* (2012)
Chitosan–glycerol phosphate + blood clot	Sheep	Full thickness + microfracture/femoral condyle, trochlea	Marrow cells, microfracture	6 months	Hoemann *et al.* (2005)
Type I + type II + type III collagen	Sheep	Full thickness + microfracture/medial condyle	Chondrocytes + microfracture	16 weeks	Dorotka *et al.* (2005b)
β-Tricalcium phosphate	Sheep	Full thickness/medial condyle	Mesenchymal stem cells	24 weeks	Guo *et al.* (2004)
Cell/matrix layer + calcium polyphosphate	Sheep	Full thickness/trochlear grove	Chondrocytes	9 months	Kandel *et al.* (2006)
Polyglycolic acid/polylactic acid	Pig	Osteochondral/trochlea	Mesenchymal stem cells	6 months	Zhou *et al.* (2006)
Scaffold-free	Pig	Partial thickness/medial condyle	Mesenchymal stem cell aggregate	6 months	Ando *et al.* (2007)
Poly(D,L-lactic acid-*co*-glycolide) + β-tricalcium phosphate	Pig	Osteochondral/condyle	Chondrocytes	6 months	Jiang *et al.* (2007)
Electrospun polycaprolactone + polycaprolactone + tricalcium phosphate	Pig	Osteochondral/medial condyle, petellar grove	Mesenchymal stem cells	6 months	Ho *et al.* (2010)
Type I collagen–GAG copolymer, type II collagen–GAG copolymer	Dog	Full thickness/trochlear grove	Chondrocytes	15 weeks	Nehrer *et al.* (1998)

Table 27.2 (cont.)

Biomaterial	Species	Defect type/location	Cells seeded	Study duration	Reference
Decellularized cartilage/decellularized bone matrix	Dog	Osteochondral/femoral condyles	MSCs	6 months	Yang *et al.* (2011)
Periosteum covering	Dog	Full thickness/medial femoral condyle	No additional cells	16 weeks	Sung *et al.* (2011)
Atelocollagen gel	Dog	Full thickness/femoral condyle	MSCs	10 weeks	Yamazoe *et al.* (2007)

(Mainil-Varlet *et al.*, 2010) and the O'Driscoll (O'Driscoll *et al.*, 2001) system can be used to evaluate tissue quality, surface appearance, cell morphology and number, integration, and subchondral bone quality in a semi-quantitative fashion. Concomitantly, the International Cartilage Repair Society (Hoemann *et al.*, 2011) suggests immunostaining of collagen type I and type II, in addition to polarized light microscopy to evaluate collagen type and organization.

Outcome measures that provide more information regarding the function of the repair tissue include biochemical quantification of the matrix constituents and mechanical evaluation of material properties of the regenerated articular cartilage. Of particular biochemical interest is the quantification of proteoglycans and collagens (preferentially type II) in the tissue. These molecules are particularly important for mechanical function. Common mechanical testing modalities of native cartilage and repair tissue include confined and unconfined compression, indentation, tension, shear, and push-out tests; however, confined compression stress relaxation and creep tests as described by Mow *et al.* (1980) are preferred in the ASTM standards as means to characterize the viscoelastic nature of the tissue, enabling calculation of the aggregate modulus and tissue permeability. These tests can be difficult to perform, however, insofar as they require the excision and preparation of a sample of uniform and consistent geometry. For this reason, indentation testing, coupled with finite-element analyses, is commonly performed at the intact defect site.

By far the most important, yet most difficult, issue with respect to cartilage repair outcomes is that of how to assess functional success and pain reduction. Score systems used for the clinical assessment of pain reduction and functional gain after cartilage repair include the International Knee Documentation Committee Score (IKDC) (Irrgang *et al.*, 2001), magnetic resonance observation of cartilage repair tissue (MOCART) (Marlovits *et al.*, 2004, 2006), Lysholm and Tegner scores (Kocher *et al.*, 2004; Smith *et al.*, 2009; Tegner and Lysholm, 1985), and the Visual Analogue Pain Score (VAS). For the assessment of pain in animal models, researchers must focus on behavior and physiological changes such as alterations in gait patterns, weight bearing, and changes in muscle mass, though, to date, such measures remain to be formalized in a widely accepted grading system.

27.5 Clinical studies and biomaterials for cartilage repair

Given the moderate success of cell-based therapies, such as ACI and microfracture, biomaterial-based therapies have continued to be developed with the goal of addressing the limitations associated with these techniques. In this section, we will highlight some of the biomaterial-based therapies actively being used in the clinic, as well as several emerging technologies now in clinical and pre-clinical trials.

One such therapy being used clinically, the MACI® Implant, is a matrix-associated derivative of Genzyme's Carticel treatment and is currently being marketed in Europe, Asia, and Australia, although it is not yet available in the USA. MACI utilizes a base collagen scaffold on which the isolated and expanded chondrocytes are seeded. This cell-seeded collagen membrane is then secured in the cartilage defect with the use of fibrin glue. The collagen membrane securely localizes the chondrocytes within the defect site and overcomes the need for a periosteal flap as used for ACI. Similar repair strategies to MACI include BioCart™ (ProChon Biotech Ltd), where chondrocytes are expanded in a proprietary growth factor cocktail and then seeded onto 3D human-derived scaffold sponges before being implanted into the defect site; Histogenics' Neo-Cart®, consisting of ex-vivo cultured chondrocytes and a collagen scaffold; and VeriCart™, an acellular collagen scaffold implant.

Although, in tissue engineering, biomaterials are often regarded as synthetic materials used for the scaffold component of a replacement, de-novo formation of matrix by cells may also be considered an implantable biomaterial. Products such as DeNovo ET (Zimmer and ISTO), the apparent derivative of Zimmer's Chondrofix and juvenile allograft DeNovo NT, make use of scaffold-less tissue development to create a de-novo chondrocyte-based tissue for implantation. An additional treatment, the co.don chondrosphere® (co.don AG), also creates a scaffold-less tissue replacement; however, cell culture is conducted in a cell aggregate to create dense chondrocyte spheroids.

Finally, biomaterials have been used in an attempt to increase the success of cartilage formed from marrow-derived cells. Some materials such as BST-CarGel, a chitosan gel, and ChonDux, a photo-crosslinkable gel of PEG and hyaluronic acid, are intended for the stabilization of clots formed during microfracture procedures. A slightly more complex system, INSTRUCT (Cell), aims to develop a contained system for clinical use that involves the infiltration of autologous chondrocytes and bone marrow cells into a mechanically functional scaffold that is then implanted into the patient in a single surgical procedure.

27.6 Summary – The future of cartilage repair

To date, there has been limited success in long-term clinical repair of cartilage defects, and the door remains wide open for the development of a successful, biologically based repair technique. It is likely that the future of cartilage repair will involve the delivery of chondrocytes, chondro-progenitor cells, or stem cells, in combination with a biocompatible scaffold and growth factors. On the cusp of pre-clinical and clinical models, there exists an array of biomaterials that support cartilage matrix elaboration. For example, there has been much success in the in-vitro development of cartilage constructs with mechanical properties that are similar to native tissue using adult stem cells (bovine bone-marrow-derived) encapsulated in hyaluronic acid hydrogels (Erickson *et al.*, 2012). Additionally, in-vivo implantation of pre-differentiated mesenchymal stem cells encapsulated in a collagen hydrogel has resulted in moderate improvement in comparison with untreated or chondrocyte controls after a year of follow-up in an ovine model (Figure 27.10) (Marquass *et al.*, 2011). In a porcine model, a synthetic oligo[poly(ethylene glycol)fumarate] scaffold was used for the treatment of osteochondritis dissecans (Hui *et al.*, 2012). In years to come, the pre-clinical success of these and similar treatments may result in total joint arthroplasty becoming an archaic technique. Such an eventuality would transform the chronic and one-way progression of osteoarthritis into a treatable condition wherein biological regeneration of joint surfaces restores mobility and function to the large and growing population suffering from articular cartilage pathology.

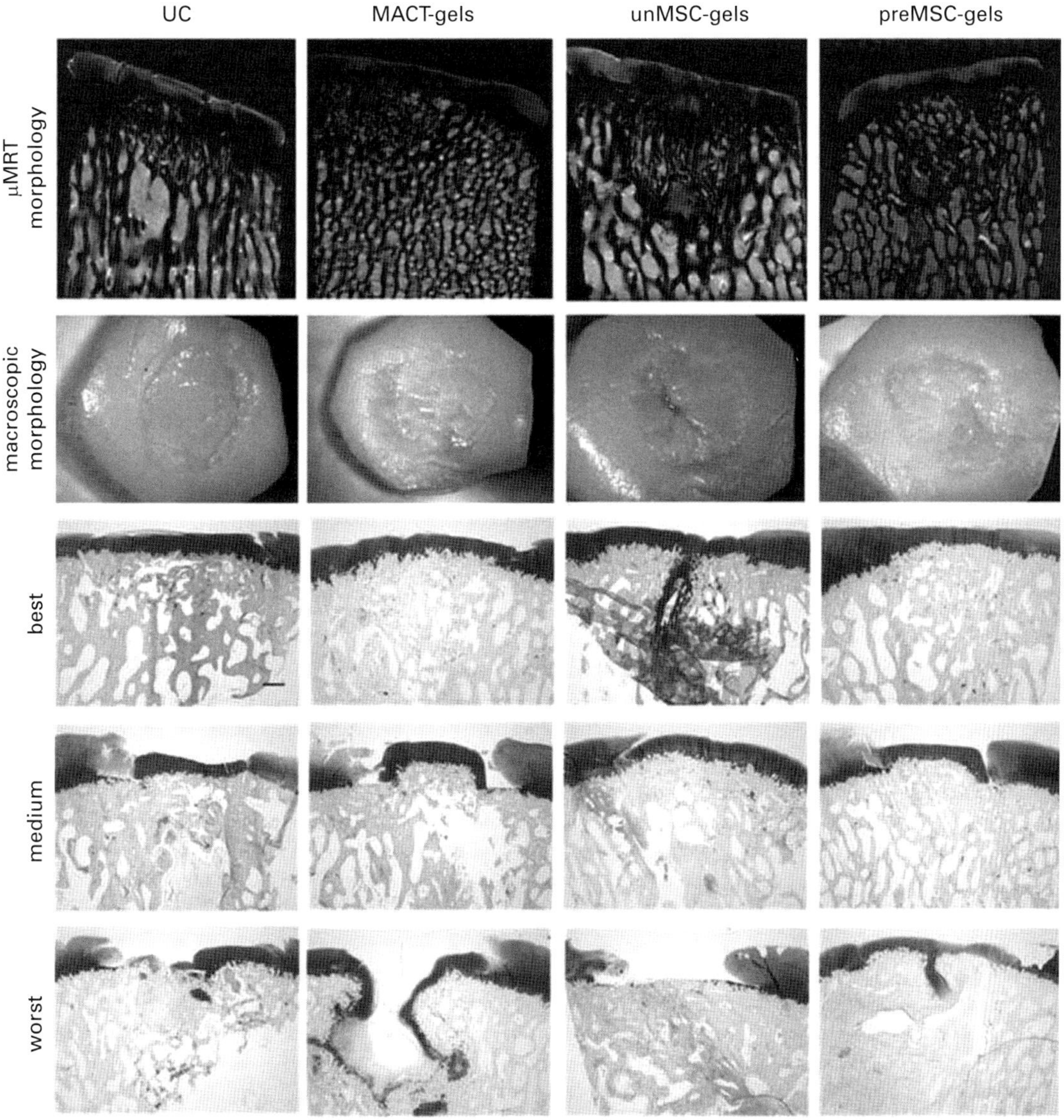

Figure 27.10 Microradiographic images (top), gross appearance (middle), and toluidine blue staining (bottom, proteoglycan) of unfilled controls, matrix-associated chondrocyte transplantation (MACT), and undifferentiated (unMSC) and pre-differentiated (preMSC) mesenchymal stem cells in a type I collagen hydrogel one year after implantation in an ovine model. Scale bar = 1 mm. Adapted from Marquass *et al.* (2011) with permission.

ACKNOWLEDGEMENTS

This work was supported by the National Institutes of Health (R01 EB008722) and the Penn Center for Musculoskeletal Disorders. The authors would like to thank Dr. Matt Fisher and Dr. Lachlan Smith for their critical reading of this work.

REFERENCES

Adesida, A. B., Mulet-Sierra, A. and Jomha, N. M. 2012. Hypoxia mediated isolation and expansion enhances the chondrogenic capacity of bone marrow mesenchymal stromal cells. *Stem Cell Res. Ther.*, **3**, 9.

Ahern, B. J., Parvizi, J., Boston, R. and Schaer, T. P. 2009. Preclinical animal models in single site cartilage defect testing: a systematic review. *Osteoarthritis Cartilage*, **17**, 705–13.

Ahmed, T. A., Dare, E. V. and Hincke, M. 2008. Fibrin: a versatile scaffold for tissue engineering applications. *Tissue Eng. Part B Rev.*, **14**, 199–215.

Ando, W., Tateishi, K., Hart, D. A. *et al.* 2007. Cartilage repair using an in vitro generated scaffold-free tissue-engineered construct derived from porcine synovial mesenchymal stem cells. *Biomaterials*, **28**, 5462–70.

Armstrong, C. G. and Mow, V. C. 1982. Variations in the intrinsic mechanical properties of human articular cartilage with age, degeneration, and water content. *J. Bone Joint Surg. Am.*, **64**, 88–94.

ASTM 2010. *Standard Guide for* in vivo *Assessment of Implantable Devices Intended to Repair or Regenerate Articular Cartilage.* West Conshohocken, PA: ASTM International.

Athanasiou, K. A., Rosenwasser, M. P., Buckwalter, J. A., Malinin, T. I. and Mow, V. C. 1991. Interspecies comparisons of *in situ* intrinsic mechanical properties of distal femoral cartilage. *J. Orthop. Res.*, **9**, 330–40.

Baker, B. M., Gee, A. O., Metter, R. B. *et al.* 2008. The potential to improve cell infiltration in composite fiber-aligned electrospun scaffolds by the selective removal of sacrificial fibers. *Biomaterials*, **29**, 2348–58.

Barnewitz, D., Endres, M., Kruger, I. *et al.* 2006. Treatment of articular cartilage defects in horses with polymer-based cartilage tissue engineering grafts. *Biomaterials*, **27**, 2882–9.

Barry, F., Boynton, R. E., Liu, B. and Murphy, J. M. 2001. Chondrogenic differentiation of mesenchymal stem cells from bone marrow: differentiation-dependent gene expression of matrix components. *Exp. Cell Res.*, **268**, 189–200.

Basić, N., Basić, V., Bulić, K. *et al.* 1996. TGF-β and basement membrane matrigel stimulate the chondrogenic phenotype in osteoblastic cells derived from fetal rat calvaria. *J. Bone Miner. Res.*, **11**, 384–91.

Benya, P. D. and Shaffer, J. D. 1982. Dedifferentiated chondrocytes reexpress the differentiated collagen phenotype when cultured in agarose gels. *Cell*, **30**, 215–24.

Bhardwaj, N., Nguyen, Q. T., Chen, A. C. *et al.* 2011. Potential of 3-D tissue constructs engineered from bovine chondrocytes/silk fibroin-chitosan for in vitro cartilage tissue engineering. *Biomaterials*, **32**, 5773–81.

Bian, L., Zhai, D. Y., Tous, E. 2011. Enhanced MSC chondrogenesis following delivery of TGF-β_3 from alginate microspheres within hyaluronic acid hydrogels in vitro and in vivo. *Biomaterials*, **32**, 6425–34.

Bowles, R. D., Gebhard, H. H., Hartl, R. and Bonassar, L. J. 2011. Tissue-engineered intervertebral discs produce new matrix, maintain disc height, and restore biomechanical function to the rodent spine. *Proc. Nat. Acad. Sci. USA*, **108**, 13106–11.

Bradham, D. M., Passaniti, A. and Horton, W. E. Jr. 1995. Mesenchymal cell chondrogenesis is stimulated by basement membrane matrix and inhibited by age-associated factors. *Matrix Biol.*, **14**, 561–71.

Brodin, H. 1955. Paths of nutrition in articular cartilage and intervertebral discs. *Acta Orthop. Scand.*, **24**, 177–83.

Buckley, C. T., Meyer, E. G. and Kelly, D. J. 2012. The influence of construct scale on the composition and functional properties of cartilaginous tissues engineered using bone marrow-derived mesenchymal stem cells. *Tissue Eng. Part A*, **18**, 382–96.

Cals, F. L., Hellingman, C. A., Koevoet, W., Baatenburg de Jong, R. J. and van Osch, G. J. 2012. Effects of transforming growth factor-β subtypes on in vitro cartilage production and mineralization of human bone marrow stromal-derived mesenchymal stem cells. *J. Tissue Eng. Regen. Med.*, **6**, 68–76.

Carr, A. J., Robertsson, O., Graves, S. *et al.* 2012 Knee replacement. *Lancet*, **379**, 1331–40.

Chang, N. J., Jhung, Y. R., Yao, C. K. and Yeh, M. L. 2012. Hydrophilic gelatin and hyaluronic acid-treated PLGA scaffolds for cartilage tissue engineering. *J. Appl. Biomater. Function. Mater.*, **11**(1), e45–52.

Chu, C. R., Szczodry, M. and Bruno, S. 2010. Animal models for cartilage regeneration and repair. *Tissue Eng. Part B Rev.*, **16**, 105–15.

Chung, C., Erickson, I. E., Mauck, R. L. and Burdick, J. A. 2008. Differential behavior of auricular and articular chondrocytes in hyaluronic acid hydrogels. *Tissue Eng. Part A*, **14**, 1121–31.

Coates, E. E., Riggin, C. N. and Fisher, J. P. 2012. Matrix molecule influence on chondrocyte phenotype and proteoglycan 4 expression by alginate-embedded zonal chondrocytes and mesenchymal stem cells. *J. Orthop. Res.*, **30**(12), 1886–97.

Custers, R. J., Dhert, W. J., Saris, D. B. *et al.* 2010. Cartilage degeneration in the goat knee caused by treating localized cartilage defects with metal implants. *Osteoarthritis Cartilage*, **18**, 377–88.

Custers, R. J., Saris, D. B., Dhert, W. J. *et al.* 2009. Articular cartilage degeneration following the treatment of focal cartilage defects with ceramic metal implants and compared with microfracture. *J. Bone Joint Surg. Am.*, **91**, 900–10.

Davidson, D., Blanc, A., Filion, D. *et al.* 2005. Fibroblast growth factor (FGF) 18 signals through FGF receptor 3 to promote chondrogenesis. *J. Biol. Chem.*, **280**, 20509–15.

Degala, S., Williams, R., Zipfel, W. and Bonassar, L. J. 2012. Calcium signaling in response to fluid flow by chondrocytes in 3D alginate culture. *J. Orthop. Res.*, **30**, 793–9.

Denker, A. E., Nicoll, S. B. and Tuan, R. S. 1995. Formation of cartilage-like spheroids by micromass cultures of murine C3H10T1/2 cells upon treatment with transforming growth factor-β_1. *Differentiation*, **59**, 25–34.

Deponti, D., Di Giancamillo, A., Mangiavini, L. *et al.* 2012. Fibrin-based model for cartilage regeneration: tissue maturation from in vitro to in vivo. *Tissue Eng. Part A*, **18**, 1109–22.

Dickhut, A., Gottwald, E., Steck, E., Heisel, C. and Richter, W. 2008. Chondrogenesis of mesenchymal stem cells in gel-like biomaterials in vitro and in vivo. *Front. Biosci.*, **13**, 4517–28.

Dorotka, R., Bindreiter, U., Vavken, P. and Nehrer, S. 2005a. Behavior of human articular chondrocytes derived from nonarthritic and osteoarthritic cartilage in a collagen matrix. *Tissue Eng.*, **11**, 877–86.

Dorotka, R., Windberger, U., Macfelda, K. *et al.* 2005b. Repair of articular cartilage defects treated by microfracture and a three-dimensional collagen matrix. *Biomaterials*, **26**, 3617–29.

El Tamer, M. K. and Reis, R. L. 2009. Progenitor and stem cells for bone and cartilage regeneration. *J. Tissue Eng. Regen. Med.*, **3**, 327–37.

Erickson, I. E., Huang, A. H., Chung, C. *et al.* 2009. Differential maturation and structure–function relationships in mesenchymal stem cell- and chondrocyte-seeded hydrogels. *Tissue Eng. Part A*, **15**, 1041–52.

Erickson, I. E., Kestle, S. R., Zellars, K. H. *et al.* 2012. High mesenchymal stem cell seeding densities in hyaluronic acid hydrogels produce engineered cartilage with native tissue properties. *Acta Biomater.*, **8**, 3027–34.

Estes, B. T., Diekman, B. O., Gimble, J. M. and Guilak, F. 2010. Isolation of adipose-derived stem cells and their induction to a chondrogenic phenotype. *Nature Protoc.*, **5**, 1294–311.

Farrell, M. J., Comeau, E. S. and Mauck, R. L. 2012. Mesenchymal stem cells produce functional cartilage matrix in three-dimensional culture in regions of optimal nutrient supply. *Eur. Cell Mater.*, **23**, 425–40.

Fening, S. D., Mihnovets, J., Jones, M. H., Midura, R. J. and Miniaci, A. 2011. The effect of storage medium tonicity on osteochondral autograft plug diameter. *Arthroscopy*, **27**, 188–93.

Flandry, F. and Hommel, G. 2011. Normal anatomy and biomechanics of the knee. *Sports Med. Arthrosc.*, **19**, 82–92.

Freeman, M. A. R. 1979. *Adult Articular Cartilage*. Tunbridge Wells: Pitman Medical.

Freyria, A. M. and Mallein-Gerin, F. 2012. Chondrocytes or adult stem cells for cartilage repair: the indisputable role of growth factors. *Injury*, **43**, 259–65.

Frisbie, D. D., Cross, M. W. and McIlwraith, C. W. 2006. A comparative study of articular cartilage thickness in the stifle of animal species used in human pre-clinical studies compared to articular cartilage thickness in the human knee. *Vet. Comp. Orthop. Traumatol.*, **19**, 142–6.

Gill, T. J., McCulloch, P. C., Glasson, S. S., Blanchet, T. and Morris, E. A. 2005. Chondral defect repair after the microfracture procedure: a nonhuman primate model. *Am. J. Sports Med.*, **33**, 680–5.

Girdler, N. M. 1997. The role of mandibular condylar cartilage in articular cartilage repair. *Ann. R. Coll. Surg. Engl.*, **79**, 28–37.

Gomoll, A. H. 2012. Microfracture and augments. *J. Knee Surg.*, **25**, 9–15.

Gomoll, A. H., Farr, J., Gillogly, S. D., Kercher, J. and Minas, T. 2010. Surgical management of articular cartilage defects of the knee. *J. Bone Joint Surg. Am.*, **92**, 2470–90.

Gomoll, A. H. and Minas, T. 2011. Debridement, microfracture, and osteochondral autograft transfer for treatment of cartilage defects. In Minas, T., editor. *A Primer in Cartilage Repair and Joint Preservation of the Knee*. Philadelphia, PA: Saunders, pp. 48–53.

Gotterbarm, T., Breusch, S. J., Schneider, U. and Jung, M. 2008. The minipig model for experimental chondral and osteochondral defect repair in tissue engineering: retrospective analysis of 180 defects. *Lab. Anim.*, **42**, 71–82.

Gray, H. and Goss, C. M. 1973. *Anatomy of the Human Body*. Philadelphia, PA: Lea & Febiger.

Guenther, H. L., Guenther, H. E., and Froesch, E. R. and Fleisch, H. 1982. Effect of insulin-like growth factor on collagen and glycosaminoglycan synthesis by rabbit articular chondrocytes in culture. *Experientia*, **38**, 979–81.

Guo, X., Wang, C., Zhang, Y. *et al.* 2004. Repair of large articular cartilage defects with implants of autologous mesenchymal stem cells seeded into β-tricalcium phosphate in a sheep model. *Tissue Eng.*, **10**, 1818–29.

Hangody, L., Vasarhelyi, G., Hangody, L. R. *et al.* 2008. Autologous osteochondral grafting - technique and long-term results. *Injury*, **39**(Suppl. 1), S32–9.

Harrington, E. K., Lunsford, L. E. and Svoboda, K. K. 2004. Chondrocyte terminal differentiation, apoptosis, and type X collagen expression are downregulated by parathyroid hormone. *Anat. Rec. A Discov. Molec. Cell Evol. Biol.*, **281**, 1286–95.

Heir, S., Nerhus, T. K., Rotterud, J. H. *et al.* 2010. Focal cartilage defects in the knee impair quality of life as much as severe osteoarthritis: a comparison of knee injury and osteoarthritis outcome score in 4 patient categories scheduled for knee surgery. *Am. J. Sports Med.*, **38**, 231–7.

Hellingman, C. A., Koevoet, W., Kops, N. *et al.* 2010. Fibroblast growth factor receptors in in vitro and in vivo chondrogenesis: relating tissue engineering using adult mesenchymal stem cells to embryonic development. *Tissue Eng. Part A*, **16**, 545–56.

Hendrickson, D. A., Nixon, A. J., Grande, D. A. *et al.* 1994. Chondrocyte-fibrin matrix transplants for resurfacing extensive articular cartilage defects. *J. Orthop. Res.*, **12**, 485–97.

Heywood, H. K. and Lee, D. A. 2010. Low oxygen reduces the modulation to an oxidative phenotype in monolayer-expanded chondrocytes. *J. Cell Physiol.*, **222**, 248–53.

Ho, S. T., Hutmacher, D. W., Ekaputra, A. K., Hitendra, D. and Hui, J. H. 2010. The evaluation of a biphasic osteochondral implant coupled with an electrospun membrane in a large animal model. *Tissue Eng. Part A*, **16**, 1123–41.

Hoemann, C. D., Hurtig, M., Rossomacha, E. *et al.* 2005. Chitosan-glycerol phosphate/blood implants improve hyaline cartilage repair in ovine microfracture defects. *J. Bone Joint Surg. Am.*, **87**, 2671–86.

Hoemann, C. D., Kandel, R. A., Roberts, S. *et al.* 2011. International Cartilage Repair Society (ICRS) recommended guidelines for histological endpoints for cartilage repair in animal studies in animal models and clinical trials. *Cartilage*, **2**, 153–72.

Hsieh-Bonassera, N. D., Wu, I., Lin, J. K. *et al.* 2009. Expansion and redifferentiation of chondrocytes from osteoarthritic cartilage: cells for human cartilage tissue engineering. *Tissue Eng. Part A*, **15**, 3513–23.

Hu, J. C. and Athanasiou, K. A. 2006. Chondrocytes from different zones exhibit characteristic differences in high density culture. *Connect. Tissue Res.*, **47**, 133–40.

Huang, A. H., Farrell, M. J., Kim, M. and Mauck, R. L. 2010. Long-term dynamic loading improves the mechanical properties of chondrogenic mesenchymal stem cell-laden hydrogel. *Eur. Cell Mater.*, **19**, 72–85.

Huang, C. Y., Stankiewicz, A., Ateshian, G. A. and Mow, V. C. 2005. Anisotropy, inhomogeneity, and tension-compression nonlinearity of human glenohumeral cartilage in finite deformation. *J. Biomech.*, **38**, 799–809.

Huang, Q., Goh, J. C., Hutmacher, D. W. and Lee, E. H. 2002. In vivo mesenchymal cell recruitment by a scaffold loaded with transforming growth factor β_1 and the potential for *in situ* chondrogenesis. *Tissue Eng.*, **8**, 469–82.

Hui, J. H., Ren, X., Afizah, M. H., Chian, K. S. and Mikos, A. G. 2013. Oligo[poly(ethylene glycol)fumarate] hydrogel enhances osteochondral repair in porcine femoral condyle defects. *Clin. Orthop. Relat. Res.*, **471**(4), 1174–85.

Huntley, J. S., Bush, P. G., McBirnie, J. M., Simpson, A. H. and Hall, A. C. 2005. Chondrocyte death associated with human femoral osteochondral harvest as performed for mosaicplasty. *J. Bone Joint Surg. Am.*, **87**, 351–60.

Hurtig, M. B., Buschmann, M. D., Fortier, L. A. *et al.* 2011. Preclinical studies for cartilage repair: recommendations from the International Cartilage Repair Society. *Cartilage*, **2**, 137–59.

Hwang, N. S., Varghese, S., Li, H. and Elisseeff, J. 2011. Regulation of osteogenic and chondrogenic differentiation of mesenchymal stem cells in PEG-ECM hydrogels. *Cell Tissue Res.*, **344**, 499–509.

Ionescu, L. C., Lee, G. C., Huang, K. L. and Mauck, R. L. 2012. Growth factor supplementation improves native and engineered meniscus repair in vitro. *Acta Biomater.*, **8**(10), 3687–94.

Irrgang, J. J., Anderson, A. F., Boland, A. L. *et al.* 2001. Development and validation of the international knee documentation committee subjective knee form. *Am. J. Sports Med.*, **29**, 600–13.

Jackson, D. W., Lalor, P. A., Aberman, H. M. and Simon, T. M. 2001. Spontaneous repair of full-thickness defects of articular cartilage in a goat model. A preliminary study. *J. Bone Joint Surg. Am.*, **83A**, 53–64.

Jiang, C. C., Chiang, H., Liao, C. J. *et al.* 2007. Repair of porcine articular cartilage defect with a biphasic osteochondral composite. *J. Orthop. Res.*, **25**, 1277–90.

Jiang, J., Tang, A., Ateshian, G. A. *et al.* 2010. Bioactive stratified polymer ceramic-hydrogel scaffold for integrative osteochondral repair. *Ann. Biomed. Eng.*, **38**, 2183–96.

Johnstone, B., Hering, T. M., Caplan, A. I., Goldberg, V. M. and Yoo, J. U. 1998. In vitro chondrogenesis of bone marrow-derived mesenchymal progenitor cells. *Exp. Cell Res.*, **238**, 265–72.

Jones, B. A. and Pei, M. 2012. Synovium-derived stem cells: a tissue-specific stem cell for cartilage engineering and regeneration. *Tissue Eng. Part B Rev.*, **18**(4), 301–11.

Jones, R. S., Keene, G. C., Learmonth, D. J. *et al.* 1996. Direct measurement of hoop strains in the intact and torn human medial meniscus. *Clin. Biomech.*, **11**, 295–300.

Jurgens, W. J., Lu, Z., Zandieh-Doulabi, B. *et al.* 2012. Hyperosmolarity and hypoxia induce chondrogenesis of adipose-derived stem cells in a collagen type 2 hydrogel. *J. Tissue Eng. Regen. Med.*, **6**, 570–78.

Kandel, R. A., Grynpas, M., Pilliar, R. *et al.* 2006. Repair of osteochondral defects with biphasic cartilage-calcium polyphosphate constructs in a sheep model. *Biomaterials*, **27**, 4120–31.

Kaplonyi, G., Zimmerman, I., Frenyo, A. D., Farkas, T. and Nemes, G. 1988. The use of fibrin adhesive in the repair of chondral and osteochondral injuries. *Injury*, **19**, 267–72.

Karagianes, M. T., Wheeler, K. R. and Nilles, J. L. 1975. Cartilage repair over porous metal implants. *Arch. Pathol.*, **99**, 398–400.

Kim, H. J. and Im, G. I. 2009. Combination of transforming growth factor-β_2 and bone morphogenetic protein 7 enhances chondrogenesis from adipose tissue-derived mesenchymal stem cells. *Tissue Eng. Part A*, **15**, 1543–51.

Kim, M., Kraft, J. J., Volk, A. C. *et al.* 2011. Characterization of a cartilage-like engineered biomass using a self-aggregating suspension culture model: molecular composition using FT-IRIS. *J. Orthop. Res.*, **29**, 1881–87.

Kim, T. K., Sharma, B., Williams, C. G. *et al.* 2003. Experimental model for cartilage tissue engineering to regenerate the zonal organization of articular cartilage. *Osteoarthritis Cartilage*, **11**, 653–64.

Klein, T. J., Chaudhry, M., Bae, W. C. and Sah, R. L. 2007. Depth-dependent biomechanical and biochemical properties of fetal, newborn, and tissue-engineered articular cartilage. *J. Biomech.*, **40**, 182–90.

Kocher, M. S., Steadman, J. R., Briggs, K. K., Sterett, W. I. and Hawkins, R. J. 2004. Reliability, validity, and responsiveness of the Lysholm knee scale for various chondral disorders of the knee. *J. Bone Joint Surg. Am.*, **86A**, 1139–45.

Kon, E., Filardo, G., Tschon, M. *et al.* 2012. Tissue engineering for total meniscal substitution: animal study in sheep model – Results at 12 months. *Tissue Eng. Part A*, **18**(15–16), 1573–82.

Kon, E., Mutini, A., Arcangeli, E. *et al.* 2010. Novel nanostructured scaffold for osteochondral regeneration: pilot study in horses. *J. Tissue Eng. Regen. Med.*, **4**, 300–8.

Lahiji, A., Sohrabi, A., Hungerford, D. S. and Frondoza, C. G. 2000. Chitosan supports the expression of extracellular matrix proteins in human osteoblasts and chondrocytes. *J. Biomed. Mater. Res.*, **51**, 586–95.

LaPrade, R. F., Bursch, L. S., Olson, E. J., Havlas, V. and Carlson, C. S. 2008. Histologic and immunohistochemical characteristics of failed articular cartilage resurfacing procedures for osteochondritis of the knee: a case series. *Am. J. Sports Med.*, **36**, 360–8.

Lawrence, R. C., Felson, D. T., Helmick, C. G. *et al.* 2008. Estimates of the prevalence of arthritis and other rheumatic conditions in the United States. Part II. *Arthritis Rheum.*, **58**, 26–35.

Lee, C. H., Cook, J. L., Mendelson, A. *et al.* 2010. Regeneration of the articular surface of the rabbit synovial joint by cell homing: a proof of concept study. *Lancet*, **376**, 440–8.

Li, X. A., Iyer, S., Cross, M. B. and Figgie, M. P. 2012. Total joint replacement in adolescents: literature review and case examples. *Curr. Opin. Pediatr.*, **24**, 57–63.

Lima, E. G., Bian, L., Ng, K. W. *et al.* 2007. The beneficial effect of delayed compressive loading on tissue-engineered cartilage constructs cultured with TGF-β_3. *Osteoarthritis Cartilage*, **15**, 1025–33.

Lind, M., Larsen, A., Clausen, C., Osther, K. and Everland, H. 2008. Cartilage repair with chondrocytes in fibrin hydrogel and MPEG polylactide scaffold: an in vivo study in goats. *Knee Surg. Sports Traumatol. Arthrosc.*, **16**, 690–8.

Liu, X., Jin, X. and Ma, P. X. 2011 Nanofibrous hollow microspheres self-assembled from star-shaped polymers as injectable cell carriers for knee repair. *Nature Mater.*, **10**, 398–406.

Macchiarini, P., Jungebluth, P., Go, T. *et al.* 2008. Clinical transplantation of a tissue-engineered airway. *Lancet*, **372**, 2023–30.

Maher, S. A., Mauck, R. L., Rackwitz, L. and Tuan, R. S. 2010. A nanofibrous cell-seeded hydrogel promotes integration in a cartilage gap model. *J. Tissue Eng. Regen. Med.*, **4**, 25–9.

Mainil-Varlet, P., Van Damme, B., Nesic, D. *et al.* 2010. A new histology scoring system for the assessment of the quality of human cartilage repair: ICRS II. *Am. J. Sports Med.*, **38**, 880–90.

Makris, E. A., Hadidi, P. and Athanasiou, K. A. 2011. The knee meniscus: structure–function, pathophysiology, current repair, techniques, and prospects for regeneration. *Biomaterials*, **32**, 7411–31.

Malda, J., Martens, D. E., Tramper, J., van Blitterswijk, C. A. and Riesle, J. 2003. Cartilage tissue engineering: controversy in the effect of oxygen. *Crit. Rev. Biotechnol.*, **23**, 175–94.

Mandal, B. B., Park, S. H., Gil, E. S. and Kaplan, D. L. 2011. Stem cell-based meniscus tissue engineering. *Tissue Eng. Part A*, **17**, 2749 61.

Mardones, R. M., Reinholz, G. G., Fitzsimmons, J. S. *et al.* 2005. Development of a biologic prosthetic composite for cartilage repair. *Tissue Eng.*, **11**, 1368–78.

Marlovits, S., Singer, P., Zeller, P. *et al.* 2006. Magnetic resonance observation of cartilage repair tissue (MOCART) for the evaluation of autologous chondrocyte transplantation: determination of interobserver variability and correlation to clinical outcome after 2 years. *Eur. J. Radiol.*, **57**, 16–23.

Marlovits, S., Striessnig, G., Resinger, C. T. *et al.* 2004. Definition of pertinent parameters for the evaluation of articular cartilage repair tissue with high-resolution magnetic resonance imaging. *Eur. J. Radiol.*, **52**, 310–19.

Marquass, B., Schulz, R., Hepp, P. *et al.* 2011. Matrix-associated implantation of predifferentiated mesenchymal stem cells versus articular chondrocytes: in vivo results of cartilage repair after 1 year. *Am. J. Sports Med.*, **39**, 1401–12.

Matricali, G. A., Dereymaeker, G. P. and Luyten, F. P. 2010. Donor site morbidity after articular cartilage repair procedures: a review. *Acta Orthop. Belg.*, **76**, 669–74.

Mauck, R. L., Yuan, X. and Tuan, R. S. 2006. Chondrogenic differentiation and functional maturation of bovine mesenchymal stem cells in long-term agarose culture. *Osteoarthritis Cartilage*, **14**, 179–89.

McCormick, F., Yanke, A., Provencher, M. T. and Cole, B. J. 2008. Minced articular cartilage – basic science, surgical technique, and clinical application. *Sports Med. Arthrosc.*, **16**, 217–20.

Mease, P. J., Hanna, S., Frakes, E. P. and Altman, R. D. 2011. Pain mechanisms in osteoarthritis: understanding the role of central pain and current approaches to its treatment. *J. Rheumatol.*, **38**, 1546–51.

Minas, T. 2001. Autologous chondrocyte implantation for focal chondral defects of the knee. *Clin. Orthop. Relat. Res.*, S349–61.

Minas, T. 2011. Autologous chondrocyte implantation. In Minas, T., editor. *A Primer in Cartilage Repair and Joint Preservation of the Knee.* Philadelphia, PA: Saunders, pp. 65–119.

Miot, S., Brehm, W., Dickinson, S. *et al.* 2012. Influence of in vitro maturation of engineered cartilage on the outcome of osteochondral repair in a goat model. *Eur. Cell Mater.*, **23**, 222–36.

Mithoefer, K., McAdams, T., Williams, R. J., Kreuz, P. C. and Mandelbaum, B. R. 2009. Clinical efficacy of the microfracture technique for articular cartilage repair in the knee: an evidence-based systematic analysis. *Am. J. Sports Med.*, **37**, 2053–63.

Moutos, F. T., Freed, L. E. and Guilak, F. 2007. A biomimetic three-dimensional woven composite scaffold for functional tissue engineering of cartilage. *Nature Mater.*, **6**, 162–7.

Moutos, F. T. and Guilak, F. 2010. Functional properties of cell-seeded three-dimensionally woven poly(ε-caprolactone) scaffolds for cartilage tissue engineering. *Tissue Eng. Part A*, **16**, 1291–301.

Mow, V. C., and Huiskes, R. 2005. *Basic Orthopaedic Biomechanics & Mechanobiology.* Philadelphia, PA: Lippincott Williams & Wilkins.

Mow, V. C., Kuei, S. C., Lai, W. M. and Armstrong, C. G. 1980. Biphasic creep and stress relaxation of articular cartilage in compression? Theory and experiments. *J. Biomech. Eng.*, **102**, 73–84.

Mrosek, E. H., Schagemann, J. C., Chung, H. W. *et al.* 2010. Porous tantalum and poly-ε-caprolactone biocomposites for osteochondral defect repair: preliminary studies in rabbits. *J. Orthop. Res.*, **28**, 141–8.

Mulhall, K. J., Ghomrawi, H. M., Scully, S., Callaghan, J. J. and Saleh, K. J. 2006. Current etiologies and modes of failure in total knee arthroplasty revision. *Clin. Orthop. Relat. Res.*, **446**, 45–50.

Natoli, R. M., Revell, C. M. and Athanasiou, K. A. 2009. Chondroitinase ABC treatment results in greater tensile properties of self-assembled tissue-engineered articular cartilage. *Tissue Eng. Part A*, **15**, 3119–28.

Nehrer, S., Breinan, H. A., Ramappa, A. *et al.* 1998. Chondrocyte-seeded collagen matrices implanted in a chondral defect in a canine model. *Biomaterials*, **19**, 2313–28.

Nehrer, S., Spector, M. and Minas, T. 1999. Histologic analysis of tissue after failed cartilage repair procedures. *Clin. Orthop. Relat. Res.*, 149–62.

Nerurkar, N. L., Sen, S., Huang, A. H., Elliott, D. M. and Mauck, R. L. 2010. Engineered disc-like angle-ply structures for intervertebral disc replacement. *Spine*, **35**, 867–73.

Nettles, D. L., Kitaoka, K., Hanson, N. A. *et al.* 2008. *In situ* crosslinking elastin-like polypeptide gels for application to articular cartilage repair in a goat osteochondral defect model. *Tissue Eng. Part A*, **14**, 1133–40.

Ng, K. W., Ateshian, G. A. and Hung, C. T. 2009. Zonal chondrocytes seeded in a layered agarose hydrogel create engineered cartilage with depth-dependent cellular and mechanical inhomogeneity. *Tissue Eng. Part A*, **15**, 2315–24.

Nguyen, Q. T., Hwang, Y., Chen, A. C., Varghese, S. and Sah, R. L. 2012. Cartilage-like mechanical properties of poly(ethylene glycol)-diacrylate hydrogels. *Biomaterials*, **33**, 6682–90.

Niederauer, G. G., Slivka, M. A., Leatherbury, N. C. *et al.* 2000. Evaluation of multiphase implants for repair of focal osteochondral defects in goats. *Biomaterials*, **21**, 2561–74.

O'Driscoll, S. W., Marx, R. G., Beaton, D. E. *et al.* 2001. Validation of a simple histological-histochemical cartilage scoring system. *Tissue Eng.*, **7**, 313–20.

Ogston, A. G., and Stanier, J. E. 1953. The physiological function of hyaluronic acid in synovial fluid; viscous, elastic and lubricant properties. *J. Physiol.*, **119**, 244–52.

Pallante, A. L., Bae, W. C., Chen, A. C. *et al.* 2009. Chondrocyte viability is higher after prolonged storage at 37 degrees C than at 4 degrees C for osteochondral grafts. *Am. J. Sports Med.*, **37**(Suppl. 1), 24S–32S.

Park, S. H., Gil, E. S. and Cho, H. 2012. Intervertebral disk tissue engineering using biphasic silk composite scaffolds. *Tissue Eng. Part A*, **18**, 447–58.

Pelttari, K., Winter, A., Steck, E. *et al.* 2006. Premature induction of hypertrophy during in vitro chondrogenesis of human mesenchymal stem cells correlates with calcification and vascular invasion after ectopic transplantation in SCID mice. *Arthritis Rheum.*, **54**, 3254–66.

Pittenger, M. F., Mackay, A. M., Beck, S. C. *et al.* 1999. Multilineage potential of adult human mesenchymal stem cells. *Science*, **284**, 143–7.

Re'em, T., Witte, F., Willbold, E., Ruvinov, E. and Cohen, S. 2012. Simultaneous regeneration of articular cartilage and subchondral bone induced by spatially presented TGF-β and BMP-4 in a bilayer affinity binding system. *Acta Biomater.*, **8**, 3283–93.

Reimann, I. 1976. Pathological human synovial fluids. Viscosity and boundary lubricating properties. *Clin. Orthop. Relat. Res.*, 237–41.

Reinholz, G. G., Lu, L., Saris, D. B., Yaszemski, M. J. and O'Driscoll, S. W. 2004. Animal models for cartilage reconstruction. *Biomaterials*, **25**, 1511–21.

Robinson, P. D. 1993. Histologic study of articular cartilage repair in the marmoset condyle. *J. Oral Maxillofac. Surg.*, **51**, 1088–94; discussion 1094–5.

Ropes, M. W., Bennett, G. A. and Bauer, W. 1939. The origin and nature of normal synovial fluid. *J. Clin. Invest.*, **18**, 351–72.

Sage, A., Chang, A. A., Schumacher, B. L. Sah, R. L. and Watson, D. 2009. Cartilage outgrowth in fibrin scaffolds. *Am. J. Rhinol. Allergy*, **23**, 486–91.

Sams, A. E., and Nixon, A. J. 1995. Chondrocyte-laden collagen scaffolds for resurfacing extensive articular cartilage defects. *Osteoarthritis Cartilage*, **3**, 47–59.

Schatti, O., Grad, S., Goldhahn, J. *et al.* 2011. A combination of shear and dynamic compression leads to mechanically induced chondrogenesis of human mesenchymal stem cells. *Eur. Cell Mater.*, **22**, 214–25.

Schek, R. M., Taboas, J. M., Segvich, S. J., Hollister, S. J. and Krebsbach, P. H. 2004. Engineered osteochondral grafts using biphasic composite solid free-form fabricated scaffolds. *Tissue Eng.*, **10**, 1376–85.

Schiltz, J. R., Mayne, R. and Holtzer, H. 1973. The synthesis of collagen and glycosaminoglycans by dedifferentiated chondroblasts in culture. *Differentiation*, **1**, 97–108.

Schinagl, R. M., Gurskis, D., Chen, A. C. and Sah, R. L. 1997. Depth-dependent confined compression modulus of full-thickness bovine articular cartilage. *J. Orthop. Res.*, **15**, 499–506.

Schinhan, M., Gruber, M., Vavken, P. *et al.* 2012. Critical-size defect induces unicompartmental osteoarthritis in a stable ovine knee. *J. Orthop. Res.*, **30**, 214–20.

Schulz, R. M., Zscharnack, M., Hanisch, I. *et al.* 2008. Cartilage tissue engineering by collagen matrix associated bone marrow derived mesenchymal stem cells. *Biomed. Mater. Eng.*, **18**, S55–70.

Schumacher, B. L., Block, J. A., Schmid, T. M., Aydelotte, M. B. and Kuettner, K. E. 1994. A novel proteoglycan synthesized and secreted by chondrocytes of the superficial zone of articular cartilage. *Arch. Biochem. Biophys.*, **311**, 144–52.

Sechriest, V. F., Miao, Y. J., Niyibizi, C. *et al.* 2000. GAG-augmented polysaccharide hydrogel: a novel biocompatible and biodegradable material to support chondrogenesis. *J. Biomed. Mater. Res.*, **49**, 534–41.

Shahin, K. and Doran, P. M. 2011. Improved seeding of chondrocytes into polyglycolic acid scaffolds using semi-static and alginate loading methods. *Biotechnol. Prog.*, **27**, 191–200.

Shortkroff, S., Barone, L., Hsu, H. P. *et al.* 1996. Healing of chondral and osteochondral defects in a canine model: the role of cultured chondrocytes in regeneration of articular cartilage. *Biomaterials*, **17**, 147–54.

Skaalure, S. C., Milligan, I. L. and Bryant, S. J. 2012. Age impacts extracellular matrix metabolism in chondrocytes encapsulated in degradable hydrogels. *Biomed. Mater.*, **7**, 024111.

Smith, H. J., Richardson, J. B. and Tennant, A. 2009. Modification and validation of the Lysholm Knee Scale to assess articular cartilage damage. *Osteoarthritis Cartilage*, **17**, 53–8.

Solorio, L. D., Vieregge, E. L., Dhami, C. D., Dang, P. N. and Alsberg, E. 2012. Engineered cartilage via self-assembled hMSC sheets with incorporated biodegradable gelatin microspheres releasing transforming growth factor-β_1. *J. Control. Release*, **158**, 224–32.

Spiller, K. L., Holloway, J. L., Gribb, M. E. and Lowman, A. M. 2011. Design of semi-degradable hydrogels based on poly(vinyl alcohol) and poly(lactic-*co*-glycolic acid) for cartilage tissue engineering. *J. Tissue. Eng. Regen. Med.*, **5**, 636–47.

Spiller, K. L., Laurencin, S. J. and Lowman, A. M. 2009. Characterization of the behavior of porous hydrogels in model osmotically-conditioned articular cartilage systems. *J. Biomed. Mater. Res. B Appl. Biomater.*, **90**, 752–9.

Starkman, B. G., Cravero, J. D., Delcarlo, M. and Loeser, R. F. 2005. IGF-I stimulation of proteoglycan synthesis by chondrocytes requires activation of the PI 3-kinase pathway but not ERK MAPK. *Biochem. J.*, **389**, 723–9.

Strangeways, T. S. 1920. Observations on the nutrition of articular cartilage. *Br. Med. J.*, **1**, 661–3.

Sung, M. S., Jeong, C. H., Lim, Y. S. *et al.* 2011. Periosteal autograft for articular cartilage defects in dogs: MR imaging and ultrasonography of the repair process. *Acta Radiol.*, **52**, 181–90.

Swann, D. A., Silver, F. H., Slayter, H. S., Stafford, W. and Shore, E. 1985. The molecular structure and lubricating activity of lubricin isolated from bovine and human synovial fluids. *Biochem. J.*, **225**, 195–201.

Tampieri, A., Sandri, M., Landi, E. *et al.* 2008. Design of graded biomimetic osteochondral composite scaffolds. *Biomaterials*, **29**, 3539–46.

Tanaka, T., Komaki, H., Chazono, M. and Fujii, K. 2005. Use of a biphasic graft constructed with chondrocytes overlying a β-tricalcium phosphate block in the treatment of rabbit osteochondral defects. *Tissue Eng.*, **11**, 331–9.

Tegner, Y. and Lysholm, J. 1985. Rating systems in the evaluation of knee ligament injuries. *Clin. Orthop. Relat. Res.*, 43–9.

Terada, S., Yoshimoto, H., Fuchs, J. R. *et al.* 2005. Hydrogel optimization for cultured elastic chondrocytes seeded onto a polyglycolic acid scaffold. *J. Biomed. Mater. Res. A*, **75**, 907–16.

Thomopoulos, S., Williams, G. R., Gimbel, J. A., Favata, M. and Soslowsky, L. J. 2003. Variation of biomechanical, structural, and compositional properties along the tendon to bone insertion site. *J. Orthop. Res.*, **21**, 413–19.

Thoms, R. J. and Marwin, S. E. 2009. The role of fibrin sealants in orthopaedic surgery. *J. Am. Acad. Orthop. Surg.*, **17**, 727–36.

Toh, W. S., Lee, E. H. and Cao, T. 2011. Potential of human embryonic stem cells in cartilage tissue engineering and regenerative medicine. *Stem Cell Rev.*, **7**, 544–59.

Toh, W. S., Lim, T. C., Kurisawa, M. and Spector, M. 2012. Modulation of mesenchymal stem cell chondrogenesis in a tunable hyaluronic acid hydrogel microenvironment. *Biomaterials*, **33**, 3835–45.

Tran-Khanh, N., Hoemann, C. D., McKee, M. D., Henderson, J. E. and Buschmann, M. D. 2005. Aged bovine chondrocytes display a diminished capacity to produce a collagen-rich, mechanically functional cartilage extracellular matrix. *J. Orthop. Res.*, **23**, 1354–62.

Treppo, S., Koepp, H., Quan, E. C. *et al.* 2000. Comparison of biomechanical and biochemical properties of cartilage from human knee and ankle pairs. *J. Orthop. Res.*, **18**, 739–48.

Van Assche, D., Staes, F., Van Caspel, D. *et al.* 2010. Autologous chondrocyte implantation versus microfracture for knee cartilage injury: a prospective randomized trial, with 2-year follow-up. *Knee Surg. Sports Traumatol. Arthrosc.*, **18**, 486–95.

Watanabe, H., de Caestecker, M. P. and Yamada, Y. 2001. Transcriptional cross-talk between Smad, ERK1/2, and p38 mitogen-activated protein kinase pathways regulates transforming growth factor-β-induced aggrecan gene expression in chondrogenic ATDC5 cells. *J. Biol. Chem.*, **276**, 14466–73.

Weiss, S., Hennig, T., Bock, R., Steck, E. and Richter, W. 2010. Impact of growth factors and PTHrP on early and late chondrogenic differentiation of human mesenchymal stem cells. *J. Cell Physiol.*, **223**, 84–93.

Williamson, A. K., Chen, A. C. and Sah, R. L. 2001. Compressive properties and function-composition relationships of developing bovine articular cartilage. *J. Orthop. Res.*, **19**, 1113–21.

Wong, J. M., and Khan, W. S., Chimutengwende-Gordon, M. and Dowd, G. S. 2011. Recent advances in designs, approaches and materials in total knee replacement: literature review and evidence today. *J. Perioper. Pract.*, **21**, 165–71.

Xerogeanes, J. W., Fox, R. J., Takeda, Y. *et al.* 1998. A functional comparison of animal anterior cruciate ligament models to the human anterior cruciate ligament. *Ann. Biomed. Eng.*, **26**, 345–52.

Yamazoe, K., Mishima, H., Torigoe, K. *et al.* 2007. Effects of atelocollagen gel containing bone marrow-derived stromal cells on the repair of osteochondral defects in a dog. *J. Vet. Med. Sci.*, **69**, 835–9.

Yang, Q., Peng, J., Lu, S. B. *et al.* 2011. Evaluation of an extracellular matrix-derived acellular biphasic scaffold/cell construct in the repair of a large articular high-load-bearing osteochondral defect in a canine model. *Chin. Med. J. (Engl.)*, **124**, 3930–8.

Yokota, M., Yasuda, K., Kitamura, N. *et al.* 2011. Spontaneous hyaline cartilage regeneration can be induced in an osteochondral defect created in the femoral condyle using a novel double-network hydrogel. *BMC Musculoskelet. Disord.*, **12**, 49.

Youn, I., Choi, J. B., Cao, L., Setton, L. A. and Guilak, F. 2006. Zonal variations in the three-dimensional morphology of the chondron measured *in situ* using confocal microscopy. *Osteoarthritis Cartilage*, **14**, 889–97.

Yuan, T., Zhang, L., Feng, L., Fan, H. and Zhang, X. 2010. Chondrogenic differentiation and immunological properties of mesenchymal stem cells in collagen type I hydrogel. *Biotechnol. Prog.*, **26**, 1749–58.

Zhou, G., Liu, W., Cui, L. *et al.* 2006. Repair of porcine articular osteochondral defects in non-weightbearing areas with autologous bone marrow stromal cells. *Tissue Eng.*, **12**, 3209–21.

Zhou, S., Cui, Z. and Urban, J. P. 2004. Factors influencing the oxygen concentration gradient from the synovial surface of articular cartilage to the cartilage-bone interface: a modeling study. *Arthritis Rheum.*, **50**, 3915–24.

28

Engineering tissue-to-tissue interfaces

Nora T. Khanarian, Nancy M. Lee, Marissa R. Solomon and Helen H. Lu

28.1 Introduction

Orthopedic injuries and diseases commonly affect soft tissues, including cartilage, which line the surface of articulating joints, as well as ligaments and tendons, which connect bone to bone and muscle to bone, respectively. Continued developments in tissue engineering have led to advancements in the regeneration of these tissues, while recently emphasis has been placed on the regeneration of the interfaces or insertion sites that connect these soft tissues to bone, which are characterized by a gradient of structural and mechanical properties [1]. The integrity of these regions is essential to facilitating synchronized joint motion, mediating load transfer between distinct tissue types, and sustaining heterotypic cellular communications necessary for interface function and homeostasis [2–4]. These critical junctions are also prone to injury, and healing is typically incomplete after surgical repair. The need for functional interface regeneration is highlighted by the fact that failure to restore the intricate tissue-to-tissue interface has been reported to compromise graft stability and long-term clinical outcome [5, 6].

Fundamentally, tissue engineering involves the use of cells, growth factors, and/or biomaterial scaffolds in a variety of ways to engineer tissues in vitro and in vivo. The principles of tissue engineering have been applied for the successful formation of connective tissues, including bone, cartilage, ligament, and tendon. Recently the focus in the field has shifted from tissue formation to tissue function [7], specifically to imparting physiologically relevant functionality to tissue-engineered grafts. One of the most significant challenges to clinical application is achieving *biological fixation* of musculoskeletal grafts with each other as well as to the native host environment [8].

This chapter reviews current biological fixation strategies aimed at engineering the junction between soft tissue and bone. The interface tissue engineering challenge is rooted in the complexity of the musculoskeletal system and the structural intricacy of both hard and soft tissues. Although these tissues are comprised of a distinct cellular population, both must operate in unison to facilitate physiological function and homeostasis. Interfaces often exhibit a unique biochemical composition, which is distinct from that of the tissues they connect. Furthermore, the transition between various tissue types is characterized by a high level of heterogeneous structural organization. For example, ligaments with direct insertions into subchondral bone exhibit a multitissue transition consisting of three distinct, yet continuous, regions of ligament, fibrocartilage, and bone [2, 9, 10]. The fibrocartilage region is further divided into non-calcified and calcified regions. In light of this complexity, functional tissue engineering must incorporate *strategic biomimicry* in order to facilitate the formation of the tissue-to-tissue interface and enable seamless graft integration.

In additional to developmental and reparative cues, studies characterizing the structure–function relationship at the soft-tissue-to-bone insertion have revealed remarkable organizational similarities between many tissue-to-tissue interfaces [2, 4, 11–17]. These regions are characterized by multitissue transitions, between bone and ligaments or tendons, as well as containing a controlled distribution of non-mineralized and mineralized cartilaginous interface regions that, together with other structural parameters such as collagen fiber organization, have been reported to be responsible for the gradual transition in mechanical properties observed in the progression from soft tissue to bone. These observations have inspired the design of biomimetic scaffolds, with a multiphased structure intended to recapitulate the multitissue organization of the soft-tissue-to-bone interface. These multiphased scaffolds can be fabricated to contain either a continuous gradient or a distinct stratification of composition and/or scaffold organization. Multiphased scaffolds should exhibit phase-specific structural and material properties, with an increase in mechanical strength across the scaffold phases. Furthermore, the formation of stress concentrations can be minimized by imparting scaffold heterogeneity through control of the spatial mineral distribution on a multiphased scaffold. Compared with a homogeneous structure, a stratified scaffold with phase-specific matrix heterogeneity can better transmit and thus sustain the distribution of complex loads at the multitissue interface [9, 18, 19]. A key consideration in the fabrication of stratified scaffolds is that each phase must be interconnected and pre-integrated with the others, in effect supporting the formation of distinct yet continuous multitissue regions. Furthermore, precise control over the spatial distribution of interface-relevant cell populations is also critical for multitissue formation and interface regeneration [20–22]. Interactions between these cell populations serve important functions in the formation, maintenance, and repair of interfacial tissue. Consideration of these biomimetic parameters will collectively enable the design of scaffolds optimized for promoting the regeneration and homeostasis of controlled matrix heterogeneity and tissue-to-tissue integration.

This chapter highlights current tissue engineering efforts in the regeneration of three common soft-tissue-to-bone interfaces, namely ligament-to-bone, tendon-to-bone, and cartilage-to-bone. Emphasis will be placed on the design of biomimetic scaffolds and the utilization of biomaterials and cell-based strategies to engineer a functional gradient of mechanical and biochemical properties to mimic that of the native tissue. Each section will begin with a brief overview of the scaffold design requirements, which are derived from the characterization and known structure–function relationships of the native interface. A review of stratified and gradient-based scaffold designs currently utilized for soft-tissue-to-bone interface tissue engineering will then be presented. Lastly, potential challenges and future directions in this rapidly expanding area of functional tissue engineering will be discussed.

28.1.1 Interface scaffold design for ligament-to-bone interface tissue engineering

The site of anterior cruciate ligament (ACL) insertion into bone is a classic example of a complex soft-tissue-to-bone interface consisting of spatial variations in cell type and matrix composition resulting in three distinct yet continuous regions of ligament, fibrocartilage, and bone [2, 9, 10], whereby the fibrocartilage region is further divided into mineralized and non-mineralized regions. The complex organization of this interface is likely attributable to the nature and distribution of mechanical stress experienced in this region. It has been reported that matrix organization at the insertion is optimized to sustain both tensile and compressive stresses [4, 11]. These region-specific mechanical properties facilitate a gradual transition in strain across the insertion and provide valuable cues for ligament-to-bone interface scaffold design.

The regeneration of the ligament-to-bone insertion site presents a significant challenge for functional ligament engineering. Rodeo *et al.* demonstrated that surgically juxtaposing soft tissue to bone does not spontaneously result in the regeneration of the fibrocartilaginous interface [23]. Furthermore, without the formation of an anatomical interface, the mechanical stability of the graft-to-bone junction is limited [6, 24, 25]. Initial attempts to improve graft-to-bone fixation during ACL reconstruction involved augmenting the surgical graft with materials that would encourage bone tissue ingrowth within the bone tunnel [26–31]. In a rabbit study, Tien *et al.* filled the interface between the ACL reconstruction graft and bone tunnel with calcium phosphate cement. It was noted that the addition of ceramic helped to augment bone tissue growth and organization [26]. In a similar study, the injection of tricalcium phosphate (TCP) cement into the bone tunnel in a canine ACL reconstruction model resulted in more organized bone tissue formation than occurred in the uncemented control [27]. As an alternative approach to improving graft-to-bone attachment, Mutsuzaki *et al.* soaked tendon-based ACL reconstruction grafts in a series of solutions, which facilitated the formation of a calcium phosphate layer prior to implantation [32]. The pre-soaked grafts were evaluated in a rabbit model, and, after 3 weeks, direct bonding between the implanted graft and the surrounding bone was observed. In contrast, untreated controls developed fibrous tissue only at the interface. Other approaches to improve bone tunnel osteointegration include the addition of periosteum wraps to the region of the graft that interacts with bone [33–37] as well as growth factors such as BMP-2 [24, 38–41], BMP-7 [42] and granulocyte colony-stimulating factor [43]. Additionally, several groups have also investigated the direct application of multipotent mesenchymal stem cells as a method to improve graft-to-bone integration [44–48]. While these strategies have succeeded in enhancing graft-to-bone fixation as revealed by biomechanical testing and histology, none resulted in the regeneration of the anatomic fibrocartilaginous interface. Moreover, it is known that the complex graft-to-bone healing process involves a controlled cascade of growth factors and cytokines. To this end, using biomimetic stratified scaffolds with controlled design of the multitissue layers characteristic of the ligament-to-bone interface may overcome the shortcomings of these previous approaches.

Both biochemical and mechanical design parameters must be considered in the ideal scaffold design. The scaffold should function in supporting the growth and differentiation of the relevant cell populations, directing cellular interactions, and promoting the formation and maintenance of controlled extracellular matrix heterogeneity. The scaffold must also exhibit a gradient in mechanical properties that mimics that of the native insertion site, with magnitudes comparable to those of the ligament-to-bone interface. An additional consideration is that the scaffold must be biodegradable on a relevant time scale in order to be gradually replaced by living tissue. Finally, in order to be clinically relevant, the engineered graft must be easily adaptable with current ACL reconstruction grafts, or must be pre-incorporated into the design of the ligament replacement grafts.

Traditional efforts for developing tissue-engineered grafts for ACL reconstruction have centered on regenerating the ligament proper [49–51], with more recent studies (Table 28.1) focussing on ligament-to-bone integration [52–55]. Cooper *et al.* reported on the design of a synthetic multi-phased ACL graft fabricated from three-dimensional (3D) braiding of polylactide-*co*-glycolide fibers into a ligament proper and two bony regions [52]. In-vitro [55] and in-vivo [54] evaluation demonstrated scaffold biocompatibility, healing, and mechanical strength in a rabbit model. Ma *et al.* reported that by using a cell-based approach it is possible to form bone–ligament–bone constructs by introducing engineered bone segments into ligament monolayer cultures [56]. The monolayer attached to bone, resulting in the self-assembly of a ligament–bone–ligament-like construct. Paxton *et al.* utilized a similar methodology when evaluating the use of a poly(ethylene glycol) hydrogel, incorporating hydroxyapatite (HA) and the RGD adhesion peptide to engineer functional ligament-to-bone attachments [57]. These novel ACL graft designs represent significant improvement over single-phased ACL grafts. On the other hand, the challenge of biological fixation must still be addressed; a potential strategy toward achieving this is by incorporating a region for the fibrocartilage interface into the ACL scaffold design.

Focussing on ligament-to-bone integration, Spalazzi *et al.* pioneered the design of a triphasic scaffold for the ACL-to-bone interface [21, 22]. The scaffold, which was modeled after the native insertion, consists of three distinct yet continuous phases, Phase A (PLGA 10:90) for fibroblast culture and ligament formation, Phase B (sintered PLGA 85:15 microspheres) for the interface region intended for fibrochondrocyte culture, and Phase C, comprised of sintered PLGA (85:15) and 45S5 bioactive glass composite microspheres, for bone

Table 28.1 Scaffolds for ligament-to-bone tissue engineering

Study	Scaffold design	Study model/time point	Outcomes
Dunn *et al.* (1992) [51]	Collagen fibers with PMMA bone fixation plugs	In vivo/rabbit model/4 and 20 weeks	Supported development of neoligament tissue
Bitar *et al.* (2005) [117]	Phosphate-based glass fibers	In vitro/human osteoblasts and fibroblasts	Cell differentiation maintained by both cell types and strongly related to fiber composition
Lu *et al.* (2005) [55]	Multiregion knitted PLLA fiber scaffold	In vitro/rabbit ACL cells	Supported long-term matrix deposition
Cooper *et al.* (2007) [54]	Multiregion knitted PLLA fiber scaffold	In vivo/rabbit model with primary ACL cells/4 and 12 weeks	Demonstrated scaffold healing and mechanical strength
Spalazzi *et al.* (2006) [118]	Triphasic: Phase A, PLGA mesh; Phase B, PLGA (85:15) microspheres; Phase C, PLGA-bioglass composite	In vitro/bovine fibroblast (phase A), osteoblast (phase C) co-culture	Supported cell proliferation and matrix production while maintaining distinct cellular regions
Spalazzi *et al.* (2008a) [119]	Triphasic: Phase A, PLGA mesh; Phase B, PLGA (85:15) microspheres; Phase C, PLGA-bioglass composite	In vivo/rat model with bovine fibroblast, chondrocyte, osteoblast triculture/4 and 8 weeks	Interface-like matrix heterogeneity maintained
Spalazzi *et al.* (2008b) [60]	PLGA (85:15) nanofibers, PLGA (85:15) microspheres	In vitro/bovine patellar tendon graft	Up-regulation of fibrocartilage markers after 7 days of tendon compression with mechanoactive collar
Phillips *et al.* (2008) [83]	3D poly(L-lysine) retrovirus gradient	In vitro/rat dermal fibroblasts	Cells displayed spatial patterns of transcription factor expression, differentiation and matrix deposition
Ma *et al.* (2009) [56]	Ligament-bone constructs from rat BMSCs	In vivo/rat model/2 months	Tissues grew and remodeled quickly, with partial restoration of knee function
Paxton *et al.* (2009) [57]	Poly(ethylene glycol) hydrogel with HA	In vitro/rat Achilles tendon fibroblasts	Inclusion of HA in PEG hydrogel enhanced mechanical strength and cell attachment
Paxton *et al.* (2010a, 2010b) [120, 121]	Brushite cement anchors with cell-seeded fibrin gels	In vitro/rat Achilles tendon fibroblasts	Anchor shape altered longevity and strength of the bone-cement-ligament-tissue interface
Lee *et al.* (2011) [59]	Poly(L-lactide-*co*-ε-caprolactone) (60:40 mol%) scaffold with (1) fibrochondrocyte and BMP2 delivered via heparin hydrogel and (2) fibroblast regions	In vitro/rabbit patella ligament fibroblasts and meniscal fibrochondrocytes In vivo/subcutaneous murine model with rabbit fibroblasts and fibrochondrocytes/4 and 8 weeks	Results from in-vitro and in-vivo studies confirm increases in calcium and GAG production and improvements in mechanical properties of hydrogel-containing scaffold.

formation [58]. Heterotypic cellular interactions on the triphasic scaffold were assessed both in vitro [21] and in vivo [22]. To form the ligament and bone regions, fibroblasts and osteoblasts were seeded onto Phase A and Phase C, respectively. This controlled cell distribution resulted in the elaboration of cell-type-specific matrix on each phase of the scaffold in vitro, with a mineralized matrix detected only on Phase C, and an extensive type I collagen matrix found on both Phases A and B. In-vivo evaluation [22] of the co-cultured scaffold revealed extensive tissue infiltration and abundant matrix deposition on Phase A and Phase C. Cell migration, increased matrix production, and vascularization were observed on Phase B, the interface region. Moreover, tissue continuity was maintained across all three scaffold phases. Interestingly, extracellular matrix production compensated for the decrease in mechanical strength accompanying scaffold degradation, and the phase-specific controlled matrix heterogeneity was maintained in vivo [22].

To promote the formation of a fibrocartilage region at the interface phase of the triphasic scaffold, Spalazzi *et al.* extended the above scaffold system to triculture [21, 22]. Specifically, articular chondrocytes were encapsulated in a hydrogel matrix and loaded into Phase B of the scaffold, while ligament fibroblasts and osteoblasts were pre-seeded onto Phase A and Phase C, respectively. The scaffold was implanted subcutaneously in a rat model, and, two months after implantation, an extensive collagen-rich matrix was prevalent in all three phases of the tricultured scaffolds. Moreover, a fibrocartilaginous region of chondrocyte-like cells embedded within a matrix of types I and II collagen as well as glycosaminoglycans was observed. Interestingly, both the cell shape and the matrix morphology of the neo-fibrocartilage resembled those of the neonatal ligament-to-bone interface [10]. Moreover, the neo-fibrocartilage formed was continuous with the ligament-like tissue observed in Phase A as well as the bone-like tissue found in Phase C [22].

Recently, Lee *et al.* investigated the efficacy of the local delivery of fibrocondrocytes and BMP-2 using a heparin-based hydrogel [59]. Cylindrical poly-L-lactide-ploy-ε-caprolactone (PLCL) scaffolds were fabricated to contain separate fibrocartilage and ligament regions; fibrochondrocytes and BMP2 were delivered via the heparin hydrogel to the fibrocartilage region, and fibroblasts were seeded in the ligament region. Both in-vitro and in-vivo analysis demonstrated that significant matrix deposition translated into enhanced mechanical strength.

These results collectively demonstrate the potential that multiphased biomimetic scaffolds coupled with the spatial control of interface-relevant cell types have in the regeneration of multiple tissue types using a single scaffold system. In terms of clinical application, the triphasic scaffold can be used to guide the re-establishment of an anatomic fibrocartilage interfacial region directly on soft tissue grafts. Specifically, the scaffold can be utilized as a graft collar during ACL reconstruction. The feasibility of such an approach was recently demonstrated with a mechanoactive scaffold based on a composite of PLGA 85:15 nanofibers and sintered microspheres [60]. It was observed that scaffold-induced compression of tendon grafts resulted in significant matrix remodeling and the up-regulation of fibrocartilage interface-related markers such as type II collagen, aggrecan, and transforming growth factor-β_3 (TGF-β_3). These results suggest that the stratified scaffold can be used to induce the formation of an anatomic fibrocartilage interface directly on biological ACL reconstruction grafts.

In summary, a promising strategy for achieving ligament-to-bone interface regeneration is to first address the difficult problem of soft-tissue-to-bone integration ex vivo by pre-engineering the multitissue interface through a stratified scaffold design and then focussing on the relatively less challenging task of bone-to-bone integration in vivo. In the design of such complex scaffolds one must consider that each region of the scaffold needs to be engineered with physiologically relevant mechanical properties. Interface-relevant cell types, and bioactive molecules, such as growth factors and cytokines, can also be integrated into the stratified scaffold as efforts to recapitulate the complex nanoscale-to-microscale organization of the native ligament-to-bone interface.

Table 28.2 Scaffolds for tendon-to-bone tissue engineering

Study	Scaffold design	Study model/time point	Outcomes
Chang *et al.* (2009) [67]	Periosteum attached to end of transected tendon	In vivo/infraspinatus tendon-to-bone repair in rabbit model/4, 8, and 12 weeks	Extensive fibrocartilage and bone formation at interface; significant increase in failure load at interface region over time
Li *et al.* (2009) [19]	PLGA and PCL nanofibers (unaligned) with a gradient of calcium phosphate across scaffold	In vitro/MC3T3 cells (mouse preosteoblasts)	Gradation in mineral across scaffold produced a gradient in stiffness; gradient in cell density observed, with density being greater in regions of higher mineral concentration
Sundar *et al.* (2009) [68]	Demineralized bone matrix (DBM) interposed between tendon and bone	In vivo/patellar tendon-to-bone repair in ovine model/12 weeks	Augmentation with DBM increased area of fibrocartilage and mineralized fibrocartilage found at interface
Moffat *et al.* (2009) [77]	PLGA (85:15) nanofiber scaffolds (aligned and unaligned)	In vitro/human rotator cuff tendon fibroblasts	Tendon fibroblasts organized and produced matrix oriented according to the underlying nanofiber organization; matrix deposition and scaffold mechanical properties mimicked those of human rotator cuff tendons
Moffat *et al.* (2010) [81]	Biphasic nanofiber-based scaffold (aligned): Phase A, PLGA (85:15); Phase B, PLGA + HA	In vitro and in vivo/bovine full-thickness articular chondrocytes in athymic rat model/3 and 8 weeks	Scaffold mineral distribution mimics that of native insertion sites; synthesis of fibrocartilage-like matrix on Phase A and Phase B; regional mineral distribution maintained; increase in mineral density and osteointegration over time
Xie *et al.* (2010) [82]	PLGA (50:50) nanofiber scaffold with an aligned-to-random gradient in structure	In vitro/rat tendon fibroblasts	Both scaffold regions supported cell proliferation and deposition of collagen type I; cell morphology and matrix deposition oriented according to nanofiber organization

28.1.2 Scaffold design for tendon-to-bone interface tissue engineering

The tendon-to-bone interface displays a zonal distribution of cells and extracellular matrix components, which is similar to that of the ligament-to-bone interface [2, 61]. While the tendon-to-bone and ligament-to-bone insertion sites are physiologically structurally similar, differences in properties and biochemical composition do arise given the distinct loading environment, mineral distribution, and functionality of each type of soft tissue. Current efforts in tendon-to-bone interface tissue engineering have centered on rotator cuff repair (Table 28.2), which is the most common type of shoulder injury. There is a clear clinical need for functional solutions to integrative tendon-to-bone repair, since existing surgical strategies and mechanical fixation methods for rotator cuff repair often result in the incomplete healing of these complex tissues, and are associated with a high incidence of failure [62–65]. Graft solutions designed to target interface formation and biological fixation are thus necessary in order to address this challenge. Several groups have evaluated the feasibility of integrating tendon with bone or biomaterials through the formation of an anatomic insertion site. By surgically reattaching tendon to bone using a rat Achilles tendon avulsion model, Fujioka *et al.* induced cellular reorganization at the reattachment site, together with the formation of calcified and non-calcified fibrocartilage-like regions [66]. Additionally, periosteum [67] and demineralized bone matrix [68] have been investigated as materials for tendon-to-bone interface regeneration. The periosteum is known to be a source of multipotent stem cells that have the potential to differentiate into osteogenic and chondrogenic lineages. Chang *et al.* sutured a periosteal flap between the torn end of the rabbit infraspinatus tendon and bone [67]. At 4 weeks, fibrous tissue was observed at the interface between the rotator cuff tendon and bone, which later remodeled into a fibrocartilage-like matrix after 12 weeks. A significant increase in failure load over time indicated a progressive increase in the tendon-to-bone integration with healing. Demineralized bone matrix (DBM), which has been reported to exhibit osteogenic and chondrogenic properties, was used by Sundar *et al.* in a patellar tendon ovine model whereby DBM was interposed between patellar tendon and osteotomized bone [68]. Significantly improved functional weight bearing, as well as increased matrix deposition versus the control at the tendon-to-bone interface, were reported.

The delivery of osteoinductive growth factors [69] and the inhibition of matrix metalloproteinases (MMPs) during the healing process [70, 71] have also been tried as means to improve tendon-to-bone integration. Rodeo *et al.* [69] utilized a type I collagen sponge to deliver a mixture of osteoinductive growth factors, which had been harvested from platelet-rich plasma, to the infraspinatus tendon-to-bone interface in an ovine model. Enhanced bone, soft tissue, and fibrocartilage formation, as well as an increase in tendon attachment strength, were noted in the growth-factor-treated groups. Bedi *et al.* [71] investigated the effect of MMP inhibition on tendon-to-bone healing and insertion site regeneration in a rat rotator cuff model. Recombinant α-2-macroglobulin protein, a universal MMP inhibitor, was applied at the tendon-to-bone interface, resulting in enhanced fibrocartilage formation, greater collagen organization, and less collagen degradation.

In addition to biological grafts and cytokines, synthetic biomaterials have been investigated for tendon-to-bone integration. Implantation of a polyglycolide microfiber mesh in a rat model was shown to lead to the formation of an organized fibrovascular matrix at the infraspinatus tendon-to-bone junction [72]. Recently, nanofiber scaffolds have been investigated for tendon-to-bone interface tissue engineering, largely due to their biomimetic potential and physiological relevance. Through modification of fabrication methods, these scaffolds can be designed to match the native tendon matrix, with controlled alignment, high surface-area-to-volume ratio, permeability, and porosity [73–76]. Moffat *et al.* evaluated the effects of PLGA nanofiber organization (aligned vs. unaligned) on human tendon fibroblast attachment and matrix deposition [77]. Nanofiber alignment was found to be the primary factor guiding tendon fibroblast morphology, alignment, and integrin expression. Types I and III collagen, the dominant collagen types of the supraspinatus tendon, were synthesized on the nanofiber scaffolds, and it was shown that their deposition was also controlled by the underlying fiber orientation. Furthermore, scaffold mechanical strength, which was directly related to fiber alignment, decreased as the polymer degraded but remained within the range reported for the native supraspinatus tendon [78].

Building upon these promising results, Moffat *et al.* designed a stratified, composite nanofiber system consisting of distinct yet continuous non-calcified and calcified regions intended to mimic the organization of native tendon-to-bone insertion [79]. The biphasic scaffold is produced by layered electrospinning, with Phase A comprised of aligned PLGA nanofibers to support the regeneration of the non-mineralized fibrocartilage region, and Phase B based on aligned PLGA nanofibers embedded with nanoparticles of hydroxyapatite (PLGA–HA) to support the regeneration of the mineralized fibrocartilage region. The stratified scaffold design was evaluated both in vitro [80] and in vivo [81]. It was observed that a fibrocartilage-like extracellular matrix was found on each scaffold phase, while mineral distribution was maintained, with a calcified fibrocartilage formed on Phase B, through which the biphasic scaffold can functionally integrate with surrounding bone tissue.

Nanofiber scaffolds with gradients in mineral content [19] and structure, specifically fiber alignment [82], have also been investigated for tendon-to-bone interface regeneration. As discussed previously, the natural tendon-to-bone attachment relies on a gradient in structure and composition, resulting in a spatial variation of mechanical properties. By varying the immersion time in concentrated simulated body fluid, Li *et al.* formed a continuously graded calcium phosphate coating that spanned a distance of 12 mm on PLGA and PCL nanofiber scaffolds. The mineral gradient resulted in a gradation in mechanical properties along the length of the scaffold, with lower strains and higher elastic moduli corresponding to areas of higher calcium phosphate concentration. To mimic the change in fiber orientation that exists at the tendon-to-bone insertion site, Xie *et al.* fabricated aligned-to-random electrospun PLGA nanofiber scaffolds using a custom-designed collector [82]. Rat tendon fibroblast cultured on the scaffolds as well as collagen type I deposited on the scaffolds exhibited organized and disorganized morphologies on the aligned and random portions, respectively. Alternatively, Phillips *et al.* employed a novel, cell-based approach toward engineering a graded tissue interface [83], whereby collagen scaffolds with a compositional gradient of retroviral coating for the osteogenic transcription factor RUNX2 induced fibroblasts to produce a gradient of mineralized matrix both in vitro and in vivo. Thus scaffold systems containing interfacial zones of graded mineral content hold significant promise for biomimetic tendon-to-bone interface regeneration.

Since the primary function of the tendon is to connect muscle to bone, the myotendinous junction (MTJ) is an important interface in the musculoskeletal system, serving as a mechanical bridge distributing loads between skeletal muscle and bone [84]. While regeneration/reinforcement of this junction is also critical for functional rotator cuff repair, especially in cases where muscle atrophy has occurred, the MTJ has not been studied extensively. It is known that the interface consists of interdigitating tissue that connects the dense collagen fibers of the tendon to the more elastic muscle fibers while also displaying a gradient of structural properties [85]. Current tissue engineering approaches, as demonstrated by Swasdison *et al.*, include the culturing of myoblasts in collagen gels in vitro to form contractile muscle constructs with fibrils that terminate in a manner similar to the native MTJ [86, 87]. Adopting a cell-based approach, Larkin *et al.* evaluated a novel self-organizing system for in-vitro myotendinous junction formation by co-culturing skeletal muscle constructs with engineered tendon constructs. Interestingly, up-regulation of paxillin was observed at the neo-interface, and the MTJ formed was able to sustain tensile loading beyond the physiological strain range [88].

These results collectively demonstrate the importance of regenerating both the tendon-to-bone interface and the muscle–tendon junction, highlighting the promise of different tissue engineering methodologies for achieving tissue-to-tissue healing and integration. Specifically, functional tendon-to-bone interface tissue engineering focusses on the design of biomimetic scaffolds that are pre-engineered to recapitulate the inherent structural, mechanical, and biochemical heterogeneity of the native interface. Most MTJ regeneration strategies have focussed on elucidating cell–scaffold and cell–cell interaction, but, as research on this musculoskeletal interface matures, it is envisioned that many of the scaffold design strategies utilized for tendon-to-bone interface tissue engineering will also be applied to the MTJ. Biomaterials, combined with physiologically relevant growth factors and cytokines to guide cellular differentiation, have shown promise and hold immense potential for enhancing tendon-to-tissue integration.

28.1.3 Interface scaffold design for cartilage-to-bone tissue engineering

Another interface of the musculoskeletal system is the osteochondral interface which is found between articular cartilage and subchondral bone. The articular cartilage proper consists of the tangential (surface) zone, transitional (middle) zone, and radial (deep) zone; furthermore, directly below the deep zone is the osteochondral interface, which consists of hypertrophic chondrocytes embedded in a mineralized collagen- and proteoglycan-containing matrix [14, 89–91]. This interface serves two critical roles. Its mechanical functions are to provide tissue-to-tissue integration, distribute load from soft to hard tissue, and facilitate the pressurization of articular cartilage [92–94]. Calcified cartilage also regulates transport and vascularization across the interface, thereby maintaining the integrity of cartilage tissue above bone [15]. Hunziker *et al.* elegantly demonstrated the importance of a barrier between cartilage and bone during healing in vivo of full-thickness defects treated with a fibrinogen matrix [95]. It was found that a structural barrier placed between the cartilage and bone compartments, in place of the calcified cartilage layer, was necessary in order to maintain the integrity of the newly formed cartilage by preventing vasculature upgrowth and subsequent ectopic mineralization. The regeneration of the osteochondral interface is therefore critical for integrative and functional cartilage tissue engineering.

Stratified scaffold design has been extensively researched for osteochondral tissue engineering, with the first generation of scaffolds consisting of two distinct cartilage or bone regions joined together using either sutures or sealants (Table 28.3). Schaefer *et al.* seeded articular chondrocytes on polyglycolic acid (PGA) meshes and periosteal cells on poly(lactic-*co*-glycolic acid) (PLGA)–polyethylene glycol foams, and sutured the constructs together one or four weeks after seeding [96]. Integration between the two scaffolds was enhanced when they were brought together after one week, suggesting the importance of immediate osteoblast–chondrocyte interactions for phase-to-phase integration. Gao *et al.* seeded mesenchymal stem cells (MSCs) stimulated with transforming growth factor β_1 (TGF-β_1) for chondrogenic differentiation on a hyaluronan sponge, and stimulated the MSCs with osteogenic media on a porous calcium phosphate scaffold [97]. These scaffolds were then joined by a fibrin sealant and evaluated in a subcutaneous model. Continuous collagen fibers were observed between the two scaffolds after six weeks. Utilizing sequential photo-polymerization, Alhadlaq *et al.* formed a bilayered mandibular condyle-shaped osteochondral construct from a polyethylene glycol-diacrylate hydrogel. The top layer contained MSC-derived chondrocytes while the bottom layer contained MSC-derived osteoblasts [98]. After 12 weeks in vivo, distinct cartilaginous and osseous regions were observed, with histological integration evident between them. Similar observations have been reported for MSCs cultured on biphasic scaffolds [99–101]. Collectively, these studies demonstrate the feasibility of achieving multitissue formation on multiphased scaffolds.

Scaffolds with compositional gradients have been investigated too. Sherwood *et al.* designed a continuous biphasic scaffold using 3D printing and evaluated chondrocyte response to the scaffold [102]. The upper, cartilage region was composed of PLGA/polylactide (PLA), with macroscopic staggered channels to facilitate cell seeding. The lower, bone, portion was characterized by a lower porosity and consisted of PLGA and tricalcium phosphate. Most importantly, there was a transition region with a gradient of composition and porosity. Similarly, a composite polymer scaffold was fabricated from polysulfone and bioactive glass with a dense top layer and porous bottom layer [103]. It was also demonstrated that scaffold microstructure and mechanical properties were tunable by varying the glass and polymer content. Harley *et al.* designed an osteochondral scaffold composed of an unmineralized type II collagen–glycosaminoglycan suspension and a mineralized type I collagen–glycosaminoglycan suspension [104]. The resulting scaffold consisted of cartilage and bone regions, as well as a continuous osteochondral interface-like region in between these two phases. Gradient collagen–HA scaffolds consisting of an upper layer of 100% type I collagen, an intermediate layer of 60% type I collagen and 40% HA, and a lower layer of 30% type I collagen and 70% HA have also been developed [105]. This type of biomimetic scaffold was then tested in an equine osteochondral defect, and it was found that distinct unmineralized and mineralized regions were present.

In addition to compositional gradients, chemical gradients have also been incorporated into osteochondral scaffolds. In a study by Dormer *et al.*,

Table 28.3 Scaffolds for cartilage-to-bone tissue engineering

Study	Scaffold design	Study model/time point	Outcomes
Kandel *et al.* (1997) [122]	Chondrocytes seeded on filters and cultured in mineralizing media	In vitro/bovine articular chondrocytes (deep-zone chondrocytes)	Formation of calcified cartilage matrix, including proteoglycan, collagen II, and collagen X
Schaefer *et al.* (2000) [96]	PGA mesh sutured to PLGA–PEG foam	In vitro/bovine articular chondrocytes and periosteal cells	Improved integration (tissue-to-tissue contact) of cartilage and bone regions with decreased pre-culture time
Gao *et al.* (2001) [97]	Hyaluronan sponge and porous calcium phosphate scaffold joined with fibrin sealant	In vivo/subcutaneous rat model (MSCs + TGF-β_1)/ 3 and 6 weeks	Supports MSC differentiation and continuous fibrocartilage and bone regions
Sherwood *et al.* (2002) [102]	90% porous D,L-PLGA/L-PLA and 55% L-PLGA/TCP composite	In vitro/ovine articular chondrocytes	Gradient of material properties and porosity prevents delamination in transition region
Zhang *et al.* (2002) [103]	Porous composite of polysulfone and BG	Acellular scaffold fabrication	Biomimetic gradient in mechanical properties and porosity of scaffold properties
Alhadlaq *et al.* (2005) [98]	Bilayered PEG hydrogel	In vivo/subcutaneous mouse model (MSCs + TGF-β_1)/ 4 weeks	Supports MSC differentiation and stratified cartilage- and bone-like regions
Allan *et al.* (2007) [112]	Chondrocytes seeded directly above calcium phosphate substrate	In vitro/bovine chondrocytes (deep-zone chondrocytes)	Formation of calcified cartilage matrix in presence of mineralizing media
Swieszkowski *et al.* (2007) [99]	PCL and PCL/TCP composite	In vivo/osteochondral rabbit model (MSCs)/3 and 6 months	Promotes bone filling and regeneration
Heymer *et al.* (2009) [108]	Collagen fiber cartilage scaffold and mineralized PLA bone scaffold, addition of hyaluronan used to make cartilage and bone hydrophilic with hydrophobic region at interface	In vitro/human MSCs + TGF-β_1	Chondrogenic differentiation restricted to upper third of scaffold
Harley *et al.* (2010) [104]	Mineralized collagen I/GAG and nonmineralized collagen II/GAG with interdiffused interface region	Acellular scaffold fabrication	Biomimetic gradient of scaffold mechanical properties, porosity, and composition
Dormer *et al.* (2010) [106]	PLGA microsphere scaffold with opposing BMP-2 and TGF-β_1 gradients	In vitro/human MSCs + TGF-β_1	Gradient scaffold produces cartilage- and bone-like matrices on single scaffold
Jiang *et al.* (2010) [123]	Agarose hydrogel and PLGA/BG composite	In vitro/bovine chondrocytes and osteoblasts	Supports region-specific co-culture of chondrocytes and osteoblasts, which can lead to the production of distinct yet continuous regions of cartilage, calcified cartilage-like, and bone-like matrices
Kon *et al.* (2010) [124]	100% collagen, 60% collagen/40% HA, 30% collagen/70% HA trilayered scaffold	In vivo/osteochondral horse model/6 months	Regeneration of fibrocartilage and bone tissue with tidemark at interface

Table 28.3 (cont.)

Study	Scaffold design	Study model/time point	Outcomes
Cheng *et al.* (2011) [110]	Cells encapsulated in collagen microspheres and then aggregated to form chondrogenic and osteogenic layers of the osteochondral scaffold, with a middle layer of undifferentiated cells	In vitro/rabbit MSCs + TGF-β_1	Formation of an intact and continuous calcified cartilage zone separating an upper non-calcified chondrongenic layer and an underlying osteogenic layer
Erisken *et al.* (2011) [107]	PCL nanofiber scaffolds with insulin and β-GP gradients	In vitro/human adipose-derived stem cells	Insulin promotes chondrogenic differentiation and β-GP promotes mineralization
Khanarian *et al.* (2011) [115]	Composite 2% alginate hydrogel with 1.5 wt/vol% HA (25 μm)	In vitro/bovine chondrocytes (deep-zone chondrocytes)	HA presence promotes deep-zone chondrocyte hypertrophy and collagen deposition
Khanarian *et al.* (2012) [116]	Composite 2% agarose hydrogel with 1.5–6 wt/vol% HA (200 nm and 25 μm)	In vitro/bovine chondrocytes (deep-zone chondrocytes and induced hypertrophic chondrocytes)	Addition of 3 wt/vol% micro-HA promotes highest mineralization potential, matrix deposition, and scaffold mechanical strength

chondrogenic and osteogenic growth factors were added to a PLGA microsphere-based scaffold in opposing gradients [106]. This scaffold was then seeded with human MSCs, and it was found that there was a corresponding gradient from cartilage-like to bone-like matrices. Using a novel twin-screw extrusion and electrospinning method, gradients of insulin and β-glycerophosphate (β-GP) have also been added to poly(ε-caprolactone) nanofiber mesh [107]. These scaffolds were then seeded with human adipose-derived stromal cells, and it was found that chondrogenic differentiation of the stem cells increased at insulin-rich locations and mineralization increased at β-GP-rich locations. These results clearly demonstrate the feasibility of forming unmineralized and mineralized tissue, but the challenge of finding out how to consistently regenerate a distinct calcified cartilage layer at the soft-to-hard-tissue junction, after cartilage repair, still remains. One approach, inspired by the classic barrier study by Hunziker *et al.* [95], was to introduce an acellular barrier between the cartilage and bone regions. To this end, Heymer *et al.* utilized a hydrophobic interface to separate the cartilage and subchondral bone portions of a composite scaffold, which was comprised of collagen I fibers and mineral containing-polylactic acid [108]. To initially demonstrate the feasibility of the scaffold, MSCs were seeded in the collagen I matrix, and chondrogensis and abundant glycosaminoglycan deposition were observed. The formation of cartilage-like tissue, which was confined to the top portion of the composite scaffold, demonstrated the promise of the construct for osteochondral repair.

The importance of cell–cell interactions has also been a focus of interface regeneration. A novel scaffold design by Jiang *et al.* consisted of an agarose hydrogel layered above composite microspheres of PLGA and 45S5 bioactive glass [109]. It was observed that the stratified scaffold supported the region-specific co-culture of chondrocytes and osteoblasts which can lead to the production of three distinct yet continuous regions of cartilage, calcified cartilage, and bone-like matrices. More recently, in a study by Cheng *et al.*, MSCs cultured in collagen microspheres were pre-differentiated into chondrocytes and osteoblasts using a novel collagen microencapsulation technology [110].

These microspheres were then aggregated to form chondrogenic and osteogenic layers of the osteochondral scaffold, with a middle layer of undifferentiated MSCs. Formation of a calcified cartilage interface layer occurred only in the triculture group with all three layers, whereas no interface was observed when undifferentiated MSCs were cultured on bilayered scaffolds with either chondrogenic or osteogenic layers. These results highlight the importance of cell-to-cell interactions for interface formation.

The ideal scaffold for an osteochondral interface should support chondrocyte viability and the interface-relevant hypertrophic phenotype. Secondly, the scaffold should support comparable proteoglycan and collagen deposition to that of deep-zone cartilage, with interface-relevant mechanical properties. Furthermore, the scaffold should support formation of calcified cartilage and prohibit ectopic mineralization. Finally, the interface scaffold must be osteointegrative. Most of the published approaches toward regenerating the osteochondral interface have been largely cell-based, with chondrocytes cultured in a mineralizing medium and/or seeded directly on a calcium phosphate substrate. Kandel *et al.* first seeded deep-zone chondrocytes on filter inserts that had been pre-coated with collagen II and also cultured in a mineralizing medium containing 10 mM β-GP [111]. It was found that mineralized cartilage formed in the region directly adjacent to the insert. More recently, Allan *et al.* seeded interface-relevant deep-zone chondrocytes directly above a calcium polyphosphate scaffold and formed a calcified cartilage-like zone above the ceramic in a mineralization medium [112]. The mineral formed in vitro was shown to be biomimetic, and the interfacial mechanical properties were also found to be superior to those of scaffolds cultured without mineralizing media, which lacked the mineralized cartilage zone [113].

Biomimetic hydrogel–ceramic composite scaffolds have recently been investigated for calcified cartilage regeneration. Hydrogel scaffolds are commonly used for chondrocyte culture and cartilage tissue engineering applications since these scaffolds have been shown to maintain the chondrocyte phenotype and biosynthetic activity. The ceramic phase within the scaffold consists of HA particles that have similar chemistry to that found in calcified cartilage [114]. In comparison with scaffold-free osteochondral interface engineering approaches where chondrocytes are seeded above ceramic substrates, relatively fewer chondrocytes are needed to seed hydrogel–ceramic scaffolds. Additionally, ceramic can be directly incorporated into the scaffold, which decreases the need for cell-mediated mineralization. Hydrogel-based scaffolds can also integrate with hydrogel-based cartilage grafts for integrative cartilage repair (Figure 28.1).

In a study by Khanarian *et al.*, a hybrid scaffold of HA and alginate hydrogel was evaluated for the regeneration of the osteochondral interface [115]. It was observed that the HA phase of the composite scaffold promoted the formation of a proteoglycan and type II collagen-rich matrix when seeded with deep-zone chondrocytes. More importantly, the elevated biosynthesis translated into significant increases in both compressive and shear moduli relative to those of the ceramic-free control. The presence of HA also promoted chondrocyte hypertrophy and deposition of type X collagen. In a subsequent study optimizing the ceramic phase of an agarose–HA composite scaffold, it was determined that hypertrophic chondrocytes also exhibited higher matrix deposition and mineralization potential with the addition of HA [116]. While cell hypertrophy was observed to be independent of ceramic size, matrix deposition increased only with the addition of micron-sized ceramic particles. In addition, the highest matrix content, mechanical strength, and mineralization potential were found in scaffolds with 3% micro-HA, which approximates both the mineral aggregate size and the content of the native interface. These observations suggest that a biomimetic hydrogel–ceramic composite is optimal for calcified cartilage formation, and that its use is a promising design strategy for osteochondral interface regeneration. It is expected that the ceramic phase of the scaffold would promote osteointegration with bone, while the hydrogel phase can facilitate integration with other hydrogel-based cartilage grafts.

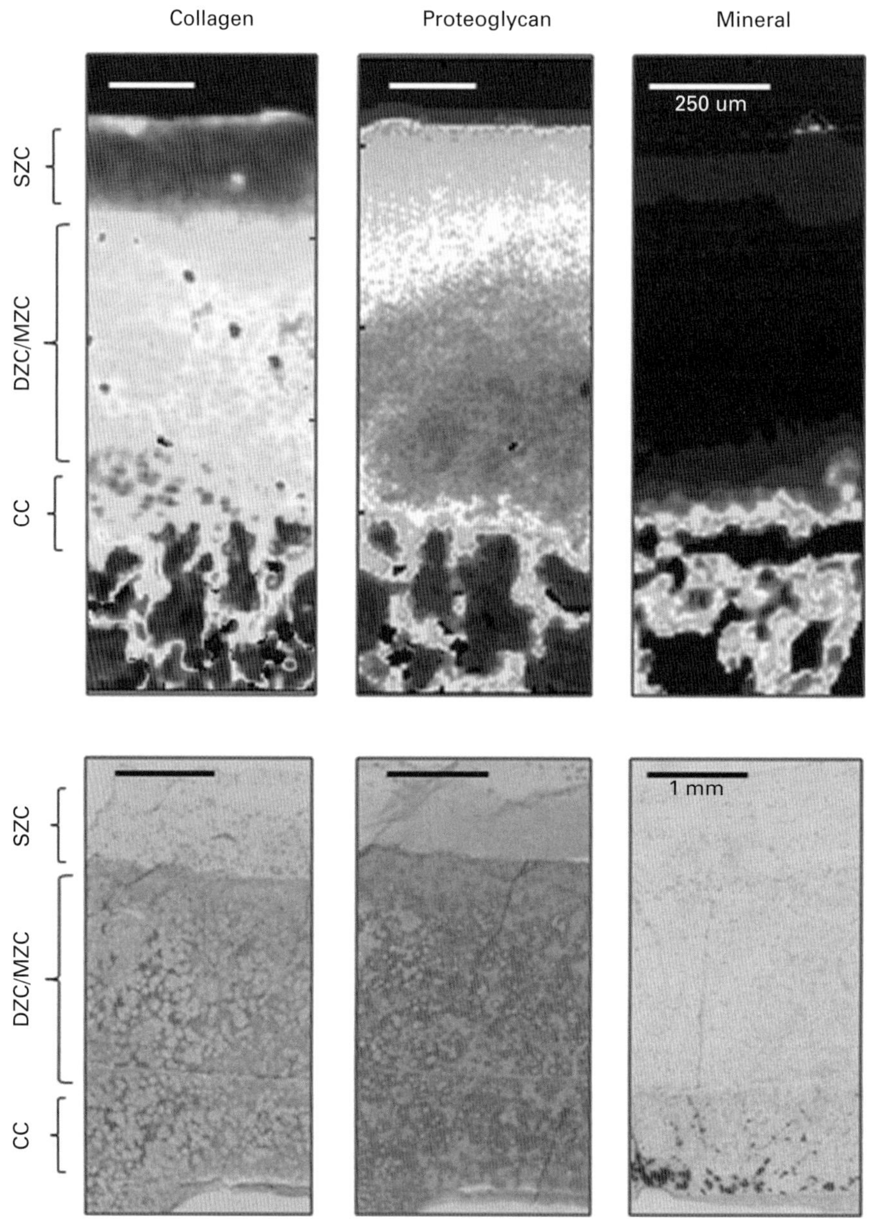

Figure 28.1 Biomimetic cartilage-to-bone scaffold design. The distribution of collagen, proteoglycan, and mineral across the osteochondral interface has been determined using Fourier-transform infrared imaging. The calcified cartilage (CC) region is characterized by mineral presence and high matrix content. A hydrogel-based scaffold can be used to mimic the matrix and mineral transition from soft to hard tissue, with stratified surface (SZC), middle-zone (MZC), and deep-zone chondrocytes (DZC) seeded in ceramic-free agarose above the CC layer comprised of DZC in hydroxyapatite-containing agarose. As in the native tissue, matrix and mineral staining is lowest at the articular surface, followed by mineral-free and matrix-rich deep-zone cartilage, and finally, mineral-rich and matrix-rich calcified cartilage.

In summary, results from these studies collectively highlight the importance of the cartilage-to-bone interface for functional cartilage repair, as well as the unique tissue engineering challenges faced, such as how to control and take advantage of cell–cell and cell–scaffold interactions. The use of scaffolds designed with multiple phases or a gradient of properties that mimic the compositional and chemical gradients present in the native interface, in conjunction with the use of relevant cell populations, constitutes a promising approach toward engineering the osteochondral interface and achieving cartilage-to-bone integration.

28.2 Summary and future directions

Interface tissue engineering, which focusses on the functional regeneration of the anatomic interface between distinct tissue types, is essential for musculoskeletal function. It aims to develop innovative technologies for the formation of complex tissue systems, with the broader goal of achieving the biological fixation of biological or tissue-engineered grafts with the host environment. Biomimetic scaffolds developed to mimic the structure and function of the native soft-tissue-to-bone interface have been designed to contain a gradient in mechanical and structural properties. Furthermore, imparting control over the spatial distribution of interface-relevant cell populations has also been shown to support the formation of integrated multitissue systems. The vast potential of multiphased scaffold systems is evident from the in-vitro and in-vivo evaluations described in this chapter for the integrative repair of major soft-tissue injuries. Moreover, these novel scaffolds can be further refined by incorporating well-controlled gradients in composition, growth factors, and other bioactive molecules, as well as through the use of biochemical and biomechanical stimulation to encourage tissue growth and maturation. Clinically, the use of stratified scaffolds would significantly improve current soft-tissue repair strategies by encouraging functional integration with host tissue, and stimulating interface formation while also enabling biological fixation.

It is clear that interface tissue engineering will be instrumental for the ex-vivo development and in-vivo regeneration of functionally integrated musculoskeletal tissue systems, but there remains a number of challenges in this exciting area. These include the need for a greater understanding of the structure–function relationship existing at the native tissue-to-tissue interface as well as of how the graded structures between different types of connective tissues are formed and re-established after injury. Further research on long-term interface maintenance is also needed. Moreover, the effects of biological, physical, and chemical stimulation on interface formation and regeneration also remain to be explored. Physiologically relevant in-vivo models are also needed in order to determine the clinical potential of the designed scaffolds.

As is evident in many of the reported studies, selection of multiple cell sources is typically necessary in order to ensure or promote heterogeneous tissue formation. Clinical implementation of these scaffolds will ultimately require identifying an optimal cell source that is both readily available and highly expandable. Mesenchymal stem cells are an expandable, attractive alternative cell source for interface regeneration. While interface-relevant cells must be surgically obtained from the patient or from a donor, adult stem cells can be isolated from the patient's own bone marrow, adipose tissue or blood via minimally invasive outpatient procedures. When stimulated with appropriate signals, stem cells can be guided to differentiate into multiple cell types, including fibroblasts, osteoblasts, chondrocytes, hypertrophic chondrocytes, and fibrochondrocytes.

In summary, strategic biomimicry provides the inspiration for the design of novel interface scaffolds and for achieving biological fixation and integrative soft-tissue repair. It is anticipated that these efforts will lead to the development of a new generation of functional fixation devices for soft-tissue repair as well as augmenting the clinical translation potential of tissue-engineered grafts. Moreover, by bridging distinct types of tissue, interface tissue engineering will be instrumental for the development of integrated musculoskeletal tissue systems with biomimetic complexity and functionality.

REFERENCES

[1] Lu, H. H., Subramony, S. D., Boushell, M. K. and Zhang, X. 2010. Tissue engineering strategies for the regeneration of orthopedic interfaces. *Ann. Biomed. Eng.*, **38**(6), 2142–54.

[2] Benjamin, M., Evans, E. J. and Copp, L. 1986. The histology of tendon attachments to bone in man. *J. Anat.*, **149**, 89–100.

[3] Lu, H. H. and Jiang, J. 2006. Interface tissue engineering and the formulation of multiple-tissue systems. *Adv. Biochem. Eng. Biotechnol.*, **102**, 91–111.

[4] Woo, S. L., Maynard, J., Butler, D. L. *et al.* 1988. Ligament, tendon, and joint capsule insertions to bone. In Woo, S. L.-Y. and Buckwalter, J. A., editors. *Injury and Repair of Musculoskeletal Soft Tissues.* Chicago, IL: American Academy of Orthopaedic Surgeons, pp. 133–66.

[5] Friedman, M. J., Sherman, O. H., Fox, J. M. *et al.* 1985. Autogeneic anterior cruciate ligament (ACL) anterior reconstruction of the knee. A review. *Clin. Orthop.*, **196**, 9–14.

[6] Robertson, D. B., Daniel, D. M. and Biden, E. 1986. Soft tissue fixation to bone. *Am. J. Sports Med.*, **14**(5), 398–403.

[7] Butler, D. L., Goldstein, S. A. and Guilak, F. 2000. Functional tissue engineering: the role of biomechanics. *J. Biomech. Eng.*, **122**(6), 570–5.

[8] Moffat, K. L., Wang, I. N., Rodeo, S. A. and Lu, H. H. 2009. Orthopedic interface tissue engineering for the biological fixation of soft tissue grafts. *Clin. Sports Med.*, **28**(1), 157–76.

[9] Cooper, R. R. and Misol, S. 1970. Tendon and ligament insertion. A light and electron microscopic study. *J. Bone Joint Surg. Am.*, **52**(1), 1–20.

[10] Wang, I. E., Mitroo, S., Chen, F. H., Lu, H. H. and Doty, S. B. 2006. Age-dependent changes in matrix composition and organization at the ligament-to-bone insertion. *J. Orthop. Res.*, **24**(8), 1745–55.

[11] Matyas, J. R., Anton, M. G., Shrive, N. G. and Frank, C. B. 1995. Stress governs tissue phenotype at the femoral insertion of the rabbit MCL. *J. Biomech.*, **28** (2), 147–57.

[12] Spalazzi, J. P., Costa, K. D., Doty, S. B. and Lu, H. H. 2004. Characterization of the mechanical properties, structure, and composition of the anterior cruciate ligament-bone insertion site. *Trans. Orthopaedic Res. Soc.*, **29**, Poster #1271.

[13] Moffat, K. L., Sun, W. H., Pena, P. E. *et al.* 2008. Characterization of the structure-function relationship at the ligament-to-bone interface. *Proc. Nat. Acad. Sci. USA*, **105**(23), 7947–52.

[14] Bullough, P. G. and Jagannath, A. 1983. The morphology of the calcification front in articular cartilage. Its significance in joint function. *J. Bone Joint Surg. Br.*, **65**(1), 72–8.

[15] Oegema, T. R. Jr. and Thompson, R. C. Jr. 1992. The zone of calcified cartilage. Its role in osteoarthritis. In Kuettner, K. E., Schleyerbach, R., Peyron, J. G. and Hascall, V. C., editors. *Articular Cartilage and Osteoarthritis.* New York: Raven Press, pp. 319–31.

[16] Thomopoulos, S., Williams, G. R., Gimbel J. A., Favata, M. and Soslowsky, L. J. 2003. Variations of biomechanical, structural, and compositional properties along the tendon to bone insertion site. *J. Orthop. Res.*, **21**(3), 413–19.

[17] Ralphs, J. R., Benjamin, M., Waggett, A. D. *et al.* 1998. Regional differences in cell shape and gap junction expression in rat Achilles tendon: relation to fibrocartilage differentiation. *J. Anat.*, **193**(Part 2), 215–22.

[18] Ladd, M. R., Lee, S. J., Stitzel, J. D., Atala, A. and Yoo, J. J. 2011. Co-electrospun dual scaffolding system with potential for muscle-tendon junction tissue engineering. *Biomaterials*, **32**(6), 1549–59.

[19] Li, X. R., Xie, J. W., Lipner, J. *et al.* 2009. Nanofiber scaffolds with gradations in mineral content for mimicking the tendon-to-bone insertion site. *Nano Lett.*, **9**(7), 2763–8.

[20] Wang, I. E., Shan, J., Choi, R. *et al.* 2007. Role of osteoblast-fibroblast interactions in the formation of the ligament-to-bone interface. *J. Orthop. Res.*, **25**(12), 1609–20.

[21] Spalazzi, J. P., Doty, S. B., Moffat, K. L., Levine, W. N. and Lu, H. H. 2006. Development of controlled matrix heterogeneity on a triphasic scaffold for orthopedic interface tissue engineering. *Tissue Eng.*, **12**(12), 3497–508.

[22] Spalazzi, J. P., Dagher, E., Doty, S. B. *et al.* 2008. In vivo evaluation of a multiphased scaffold designed for orthopaedic interface tissue engineering and soft tissue-to-bone integration. *J. Biomed. Mater. Res. Part A*, **86**(1), 1–12.

[23] Rodeo, S. A., Arnoczky, S. P., Torzilli, P. A., Hidaka, C. and Warren, R. F. 1993. Tendon-healing in a bone tunnel. A biomechanical and histological study in the dog. *J. Bone Joint Surg. Am.*, **75**(12), 1795–803.

[24] Rodeo, S. A., Suzuki, K., Deng, X. H., Wozney, J. and Warren, R. F. 1999. Use of recombinant human bone morphogenetic protein-2 to enhance tendon healing in a bone tunnel. *Am. J. Sports Med.*, **27**(4), 476–88.

[25] Kurosaka, M., Yoshiya, S. and Andrish, J. T. 1987. A biomechanical comparison of different surgical techniques of graft fixation in anterior cruciate ligament reconstruction. *Am. J. Sports Med.*, **15**(3), 225–9.

[26] Tien, Y. C., Chih, T. T., Lin, J. H., Ju, C. P. and Lin, S. D. 2004. Augmentation of tendon–bone healing by the use of calcium-phosphate cement. *J. Bone Joint Surg. Br.*, **86**(7), 1072–6.

[27] Huangfu, X. and Zhao, J. 2007. Tendon–bone healing enhancement using injectable tricalcium phosphate in a dog anterior cruciate ligament reconstruction model. *Arthroscopy*, **23**(5), 455–62.

[28] Gulotta, L. V., Kovacevic, D., Ying, L. *et al.* 2008. Augmentation of tendon-to-bone healing with a magnesium-based bone adhesive. *Am. J. Sports Med.*, **36**(7), 1290–7.

[29] Robertson, W. J., Hatch, J. D. and Rodeo, S. A. 2007. Evaluation of tendon graft fixation using α-BSM calcium phosphate cement. *Arthroscopy*, **23**(10), 1087–92.

[30] Ishikawa, H., Koshino, T., Takeuchi, R. and Saito, T. 2001. Effects of collagen gel mixed with hydroxyapatite powder on interface between newly formed bone and grafted Achilles tendon in rabbit femoral bone tunnel. *Biomaterials*, **22**(12), 1689–94.

[31] Shen, H., Qiao, G., Cao, H. and Jiang, Y. 2010. An histological study of the influence of osteoinductive calcium phosphate ceramics on tendon healing pattern in a bone tunnel with suspensory fixation. *Int. Orthop.*, **34**(6), 917–24.

[32] Mutsuzaki, H., Sakane, M., Nakajima, H. *et al.* 2004. Calcium-phosphate-hybridized tendon directly promotes regeneration of tendon–bone insertion. *J. Biomed. Mater. Res. A*, **70**(2), 319–27.

[33] Chen, C. H., Chen, W. J., Shih, C. H. *et al.* 2003. Enveloping the tendon graft with periosteum to enhance tendon–bone healing in a bone tunnel: a biomechanical and histologic study in rabbits. *Arthroscopy*, **19**(3), 290–6.

[34] Youn, I., Jones, D. G., Andrews, P. J., Cook, M. P. and Suh, J. K. 2004. Periosteal augmentation of a tendon graft improves tendon healing in the bone tunnel. *Clin. Orthop. Relat. Res.*, **419**, 223–31.

[35] Ohtera, K., Yamada, Y., Aoki, M., Sasaki, T. and Yamakoshi, K. 2000. Effects of periosteum wrapped around tendon in a bone tunnel: a biomechanical and histological study in rabbits. *Crit. Rev. Biomed. Eng.*, **28**(1–2), 115–18.

[36] Kyung, H. S., Kim, S. Y., Oh, C. W. and Kim, S. J. 2003. Tendon-to-bone tunnel healing in a rabbit model: the effect of periosteum augmentation at the tendon-to-bone interface. *Knee Surg. Sports Traumatol. Arthrosc.*, **11**(1), 9–15.

[37] Karaoglu, S., Celik, C. and Korkusuz, P. 2009. The effects of bone marrow or periosteum on tendon-to-bone tunnel healing in a rabbit model. *Knee Surg. Sports Traumatol. Arthrosc.*, **17**(2), 170–8.

[38] Hashimoto, Y., Yoshida, G., Toyoda, H. and Takaoka, K. 2007. Generation of tendon-to-bone interface "enthesis" with use of recombinant BMP-2 in a rabbit model. *J. Orthop. Res.*, **25**(11), 1415–24.

[39] Ma, C. B., Kawamura, S., Deng, X. H. *et al.* 2007. Bone morphogenetic proteins-signaling plays a role in tendon-to-bone healing: a study of rhBMP-2 and noggin. *Am. J. Sports Med.*, **35**(4), 597–604.

[40] Martinek, V., Latterman, C., Usas, A. *et al.* 2002. Enhancement of tendon–bone integration of anterior cruciate ligament grafts with bone morphogenetic protein-2 gene transfer: a histological and biomechanical study. *J. Bone Joint Surg. Am.*, **84A**(7), 1123–31.

[41] Chen, C. H., Liu, H. W., Tsai, C. L. *et al.* 2008. Photoencapsulation of bone morphogenetic protein-2 and periosteal progenitor cells improve tendon graft healing in a bone tunnel. *Am. J. Sports Med.*, **36**(3), 461–73.

[42] Mihelić, R., Pečina, M., Jelić, M. *et al.* 2004. Bone morphogenetic protein-7 (osteogenic protein-1) promotes tendon graft integration in anterior cruciate ligament reconstruction in sheep. *Am. J. Sports Med.*, **32**(7), 1619–25.

[43] Sasaki, K., Kuroda, R., Ishida, K. *et al.* 2008. Enhancement of tendon–bone osteointegration of anterior cruciate ligament graft using granulocyte colony-stimulating factor. *Am. J. Sports Med.*, **36**(8), 1519–27.

[44] Soon, M. Y., Hassan, A., Hui, J. H., Goh, J. C. and Lee, E. H. 2007. An analysis of soft tissue allograft anterior cruciate ligament reconstruction in a rabbit model: a short-term study of the use of mesenchymal stem cells to enhance tendon osteointegration. *Am. J. Sports Med.*, **35**(6), 962–71.

[45] Fan, H., Liu, H., Wong, E. J., Toh, S. L. and Goh, J. C. 2008. In vivo study of anterior cruciate ligament regeneration using mesenchymal stem cells and silk scaffold. *Biomaterials*, **29**(23), 3324–37.

[46] Ju, Y. J., Muneta, T., Yoshimura, H., Koga, H. and Sekiya, I. 2008. Synovial mesenchymal stem cells accelerate early remodeling of tendon-bone healing. *Cell Tissue Res.*, **332**(3), 469–78.

[47] Lim, J. K., Hui, J., Li, L. *et al.* 2004. Enhancement of tendon graft osteointegration using mesenchymal stem cells in a rabbit model of anterior cruciate ligament reconstruction. *Arthroscopy*, **20**(9), 899–910.

[48] Ouyang, H. W., Goh, J. C. and Lee, E. H. 2004. Use of bone marrow stromal cells for tendon graft-to-bone healing: histological and immunohistochemical studies in a rabbit model. *Am. J. Sports Med.*, **32**(2), 321–7.

[49] Dunn, M. G., Liesch, J. B., Tiku, M. L. and Zawadsky, J. P. 1995. Development of fibroblast-seeded ligament analogs for ACL reconstruction. *J. Biomed. Mater. Res.*, **29**(11), 1363–71.

[50] Altman, G. H., Horan, R. L., Lu, H. H. *et al.* 2002. Silk matrix for tissue engineered anterior cruciate ligaments. *Biomaterials*, **23**(20), 4131–41.

[51] Dunn, M. G., Tria, A. J., Kato, Y. P. *et al.* 1992. Anterior cruciate ligament reconstruction using a composite collagenous prosthesis. A biomechanical and histologic study in rabbits. *Am. J. Sports Med.*, **20**(5), 507–15.

[52] Cooper, J. A., Lu, H. H., Ko, F. K., Freeman, J. W. and Laurencin, C. T. 2005. Fiber-based tissue-engineered scaffold for ligament replacement: design considerations and in vitro evaluation. *Biomaterials*, **26**(13), 1523–32.

[53] Inoue, N., Ikeda, K., Aro, H. T. *et al.* 2002. Biologic tendon fixation to metallic implant augmented with autogenous cancellous bone graft and bone marrow in a canine model. *J. Orthop. Res.*, **20**(5), 957–66.

[54] Cooper, J. A. Jr., Sahota, J. S., Gorum, W. J. *et al.* 2007. Biomimetic tissue-engineered anterior cruciate ligament replacement. *Proc. Nat. Acad. Sci. USA*, **104**(9), 3049–54.

[55] Lu, H. H., Cooper, J. A. Jr., Manuel, S. *et al.* 2005. Anterior cruciate ligament regeneration using braided biodegradable scaffolds: in vitro optimization studies. *Biomaterials*, **26**(23), 4805–16.

[56] Ma, J., Goble, K., Smietana, M. *et al.* 2009. Morphological and functional characteristics of three-dimensional engineered bone-ligament-bone constructs following implantation. *J. Biomech. Eng.*, **131**(10), 101017.

[57] Paxton, J. Z., Donnelly, K., Keatch, R. P. and Baar, K. 2009. Engineering the bone-ligament interface using polyethylene glycol diacrylate incorporated with hydroxyapatite. *Tissue Eng. Part A*, **15**(6), 1201–9.

[58] Lu, H. H., El Amin, S. F., Scott, K. D. and Laurencin, C. T. 2003. Three-dimensional, bioactive, biodegradable, polymer-bioactive glass composite scaffolds with improved mechanical properties support collagen synthesis and mineralization of human osteoblast-like cells in vitro. *J. Biomed. Mater. Res.*, **64A**(3), 465–74.

[59] Lee, J., Il Choi, W., Tae, G. *et al.* 2011. Enhanced regeneration of the ligament-bone interface using a poly (L-lactide-*co*-ε-caprolactone) scaffold with local delivery of cells/BMP-2 using a heparin-based hydrogel. *Acta Biomater.*, **7**(1), 244–57.

[60] Spalazzi, J. P., Vyner, M. C., Jacobs, M. T., Moffat, K. L. and Lu, H. H. 2008. Mechanoactive scaffold induces tendon remodeling and expression of fibrocartilage markers. *Clin. Orthopaedics Related Res.*, **466**(8), 1938–48.

[61] Blevins, F. T., Djurasovic, M., Flatow, E. L. and Vogel, K. G. 1997. Biology of the rotator cuff tendon. *Orthop. Clin. North Am.*, **28**(1), 1–16.

[62] Galatz, L. M., Ball, C. M., Teefey, S. A., Middleton, W. D. and Yamaguchi, K. 2004. The outcome and repair integrity of completely arthroscopically repaired large and massive rotator cuff tears. *J. Bone Joint Surg. Am.*, **86A**(2), 219–24.

[63] Coons, D. A. and Alan, B. F. 2006. Tendon graft substitutes-rotator cuff patches. *Sports Med. Arthrosc.*, **14**(3), 185–90.

[64] Derwin, K. A., Baker, A. R., Spragg, R. K., Leigh, D. R. and Iannotti, J. P. 2006. Commercial extracellular matrix scaffolds for rotator cuff tendon repair. Biomechanical, biochemical, and cellular properties. *J. Bone Joint Surg. Am.*, **88**(12), 2665–72.

[65] Iannotti, J. P., Codsi, M. J., Kwon, Y. W. *et al.* 2006. Porcine small intestine submucosa augmentation of surgical repair of chronic two-tendon rotator cuff tears. A randomized, controlled trial. *J. Bone Joint Surg. Am.*, **88**(6), 1238–44.

[66] Fujioka, H., Thakur, R., Wang, G. J. *et al.* 1998. Comparison of surgically attached and non-attached repair of the rat Achilles tendon-bone interface. Cellular organization and type X collagen expression. *Connect. Tissue Res.*, **37**(3-4), 205–18.

[67] Chang, C. H., Chen, C. H., Su, C. Y., Liu, H. T. and Yu, C. M. 2009. Rotator cuff repair with periosteum for enhancing tendon-bone healing: a biomechanical and histological study in rabbits. *Knee Surg. Sports Traumatol. Arthrosc.*, **17**(12), 1447–53.

[68] Sundar, S., Pendegrass, C. J. and Blunn, G. W. 2009. Tendon bone healing can be enhanced by demineralized bone matrix: a functional and histological

study. *J. Biomed. Mater. Res. B Appl. Biomater.*, **88**(1), 115–22.

[69] Rodeo, S. A., Potter, H. G., Kawamura, S. *et al.* 2007. Biologic augmentation of rotator cuff tendon-healing with use of a mixture of osteoinductive growth factors. *J. Bone Joint Surg. Am.*, **89**(11), 2485–97.

[70] Gulotta, L. V., Kovacevic, D., Montgomery, S. *et al.* 2010. Stem cells genetically modified with the developmental gene MT1-MMP improve regeneration of the supraspinatus tendon-to-bone insertion site. *Am. J. Sports Med.*, **38**(7), 1429–37.

[71] Bedi, A., Kovacevic, D., Hettrich, C. *et al.* 2010. The effect of matrix metalloproteinase inhibition on tendon-to-bone healing in a rotator cuff repair model. *J. Shoulder. Elbow. Surg.*, **19**(3), 384–91.

[72] Yokoya, S., Mochizuki, Y., Nagata, Y., Deie, M. and Ochi, M. 2008. Tendon–bone insertion repair and regeneration using polyglycolic acid sheet in the rabbit rotator cuff injury model. *Am. J. Sports Med.*, **36**(7), 1298–309.

[73] Ma, Z., Kotaki, M., Inai, R. and Ramakrishna, S. 2005. Potential of nanofiber matrix as tissue-engineering scaffolds. *Tissue Eng.*, **11**(1–2), 101–9.

[74] Li, W. J., Laurencin, C. T., Caterson, E. J., Tuan, R. S. and Ko, F. K. 2002. Electrospun nanofibrous structure: a novel scaffold for tissue engineering. *J. Biomed. Mater. Res.*, **60**(4), 613–21.

[75] Pham, Q. P., Sharma, U. and Mikos, A. G. 2006. Electrospinning of polymeric nanofibers for tissue engineering applications: a review. *Tissue Eng.*, **12**(5), 1197–211.

[76] Li, W. J., Mauck, R. L., Cooper, J. A., Yuan, X. and Tuan, R. S. 2007. Engineering controllable anisotropy in electrospun biodegradable nanofibrous scaffolds for musculoskeletal tissue engineering. *J. Biomech.*, **40**(8), 1686–93.

[77] Moffat, K. L., Kwei, A. S., Spalazzi, J. P. *et al.* 2009. Novel nanofiber-based scaffold for rotator cuff repair and augmentation. *Tissue Eng. Part A*, **15**(1), 115–26.

[78] Itoi, E., Berglund, L. J., Grabowski, J. J. *et al.* 1995. Tensile properties of the supraspinatus tendon. *J. Orthop. Res.*, **13**(4), 578–84.

[79] Moffat, K. L., Levine, W. N. and Lu, H. H. 2008. In vitro evaluation of rotator cuff tendon fibroblasts on aligned composite scaffold of polymer nanofibers and hydroxyapatite nanoparticles. In *Transactions of the 54th Annual Meeting of the Orthopaedic Research Society.*

[80] Moffat, K. L. 2010. Biomimetic nanofiber scaffold design for tendon-to-bone interface tissue engineering. Ph.D. Thesis, Columbia University.

[81] Moffat, K. L., Cassilly, R. T., Subramony, S. D. *et al.* 2010. In vivo evalution of a bi-phasic nanofiber-based scaffold for integrative rotator cuff repair. In *Transactions of the 56th Annual Meeting of the Orthopaedic Research Society.*

[82] Xie, J., Li, X., Lipner, J. *et al.* 2010. "Aligned-to-random" nanofiber scaffolds for mimicking the structure of the tendon-to-bone insertion site. *Nanoscale*, **2**(6), 923–6.

[83] Phillips, J. E., Burns, K. L., Le Doux, J. M., Guldberg, R. E. and Garcia, A. J. 2008. Engineering graded tissue interfaces. *Proc. Nat. Acad. Sci. USA*, **105**(34), 12170–5.

[84] Yang, P. J. and Temenoff, J. S. 2009. Engineering orthopedic tissue interfaces. *Tissue Eng. Part B Rev.*, **15**(2), 127–41.

[85] Tidball, J. G. 1991. Myotendinous junction injury in relation to junction structure and molecular composition. *Exerc. Sport Sci. Rev.*, **19**, 419–45.

[86] Swasdison, S. and Mayne, R. 1991. In vitro attachment of skeletal muscle fibers to a collagen gel duplicates the structure of the myotendinous junction. *Exp. Cell Res.*, **193**(1), 227–31.

[87] Swasdison, S. and Mayne, R. 1992. Formation of highly organized skeletal muscle fibers in vitro. Comparison with muscle development in vivo. *J. Cell Sci.*, **102**(Part 3), 643–52.

[88] Larkin, L. M., Calve, S., Kostrominova, T. Y. and Arruda, E. M. 2006. Structure and functional evaluation of tendon–skeletal muscle constructs engineered in vitro. *Tissue Eng.*, **12**(11), 3149–58.

[89] Fawns, H. T. and Landells, J. W. 1953. Histochemical studies of rheumatic conditions. I. Observations on the fine structures of the matrix of normal bone and cartilage. *Ann. Rheum. Dis.*, **12**(2), 105–13.

[90] Oegema, T. R. Jr. and Thompson, R. C. Jr. 1990. Cartilage–bone interface (tidemark). In Brandt, K. D., editor. *Cartilage Changes in Osteoarthritis.* Bloomington, IN: Indiana University Press, pp. 43–52.

[91] Lyons, T. J., Stoddart, R. W., McClure, S. F. and McClure, J. 2005. The tidemark of the chondro-osseous junction of the normal human knee joint. *J. Molec. Histol.*, **36**(3), 207–15.

[92] Collins, D. H. 1950. *The Pathology of Articular and Spinal Diseases.* Baltimore, MD: Lippincott Williams & Wilkins.

[93] Redler, I., Mow, V. C., Zimny, M. L. and Mansell, J. 1975. The ultrastructure and biomechanical significance of the tidemark of articular cartilage. *Clin. Orthop. Relat. Res.*, **112**, 357–62.

[94] Mow, V. C., Proctor, C. S. and Kelly, M. A. 1989. Biomechanics of articular cartilage. In Nordin, M. and Frankel, V. H., editors. *Basic Biomechanics of the Musculoskeletal System*, 2nd edn. Baltimore, MD: Lippincott Williams & Wilkins, pp. 31–58.

[95] Hunziker, E. B., Driesang, I. M. and Saager, C. 2001. Structural barrier principle for growth factor-based articular cartilage repair. *Clin. Orthop. Relat. Res.*, **391** (Suppl.), S182–9.

[96] Schaefer, D., Martin, I., Shastri, P. *et al.* 2000. In vitro generation of osteochondral composites. *Biomaterials*, **21**(24), 2599–606.

[97] Gao, J., Dennis, J. E., Solchaga, L. A. *et al.* 2001. Tissue-engineered fabrication of an osteochondral composite graft using rat bone marrow-derived mesenchymal stem cells. *Tissue Eng.*, **7**(4), 363–71.

[98] Alhadlaq, A. and Mao, J. J. 2005. Tissue-engineered osteochondral constructs in the shape of an articular condyle. *J. Bone Joint Surg. Am.*, **87**(5), 936–44.

[99] Swieszkowski, W., Tuan, B. H. S., Kurzydlowski, K. J. and Hutmacher, D. W. 2007. Repair and regeneration of osteochondral defects in the articular joints. *Biomolec. Eng.*, **24**(5), 489–95.

[100] Chen, G., Sato, T., Tanaka, J. and Tateishi, T. 2006. Preparation of a biphasic scaffold for osteochondral tissue engineering. *Mater. Sci. Eng. C*, **26**(1), 118–23.

[101] Shao, X., Goh, J. C., Hutmacher, D. W., Lee, E. H. and Zigang, G. 2006. Repair of large articular osteochondral defects using hybrid scaffolds and bone marrow-derived mesenchymal stem cells in a rabbit model. *Tissue Eng.*, **12**(6), 1539–51.

[102] Sherwood, J. K., Riley, S. L., Palazzolo, R. *et al.* 2002. A three-dimensional osteochondral composite scaffold for articular cartilage repair. *Biomaterials*, **23**(24), 4739–51.

[103] Zhang, K., Ma, Y. and Francis, L. F. 2002. Porous polymer/bioactive glass composites for soft-to-hard tissue interfaces. *J. Biomed. Mater. Res.*, **61**(4), 551–63.

[104] Harley, B. A., Lynn, A. K., Wissner-Gross, Z. *et al.* 2010. Design of a multiphase osteochondral scaffold III: Fabrication of layered scaffolds with continuous interfaces. *J. Biomed. Mater. Res. A*, **92**(3), 1078–93.

[105] Kon, E., Mutini, A., Arcangeli, E. *et al.* 2010. Novel nanostructured scaffold for osteochondral regeneration: pilot study in horses. *J. Tissue Eng. Regen. Med.*, **4**(4), 300–8.

[106] Dormer, N. H., Singh, M., Wang, L., Berkland, C. J. and Detamore, M. S. 2010. Osteochondral interface tissue engineering using macroscopic gradients of bioactive signals. *Ann. Biomed. Eng.*, **38**(6), 2167–82.

[107] Erisken, C., Kalyon, D. M., Wang, H. J., Ornek-Ballanco, C. and Xu, J. H. 2011. Osteochondral tissue formation through adipose-derived stromal cell differentiation on biomimetic polycaprolactone nanofibrous scaffolds with graded insulin and β-glycerophosphate concentrations. *Tissue Eng. Part A*, **17**(9–10), 1239–52.

[108] Heymer, A., Bradica, G., Eulert, J. and Noth, U. 2009. Multiphasic collagen fibre–PLA composites seeded with human mesenchymal stem cells for osteochondral defect repair: an in vitro study. *J. Tissue Eng. Regen. Med.*, **3**(5), 389–97.

[109] Jiang, J., Tang, A., Ateshian, G. A. *et al.* 2010. Bioactive stratified polymer ceramic–hydrogel scaffold for integrative osteochondral repair. *Ann. Biomed. Eng.*, **38**(6), 2183–96.

[110] Cheng, H. W., Luk, K. D., Cheung, K. M. and Chan, B. P. 2011. In vitro generation of an osteochondral interface from mesenchymal stem cell–collagen microspheres. *Biomaterials*, **32**(6), 1526–35.

[111] Kandel, R. A., Hurtig, M. and Grynpas, M. 1999. Characterization of the mineral in calcified articular cartilagenous tissue formed in vitro. *Tissue Eng.*, **5**(1), 25–34.

[112] Allan, K. S., Pilliar, R. M., Wang, J., Grynpas, M. D. and Kandel, R. A. 2007. Formation of biphasic constructs containing cartilage with a calcified zone interface. *Tissue Eng.*, **13**(1), 167–77.

[113] St-Pierre, J. P., Gan, L., Wang, J. *et al.* 2012. The incorporation of a zone of calcified cartilage improves the interfacial shear strength between in vitro-formed cartilage and the underlying substrate. *Acta Biomater.*, **8**(4), 1603–15.

[114] Duer, M. J., Friscic, T., Murray, R. C., Reid, D. G. and Wise, E. R. 2009. The mineral phase of calcified cartilage: its molecular structure and interface with the organic matrix. *Biophys. J.*, **96**(8), 3372–8.

[115] Khanarian, N. T., Jiang, J., Wan, L. Q., Mow, V. C. and Lu, H. H. 2012 A hydrogel–mineral composite scaffold for osteochondral interface tissue engineering. *Tissue Eng. Part A*, **18**(5–6), 533–45.

[116] Khanarian, N. T., Haney, N. M., Burga, R. A. and Lu, H. H. 2012. A functional agarose–hydroxyapatite scaffold for osteochondral interface regeneration. *Biomaterials*, **33**(21), 5247–58.

[117] Bitar, M., Knowles, C., Lewis, M. P. and Salih, V. 2005. Soluble phosphate glass fibres for repair of bone–ligament interface. *J. Mater. Sci. Mater. Med.*, **16**(12), 1131–6.

[118] Spalazzi, J. P., Doty, S. B., Moffat, K. L., Levine, W. N. and Lu, H. H. 2006. Development of controlled matrix heterogeneity on a triphasic scaffold for orthopedic interface tissue engineering. *Tissue Eng.*, **12**(12), 3497 508.

[119] Spalazzi, J. P., Dagher, E., Doty, S. B. *et al.* 2008. In vivo evaluation of a multiphased scaffold designed for orthopaedic interface tissue engineering and soft tissue-to-bone integration. *J. Biomed. Mater. Res. A*, **86**(1), 1-12.

[120] Paxton, J. Z., Grover, L. M. and Baar, K. 2010. Engineering an in vitro model of a functional ligament from bone to bone. *Tissue Eng. Part A*, **16**(11), 3515-25.

[121] Paxton, J. Z., Donnelly, K., Keatch, R. P., Baar, K. and Grover, L. M. 2010. Factors affecting the longevity and strength in an in vitro model of the bone-ligament interface. *Ann. Biomed. Eng.*, **38**(6), 2155-66.

[122] Kandel, R. A., Boyle, J., Gibson, G., Cruz, T. and Speagle, M. 1997. In vitro formation of mineralized cartilagenous tissue by articular chondrocytes. *In Vitro Cell Dev. Biol. Anim.*, **33**(3), 174-81.

[123] Jiang, J., Tang, A., Ateshian, G. A. *et al.* 2010. Bioactive stratified polymer ceramic-hydrogel scaffold for integrative osteochondral repair. *Ann. Biomed. Eng.*, **38**(6), 2183-96.

[124] Kon, E., Delcogliano, M., Filardo, G. *et al.* 2010. A novel nano-composite multi-layered biomaterial for treatment of osteochondral lesions: technique note and an early stability pilot clinical trial. *Injury*, **41**(7), 778-86.

29

Models of composite bone and soft-tissue limb trauma

Brent A. Uhrig, Mon-Tzu A. Li, Nick J. Willett and Robert E. Guldberg

29.1 Introduction

Severe limb trauma often results in substantial injuries to multiple tissue types, including bone, skeletal muscle, nerve, and vasculature. These injuries generally present increased clinical challenges and frequently cannot be managed with conventional reconstruction techniques. Furthermore, due to the complex nature of these injuries, there is no real consensus on intervention strategies [1–3]. Given the inherent severe and pervasive tissue damage, multistage treatment is routinely required, and patients are typically encumbered with diminished long-term function even if limb salvage and reconstruction are successful [4, 5].

Extremity trauma remains the predominant type of combat casualty for US armed forces members engaged in ongoing military conflicts, a continuation of historical trends. Explosive munitions are the primary cause of these injuries [6, 7], resulting in penetrating blast wounds with large zones of injury that encompass multiple tissue types, and, notably, a high incidence of bone and soft-tissue trauma [6] (Figure 29.1). High-energy trauma incidents, such as motor vehicle collisions, produce an additional civilian patient population. Although passenger survival in these incidents has increased with improved engineering of safety features, severe extremity trauma remains common [8, 9].

The clinical gold standard for many tissue defect reconstruction procedures, including large bone defects, volumetric muscle loss, peripheral nerve gaps, and blood vessel repair, remains autologous tissue grafting. Although autograft interventions currently provide the best treatment outcomes, these procedures possess inherent limitations due to the volume of tissue available for grafting and the associated donor-site morbidity. Considerable resources have been devoted to the investigation of tissue engineering and regenerative medicine (TE/RM) therapeutics to overcome the unmet clinical needs of reconstruction, but, to date, few products are commercially available. Developing effective TE/RM therapies and successful translation to clinical practice will first require establishing rigorous, well-characterized pre-clinical models with quantitative outcome measures of functional restoration to use as test beds for evaluating emerging technologies.

Currently, the vast majority of musculoskeletal trauma models used for evaluating therapeutics consist of single-tissue defects. Such models have an undeniable place as regenerative medicine research tools, but possess only limited utility for investigating therapeutic strategies for the repair of large, multiple-tissue defects. Furthermore, they offer little potential for insight into endogenous interactions between healing tissues. Accordingly, there exists a need for established animal models of composite tissue limb trauma that more closely resemble clinical conditions. This chapter reviews relevant models of composite bone and soft-tissue extremity injuries published to date, and provides motivation and direction for future work.

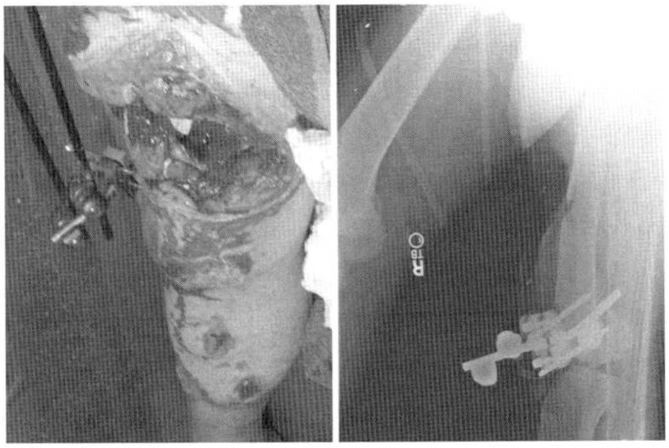

Figure 29.1 A clinical case of composite tissue limb trauma. Severe damage to the skeletal system and the surrounding vasculature is evident both in the photograph (left) and in the radiograph (right). (Adapted with permission from SLACK Incorporated: V. J. Mase, Jr., J. R. Hsu, S. E. Wolf, J. C. Wenke, D. G. Baer, J. Owens, S. F. Badylak, and T. J. Walters, Clinical application of an acellular biologic scaffold for surgical repair of a large, traumatic quadriceps femoris muscle defect. *Orthopedics*, **33**:7 (2010), 511.)

29.2 Composite bone and vascular injury models

Although the importance of blood vessels in skeletal system physiology has been documented for well over 200 years [10, 11], complexities in this relationship continue to be discovered. Healthy bones are highly vascularized, with long bones receiving blood supply from the intramedullary nutrient artery (or arteries), arteries in the periosteum, and metaphyseal and epiphyseal arteries that enter near bone ends. The branching of these arterial sources, such as the supply to Volkmann's canals, is abundant and complex, with significant anastomosis. During skeletal development, blood vessel invasion is a critical step in the conversion of the cartilage intermediate to bone in the endochondral bone formation process [12–14]. Post-natal skeletal repair is also tightly coupled to, and dependent on, vascular supply and angiogenesis [15, 16]. Sufficient vascular supply is imperative for bone healing due to its physiological role in oxygen and nutrient transport, but it also serves as a conduit for migrating inflammatory and progenitor cells as well as soluble factors. In addition, disrupted blood perfusion may have potential consequences for local cell fate in the region of bone repair [17]. Clinical risk factors for delayed or non-union fracture healing include diminished blood supply [18] and concomitant vascular injury [19, 20]. Furthermore, lower limb fractures with vascular injuries are associated with higher rates of amputation [21].

29.2.1 Existing models

Despite the established links between vasculature and bone healing, few models of composite bone and vascular injuries can be found in the literature (Figure 29.2). Kase *et al.* incorporated transient, acute hindlimb ischemia (via tourniquet and microvascular clip application) into a rat tibial fracture model to investigate how bone healing was affected [22]. Interestingly, no differences in fracture healing were found radiographically or in three-point-bending mechanical testing. Labeled microspheres were used to evaluate blood perfusion to the tibia and surrounding muscles, with no differences between ischemic and control groups being found. While surprising, the observed lack of differences in bone healing may be due to insufficient ischemia having been produced by the transient, acute ischemia–reperfusion procedure, or the lack of quantitative outcome measures of tissue composition at the fracture site. In a mouse model, Lu *et al.* found that ischemia induced by resection of the femoral artery impaired healing of non-stabilized tibial fractures [23]. At early time points, reduced numbers of blood vessels were present in and around fractures in ischemic legs. Ischemic fractures also displayed decreased cell proliferation, increased cell death, and delayed chondrocyte maturation at early time points. Fracture calluses in ischemic limbs were smaller than those in controls, and possessed less bone and cartilage. Nearly all ischemic fractures failed to achieve bony bridging, whereas all control fractures proceeded normally to bridging.

While there have been few studies using definitive models of composite bone and vascular injuries, a significant amount of work has focussed on the intimate relationship between angiogenesis and bone repair. Most relevant to this chapter is the research

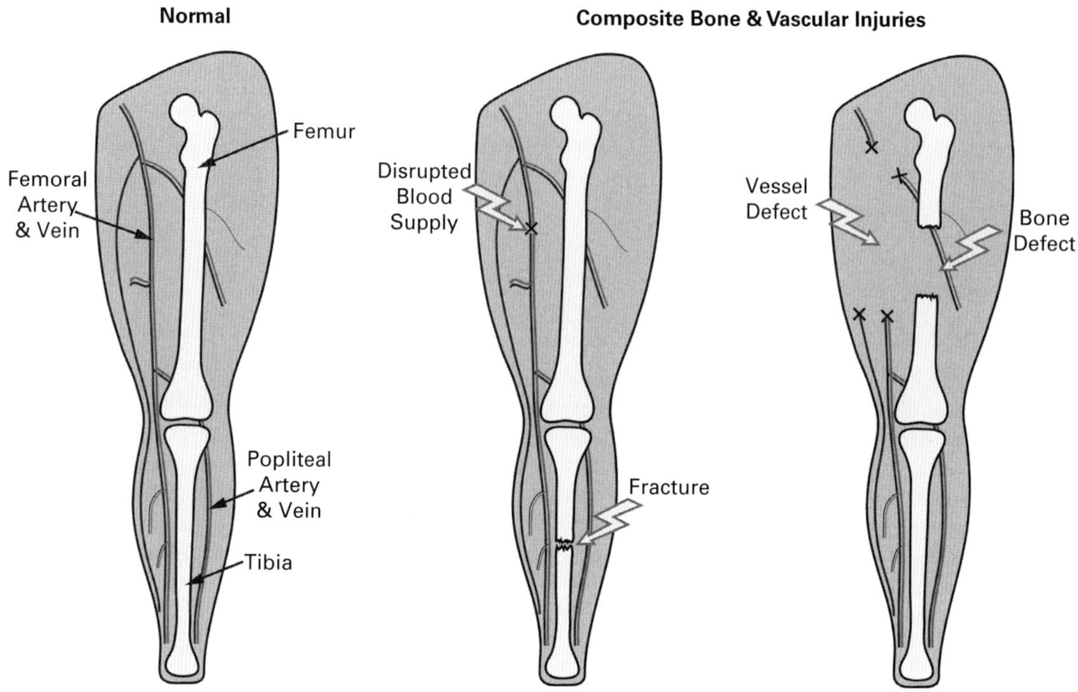

Figure 29.2 Examples of composite bone and vascular injury models. Research models of these injuries might be inclusive of a bone fracture with disrupted blood supply due to proximal injury (center), or segmental bone loss with local vascular damage (right). Normal anatomy is shown for reference (left). An anterior point of view of a coronal plane is depicted.

incorporating interventions to impair angiogenesis in an effort to determine what effect this decoupling has on bone repair. Street *et al.* used murine models for femoral fracture healing and tibial cortical defects to demonstrate that inhibition of angiogenesis will disrupt endochondral and intramembranous bone repair, respectively [24]. In fracture repair, angiogenesis was shown to be a mediator of both soft-callus formation and calcification of the hard callus. In cortical defects, where repair proceeds primarily through intramembranous ossification, the effects of angiogenesis inhibition were more prominent at early time points than they were later. Similar results have been reported by Hausman *et al.* in a rat femoral fracture model, where administration of a pharmaceutical angiogenesis inhibitor impaired both the endochondral and the intramembranous osteogenic pathways [25]. Fractures in the treatment group developed little to no bony callus, displayed minimal periosteal woven bone formation, and typically proceeded to non-union. Additionally, the treatment group fractures had less mechanical strength than did control fractures when tested in torsion. Wan *et al.* used a transgenic mouse model to impair angiogenesis at the level of gene expression during distraction osteogenesis in the tibia [26]. Compared with wild-type controls, the transgenic mice displayed lower vascularity in the distraction region and subsequently less bone regeneration. Administration of a pharmaceutical angiogenesis inhibitor (the same as that used by Hausman *et al.*) was used by Fang *et al.* in a mandibular distraction osteogenesis model in rats to investigate the effect on bone regeneration [27]. Once again, inhibition of angiogenesis was shown to preclude successful bone formation in the distraction region, giving way to fibrous scar tissue. Although this study did not use a limb injury model, the authors reported the particularly interesting finding that both an osteogenic mechanical environment and angiogenic gene expression are necessary conditions for the formation of a vascular network to support bone regeneration, and that either stimulus alone is insufficient.

An ability of the mechanical environment to influence formation of vascular networks, and ultimately bone healing, has been reported by several investigators. Wallace *et al.* investigated the difference between rigid and semi-rigid axial fixation stiffness in an ovine tibial osteotomy model with external fixation [28]. The semi-rigid fixation group experienced transiently increased micromovement at the osteotomy site and increased corticomedullary blood flow compared with the group subjected to rigid fixation. While differences in blood flow and interfragmentary movement did not persist at later time points, differences were apparent in the morphology of healing bones, insofar as the semi-rigid group displayed increased callus perimeter and cross-sectional area with decreased cortical porosity. In a similar design, Lienau *et al.* used external fixators of rigid or semi-rigid bending stiffness in an ovine tibial osteotomy model to study vascularization and tissue differentiation [29]. Larger interfragmentary movement was observed in the semi-rigid group at early time points, and was accompanied by an initially reduced number of blood vessels compared with the group subjected to rigid fixation. Differences in callus size and tissue composition at later time points were indicative of semi-rigid fixation leading to delayed healing.

The effects of interfragmentary movement on vascularity reported by Lienau *et al.* [29] are in contrast to those previously reported by Wallace *et al.* [28]. Clearly, altering fixation bending stiffness as opposed to axial stiffness may be the source of the discrepancy. It may also be in part due to differences in evaluation methods and in the regions analyzed. Wallace *et al.* measured blood flow to the bone 10 mm proximally and distally to the osteotomy in terms of the accumulation of systemically delivered labeled microspheres, whereas Lienau *et al.* histomorphometrically quantified blood vessels in the region that extended only 6 mm proximally and distally. Additionally, Wallace *et al.* were unable to distinguish whether the increase in blood flow was due to increased perfusion to existing vessels, new vessel formation, or a combination thereof.

Boerckel *et al.* used a critically sized rat femoral defect model and contrast-enhanced three-dimensional (3D) vascular imaging to demonstrate that the timing of load initiation had an effect on vascular growth and remodeling during bone repair [30]. Whereas application of early axial mechanical loading resulted in decreased vascularity in the defect and attenuated bone regeneration compared with unloaded controls, delayed loading enhanced bone regeneration and was associated with apparent vascular remodeling, exhibiting a decrease in the number of small vessels and an increase in the number of large vessels. When taken together with the results from the ovine model studies, the evidence for an effect of mechanical loading on blood vessel network formation and bone healing is both compelling and complex. If applied too soon or in excess, mechanical loading has the potential to disrupt vascular ingrowth and negatively influence bone healing, whereas, when applied with the appropriate timing and magnitude, mechanical signals can have stimulatory effects.

29.2.2 Mechanisms of interaction

The molecular coupling of angiogenesis and osteogenesis by a "vascular stimulating factor" was first proposed by Trueta in 1963 [31]. Since then, a variety of growth factor and cytokine molecular players have been implicated, including members of the transforming growth factor β (TGF-β), bone morphogenetic protein (BMP), platelet-derived growth factor (PDGF), vascular endothelial growth factor (VEGF), fibroblast growth factor (FGF), and insulin-like growth factor (IGF) families, as well as systemic regulators (e.g. vitamin D and parathyroid hormone) [16, 32]. Of these, VEGF has been perhaps the most thoroughly studied. VEGF-mediated angiogenesis is an essential component for coordinating conversion of cartilaginous anlage to bone during endochondral bone formation in skeletal development [12, 13]. Endogenous VEGF is also necessary for normal bone healing in both intramembranous and endochondral ossification, and delivery of exogenous VEGF enhances fracture and segmental bone defect repair [24]. This augmentation of bone repair is, at least in part, controlled at the gene expression level by hypoxia-inducible transcription factor 1α (HIF-1α), an angiogenic transcription factor under inhibitory control in normoxic conditions. During skeletal development, the HIF-1α/VEGF pathway couples angiogenesis and osteogenesis [33, 34]. HIF-1α is also a mediator of post-natal skeletal repair, insofar as constitutively active osteoblast HIF-1α via genetic mutation has been shown to enhance angiogenesis and bone regeneration in a VEGF-dependent process, whereas osteoblast-specific knock out of the HIF-1α gene resulted in impaired angiogenesis and bone regeneration [26]. Furthermore, pharmacological small-molecule activation of HIF-1α has been shown to effectively augment vascularity and bone repair in models of fracture healing [35], distraction osteogenesis [26], and segmental defect repair [36].

Another important source of molecular crosstalk between bone and vasculature is provided by members of the BMP family of proteins. Given their osteoinductive capacity [37], BMPs play a vital role in osteogenesis; however, they also provide an important contribution to the angiogenesis–osteogenesis interaction by stimulating osteoblast VEGF production and increasing blood vessel formation [38, 39]. BMPs may also act directly on endothelial progenitor cells to promote angiogenesis [40]. Furthermore, sequential co-delivery of exogenous VEGF followed by BMP-2 was reported to enhance bone formation [41], whereas delivery of stem cells engineered to co-express VEGF and BMP-4 led to synergistic enhancement of bone regeneration in a calvarial defect model [42]. In a follow-up to previous work in a mouse model of ischemic tibial fractures [23], rhBMP-7 treatment appeared sufficient to overcome the limitations of diminished blood supply, providing enhanced healing in fractures that would otherwise proceed to delayed union or non-union [43]. Another potential contributor to vascularization and bone repair is the extracellular matrix

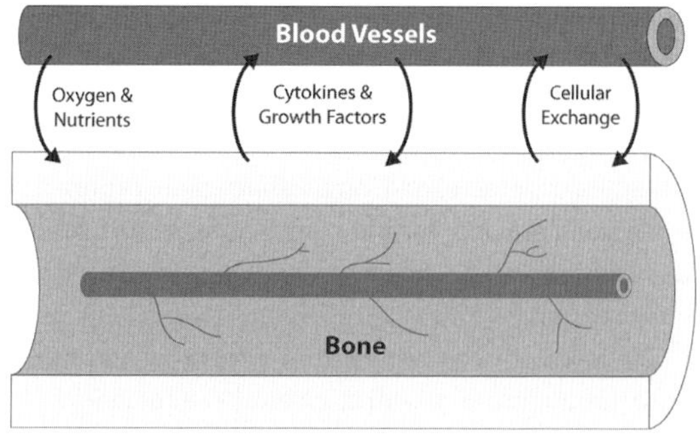

Figure 29.3 Mechanisms of interaction between bone and vasculature. In addition to providing oxygen and nutrients, blood vessels provide a conduit for transport of soluble factors and cellular exchange.

(ECM) protein osteopontin (OPN). Duvall *et al.* demonstrated that OPN is involved in regulating several aspects of fracture healing, including ECM organization, angiogenesis, callus formation, bone remodeling, and, ultimately, mechanical strength [44].

29.2.3 Conclusions and future considerations

As reviewed, few models of composite bone and vascular trauma currently exist. To date, research has primarily focussed on the basic biological coupling of angiogenesis and osteogenesis, or how the mechanical environment influences the formation of blood vessel networks to support bone repair. Means of interaction between bones and their vascular supply extend beyond the delivery of oxygen and nutrients, since the vessels also serve as a conduit for soluble factors and cellular exchange (Figure 29.3). The sparse amount of published work on bone repair with concomitant vascular injury is surprising given the known clinical complications and poor healing outcomes for patients with these injuries. Accordingly, this is a clear area for future investigation to advance our understanding of this complex relationship and to develop TE/RM therapies to improve patient outcomes. In the two published models of composite bone and vascular injuries, both groups studied ischemic tibial fracture healing, with conflicting results. Whereas Lu *et al.* reported finding impaired healing [23], Kase *et al.*

reported finding no effect [22]. The latter result is potentially attributable to the acute, transient ischemia used and the lack of quantitative outcome measures of tissue composition at the fracture site. In each study some degree of analysis of vascularity was performed, but neither group incorporated 3D, quantitative evaluation of the volume or morphology of blood vessels at the site of bone repair or in the surrounding tissues. No segmental bone defect model with concomitant vascular injury has been presented in the literature to date. These injuries present unique and significant clinical challenges to surgeons, and the lack of an established model is a clear deficiency in the field of orthopedic research.

As with all in-vivo research, selection of the appropriate animal model for the desired objectives is paramount. Rat and mouse models present attractive choices for composite bone and vascular tissue trauma research for a variety of reasons, but consideration should be given to the specific limitations of models in these species. Undoubtedly, small-animal composite injury models are more representative of clinical trauma conditions than their single-tissue injury counterparts, and are capable of providing new insight into interactions between angiogenesis and osteogenesis beyond the scope of normal bone healing. However, interpretation of data from small-animal models must take into consideration the robust neovascularization response in these species and differences in mass transport due to reduced size scale. This may be of particular importance when developing therapies to overcome the increased clinical challenges associated with diminished blood supply. Evaluation of therapeutic angiogenesis strategies in models where revascularization is not a limiting factor is unlikely to reveal positive effects. Location of the orthopedic injury is another important consideration. For example, the bones of the lower leg have substantially less surrounding skeletal muscle mass. As such, they are likely more susceptible to local tissue ischemia, and healing may be more strongly influenced by concomitant vascular injury. With sufficient consideration given to experimental design and intrinsic limitations, animal models of composite bone and vascular injuries offer a unique platform to obtain valuable insight for bone repair in instances with compromised vasculature, to advance our understanding of the intimate angiogenesis–osteogenesis coupling, and ultimately to improve outcomes for trauma patients.

29.3 Composite bone and nerve injury models

The innervation of the skeletal system has long been established, both clinically and experimentally [45, 46]; however, the anatomical distribution has yet to be thoroughly characterized, and the physiological implications of innervation remain incompletely understood. In general, the periosteum is densely innervated, and nerves predominantly enter bones alongside arterial blood supply, after which they branch to Haversian canals, bone marrow, and even mineralized bone tissue [47, 48]. Nerve growth factor (NGF), a neurotrophin modulating sensory and sympathetic innervations, has also been shown to be present in developing skeletal tissues [49]. A growing body of work continues to elucidate neurotransmitter and neuropeptide signaling pathways in the skeletal system and a neuronal arm contributing to the regulation of bone modeling and remodeling [50–52]. Notably, Ducy *et al.* demonstrated a leptin-mediated central nervous system control of bone mass [53]. In addition, others have reported a neural contribution in the regulation of functional adaptation to loading [54], which is at least partially mediated via the sympathetic nervous system [55, 56], and that the neuropathy-induced reduction in bone mineral density is not strictly a result of reduced load bearing [57]. During fracture healing, regenerating nerve fibers have experimentally been shown to be present in the hematoma at early stages, followed by presence in the fracture callus, periosteum, fibrocartilage, and ultimately new woven bone at later time points [58]. Immunological characterization of tissue samples from non-infected, human diaphyseal fractures that experienced delayed or non-union revealed a virtually non-existent presence of peripheral nerve fibers [59]. Furthermore, clinical observation of enhanced osteogenic activity in fracture patients with head injuries provides anecdotal

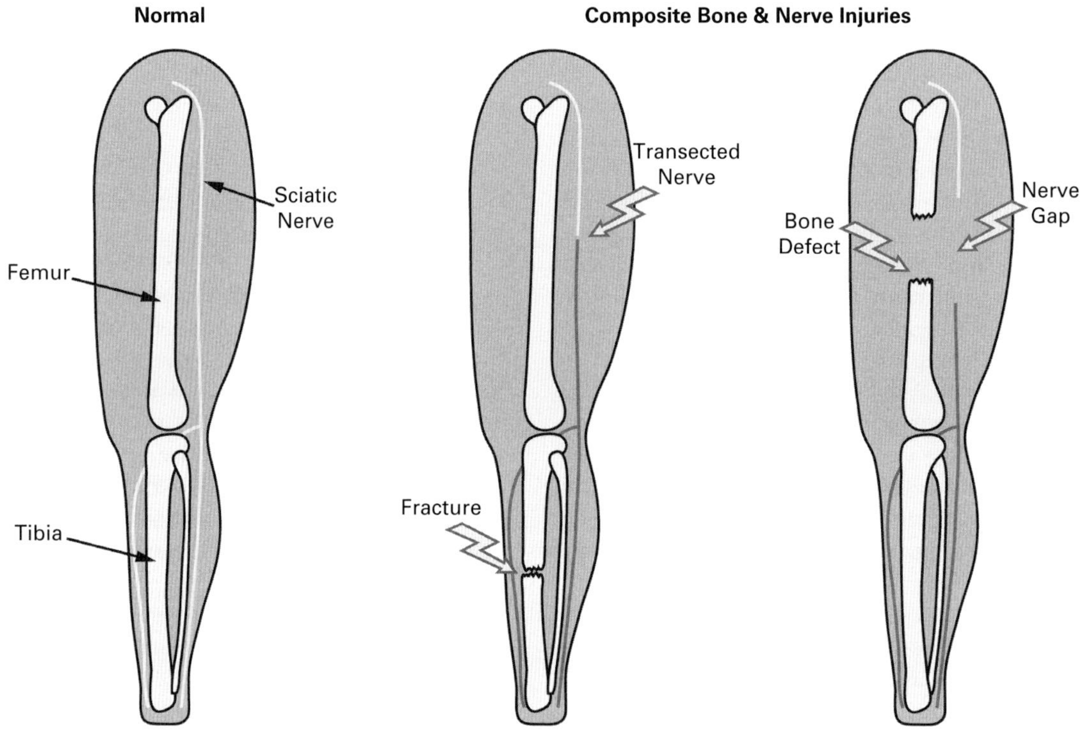

Figure 29.4 Examples of composite bone and nerve injury models. Research models of these injuries might be inclusive of a bone fracture with disrupted innervation due to proximal nerve transection (center), or segmental bone loss with an associated peripheral nerve gap (right). Normal anatomy is shown for reference (left). A lateral point of view of a sagittal plan is depicted.

evidence for the role of the nervous system in bone physiology [60–62]. However, it remains controversial whether this increase in osteogenesis is an actual acceleration of fracture healing, or rather a form of heterotopic ossification [63, 64].

29.3.1 Existing models

While increasing effort is being devoted to investigating the complexity of crosstalk between the nervous and skeletal systems, interactions in instances of composite bone and nerve injuries have largely been left unexplored (Figure 29.4). Among the experiments that have been performed, the primary model employed has been disrupted innervation in tibial fracture healing by way of sciatic nerve transection. Aro *et al.* studied the effect of sciatic nerve transection, spinal cord transection, or both on tibial fracture healing in a rat model [65]. Weight-bearing controls (fracture alone) and non-weight-bearing controls (fracture with hip dislocations) were included. Groups with disrupted innervation displayed more frequent fracture union at early time points, but possessed noticeably less dense calluses than did control groups. By the study end point, all fractures had achieved union; however, irregularities in shape and/or density were reported for fracture calluses with denervation. While tensile testing of specimens indicated that there was a greater load to failure at early time points for fracture groups with disrupted innervations than for control groups, this method of loading is of minimal physiological relevance. In a subsequent study, Aro again used transection of the sciatic nerve to further study the effect of nerve injury on fracture healing and callus formation in the rat [66]. In this study, no attempt was made to control for unequal weight-bearing in groups with or without nerve injury. In confirmation of previous findings, radiographs and histology indicated more rapid bridging in fractures with nerve transection, but smaller, less dense calluses. A smaller amount of collagenous matrix was also reported for denervated fracture calluses than for controls.

Nordsletten *et al.* also used a rat model to study the effect of sciatic nerve resection on tibial fracture healing, but included cast-immobilization of the fractured limbs to control for differences in weight-bearing between denervated animals and controls [67]. Larger fracture calluses were reported for the nerve resection group than for controls. In fact, radiographs of control fractures indicated that very little callus formation had occurred. Furthermore, nerve resection fractures possessed significantly higher bone mineral content. The larger, more mineralized nerve resection fracture calluses did not demonstrate better mechanical properties, however, when evaluated in three-point bending. A parallel experiment by these authors using histological techniques to study the growth of neural fibers into fracture calluses in this model corroborated the observed radiographic results [68]. In a follow-up to this study, Madsen *et al.* investigated fracture healing and callus innervation after resection both of the sciatic and of the femoral nerve [69]. Again, cast-immobilization was used to control for differences in weight-bearing. When assessed radiographically, calluses from the nerve resection group were larger than those in controls. Immunostaining of the fracture callus for nerve fibers and neuropeptides indicated that the pattern of innervation is altered following nerve resection, but total denervation is not experienced. Mechanical testing of the femora in three-point bending demonstrated that there was a lower mechanical strength for nerve resection fractures. These results suggest that maturation of the fracture callus may be dependent on the innervation status of the bone.

The discrepancies in callus formation and bone healing results for fractures with sciatic nerve transection from seemingly similar surgical models may be explained by invoking differences in fixation stability. All experiments used intramedullary nailing for internal fixation; however, Nordsletten *et al.* [67], Hukkanen *et al.* [68], and Madsen *et al.* [69] attempted to control for unequal weight-bearing between groups by immobilizing fractured limbs in casts, whereas the work by Aro *et al.* [65, 66] allowed for weight-bearing on fractured limbs. Although cast-immobilization may prevent unequal load-bearing during ambulation, it also precludes functional mechanical stimulation of the healing fracture, a factor known to influence bone modeling and remodeling. Thus, it is possible that cast-immobilized control fractures were stable enough to proceed through primary fracture healing, which would explain the absence of callus formation. If true, this may suggest that modulation of fracture healing occurs via sensory innervation feedback on fracture stability. Consideration should also be given to the physiological loading imparted by skeletal muscle. While immobilization can attempt to tease out effects of load bearing, it cannot account for disruption of the resting muscle tone in the lower limb as a result of nerve transection.

While sciatic nerve transection in combination with tibial fracture is the predominant composite bone and nerve injury model found in the literature, other models have been described. Frymoyer and Pope used a rat model of fibular fractures without fixation to study the effect of sciatic nerve resection on healing [70]. No attempt was made to control for possible differences in weight-bearing due to sciatic nerve injury. Histological scoring of fracture healing was performed at multiple time points, with no differences observed except in one instance, at which time fractures from the sciatic nerve injury group displayed better healing than did those in controls. Differences in mechanical properties from tensile testing of samples were reported, with denervated fractures outperforming controls, but are of questionable relevance to physiological loading conditions. Others have taken an additional step with this model and investigated the effect of sciatic nerve transection on fibular fracture healing, including the surgical removal of periosteal neural mechanoreceptors located in the distal portion of the rat fibula [71]. In relative agreement with Frymoyer and Pope, in this study Aro *et al.* found that fibular fracture healing proceeded undisturbed by transection of the sciatic nerve. However, surgical stripping of mechanoreceptors was associated with fracture non-union that, at times, became atrophic. Inclusion of sciatic nerve transection exacerbated this effect, with all fractures going on to atrophic non-union. Histological analysis of atrophic fragments indicated that they were active sites of osteoclastic bone resorption. Interestingly, two control samples with stripped mechanoreceptors and intact sciatic nerves presented hypertrophic non-unions in the distal fibula, visible as early as one month after surgery. No such instances were observed in intact control fibulae with stripped mechanoreceptors and transected sciatic nerves, but a thinner appearance, potentially attributable to altered weight-bearing in response to the sciatic nerve injury, was noted. Recently, Apel *et al.* used neurotoxin injection at the cortex of the femur to model fracture healing in instances of local sensory denervation [72]. Intramedullary rods were used for fixation, and no attempt was made to control for weight-bearing in this model. Sensory denervation resulted in decreased deposition of type I and II collagen during early fracture healing, but an eventual increase in the size of the fracture callus when evaluated histologically and via microcomputed tomography. Despite their larger fracture calluses, sensory-denervated samples failed at lower loads in three-point bending.

Although not specifically a composite limb injury model, Boes *et al.* recently investigated experimental fracture healing with associated traumatic brain injury in a reproducible rat model [73]. To do so, a standard closed femoral fracture with intramedullary fixation was combined with a model of traumatic brain injury produced from an impact acceleration system. Rats in the brain-injury group had smaller fracture calluses with greater torsional stiffness than did rats subjected to fracture alone, which may suggest that an enhanced of progression through the remodeling stage of fracture healing was achieved. Further, to investigate possible systemic mitogenic differences between groups, serum collected at euthanasia was used to supplement in-vitro cell culture media. Greater proliferation was observed in a mesenchymal stem cell line when supplemented with serum from the brain-injury group rather than with serum from the fracture-only group, but enhanced proliferation was not observed in osteoblastic or fibroblastic cell lines.

29.3.2 Mechanisms of interaction

Given the relative paucity of research in this area to date, the cellular and molecular mechanisms involved are far from completely understood. Results from several studies have implicated sensory neuropeptide calcitonin gene-related peptide (CGRP) as a potential agent exerting a neural influence on bone repair. CGRP-immunoreactive sensory fibers are known to innervate normal bone tissue [48, 74, 75]. Additionally, CGRP-immunoreactive fibers have been reported to sprout and proliferate in bone tissue during normal fracture healing [75], but exhibit a reduced presence in tibial fracture healing when innervation to the lower limb has been disrupted by sciatic nerve resection [68]. Modulation of skeletal repair by CGRP could occur directly, since CGRP has been shown to have osteogenic capacity in vitro, with CGRP-supplemented media increasing bone-forming colonies in a dose-dependent manner [76], and in vivo, as CGRP expression in osteoblasts gives way to a skeletal phenotype with increased bone density in mice [77]. The influence may also be exerted via an indirect route through the vasculature given the potent vasodilator action of CGRP [78] and its ability to stimulate endothelial cell proliferation [79]. An effect of denervation on fracture healing may also be modulated by changes in blood perfusion and hemodynamics in the surrounding skeletal muscle. Transection of the sciatic or femoral nerves has been shown to result in transient hyperemia in the muscles of the hind limb [80]. Others have reported that denervation of a muscle flap produces an acute increase in arteriole diameters and a more sustained increase in perfused capillaries than in innervated controls [81]. An increase in blood flow in the bones of the lower leg was also observed with transection of the sciatic nerve [82]. The coupling of tissue blood perfusion in response to nerve injuries is most likely explained, at least in

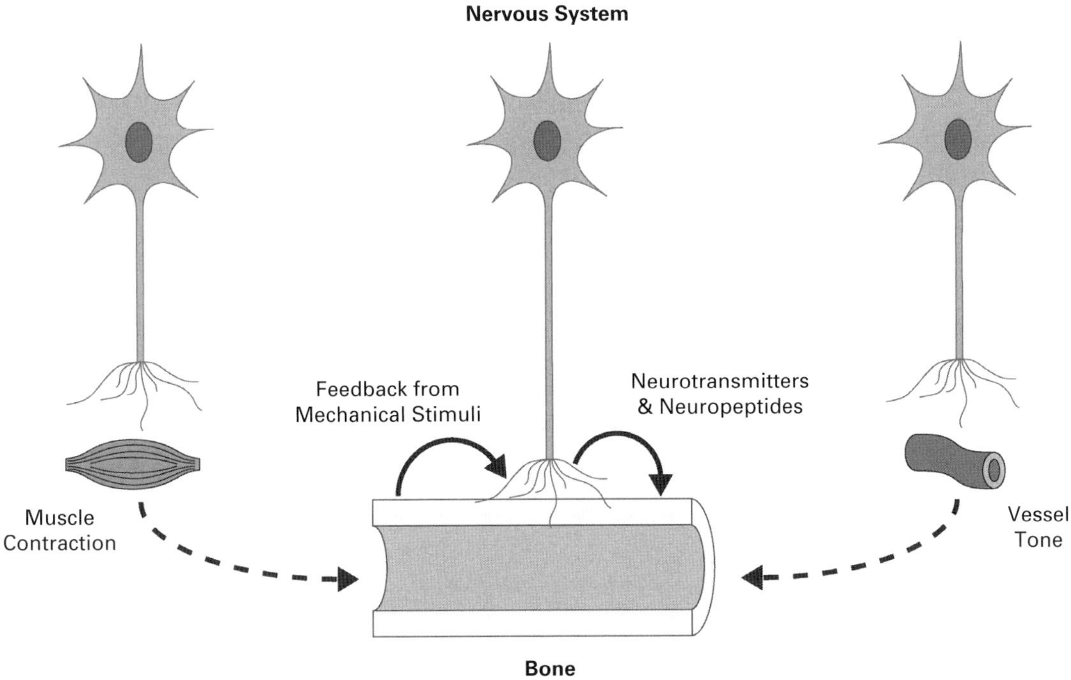

Figure 29.5 Mechanisms of interaction between bone and the nervous system. Neurotransmitter and neuropeptides offer pathways for direct signaling, and the nervous system has a regulatory role in loading-induced bone metabolism. Indirect interactions (shown with dotted lines) are also exerted via nervous system control of muscle contractions and blood vessel tone.

part, by sympathetic nervous system control of vascular tone.

29.3.3 Conclusions and future considerations

The composite bone and nerve injury models currently described in the literature are primarily designed to assess what effect disrupted peripheral innervation has on fracture healing, with somewhat inconsistent results. When these are taken together with clinical reports, it seems clear that concomitant neural insult is at least associated with altered fracture healing or osteogenic response. The exact effect a specific neural insult imparts on bone healing has yet to be completely understood, let alone the precise mechanisms through which it may act. Several means of interaction between bones and the nervous system exist, including a regulatory arm in bone metabolism and neuropeptide/neurotransmitter signaling pathways (Figure 29.5). The apparently confounding fracture healing results from similar experimental models may be attributable to the varying degrees of fracture stabilization employed across the studies, which precludes the ability to interpret the findings collectively. Further confounding the results is the heavy reliance on qualitative radiographic evaluation of bone healing. Also yet to be determined is how the loss of muscle tone mechanical stimuli due to nerve injury affects the repair process. To date, no published models have included large peripheral nerve gaps undergoing treatment, opting instead for untreated nerve resection. While relevant for studying the effect of disrupted innervation skeletal repair, models treating both tissue injuries would be more relevant to clinical practice. Clearly, this deficiency is an area to address with future work.

Model selection should ultimately depend on the type of injury of interest or the scientific question under investigation. Concomitant femur and sciatic nerve injuries would present a relevant model of upper-leg composite tissue trauma, perhaps representative of a penetrating blast wound. Such a model would be of use for investigating local interactions between the healing bone and nerve tissues, or the overall effect on limb function. However, it would likely not be as applicable for studying the direct effects of innervation status on bone healing given that the sciatic nerve innervates the lower limb. A more prudent model for these investigations would consist of nerve injury proximal to the bone injury (as has been done previously with sciatic nerve injury and tibial fractures), or possibly local denervation at the fracture by way of neurotoxin administration. Careful consideration should also be given to the degree of load-bearing allowed and whether muscle tone in surrounding tissue has been disrupted, since both may influence the healing response observed in experimental and control groups, and ultimately the interpretation of results. There also exist ethical considerations specific to rodent strain selection for peripheral nerve injury models. Differences in the degree of autotomy/autophagia (i.e. self-mutilation) have been reported amongst rat strains following sciatic nerve transection, ranging from a complete absence to severe complications [83]. Although a growing amount of research is being devoted to studying interactions between the nervous and skeletal systems, the complexities are far from being completely understood. With proper design considerations, composite bone and nerve injury models can provide a novel avenue to explore the degree of crosstalk and the specific pathways involved.

29.4 Composite bone and muscle injury models

An intimate relationship between bone and muscle tissue is intuitive given their anatomical arrangement and cumulative physiological locomotive function, yet much is still unknown in regard to how the tissues interact during healing. Normal muscle contraction provides a mechanical stimulus that is required for bone health and modeling/remodeling. During embryonic development, muscle-induced mechanical loads significantly contribute to structural and mineral changes in bone [84], and muscle tissue functions as a determinant of bone geometry, density, and strength during post-natal growth [85]. In instances of impaired muscle function, such as those experienced by Duchenne muscular dystrophy, myasthenia gravis, and cerebral palsy patients, negative bone physiology consequences are routinely presented, often leading to osteoporosis and increased fracture risk [86]. Beyond biomechanical function, the close anatomical relationship of bones and skeletal muscle lends credence to the idea that muscle contributes to bone healing as a source of blood vessels, growth factors, and progenitor cells [87]. Sufficient muscle coverage has long been considered an integral component for promoting bone healing and is strongly advocated for severe tibial fractures in the clinical field [88]. The clinical gold standard for treating open fractures consists of muscular flaps used to cover the bone and occupy empty space in order to reduce complications. Use of the muscle flap is known to be vital in treating lower-extremity composite injuries and has been shown to increase bone union rate [89]; however, the percentage of complications remains high [90], with the authors of one 15-year study reporting 58% non-union and 11% amputation [91]. In addition, even when results show high rates of bone union and integration of the soft tissue flaps, patients often do not regain normal function of their extremity [92]. Through careful observation of callus formation after tibial fractures in rats, rabbits, and sheep, Stein *et al.* noted that the callus forms between the fracture and the intact muscle bed adjacent to it [93]. This adjacent muscle acts almost as a "secondary periosteum" that can provide osteoprogenitors, especially when the periosteum itself, which is normally a good source of osteogenic cells, is damaged [94].

29.4.1 Existing models

Although the negative consequences of concomitant skeletal muscle injury on bone repair appear widely accepted and supported by clinical evidence, relatively

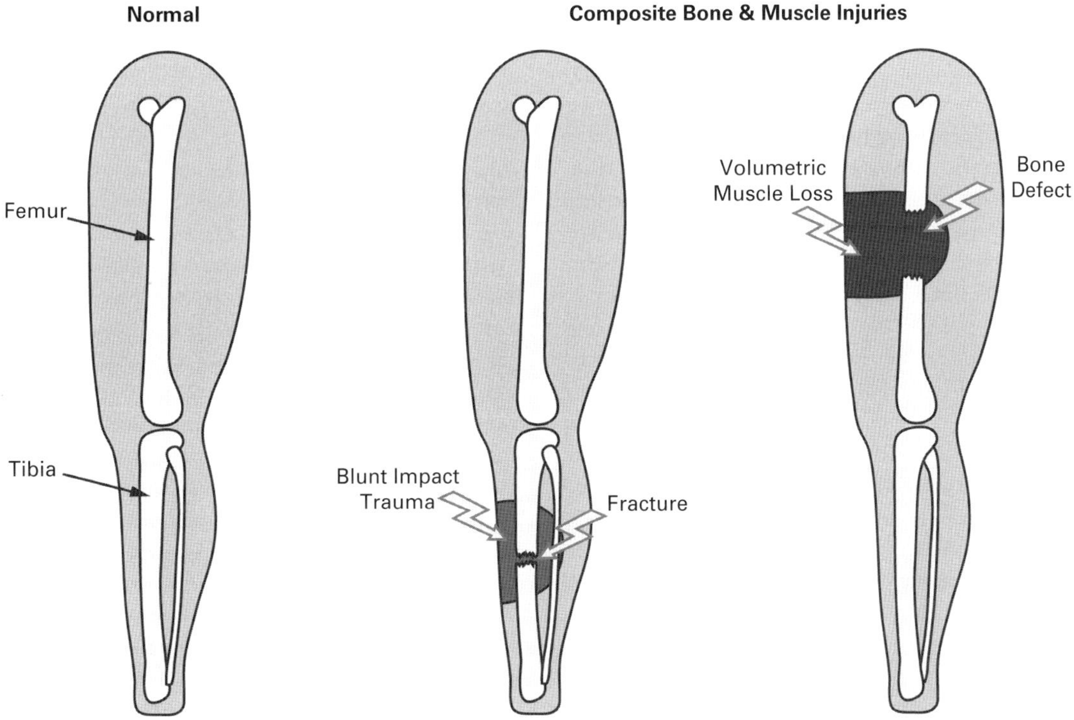

Figure 29.6 Examples of composite bone and muscle injury models. Research models of these injuries might be inclusive of a bone fracture with associated blunt impact trauma (center), or a more severe segmental bone loss with concomitant volumetric muscle loss (right). Normal anatomy is shown for reference (left). A lateral point of view of a sagittal plane is depicted.

few established animal models of these conditions appear in the published literature (Figure 29.6). Augat and colleagues incorporated blunt-impact soft-tissue trauma to the lower leg into a rat closed tibial fracture model to study the influence of muscle injury on revascularization during fracture healing [95, 96]. Compared with the fracture control group, fractures with soft-tissue trauma displayed little periosteal bone formation during the early stage of healing. Using a rat tibial cortical defect model, Landry *et al.* incorporated a tibialis anterior muscle injury to investigate the inflammatory and cellular response in periosteally mediated bone repair [97, 98]. In some animals, approximately 10% (by weight) of the tibialis anterior muscle was removed to create an additional soft-tissue injury. Addition of the muscle injury significantly increased the number of proliferating cells in the periosteum compared with the number for the cortical defect-only group, albeit only transiently. While the osteoblast concentration in the inner periosteal layer was increased by inclusion of the muscle injury, callus formation, as measured by histology, did not reveal a significant difference between groups.

The lack of a sustained effect on bone healing in the above studies may be attributable to insufficient severity of the concomitant muscle injury. Utvag *et al.* investigated the effect of increasing muscle injury severity on bone healing in a rat tibial osteotomy model. Three levels of soft-tissue damage were tested: intact muscle (control), moderate muscle injury (muscle crush), and severe muscle injury (resection of muscles from the anterolateral compartment) [99]. A significantly lower callus cross-sectional area was found in the group with severe muscle injury than in the control group, which was associated with a significantly lower maximum load in three-point bending. Surprisingly, the group with moderate muscle injury did not differ significantly from the control group in terms of these two parameters. In the same rat tibial osteotomy model, it was demonstrated that the impaired fracture healing associated with an extensive muscle defect can be treated by autologous muscle flap coverage [100]. In one group, the anterolateral compartment muscles were detached from the bone but left intact (*in situ* muscle flap). In another, an extensive muscle defect was created next to the osteotomy site by excising the anterolateral compartment muscles and connecting periosteum. In a third group, the muscle compartment was excised, after which the superficial gluteal muscle was transposed as a muscle flap with arterial blood supply intact. Results showed a significantly lower bending moment at fracture and bending rigidity in the empty muscle defect group than for groups with both muscle flap treatments. However, no differences in bone healing were noted between the two muscle flap treatments.

Others have investigated healing outcomes based on the soft tissue used for coverage. In a series of canine studies, Richards *et al.* compared the effect of skin coverage versus a local muscle flap on bone repair in a model of devascularized segmental grafting in the tibia [101–104]. Muscle flap coverage promoted superior bone repair [101] and enhanced mechanical properties [103] than did skin coverage. Further study showed that the muscle flap group had greater intracortical blood flow, which correlated with greater cortical porosity, a measure of bone turnover [104]. In a similar study in mice, Harry *et al.* investigated the effect of different soft-tissue coverage for open tibial fractures [105]. An inert polymer insert was used for selective tissue exclusion either directly between the bone and the anterior skin/fascia or between the bone and the posterior muscle. A tibial fracture group with no additional treatment served as a control. Muscle coverage (fasciocutaneous separation) yielded histomorphometrically similar results to those for the fracture control group and performed equally well in four-point bending. However, the group with fasciocutuaneous coverage (muscle exclusion) had an impaired healing response, with a significantly lower load to failure, bone mineral content, bone mineral density, and bone volume than the fracture control and muscle coverage groups.

Although not constituting a definitive composite injury model, Kaufman *et al.* modified a rat tibial fracture model to investigate contributions of the surrounding skeletal muscle to bone repair by physically separating the two tissues with a nitrocellulose membrane wrapped around the fractured bone [106]. Experimental groups were designated according to the membrane pore cut-off size (3.5, 12–14, or 50 kDa), and a control group received the fracture without a membrane. Bone healing was attenuated in all membrane groups compared with that in the membrane-free control group. The attenuated bone formation in membrane groups was accompanied by increased type II collagen expression at the fracture site. While the membrane-free control group exhibited very low levels of type II collagen, expression was both more abundant and more persistent the smaller the pore size, indicating a delay in bone healing or a repair site more conducive to cartilage synthesis. Although this study provided interesting insight into selective exclusion of muscle-derived cytokines from the fracture site, the authors did not attempt to account for disruption of cellular exchange or vascular ingrowth due to the presence of a membrane. Kolambkar *et al.* reported similar findings when using a hybrid nanofiber mesh–alginate hydrogel system for the treatment of critically sized femoral defects in a rat model [107]. Perforations in the nanofiber mesh placed around the bone defect accelerated BMP-2-mediated bone healing compared with perforation-free constructs, and yielded restoration of torsional mechanical properties to the level of intact controls.

29.4.2 Mechanisms of interaction

Taken together with clinical observations, results from these studies provide compelling evidence for the role of skeletal muscle in bone health and repair. Although the exact mechanisms have yet to be entirely understood, several important means of interaction have been identified. Specifically, the skeletal muscle envelope may serve as a source for blood vessel networks to support bone repair. Concomitant muscle injury might then diminish blood supply to sites of active bone repair, with negative consequences for healing outcomes. The microvasculature within the periosteum of intact bone was reported to be reduced in extent for several weeks following a soft-tissue injury [108], and blunt-impact trauma to the skeletal muscle surrounding tibial fractures was associated with transiently decreased blood flow within and around the fracture site compared with fractures without soft-tissue trauma [95, 96]. Furthermore, in a model of devascularized segmental grafting in the tibia, coverage with a local muscle flap promoted increased blood flow to the bone and enhanced healing compared with coverage with skin [102, 104].

Beyond providing a vascular supply, skeletal muscle likely offers a source of progenitor cells and growth factors that contribute to the bone healing, as suggested by previously discussed work from Kaufman *et al.* [106] and Kolambkar *et al.* [107]. Although much of the specifics regarding interaction pathways has yet to be identified, various factors that may aid in muscle and bone crosstalk have been proposed [109], with IGF-1 and FGF-2 the most studied to date. Receptors for IGF-1 and FGF-2, two soluble factors secreted by and abundantly present in skeletal muscle adjacent to bone, are highly expressed along the bone periosteum [110]. In addition, FGF-2 is known to play an important role in osteoblast growth and proliferation [111], whereas IGF-1 has the capacity to directly regulate bone growth [112].

Molecular signaling between muscle and bone is unlikely to be confined to anabolic pathways. The discovery of myostatin (GDF-8) and its negative regulation of muscle mass brought to light another potential skeletal muscle molecule with the capacity to modulate bone physiology [113]. Given that impaired muscle function and reduced mass are known to also significantly reduce bone density [86], myostatin may have pronounced effects on bone physiology, directly or indirectly. In support of this hypothesis, the muscle mass increase in a myostatin-deficient mouse model was associated with an increase in bone mineral density in all long bones and the spine [114]. Although a sharp shift in skeletal phenotype is evident, the exact mechanisms by which myostatin acts are not well understood. While myostatin may regulate bone mineral density solely via indirect regulation of muscle mass and contraction-induced mechanical stimuli, it may possibly directly affect bone. In-vitro osteogenic differentiation of bone-marrow-derived mesenchymal stem cells obtained from myostatin-deficient mice was greater than that in wild-type controls; but, surprisingly, the addition of recombinant myostatin to the culture media of these cells did not attenuate this osteogenic potential, and the exact effects on in-vivo differentiation remain unclear [115]. Additionally, in a fibular osteotomy model, myostatin-deficient mice demonstrated an increase in fracture callus size compared with wild-type controls (including when normalized with respect to intact fibular shaft diameter) that was accompanied by enhanced callus strength in three-point bending, suggesting an implication of myostatin in the fracture healing process [116]. Irrespective of the mechanism, inhibition of myostatin, via delivery of recombinant myostatin propeptide, has shown some therapeutic potential in a murine composite bone and muscle injury model consisting of a fibular osteotomy in combination with severing of the lateral calf compartment muscles [117]. Compared with a saline-treated control group, the myostatin propeptide-treated group showed improved bridging of the osteotomy site, with an increase in the size of the fracture callus and a greater amount of mineralized tissue. The improved bone healing of the propeptide-treated group was also accompanied by less fibrosis at the muscle injury site than in controls.

Beyond the potential for muscle-derived soluble factors to affect bone healing, skeletal muscle may serve as a source of cells to participate in bone repair. Spontaneous and post-traumatic heterotopic ossification phenomena suggest that resident cells within skeletal muscle possess an osteogenic capacity. A population of mesenchymal progenitor cells isolated from debrided traumatized human muscle tissue exhibits a similar phenotype to bone-marrow-derived mesenchymal stem cells, including a capability for osteogenic, chondrogenic, and adipogenic differentiation [118, 119].

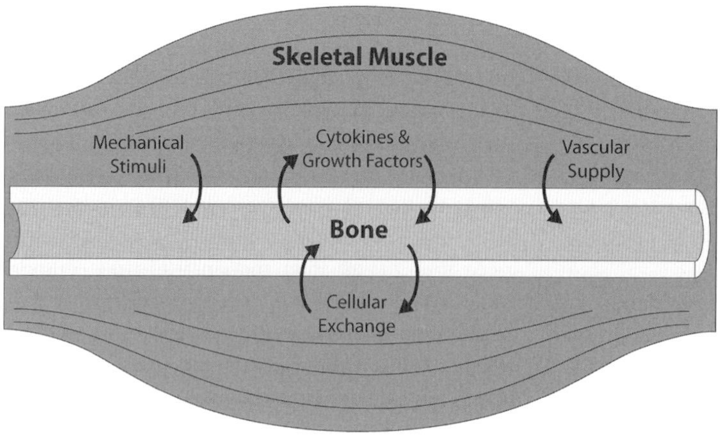

Figure 29.7 Mechanisms of interaction between bone and skeletal muscle. The skeletal muscle envelope of bones provides contraction-induced mechanical stimuli due to its physiological function, but also serves as a source of vascular supply, soluble factors, and cellular exchange.

Muscle-derived stem cells (MDSCs) isolated from healthy skeletal muscle have also shown the ability to differentiate into multiple lineages, including myogenic and osteoblastic [120]. These cells differentiate into myogenic cells in vitro under low-serum conditions and into osteogenic cells when cultured with BMP-2, -4, and -7 [121, 122]. Further enrichment and engineering of a population of MDSCs yielded accelerated bone healing when they were transplanted into a calvarial defect model [123]. Additionally, skeletal myoblasts engineered for osteogenic gene expression are capable of osteoblastic differentiation both in vitro and in vivo [124].

29.4.3 Conclusions and future considerations

Although relatively few composite bone and muscle injury models have been established in the literature compared with their single-injury counterparts, collective interpretation of the results together with clinical reports provides a compelling body of evidence for the role of concomitant injury to the soft-tissue envelope in the process of bone repair. Unsurprisingly, the influence of muscle injury on bone healing appears to depend on the severity of the soft-tissue trauma, which is an important consideration when designing experiments and interpreting results. Interactions between skeletal muscle and the bones it envelops extend beyond physiological biomechanical stimuli. Initial studies have identified skeletal muscle as a source of vascular supply to intact and healing bone, as well as indicating that it is a possible reservoir of soluble factors and progenitor cells capable of participating in, and influencing the outcome of, bone healing (Figure 29.7). Yet, much remains unknown in regard to the specific pathways of interaction. While the importance of muscle-derived growth factors to bone healing has been noted, the key myokines that affect bone growth and regeneration have only begun to be elucidated. Of the few composite bone and muscle injury models described in the literature, none include segmental bone defects in combination with volumetric muscle loss. There is a clear need for future investigation, given the high probability of extensive muscle damage in instances of severe bone trauma, and the formidable challenges such injuries present for limb salvage, reconstruction, and functional recovery. Furthermore, hardly any of the work to date has studied temporal muscle regeneration in parallel with bone healing, including quantitative analysis of muscle function. Also yet to be investigated is what effect, if any, concomitant bone injury may have on muscle repair. Composite bone and muscle injury models offer a promising means to probe many of the unanswered questions on the intimate interactions between the bones of the musculoskeletal system and their enveloping skeletal muscle. Ultimately, a better understanding of these relationships may yield improved treatment and healing for musculoskeletal trauma patients.

29.5 Summary

Improving structural and functional intervention outcomes for extremity trauma patients remains a pressing, unmet clinical need. Doing so likely requires advancing our understanding of the biological interactions between damaged tissues. While TE/RM therapeutics offer promising potential to overcome the status-quo limitations of surgical reconstruction, very few products have transitioned to clinical practice. Currently, the majority of musculoskeletal trauma models used for evaluating new TE/RM technologies consist of single-tissue defects. While these models have a place as valuable research tools, they inherently possess limited utility for investigating therapeutic strategies for the repair of large, multiple-tissue defects and afford little potential for insight into endogenous interactions between healing tissues. Additionally, while a given therapeutic intervention may produce the desired healing response in one tissue of interest, single-injury models are unable to detect unwanted negative consequences in other damaged tissues. Models of composite tissue trauma are uniquely positioned to bridge this knowledge gap and advance the TE/RM field.

As with all in-vivo research, selection of the appropriate animal model for the research questions of interest is paramount. Considerations specific to bone–vascular, bone–nerve, and bone–muscle models have been discussed at the end of each section. In general, the ramifications of species selection should be considered when designing research questions and when interpreting experimental results. Furthermore, the location of the musculoskeletal injury should be carefully considered due to anatomical and physiological differences between the upper and lower portions of extremities. For effective comparisons of therapeutics, the model must present a challenging tissue defect in which a regenerative intervention is required for full recovery. In all models, quantitative outcome measures should be included for evaluation of tissue regeneration and composition, with 3D analysis whenever possible. When evaluating therapeutics, functional assessments should be performed for the regenerated tissue, including comparisons with intact or autograft controls. Additionally, when practical, outcome measures should be included in order to evaluate the degree of functional restoration in the limb in vivo.

The material covered here is certainly not exhaustive of all possible composite limb injury models, and was focussed on those with an aspect of bone trauma. Moreover, the models covered here are primarily representative of injuries to just two tissue types. While these models are undeniably more representative of clinical conditions, the most accurate model of extremity trauma would be inclusive of bone, skeletal muscle, vascular, neural, and adipocutaneous injuries. Such a model would certainly present its own set of limitations, however, most notably the feasibility of implementation. Beyond pre-clinical mammalian models, additional future insight may be gleaned from ongoing work on vertebrate species such as salamanders that possess the inherent capacity to regenerate entire limbs [125, 126]. This chapter has highlighted an emerging set of novel research tools for the TE/RM field with motivation for future work. Successful leverage of models of composite tissue limb trauma will advance the understanding of tissue repair biology, and, ultimately, may improve limb salvage and reconstruction outcomes for extremity trauma patients.

REFERENCES

[1] Yazar, S., Lin, C. H. and Wei, F. C. 2004. One-stage reconstruction of composite bone and soft-tissue defects in traumatic lower extremities. *Plast. Reconstr. Surg.*, **114**(6), 1457–66.

[2] DeFranco, M. J. and Lawton, J. N. 2006. Radial nerve injuries associated with humeral fractures. *J. Hand Surg. Am.*, **31**(4), 655–63.

[3] Nauth, A., McKee, M. D., Einhorn, T. A. *et al.* 2011. Managing bone defects. *J. Orthop. Trauma*, **25**(8), 462–6.

[4] Bosse, M. J., MacKenzie, E. J., Kellam, J. F. *et al.* 2002. An analysis of outcomes of reconstruction or amputation after leg-threatening injuries. *N. Engl. J. Med.*, **347**(24), 1924–31.

[5] MacKenzie, E. J., Bosse, M. J., Pollak, A. N. *et al.* 2005. Long-term persistence of disability following severe lower-limb trauma. Results of a seven-year follow-up. *J. Bone Joint Surg. Am.*, **87**(8), 1801–9.

[6] Owens, B. D., Kragh, J. F. Jr., Macaitis, J., Svoboda, S. J. and Wenke, J. C. 2007. Characterization of extremity wounds in Operation Iraqi Freedom and Operation Enduring Freedom. *J. Orthop. Trauma*, **21**(4), 254–7.

[7] Owens, B. D., Kragh, J. F. Jr., Wenke, J. C. *et al.* 2008. Combat wounds in operation Iraqi Freedom and operation Enduring Freedom. *J. Trauma*, **64**(2), 295–9.

[8] Burgess, A. R., Dischinger, P. C., O'Quinn, T. D. and Schmidhauser, C. B. 1995. Lower extremity injuries in drivers of airbag-equipped automobiles: clinical and crash reconstruction correlations. *J. Trauma*, **38**(4), 509–16.

[9] Richter, M., Pape, H. C., Otte, D. and Krettek, C. 2005. Improvements in passive car safety led to decreased injury severity – a comparison between the 1970s and 1990s. *Injury*, **36**(4), 484–8.

[10] Haller, A. 1763. Experimentorum de ossium formatione. In *Opera minora*. Lausanne: Francisci Grasset.

[11] Hunter, J. 1794. *A Treatise on the Blood, Inflammation, and Gun-Shot Wounds*. London: G. Nicol.

[12] Gerber, H. P., Vu, T. H., Ryan, A. M. *et al.* 1999. VEGF couples hypertrophic cartilage remodeling, ossification and angiogenesis during endochondral bone formation. *Nature Med.*, **5**(6), 623–8.

[13] Ferguson, C., Alpern, E., Miclau, T. and Helms, J. A. 1999. Does adult fracture repair recapitulate embryonic skeletal formation? *Mech. Dev.*, **87**(1–2), 57–66.

[14] Kronenberg, H. M. 2003. Developmental regulation of the growth plate. *Nature*, **423**(6937), 332–6.

[15] Glowacki, J. 1998. Angiogenesis in fracture repair. *Clin. Orthop. Relat. Res.*, **355**(Suppl.), S82–9.

[16] Carano, R. A. and Filvaroff, E. H. 2003. Angiogenesis and bone repair. *Drug Discov. Today*, **8**(21), 980–9.

[17] Muschler, G. F., Nakamoto, C. and Griffith, L. G. 2004. Engineering principles of clinical cell-based tissue engineering. *J. Bone Joint Surg. Am.*, **86A**(7), 1541–58.

[18] Einhorn, T. A. 1995. Enhancement of fracture-healing. *J. Bone Joint Surg. Am.*, **77**(6), 940–56.

[19] Brinker, M. R. and Bailey, D. E. Jr. 1997. Fracture healing in tibia fractures with an associated vascular injury. *J. Trauma*, **42**(1), 11–9.

[20] Dickson, K., Katzman, S., Delgado, E. and Contreras, D. 1994. Delayed unions and nonunions of open tibial fractures. Correlation with arteriography results. *Clin. Orthop. Relat. Res.*, **302**, 189–93.

[21] Glass, G. E., Pearse, M. F. and Nanchahal, J. 2009. Improving lower limb salvage following fractures with vascular injury: a systematic review and new management algorithm. *J. Plast. Reconstr. Aesthet. Surg.*, **62**(5), 571–9.

[22] Kase, T., Skjeldal, S., Nordsletten, L. and Reikeras, O. 1998. Healing of tibial fractures is not impaired after acute hindlimb ischemia in rats. *Arch. Orthop. Trauma Surg.*, **117**(4–5), 273–6.

[23] Lu, C., Miclau, T., Hu, D. and Marcucio, R. S. 2007. Ischemia leads to delayed union during fracture healing: a mouse model. *J. Orthop. Res.*, **25**(1), 51–61.

[24] Street, J., Bao, M., deGuzman, L. *et al.* 2002. Vascular endothelial growth factor stimulates bone repair by promoting angiogenesis and bone turnover. *Proc. Nat. Acad. Sci. USA*, **99**(15), 9656–61.

[25] Hausman, M. R., Schaffler, M. B. and Majeska, R. J. 2001. Prevention of fracture healing in rats by an inhibitor of angiogenesis. *Bone*, **29**(6), 560–4.

[26] Wan, C., Gilbert, S. R., Wang, Y. *et al.* 2008. Activation of the hypoxia-inducible factor-1α pathway accelerates bone regeneration. *Proc. Nat. Acad. Sci. USA*, **105**(2), 686–91.

[27] Fang, T. D., Salim, A., Xia, W. *et al.* 2005. Angiogenesis is required for successful bone induction during distraction osteogenesis. *J. Bone Miner. Res.*, **20**(7), 1114–24.

[28] Wallace, A. L., Draper, E. R., Strachan, R. K., McCarthy, I. D. and Hughes, S. P. 1994. The vascular response to fracture micromovement. *Clin. Orthop. Relat. Res.*, **301**, 281–90.

[29] Lienau, J., Schell, H., Duda, G. N. *et al.* 2005. Initial vascularization and tissue differentiation are influenced by fixation stability. *J. Orthop. Res.*, **23**(3), 639–45.

[30] Boerckel, J. D., Uhrig, B. A., Willett, N. J., Huebsch, N. and Guldberg, R. E. 2011. Mechanical regulation of vascular growth and tissue regeneration in vivo. *Proc. Nat. Acad. Sci. USA*, **108**(37), E674–80.

[31] Trueta, J. 1963. The role of the vessels in osteogenesis. *J. Bone Joint Surg. – Brit. Vol.*, **45**(2), 402–18.

[32] Kempen, D. H., Creemers, L. B., Alblas, J. *et al.* 2010. Growth factor interactions in bone regeneration. *Tissue Eng. Part B Rev.*, **16**(6), 551–66.

[33] Wang, Y., Wan, C., Deng, L. *et al.* 2007. The hypoxia-inducible factor α pathway couples angiogenesis to osteogenesis during skeletal development. *J. Clin. Invest.*, **117**(6), 1616–26.

[34] Araldi, E. and Schipani, E. 2010. Hypoxia, HIFs and bone development. *Bone*, **47**(2), 190–6.

[35] Shen, X., Wan, C., Ramaswamy, G. *et al.* 2009. Prolyl hydroxylase inhibitors increase neoangiogenesis and callus formation following femur fracture in mice. *J. Orthop. Res.*, **27**(10), 1298–305.

[36] Stewart, R., Goldstein, J., Eberhardt, A., Chu, G. T. and Gilbert, S. 2011. Increasing vascularity to improve healing of a segmental defect of the rat femur. *J. Orthop. Trauma*, **25**(8), 472–6.

[37] Urist, M. R. 1965. Bone: formation by autoinduction. *Science*, **150**(698), 893–9.

[38] Deckers, M. M., van Bezooijen, R. L., van der Horst, G. *et al.* 2002. Bone morphogenetic proteins stimulate angiogenesis through osteoblast-derived vascular endothelial growth factor A. *Endocrinology*, **143**(4), 1545–53.

[39] Zhang, F., Qiu, T., Wu, X. *et al.* 2009. Sustained BMP signaling in osteoblasts stimulates bone formation by promoting angiogenesis and osteoblast differentiation. *J. Bone Miner. Res.*, **24**(7), 1224–33.

[40] Smadja, D. M., Bieche, I., Silvestre, J. S. *et al.* 2008. Bone morphogenetic proteins 2 and 4 are selectively expressed by late outgrowth endothelial progenitor cells and promote neoangiogenesis. *Arterioscler. Thromb. Vasc. Biol.*, **28**(12), 2137–43.

[41] Kempen, D. H., Lu, L., Heijink, A. *et al.* 2009. Effect of local sequential VEGF and BMP-2 delivery on ectopic and orthotopic bone regeneration. *Biomaterials*, **30**(14), 2816–25.

[42] Peng, H., Wright, V., Usas, A. *et al.* 2002. Synergistic enhancement of bone formation and healing by stem cell-expressed VEGF and bone morphogenetic protein-4. *J. Clin. Invest.*, **110**(6), 751–9.

[43] Lu, C., Xing, Z., Yu, Y. Y. *et al.* 2010. Recombinant human bone morphogenetic protein-7 enhances fracture healing in an ischemic environment. *J. Orthop. Res.*, **28**(5), 687–96.

[44] Duvall, C. L., Taylor, W. R., Weiss, D., Wojtowicz, A. M. and Guldberg, R. E. 2007. Impaired angiogenesis, early callus formation, and late stage remodeling in fracture healing of osteopontin-deficient mice. *J. Bone Miner. Res.*, **22**(2), 286–97.

[45] Hurrell, D. J. 1937. The nerve supply of bone. *J. Anat.*, **72**(1), 54–61.

[46] Sherman, M. S. 1963. The nerves of bone. *J. Bone Joint Surg. – Am. Vol.*, **45**(3), 522–8.

[47] Serre, C. M., Farlay, D., Delmas, P. D. and Chenu, C. 1999. Evidence for a dense and intimate innervation of the bone tissue, including glutamate-containing fibers. *Bone*, **25**(6), 623–9.

[48] Mach, D. B., Rogers, S. D., Sabino, M. C. *et al.* 2002. Origins of skeletal pain: sensory and sympathetic innervation of the mouse femur. *Neuroscience*, **113**(1), 155–66.

[49] Frenkel, S. R., Guerra, L. A., Mitchell, O. G. and Singh, I. J. 1990. Nerve growth factor in skeletal tissues of the embryonic chick. *Cell Tissue Res.*, **260**(3), 507–11.

[50] Imai, S. and Matsusue, Y. 2002. Neuronal regulation of bone metabolism and anabolism: calcitonin gene-related peptide-, substance P-, and tyrosine hydroxylase-containing nerves and the bone. *Microsc. Res. Tech.*, **58**(2), 61–9.

[51] Spencer, G. J., Hitchcock, I. S. and Genever, P. G. 2004. Emerging neuroskeletal signalling pathways: a review. *FEBS Lett.*, **559**(1–3), 6–12.

[52] Elefteriou, F. 2008. Regulation of bone remodeling by the central and peripheral nervous system. *Arch. Biochem. Biophys.*, **473**(2), 231–6.

[53] Ducy, P., Amling, M., Takeda, S. *et al.* 2000. Leptin inhibits bone formation through a hypothalamic relay: a central control of bone mass. *Cell*, **100**(2), 197–207.

[54] Sample, S. J., Behan, M., Smith, L. *et al.* 2008. Functional adaptation to loading of a single bone is neuronally regulated and involves multiple bones. *J. Bone Miner. Res.*, **23**(9), 1372–81.

[55] Kondo, H., Nifuji, A., Takeda, S. *et al.* 2005. Unloading induces osteoblastic cell suppression and osteoclastic cell activation to lead to bone loss via sympathetic nervous system. *J. Biol Chem.*, **280**(34), 30192–200.

[56] Nagao, M., Feinstein, T. N., Ezura, Y. *et al.* 2011. Sympathetic control of bone mass regulated by osteopontin. *Proc. Nat. Acad. Sci. USA*, **108**(43), 17767–72.

[57] Whiteside, G. T., Boulet, J. M., Sellers, R., Bunton, T. E. and Walker, K. 2006. Neuropathy-induced osteopenia in rats is not due to a reduction in weight born on the affected limb. *Bone*, **38**(3), 387–93.

[58] Li, J., Ahmad, T., Spetea, M., Ahmed, M. and Kreicbergs, A. 2001. Bone reinnervation after fracture: a study in the rat. *J. Bone Miner. Res.*, **16**(8), 1505–10.

[59] Santavirta, S., Konttinen, Y. T., Nordstrom, D. *et al.* 1992. Immunologic studies of nonunited fractures. *Acta Orthop. Scand.*, **63**(6), 579–86.

[60] Perkins, R. and Skirving, A. P. 1987. Callus formation and the rate of healing of femoral fractures in patients with head injuries. *J. Bone Joint Surg. – Brit. Vol.*, **69**(4), 521–4.

[61] Spencer, R. F. 1987. The effect of head injury on fracture healing. A quantitative assessment. *J. Bone Joint Surg. - Brit.* Vol., **69**(4), 525–8.

[62] Garland, D. E. 1988. Clinical observations on fractures and heterotopic ossification in the spinal cord and raumatic brain injured populations. *Clin. Orthop. Relat. Res.*, **233**, 86–101.

[63] Kushwaha, V. P. and Garland, D. G. 1998. Extremity fractures in the patient with a traumatic brain injury. *J. Am. Acad. Orthop. Surg.*, **6**(5), 298–307.

[64] Morley, J., Marsh, S., Drakoulakis, E., Pape, H. C. and Giannoudis, P. V. 2005. Does traumatic brain injury result in accelerated fracture healing? *Injury*, **36**(3), 363–8.

[65] Aro, H., Eerola, E., Aho, A. J. and Penttinen, R. 1981. Healing of experimental fractures in the denervated limbs of the rat. *Clin. Orthop. Relat. Res.*, **155**, 211–17.

[66] Aro, H. 1985. Effect of nerve injury on fracture healing. Callus formation studied in the rat. *Acta Orthop. Scand.*, **56**(3), 233–7.

[67] Nordsletten, L., Madsen, J. E., Almaas, R. *et al.* 1994. The neuronal regulation of fracture healing. Effects of sciatic nerve resection in rat tibia. *Acta Orthop. Scand.*, **65**(3), 299–304.

[68] Hukkanen, M., Konttinen, Y. T., Santavirta, S. *et al.* 1995. Effect of sciatic nerve section on neural ingrowth into the rat tibial fracture callus. *Clin. Orthop. Relat. Res.*, **311**, 247–57.

[69] Madsen, J. E., Hukkanen, M., Aune, A. K. *et al.* 1998. Fracture healing and callus innervation after peripheral nerve resection in rats. *Clin. Orthop. Relat. Res.*, **351**, 230–40.

[70] Frymoyer, J. W. and Pope, M. H. 1977. Fracture healing in the sciatically denervated rat. *J. Trauma*, **17**(5), 355–61.

[71] Aro, H., Eerola, E. and Aho, A. J. 1985. Development of nonunions in the rat fibula after removal of periosteal neural mechanoreceptors. *Clin. Orthop. Relat. Res.*, **199**, 292–9.

[72] Apel, P. J., Crane, D., Northam, C. N. *et al.* 2009. Effect of selective sensory denervation on fracture-healing: an experimental study of rats. *J. Bone Joint Surg. Am.*, **91**(12), 2886–95.

[73] Boes, M., Kain, M., Kakar, S. *et al.* 2006. Osteogenic effects of traumatic brain injury on experimental fracture-healing. *J. Bone Joint Surg. Am.*, **88**(4), 738–43.

[74] Bjurholm, A., Kreicbergs, A., Brodin, E. and Schultzberg, M. 1988. Substance P- and CGRP-immunoreactive nerves in bone. *Peptides*, **9**(1), 165–71.

[75] Hukkanen, M., Konttinen, Y. T., Santavirta, S. *et al.* 1993. Rapid proliferation of calcitonin gene-related peptide-immunoreactive nerves during healing of rat tibial fracture suggests neural involvement in bone growth and remodelling. *Neuroscience*, **54**(4), 969–79.

[76] Bernard, G. W. and Shih, C. 1990. The osteogenic stimulating effect of neuroactive calcitonin gene-related peptide. *Peptides*, **11**(4), 625–32.

[77] Ballica, R., Valentijn, K., Khachatryan, A. *et al.* 1999. Targeted expression of calcitonin gene-related peptide to osteoblasts increases bone density in mice. *J. Bone Miner. Res.*, **14**(7), 1067–74.

[78] Brain, S. D., Williams, T. J., Tippins, J. R., Morris, H. R. and MacIntyre, I. 1985. Calcitonin gene-related peptide is a potent vasodilator. *Nature*, **313**(5997), 54–6.

[79] Haegerstrand, A., Dalsgaard, C. J., Jonzon, B., Larsson, O. and Nilsson, J. 1990. Calcitonin gene-related peptide stimulates proliferation of human endothelial cells. *Proc. Nat. Acad. Sci. USA*, **87**(9), 3299–303.

[80] Midrio, M., Corsi, A. and Granata, A. L. 1968. Early effects of nerve section on the blood flow of skeletal muscle. *Am. J. Physiol.*, **214**(2), 287–93.

[81] Siemionow, M., Andreasen, T., Chick, L. and Lister, G. 1994. Effect of muscle flap denervation on flow hemodynamics: a new model for chronic in vivo studies. *Microsurgery*, **15**(12), 891–4.

[82] Shim, S. S., Copp, D. H. and Patterson, F. P. 1966. Bone blood flow in the limb following complete sciatic nerve section. *Surg. Gynecol. Obstet.*, **123**(2), 333–5.

[83] Carr, M. M., Best, T. J., Mackinnon, S. E. and Evans, P. J. 1992. Strain differences in autotomy in rats undergoing sciatic nerve transection or repair. *Ann. Plast. Surg.*, **28**(6), 538–44.

[84] Sharir, A., Stern, T., Rot, C., Shahar, R. and Zelzer, E. 2011. Muscle force regulates bone shaping for optimal load-bearing capacity during embryogenesis. *Development*, **138**(15), 3247–59.

[85] Macdonald, H., Kontulainen, S., Petit, M., Janssen, P. and McKay, H. 2006. Bone strength and its determinants in pre- and early pubertal boys and girls. *Bone*, **39**(3), 598–608.

[86] Gross, T. S., Poliachik, S. L., Prasad, J. and Bain, S. D. 2010. The effect of muscle dysfunction on bone mass and morphology. *J. Musculoskelet. Neuronal Interact.*, **10**(1), 25–34.

[87] Duda, G. N., Taylor, W. R., Winkler, T. *et al.* 2008. Biomechanical, microvascular, and cellular factors promote muscle and bone regeneration. *Exerc. Sport Sci. Rev.*, **36**(2), 64–70.

[88] Gopal, S., Majumder, S., Batchelor, A. G. *et al.* 2000. Fix and flap: the radical orthopaedic and plastic treatment of severe open fractures of the tibia. *J. Bone Joint Surg. – Brit. Vol.*, **82**(7), 959–66.

[89] Will, R. E., Fleming, M. E., Lafferty, P. M., Fletcher, J. W. and Cole, P. A. 2011. Low complication rate associated with raising mature flap for tibial nonunion reconstruction. *J. Trauma*, **71**(6), 1709–14.

[90] Franken, J. M., Hupkens, P. and Spauwen, P. H. 2010. The treatment of soft-tissue defects of the lower leg after a traumatic open tibial fracture. *Eur. J. Plastic Surg.*, **33**(3), 129–33.

[91] Choudry, U., Moran, S. and Karacor, Z. 2008. Soft-tissue coverage and outcome of gustilo grade IIIB midshaft tibia fractures: a 15-year experience. *Plastic Reconstruct. Surg.*, **122**(2), 479–85.

[92] Jupiter, J. B., Gerhard, H. J., Guerrero, J., Nunley, J. A. and Levin, L. S. 1997. Treatment of segmental defects of the radius with use of the vascularized osteoseptocutaneous fibular autogenous graft. *J. Bone Joint Surg. Am. Vol.*, **79**(4), 542–50.

[93] Stein, H., Perren, S. M., Cordey, J. *et al.* 2002. The muscle bed – a crucial factor for fracture healing: a physiological concept. *Orthopedics*, **25**(12), 1379–83.

[94] Liu, R., Schindeler, A. and Little, D. G. 2010. The potential role of muscle in bone repair. *J. Musculoskelet. Neuronal Interact.*, **10**(1), 71–6.

[95] Claes, L., Maurer-Klein, N., Henke, T. *et al.* 2006. Moderate soft tissue trauma delays new bone formation only in the early phase of fracture healing. *J. Orthop. Res.*, **24**(6), 1178–85.

[96] Melnyk, M., Henke, T., Claes, L. and Augat, P. 2008. Revascularisation during fracture healing with soft tissue injury. *Arch. Orthop. Trauma Surg.*, **128**(10), 1159–65.

[97] Landry, P. S., Marino, A. A., Sadasivan, K. K. and Albright, J. A. 1996. Bone injury response. An animal model for testing theories of regulation. *Clin. Orthop. Relat. Res.*, **332**, 260–73.

[98] Landry, P. S., Marino, A. A., Sadasivan, K. K. and Albright, J. A. 2000. Effect of soft-tissue trauma on the early periosteal response of bone to injury. *J. Trauma*, **48**(3), 479–83.

[99] Utvag, S. E., Grundnes, O., Rindal, D. B. and Reikeras, O. 2003. Influence of extensive muscle injury on fracture healing in rat tibia. *J. Orthop. Trauma*, **17**(6), 430–5.

[100] Utvag, S. E., Iversen, K. B., Grundnes, O. and Reikeras, O. 2002. Poor muscle coverage delays fracture healing in rats. *Acta Orthop. Scand.*, **73**(4), 471–4.

[101] Richards, R. R., Orsini, E. C., Mahoney, J. L. and Verschuren, R. 1987. The influence of muscle flap coverage on the repair of devascularized tibial cortex: an experimental investigation in the dog. *Plast. Reconstr. Surg.*, **79**(6), 946–58.

[102] Richards, R. R. and Schemitsch, E. H. 1989. Effect of muscle flap coverage on bone blood flow following devascularization of a segment of tibia: an experimental investigation in the dog. *J. Orthop. Res.*, **7**(4), 550–8.

[103] Richards, R. R., McKee, M. D., Paitich, C. B., Anderson, G. I. and Bertoia, J. T. 1991. A comparison of the effects of skin coverage and muscle flap coverage on the early strength of union at the site of osteotomy after devascularization of a segment of canine tibia. *J. Bone Joint Surg. Am.*, **73**(9), 1323–30.

[104] Schemitsch, E. H., Weinberg, J. A., McKee, M. D. and Richards, R. R. 1997. The relative importance of intramedullary, intracortical, and extraosseous soft-tissue blood flow to the repair of devascularized canine tibial cortex. *Ann. Plast. Surg.*, **38**(6), 623–31.

[105] Harry, L. E., Sandison, A., Paleolog, E. M. *et al.* 2008. Comparison of the healing of open tibial fractures covered with either muscle or fasciocutaneous tissue in a murine model. *J. Orthop. Res.*, **26**(9), 1238–44.

[106] Kaufman, H., Reznick, A., Stein, H., Barak, M. and Maor, G. 2008. The biological basis of the bone-muscle inter-relationship in the algorithm of fracture healing. *Orthopedics*, **31**(8), 751.

[107] Kolambkar, Y. M., Dupont, K. M., Boerckel, J. D. *et al.* 2011. An alginate-based hybrid system for growth factor delivery in the functional repair of large bone defects. *Biomaterials*, **32**(1), 65–74.

[108] Schaser, K. D., Zhang, L., Haas, N. P. *et al.* 2003. Temporal profile of microvascular disturbances in rat tibial periosteum following closed soft tissue trauma. *Langenbeck's Arch. Surg./Deutsche Gesellschaft Chirurg.*, **388**(5), 323–30.

[109] Hamrick, M. W. 2011. A role for myokines in muscle – bone interactions. *Exerc. Sport Sci. Rev.*, **39**(1), 43–7.

[110] Hamrick, M. W., McNeil, P. L. and Patterson, S. L. 2010. Role of muscle-derived growth factors in bone formation. *J. Musculoskelet. Neuronal Interact.*, **10**(1), 64–70.

[111] Hughes-Fulford, M. and Li, C. F. 2011. The role of FGF-2 and BMP-2 in regulation of gene induction, cell proliferation and mineralization. *J. Orthop. Surg. Res.*, **6**, 8.

[112] Yakar, S., Rosen, C. J., Beamer, W. G. *et al.* 2002. Circulating levels of IGF-1 directly regulate bone growth and density. *J. Clin. Invest.*, **110**(6), 771–81.

[113] McPherron, A. C., Lawler, A. M. and Lee, S. J. 1997. Regulation of skeletal muscle mass in mice by a new TGF-β superfamily member. *Nature*, **387**(6628), 83–90.

[114] Elkasrawy, M. N. and Hamrick, M. W. 2010. Myostatin (GDF-8) as a key factor linking muscle mass and bone structure. *J. Musculoskelet. Neuronal Interact.*, **10**(1), 56–63.

[115] Hamrick, M. W., Shi, X., Zhang, W. *et al.* 2007. Loss of myostatin (GDF8) function increases osteogenic differentiation of bone marrow-derived mesenchymal stem cells but the osteogenic effect is ablated with unloading. *Bone*, **40**(6), 1544–53.

[116] Kellum, E., Starr, H., Arounleut, P. *et al.* 2009. Myostatin (GDF-8) deficiency increases fracture callus size, Sox-5 expression, and callus bone volume. *Bone*, **44**(1), 17–23.

[117] Hamrick, M. W., Arounleut, P., Kellum, E. *et al.* 2010. Recombinant myostatin (GDF-8) propeptide enhances the repair and regeneration of both muscle and bone in a model of deep penetrant musculoskeletal injury. *J. Trauma*, **69**(3), 579–83.

[118] Nesti, L. J., Jackson, W. M., Shanti, R. M. *et al.* 2008. Differentiation potential of multipotent progenitor cells derived from war-traumatized muscle tissue. *J. Bone Joint Surg. Am.*, **90**(11), 2390–8.

[119] Jackson, W. M., Aragon, A. B., Djouad, F. *et al.* 2009. Mesenchymal progenitor cells derived from traumatized human muscle. *J. Tissue Eng. Regen. Med.*, **3**(2), 129–38.

[120] Peng, H. and Huard, J. 2004. Muscle-derived stem cells for musculoskeletal tissue regeneration and repair. *Transpl. Immunol.*, **12**(3–4), 311–19.

[121] Asakura, A., Komaki, M. and Rudnicki, M. 2001. Muscle satellite cells are multipotential stem cells that exhibit myogenic, osteogenic, and adipogenic differentiation. *Differentiation*, **68**(4–5), 245–53.

[122] Wada, M. R., Inagawa-Ogashiwa, M., Shimizu, S., Yasumoto, S. and Hashimoto, N. 2002. Generation of different fates from multipotent muscle stem cells. *Development*, **129**(12), 2987–95.

[123] Lee, J. Y., Qu-Petersen, Z., Cao, B. *et al.* 2000. Clonal isolation of muscle-derived cells capable of enhancing muscle regeneration and bone healing. *J. Cell Biol.*, **150**(5), 1085–100.

[124] Gersbach, C. A., Guldberg, R. E. and Garcia, A. J. 2007. In vitro and in vivo osteoblastic differentiation of BMP-2- and Runx2-engineered skeletal myoblasts. *J. Cell Biochem.*, **100**(5), 1324–36.

[125] Brockes, J. P. and Kumar, A. 2005. Appendage regeneration in adult vertebrates and implications for regenerative medicine. *Science*, **310**(5756), 1919–23.

[126] Nacu, E. and Tanaka, E. M. 2011. Limb regeneration: a new development? *Ann. Rev. Cell Dev. Biol.*, **27**, 409–40.

30

Tooth development and regeneration

Weibo Zhang and Pamela C. Yelick

30.1 Tooth development

Each tooth, even though it looks simple, is an organ with complex structure and consists of multiple types of tissues (Ten Cate, 1998). Dentin is the main component, which is a hard and avascular tissue with a small hollow tubular inside. Enamel is the hardest tissue of the whole living body, protecting the dentin underneath by covering the crown dentin. Cementum, including cellular and acellular cementum, is present on the surface of root dentin. Other than those three types of hard tissue, a tooth also contains dental pulp, the highly vascularized soft tissue that acts as nutrition source and biosensor, as well as periodontal ligament (PDL), the tissue with well-organized collagen bundles that anchors the tooth to the surrounding alveolar bone. Among those tissues, only enamel is from the epithelium. The rest of the dental tissues are all from the neural crest-cell-derived mesenchyme (Nanci, 2007). The sequential and reciprocal interactions between the oral epithelium and the cranial neural crest-derived mesenchyme are essential to control tooth formation, including their size, number, and shape (Thesleff and Nieminen, 1996).

Similarly to the development of other ectodermal organs such as hair, nails, and glands, tooth formation starts from epithelial thickenings and the condensation of mesenchymal cells underneath at the position of the future teeth (Driessens and Wöltgens, 1986). The thickened epithelium and mesenchyme below form a bud structure called a tooth bud (TB). Each TB then goes through bud, cap, bell, and crown stages and forms one tooth eventually (Nanci, 2007). Histologically, there are three components of the tooth bud – the enamel organ from the dental epithelium (DE), the dental papilla, and the dental follicle from dental mesenchyme (DM) (Figure 30.1). The DE and the DM are separated by a layer of basement membrane. The DE cells adjacent to the basement membrane give rise to ameloblasts, which elaborate enamel. Enamel-organ-derived cells at the edge of the enamel organ form a structure called the cervical loop, which differentiates to form Hertwig's epithelial root sheath (HERS), which directs tooth root formation. The DM cells right below the basement membrane differentiate into odontoblasts that produce dentin. The DM cells within the dental follicle contribute to the formation of PDL, differentiating into cementoblasts that form cementum, as well as osteoblasts that generate the alveolar bone which surrounds and supports the teeth (Figure 30.1). The DM encapsulated in the dentin differentiates and forms the dental pulp (Melfi and Permar, 1988). During root formation, the tooth gradually erupts and becomes visible. After the completion of enamel formation, the DE cells undergo apoptosis and disappear. No DE cells are present in the erupted tooth (Vaahtokari *et al.*, 1996).

Even the mechanism of tooth formation is not fully understood, but it is widely accepted that numerous signaling molecules are involved in controlling all steps of tooth formation, including cell proliferation, differentiation, and mineralization. Furthermore, it has been shown that tooth shape is determined by the enamel knot (EK), a signaling center formed by dental epithelial cells (Jernvall and Jung, 2000). The array of molecules secreted by the EK signaling center can

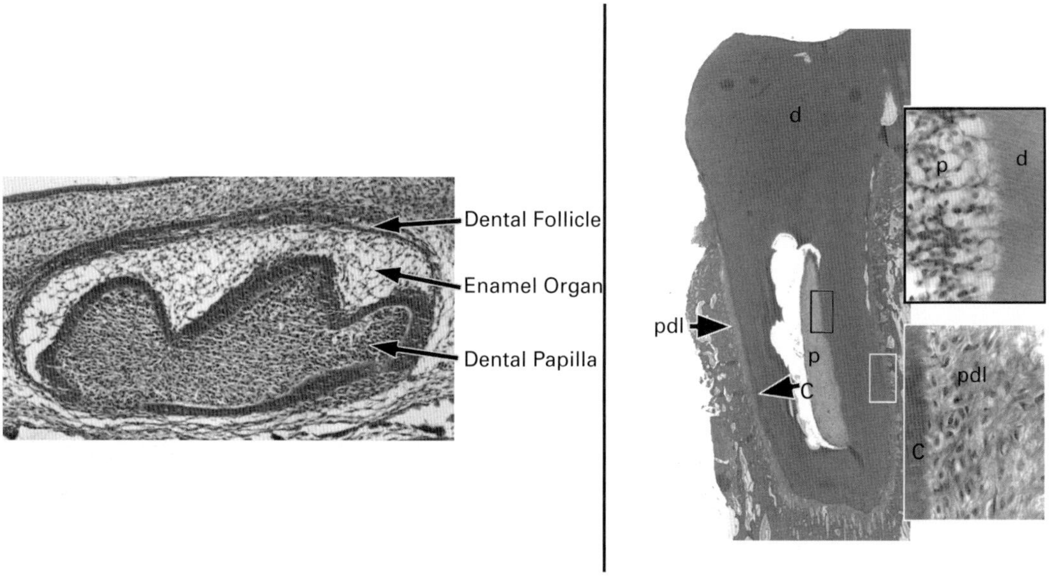

Figure 30.1. Tooth maturation.

direct the growth and differentiation of DE and DM cells, and eventually directs tooth morphology (Thesleff *et al.*, 2001; Cho *et al.*, 2007). The main molecules that are involved in tooth development belong to five signaling pathways: Notch, bone morphogenetic protein (BMP), fibroblast growth factor (FGF), sonic hedgehog (Shh), and wingless/integration 1 (Wnt) (Mitsiadis and Luder, 2011). Each signaling pathway involves several molecules, such as transcription factors and correlated receptors. During the different stages of tooth development, production of the same molecules is repetitively upgraded or downgraded in a precise time-depended manner (Figure 30.2) (Thesleff, 2003). Fully understanding the interactions among those signals would provide valuable guidance for tooth regeneration.

It is difficult to analyze tooth development using a human model. Luckily, although many different species have various kinds of teeth, tooth development is quite conservative among species. Numerous regulatory genes that have been primarily found in organisms such as Drosophila, zebrafish, xenopus, and mouse also play important roles in human tooth formation. Compared with the years-to-decades-long process of human tooth formation, the same process with identical mineral formulation in takes months the mouse, and in zebrafish teeth form within a few days (Arnold *et al.*, 2008).

The mouse is one of the most commonly used animal models (Chai *et al.*, 1998; Peterkova *et al.*, 2002). The molecular signals that control the DE–DM interaction can be analyzed using a wild-type mouse line. Also, transgenic mouse lines with different genetic mutations serve as important tools to determine the roles of specific genes in tooth development (Song *et al.*, 2008; Chai *et al.*, 1998). Furthermore, teeth were lost from Aves almost 100 million years ago. Mouse-mesenchyme–chicken-epithelium recombinations also help one to understand the interaction between DE and DM layers (Cai *et al.*, 2009; Harris *et al.*, 2006)

The zebrafish is another useful animal model for tooth development. Zebrafish have only pharyngeal teeth, with no dentition in the oral cavity. On each side of both pharyngeal jaws, there are three rows of teeth with 11 teeth in total (Van der Heyden *et al.*, 2001). The basic morphology of these pharyngeal teeth is similar

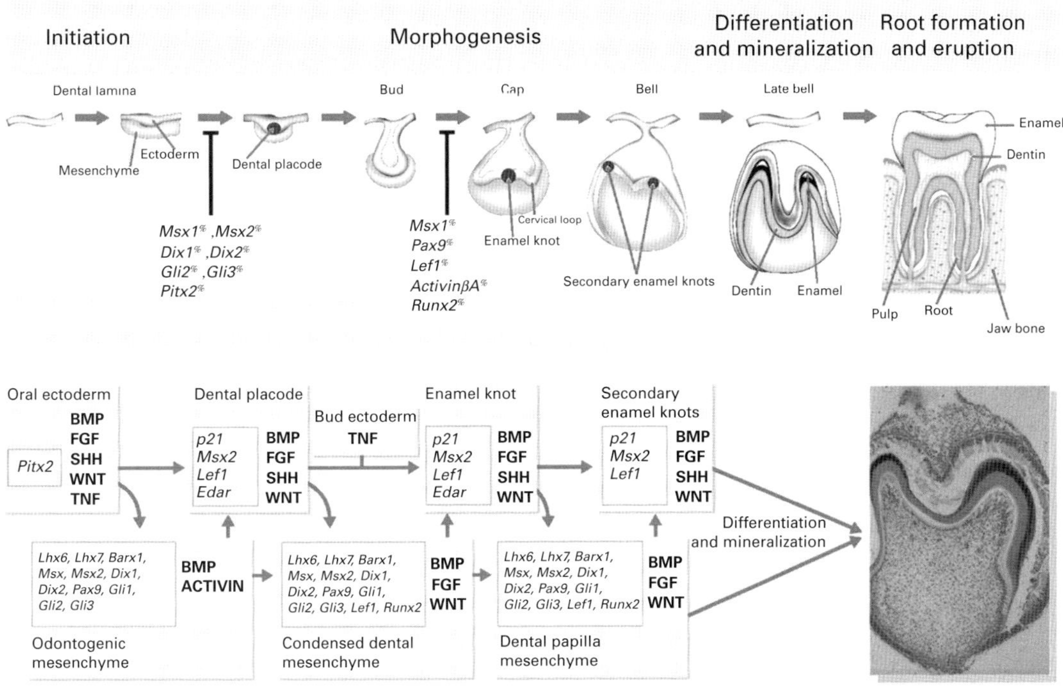

Figure 30.2. Signaling in tooth development. (From Irma Thesleff, signalling in tooth development. *Journal of Cell Science*, 2003, **116**, 1647–8).

to the morphology of most vertebrate teeth, with tubular dentin surrounding a pulp chamber with odontoblasts and pulp cells (Van der Heyden and Huysseune, 2000). Also, these pharyngeal teeth are replaced continuously within 11–13 days throughout the whole lifespan of the fish (Van der Heyden *et al.*, 2001). Those qualities make the zebrafish a good model to study tooth development and biomineralization of enamel and dentin (Huysseune and Sire, 2004; Bartlett *et al.*, 2005). The main difference between zebrafish and vertebrate teeth is that the tooth epithelium of the pharyngeal teeth may be of endodermal origin. Therefore, the tooth crown is covered by a thin layer of enameloid, which is different from the enamel of vertebrate teeth (Huysseune *et al.*, 1998). The root is attached to the underlying branchial bone by a specialized bone of attachment. The process of tooth eruption and ankylosis of the pharyngeal teeth is completed before the completion of dentin mineralization (Huysseune and Sire, 2004; Huysseune, 2006).

These signaling molecules, together with specific transcription factors, constitute a unique molecular imprint for odontogenesis, and contribute to the generation of teeth with various and function-specific shapes. However, the cell biology of the formation of teeth is still not fully understood, and the assembly process for the construction of a whole tooth remains largely unknown.

30.2 Tooth regeneration

Tissue engineering research has grown exponentially because accumulated evidence has proved that stem-cell-based therapies have the potential to repair damaged tissues, such as the brain (Heile and Brinker, 2011; Hwang *et al.*, 2011), heart (Hwang *et al.*, 2011; Strauer and Steinhoff, 2011), and bone (Khaled *et al.*, 2011; Khosla *et al.*, 2010). Allogeneic and autologous transplantations of bone-marrow-derived hematopoietic stem cells are widely used in the clinic to treat diseases such as leukemias (Haurani *et al.*, 1960), lymphomas (van Besien, 2009), aplastic anemia (Peinemann *et al.*, 2009), immune deficiency disorders (Rappeport *et al.*, 2010), and some solid tumor cancers (Demirer *et al.*, 2008; Bregni *et al.*, 2011). Clinical treatments for Alzheimer's, cardiac ischemia, or bone loss using stem-cell-based therapies will improve the quality of life of patients (Schwarz and Schwarz, 2010; Matoba *et al.*, 2008).

The main function of teeth is to masticate food in order to facilitate digestion. Other functions include helping speech and facial aesthetics. Dental tissue damage, even tooth loss, is not life-threatening. Nonetheless, it can severely affect the quality of life both physically and mentally (Brennan *et al.*, 2008). Humans have only two sets of dentition, deciduous and permanent. Permanent teeth erupt to replace the lost function of the accordant deciduous teeth, but there is no replacement for permanent teeth if they get damaged or lost (Linden and Duterloo, 1976). Conventional therapies for tooth loss are prostheses, such as dentures and implants. Synthetic materials have no capacity for self-repair (Mjör and Ferrari, 2002). Regeneration is defined as the restoration of a tissue defect to its original form and function by biological substitutes (Stappenbeck and Miyoshi, 2009). Regeneration of dental tissues would provide a better means for vital, long-term tooth repair or replacement.

The stem cell is the key component for tissue regeneration (Just and Cross, 2008). Stem cells are characterized as undifferentiated cells with the capacity for self-renewal and the potential to differentiate into specialized cell types (Langer and Vacanti, 1993). Autologous stem cells can be transplanted back into the individual from which they were extracted, thereby eliminating the complications associated with immune rejection (Lee *et al.*, 2010). Other than the stem cells derived from dental pulp and PDL, the dental tissues originating from post-natal stem cells (PSCs) also include stem cells from the apical papilla, dental epithelial, and tooth bud (Huang *et al.*, 2009). Bone-marrow-derived mesenchymal stem cells, ESCs, and iPS cells are non-dental tissue stem cells.

30.2.1 Stem cells for dental tissue regeneration

30.2.1.1 Dental pulp stem cells (DPSCs)

Odontoblasts, the most characterized cells within the dental pulp, are terminally differentiated cells that exhibit the ability to synthesize dentin. Under healthy conditions or mild stimulus, odontoblasts within the dental pulp can retain their function to repair dentin. However, under strong stimulus, such as caries, trauma, and erosion, odontoblasts can be easily damaged and DPSCs are required for tissue regeneration (Bjorndal and Mjör, 2001; Heyeraas *et al.*, 2001). The formation of reparative dentin under such circumstances demonstrates the presence in dental pulp of DPSCs, which can be induced to differentiate into odontoblasts (Goldberg *et al.*, 2008).

DPSCs have been isolated from post-natal human dental pulp (Gronthos *et al.*, 2000) and from human deciduous teeth; these were named "stem cells from human exfoliated deciduous teeth" (SHED) (Miura *et al.*, 2003). Both types of cell could form a dentin/pulp-like complex with a well-defined layer of odontoblast-like cells, dentin, and highly vascularized pulp tissue at the center, after being transplanted into immunocompromised mice (Miura *et al.*, 2003; Gronthos *et al.*, 2000). DPSCs have also been shown to be capable of neuronal cell differentiation when cultured in the neurogenic medium in vitro (Zhang *et al.*, 2006a) and transplanted in vivo (Nosrat *et al.*, 2001). Like their adult tooth counterpart, SHED also exhibit neurogenic potential (Nourbakhsh *et al.*, 2011). DPSCs can be isolated from teeth that have to be removed in the clinic, and SHED can be isolated from the deciduous teeth. Therefore, it is easy to obtain autologous PSCs from dental pulp (Karaoz *et al.*, 2010).

30.2.1.2 Stem cells from PDL (PDSLs)

PDL has the ability of self-healing after damage, and remodeling in response to the orthodontic force. The guided tissue regeneration (GTR) stem cells obtained from PDL tissues (PDLSCs) exhibit the characteristic ability to form cementum/PDL-like structures in nude mice (Trubiani *et al.*, 2008). PDSLs can differentiate into all the main cell types of periodontium, such as osteoblasts and cementoblasts (Wang *et al.*, 2011). No in-vivo result showed PDLSCs to have the potential to generate dentin/pulp-like complex.

30.2.1.3 Stem cells from apical papilla (SCAP)

Continuing tooth root formation of immature teeth after endodontic treatment suggested the existence of a stem cell population at the tooth root apex (Selden, 2002). Those stem cells has been isolated from the dental apical region and named "stem cells from the apical papilla" (SCAP). When transplanted in vivo, SCAP were capable of differentiation into odontoblast-like cells, and produce dentin–pulp complex with similar histology to that generated by DPSCs or SHED (Sonoyama *et al.*, 2006; Abe *et al.*, 2008). This observation not only shows the importance of preserving the peri-apical tissue containing SCAP during root canal treatment, but also suggests the possibility of tooth regeneration by SCAP. Cells from the apical region can also differentiate into a vascularized pulp tissue (Trope, 2010). Also, when combined with PDLSCs, SCAP formed a root–periodontal complex around a porcelain crown, which resulted in normal tooth function (Sonoyama *et al.*, 2006).

30.2.1.4 Stem cells from dental epithelium

Ameloblasts are the only type of cell that can generate enamel. Rodents, such as the mouse and rat, have continuously growing incisors throughout their lives because of the dental epithelial stem cell niche located at the cervical loop. The isolated stem cells were able to differentiate into enamel-forming ameloblasts (Kawano *et al.*, 2004). Unfortunately, human dental epithelium cells undergo apoptosis once they have finished amelogensis, and are not present in the erupted tooth. Using synthetic material is the only possible way to repair human enamel when it gets damaged (Yamagishi *et al.*, 2005).

30.2.1.5 Dental tooth bud cells

Naturally formed teeth have two types of tooth buds in terms of their developmental stages - embryonic and post-natal tooth buds. Embryonic tooth buds contain all cell types required to regenerate the whole tooth, and re-aggregated tooth bud can form anatomically correct bioengineered tooth-crown teeth (Hu *et al.*, 2006a; Honda *et al.*, 2008). Recognizable dental tissues, including dentin, pulp, and enamel, were also observed in dental implants generated from dissociated post-natal tooth bud cells (Young *et al.*, 2002). The study of embryonic tooth bud cell characterizations provides valuable information about the mechanism of tooth regeneration.

The dental follicle is the tooth sac derived from ectomesenchymal tissue surrounding the developing tooth. The presence of stem cells in dental follicle, known as dental follicle stem cells (DFSCs), has been confirmed (Yao *et al.*, 2008). DFSCs have been shown to be able to differentiate into osteoblasts/cementoblasts, adipocytes, and neurons. DFSCs isolated from human wisdom teeth expressed the putative stem cell markers Notch-1 and Nestin, and produced compact calcified nodules in vitro (Morsczeck *et al.*, 2005).

As yet, no autologous human embryonic tooth bud is available, which makes these studies of limited use for widely applicable tooth regeneration strategies in humans.

30.2.1.6 Non-dental stem cells for dental tissue regeneration

Embryonic stem cells (ESCs), the stem cells derived from the inner cell mass of the blastocyst, are the most versatile of all stem cell types (Thomson *et al.*, 1998). Theoretically, they have the ability to differentiate into cells of all three germ layers, including dental-related cells. However, the ethical debate, immune rejection, and possible teratoma formation severely limit their clinical usage. Therefore, there have been only a few reports about using ESCs in tooth regeneration. Inanc's group reported that human ESCs can facilitate periodontal tissue regeneration in vitro when co-cultured with periodontal ligament fibroblastic cells (Inanc *et al.*, 2009). Another report demonstrated that mouse ESCs were able to differentiate into ameloblasts when cultured in conditioned media from mouse embryonic tooth bud culture (Ning *et al.*, 2010).

Bone marrow stem cells (BMSCs) are non-hematopoietic mesenchymal stem cells isolated from the bone marrow (Chamberlain *et al.*, 2007). So far, BMSCs are the most well-studied and commonly used stem cells because they can differentiate into a wide range of specific cell types. BMSCs have been used for alveolar bone regeneration. Also, BMSCs have the potential to differentiate into ameloblast-like cells after c-Kit$^+$ enrichment (Hu *et al.*, 2006b).

Amniotic-fluid-derived stem cells (AFSCs) can be isolated from aspirates of amniocentesis during genetic screening without any tissue damage (Sessarego *et al.*, 2008). Accumulating data have demonstrated that AFSCs have the capacity for remarkable proliferation and differentiation into multiple lineages, such as chondrocytes, adipocytes, osteoblasts, myocytes, endothelial cells, neuron-like cells, and live cells (Prusa and Hengstschlager, 2002). Umbilical cord stem cells (UCSCs) derive from the blood of the umbilical cord. There is growing interest in their capacity for self-replication and multilineage differentiation (Laughlin *et al.*, 2001; Zhao *et al.*, 2010). There has been no reported of usage AFSCs and UCSCs in the dental field, but their ability to undergo multilineage differentiation suggests their potential for dental tissue regeneration.

30.2.1.7 Induced pluripotent stem (iPS) cells from dental or non-dental origin

Recently, another type of stem cells with great differentiation potency, induced pluripotent stem (iPS) cells, has been created by over-expression of key factors in somatic cells via viral modification (Takahashi *et al.*, 2007; Takahashi and Yamanaka, 2006; Yu *et al.*, 2007). Different non-viral-related methods have been developed for generation of iPS cells to facilitate their clinical application (Okita *et al.*, 2007). It has been proved that iPS cells have comparable differentiation potential to that of ESCs. Since iPS cells can be generated from autologous differentiated cells, they show great clinical potential for dental tissue regeneration.

Huang's group tested viral transfection of Lin28/Nanog/Oct4/Sox2 or c-Myc/Klf4/Oct4/Sox2 into hDPCs, pulp cells harvested from exfoliated deciduous (baby) teeth, and SCAP. They observed that all three cell lines were efficiently reprogrammed into iPS cells (Yan *et al.*, 2010). Tezuka's group infected six lines of hDPCs with retroviruses expressing Oct3/4, Sox2, Kl4, and c-Myc, and established iPS cells from five of them (Tamaoki *et al.*, 2010).

30.2.2 Dental tissue regeneration

Tooth regeneration can be divided into two main areas. One is dental tissue regeneration when only one or several types of tissues would have been partly or fully damaged, and the other one is whole-tooth regeneration, the formation of an entire tooth with all types of anatomically correct dental tissues.

Dental tissue regeneration has been successfully used in the clinic for a long time. Clinicians have been attempting to regenerate damaged dentin–pulp complex (Zander, 1939; Glass and Zander, 1949) and periodontium (Kronfeld, 1935; Goldman, 1950) for 70 years. Currently, pulp capping for generation of the dentin–pulp complex and Glass and Zander, 1949 GTR for periodontium generation are widely used in the clinic and retain their pioneering positions in this area (Quinones *et al.*, 1996; Mulligan and Niemiec, 2001). As we described above, the explanation for the limited regeneration property of dental tissue is the presence of only a small population of stem cells within dental pulp and PDL. Those stem cells, like the other PSCs, are able to differentiate into tissue-specific cells and repair the lost function.

30.2.2.1 Dental tissue regeneration

The most commonly studied types of dental tissue regeneration are pulp regeneration and periodontium regeneration.

Dentin and pulp are two different tissues, but they are always regarded as belonging together because of their close relationship in what is termed the dentin–pulp complex. The immature tooth has an incomplete root with ample blood supply to the pulp. Therefore, preserving the tissue with stem cells, especially SCAP, is the main purpose when treating the immature tooth. Since the dental pulp of the matured tooth is fully enclosed in hard dentin, it is difficult to insure the complete removal of inflammatory pathogens caused by infection. Therefore, endodontic therapy, also known as root canal treatment, is always considered to treat pulpitis (West, 2006). Endodontic therapy replaces the vital pulp with synthetic materials. Synthetic material lacks the ability to sense stimuli from the environment or provide nutrition to the treated tooth. Autologous pulp transplantation has been tried in one of the first attempts at vital pulp therapy (Takei *et al.*, 1988). Although animal studies produced good results, it is not really applicable to humans (Inoue *et al.*, 1993).

One of the main obstacles to pulp regeneration is the limited blood supply because of the anatomical structure of pulp. The small root apexes are the only openings of pulp to surrounding tissue. Therefore, it is important to ensure revascularization in order to provide enough blood supply to the engineered pulp.

DPSCs and SHED can differentiate into odontoblasts, neural cells, and vascular endothelial cells to restore the damaged dentin–pulp complex. Full pulp regeneration with stem cells is a possible solution to fully recover the function of dental pulp. Human pulp cells have been seeded onto a three-dimensional (3D) PGA matrix and formed new tissue with a cellularity similar to that of native pulp in vitro (Mooney *et al.*, 1996). Gotlieb's group have transplanted SHED-seeded synthetic D,D-L,L-polylactic acid (PLGA) scaffolds into extracted endodontically treated human teeth and observed the formation of living pulp (Gotlieb *et al.*, 2008). The combination of SCAP and DPSCs was seeded onto synthetic scaffolds consisting of poly-D,L-lactide/glycolide, inserted into an artificial tooth root canal, and transplanted into nude mice. De-novo regeneration of dentin–pulp complex was observed (Cordeiro *et al.*, 2008; Huang *et al.*, 2010).

For dental pulp tissue engineering, the tooth slice/scaffold model can provide valuable information when cultured both in vitro and in vivo (Nör *et al.*, 2001). The tooth slice/scaffold model of dental pulp tissue engineering allows the generation of a pulp-like tissue within the artificial pulp chamber with a layer of dentin along the surface of the tooth slice/scaffold. SHED seeded onto tooth slices containing a poly-L-lactic acid (PLLA) polymer scaffold packed into the pulp cavity also resulted in the formation of dentin–pulp complex with the differentiation of odontoblast- and endothelial-like (Cordeiro *et al.*, 2008).

Other than transplanting the stem cell into the pre-prepared root canal, it is possible to induce SCAP cells from the apical papilla into the root canal with peripheral blood. For endodontic treatment, a blood clot is always created after removal of the contaminated tissue and infection control treatment (Shah *et al.*, 2008). Blood can deliver abundant growth factors within the blood clot, which acts as a natural scaffold for tissue revascularization.

Currently, GTR is the gold-standard surgery for periodontal tissue regeneration. This procedure is aiming at regeneration of periodontium, including PDL, cementum, and alveolar bone. After removing the pathogen and infected tissues, biocompatible membranes are inserted along the root surface to direct the growth of new tissue. Stimulating the remaining PDSLs is the essential point of this procedure.

Dental implants are becoming ever more popular as a means to treat tooth loss because it has been proved that the prognosis for dental implant therapy is fairly stable (Shalabi *et al.*, 2007; Atieh *et al.*, 2010). Osseointegration, meaning solid bone integration, is commonly observed at the interface between bone and dental implant (Branemark *et al.*, 1977). The rigid osseintegration can cause damage and absorption of the surrounding bone, resulting in implant failure (Rinaldi and Arana-Chavez, 2010). Moreover, without the PDL, it is difficult, if not impossible, to adjust the position of the implant (Devlin and Sloan, 2002). Regeneration of cushion tissue around the implant, like the natural PDL, will help to solve the problem. There are two possible ways to facilitate the regeneration of PDL around implants; one is transplantation

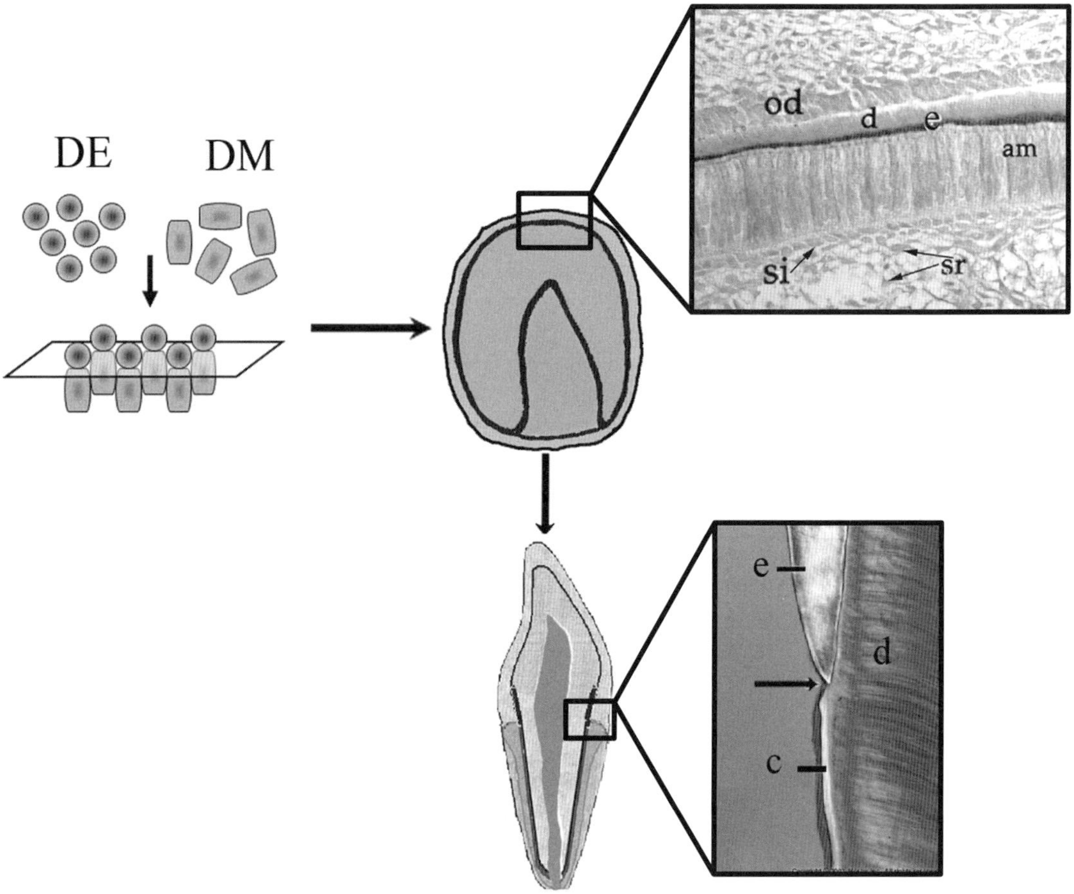

Figure 30.3. A scheme for whole-tooth regeneration.

of autologous stem cells with dental implants, and the other is to modify the implants to attract the surrounding stem cells and then induce them to differentiate into cells for PDL generation.

30.2.2.2 Whole-tooth regeneration

The ultimate goal of whole-tooth regeneration is to regenerate full-sized, functional teeth. In order to achieve that, the essential step is to regenerate the proper spatial and reciprocal interactions between epithelial and mesenchymal dental cells during natural tooth development (Figure 30.3). Since no human dental epithelial cells are available, methods to induce non-dental epithelial cells, such as oral epithelial cells, for example, to differentiate into enamel-producing ameloblast cells could help to overcome this barrier to enamel-regeneration therapies.

There are two basic methods for whole-tooth regeneration, namely tooth bud regeneration and *in situ* tissue regeneration. A tooth bud regeneration approach is to bioengineer an early-forming tooth bud with the proper epithelial–mesenchymal cell layer interactions. The bioengineered tooth bud could then be cultured in vitro or implanted in vivo for further development. The second method can be called "*in situ* tissue regeneration," or "cell homing," whereby an engineered scaffold would be implanted directly into the repair site, in order to attract and simulate cells for local tissue regeneration.

An artificial tooth bud model has been successfully developed to generate fully functional tooth using embryonic tooth bud cells (Ikeda *et al.*, 2009). In this model, DE and DM cell layers were generated separately and sandwiched together to form an artificial tooth bud. An intact or dissociated embryonic DE layer is the most important part of this model, to ensure the successful generation of tooth. Tooth formation was observed when the DE layer was combined with dissociated DM cells or a mixture of embryonic neural stem cells from embryo spinal cords, and embryonic bone marrow cell (Yamamoto *et al.*, 2003; Ohazama *et al.*, 2004). However, successful results were obtained only using cells from mouse embryonic tooth buds, by seeding dental epithelial and mesenchymal cells adjacently at high density (Nakao *et al.*, 2007). There has been no report of successful formation of tooth using post-natal cells (Zhang *et al.*, 2010).

Enzymatically dissociated post-natal pig tooth bud cells were seeded onto a tooth-shaped, 3D mold and transplanted into the omentum of athymic rats. Multiple small but anatomically correct tooth crowns including dentin, odontoblasts, pulp, and enamel were detected (Young *et al.*, 2002; Honda *et al.*, 2007). Later, a tooth bud–bone hybrid construct was developed from a tooth bud with DM core wrapped in DE scaffold and combined with bioengineered bone constructs. The bone–tooth structure formed well-organized dental tissues that closely integrated to the surrounding newly formed bone tissues after implantation in rat or pig jaws (Duailibi *et al.*, 2008; Abukawa *et al.*, 2009; Zhang *et al.*, 2009). The formation of small and aberrant cusps suggests that the correct but random interaction between epithelium and mesenchyme has been attained in this model.

The biggest obstacle to applying this method of tooth bud regeneration clinically is the lack of appropriate sources of human DE cells. As discussed above, the most promising cell source may be the autologous iPS cell.

The other method for whole-tooth generation is *in situ* tooth regeneration, also known as cell homing. This technique requires biomaterials that can release bioactive molecules to attract stem cells in surrounding tissues to stimulate the generation of new tissues (Karp and Leng Teo, 2009), which is new in the dental field. Mao's group filled the pulp chambers and root canals of endodontically treated teeth with growth factors, including vascular endothelial growth factor (VEGF-2), fibroblast growth factor (bFGF), platelet-derived growth factor (PDGF), nerve growth factor (NGF), and bone morphogenetic protein-7 (BMP-7) (Kim *et al.*, 2010a). Pre-treated human teeth were then subcutaneously transplanted into mice, and pulp-like tissue with erythrocyte-filled blood vessels was observed after 3 weeks. The same group also manufactured polycaprolactone (PDL)–hydroxyapatite (HA) tooth scaffolds containing stromal-derived factor-1 (SDF-1) and BMP-7, and implanted them subcutaneously or into the jaw bone of the rat. Distinct periodontal ligament and new bone, but no dentin or enamel tissues, were regenerated (Kim *et al.*, 2010b). Even though the possibility of formation of ameloblasts or enamel, has not been demonstrated cell homing is still regarded as the possible way to achieve whole-tooth regeneration, because it aims at the regeneration of all other dental tissues. Also, no additional cells are required, let alone the epithelial–mesenchymal interaction.

30.2.3 Problems related to tooth regeneration

For successful tooth regeneration, the essential concern is to generate appropriate interactions among cells, scaffold materials, and growth factors using information derived from natural tooth development. Still, some issues need to be solved if tooth regeneration is to become feasible for clinical application.

One issue is related to the identification and isolation of appropriate dental stem cell populations. Just like with the other MSCs, the exact origin of dental stem cells remains uncertain because there is no identified single marker for stem cells. One of the arguments is that MSCs are actually pericytes, because pericytes, like MSCs, reside in close proximity to endothelial cells in capillaries and express similar cell markers (Andreeva *et al.*, 1998; Shi and Gronthos,

2003). A recent publication showed by using genetic lineage tracing that pericytes were able to differentiate into odontoblasts during tooth growth and in response to damage in vivo, but there were other MSCs of non-pericyte origin that also play the same role (Feng *et al.*, 2011).

Methods for the isolation of dental stem cells can only achieve heterogeneous cell populations with no more than 0.01%–1% of real stem cells. Fluorescence-activated cell sorting (FACS) can be used to obtain a more concentrated population of stem cells. Furthermore, ex-vivo expansion is necessary in order to obtain sufficiently large stem cell populations for dental tissue regeneration. In order to eliminate the potential risk of transmitting animal diseases, serum-free medium is recommended for cell expansion. There have been only a few publications on serum-free medium for culture of human SHEDs and PDLSCs (Tarle *et al.*, 2011; Hirata *et al.*, 2010). Still, further analyses are required in order to assess whether the cells cultured in serum-free medium retain their ability to regenerate dental tissues.

Selection of carrier materials is another issue related to successful dental tissue regeneration. Different materials have been tested in the dental field, including collagen, HA, and polymers (Zhang *et al.*, 2006b; Gronthos *et al.*, 2000; Duailibi *et al.*, 2004). The question of the ideal material for dental tissue regeneration is still under investigation. So far, the only functional whole tooth was regenerated by a collagen-drop method. For this method, both epithelial and mesenchymal tooth bud cells will be injected adjacently into a collagen drop. In this case, the function of collagen is more like that of a supporter. There is no direct interaction between the material and seeded cells. Collagen was selected because it is highly biocompatible, easy to handle, and cheap. Other materials that have similar physical and biochemical properties should be appropriate for this application. However, the size of the teeth generated in this way is limited by the amount of cells that can be supported by the surrounding materials.

Growth factors that can benefit dental tissue regeneration have been identified. Some dental pulp cells express the growth factors, including TGF and BMP, and accordingly receptors, under both healthy and pathological conditions (Tran-Hung *et al.*, 2008). Those pulp supportive cells (all non-progenitor cells) can be regarded as acting cells in the sequence of events regulating dentinogenesis, vasculature, and innervation of the dental pulp (About, 2011). It also was revealed that human pulp fibroblasts harvested from third molar teeth expressed two important pro-angiogenic factors, namely vascular endothelial growth factor (VEGF) and basic fibroblast growth factor (FGF-2) (Tran-Hung *et al.*, 2006). During tooth development, the odontoblasts can secrete different types of growth factors, which then *sequester* in the calcified dentin (Roberts-Clark and Smith, 2000; Cassidy *et al.*, 1997). Those growth factors can be released when the mineralized dentin is dissolved in an acidic environment, such as a carious one. The released factors include TGF-β_1, TGF-β_3, and BMP-7, which can stimulate the underlying odontoblasts to secrete reactionary dentin locally (Sloan and Smith, 1999; Zhao *et al.*, 2000). Integration of those growth factors into the tooth regeneration model will benefit tissue generation. However, the missing information is how to understand and replicate the interaction of those growth factors between DE and DM layers.

30.3 Conclusion

Partial dental tissue regeneration, including of the dentin–pulp complex and PDL, has been achieved in the dental clinic and is on the way to becoming a routine treatment. However, whole-tooth regeneration is still at its cradle stage. The lack of human embryonic-stage dental epithelial cells that can initiate the proper epithelial–mesenchymal interaction is the main obstacle. Another problem is that the outcome of dental epithelial–mesenchymal interaction should reach a certain size in order to ensure the generation of a full-size tooth. Furthermore, for a fully functional tooth one requires the formation of mineralized dental tissues, especially dental root, which should occur automatically if a whole tooth bud is regenerated. Still, no large-animal study has been performed to support this theory so far.

Stem-cell-based tissue engineering approaches provide the most promising solutions for dental tissue engineering strategies. Translation of the relevant information to the clinic requires the partnership of researchers and skilled clinicians who can effectively apply advances in knowledge to appropriate clinical cases and develop novel therapies that can realistically be introduced into the clinic.

REFERENCES

Abe, S., Yamaguchi, S., Watanabe, A., Hamada, K. and Amagasa, T. 2008. Hard tissue regeneration capacity of apical pulp derived cells (APDCs) from human tooth with immature apex. *Biochem. Biophys. Res. Commun.*, **371**, 90–3.

About, I. 2011. Dentin regeneration in vitro: the pivotal role of supportive cells. *Adv. Dent. Res.*, **23**, 320–4.

Abukawa, H., Zhang, W., Young, C. S. *et al.* 2009. Reconstructing mandibular defects using autologous tissue-engineered tooth and bone constructs. *J. Oral. Maxillofac. Surg.*, **67**, 335–47.

Andreeva, E. R., Pugach, I. M., Gordon, D. and Orekhov, A. N. 1998. Continuous subendothelial network formed by pericyte-like cells in human vascular bed. *Tissue Cell*, **30**, 127–35.

Arnold, W. H., Naumova, K. I., Naumova, E. A. and Gaengler, P. 2008. Comparative qualitative and quantitative assessment of biomineralization of tooth development in man and zebrafish (*Danio rerio*). *Anat. Rec. (Hoboken)*, **291**, 571–6.

Atieh, M. A., Payne, A. G., Duncan, W. J., De Silva, R. K. and Cullinan, M. P. 2010. Immediate placement or immediate restoration/loading of single implants for molar tooth replacement: a systematic review and meta-analysis. *Int. J. Oral Maxillofac. Implants*, **25**, 401–15.

Bartlett, J. D., Dwyer, S. E., Beniash, E., Skobe, Z. and Payne Ferreira, T. L. 2005. Fluorosis: a new model and new insights. *J. Dent. Res.*, **84**, 832–6.

Bjorndal, L. and Mjör, I. A. 2001. Pulp–dentin biology in restorative dentistry. Part 4: dental caries – characteristics of lesions and pulpal reactions. *Quintessence Int.*, **32**, 717–36.

Branemark, P. I., Hansson, B. O., Adell, R. *et al.* 1977. Osseointegrated implants in the treatment of the edentulous jaw. Experience from a 10-year period. *Scand. J. Plast. Reconstr. Surg. Suppl.*, **16**, 1–132.

Bregni, M., Ciceri, F. and Peccatori, J. 2011. Allogeneic stem cell transplantation for metastatic renal cell cancer (RCC). *J. Cancer*, **2**, 347–9.

Brennan, D. S., Spencer, A. J. and Roberts-Thomson, K. F. 2008. Tooth loss, chewing ability and quality of life. *Qual. Life Res.*, **17**, 227–35.

Cai, J., Cho, S. W., Ishiyama, M. *et al.* 2009. Chick tooth induction revisited. *J. Exp. Zool. B. Molec. Dev. Evol.*, **312**, 465–72.

Cassidy, N., Fahey, M., Prime, S. S. and Smith, A. J. 1997. Comparative analysis of transforming growth factor-β isoforms 1–3 in human and rabbit dentine matrices. *Arch. Oral Biol.*, **42**, 219–23.

Chai, Y., Bringas, P., Jr., Shuler, C. *et al.* 1998. A mouse mandibular culture model permits the study of neural crest cell migration and tooth development. *Int. J. Dev. Biol.*, **42**, 87–94.

Chamberlain, J., Yamagami, T., Colletti, E. *et al.* 2007. Efficient generation of human hepatocytes by the intrahepatic delivery of clonal human mesenchymal stem cells in fetal sheep. *Hepatology*, **46**, 1935–45.

Cho, S. W., Lee, H. A., Cai, J. *et al.* 2007. The primary enamel knot determines the position of the first buccal cusp in developing mice molars. *Differentiation*, **75**, 441–51.

Cordeiro, M. M., Dong, Z., Kaneko, T. *et al.* 2008. Dental pulp tissue engineering with stem cells from exfoliated deciduous teeth. *J. Endod.*, **34**, 962–9.

Demirer, T., Barkholt, L., Blaise, D. *et al.* 2008. Transplantation of allogeneic hematopoietic stem cells: an emerging treatment modality for solid tumors. *Nat. Clin. Pract. Oncol.*, **5**, 256–67.

Devlin, H. and Sloan, P. 2002. Early bone healing events in the human extraction socket. *Int. J. Oral Maxillofac. Surg.*, **31**, 641–5.

Driessens, F. C. M. and Wöltgens, J. H. M. 1986. *Tooth Development and Caries*. Boca Raton, FL: CRC Press.

Duailibi, M. T., Duailibi, S. E., Young, C. S. *et al.* 2004. Bioengineered teeth from cultured rat tooth bud cells. *J. Dent. Res.*, **83**, 523–8.

Duailibi, S. E., Duailibi, M. T., Zhang, W. *et al.* 2008. Bioengineered dental tissues grown in the rat jaw. *J. Dent. Res.*, **87**, 745–50.

Feng, J., Mantesso, A., De Bari, C., Nishiyama, A. and Sharpe, P. T. 2011. Dual origin of mesenchymal stem cells contributing to organ growth and repair. *Proc. Nat. Acad. Sci. USA*, **108**, 6503–8.

Glass, R. L. and Zander, H. A. 1949. Pulp healing. *J. Dent. Res.*, **28**(2), 97–110.

Goldberg, M., Farges, J. C., Lacerda-Pinheiro, S. *et al.* 2008. Inflammatory and immunological aspects of dental pulp repair. *Pharmacol. Res.*, **58**, 137–47.

Goldman, H. M. 1950. The development of physiologic gingival contours by gingivoplasty. *Oral Surg. Oral Med. Oral Pathol.*, **3**, 879–88.

Gotlieb, E. L., Murray, P. E., Namerow, K. N., Kuttler, S. and Garcia-Godoy, F. 2008. An ultrastructural investigation of tissue-engineered pulp constructs implonted within endoscopically treated teeth. *J. Am. Dent. Assoc.*, **139**(4), 457–65.

Gronthos, S., Mankani, M., Brahim, J., Robey, P. G. and Shi, S. 2000. Post-natal human dental pulp stem cells (DPSCs) in vitro and in vivo. *Proc. Nat. Acad. Sci. USA*, **97**, 13625–30.

Harris, M. P., Hasso, S. M., Ferguson, M. W. and Fallon, J. F. 2006. The development of archosaurian first-generation teeth in a chicken mutant. *Curr. Biol.*, **16**, 371–7.

Haurani, F. I., Repplinger, E. and Tocantins, L. M. 1960. Attempts at tranplantation of human bone marrow in patients with acute leukemia and other marrow depletion disorders. *Am. J. Med.*, **28**, 794–806.

Heile, A. and Brinker, T. 2011. Clinical translation of stem cell therapy in traumatic brain injury: the potential of encapsulated mesenchymal cell biodelivery of glucagon-like peptide-1. *Dialogues Clin. Neurosci.*, **13**, 279–86.

Heyeraas, K. J., Sveen, O. B. and Mjor, I. A. 2001. Pulp–dentin biology in restorative dentistry. Part 3: pulpal inflammation and its sequelae. *Quintessence Int.*, **32**, 611–25.

Hirata, T. M., Ishkitiev, N., Yaegaki, K. *et al.* 2010. Expression of multiple stem cell markers in dental pulp cells cultured in serum-free media. *J. Endod.*, **36**, 1139–44.

Honda, M. J., Fong, H., Iwatsuki, S., Sumita, Y. and Sarikaya, M. 2008. Tooth-forming potential in embryonic and postnatal tooth bud cells. *Med. Molec. Morphol.*, **41**, 183–92.

Honda, M. J., Tsuchiya, S., Sumita, Y., Sagara, H. and Ueda, M. 2007. The sequential seeding of epithelial and mesenchymal cells for tissue-engineered tooth regeneration. *Biomaterials*, **28**, 680–9.

Hu, B., Nadiri, A., Kuchler-Bopp, S. *et al.* 2006a. Tissue engineering of tooth crown, root, and periodontium. *Tissue Eng.*, **12**, 2069–75.

Hu, B., Unda, F., Bopp-Kuchler, S. *et al.* 2006b. Bone marrow cells can give rise to ameloblast-like cells. *J. Dent. Res.*, **85**, 416–21.

Huang, G. T., Gronthos, S. and Shi, S. 2009. Mesenchymal stem cells derived from dental tissues vs. those from other sources: their biology and role in regenerative medicine. *J. Dent. Res.*, **88**, 792–806.

Huang, G. T., Yamaza, T., Shea, L. D. *et al.* 2010. Stem/progenitor cell-mediated de novo regeneration of dental pulp with newly deposited continuous layer of dentin in an in vivo model. *Tissue Eng. Part A*, **16**, 605–15.

Huysseune, A. 2006. Formation of a successional dental lamina in the zebrafish (*Danio rerio*): support for a local control of replacement tooth initiation. *Int. J. Dev. Biol.*, **50**, 637–43.

Huysseune, A. and Sire, J. Y. 2004. The role of epithelial remodelling in tooth eruption in larval zebrafish. *Cell Tissue Res.*, **315**, 85–95.

Huysseune, A., Van Der Heyden, C. and Sire, J. Y. 1998. Early development of the zebrafish (*Danio rerio*) pharyngeal dentition (Teleostei, Cyprinidae). *Anat. Embryol. (Berlin)*, **198**, 289–305.

Hwang, D. H., Jeong, S. R. and Kim, B. G. 2011. Gene transfer mediated by stem cell grafts to treat CNS injury. *Expert Opin. Biol. Ther.*, **11**, 1599–610.

Ikeda, E., Morita, R., Nakao, K. *et al.* 2009. Fully functional bioengineered tooth replacement as an organ replacement therapy. *Proc. Nat. Acad. Sci. USA*, **106**, 13475–80.

Inanc, B., Elcin, A. E. and Elcin, Y. M. 2009. In vitro differentiation and attachment of human embryonic stem cells on periodontal tooth root surfaces. *Tissue Eng. Part A*, **15**, 3427–35.

Inoue, T., Osada, H., Shiigai, T., Fujiseki, M. and Shimono, M. 1993. An experimental study of osteogenesis by autografted dental pulp, periodontal ligament, and bone marrow in vivo. *Bull Tokyo Dent. Coll.*, **34**, 183–90.

Jernvall, J. and Jung, H. S. 2000. Genotype, phenotype, and developmental biology of molar tooth characters. *Am. J. Phys. Anthropol., Suppl.*, **31**, 171–90.

Just, U. and Cross, M. 2008. Stem cells, tissue regeneration and repair. *Cells Tissues Organs*, **188**, 5.

Karaoz, E., Dogan, B. N., Aksoy, A. *et al.* 2010. Isolation and in vitro characterisation of dental pulp stem cells from natal teeth. *Histochem. Cell Biol.*, **133**, 95–112.

Karp, J. M. and Leng Teo, G. S. 2009. Mesenchymal stem cell homing: the devil is in the details. *Cell Stem Cell*, **4**, 206–16.

Kawano, S., Saito, M., Handa, K. *et al.* 2004. Characterization of dental epithelial progenitor cells derived from cervical-loop epithelium in a rat lower incisor. *J. Dent Res.*, **83**, 129–33.

Khaled, E. G., Saleh, M., Hindocha, S., Griffin, M. and Khan, W. S. 2011. Tissue engineering for bone production – stem cells, gene therapy and scaffolds. *Open Orthop. J.*, **5**(Suppl. 2), 289–95.

Khosla, S., Westendorf, J. J. and Modder, U. I. 2010. Insights from normal bone remodeling and stem cell-based therapies for bone repair. *Stem Cells*, **28**, 2124–8.

Kim, J. Y., Xin, X., Moioli, E. K. *et al.* 2010a. Regeneration of dental-pulp-like tissue by chemotaxis-induced cell homing. *Tissue Eng. Part A*, **16**, 3023–31.

Kim, K., Lee, C. H., Kim, B. K. and Mao, J. J. 2010b. Anatomically shaped tooth and periodontal regeneration by cell homing. *J. Dent Res.*, **89**, 842–7.

Kronfeld, R. J. 1935. Condition of the bone tissue of the alveolar process below the periodontal pockets. *J. Periodontol.*, **6**, 22–9.

Langer, R. and Vacanti, J. P. 1993. Tissue engineering. *Science*, **260**, 920–6.

Laughlin, M. J., Barker, J., Bambach, B. *et al.* 2001. Hematopoietic engraftment and survival in adult recipients of umbilical-cord blood from unrelated donors. *N. Engl. J. Med.*, **344**, 1815–22.

Lee, J. S., Hong, J. M., Moon, G. J. *et al.* 2010. A long-term follow-up study of intravenous autologous mesenchymal stem cell transplantation in patients with ischemic stroke. *Stem Cells*, **28**, 1099–106.

Linden, F. P. G. M. V. D. and Duterloo, H. S. 1976. *Development of the Human Dentition: An Atlas*, Hagerstown, MD: Harper and Row.

Matoba, S., Tatsumi, T., Murohara, T. *et al.* 2008. Long-term clinical outcome after intramuscular implantation of bone marrow mononuclear cells (Therapeutic Angiogenesis by Cell Transplantation [TACT] trial) in patients with chronic limb ischemia. *Am. Heart J.*, **156**, 1010–18.

Melfi, R. C. and Permar, D. 1988. *Permar's Oral Embryology and Microscopic Anatomy: A Textbook for Students in Dental Hygiene*. Philadelphia, PA: Lea and Febiger.

Mitsiadis, T. and Luder, H. 2011. Genetic basis for tooth malformations: from mice to men and back again. *Clin Genet.*, **80**(4), 319–29.

Miura, M., Gronthos, S., Zhao, M. 2003. SHED: stem cells from human exfoliated deciduous teeth. *Proc. Nat. Acad. Sci. USA*, **100**, 5807–12.

Mjör, I. A. and Ferrari, M. 2002. Pulp-dentin biology in restorative dentistry. Part 6: reactions to restorative materials, tooth-restoration interfaces, and adhesive techniques. *Quintessence Int.*, **33**, 35–63.

Mooney, D. J., Powell, C., Piana, J. and Rutherford, B. 1996. Engineering dental pulp-like tissue in vitro. *Biotechnol. Prog.*, **12**, 865–8.

Morsczeck, C., Moehl, C., Gotz, W. *et al.* 2005. In vitro differentiation of human dental follicle cells with dexamethasone and insulin. *Cell Biol. Int.*, **29**, 567–75.

Mulligan, T. W. and Niemiec, B. A. 2001. Endodontic treatment of vital pulp tissue. *Clin. Tech. Small Anim. Pract.*, **16**, 159–67.

Nakao, K., Morita, R., Saji, Y. 2007. The development of a bioengineered organ germ method. *Nature Methods*, **4**, 227–30.

Nanci, A. 2007. *Ten Cate's Oral Histology: Development, Structure, and Function*. St. Louis, MO: Mosby, Inc.

Ning, F., Guo, Y., Tang, J. *et al.* 2010. Differentiation of mouse embryonic stem cells into dental epithelial-like cells induced by ameloblasts serum-free conditioned medium. *Biochem. Biophys. Res. Commun.*, **394**, 342–7.

Nör, J. E., Peters, M. C., Christensen, J. B. *et al.* 2001. Engineering and characterization of functional human microvessels in immunodeficient mice, *Lab. Invest.*, **81**, 453–63.

Nosrat, I. V., Widenfalk, J., Olson, L. and Nosrat, C. A. 2001. Dental pulp cells produce neurotrophic factors, interact with trigeminal neurons in vitro, and rescue motoneurons after spinal cord injury. *Dev. Biol.*, **238**, 120–32.

Nourbakhsh, N., Soleimani, M., Taghipour, Z. *et al.* 2011. Induced in vitro differentiation of neural-like cells from human exfoliated deciduous teeth-derived stem cells. *Int. J. Dev. Biol.*, **55**, 189–95.

Ohazama, A., Modino, S. A., Miletich, I. and Sharpe, P. T. 2004. Stem-cell-based tissue engineering of murine teeth. *J. Dent. Res.*, **83**, 518–22.

Okita, K., Ichisaka, T. and Yamanaka, S. 2007. Generation of germline-competent induced pluripotent stem cells. *Nature*, **448**, 313–17.

Peinemann, F., Grouven, U., Kroger, N. *et al.* 2009. Unrelated donor stem cell transplantation in acquired severe aplastic anemia: a systematic review. *Haematologica*, **94**, 1732–42.

Peterkova, R., Peterka, M., Viriot, L. and Lesot, H. 2002. Development of the vestigial tooth primordia as part of mouse odontogenesis. *Connect. Tissue Res.*, **43**, 120–8.

Prusa, A. R. and Hengstschlager, M. 2002. Amniotic fluid cells and human stem cell research: a new connection. *Med. Sci. Monit.*, **8**, RA253–7.

Quinones, C. R., Casellas, J. C. and Caffesse, R. G. 1996. Guided periodontal tissue regeneration (GPTR): an update. *Pract. Periodontics Aesthet. Dent.*, **8**, 169–80; quiz 182.

Rappeport, J. M., O'Reilly, R. J., Kapoor, N. and Parkman, R. 2010. Hematopoietic stem cell transplantation for severe combined immune deficiency or what the children have taught us. *Immunol. Allergy Clin. North Am.*, **30**, 17–30.

Rinaldi, J. C. and Arana-Chavez, V. E. 2010. Ultrastructure of the interface between periodontal tissues and titanium mini-implants. *Angle Orthod.*, **80**, 459–65.

Roberts-Clark, D. J. and Smith, A. J. 2000. Angiogenic growth factors in human dentine matrix. *Arch. Oral Biol.*, **45**, 1013–16.

Schwarz, S. C. and Schwarz, J. 2010. Translation of stem cell therapy for neurological diseases. *Transl. Res.*, **156**, 155–60.

Selden, H. S. 2002. Apexification: an interesting case. *J. Endod.*, **28**, 44–5.

Sessarego, N., Parodi, A., Podesta, M. *et al.* 2008. Multipotent mesenchymal stromal cells from amniotic fluid: solid perspectives for clinical application. *Haematologica*, **93**, 339–46.

Shah, N., Logani, A., Bhaskar, U. and Aggarwal, V. 2008. Efficacy of revascularization to induce apexification/apexogenesis in infected, nonvital, immature teeth: a pilot clinical study. *J. Endod.*, **34**, 919–25; discussion 1157.

Shalabi, M. M., Wolke, J. G., Cuijpers, V. M. and Jansen, J. A. 2007. Evaluation of bone response to titanium-coated polymethyl methacrylate resin (PMMA) implants by X-ray tomography. *J. Mater. Sci. Mater. Med.*, **18**, 2033–9.

Shi, S. and Gronthos, S. 2003. Perivascular niche of postnatal mesenchymal stem cells in human bone marrow and dental pulp. *J. Bone. Miner. Res.*, **18**, 696–704.

Sloan, A. J. and Smith, A. J. 1999. Stimulation of the dentine-pulp complex of rat incisor teeth by transforming growth factor-β isoforms 1-3 in vitro. *Arch. Oral Biol.*, **44**, 149–56.

Song, Y., Yan, M., Muneoka, K. and Chen, Y. 2008. Mouse embryonic diastema region is an ideal site for the development of ectopically transplanted tooth germ. *Dev. Dyn.*, **237**, 411–16.

Sonoyama, W., Liu, Y., Fang, D. *et al.* 2006. Mesenchymal stem cell-mediated functional tooth regeneration in swine. *PLoS One*, **1**, e79.

Stappenbeck, T. S. and Miyoshi, H. 2009. The role of stromal stem cells in tissue regeneration and wound repair. *Science*, **324**, 1666–9.

Strauer, B. E. and Steinhoff, G. 2011. 10 years of intracoronary and intramyocardial bone marrow stem cell therapy of the heart: from the methodological origin to clinical practice. *J. Am. Coll. Cardiol.*, **58**, 1095–104.

Takahashi, K., Okita, K., Nakagawa, M. and Yamanaka, S. 2007. Induction of pluripotent stem cells from fibroblast cultures. *Nature Protoc.*, **2**, 3081–9.

Takahashi, K. and Yamanaka, S. 2006. Induction of pluripotent stem cells from mouse embryonic and adult fibroblast cultures by defined factors. *Cell*, **126**, 663–76.

Takei, K., Inoue, T., Shimono, M. and Yamamura, T. 1988. An experimental study of dentinogenesis in autografted dental pulp in rats. *Bull. Tokyo Dent. Coll.*, **29**, 9–19.

Tamaoki, N., Takahashi, K., Tanaka, T. *et al.* 2010. Dental pulp cells for induced pluripotent stem cell banking. *J. Dent. Res.*, **89**, 773–8.

Tarle, S. A., Shi, S. and Kaigler, D. 2011. Development of a serum-free system to expand dental-derived stem cells: PDLSCs and SHEDs. *J. Cell. Physiol.*, **226**, 66–73.

Ten Cate, A. R. 1998. *Oral Histology: Development, Structure, and Function*, St. Louis, MO: Mosby.

Thesleff, I. 2003. Epithelial–mesenchymal signalling regulating tooth morphogenesis. *J. Cell Sci.*, **116**, 1647–8.

Thesleff, I., Keranen, S. and Jernvall, J. 2001. Enamel knots as signaling centers linking tooth morphogenesis and odontoblast differentiation. *Adv. Dent. Res.*, **15**, 14–18.

Thesleff, I. and Nieminen, P. 1996. Tooth morphogenesis and cell differentiation. *Curr. Opin. Cell. Biol.*, **8**, 844–50.

Thomson, J. A., Itskovitz-Eldor, J., Shapiro, S. S. *et al.* 1998. Embryonic stem cell lines derived from human blastocysts. *Science*, **282**, 1145–7.

Tran-Hung, L., Laurent, P., Camps, J. and About, I. 2008. Quantification of angiogenic growth factors released by human dental cells after injury. *Arch. Oral Biol.*, **53**, 9–13.

Tran-Hung, L., Mathieu, S. and About, I. 2006. Role of human pulp fibroblasts in angiogenesis. *J. Dent. Res.*, **85**, 819–23.

Trope, M. 2010. Treatment of the immature tooth with a non-vital pulp and apical periodontitis. *Dent. Clin. North Am.*, **54**, 313–24.

Trubiani, O., Orsini, G., Zini, N. *et al.* 2008. Regenerative potential of human periodontal ligament derived stem cells on three-dimensional biomaterials: a morphological report. *J. Biomed. Mater. Res. A.*, **87**, 986–93.

Vaahtokari, A., Aberg, T. and Thesleff, I. 1996. Apoptosis in the developing tooth: association with an embryonic signaling center and suppression by EGF and FGF-4. *Development*, **122**, 121–9.

Van Besien, K. 2009. Allogeneic stem cell transplantation in follicular lymphoma: recent progress and controversy. *Hematol. Am. Soc. Hematol. Educ. Program*, 610–18.

Van der Heyden, C. and Huysseune, A. 2000. Dynamics of tooth formation and replacement in the zebrafish (*Danio rerio*) (Teleostei, Cyprinidae). *Dev. Dyn.*, **219**, 486–96.

Van der Heyden, C., Wautier, K. and Huysseune, A. 2001. Tooth succession in the zebrafish (*Danio rerio*). *Arch. Oral Biol.*, **46**, 1051–8.

Wang, L., Shen, H., Zheng, W. *et al.* 2011. Characterization of stem cells from alveolar periodontal ligament. *Tissue Eng. Part A*, **17**, 1015–26.

West, J. 2006. Endodontic update 2006. *J. Esthet. Restor. Dent.*, **18**, 280–300.

Yamagishi, K., Onuma, K., Suzuki, T. *et al.* 2005. Materials chemistry: a synthetic enamel for rapid tooth repair. *Nature,* **433**, 819.

Yamamoto, H., Kim, E. J., Cho, S. W. and Jung, H. S. 2003. Analysis of tooth formation by reaggregated dental mesenchyme from mouse embryo. *J. Electron Microsc. (Tokyo),* **52**, 559–66.

Yan, X., Qin, H., Qu, C. *et al.* 2010. iPS cells reprogrammed from human mesenchymal-like stem/progenitor cells of dental tissue origin. *Stem Cells Dev.,* **19**, 469–80.

Yao, S., Pan, F., Prpic, V. and Wise, G. E. 2008. Differentiation of stem cells in the dental follicle. *J. Dent. Res.,* **87**, 767–71.

Young, C. S., Terada, S., Vacanti, J. P. *et al.* 2002. Tissue engineering of complex tooth structures on biodegradable polymer scaffolds. *J. Dent. Res.,* **81**, 695–700.

Yu, J., Vodyanik, M. A., Smuga-Otto, K. *et al.* 2007. Induced pluripotent stem cell lines derived from human somatic cells. *Science,* **318**, 1917–20.

Zander, H. A. 1939. Reaction of the pulp to calcium hydroxide. *J. Dent. Res.* **18**, 373–437.

Zhang, W., Abukawa, H., Troulis, M. J. *et al.* 2009. Tissue engineered hybrid tooth-bone constructs. *Methods,* **47**, 122–8.

Zhang, W., Ahluwalia, I. P. and Yelick, P. C. 2010. Three dimensional dental epithelial-mesenchymal constructs of predetermined size and shape for tooth regeneration. *Biomaterials,* **31**, 7995–8003.

Zhang, W., Walboomers, X. F., Shi, S., Fan, M. and Jansen, J. A. 2006a. Multilineage differentiation potential of stem cells derived from human dental pulp after cryopreservation. *Tissue Eng.,* **12**, 2813–23.

Zhang, W., Walboomers, X. F., Van Kuppevelt, T. H. *et al.* 2006b. The performance of human dental pulp stem cells on different three-dimensional scaffold materials. *Biomaterials,* **27**, 5658–68.

Zhao, L., Weir, M. D. and Xu, H. H. 2010. An injectable calcium phosphate-alginate hydrogel-umbilical cord mesenchymal stem cell paste for bone tissue engineering. *Biomaterials,* **31**, 6502–10.

Zhao, S., Sloan, A. J., Murray, P. E., Lumley, P. J. and Smith, A. J. 2000. Ultrastructural localisation of TGF-β exposure in dentine by chemical treatment. *Histochem. J.,* **32**, 489–94.

31

Dentin–pulp tissue engineering and regeneration

Jing Wang, Xiaobing Jin and Peter X. Ma

31.1 Introduction

The dentin–pulp complex is the principal inner component of the tooth beneath the superficial enamel layer in the tooth crown, and comprises the entire tooth root outlined with a thin cementum layer. The highly mineralized dentin confers structural integrity and insulative properties to the tooth and surrounds the pulp chamber and canals, which confer vitality to the tooth and whose neurovascular supplies exit through constricted foramina at the root apices. The pulp also has reparative mechanisms, activated by insults to the overlying dentin by noxious stimuli such as attrition, trauma, and caries. Together, the dentin–pulp complex plays a crucial role in tooth health.

The aforementioned noxious stimuli may lead to dentinal damage, as well as pulpal inflammation or necrosis. Such external damage to the dentin renders the pulp vulnerable to external invasion if the extent of the insult extends throughout the thickness of the dentin layer in question. Given the pulp's solely apical blood supply and limited self-healing capacity, recovery from insult to pulp tissue is difficult, and the resulting inflammation is often irreversible. Currently, complete pulpal resection (root canal therapy) is the default treatment for necrosed or irreversibly inflamed pulp of a tooth that is otherwise restorable. Such teeth are restored first by obturating the pulp canals with an inert material, usually Gutta-Percha; then, direct restorative materials (such as silver amalgam or resin-based composites) and/or full-coverage crowns (metal/porcelain/combination) are used to restore the remainder of the tooth. Although these traditional restorative materials and methods have proven to be adequately effective in conserving teeth, they may render the remaining natural tooth structure mechanically compromised [1], and are incapable of repairing the tissue exposed to harmful stimuli [1, 2].

Recent progress in tissue engineering technology has led to a growing interest in the development of a regenerative dentin–pulp structure, which could provide natural replacement or repair of damaged tooth tissues, and has the potential of creating a more seamless interface between existing tooth structure and newly generated tissue, in contrast to the non-ideal biomechanical properties of current restorative methods [2]. The three key ingredients for successful dentin–pulp tissue engineering are the seeded cells, the scaffold, and the morphogens [3–5]. This chapter will begin by briefly introducing the dentin–pulp complex and the basic principles of dentin–pulp tissue engineering. We will then focus on the current applications of stem cells, growth/differentiation factors, and scaffolds involved in dentin–pulp regeneration.

31.2 The dentin–pulp complex

Despite the stark differences between tissue properties of dentin, which is highly mineralized hard tissue, and pulp, which is soft connective tissue, they both originate from the mesenchymally derived dental papilla. In other words, dentin and pulp are closely related in embryonic development and histogenesis. The close link between the inner dental pulp and the surrounding dentin makes dentin and pulp a functional unit, i.e. the "dentin-pulp complex" [6].

Dentin, which possesses a unique tubular structure, comprises the bulk of the tooth. By weight, dentin is roughly 70% hydroxyapatite, 20% organic material, and 10% water [7]. Type I collagen accounts for 80%–90% of the organic non-mineralized component of dentin's extracellular matrix (ECM) and is closely associated with dentin formation [8]. Dentin consists of dentinal tubules, which contain fluid and cellular structures. The three types of dentin, classified in terms of the timing or stimulus of deposition, are primary, secondary, and tertiary. Primary dentin is the outermost layer of dentin and is connected with the enamel, which is deposited during tooth development. Secondary dentin is deposited on the primary dentin after the root of the tooth has completely formed. Tertiary dentin is formed in response to stimuli, such as attrition, trauma, or caries. In contrast to dentin, the pulp, comprising the center of the tooth with soft connective tissue, consists of a variety of cells, nerves, blood vessels, and ECM. A layer of odontoblast cells lines the outer part of the pulp cavity, with the principal function of producing and depositing dentin throughout life. As the production of dentin progresses, each odontoblastic process becomes embedded in a single dentinal tubule. The close relationship between dentin and the odontoblasts renders dentin a vital tissue. Dentin has a degree of permeability, which can increase the sensation of pain and the rate of tooth decay.

The pulp is known to have limited self-reparative abilities. It possesses a distinctive anatomical structure, which is embraced with unyielding dentin, and is limited, with a source of blood supply through the tooth apex or apices. Once infected or exposed to the external environment, recovery is difficult, owing to the lack of a collateral blood supply. However, if the pulp is not infected or irreversibly inflamed, the cells of the odontoblast layer are capable of depositing reactionary dentin peripheral to the pulp with age or in response to noxious stimuli such as attrition, trauma, and caries [9, 10]. Additionally, pulpal progenitor cells (dental pulp stem cells) are able to differentiate into dentin-depositing odontoblast-like cells if the stimuli are potent enough to kill native odontoblasts [11].

31.3 Principles of dentin-pulp regeneration

Tissue engineering technology provides an approach to achieve dentin-pulp regeneration to potentially replace or repair the impaired dentin-pulp tissues. A tooth is a small but complex organ, which is derived from both ectoderm and mesoderm. Tooth tissue engineering is ultimately aimed at the reconstruction of the entire tooth. In a recent study, an entire tooth with proper anatomical configuration was regenerated and successfully integrated into native alveolar bone with a periodontal ligament in a rat model [12]. Although the approach of engineering an entire tooth shows promise in restoring missing teeth and replacing artificial dental implants [13–15], it is still in a preliminary stage and there are significant technical difficulties, obstacles, and limitations to overcome before it can be translated into a feasible therapeutic modality. Whereas the replacement of whole tooth remains a challenge, the partial regeneration of tooth structure, such as dentin-pulp tissue, might be a relatively more feasible goal in preserving the tooth in question. To regenerate new dentin-pulp tissue, it is necessary to understand the molecular mechanisms of tooth development and to develop advanced technologies of tissue engineering. Similarly to the construction of other tissues, the triad of seeding cells, morphogens including growth and differentiation factors, and scaffolds is needed for dental pulp tissue engineering [3–5]. The isolation of dental stem cells from a variety of oral tissues provides needed stem cell sources for dentin-pulp tissue regeneration [16–19]. In addition, to fulfill the diverse needs in tissue engineering, various materials have been exploited as scaffolds for tissue regeneration, including for dentin-pulp tissue regeneration. Moreover, scaffolds are transitioning from passive cell delivery systems to biomolecule-containing bioactive matrices, providing the microenvironment for regenerative cells, supporting cell attachment, proliferation, differentiation, and genesis of new tissue [20, 21]. With the application of dental stem cells, novel scaffolding materials, and growth/differentiation factors, the regeneration of the dental-pulp tissue complex is well under way.

31.4 Dental-pulp-related stem cells

It was reported a decade ago by Shi's group that post-natal stem cells could be isolated from an easily accessible tissue – the pulp of extracted wisdom teeth [16]. This was the first line of dental stem cells, which are termed dental pulp stem cells (DPSCs) due to their origin from adult dental pulp. DPSCs were demonstrated to possess features of mesenchymal stem cells (MSCs), such as self-renewal and multilineage differentiation capacity. They also exhibited the ability to form dentin–pulp complex-like structures in immunocompromised mice with hydroxyapatite/tricalcium phosphate powder [16, 22]. This research shed new light on the possibility of regenerating dentin–pulp tissue for clinical applications.

DPSCs were found to home in the perivascular regions by using STRO-1 as the marker [23]. Further research demonstrated that subpopulations of DPSCs expressing embryonic neural-crest cell markers appear to exist and possess multipotent differentiation capacity [24]. Since then, several other types of stem cells for dentin–pulp regeneration have been isolated from dental tissues. These dental stem cells include those from human exfoliated deciduous teeth (SHED) [17], apical papilla (SCAP) [18], and dental follicle progenitor cells [19]. Like DPSCs, all these dental stem cells have MSC-like characteristics, expressing STRO-1 and displaying the potential to differentiate into distinct cell lineages: odontoblasts, osteoblasts, adipocytes, and neural cells [16–19]. However, differences between the dental stem cells and MSCs have been reported. Dental stem cells have been reported to seem more inclined toward odontogenic rather than osteogenic differentiation [16]. A study demonstrated that, compared with MSCs, both DPSCs and SHED showed 30%–50% higher proliferation rates and greater population doublings [17]. Distinct gene expression patterns of DPSCs compared with those of MSCs have been revealed by microarray analysis [25].

Meanwhile, further research has been focussing on comparing the characteristics as well as the regeneration potentials of different dental stem cells. Both SHED and DPSCs were observed to express osteogenic and odontogenic markers and form mineralized nodules when cultured in inductive medium [16, 17]. They were also observed to exhibit chondrogenic, adipogenic, and neurogenic potential [16, 17]. SCAP from apical papilla are responsible for the formation of root dentin. It has been demonstrated that SCAP, as stem cells from a developing tissue, are relatively more robust than DPSCs in terms of population-doubling capacity, proliferation rate, telomerase activity, and cell migration ability. Like DPSCs, they showed a high capacity for dentin regeneration and formed dentin–pulp complex tissue when transplanted into immunocompromised mice [18]. A recent, highly promising approach for tissue regeneration is to reprogram somatic cells into induced pluripotent stem cells. Dental pulp cells have been shown to be an ideal source to generate induced pluripotent stem cells. These induced pluripotent stem cells acquired ESC-like morphology, expressed pluripotent markers, possessed stable, normal karyotypes, and demonstrated the ability to differentiate in vitro and in vivo [26, 27].

31.5 Growth/differentiation factors for dentin–pulp regeneration

Another key element for the success of dentin–pulp regeneration is the induction by morphogenic factors. Such morphogens are inductive signals that induce and facilitate odontoblast differentiation and reparative dentin formation. Most of the growth factors are secreted by odontoblasts and deposited within the dentin matrix [28, 29], where they remain in an active condition. Among these growth factors, the TGF-β family plays an important part in cellular signaling, odontoblast differentiation, and dentin tissue regeneration [28]. It was reported that millipore filters containing TGF-β_1 implanted into pulp cavity could induce odontoblast differentiation and reparative dentin formation surrounding the implants [30]. TGF-β_1 combined with inactive total EDTA-soluble fraction of dentin proteins stimulated dental papillae cells to differentiate to odontoblasts [31]. The similar effects of TGF-β_1 and TGF-β_3 have also been demonstrated in cultured tooth slices [32]. Bone morphogenetic proteins (BMPs) are also very important in tooth development and regeneration. BMPs were originally isolated from demineralized bone matrix. It is reported that recombinant human BMP-2 stimulated the differentiation of DPSCs into odontoblast-like cells both in monolayer cultures [33, 34] and in three-dimensional (3D) pellet cultures [35]. BMP-7 has also been examined as a pulp-capping agent in monkeys, miniature swine, and ferrets [36–38]. Recombinant BMP-2 and BMP-4 induce formation of reparative dentin in vivo [39, 40]. Another growth factor, recombinant human insulin-like growth factor-1 (IGF-1), has been found to induce dentin bridging and tubular dentin formation [41]. Application of IGF-1 to mechanically exposed pulp appeared to reduce inflammation, preserve pulp vitality, and promote dentin–pulp regeneration in the rabbit [42].

Besides growth factors, matrix proteins and other biomolecules have displayed potential to promote pulp progenitor/dental stem cell differentiation and dentin–pulp regeneration. Dentin matrix protein-1 (Dmp-1), which contains a complex mixture of bioactive molecules involved in the mineralization process, induced differentiation of pulp progenitor cells into odontoblast-like cells, collagen production, formation of calcified deposits, and reparative dentin formation in vivo [43, 44]. Application of mineral trioxide aggregate (a material used to fill root canals), bone sialoprotein, or amelogenin gene splice products for dentin–pulp regeneration resulted in ectopic formation of bone-like material [45–47]. Dexamethasone (DXM), a synthetic glucocorticoid, reduced cell proliferation and induced expression of alkaline phosphatase and dentin sialophosphoprotein in primary human pulp cells [48, 49]. The addition of β-glycerophosphate to the culture medium of human tooth explants induced cell morphology change, collagen synthesis, and mineral formation [50]. Further research demonstrated that the combination of multiple inductive factors could better promote the differentiation of dental stem cells and regeneration of dentin–pulp tissue. Combinations of DXM with inorganic phosphates have been widely applied as a mineralization inducer for dentin formation [51–53]. The combination of BMP-7 and DXM induced the odontogenic differentiation more effectively than DXM alone and provided excellent environment for DPSCs to regenerate dentin [54]. A combination of stromal-derived factor-1 (SDF-1) and BMP-7, delivered from an orthotopically implanted scaffold for the regeneration of an entire rat tooth, enhanced angiogenesis and endogenous cell recruitment compared with growth factor-free control scaffolds [12].

Although a variety of inductive factors have adequately induced odontoblast differentiation in vitro, these directly applied factors have limitations in terms of sustaining physiological levels required for tissue regeneration in vivo. Moreover, supraphysiological concentrations of inductive factors might give rise to apoptosis of the cells [55]. Other methods such as gene therapy and controlled-release technology have been utilized to overcome these disadvantages. Some groups have investigated the use of gene therapy in dentin–pulp regeneration. Transfer of BMP-7 ex vivo transduced autologous dermal fibroblasts in a collagen hydrogel, inducing dentin–pulp tissue formation in the exposed pulp with reversible pulpitis [36]. The Gdf11 gene transfer, utilizing ultrasound-generated microbubbles, also induced differentiation of dental pulp cells into odontoblasts in vitro and reparative dentin formation in vivo [56]. Gdf11-electrotransfected pulp stem cells stimulated initially formation of osteodentin and subsequently tubular dentin formation in the exposed pulp [57]. In another study, STRO-1-selected rat dental pulp-derived stem cells, when transduced with human BMP-2 gene using adenoviral vector, showed the ability to differentiate into the odontoblast phenotype and to produce a calcified extracellular matrix, even without the addition of odontogenic supplements to the medium [58]. Moreover, plasmid DNA-loaded calcium phosphate nanoparticles have been reported to work as a non-viral vector for BMP-2 gene transfection to enhance odontogenic differentiation [59]. However, the main challenge for gene therapy will be the requirement to demonstrate that gene therapy can provide cost-effective and safe long-term treatments for conditions that would otherwise lead to significant pulp necrosis. Another promising alternative might be controlled release using microspheres. A rat subcutaneous implantation model has been successfully used for bone regeneration with

BMP-7-loaded nanospheres incorporated into a nanofibrous PLLA scaffold. The results indicated that incorporation of BMP-7 into nanospheres, which were then immobilized onto a scaffold, preserved the biological activity of BMP-7 and could prolong the duration of its action to induce ectopic bone formation [60].

31.6 Scaffolds for dentin–pulp tissue engineering

Scaffolds play a vital role in tissue engineering. They serve as 3D tissue templates and are intended to provide synthetic ECM microenvironments for cell attachment, proliferation, differentiation, and new tissue genesis [20]. Ideally, they should be fabricated to form any desired shape and carry required growth factors to guide the process of cell differentiation and tissue formation. In addition, scaffolds should biodegrade at the same rate as the new tissue formation and should be biocompatible and non-toxic. Scaffolds for dentin-pulp applications have been fabricated from a variety of biomaterials. The scaffolds for dentin–pulp regeneration are made from various natural, naturally derived, and synthetic biomaterials.

The main natural scaffolds used in dentin–pulp regeneration are natural polymers (collagen, gelatin, alginate, chitosan, etc.), as well as bioceramic materials (hydroxyapatite, tricalcium phosphate, etc.). Results of previous studies demonstrated that collagen matrix promoted odontogenic differentiation and mineralization, and it has been used widely as a scaffold in tooth tissue engineering [61–63]. In one study, collagen was applied as a scaffold to carry DPSCs combined with DMP-1, and a dental pulp-like tissue was generated after subcutaneous transplantation into immunocompromised mice [64]. In another study, a comparison of different biomaterials (collagen I and III, alginate, and chitosan) demonstrated that collagen I could better promote proliferation and mineralization of dental pulp cells than the other biomaterials [63]. Although collagen is biocompatible and degradable by enzymes, there are concerns over potential pathogen transmission, immune reactions, and the poor mechanical properties of collagen. Moreover, research showed that dental pulp cells seeded into collagen gel caused dramatic contraction, and the level of contraction is proportional to the density of cells seeded [65]. Hydroxyapatite (HA), which is the main component of hard tissues, has good biocompatibility and osteoconductivity, and therefore has been widely studied as a naturally derived scaffold in dental tissue engineering [16, 17, 22, 53, 66, 67]. It was reported that, when DPSCs and SHED were mixed with HA/tricalcium phosphate (HA/TCP), the formation of dentin, bone, and dentin–pulp-like complexes was observed [16, 17]. When DPSCs were seeded onto different 3D scaffold materials (i.e. a spongy collagen, a porous ceramic, and a fibrous titanium mesh), the characteristics of the tissues formed in all scaffolds more closely resembled connective tissue than a dentin-like tissue; limited calcification of the ECM was seen only in the ceramic scaffold [67]. However, most of the bioceramics have poor biodegradability and processability into highly porous structures, and they are often brittle.

Compared with natural biomaterials, synthetic polymers have advantages in terms of their stability, controllable degradation rate, and flexible molecular/structural design. These features allow a polymer scaffold to be integrated into biological systems and tailored to specific needs. Moreover, synthetic polymers such as polylactic acid (PLA), polyglycolic acid (PGA), and their copolymer poly(lactic-*co*-glycolic acid) (PLGA) have gained FDA approval; therefore, they have been extensively studied in various tissue engineering applications, including tooth tissue engineering [68–70]. It was reported that, when human dental pulp cells were seeded onto PGA fibers, the cells proliferated and formed tissue similar to native dental pulp [71, 72]. In another study, SHED cells were seeded onto PLLA scaffolds within tooth slices, and then cell–scaffold/tooth-slice constructs were transplanted into immunocompromised mice. It was reported that odontoblast-like cells, vascularized pulp-like tissue, and newly generated tubular dentin grew toward the existing dentin walls of the tooth slices [73]. Similarly, when DPSCs and SCAP were cultured onto PLGA scaffolds in empty root-canal space, and then transplanted into nude mice subcutaneously,

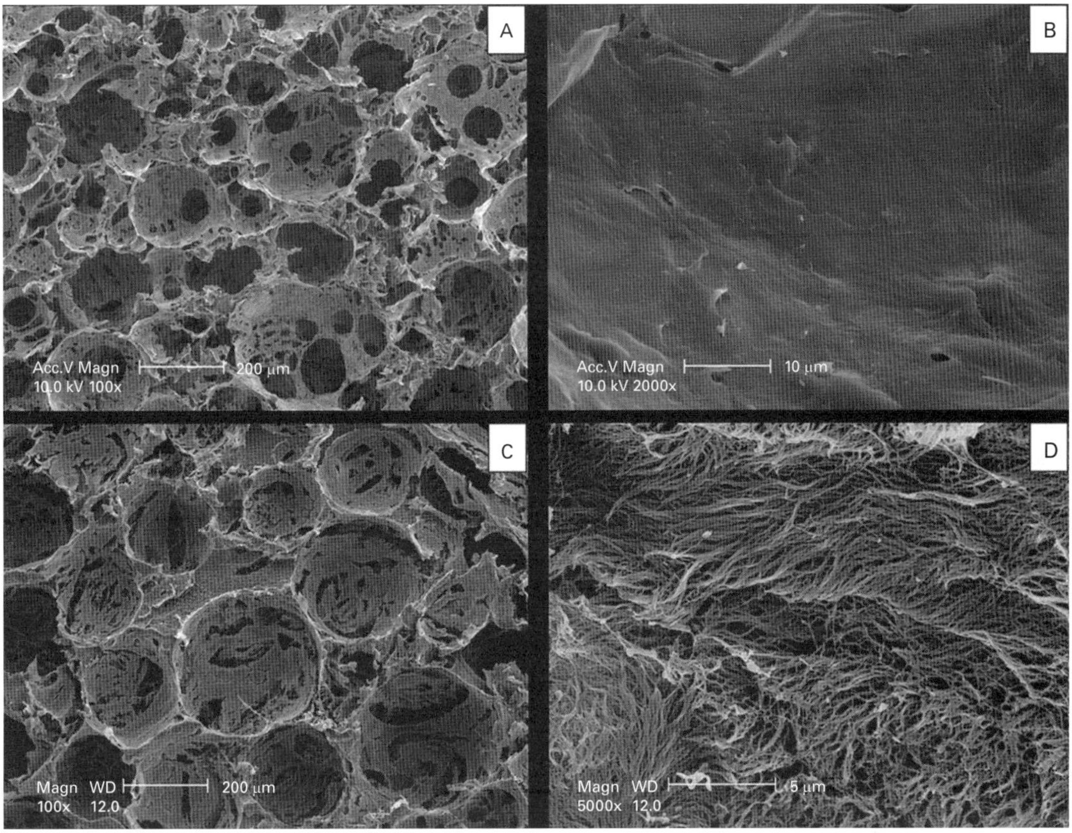

Figure 31.1 SEM images of SW-PLLA and NF-PLLA scaffolds: (A) macroporous structure of SW-PLLA scaffolds at low magnification; (B) solid-walled architecture of SW-PLLA scaffolds at high magnification; (C) macroporous structure of NF-PLLA scaffolds at low magnification; and (D) nanofibrous architecture of NF-PLLA scaffolds at high magnification. (Reprinted from *Biomaterials*, 32, Jing Wang, Haiyun Ma, Xiaobing Jin, Jiang Hu, Xiaohua Liu, Longxi Ni, and Peter X. Ma, The effect of scaffold architecture on odontogenic differentiation of human dental pulp stem cells, 7822–30, Copyright (2011), with permission from Elsevier.)

newly generated vascularized pulp-like tissue filled up the canal space, and a layer of new dentin tissue was deposited onto the root dentin walls [74].

The ECM is a nanofibrous protein network, which is surrounded by cells of different tissues to support their physiological functions [75]. Although various synthetic scaffolds have been applied in tissue engineering, none possesses all the structural features and properties of the natural ECM. It is often beneficial for a synthetic scaffold to mimic the structural features of ECM to enhance cell attachment, proliferation, migration, differentiation, and neo-tissue genesis [20]. To generate a structure similar to ECM, three main techniques are used to fabricate nanofibrous scaffolds in tissue engineering: electrospinning, self-assembly, and phase separation. Electrospinning is commonly used for many synthetic and natural polymers, due to its ease and compatibility with numerous dissolvable polymers. The electrospun nanofibrous polymer scaffolds have been used in dentin–pulp tissue engineering. It has been reported that electrospun nanofibers supported cell adhesion and enhanced odontogenic differentiation of DPSCs [76–78]. However, one of the limitations of electronspinning is that designed 3D pore structures are difficult to achieve in the electrospun scaffolds. Moreover, electrospinning often cannot produce true nanofibers that are on the 100-nm scale with frequently used biodegradable polymers. Besides electrospun nanofibers, peptide-based nanofibers are attractive to many scientists [79, 80]. The natural self-assembly processes can be mimicked to form nanofibrous polymer scaffolds from engineered self-assembling peptides. Molecular self-assembly can often result in the formation of hydrogels containing nanofibers of a much smaller diameter than electrospun fibers. In the dental field, SHED and DPSCs were tested for compatibility with a self-assembling peptide hydrogel, which offers manifold possibilities to modify the matrix and generate a custom-made system [81]. The optimization of a peptide sequence through the incorporation of the cell-adhesion motif RGD (arginine-glycine-aspartic acid) and a matrix metalloproteinase-2-specific enzyme-cleavable site led to increased proliferation rates and the migration of SHED and DPSCs into the matrix [81]. However, self-assembled hydrogels do not allow one to exert control over the internal pore shape, and have poor mechanical strength. They are also susceptible to enzymatic degradation, which can affect the scaffold degradation rate in an uncontrolled manner.

Collagen type I accounts for 80%–90% of the organic substance of non-mineralized dentin ECM and is correlated closely with dentin formation [8]. A phase-separation technique has been developed to fabricate NF-PLLA scaffolds to mimic Col I fiber structure [82–84]. By using this fabrication process, the physical architecture of the scaffolds can be more accurately controlled on several size scales [84, 85], including the scaffold shape on the macroscale, the spherical pore size on the microscale, and the fiber diameter on the nanoscale (50–500 nm) (Figure 31.1). When DPSCs were seeded onto phase-separated nanofibrous PLLA scaffolds, nanofibers promoted attachment and proliferation of human DPSCs in vitro [54, 86] (Figure 31.2). The alkaline phosphatase (ALP) activity and the expression of odontogenic genes of human DPSCs

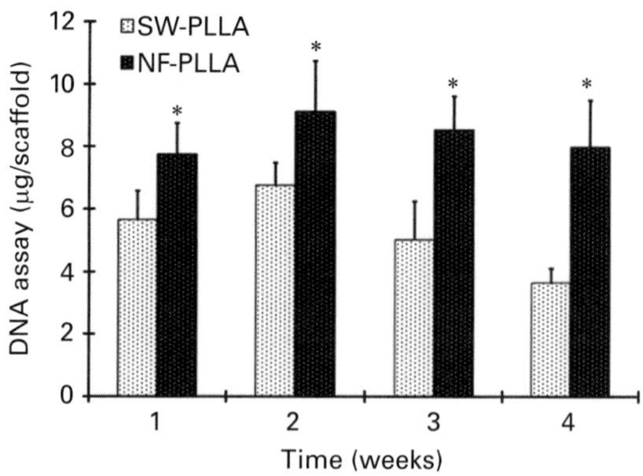

Figure 31.2 The proliferation of human DPSCs cultured on SW-PLLA and NF-PLLA scaffolds. The error bars represent means ± SD ($n = 3$). When the NF-PLLA group and the SW-PLLA group are compared, * indicates $p < 0.05$. (Reprinted from *Biomaterials*, 32, Jing Wang, Haiyun Ma, Xiaobing Jin, Jiang Hu, Xiaohua Liu, Longxi Ni, and Peter X. Ma, The effect of scaffold architecture on odontogenic differentiation of human dental pulp stem cells, 7822–30, Copyright (2011), with permission from Elsevier.)

were increased on nanofibrous PLLA scaffolds compared with those on solid-walled scaffolds [86] (Figure 31.3). Consistently with the results from in-vitro studies, the nanofibrous PLLA scaffolds could better promote collagen matrix deposition, dentin sialoprotein secretion, blood vessel ingrowth, and mineralization in nude mice then could solid-walled scaffolds [86] (Figure 31.4). Several factors might have contributed to the enhanced odontogenic differentiation and mineralization of human DPSCs on the nanofibrous PLLA scaffolds. Previous results demonstrated that nanofibrous PLLA scaffolds adsorbed greater quantities of cell-adhesion proteins (such as fibronectin) than did solid-walled scaffolds [87]. In dentin tissue, fibronectin enhances the differentiation of odontoblasts and dentin formation [88, 89]. A fibronectin-rich matrix may serve as a reservoir of growth factors, which are known to have participated in the differentiation of odontoblasts [90, 91]. These findings suggested that the nanofibrous architecture of PLLA scaffolds exhibited certain characteristics similar to those of natural collagen fibers, thereby facilitating

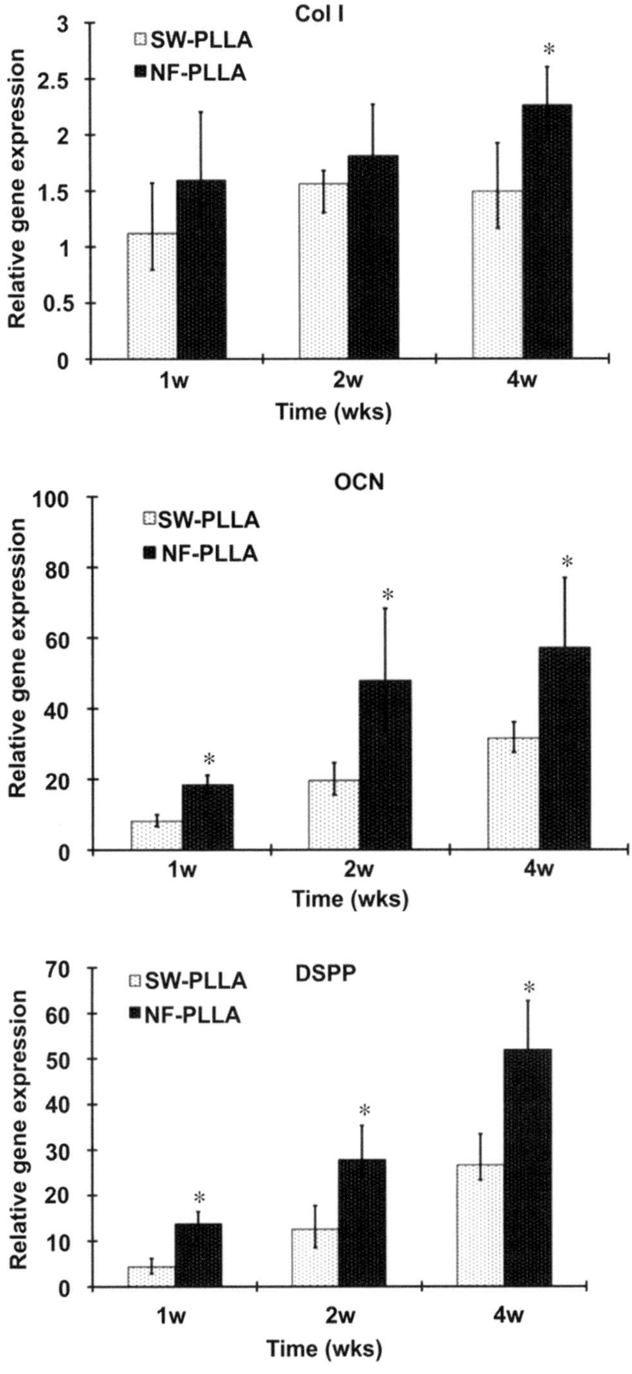

Figure 31.3 Real-time PCR quantification of gene expression of human DPSCs grown on the SW-PLLA and NF-PLLA scaffolds for 1, 2, and 4 weeks. The Col I, OCN, and DSPP genes were up-regulated on NF-PLLA scaffolds in comparison with those on SW-PLLA scaffolds at the time points examined. When the NF-PLLA group and the SW-PLLA group are compared, * indicates $p < 0.05$. (Reprinted from *Biomaterials*, 32, Jing Wang, Haiyun Ma, Xiaobing Jin, Jiang Hu, Xiaohua Liu, Longxi Ni, and Peter X. Ma, The effect of scaffold architecture on odontogenic differentiation of human dental pulp stem cells, 7822–30, Copyright (2011), with permission from Elsevier.)

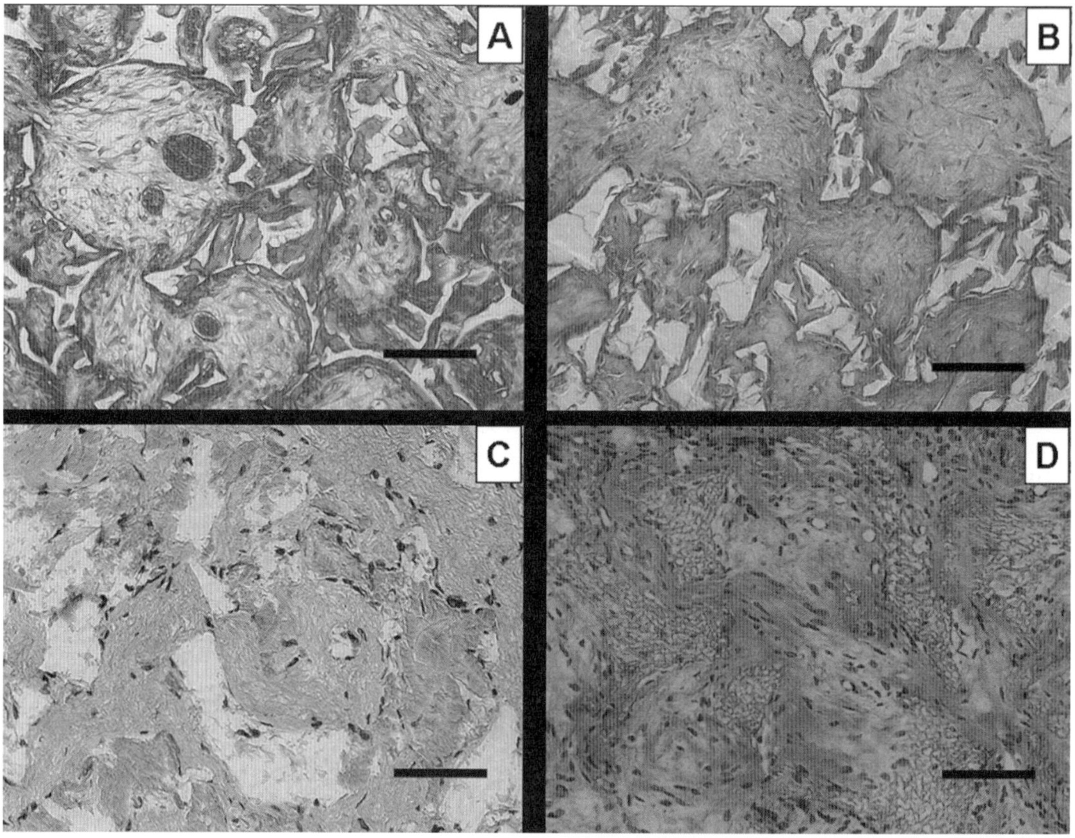

Figure 31.4 Masson's trichrome staining and immunohistochemical staining for DSP of human DPSC–scaffold constructs implanted subcutaneously in nude mice for 8 weeks: (A) on SW-PLLA scaffolds (Masson's trichrome staining); (B) on NF-PLLA scaffolds (Masson's trichrome staining); (C) on SW-PLLA scaffolds (immunohistochemical staining for DSP); and (D) on NF-PLLA scaffolds (immunohistochemical staining for DSP). Scale bars represent 100 mm. (Reprinted from *Biomaterials*, 32, Jing Wang, Haiyun Ma, Xiaobing Jin, Jiang Hu, Xiaohua Liu, Longxi Ni, and Peter X. Ma, The effect of scaffold architecture on odontogenic differentiation of human dental pulp stem cells, 7822–30, Copyright (2011), with permission from Elsevier.)

the odontogenic differentiation and biomineralization of human DPSCs.

31.7 Conclusion

The dentin–pulp complex plays a crucial role in maintaining tooth health. Tissue engineering technology provides a promising approach to achieve dentin-pulp regeneration. The triad of dental stem cells, growth/differentiation factors, and scaffolds is needed for dentin–pulp tissue regeneration. Dental stem cells have been demonstrated to be a suitable cell source for dentin–pulp tissue regeneration, due to their clonogenic ability, rapid proliferation rate, and multiple differentiation potential. Growth/differentiation factors can be used to stimulate dentin–pulp regeneration, and combinations of appropriate factors may have synergistic effects. Scaffolds play important roles in tissue engineering, and have been fabricated for dentin-pulp regeneration with a variety of biomaterials. Technologies to engineer materials mimicking the nanofibrous ECM proteins have been developed and successfully applied to dentin-pulp regeneration. In the future, more investigation of optimal odontogenic factors and integration with novel biomimetic scaffolds may lead to further improved microenvironments for high quality dentin-pulp regeneration.

ACKNOWLEDGEMENTS

The authors would like to acknowledge the financial support from the National Institutes of Health (NIDCR DE015384, DE017689 and DE022327: PXM), DOD (W81XWH-12-2-0008: PXM) and NSF (DMR-1206575: PXM). The authors also thank Mr. Zubad Newaz for editing assistance.

REFERENCES

[1] Dietschi, D., Duc, O., Krejci, I. and Sadan, A. 2007. Biomechanical considerations for the restoration of endodontically treated teeth: a systematic review of the literature - Part 1. Composition and micro- and macrostructure alterations. *Quintessence Int.*, **38**(9), 733–43.

[2] Dietschi, D., Duc, O., Krejci, I. and Sadan A. 2007. Biomechanical considerations for the restoration of endodontically treated teeth: a systematic review of the literature, part II (evaluation of fatigue behavior, interfaces, and in vivo studies). *Quintessence Int.*, **39**(2), 117–29.

[3] Nakashima, M. and Reddi, A. H. 2003. The application of bone morphogenetic proteins to dental tissue engineering. *Nature Biotechnol.*, **21**(9), 1025–32.

[4] Sloan, A. J. and Smith, A. J. 2007. Stem cells and the dental pulp: potential roles in dentine regeneration and repair. *Oral Dis.*, **13**(2), 151–7.

[5] Galler, K. M., D'Souza, R. N., Hartgerink, J. D. and Schmalz, G. 2011. Scaffolds for dental pulp tissue engineering. *Adv. Dent. Res.*, **23**(3), 333–9.

[6] Ten Cate, A. R. 1992. Dentin/pulp complex reactions: a reaction. *Proc. Finn. Dent. Soc.*, **88**(Suppl. 1), 275–8.

[7] Ten Cate, A. R. 1998. *Oral Histology: Development, Structure, and Function*, 5th edn. St. Louis, MO: Mosby, p. 150.

[8] Wiesmann, H. P., Meyer, U., Plate, U. and Hohling, H. J. 2005. Aspects of collagen mineralization in hard tissue formation. *Int. Rev. Cytol.*, **242**, 121–56.

[9] Smith, A. J., Sloan, A. J., Matthews, J. B., Murray, P. E. and Lumley P J. 2000. Reparative processes in dentine and pulp. In Addy, M., Embery, G., Edgar, W. M. and Orchardson, R., editors. *Toothwear and Sensitivity.* London: Martin-Dunitz.

[10] Tziafas, D., Smith, A. J. and Lesot, H. 2000. Designing new treatment strategies in vital pulp therapy. *J. Dentistry*, **28**(2), 77–92.

[11] Cox, C. F., White, K. C., Ramus, D. L., Farmer, J. B. and Snuggs, H. M. 1992. Reparative dentin: factors affecting its deposition. *Quintessence Int.*, **23**(4), 257–70.

[12] Kim, K., Lee, C. H., Kim, B. K. and Mao, J. J. 2010. Anatomically shaped tooth and periodontal regeneration by cell homing. *J. Dental Res.*, **89**(8), 842–7.

[13] Young, C. S., Terada, S., Vacanti, J. P. *et al.* 2002. Tissue engineering of complex tooth structures on biodegradable polymer scaffolds. *J. Dental Res.*, **81**(10), 695–700.

[14] Yen, A. H. and Sharpe, P. T. 2008. Stem cells and tooth tissue engineering. *Cell Tissue Res.*, **331**(1), 359–72.

[15] Sonoyama, W., Liu, Y., Fang, D. *et al.* 2006. Mesenchymal stem cell-mediated functional tooth regeneration in swine. *PLoS One*, **1**, e79.

[16] Gronthos, S., Mankani, M., Brahim, J., Robey, P. G. and Shi, S. 2000. Postnatal human dental pulp stem cells (DPSCs) in vitro and in vivo. *Proc. Nat. Acad. Sci. USA*, **97**(25), 13625–30.

[17] Miura, M., Gronthos, S., Zhao, M. *et al.* 2003. SHED: stem cells from human exfoliated deciduous teeth. *Proc. Nat. Acad. Sci. USA*, **100**(10), 5807–12.

[18] Sonoyama, W., Liu, Y., Yamaza, T. *et al.* 2008. Characterization of the apical papilla and its residing stem cells from human immature permanent teeth: a pilot study. *J. Endod.*, **34**(2), 166–71.

[19] Morsczeck, C., Gotz, W., Schierholz, J. *et al.* 2005. Isolation of precursor cells (PCs) from human dental follicle of wisdom teeth. *Matrix Biol.*, **24**(2), 155–65.

[20] Ma, P. X. 2008. Biomimetic materials for tissue engineering. *Adv. Drug Deliv. Rev.*, **60**(2), 184–98.

[21] Langer, R. and Tirrell, D. A. 2004. Designing materials for biology and medicine. *Nature*, **428**(6982), 487–92.

[22] Gronthos, S., Brahim, J., Li, W. *et al.* 2002. Stem cell properties of human dental pulp stem cells. *J. Dental Res.*, **81**(8), 531–5.

[23] Shi, S. and Gronthos, S. 2003. Perivascular niche of postnatal mesenchymal stem cells in human bone marrow and dental pulp. *J. Bone Miner. Res.*, **18**(4), 696–704.

[24] Waddington, R. J., Youde, S. J., Lee, C. P. and Sloan, A. J. 2009. Isolation of distinct progenitor stem cell populations from dental pulp. *Cells Tissues Organs*, **189**(1–4), 268–74.

[25] Shi, S., Robey, P. G. and Gronthos, S. 2001. Comparison of human dental pulp and bone marrow stromal stem cells by cDNA microarray analysis. *Bone*, **29**(6), 532–9.

[26] Beltrão-Braga, P. I., Pignatari, G. C., Maiorka, P. C. *et al.* 2011. Feeder-free derivation of induced pluripotent stem cells from human immature dental pulp stem cells. *Cell Transplant.*, **20**(11–12), 1707–19.

[27] Tamaoki, N., Takahashi, K., Tanaka, T. *et al.* 2010. Dental pulp cells for induced pluripotent stem cell banking. *J. Dental Res.*, **89**(8), 773–8.

[28] Smith, A. J., Matthews, J. B. and Hall, R. C. 1998. Transforming growth factor-β_1 (TGF-β_1) in dentine matrix. Ligand activation and receptor expression. *Eur. J. Oral Sci.*, **106**(Suppl. 1), 179–84.

[29] Roberts-Clark, D. J. and Smith, A. J. 2000. Angiogenic growth factors in human dentine matrix. *Arch. Oral Biol.*, **45**(11), 1013–16.

[30] Tziafas, D., Alvanou, A., Papadimitriou, S., Gasic, J. and Komnenou, A. 1998. Effects of recombinant basic fibroblast growth factor, insulin-like growth factor-II and transforming growth factor-β_1 on dog dental pulp cells in vivo. *Arch. Oral Biol.*, **43**(6), 431–44.

[31] Begue-Kirn, C., Smith, A. J., Ruch, J. V. *et al.* 1992. Effects of dentin proteins, transforming growth factor β_1 (TGF β_1) and bone morphogenetic protein 2 (BMP2) on the differentiation of odontoblast in vitro. *Int. J. Dev. Biol.*, **36**(4), 491–503.

[32] Sloan, A. J. and Smith, A. J. 1999. Stimulation of the dentine–pulp complex of rat incisor teeth by transforming growth factor-β isoforms 1–3 in vitro. *Arch. Oral Biol.*, **44**(2), 149–56.

[33] Nakashima, M., Nagasawa, H., Yamada, Y. and Reddi, A. H. 1994. Regulatory role of transforming growth factor-β, bone morphogenetic protein-2, and protein-4 on gene expression of extracellular matrix proteins and differentiation of dental pulp cells. *Dev. Biol.*, **162**(1), 18–28.

[34] Saito, T., Ogawa, M., Hata, Y. and Bessho, K. 2004. Acceleration effect of human recombinant bone morphogenetic protein-2 on differentiation of human pulp cells into odontoblasts. *J. Endod.*, **30**(4), 205–8.

[35] Yang, X., van der Kraan, P. M., Bian, Z. *et al.* 2009. Mineralized tissue formation by BMP2-transfected pulp stem cells. *J. Dental Res.*, **88**(11), 1020–5.

[36] Rutherford, R. B. 2001. BMP-7 gene transfer to inflamed ferret dental pulps. *Eur. J. Oral Sci.*, **109**(6), 422–4.

[37] Rutherford, R. B., Spangberg, L., Tucker, M., Rueger, D. and Charette M. 1994. The time-course of the induction of reparative dentine formation in monkeys by recombinant human osteogenic protein-1. *Arch. Oral Biol.*, **39**(10), 833–8.

[38] Jepsen, S., Albers, H. K., Fleiner, B., Tucker, M. and Rueger, D. 1997. Recombinant human osteogenic protein-1 induces dentin formation: an experimental study in miniature swine. *J. Endod.*, **23**(6), 378–82.

[39] Nakashima, M. 1994. Induction of dentine in amputated pulp of dogs by recombinant human bone morphogenetic proteins-2 and -4 with collagen matrix. *Arch. Oral Biol.*, **39**(12), 1085–9.

[40] Nakashima, M. 1994. Induction of dentin formation on canine amputated pulp by recombinant human bone morphogenetic proteins (BMP)-2 and -4. *J. Dent. Res.*, **73**(9), 1515–22.

[41] Lovschall, H., Fejerskov, O. and Flyvbjerg, A. 2001. Pulp-capping with recombinant human insulin-like growth factor I (rhIGF-I) in rat molars. *Adv. Dent. Res.*, **15**, 108–12.

[42] Haddad, M., Lefranc, G. and Aftimos, G. 2003. Local application of IGF1 on dental pulp mechanically exposed; in vivo study on rabbit. *Bull. Groupe Int. Rech. Sci. Stomatol. Odontol.*, **45**(1), 12–17.

[43] Almushayt, A., Narayanan, K., Zaki, A. E. and George, A. 2006. Dentin matrix protein 1 induces cytodifferentiation of dental pulp stem cells into odontoblasts. *Gene Ther.*, **13**(7), 611–20.

[44] Liu, J., Jin, T., Ritchie, H. H., Smith, A. J. and Clarkson, B. H. 2005. In vitro differentiation and mineralization of human dental pulp cells induced by dentin extract. *In Vitro Cell Dev. Biol. Anim.*, **41**(7), 232–8.

[45] Andelin, W. E., Shabahang, S., Wright, K. and Torabinejad, M. 2003. Identification of hard tissue after experimental pulp capping using dentin sialoprotein (DSP) as a marker. *J. Endod.*, **29**(10), 646–50.

[46] Decup, F., Six, N., Palmier, B. *et al.* 2000. Bone sialoprotein-induced reparative dentinogenesis in the pulp of rat's molar. *Clin. Oral Investig.*, **4**(2), 110–19.

[47] Goldberg, M., Six, N., Decup, F. *et al.* 2003. Bioactive molecules and the future of pulp therapy. *Am. J. Dent.*, **16**(1), 66–76.

[48] Paino, F., Ricci, G., De Rosa, A. *et al.* 2010. Ecto-mesenchymal stem cells from dental pulp are committed to differentiate into active melanocytes. *Eur. Cell Mater.*, **20**, 295–305.

[49] Alliot-Licht, B., Bluteau, G., Magne, D. *et al.* 2005. Dexamethasone stimulates differentiation of odontoblast-like

cells in human dental pulp cultures. *Cell Tissue Res.*, **321**(3), 391–400.

[50] Couble, M. L., Farges, J. C., Bleicher, F. *et al.* 2000. Odontoblast differentiation of human dental pulp cells in explant cultures. *Calcif. Tissue Int.*, **66**(2), 129–38.

[51] Zhang, W., Walboomers, X. F., Wolke, J. G. *et al.* 2005. Differentiation ability of rat postnatal dental pulp cells in vitro. *Tissue Eng.*, **11**(3–4), 357–68.

[52] Laino, G., Graziano, A., d'Aquino, R. *et al.* 2006. An approachable human adult stem cell source for hard-tissue engineering. *J. Cell Physiol.*, **206**(3), 693–701.

[53] Zhang, W., Walboomers, X. F., van Osch, G. J., van den Dolder, J. and Jansen, J. A. 2008. Hard tissue formation in a porous HA/TCP ceramic scaffold loaded with stromal cells derived from dental pulp and bone marrow. *Tissue Eng. Part A*, **14**(2), 285–94.

[54] Wang, J., Liu, X., Jin, X. *et al.* 2010. The odontogenic differentiation of human dental pulp stem cells on nano-fibrous poly(L-lactic acid) scaffolds in vitro and in vivo. *Acta Biomater.*, **6**(10), 3856–63.

[55] Smith, A. J., Patel, M., Graham, L., Sloan, A. J. and Cooper, P. R. 2005. Dentine regeneration: key roles for stem cells and molecular signalling. *Oral Biosci. Med.*, **2**, 127–32.

[56] Nakashima, M., Tachibana, K., Iohara, K. *et al.* 2003. Induction of reparative dentin formation by ultrasound-mediated gene delivery of growth/differentiation factor 11. *Hum. Gene Ther.*, **14**(6), 591–7.

[57] Nakashima, M., Iohara, K., Ishikawa, M. *et al.* 2004. Stimulation of reparative dentin formation by ex vivo gene therapy using dental pulp stem cells electrotransfected with growth/differentiation factor 11 (Gdf11). *Hum. Gene Ther.*, **15**(11), 1045–53.

[58] Yang, X., van der Kraan, P. M., van den Dolder, J. *et al.* 2007. STRO-1 selected rat dental pulp stem cells transfected with adenoviral-mediated human bone morphogenetic protein 2 gene show enhanced odontogenic differentiation. *Tissue Eng.*, **13**(11), 2803–12.

[59] Yang, X., Walboomers, X. F., van den Dolder, J. *et al.* 2008. Non-viral bone morphogenetic protein 2 transfection of rat dental pulp stem cells using calcium phosphate nanoparticles as carriers. *Tissue Eng. Part A*, **14**(1), 71–81.

[60] Wei, G., Jin, Q., Giannobile, W. V. and Ma, P. X. 2007. The enhancement of osteogenesis by nano-fibrous scaffolds incorporating rhBMP-7 nanospheres *Biomaterials*, **28**(12), 2087–96.

[61] Mizuno, M. K. Y. 2000. Type 1 collagen matrix and β-glycerophosphate facilitates mineralized tissue formation by rat dental pulp cells. *Jap. J. Oral Biol.*, **42**, 102–8.

[62] Mizuno, M., Miyamoto, T., Wada, K., Watatani, S. and Zhang, G. X. 2003. Type I collagen regulated dentin matrix protein-1 (Dmp-1) and osteocalcin (OCN) gene expression of rat dental pulp cells. *J. Cell Biochem.*, **88**(6), 1112–19.

[63] Kim, N. R., Lee, D. H., Chung, P. H. and Yang, H. C. 2009. Distinct differentiation properties of human dental pulp cells on collagen, gelatin, and chitosan scaffolds. *Oral Surg. Oral Med. Oral Pathol. Oral Radiol. Endod.*, **108**(5), e94–100.

[64] Prescott, R. S., Alsanea, R., Fayad, M. I. *et al.* 2008. In vivo generation of dental pulp-like tissue by using dental pulp stem cells, a collagen scaffold, and dentin matrix protein 1 after subcutaneous transplantation in mice. *J. Endod.*, **34**(4), 421–6.

[65] Huang, G. T., Sonoyama, W., Chen, J. and Park, S. H. 2006. In vitro characterization of human dental pulp cells: various isolation methods and culturing environments. *Cell Tissue Res.*, **324**(2), 225–36.

[66] Yang, X., Walboomers, X. F., van den Beucken, J. J. *et al.* Hard tissue formation of STRO-1-selected rat dental pulp stem cells in vivo. *Tissue Eng. Part A*, **15**(2), 367–75.

[67] Zhang, W., Walboomers, X. F., van Kuppevelt, T. H. *et al.* 2006. The performance of human dental pulp stem cells on different three-dimensional scaffold materials. *Biomaterials*, **27**(33), 5658–68.

[68] Duailibi, M. T., Duailibi, S. E., Young, C. S. *et al.* 2004. Bioengineered teeth from cultured rat tooth bud cells. *J. Dent. Res.*, **83**(7), 523–8.

[69] Iwatsuki, S., Honda, M. J., Harada, H. and Ueda, M. 2006. Cell proliferation in teeth reconstructed from dispersed cells of embryonic tooth germs in a three-dimensional scaffold. *Eur. J. Oral Sci.*, **114**(4), 310–7.

[70] Young, C. S., Abukawa, H., Asrican, R. *et al.* 2005. Tissue-engineered hybrid tooth and bone. *Tissue Eng.*, **11**(9–10), 1599–610.

[71] Mooney, D. J., Powell, C., Piana, J. and Rutherford, B. 1996. Engineering dental pulp-like tissue in vitro. *Biotechnol. Prog.*, **12**(6), 865–8.

[72] Bohl, K. S., Shon, J., Rutherford, B. and Mooney, D. J. 1998. Role of synthetic extracellular matrix in development of engineered dental pulp. *J. Biomater. Sci. Polymer Edition*, **9**(7), 749–64.

[73] Cordeiro, M. M., Dong, Z., Kaneko, T. *et al.* 2008. Dental pulp tissue engineering with stem cells from exfoliated deciduous teeth. *J. Endod.*, **34**(8), 962–9.

[74] Huang, G. T., Yamaza, T., Shea, L. D. *et al.* 2010. Stem/progenitor cell-mediated de novo regeneration of dental pulp with newly deposited continuous layer of dentin in an in vivo model. *Tissue Eng. Part A*, **16**(2), 605–15.

[75] Ekblom, P., Vestweber, D. and Kemler, R. 1986. Cell-matrix interactions and cell adhesion during development. *Ann. Rev. Cell Biol.*, **2**, 27–47.

[76] Deng, X. L., Xu, M., Li, D. *et al.* 2007. Electrospun PLLA/MWNTs/HA hybrid nanofiber scaffolds and their potential in dental tissue engineering. *Key Eng. Mater. Bioceram.*, **19**(V330-2), 393–6.

[77] Xu, M. M., Fan, M., Li, D. *et al.* 2007. Electrospun poly(L-lacticacid)/nano-hydroxyapatite hybrid nanofibers and their potential in dental tissue engineering. *Key Eng. Mater. Bioceram.*, **19**(V330-2), 377–80.

[78] Yang, X., Yang, F., Walboomers, X. F. *et al.* 2010. The performance of dental pulp stem cells on nanofibrous PCL/gelatin/nHA scaffolds. *J. Biomed. Mater. Res. A*, **93**(1), 247–57.

[79] Hartgerink, J. D., Beniash, E. and Stupp, S. I. 2001. Self-assembly and mineralization of peptide-amphiphile nanofibers. *Science*, **294**(5547), 1684–8.

[80] Silva, G. A., Czeisler, C., Niece, K. L. *et al.* 2004. Selective differentiation of neural progenitor cells by high-epitope density nanofibers. *Science*, **303**(5662), 1352–5.

[81] Galler, K. M., Cavender, A., Yuwono, V. *et al.* 2008. Self-assembling peptide amphiphile nanofibers as a scaffold for dental stem cells. *Tissue Eng. Part A*, **14**(12), 2051–8.

[82] Ma, P. X. and Zhang, R. 1999. Synthetic nano-scale fibrous extracellular matrix. *J. Biomed. Mater. Res.*, **46**(1), 60–72.

[83] Zhang, R. and Ma, P. X. 2000. Synthetic nano-fibrillar extracellular matrices with predesigned macroporous architectures. *J. Biomed. Mater. Res.*, **52**(2), 430–8.

[84] Chen, V. J. and Ma, P. X. 2004. Nano-fibrous poly(L-lactic acid) scaffolds with interconnected spherical macropores. *Biomaterials*, **25**(11), 2065–73.

[85] Wei, G. and Ma, P. X. 2006. Macroporous and nanofibrous polymer scaffolds and polymer/bone-like apatite composite scaffolds generated by sugar spheres. *J. Biomed. Mater. Res. Part A*, **78**(2), 306–15.

[86] Wang, J., Ma, H., Jin, X. *et al.* 2011. The effect of scaffold architecture on odontogenic differentiation of human dental pulp stem cells. *Biomaterials*, **32**(31), 7822–30.

[87] Woo, K. M., Chen, V. J. and Ma, P. X. 2003. Nano-fibrous scaffolding architecture selectively enhances protein adsorption contributing to cell attachment. *J. Biomed. Mater. Res. A*, **67**(2), 531–7.

[88] Lesot, H., Fausser, J. L., Akiyama, S. K. *et al.* 1992. The carboxy-terminal extension of the collagen binding domain of fibronectin mediates interaction with a 165 kDa membrane protein involved in odontoblast differentiation. *Differentiation*, **49**(2), 109–18.

[89] Tziafas, D., Alvanou, A. and Kaidoglou, K. 1992. Dentinogenic activity of allogenic plasma fibronectin on dog dental pulp. *J. Dent. Res.*, **71**(5), 1189–95.

[90] Tziafas, D., Panagiotakopoulos, N. and Komnenou, A. 1995. Immunolocalization of fibronectin during the early response of dog dental pulp to demineralized dentine or calcium hydroxide-containing cement. *Arch. Oral Biol.*, **40**(1), 23–31.

[91] Murray, P. E., About, I., Franquin, J. C., Remusat, M. and Smith, A. J. 2001. Restorative pulpal and repair responses. *J. Am. Dent. Assoc.*, **132**(4), 482–91.

32

Dental enamel regeneration

Xanthippi Chatzistavrou and Petros Papagerakis

32.1 Introduction

32.1.1 Enamel formation

Enamel is the outermost covering of vertebrate teeth and the hardest tissue in the vertebrate body. During tooth development, ectoderm-derived ameloblast cells create enamel by synthesizing a complex protein mixture into the extracellular space where the proteins self-assemble to form a matrix that patterns the woven hydroxyapatite (Wang *et al.*, 2007; Zhu *et al.*, 2006). During enamel biomineralization, the assembly of the protein matrix precedes mineral replacement. The predominant protein of mammalian enamel is amelogenin, which is secreted from ameloblasts. It is a hydrophobic protein that self-assembles to form nanospheres that in turn influence the crystal type, organization, and packing of the crystallites (Du *et al.*, 2005). In contrast to the mesenchyme-controlled biomineralization of bone, which uses collagen and remodels both the organic and the inorganic phases over a lifetime, enamel contains no collagen and does not remodel. The mature enamel composite contains hardly any protein (Smith *et al.*, 1998) and is a tough, crack-tolerant, and abrasion-resistant tissue (White *et al.*, 2001).

The process of enamel formation, termed amelogenesis, is the end product of a series of complex, dynamic, and programmed cellular, chemical and physiological events (Simmer *et al.*, 2010). Enamel formation can be categorized into three distinct stages – the secretory, transition, and maturation stages. The secretory stage is characterized by active protein synthesis and secretion by the ameloblasts. Ameloblasts also deposit enamel crystals at oblique angles while they are moving in the direction of the future cusps to accommodate expansion of the enamel surface. The transition stage is of short duration and is characterized by extensive apoptosis and shortening of ameloblasts in preparation for their transition into the maturation stage. The maturation stage is characterized by removal of enamel organic materials and growth of hydroxyapatite crystals in thickness, as well as by regulated movement of ions into and out of the enamel matrix (Lu *et al.*, 2008; Smith *et al.*, 1998). Besides their involvement in crystal formation, ions also contribute to the color of the teeth (Yanagawa *et al.*, 2004). Enamel in humans is characterized by a large diversity of color variations.

The complexity of enamel formation represents a great challenge for the development of suitable approaches on the enamel's remineralization and/or regeneration. Cellular and material–cell-based strategies for stimulation of enamel regeneration are being studied.

32.1.2 Regenerative potential

Insofar as cell-based strategies are concerned, there is limited information about the regenerative potential of dental epithelial stem cells (DESCs), which could give rise to new ameloblasts. Undifferentiated wisdom teeth present a potential source of human dental epithelium (Honda *et al.*, 2009). The epithelial rests of Mallasez (ERM) constitute another source of human

DESCs (P. Papagerakis, unpublished data). The ERM are localized in the periodontal ligament of adult teeth and exhibit stem cell properties. The ERM can differentiate into enamel-secreting cells when co-cultured with DPSCs in humans (P. Papagerakis, unpublished data) and rodents (Shinmura *et al.*, 2008). Thus, DESCs isolated from ERM can provide a viable source of ameloblast progenitors for enamel regeneration. Alternatively, epithelial stem cells of non-dental origin (e.g. hair and skin) could be used for the formation of enamel. Therefore, dental mesenchymal stem cells that interact in vitro with dental epithelial stem cells (after recombination) might be able to form the various mesenchymal and epithelial cell populations necessary to form new enamel and dentin in a regenerated tooth.

In regard to material–cell-based strategies, research has started to emerge in the field of enamel regeneration. It is expected that strategies involving the use of tissue engineering, nanotechnology, and stem cells will play an increasing role in clinical dentistry over the next 5–20 years (Bayne *et al.*, 2005). There is evidence to support the hypothesis that tissue engineering will be the main approach for the development of new dental structures in the future of operative dentistry. Regenerative processes have already started to be used to treat dental disease in operative dentistry (Smith *et al.*, 2008). The use of calcium hydroxide to stimulate reparative dentin is an example of a regenerative therapeutic strategy (Graham *et al.*, 2006). Tissue engineering encourages dentistry to move forward in the application of regeneration as an important principle for the treatment of dental disease. It is based on fundamental approaches that involve the identification of appropriate cells, the development of conductive biomaterials, and an understanding of the morphogenic signals required in order to induce cells to regenerate the lost tissue.

In conclusion, strategies applied for enamel formation must support the three stages of enamel formation, and direct the proper cellular movement that occurs during enamel apposition. Organic material removal, vascularization, and extensive ion transport must also be achieved in the regenerated enamel. There are major issues to overcome before such strategies can be applied to clinical practice; for example, there is a lack of information regarding the role of ions in the control of color variability in human enamel, while the time required for enamel's regeneration constitutes an additional important barrier.

32.2 Making enamel

An *in situ* exclusively cell-based approach to regenerate enamel does not seem feasible in the near future, since the ameloblasts which specialize in making enamel are no longer present in teeth with complete crown development. On the other hand, the development of synthetic enamel using the principles of tissue regeneration and nanotechnology has been reported (Huang *et al.*, 2008, 2010; Khan *et al.*, 2012; Yan-Zhong *et al.*, 2011; Zhang *et al.*, 2010). Restoration and remineralization processes have already been developed and applied in clinical practice, while cell-based regeneration protocols are an open and ongoing area of research. Characteristic approaches for the development of enamel tissue are presented in the following paragraphs.

32.2.1 Restoration: remineralization with synthetic enamel fabrication

Surfactants were used as reverse micelles or microemulsions to synthesize enamel, since they can mimic the biological action of enamel proteins (Chen *et al.*, 2005). The synthesized nanoscale structures may self-assemble into "one-dimensional building blocks," leading to the development of hydroxyapatite nanorods similar to natural enamel crystals. The fabricated nanorods can potentially be applied as flowable restorative material for the restoration of lost enamel. Chen *et al.* (2006), on the basis of biological processes involved in amelogenesis, combined with new approaches in nanotechnology, fabricated enamel prism-like structures consisting of fluorapatite nanorods (Figure 32.1(a)) precipitated directly from solution under controlled chemical conditions without the use of surfactants, proteins, or cells. The fabricated nanorods present similar characteristics to those of the natural enamel crystals isolated from rat incisor enamel, as

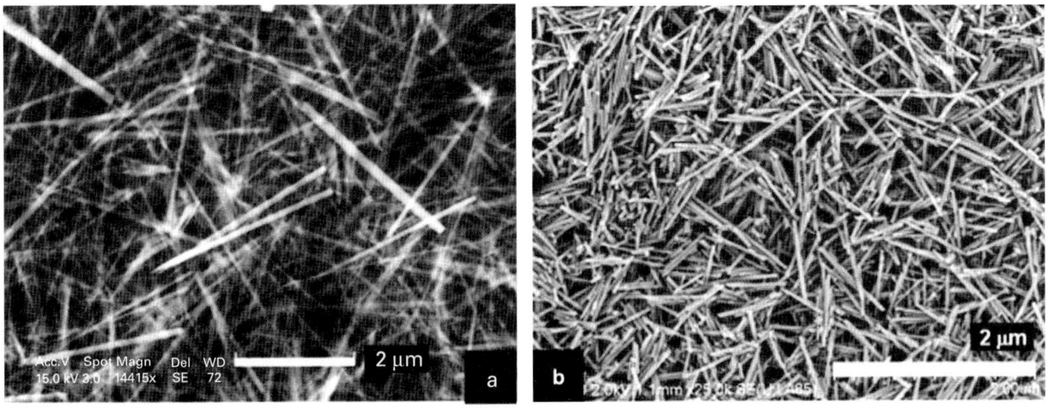

Figure 32.1 SEM images of (a) fluorapatite nanorods prepared by direct precipitation from solution and (b) enamel crystals isolated from the maturation stage of rat incisor enamel (Chen *et al.*, 2006). (Reproduced with permission from the American Chemical Society).

was confirmed by examination of the scanning electron microscope (SEM) images in Figure 32.1(b).

Another enamel-based biomaterial having the added benefit of fluorapatite incorporated intrinsically into the composition was also studied. In particular, amelogenin-driven apatite crystal growth, incorporating fluoride into the process, allowed the synthesis of elongated rod-like apatite crystals with dimensions similar to those observed in natural enamel (Iijima *et al.*, 2002).

On the other hand, Lynch *et al.* (2007) observed a differential remineralization potential depending on the depth of the demineralized area. The treatment of deep demineralized areas using supersaturated solutions containing less crystalline calcium phosphate phase was more effective, while solutions of stoichiometric amounts of hydroxyapatite were very effective to remineralize, in vitro, superficial lesions (Lynch *et al.*, 2007). Furthermore, fluoride compounds and glass ionomers are traditionally considered as remineralizing agents for damaged enamel (Gaengler *et al.*, 2009). Glass ionomers applied on etched enamel have been observed to be transformed in vitro into enamel-like material when studied with SEM and EDAX analysis (Van Duinen *et al.*, 2004). Similarly, carbon dioxide laser irradiation has been observed to enhance the formation of fluoride precipitates from titanium fluoride (TiF) and amine fluoride (AmF) onto the demineralized enamel (Wiegand *et al.*, 2010).

The role of certain milk proteins, which are thought to stabilize calcium phosphate, has also been investigated. Remineralization of enamel subsurface lesions was observed in vitro after application of a paste of casein phosphopeptide-stabilized amorphous calcium phosphate and amorphous calcium fluoride phosphate (Ranjitkar *et al.*, 2009; Walker *et al.*, 2009; Willershausen *et al.*, 2009). The remineralization, which was consistent with hydroxyapatite and fluorapatite, was found to be pH-dependent, with a maximum at pH 5.5. In the case of carbonated hydroxyapatite (CHA) nanocrystals, remineralization occurs by means of the addition of a layer of apatite similar to those of natural tissues, even if prismatic enamel structures cannot be built, whereas the application of fluoride may act by changing the chemical composition of the enamel, causing an increase in the Ca/P molar ratio (Kirkham *et al.*, 2007; Roveri *et al.*, 2009).

Furthermore, an in-vitro technique that induces the localized formation of an ordered enamel-like mineral on human teeth with tight contact to the substrate has also been introduced (Busch, 2004). The formation of parallel arrays of fluorapatite–protein composite particles up to a macroscopic length scale was observed. The method applied uses the diffusion of calcium ions

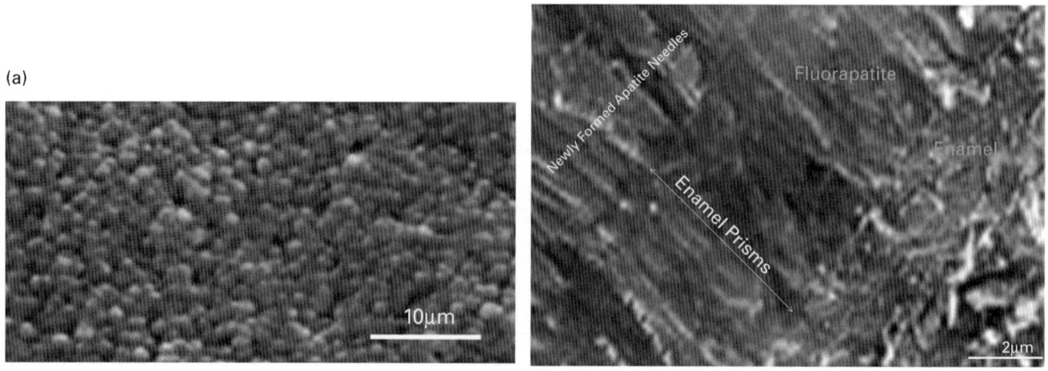

Figure 32.2 SEM images of fluorapatite layers on human enamel slices. (a) The fluorapatite layer after 10 exchange cycles. A dense layer of homogeneous crystals can be seen after the 10th exchange cycle of the gel. (b) A close-up of the borderline region between natural enamel and fluorapatite seen after the 36th exchange cycle of the gel. (Modified and reproduced with permission from Busch (2004).)

from solution in a glycerine-enriched gelatin gel at 37 °C, which contains phosphate and fluoride ions and covers the tooth surface. The ion gel was masked with another phosphate-free gel layer. To induce the mineralization of fluorapatite on the surface of the tooth, the samples prepared were immersed in a neutral calcium solution. The gel and calcium solution had to be exchanged periodically. A homogeneous enamel-like layer with a thickness depending on the number of exchange cycles developed on top of the disk. The orientation of the enamel crystals and the newly crystallized fluorapatite was parallel. The new layer, with a thickness of ~5 mm, was not fully mature after five growth cycles. Figure 32.2(a) shows a side-view SEM image of a layer grown after the 10th exchange cycle of the gel. A close-up of the enamel–fluorapatite interface (between natural enamel and fluorapatite) after the 36th exchange cycle shows the enamel prisms running perpendicular to the long axis of the newly formed apatite needles (Figure 32.2(b)). The specific approach could be considered attractive also for biomineralization issues (Busch *et al.*, 2004).

Although there has been a lot of research on engineering advanced biomaterials, from the current level of knowledge, it seems that none of the materials available today can mimic all of the physical, mechanical, and esthetic properties of enamel. This conclusion gave an important impetus toward the establishment of cell-based strategies that could stimulate enamel regeneration.

32.2.2 Regeneration: cell-based strategies

It has been suggested that extracellular matrix proteins such as fibronectin (Ruch *et al.*, 1990), laminin (Harada *et al.*, 1999), and ameloblastin (Nakashima *et al.*, 2003) not only function as a mechanical scaffold for cell attachment and survival but also provide a microenvironment for guiding cell growth and differentiation. Considering this suggestion, Huang *et al.* (2008) used an in-vitro cell and organ culture system to study the effect of artificial bioactive nanostructures on ameloblasts, with the long-term goal of developing cell-based strategies for tooth regeneration. In particular, a branched peptide amphiphile molecule containing the peptide motif Arg–Gly–Asp, or "RGD" (abbreviated BRGD-PA), which is known to self-assemble in physiological environments into a network of nanofibers, was used in order to mimic the extracellular matrix that surrounds the ameloblasts and provide the synthetic nanostructures with a biological signal. Ameloblast-like cells (line LS8) and primary

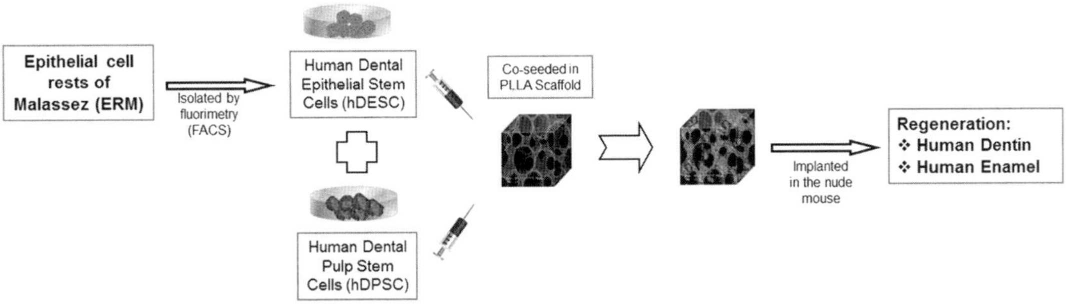

Figure 32.3 The cell-based strategy for the development of complex mineralized dental tissues by co-seeding of hDPSC and hDESC, isolated from ERM by fluorescence-activated cell sorting (FACS), within appropriate poly-L-lactide (PLLA) scaffolds.

enamel organ epithelial (EOE) cells were cultured within PA hydrogels, and the PA was injected into the enamel organ epithelia of mouse embryonic incisors. At the site of injection of the PA, EOE cell proliferation was observed, with differentiation into ameloblasts as demonstrated by the expression of enamel-specific proteins. Moreover it was shown that the nanofibers within the forming extracellular matrix, in contact with the EOE cells, were engaged in enamel formation and regeneration. Finally, it was concluded that the BRGD-PA nanofibers present together with enamel proteins participate in integrin-mediated cell binding to the matrix, with delivery of instructive signals for enamel formation (Huang *et al.*, 2008).

32.2.3 Enamel regeneration in joint structures: current research

Tissue engineering using scaffold-and-cell-aggregate methods has been suggested as a means to produce bioengineered complex dentin–enamel regeneration from dissociated cells. Shinmura *et al.* (2008) investigated the capability of the epithelial cell rests of Malassez (ERM) to regenerate dental tissues by transplanting subcultured ERM seeded onto scaffolds into the omentum of athymic rats. In particular, ERM co-seeded into collagen sponge scaffolds in combination with dental pulp cells generated enamel–dentin-complex-like structures 8 weeks after transplantation (Shinmura *et al.*, 2008). Similar results were observed with human ERM populations, isolated by fluorescence-activated cell sorting (FACS) using epithelium stem cell markers (Sato *et al.*, 2009), and subcultured under serum-free and xenon-free conditions (Chatzistavrou *et al.*, 2012). As illustrated in Figure 32.3, the collected human dental epithelial stem cells (hDESC) can generate mineralized tissue in vivo when co-seeded on poly-L-lactide (PLLA) scaffolds with human dental pulp stem cells (hDPSC) and implanted subsequently in the omentum of nude mouse. Mineralization is seen in the hDESC–hDPSC implants 10 weeks after implantation, but not in the controls (only hDESC or only hDPSC) (Chatzistavrou *et al.*, 2012). Furthermore, regeneration of complex dental tissues was investigated with different types of re-association between epithelial and mesenchymal tissues and/or cells from mouse embryos, which were cultured in-vitro before in vivo implantation (Oshima *et al.*, 2011). In vitro the re-associated tissues developed, resulted in jointed dental structures that exhibited normal epithelial histogenesis, and allowed the functional differentiation of odontoblasts and ameloblasts. After implantation, the re-associations formed roots and periodontal ligament, with the latter connected to developing bone (Hu *et al.*, 2006). However, in humans several limitations exist.

32.3 Conclusions and future trends

The regeneration of enamel is a complex task, since it requires the production and secretion of the proper amounts and types of proteins, at the right place, at the right time (Mitsiadis and Papagerakis, 2011). Otherwise, the effort to regenerate human enamel will fail. It is a long-term physiological procedure, which is difficult to simulate in vitro and in vivo. There are still many aspects to be discovered and barriers to be overcome before cell-based enamel regeneration can become a routine procedure in dentistry (Chatzistavrou *et al.*, 2012). However, a potential solution could be a material-based engineering approach. The application of appropriate advanced biological systems able to induce remineralization and create well-sealed restorations, preventing microleakages and secondary caries through the maintenance of a bacteria-free environment, is considered a promising strategy. Thus, an additional important challenge is the development of suitable carriers that can house all the necessary factors for the treatment and regeneration of lost enamel. These carriers should exhibit biocompatible, physicochemical, and mechanical properties compatible with the area of application. In conclusion, there is still a need for extended interdisciplinary research and effective collaboration between basic scientists and clinicians to eventually lead this field to the ultimate goal of enamel or joint-enamel regeneration.

REFERENCES

Bayne, S. C. 2005. Dental biomaterials: where are we and where are we going? *J. Dent. Educ.*, **69**, 571–85.

Busch, S. 2004. Biomineralization: regeneration of human tooth enamel. *Angew. Chem. Int. Edition Engl.*, **43**, 1428–31.

Chatzistavrou, X., Papagerakis, S. and Ma, P. X. and Papagerakis, P. 2012. Innovative approaches to regenerate enamel and dentin. *Int. J. Dent.*, 856470.

Chen, H., Clarkson, B. H., Sun, K. and Mansfield, J. F. 2005. Self-assembly of synthetic hydroxyapatite nanorods into an enamel prism-like structure. *J. Colloid Interface Sci.*, **288**, 97–103.

Chen, H., Sun, K., Tang, Z. *et al.* 2006. Synthesis of fluorapatite nanorods and nanowires by direct precipitation from solution. *Cryst. Growth Design*, **6**, 1504–8.

Du, C., Falini, G., Fermani, S., Abbott, C. and Moradian-Oldak, J. 2005. Supramolecular assembly of amelogenin nanospheres into birefringent microribbons. *Science*, **307**, 1450–4.

Gaengler, P., Kremniczky, T. and Arnold, W. H. 2009. In vitro effect of fluoride oral hygiene tablets on artificial caries lesion formation and remineralization in human enamel. *BMC Oral Health*, **9**, 25.

Graham, L., Cooper, P. R., Cassidy, N. *et al.* 2006. The effect of calcium hydroxide on solubilisation of bioactive dentine matrix components. *Biomaterials*, **27**, 2865–73.

Harada, H., Kettunen, P., Jung, H. S. *et al.* 1999. Localization of putative stem cells in dental epithelium and their association with Notch and FGF signaling. *J. Cell Biol.*, **147**, 105–20.

Honda, M. J., Shinmura, Y. and Shinohara, Y. 2009. Enamel tissue engineering using subcultured enamel organ epithelial cells in combination with dental pulp cells. *Cells Tissues Organs*, **189**, 261–7.

Hu, B., Nadiri, A., Kuchler-Bopp, S. *et al.* 2006. Tissue engineering of tooth crown, root, and periodontium *Tissue Eng.*, **12**, 2069–75.

Huang, Z., Sargeant, T. D., Hulvat, J. F. *et al.* 2008. Bioactive nanofibers instruct cells to proliferate and differentiate during enamel regeneration. *J. Bone Miner. Res.*, **23**, 1995–2006.

Huang, Z., Newcomb, C. J., Bringas, P. Jr., Stupp, S. I. and Snead, M. L. 2010. Biological synthesis of tooth enamel instructed by an artificial matrix. *Biomaterials*, **31**, 9202–11.

Iijima, M., Moriwaki, Y., Wen, H. B., Fincham, A. G. and Moradian-Oldak, J. 2002. Elongated growth of octacalcium phosphate crystals in recombinant amelogenin gels under controlled ionic flow. *J. Dent. Res.*, **81**, 69–73.

Khan, F., Li, W. and Habelitz, S. 2012. Biophysical characterization of synthetic amelogenin C-terminal peptides. *Eur. J. Oral Sci.*, **120**, 113–22.

Kirkham, J., Firth, A., Vernals, D. *et al.* 2007. Self-assembling peptide scaffolds promote enamel remineralization. *J. Dent. Res.*, **86**, 426–30.

Lu, Y., Papagerakis, P., Yamakoshi, Y. *et al.* 2008. Functions of KLK4 and MMP-20 in dental enamel formation. *Biol. Chem.*, **389**, 695–700.

Lynch, R. J., Mony, U. and Cate, J. M. 2007. Effect of lesion characteristics and mineralizing solution type on enamel remineralization in vitro. *Caries Res.*, **41**, 257–62.

Mitsiadis, T. and Papagerakis, P. 2011. Regenerated teeth: the future of tooth replacement? *Regen. Med.*, **6**, 135–9.

Nakashima, M. and Reddi, A. H. 2003. The application of bone morphogenetic proteins to dental tissue engineering. *Nature Biotechnol.*, **21**, 1025–32.

Oshima, M., Mizuno, M., Imamura, A. *et al.* 2001. Functional tooth regeneration using a bioengineered tooth unit as a mature organ replacement regenerative therapy. *PLoS One*, **6**, e21531.

Ranjitkar, S., Narayana, T., Kaidonis, J. A. *et al.* 2009. The effect of casein phosphopeptide–amorphous calcium phosphate on erosive dentine wear. *Aust. Dent. J.*, **54**, 101–7.

Roveri, N., Battistella, E., Bianchi, C. L. *et al.* 2009. Surface enamel remineralization: biomimetic apatite nanocrystals and fluoride ions different effects. *J. Nanomater.*, doi:10.1155/2009/746383.

Ruch, J. V. 1990. Patterned distribution of differentiating dental cells: facts and hypotheses. *J. Biol. Buccale*, **18**, 91–8.

Sato, T., Vries, R. G., Snippert, H. J. *et al.* 2009. Single Lgr5 stem cells build crypt–villus structures in vitro without a mesenchymal niche. *Nature*, **459**, 262–5.

Shinmura, Y., Tsuchiya, S., Hata, K. and Honda, M. J. 2008. Quiescent epithelial cell rests of Malassez can differentiate into ameloblastlike cells. *J. Cell Physiol.*, **217**(3), 728–38.

Simmer, J. P., Papagerakis, P., Smith, C. E. *et al.* 2010. Regulation of dental enamel shape and hardness. *J. Dent. Res.*, **89**, 1024–38.

Smith, C. E. 1998. Cellular and chemical events during enamel maturation. *Crit. Rev. Oral Biol. Med.*, **9**, 128–61.

Smith, A. J., Lumley, P. J., Tomson, P. L. and Cooper, P. R. 2008. Dental regeneration and materials – a partnership. *Clin. Oral Invest.*, **12**, 103–8.

Van Duinen, R. N., Davidson, C. L., De Gee, A. J. and Feilzer, A. J. 2004. *In situ* transformation of glass-ionomer into an enamel-like material. *Am. J. Dent.*, **17**, 223–7.

Walker, G. D., Cai, F., Shen, P. *et al.* 2009. Consumption of milk with added casein phosphopeptide–amorphous calcium phosphate remineralizes enamel subsurface lesions *in situ*. *Aust. Dent. J.*, **54**, 245–9.

Wang, L., Guan, X., Du, C., Moradian-Oldak, J. and Nancollas, G. H. 2007. Amelogenin promotes the formation of elongated microstructures in a controlled crystallization system. *J. Phys. Chem. C*, **111**, 6398–404.

White, S. N., Luo, W., Paine, M. L. *et al.* 2001. Biological organization of hydroxyapatite crystallites into a fibrous continuum toughens and controls anisotropy in human enamel. *J. Dent. Res.*, **80**, 321–6.

Wiegand, A., Magalhães, A. C., Navarro, R. S. *et al.* 2010. Effect of titanium tetrafluoride and amine fluoride treatment combined with carbon dioxide laser irradiation on enamel and dentin erosion. *Photomed. Laser Surg.*, **28**, 219–26.

Willershausen, B., Schulz-Dobrick, B. and Gleissner, C. 2009. In vitro evaluation of enamel remineralisation by a casein phosphopeptide–amorphous calcium phosphate paste. *Oral Health Prev. Dent.*, **7**(1), 13–21.

Yanagawa, T., Itoh, K., Uwayama, J. *et al.* 2004. Nrf2 deficiency causes tooth decolourization due to iron transport disorder in enamel organ. *Genes Cells*, **9**, 641–51.

Yan-Zhong, Z., Yan-Yan, H., Jun, Z. 2011. Characteristics of functionalized nano-hydroxyapatite and internalization by human epithelial cell. *Nanoscale Res. Lett.*, **6**, 600.

Zhang, J., Jiang, D., Zhang, J., Lin, Q. and Huang, Z. 2010. Synthesis of dental enamel-like hydroxyapatite through solution mediated solid-state conversion. *Langmuir*, **26**, 2989–94.

Zhu, D., Paine, M. L., Luo, W., Bringas, P. Jr. and Snead, M. L. 2006. Altering biomineralization by protein design. *J. Biol. Chem.*, **281**, 21173–82.

33

Hair follicle and skin regeneration

Makoto Takeo and Mayumi Ito

33.1 Introduction

The skin is the largest organ in the body and constitutes the interface between the body's internal organs and its external surroundings. It serves multiple functions, lending thermoregulation, structure, and insulation to the body, and preventing water loss, while also acting as a barrier against external pathogens (Elias and Friend, 1975). The skin also allows an individual to respond to the environment through the nerve endings that sense different stimuli such as touch, pressure, temperature, and pain. These functions are essential for an individual's survival and are maintained owing to the skin's ability for regeneration. Much evidence has shown that the presence of stem cells in the epidermis and hair follicles underlies skin regeneration. In this chapter, we will review how skin is maintained under homeostatic conditions and following injury, particularly focussing on the role of stem cells in the hair follicle.

33.2 Skin homeostasis

The skin epidermis (i.e. inter-follicular epidermis) is composed of keratinocytes that form stratified squamous epithelium. Throughout an individual's lifetime, epidermal cells of the skin differentiate and migrate to the superficial layer of the epidermis where they are shed, while being continuously renewed by proliferating cells of the basal layer adjacent to the basement membrane (Figure 33.1) (Mackenzie, 1970; Potten 1974; Watt 2001). Cells in the basal layer of the epidermis are a heterogeneous population in terms of their gene expression (Tani *et al.*, 2000), proliferation rate (Potten and Morris, 1988), and differentiation status (Kaur and Li, 2000). Keratin 14-expressing basal epidermal cells contain long-lived stem cells that contribute to wound healing as well as maintenance of the basal layer of the epidermis (Mascre *et al.*, 2012). However, the specific location of the stem cell niche or markers of stem cells for the inter-follicular epidermis has not yet been identified (Clayton *et al.*, 2007). The properties of epidermal stem cells, and whether stem cells play distinct roles from their progeny in the renewal of skin epidermis, remain unknown.

Unlike the constant renewal of the skin epidermis, hair follicles regenerate through cyclical phases of anagen, catagen, telogen, and exogen (Dry, 1926; Chase, 1951; Muller-Rover *et al.*, 2001) (Figure 33.2). In anagen, hair follicles develop and produce the hair shaft. The anagen hair follicle is composed of multiple types of epithelial cells that include the hair matrix, hair shaft, and inner and outer root sheaths, as well as dermal components that include the dermal papilla and the dermal sheath (Paus *et al.*, 1999) (Figure 33.3). Hair growth relies on the proliferation of hair matrix cells that are located within the lower bulb region of the hair follicle. Hair matrix cells are highly proliferative, and, as they proliferate, they give rise to distinct layers of the hair shaft (medulla, cortex, and cuticle) and the hair follicle sheath cells that surround and support the hair shaft.

The lower epithelial part of the anagen hair follicle including the matrix cells in the hair bulb degenerates after the hair has grown to a certain length, depending

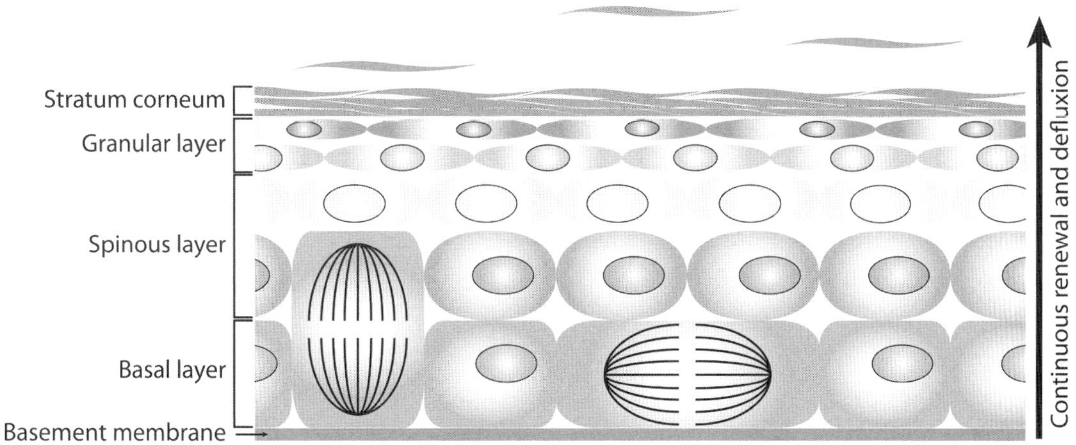

Figure 33.1 Turnover of epithelial cells. Continuous renewal of epithelial cells is achieved by proliferating cells attaching to the basement membrane throughout the subject's lifetime.

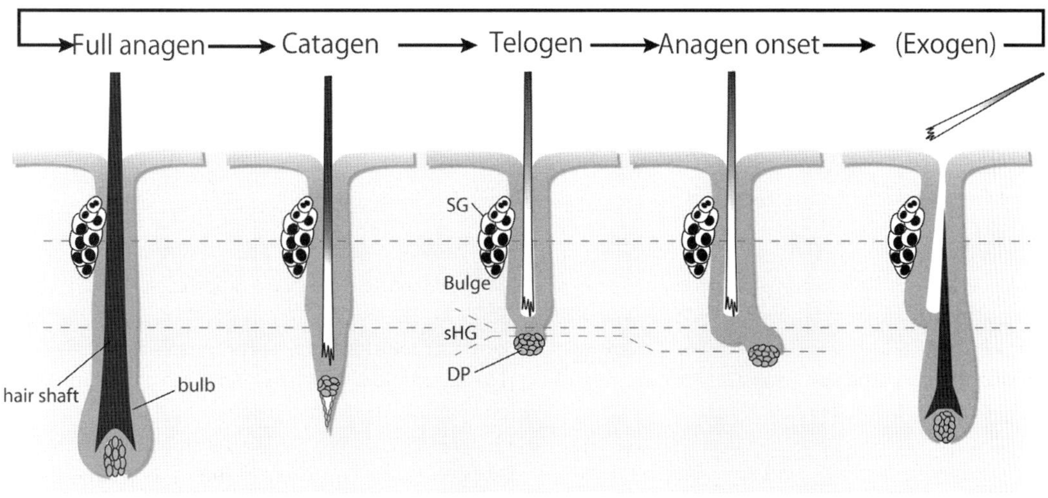

Figure 33.2 The hair follicle cycle in adult skin. Anagen, growth phase; telogen, resting phase; catagen, regression phase; exogen, shedding phase; DP, dermal papilla; SG, sebaseous gland; and sHG, secondary hair germ.

on the body site. In this degenerative phase, called the catagen phase, hair matrix cells cease proliferation, and undergo cellular apoptosis to transform into a small telogen follicle (Parrakal, 1990). The telogen phase is the resting stage of the follicle, in which there is an absence of proliferation and differentiation to produce hair, while the hair shaft is retained in the telogen follicle. The telogen follicle maintains epithelial stem cell populations and dermal papilla, specialized mesenchymal cells with the ability to induce the hair follicle (Oliver, 1967; Jahoda *et al.*, 1984). The interaction between follicular epithelial stem cells and the dermal papilla drives regeneration of the next anagen hair follicle to produce new components of the

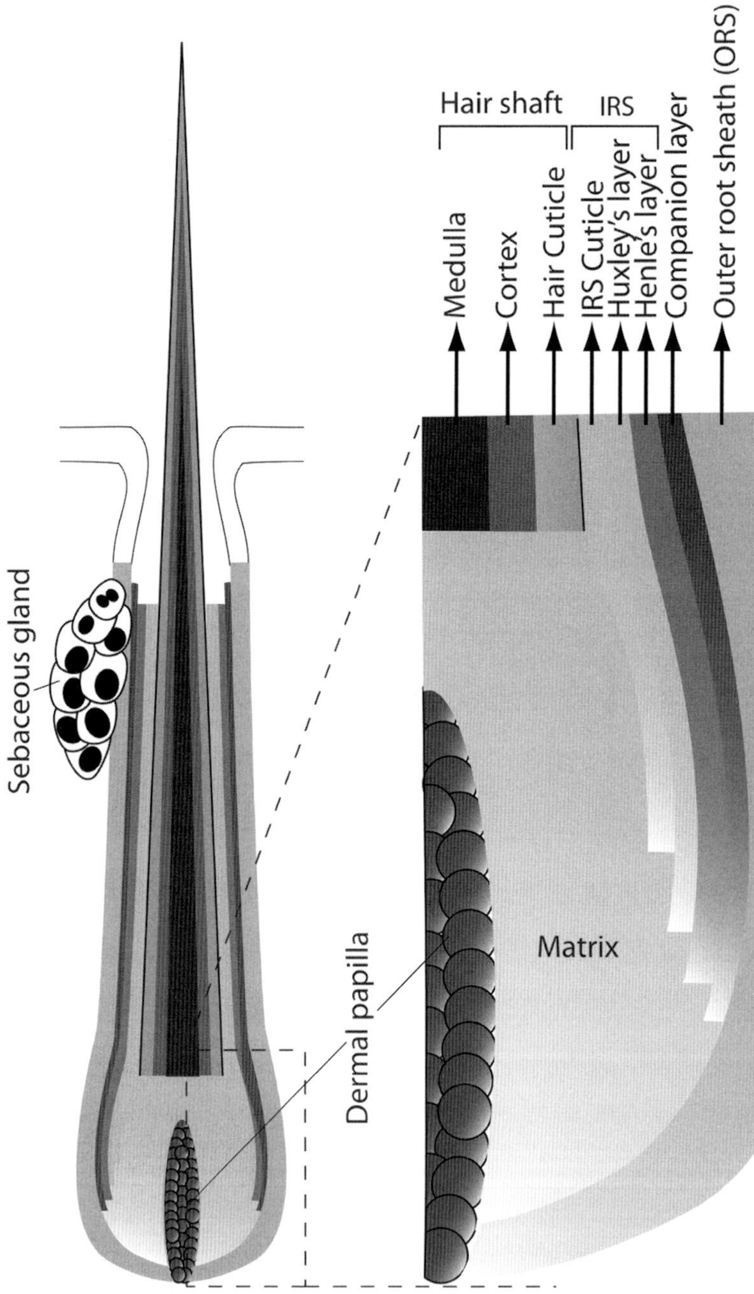

Figure 33.3 Anagen hair follicle. The hair follicle contains many distinct layers. Every time the hair follicle enters the anagen phase, epithelial stem cells regenerate the lower part of the hair follicle located below the sebaceous gland. IRS, inner root sheath.

growing follicle. The old hair which is retained by the telogen follicle eventually falls off after a certain period of time that depends on the species and type of the hair follicle. This shedding phase is called the exogen phase (Paus, 1998; Stenn, 2005). The hair follicle cycles repeatedly through the growth and resting period to replace the hair shaft, which is mediated through the interchange of signals between follicular stem cells and the underlying dermal papilla. In the human, scalp hair follicles stay in the anagen stage for 2–8 years (Paus, 1999), in the catagen stage for a few days to a few weeks, and in the telogen stage for 2–3 months (Paus, 1999). The hair cycle can be disrupted by multiple factors, including injury, infection, physiological stress, pregnancy, and chronological aging. Bald skin from patients with androgenic alopecia typically shows an increased ratio of telogen hair follicles. In the acute phase of alopecia areata, there is a 70%–90% "shift out of anagen" of the hair follicles into the catagen or telogen phase (Stefanato, 2010).

33.3 Basic characteristics of epithelial stem cells in the hair follicle

Stem cells have a self-renewing capacity to reproduce themselves; at the same time they have the ability to give rise to differentiated cells to maintain and regenerate the tissue. Epithelial stem cells have generally been thought to be dormant, in contrast to the rapidly proliferating transit amplifying cells, which undergo a limited number of cell divisions (Potten, *et al.*, 1979; Bickenbach and Mackenzie, 1984; Potten and Morris 1988). Using this theory, epithelial stem cells in the hair follicle were identified as label-retaining cells (LRCs), which were localized to a region of the follicle, known as the bulge (Cotsarelis *et al.*, 1990). The conventional method to detect LRCs involves injecting ^{3}H-thymidine or BrdU to promote uptake of the label by epithelial cells, followed by a chase period, in which transient amplifying cells dilute the label by cell division. Consequently, only slowly cycling cells are detected as LRCs. The detection of LRCs is an important means to identify the epithelial stem cells in the hair follicle. Although the stringency of the ability to distinguish LRCs and rapidly proliferating cells differs depending on the chase period, labels are typically seen in the bulge after a chase of 4–10 weeks (Cotsarelis *et al.*, 1990; Taylor *et al.*, 2000; Braun *et al.*, 2003). Importantly, when skin epidermal cells were transferred to cell culture after labeling LRCs in vivo, these LRCs were shown to have a higher proliferative capacity (Morris and Potten, 1994). Furthermore, the epidermal cells isolated from the dissected bulge area of the vibrissa follicle have a higher colony-forming potential in vitro than do those from the other regions of the hair follicle (Kobayashi *et al.*, 1993). These in-vitro assays are based upon the potential of stem cells to give rise to large number of clones in culture that can be passaged indefinitely, while more differentiated cells do not retain this ability after a finite number of cell divisions (Barrandon and Green, 1987). Additionally, the tissue regenerative potential of epithelial stem cells has been demonstrated by ex-vivo hair reconstitution assays. Typically, this experiment entails isolating specific population of epidermal cells and combining them with neonatal dermal fibroblasts, followed by implantation into the skins of immunodeficient mice (Lichti *et al.*, 1993; Liang *et al.*, 2011). Engraftments that contained bulge epithelial stem cells were shown to form hair follicles in this assay (Morris *et al.*, 2004; Blanpain *et al.*, 2004; Toyoshima *et al.*, 2012). However, it is not known whether the potential ability to regenerate hair follicles is unique to epithelial stem cells, and, if not, how well non-stem cells can be instructed to form hair follicles that are functionally equivalent to those derived from stem cells when sufficient hair follicle inductive stimuli are present. Overall, in-vitro and ex-vivo assays are useful to assess the stem cell potential in a given experimental environment, but there are limitations to these assays since the results might not faithfully reflect actual situations in vivo. Despite this caveat, these experiments, together with in-vivo characterization of stem cell behavior, have contributed significantly to our current understanding of the location and properties of epithelial stem cells in the skin.

In the past decade, the identification of biochemical markers of bulge cells including Keratin 15 (K15), CD34, S100A4, Sox9, TCF3, and NFATc1 has led to significant advances in determining the properties of hair follicle stem cells (Liu *et al.*, 2003; Lyle *et al.*, 1998; Ito *et al.*, 2002; Vidal *et al.*, 2005; Nowak *et al.*, 2008; Trempus *et al.*, 2003; Horsley *et al.*, 2008). Expression of stem cell markers that are known to detect the bulge cells of adult hair follicle does not often overlap, indicating that the epithelial cells within and around the stem cell niche are heterogeneous (Myung and Ito, 2012). The expression levels of biochemical markers in each stem cell may fluctuate within distinct stages of the hair follicle cycle. Addressing how well each marker represents the location of stem cells should ultimately rely on lineage analyses with which the fate of the cells expressing the marker can be traced for a long period of time. Lineage tracing allows us to determine whether the labeled cells can persist over time, attesting to their self-renewing capacity, and how the labeled cells contribute to the hair follicle/skin regeneration. For example, the discovery of K15 expression in the bulge led to the isolation of K15 promoter and demonstration of its utility to target epithelial bulge stem cells in transgenic mice (Liu *et al.*, 2003; Morris *et al.*, 2004). This has permitted one to definitively characterize bulge stem cell behavior utilizing in-vivo experiments that include lineage tracing as well as expression or deletion of genes in $K15^+$ epithelial stem cells. Such experiments have fueled the rapid growth of information on cellular and molecular mechanisms underlying skin homeostasis and regeneration.

33.4 Stem cell contribution to hair follicle regeneration

Stem cells responsible for cyclical regeneration of hair follicle reside in the bulge/secondary hair germ region of the hair follicle. The bulge and secondary hair germ (sHG) cells are located next to each other but are biochemically distinct populations (Ito *et al.*, 2002, 2004). LRCs are detected both in the bulge and in sHG compartments (Ito *et al.*, 2002), and they proliferate at the onset of the anagen phase, leading to an idea that these compartments may be functionally indistinguishable (Ito *et al.*, 2004). This view was challenged by careful examination of the telogen-to-anagen transition of mouse hair follicles, which demonstrated that only sHG cells initiate proliferation and mitosis at the onset of the anagen phase by interacting with dermal papilla (Greco *et al.*, 2009). According to quantitative analysis of the distribution of proliferating cells during the early anagen phase, bulge epithelial stem cells appear to begin their proliferation later, to supply more cells for the hair follicle growth. Because both bulge and sHG stem cells become highly proliferatative in early anagen (Zhang *et al.*, 2009), and exhibit the ability to form hair follicles in hair reconstitution assays ex vivo (Garza *et al.*, 2011), it is assumed that both may contribute to the regeneration of the anagen hair follicle. Interestingly, hair depilation during telogen causes cell death in the bulge, and subsequent hair follicle regeneration appears to rely on the sHG (Ito *et al.*, 2002, 2004). The precise interpretation of how the stem-progenitor population is constituted in the hair follicle and how each population contributes to the hair follicle regeneration will require lineage analyses of each cell type.

The essential role of the bulge/sHG stem cells, which are known to express K15, in maintenance of the hair follicle has been demonstrated by utilizing transgenic mice in which a suicide gene, thymidine kinase, is expressed under a K15 promoter (Ito *et al.*, 2005). This experiment demonstrated that the death of $K15^+$ epithelial stem cells causes eventual loss of hair follicles. However, it is noteworthy that the apoptosis in K15-expressing cells caused the death of animals, due to defects in the gastrointestinal tract. Thus, the requirement for bulge/sHG cells in hair follicle maintenance was demonstrated only after grafting the transgenic skin onto immunodeficient mice. Nevertheless, genetic lineage tracing that followed the fate of K15-expressing cells showed that $K15^+$ cells give rise to all layers of the anagen hair follicle (Morris *et al.*, 2004), clearly demonstrating their contribution to hair follicle regeneration in vivo. In this lineage tracing, K15-expressing cells did not appear to migrate upward to give rise to the cells within the upper follicle or skin epidermis, showing that $K15^+$ cells do not contribute to the maintenance of these compartments of skin epithelium (Ito *et al.*, 2005).

Table 33.1 Epithelial stem cells identified in the hair follicle

Marker	Expression area	Colony-forming ability	Ex-vivo hair reconstitution ability	Lineage tracing	Reference
Lgr6	Lower isthmus	Yes	Yes	Isthmus, hair follicle, hair, sebaceous gland, IFE	Snippert *et al.* (2010), Nath *et al.* (2011)
Lrig1	Isthmus junctional zone	Yes	Yes	Sebaceous gland, IFE	Jensen and Watt, (2006), Jensen *et al.* (2009)
Mts24	Entire isthmus	Yes	NA	NA	Nijhof *et al.* (2006)
Gli1	Upper bulge, bulge, sHG	NA	NA	All hair follicle lineages, IFE after wounding	Brownell *et al.* (2011)
K15	bulge, sHG	Yes	Yes	All hair follicle lineages, IFE after wounding	Cotsarelis *et al.* (1990), Morris *et al.* (2004), Ito *et al.* (2005)

NA, not applicable.

The upper follicle cells located above the bulge are constantly being renewed, just like the interfollicular epidermis. This was apparent from the experiment that showed that, following injection of BrdU, the cells in the basal layer of the upper follicle were extensively labeled with BrdU even during the telogen phase (Taylor, 2000; Ito *et al.*, 2002). Recent studies have identified novel populations of stem cells that may be responsible for maintaining these rapidly renewing areas in the skin epithelium (Table 33.1). Importantly, not all stem cells identified in the upper follicle area are claimed to be quiescent cells, unlike bulge stem cells, which were initially identified as slowly cycling label-retaining cells (Cotsarelis *et al.*, 1990). This may suggest the possibility that the high cycling rate of stem cells and their ability to self-renew need not be mutually exclusive.

33.5 Molecular mechanisms directing epithelial stem cells to regenerate hair follicles

Initial hair follicle development occurs during embryonic development through reciprocal interactions between the epithelium and underlying mesenchyme (Millar, 2002). Current theories suggest that the skin dermis supplies a “first signal” to the overlying epidermis, which leads to the development of hair follicle precursor (i.e. hair placode, hair germ) (Paus *et al.*, 1999). The molecular mechanisms regulating the interaction between inductive dermal papilla and hair germ cells during embryonic development have been extensively characterized through genetic gain and loss of function studies. Most notably, regulators of Wnt/β-catenin, EDAR, FGFR, and BMPR signaling play an important role at this stage to dictate hair follicle specification and patterning (Schmidt-Ullrich, 2005; Millar, 2002). Subsequent reciprocal signals relayed between the epithelial and mesenchymal precursors of the hair follicle coordinate the development of the hair follicle and dermal papilla.

The most fascinating characteristic of the hair follicle is its ability to cyclically undergo follicular morphogenesis through a process that partly recapitulates epithelial–mesenchymal interactions observed during embryonic development of hair follicle. Since genetic and molecular tools were developed to target and profile epithelial cell populations in adult mice (Vasioukhin, 1999; Diamond, 2000; Tumbar, 2004), it has become possible to examine whether and, if so, how, the mechanisms regulating follicular morphogenesis in the embryo are resurrected in the adult skin to regenerate anagen hair follicles.

33.5.1 Wnt signaling

Wnt signaling is activated in the sHG compartment at anagen onset, which is accompanied by up-regulation of several canonical Wnt ligands in this area (Reddy *et al.*, 2001; Greco *et al.*, 2009; Rabbani *et al.*, 2011). Several groups have observed that forced activation of the Wnt signal by expressing stabilized β-catenin in adult basal epithelial cells leads to precocious activation of hair regeneration (Van *et al.*, 2003; Lo *et al.*, 2004; Lowry *et al.*, 2005). In addition, overexpression of Wnt7a in the epidermis results in a faster hair cycling phenotype, due to a shorter telogen phase (Plikus *et al.*, 2011). In support of this, recent studies have demonstrated that Wnt7a injection into telogen skin is sufficient to induce Wnt activation in the sHG area (Rabbani *et al.*, 2011), and that Wnt ligands secreted from $K15^{+}$ epithelial stem cells are necessary for hair follicle regeneration (Myung *et al.*, 2012). These results demonstrate that Wnt/β-catenin plays a key role in signaling in the initiation of anagen follicle regeneration.

33.5.2 BMP signaling

Intriguingly, coinciding with Wnt activation, BMP signaling, which promotes quiescent status of epithelial stem cells (Kobielak *et al.*, 2007), is down-regulated in the niche. This was made evident by the up-regulation of noggin, an antagonist of BMP signaling, in the follicular epithelium and mesenchyme, and down-regulation of its receptor, BMPR-IA in the proliferating cells of the sHG at the onset of the anagen phase (Botchkarev *et al.*, 2001; Zhang *et al.*, 2006). Administration of BMP4 into mice suppresses the entry of the telogen hair follicle into the anagen phase, whereas over-expression of Noggin in transgenic mice promotes this transition (Guha *et al.*, 2004; Plikus *et al.*, 2004, 2008). These experiments established that BMP ligands expressed within (Botchkarev *et al.*, 2001; Greco *et al.*, 2009; Blanpain *et al.*, 2004), or even outside, the niche (Plikus *et al.*, 2008) may be vital factors that maintain the quiescence of bulge/SHG stem cells during telogen. Recently, TGF-β_2, which is secreted by dermal papilla at the end of the telogen phase, was identified as another activator of epithelial stem cells that functions by directly antagonizing BMP signaling in the sHG. Indeed, ablation of the TGF-β pathway significantly extends telogen duration, while intradermal injection of TGF-β_2-soaked beads results in precocious anagen initiation (Oshimori and Fuchs, 2012). This study clearly dissected how molecular signals from the dermal papilla activate adjacent epithelial stem cells, thus offering an elegant image of epithelial–mesenchymal interaction that drives hair follicle regeneration.

33.5.3 FGF signaling

Another potent inhibitor of the telogen–anagen transition is FGF18, which is expressed in the suprabasal layer and basal layer of the bulge region as well as in the dermal papilla of telogen hair follicles. Specific ablation of suprabasal cells in the bulge region that express FGF18 results in precocious anagen onset, which can be blocked by exogenous FGF18 administration (Hsu *et al.*, 2011). Furthermore, upon FGF18 deletion in epithelial cells, including those in the hair follicle, the telogen phase dramatically shortens, definitively demonstrating the potent inhibitory role of FGF18 in anagen induction (Kimura-Ueki *et al.*, 2012). Notably, several other FGF ligands have been reported to be present within and in the vicinity of the epithelial stem cells during the hair cycle transition and appear to play various roles in hair follicle regeneration. For example, injection of exogenous FGF7, which is known to be expressed by the dermal papilla at the end of telogen, into telogen skin induces sHG proliferation and anagen onset (Greco *et al.*, 2009). This may suggest that FGF7 may serve as the "first dermal signal" that activates epithelial stem cells for hair follicle regeneration. Addressing this possibility will require loss-of-function studies to deplete these FGF ligands specifically in dermal papilla cells.

It is important to note that various other genes are differentially expressed at the transition from the telogen to the anagen phase (Greco *et al.*, 2009). Currently it is not well understood how crosstalk between the different pathways, including those discussed above, cooperatively orchestrates the induction of hair follicle regeneration. Further mechanistic details of how the hair follicle cycle is regulated will provide invaluable information to identify novel cellular and molecular targets to control hair growth and regeneration.

33.6 Wound healing and stem cells

Wound healing is a complex process, which involves an inflammatory response, matrix deposition, cellular migration, and proliferation. Crosstalk among numerous types of cells, including keratinocytes, fibroblasts, platelets, macrophages, and endothelial cells, coordinates these processes involved in wound healing (Barrientos *et al.*, 2008). Since stem cells possess a robust potential for proliferation and differentiation for tissue regeneration, examination of stem cell functions during wound healing is expected to identify novel molecular targets to accelerate the wound healing process.

When homeostasis of the skin is disrupted by injury, the skin cell's behavior alters significantly in order to rapidly regenerate/repair the skin. Upon wounding, stem cells activate programs for proliferation and differentiation to repair the tissue. Migration of cells from the hair follicle toward the skin surface has been observed in wounded mouse skin in which bulge epithelial stem cells were tagged by a label-retaining technique (Taylor *et al.*, 2000; Tumbar *et al.*, 2004). Subsequently, Cre recombinase-based lineage tracing analysis has been used to label distinct epithelial populations in the hair follicle using K15 promoter (Ito *et al.*, 2005), Shh promoter (Levy *et al.*, 2005), Lgr6 promoter (Snippert *et al.*, 2010), and Gli1 promoter (Brownell *et al.*, 2011). These approaches have definitively shown that, following wound healing, epithelial stem cells residing in the hair follicle migrate to the skin epidermis. Moreover, the follicle-derived cells proliferate following the migration to the epidermis and express differentiation markers of interfollicular epidermis, indicating that these cells certainly function as skin epidermal cells (Ito *et al.*, 2005).

The molecular mechanisms of how the skin recruits follicular stem cells to contribute to epidermal healing in response to injury remain largely unknown. Importantly, studies have identified several pathways essential for controlling the differentiation fate of the bulge epithelial stem cells. For example, upon depleting the Notch signaling using transgenic mice, K15-expressing bulge cells form cysts that exhibit epidermal characteristics, showing the conversion of the hair follicle to epidermis fate (Yamamoto *et al.*, 2003; Demehri and Kopan, 2009; Vauclair *et al.*, 2005). More recently, a similar cell-fate conversion was observed in another transgenic mouse model that over-expresses DeltaNp63alpha gene, one of the isoforms of Trp63 gene, in the basal layer of skin epithelium including hair follicles (Romano *et al.*, 2010). In this mouse model, overexpression of DeltaNp63alpha in the follicular epithelium leads to the formation of epidermal cysts, adopting an inter-follicular epidermal cell identity. Whether these pathways regulate the processes of cellular movement from the hair follicle to the epidermis during wound healing is still undetermined.

33.7 Toward skin regeneration from skin repair

Whereas the skin has tremendous potential to heal, it does not regenerate in its original form during wound healing. Most strikingly, skin appendages such as sebaceous glands and hair follicles are lacking within the healed area. Only a few experimental models exist to address the question of why adult mammals typically undergo wound repair with a scar instead of "regenerative wound healing."

The possibility that new hair follicles may regenerate following wounding was raised in several early studies (Billingham *et al.*, 1956; Breedis, 1954), but has been generally disregarded due to the lack of evidence for follicular neogenesis (Straile, 1967). We have previously provided definitive evidence showing that de-novo hair follicle regeneration occurs in adult mice, offering a unique opportunity to characterize changes during skin regeneration with skin appendages at cellular and molecular levels (Ito *et al.*, 2007; Fan *et al.*,

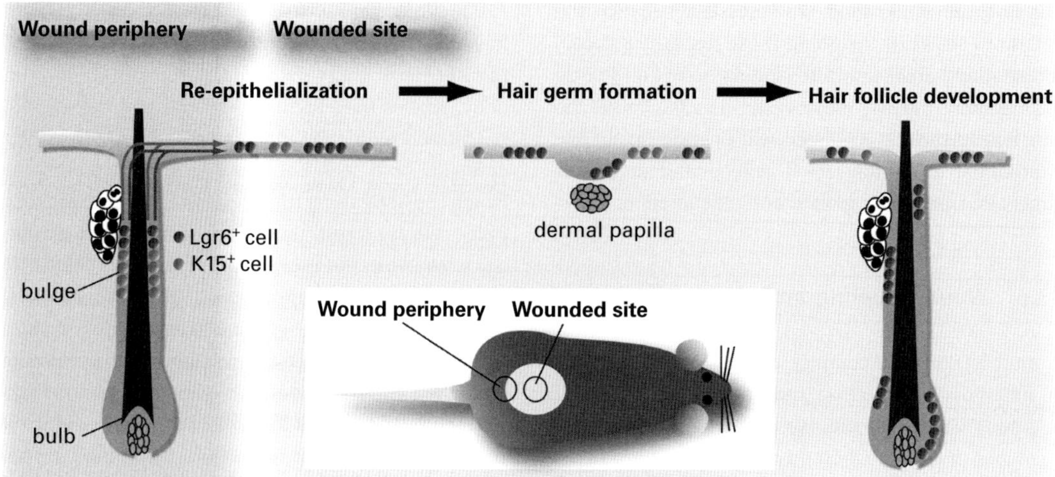

Figure 33.4 Wound-induced hair follicle neogenesis. After wounding, follicular epithelial cells contribute to the completion of the re-epithelialization process. This is followed by de-novo hair germ formation, which is associated with the development of a new dermal papilla within the center of the wound. The de-novo follicular epithelial–mesenchymal complexes then mature into functional hair follicles.

2011). In this wound-induced hair follicle neogenesis model, new hair follicle formation is induced in adult mice following large full-thickness wounds (Figure 33.4). According to the morphological characterization, neogenic hair follicles appear to form in a manner reminiscent of embryonic hair follicle development. Nascent hair germs associated with an underlying dermal dermal papilla first appear within the center of the healed wound shortly after re-epithelialization. These germs develop into mature hair follicles, whose bulge regions are populated with new stem cells that express K15. This allows them to undergo various stages of the hair cycle. K15$^+$ epithelial stem cells from peripheral intact skin do not significantly contribute to neogenic hair follicles, indicating that other epidermal cells have a plasticity to regenerate the hair follicle with a newly established stem cell niche. Recent work has shown that Lgr6$^+$ epithelial stem cells located above the bulge region have the ability to form new hair follicles following wounding (Snippert *et al.*, 2010). The cellular origin of the neogenic dermal papilla remains uncharacterized. Currently, whether or not human skin has a similar potential to regenerate new hair follicles in adult skin remains unknown. In 1950, there was an intriguing report showing that, following epidermal ablation of human adult skin, villus hair follicles, which had been removed, were regenerated in the re-epithelialized area (Kligman, 1956). This requires verification with molecular markers that detect follicular epithelium and dermal papilla before and after the skin abrasion. Nevertheless, this striking observation suggests the important possibility that human skin may also possess the regenerative potential to produce new hair follicles and that this potential may be exhibited under certain conditions.

The molecular mechanism regulating adult hair follicle neogenesis is currently under extensive investigation. Thus far, the essential role of Wnt signaling has been demonstrated by an experiment in which Dkk1, a potent inhibitor of Wnt signaling, is over-expressed in the wound epidermis. In this experiment, the epithelial Dkk1 expression inhibited the de-novo formation of hair germs and dermal papillae in the wound (Ito *et al.*, 2007). More recently, it was reported that Wnt ligand secretion from the wound epidermis is necessary for inducing hair follicle neogenesis (Myung *et al.*, 2012). Investigating the molecular mechanisms that induce formation of new hair follicles from adult skin will have direct implications for the treatment of wounds and baldness, and should help us identify strategies to induce "regenerative wound healing" instead of wound repair with a scar or fibrosis.

ACKNOWLEDGMENT

Ito M. is supported by NIH/NIAM R01AR059768.

REFERENCES

Barrandon, Y. and Green H. 1987. Three clonal types of keratinocyte with different capacities for multiplication. *Proc. Nat. Acad. Sci. USA*, **84**, 2302–6.

Barrientos, S., Stojadinovic, O., Golinko, M. S., Brem, H. and Tomic-Canic, M. 2008. Growth factors and cytokines in wound healing. *Wound Repair Regen.*, **16**, 585–601.

Bickenbach, J. R. and Mackenzie, I. C. 1984. Identification and localization of label-retaining cells in hamster epithelia. *J. Invest. Dermatol.*, **82**, 618–22.

Billingham, R. E. and Russell, P. S. 1956. Incomplete wound contracture and the phenomenon of hair neogenesis in rabbit's skin. *Nature*, **177**, 791–2.

Blanpain, C., Lowry, W. E., Geoghegan, A., Polak, L. and Fuchs, E. 2004. Self-renewal, multipotency, and the existence of two cell populations within an epithelial stem cell niche. *Cell*, **118**, 635–48.

Botchkarev, V. A., Botchkareva, N. V., Nakamura, M. *et al.* 2001. Noggin is required for induction of the hair follicle growth phase in postnatal skin. *FASEB J.*, **15**, 2205–14.

Braun, K. M., Niemann, C., Jensen, U. B. *et al.* 2003. Manipulation of stem cell proliferation and lineage commitment: visualisation of label-retaining cells in wholemounts of mouse epidermis. *Development*, **130**, 5241–55.

Breedis, C. 1954. Regeneration of hair follicles and sebaceous glands from epithelium of scars in the rabbit. *Cancer Res.*, **14**, 575–9

Brownell, I., Guevara, E., Bai, C. B., Loomis, C. A. and Joyner, A. L. 2011. Nerve-derived sonic hedgehog defines a niche for hair follicle stem cells capable of becoming epidermal stem cells. *Cell Stem Cell*, **8**, 552–65.

Chase, H. B., Rauch, R. and Smith, V. W. 1951. Critical stages of hair development and pigmentation in the mouse. *Physiol. Zool.*, **24**, 1–8.

Clayton, E., Doupe, D. P., Klein, A. M. *et al.* 2007. A single type of progenitor cell maintains normal epidermis. *Nature*, **446**, 185–9.

Cotsarelis, G., Sun, T. T. and Lavker, R. M. 1990. Label-retaining cells reside in the bulge area of pilosebaceous unit: implications for follicular stem cells, hair cycle, and skin carcinogenesis. *Cell*, **61**, 1329–37.

Demehri, S. and Kopan, R. 2009. Notch signaling in bulge stem cells is not required for selection of hair follicle fate. *Development*, **136**, 891–6.

Diamond, I., Owolabi, T., Marco, M., Lam, C. and Glick, A. 2000. Conditional gene expression in the epidermis of transgenic mice using the tetracycline-regulated transactivators tTA and rTA linked to the keratin 5 promoter. *J. Invest. Dermatol.*, **115**, 788–94.

Dry, F. W. 1926. The coat of the mouse (*Mus musculus*). *J. Genet.*, **16**, 287–340.

Elias, P. M. and Friend, D. S. 1975. The permeability barrier in mammalian epidermis. *J. Cell. Biol.*, **65**, 180–91.

Fan, C., Luedtke, M. A., Prouty, S. M. *et al.* 2011. Characterization and quantification of wound-induced hair follicle neogenesis using in vivo confocal scanning laser microscopy. *Skin Res. Technol.*, **17**, 387–97

Garza, L. A., Yang, C. C., Zhao, T. *et al.* 2011. Bald scalp in men with androgenetic alopecia retains hair follicle stem cells but lacks CD200-rich and CD34-positive hair follicle progenitor cells. *J. Clin. Invest.*, **121**, 613–22.

Greco, V., Chen, T., Rendl, M. *et al.* 2009. A two-step mechanism for stem cell activation during hair regeneration. *Cell Stem Cell*, **4**, 155–69.

Guha, U., Mecklenburg, L., Cowin, P. *et al.* 2004. Bone morphogenetic protein signaling regulates postnatal hair follicle differentiation and cycling. *Am. J. Pathol.*, **165**, 729–40.

Horsley, V., Aliprantis, A. O., Polak, L., Glimcher, L. H. and Fuchs, E. 2008. NFATc1 balances quiescence and proliferation of skin stem cells. *Cell*, **132**, 299–310.

Hsu, Y. C., Pasolli, H. A. and Fuchs, E. 2011. Dynamics between stem cells, niche, and progeny in the hair follicle. *Cell*, **144**, 92–105.

Ito, M., Kizawa, K., Hamada, K. and Cotsarelis, G. 2004. Hair follicle stem cells in the lower bulge form the secondary germ, a biochemically distinct but functionally equivalent progenitor cell population, at the termination of catagen. *Differentiation*, **72**, 548–57.

Ito, M., Kizawa, K., Toyoda, M. and Morohashi, M. 2002. Label-retaining cells in the bulge region are directed to cell death after plucking, followed by healing from the surviving hair germ. *J. Invest. Dermatol.*, **119**, 1310–16.

Ito, M., Liu, Y., Yang, Z. *et al.* 2005. Stem cells in the hair follicle bulge contribute to wound repair but not to homeostasis of the epidermis. *Nature Med.*, **11**, 1351–54.

Ito, M., Yang, Z., Andl, T. *et al.* 2007. Wnt-dependent de novo hair follicle regeneration in adult mouse skin after wounding. *Nature*, **447**, 316–20.

Jahoda, C. A. B., Horne, K. A. and Oliver, R. F. 1984. Induction of hair growth by implantation of cultured dermal papilla cells. *Nature*, **311**, 560–2.

Jensen, K. B., Collins, C. A., Nascimento, E. *et al.* 2009. Lrig1 expression defines a distinct multipotent stem cell population in mammalian epidermis. *Cell Stem Cell*, **4**, 427–39.

Jensen, K. B. and Watt, F. M. 2006. Single-cell expression profiling of human epidermal stem and transit-amplifying cells: Lrig1 is a regulator of stem cell quiescence. *Proc. Nat. Acad. Sci. USA*, **103**, 11958–63.

Jones, P. H., Simons, B. D. and Watt, F. M. 2007. *Sic transit gloria*: farewell to the epidermal transit amplifying cell? *Cell Stem Cell*, **1**, 371–81.

Jones, P. H. and Watt, F. M. 1993. Separation of human epidermal stem cells from transit amplifying cells on the basis of differences in integrin function and expression. *Cell*, **73**, 713–24.

Kaur, P. and Li, A. 2000. Adhesive properties of human basal epidermal cells: an analysis of keratinocyte stem cells, transit amplifying cells, and postmitotic differentiating cells. *J. Invest. Dermatol.*, **11**, 413–20.

Kimura-Ueki, M., Oda, Y., Oki, J. *et al.* 2012. Hair cycle resting phase is regulated by cyclic epithelial FGF18 signaling. *J. Invest. Dermatol.*, **132**, 1338–45.

Kligman, A. M. and Strauss, J. S. 1956. The formation of vellus hair follicles from human adult epidermis. *J. Invest. Dermatol.*, **27**, 19–23.

Kobielak, K., Stokes, N., de la Cruz, J., Polak, L. and Fuchs, E. 2007. Loss of a quiescent niche but not follicle stem cells in the absence of bone morphogenetic protein signaling. *Proc. Nat. Acad. Sci. USA*, **104**, 10063–8

Kobayashi, K., Rochat, A. and Barrandon, Y. 1993. Segregation of keratinocyte colony-forming cells in the bulge of the rat vibrissa. *Proc. Nat. Acad. Sci. USA*, **90**, 7391–5.

Levy, V., Lindon, C., Harfe, B. D. and Morgan, B. A. 2005. Distinct stem cell populations regenerate the follicle and interfollicular epidermis. *Dev. Cell*, **9**, 855–61.

Liang, Y., Silva, K. A., Kennedy, V. and Sundberg, J. P. 2011. Comparisons of mouse models for hair follicle reconstitution. *Exp. Dermatol.*, **20**, 1011–15

Lichti, U., Weinberg, W. C., Goodman, L. *et al.* 1993. In vivo regulation of murine: hair growth: insights from grafting defined cell populations onto nude mice. *J. Invest. Dermatol.*, **101**, 124S–129S.

Liu, Y., Lyle, S., Yang, Z. and Cotsarelis, G. 2003. Keratin 15 promoter targets putative epithelial stem cells in the hair follicle bulge. *J. Invest. Dermatol.*, **121**, 963–8.

Lo Celso, C., Prowse, D. M. and Watt, F. M. 2004. Transient activation of β-catenin signalling in adult mouse epidermis is sufficient to induce new hair follicles but continuous activation is required to maintain hair follicle tumours. *Development*, **131**, 1787–99.

Lowry, W. E., Blanpain, C., Nowak, J. A. 2005. Defining the impact of β-catenin/Tcf transactivation on epithelial stem cells. *Genes Dev.*, **19**, 1596–611.

Lyle, S., Christofidou-Solomidou, M., Liu, Y. *et al.* 1998. The C8/144B monoclonal antibody recognizes cytokeratin 15 and defines the location of human hair follicle stem cells. *J. Cell Sci.*, **111**(21), 3179–88.

Mackenzie, I. C. 1970. Relationship between mitosis and the ordered structure of the stratum corneum in mouse epidermis. *Nature*, **226**, 653–5.

Mascré, G., Dekoninck, S., Drogat, B. 2012. Distinct contribution of stem and progenitor cells to epidermal maintenance. *Nature*, **489**, 257–62.

Millar, S. E. 2002. Molecular mechanisms regulating hair follicle development. *J. Invest. Dermatol.*, **118**, 216–25.

Morris, R. J., Liu, Y., Marles, L. *et al.* 2004. Capturing and profiling adult hair follicle stem cells. *Nature Biotechnol.*, **22**, 411–17.

Morris, R. J. and Potten, C. S. 1994. Slowly cycling (label-retaining) epidermal cells behave like clonogenic stem cells in vitro. *Cell Prolif.*, **27**, 279–89.

Muller-Rover, S., Handjiski, B., van der Veen, C. *et al.* 2001. A comprehensive guide for the accurate classification of murine hair follicles in distinct hair cycle stages. *J. Invest. Dermatol.*, **117**, 3–15.

Myung, P. and Ito, M. 2012. Dissecting the bulge in hair regeneration. *J. Clin. Invest.*, **122**, 448–54.

Myung, P. S., Takeo, M., Ito, M. and Atit, R. P. 2013. Epithelial Wnt ligand secretion is required for adult hair follicle growth and regeneration. *J. Invest. Dermatol.*, **133**(1), 31–41.

Nath, M., Offers, M., Hummel, M. and Seissler, J. 2011. Isolation and in vitro expansion of Lgr6-positive multipotent hair follicle stem cells. *Cell Tissue Res.*, **344**, 435–44.

Nijhof, J. G., Braun, K. M., Giangreco, A. *et al.* 2006. The cell-surface marker MTS24 identifies a novel population of follicular keratinocytes with characteristics of progenitor cells. *Development*, **133**, 3027–37.

Nowak, J. A., Polak, L., Pasolli, H. A. and Fuchs, E. 2008. Hair follicle stem cells are specified and function in early skin morphogenesis. *Cell Stem Cell*, **3**, 33–43.

Oliver, R. F. 1967. The experimental induction of whisker growth in the hooded rat by implantation of dermal papillae. *J. Embryol. Exp. Morphol.*, **18**, 43–51.

Oshimori, N. and Fuchs, E. 2012. Paracrine TGF-β signaling counterbalances BMP-mediated repression in hair follicle stem cell activation. *Cell Stem Cell*, **10**, 63–75.

Parakkal, P. F. 1990. Catagen and telogen phases of the growth cycle. In Orfanos, C. E. and Happle, R., editors. *Hair and Hair Diseases*. Berlin: Springer-Verlag, pp. 99–116.

Paus, R. 1998. Principles of hair cycle control. *J. Dermatol.*, **25**, 793–802.

Paus, R. and Cotsarelis, G. 1999. The biology of hair follicles. *New Engl. J. Med.*, **341**, 491–7.

Paus, R., Muller-Rover, S., Van Der Veen, C. *et al.* 1999. A comprehensive guide for the recognition and classification of distinct stages of hair follicle morphogenesis. *J. Invest. Dermatol.*, **113**, 523–32.

Plikus, M., Wang, W. P., Liu, J. *et al.* 2004. Morpho-regulation of ectodermal organs: integument pathology and phenotypic variations in K14-Noggin engineered mice through modulation of bone morphogenic protein pathway. *Am. J. Pathol.*, **164**, 1099–114.

Plikus, M. V., Baker, R. E., Chen, C. C. *et al.* 2011. Self-organizing and stochastic behaviors during the regeneration of hair stem cells. *Science*, **332**, 586–9.

Plikus, M. V., Mayer, J. A., de la Cruz, D. *et al.* 2008. Cyclic dermal BMP signalling regulates stem cell activation during hair regeneration. *Nature*, **451**, 340–4.

Potten, C. S. 1974. The epidermal proliferative unit: the possible role of the central basal cell. *Cell Tissue Kinet.*, **7**, 77–88.

Potten, C. S., Hume, W. J., Reid, P. and Cairns, J. 1978. Segregation of DNA in epithelial stem-cells. *Cell*, **15**, 899–906.

Potten, C. S. and Morris, R. J. 1988. Epithelial stem cells in vivo. *J. Cell Sci. Suppl.*, **10**, 45–62.

Rabbani, P., Takeo, M., Chou, W. *et al.* 2011. Coordinated activation of Wnt in epithelial and melanocyte stem cells initiates pigmented hair regeneration. *Cell*, **145**, 941–55.

Reddy, S., Andl, T., Bagasra, A. *et al.* 2001. Characterization of Wnt gene expression in developing and postnatal hair follicles and identification of Wnt5a as a target of Sonic hedgehog in hair follicle morphogenesis. *Mech. Dev.*, **107**, 69–82.

Romano, R. A., Smalley, K., Liu, S. and Sinha, S. 2010. Abnormal hair follicle development and altered cell fate of follicular keratinocytes in transgenic mice expressing DeltaNp63alpha. *Development*, **137**, 1431–9.

Schmidt-Ullrich, R. and Paus, R. 2005. Molecular principles of hair follicle induction and morphogenesis. *Bioessays*, **27**, 247–61.

Snippert, H. J., Haegebarth, A., Kasper, M. *et al.* 2010. Lgr6 marks stem cells in the hair follicle that generate all cell lineages of the skin. *Science*, **327**, 1385–9.

Stefanato, C. M. 2010. Histopathology of alopecia: a clinicopathological approach to diagnosis. *Histopathology*, **56**, 24–38

Stenn, K. 2005. Exogen is an active, separately controlled phase of the hair growth cycle. *J. Am. Acad. Dermatol.*, **52**, 374–5.

Straile, W. E. 1967. Dermal-epithelial interactions in sensory hair follicles. In Montagna, W. and Dobson R., editors. *Advances in Biology of Skin*, Vol. 9 New York: Pergamon Press, pp. 369–91.

Tani, H., Morris, R. J. and Kaur, P. 2000. Enrichment for murine keratinocyte stem cells based on cell surface phenotype. *Proc. Nat. Acad. Sci. USA*, **26**, 10960–5.

Taylor, G., Lehrer, M. S., Jensen, P. J., Sun, T. T. and Lavker, R. M. 2000. Involvement of follicular stem cells in forming not only the follicle but also the epidermis. *Cell*, **102**, 451–61.

Toyoshima, K. E., Asakawa, K., Ishibashi, N. *et al.* 2012. Fully functional hair follicle regeneration through the rearrangement of stem cells and their niches. *Nature Commun.*, **17**, 784.

Trempus., C. S., Morris, R. J., Bortner, C. D. *et al.* 2003. Enrichment for living murine keratinocytes from the hair follicle bulge with the cell surface marker CD34. *J. Invest. Dermatol.*, **120**, 501–11.

Tumbar, T., Guasch, G., Greco, V. *et al.* 2004. Defining the epithelial stem cell niche in skin. *Science*, **303**, 359–63.

Van Mater, D., Kolligs, F. T., Dlugosz, A. A. and Fearon, E. R. 2003. Transient activation of β-catenin signaling in cutaneous keratinocytes is sufficient to trigger the active growth phase of the hair cycle in mice. *Genes Dev.*, **17**, 1219–24.

Vasioukhin, V., Degenstein, L., Wise, B. and Fuchs, E. 1999. The magical touch: genome targeting in epidermal stem cells induced by tamoxifen application to mouse skin. *Proc. Nat. Acad. Sci. USA*, **96**, 8551–6.

Vauclair, S., Nicolas, M., Barrandon, Y. and Radtke, F. 2005. Notch1 is essential for postnatal hair follicle development and homeostasis. *Dev. Biol.*, **284**, 184–93.

Vidal, V. P., Chaboissier, M. C., Lutzkendorf, S. *et al.* 2005. Sox9 is essential for outer root sheath differentiation and the formation of the hair stem cell compartment. *Curr. Biol.*, **15**, 1340–51.

Watt, F. M. 2001. Stem cell fate and patterning in mammalian epidermis. *Curr. Opin. Genet. Dev.*, **11**, 410–17.

Yamamoto, N., Tanigaki, K., Han, H., Hiai, H. and Honjo, T. 2003. Notch/RBP-J signaling regulates epidermis/hair fate determination of hair follicular stem cells. *Curr. Biol.*, **13**, 333–8.

Zhang, J., He, X. C., Tong, W. G. *et al.* 2006. Bone morphogenetic protein signaling inhibits hair follicle anagen induction by restricting epithelial stem/progenitor cell activation and expansion. *Stem Cells*, **24**, 2826–39.

Zhang, Y. V., Cheong, J., Ciapurin, N., McDermitt, D. J. and Tumbar, T. 2009. Distinct self-renewal and differentiation phases in the niche of infrequently dividing hair follicle stem cells. *Cell Stem Cell*, **53**, 267–78.

34

In-vitro blood vessel regeneration

Sashka Dimitrievska and Laura E. Niklason

34.1 Introduction

In the USA, 40% of all deaths are caused by cardiovascular disease. More than half of these incidents are a direct result of coronary artery disease [1]. In an effort to decrease the mortality from coronary heart disease, more than 500,000 coronary artery bypass procedures are performed annually [1]. The coronary artery lumen's inner diameter (ID) is about 4 mm at most, requiring a similarly small-diameter conduit to bypass the blocked artery. The most successful vascular conduit is the patient's own blood vessel, most commonly the greater saphenous vein in the leg or the internal mammary artery. However, autologous vessels are often unavailable to patients in need of a vascular graft replacement, due to prior harvesting or disease-associated vascular damage.

In search of an alternative vascular replacement, at the beginning of the twentieth century allografts were developed as the first valid vascular replacement. However allografts' limited long-term success due to aneurysm, calcification, and thrombosis, in addition to low availability and concerns relating to infectious diseases, have hindered their clinical acceptance [2, 3]. The allografts' shortcomings in small-diameter vascular applications led to the development of synthetic substitutes in the 1950s. Despite the polymers' thrombogenic surface and lack of compliance, they demonstrated acceptable long-term performance in large-diameter vessels (ID $>$ 6 mm). However, polymeric grafts are inadequate when used in medium- or small-diameter applications.

34.1.1 Biology of small-diameter vascular grafts: regeneration and failures

Although large-diameter vessel substitutes are rather successful, small-vessel replacement poses a different set of problems that is not encountered in large-caliber arterial substitutes. When blood from native vessels comes into contact with an implanted graft, a number of defense mechanisms are initiated. The most prominent defense mechanism is the coagulation system, which results in thrombus formation at the graft surface. Surface thrombus formation eventually leads to thrombotic graft failure, a failure risk that is substantially increased in small-diameter grafts. First, the increased graft-surface-to-blood-volume ratio in smaller-diameter grafts results in increased activation of blood elements. The reduced blood flow in small vessels can also cause an increase in contact time with the luminal graft surfaces. Also, mismatch between the graft's and the native blood vessel's mechanical properties creates local discontinuities in blood-flow velocity, resulting in potentially stagnant regions of blood flow, which in turn adds to the graft's thrombogenicity.

34.1.2 Human blood vessel engineering

Over the past several decades, tissue-engineered vascular grafts (TEVGs) have been studied as a means to integrate with native vasculature and maintain patency in small-diameter applications (Figure 34.1). Different approaches have resulted in important advancements of the field, all by conceptually striving to mimic similar parameters. First, the graft must offer a

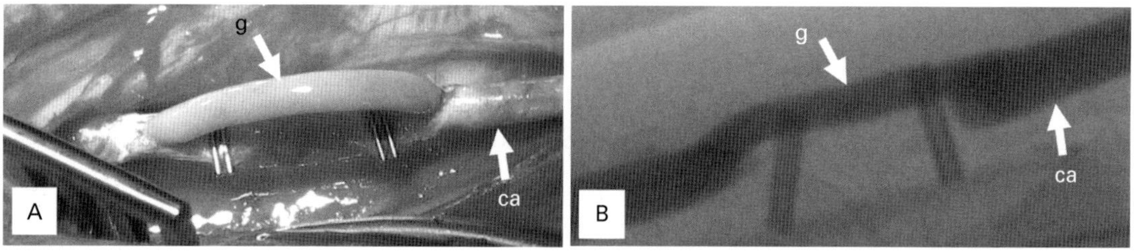

Figure 34.1 (A) A pre-clinical trial example of a canine cell-derived 3-mm TEVG implanted as a carotid bypass. The label g on the image is the demonstration that the graft was patent (open to flow), while metal clips occlude the intervening carotid artery (ca). (B) A computed tomography scan shows a patent graft (g) with no dilatation a month after implantation. (Reproduced with permission from the authors [3].)

non-thrombogenic surface and mechanical properties that match those of native vessels, while at the same time being built from native-tissue-based materials to facilitate regeneration. Second, the conduit size of the TEVG must match the diameter of the native vessel it is replacing (i.e. ID $\leq$ 6 mm). Finally, irrespective of the production strategy used, the approach must demonstrate manufacturing consistency, which can be a challenge with cell-based approaches.

This chapter is focussed on the scaffolding and cell approaches that have been developed since the inception of TEVGs. Although animal models that have demonstrated promising strategies are also discussed, the emphasis is on strategies that have resulted in clinical implementation or pre-clinical trials.

34.2 Biomaterial scaffolds for guided three-dimensional endothelial tissue-like organization

There are several approaches to developing a three-dimensional (3D) scaffold for tissue-engineered vessels. The ideal scaffold has to provide a template for smooth muscle cell (SMC) and endothelial cell (EC) growth/migration and extracellular matrix (ECM) secretion. If implanted as a structural element of the graft, the scaffold must also possess the mechanical strength and compliance necessary to withstand pulsatile pressures of the vascular system. To date, the approaches that have had most success are based on one or a combination of the following four main types of scaffold: degradable polymeric scaffolds, ECM-based scaffolds, cell sheets (which contain little or no synthetic scaffold material), and decellularized scaffolds.

34.2.1 Degradable polymeric scaffolds

The most commonly used degradable polymer scaffolds in vascular regeneration are made from polycaprolactone (PCL), polyglycolic acid (PGA), polylactic acid (PLA), and their derivatives and copolymers. Polymers are synthesized under conditions that are too harsh for cell survival (high pressures or often vacuum, high temperatures, high acidity . . .), making cellular entrapment into the scaffold during scaffold synthesis impossible. Instead, the scaffold is built from woven or non-woven polymeric fibers, and then molded into a 3D tubular hollow structure with large pore diameter. Cells are then seeded onto the 3D tubular scaffold and allowed to invade the scaffold through the large scaffold pores. Ideally, the progress of cellular invasion and tissue deposition matches the resorption of the polymer over time. In other words, the scaffold provides the initial mechanical strength for the graft in vitro until the cells have synthesized significant amounts of ECM. In comparison with the other approaches discussed in this chapter, polymer scaffolds are easily available, cheap, and have minimal batch-to-batch variation. In addition, polymeric scaffolds offer customizable control over the scaffold microstructure, mechanical properties, and resorption rates, via modulation of the chemical parameters and the 3D geometry of the polymer.

Niklason and co-workers demonstrated one of the most successful applications of this approach in 1999 [4]. A degradable PGA scaffold is wrapped around a

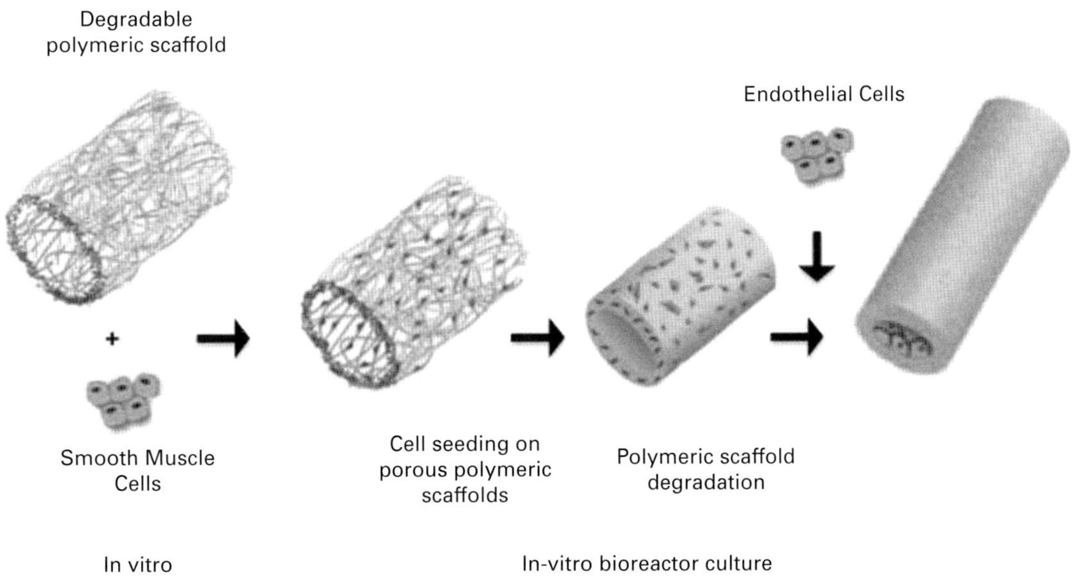

Figure 34.2 A schematic representation of vascular grafts built from degradable polymer scaffolds. Cells are seeded onto a porous polymer scaffold, and then cultured in a bioreactor inducing production of extracellular matrix proteins. The polymeric scaffold degrades with time, and the resulting tissue-based graft can be lined with endothelial cells on the luminal side prior to implantation.

distensible silicone tube inside a bioreactor, which imparts pulsatile pressures by cyclically inflating the silicone tubing. The PGA tubular grafts are seeded with SMCs and cultured for 8 weeks. The PGA scaffold initially withstands the stresses of pulsatile flow, but loses strength as it gradually degrades over the first few weeks, thereby loading the cells with physiological stresses. This stimulates the cells to synthesize substantial amounts of ECM, thereby achieving sufficient mechanical strength in the absence of the PGA scaffold. After 8 weeks of culture in a pulsatile bioreactor the silicone tubes are removed, and ECs are seeded on the luminal surface of the grafts [5]. The vessels have demonstrated promising patency rates following implantation in large-animal models [4]. This approach produced vascular grafts having burst pressures and suture retention strengths (mechanical parameters used to describe TEVGs) comparable to those of native human saphenous veins after only 8 weeks of culture. Additionally, the engineered vessels demonstrated a gross appearance identical to that of native arteries.

Multiple groups have adopted this degradable-scaffold approach, where the main advances have been modifications of the original PGA cell scaffold by copolymerization and surface modifications [6–8]. The Shin'oka team has used a degradable polymer scaffold in a similar approach for vascular reconstruction. The group designed a custom tubular scaffold composed of polycaprolactone–polylactic acid copolymer (weight ratio 1:1), reinforced with a woven PGA polymer scaffold [5]. In addition, the step of pre-culturing cells on the scaffold is entirely omitted, and instead autologous cells are simply pre-seeded onto the scaffold and directly implanted into patients with pediatric congenital heart defects in the low-pressure circulation [6]. Because of the lack of pre-cell-culture time, these implants lack the structural properties conferred by ECM at the time of implantation, making them suitable only for low-pressure vessels.

34.2.2 Extracellular matrix- and protein-based scaffolds

This approach of using purified forms of ECM proteins relies on the idea that embedding cells in ECM mimics native vasculature. The ECM scaffold provides stimuli

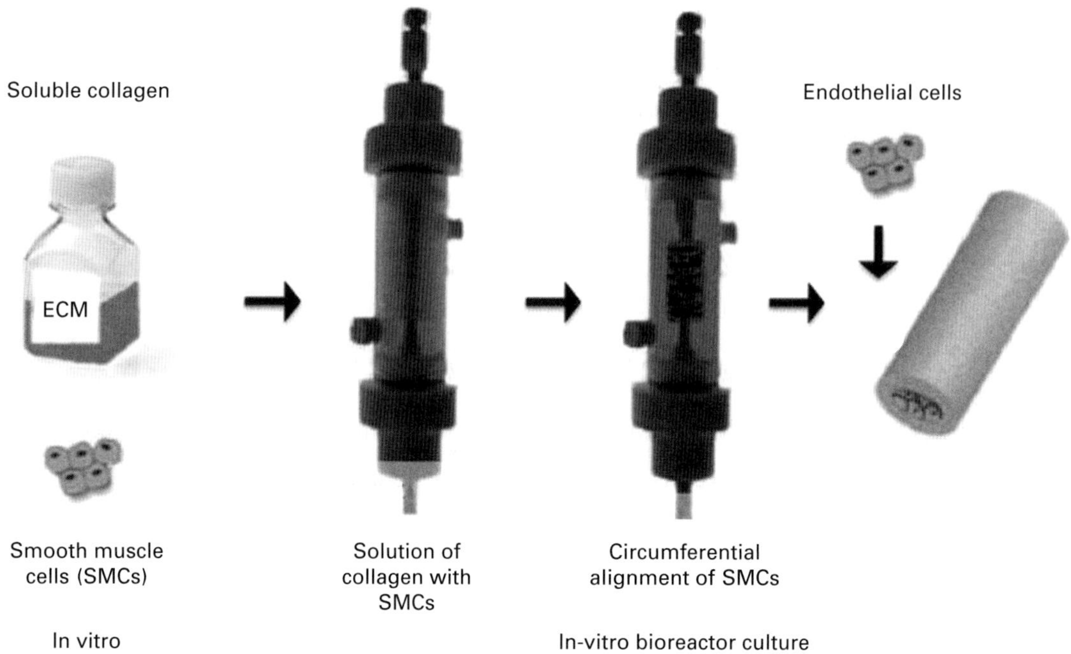

Figure 34.3 A schematic representation of TEVGs built on extracellular matrix- and protein-based scaffolds. In this example smooth muscle cells and solubilized extracellular matrix are injected into a tubular mold as a solution. The cells remodel the extracellular matrix around the tubular mold, producing a vascular tissue. Endothelial cells can be seeded on the luminal side prior to implantation.

recognized by vascular cells, allowing them to bind, migrate through the scaffold, and remodel or secrete more ECM as needed (Figure 34.2). The major structural components of native blood vessels, collagen (type I and type III) and elastin, are the main candidates for ECM scaffold approaches. However, type III collagen is difficult to isolate, and solubilized elastin does not form gels very well, making type I collagen the most popular protein for ECM scaffold construction. In comparison with polymeric scaffolds, where the cells are seeded after scaffold synthesis, ECM components are prepared in a gel-like solution, allowing direct cellularization of the ECM scaffold. This can be accomplished by injecting the cell suspension and solubilized collagen combination into a tubular mold, where the collagen-based gel solidifies under physiological conditions, thereby entrapping the cells (Figure 34.3). Although this was the first TEVG strategy (being reported in the literature by Weinberg and Bell in 1986), the low mechanical strength of collagen gels and limited ECM deposition by the cultured cells resulted in weak grafts that cannot support the physical loads of the cardiovascular system [9]. For reference, native human saphenous veins have a burst pressure of ≈2000 mm Hg, while collagen gels yield at about 40 mm Hg [10, 11].

Many strategies have been developed in attempts to improve the mechanical properties of the collagen gel scaffolds [12]. One approach has been the use of degradable mesh-like reinforcing "sleeves" that provide mechanical strength while the cells deposit appropriate amounts of ECM and gradually reabsorb the degradable polymer [12]. Other groups have attempted to replace the collagen with fibrin gels fabricated from fibrinogen and thrombin [13–15]. However, despite the multitude of attempts at strengthening the ECM-based gels through the use of glycation, crosslinking of the matrices, or dynamic

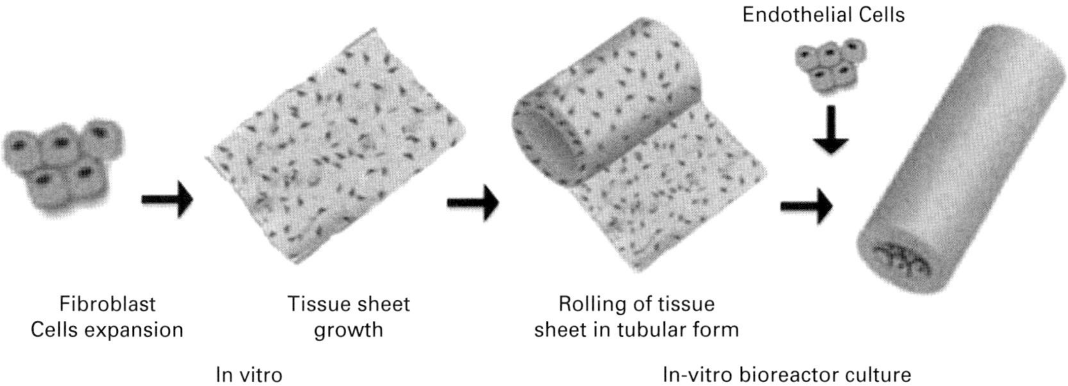

Figure 34.4 A schematic representation of TEVGs built from rolled flat sheets of fibroblast. In this example fibroblast cells sheets are produced under elevated ascorbic acid culture growth conditions. The cell sheets are then rolled around a tubular mandrel forming a tubular conduit that can be lined with endothelial cells on the luminal side prior to implantation.

mechanical stimulation in vitro, the resulting TEVGs still suffer from poor mechanical properties [16]. Irrespective of the strengthening approach used, carotid arteries have burst strengths 30–50 times higher than those of the collagen-based constructs [11, 17].

34.2.3 Cell sheets

It can be argued that the most appropriate scaffold is the one produced by the cells themselves, obviating the need for an externally supplied scaffold. L'Heureux and colleagues created a completely biological TEVG with impressive mechanical properties through a cell-sheet approach that does not use exogenous scaffolds [18] (Figure 34.4). Autologous dermal fibroblasts are grown on culture plates in the presence of an elevated concentration of ascorbic acid (to increase collagen synthesis), to produce fibroblast sheets embedded in fibrillar collagenous ECM. The sheets are then wrapped around a tubular porous mandrel, allowing the individual plies to fuse together, creating tubular structures. The tubular structures are removed from the mandrel and seeded with autologous ECs, which are harvested from a peripheral vein. Cell-sheet TEVGs underwent a first successful human clinical trial in three patients, and a second human trial in 10 patients as hemodialysis access implants [19]. Although this clinical trial did not assess the graft's efficacy at small diameters, it demonstrated the implants' initial safety and mechanical properties. However, this approach utilizes all autologous cells and requires a 6–9-month culture period. This long lead time associated with the production of an autologous cell-based vascular graft prevents the clinical use of the grafts in emergency coronary artery bypass surgery and critically ischemic limbs, both of which are common small-diameter vascular graft needs.

34.2.4 Decellularized scaffolds

An emerging trend is the development of acellular scaffold approaches that provide a native ECM, as opposed to protein-based gels. This is typically accomplished by removing the cells (i.e. decellularization) from tissues that are vascular, non-vascular (e.g. small-intestinal submucosa), or tissue-engineered in origin (Figure 34.5). Decellularization is accomplished by washing the tissues with a combination of detergents, protease inhibitors, and buffers, sparing only the ECM. When preparing the scaffold in this manner, cellular antigens that are responsible for foreign recognition are removed, creating a species-conserved and well-tolerated ECM structure [20]. The starting mechanical properties of the tissues are mostly retained, provided that the decellularization process does not alter the ECM structure and composition [3, 21].

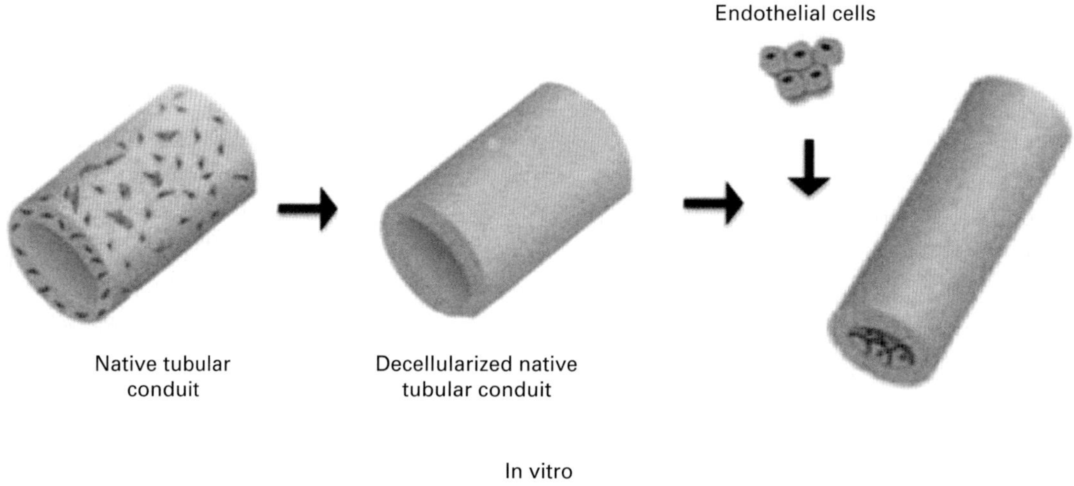

Figure 34.5 A schematic representation of TEVGs built from decellularized natural tissues to produce vascular scaffolds. A native tubular conduit (small-intestinal submucosa, artery, or vein) is decellularized, removing cellular antigens. The decellularized, tubular scaffold is then seeded with endothelial cells on the luminal side prior to implantation to prevent thrombosis.

Hence, support for decellularized vascular grafts stems from the lack of immunological reaction (if the ECM is of the same species as the recipient), the production of mechanically compliant grafts, and ready availability to patients who require expeditious intervention. This is an important advance in the vascular regeneration field, where cellular products cannot be stored in the long term and are custom-made for each patient.

In larger-diameter vessels, decellularized grafts could be implanted without cells, assuming that they will be recellularized by host cells following implantation [3]. For small-diameter applications, the thrombogenicity issue is more important. One current approach is to recellularize the "empty" tissue matrix on the luminal side with autologous ECs, creating a non-thrombogenic lumen before implantation. In 1978, Herring introduced a single-stage technique for EC seeding on prosthetic materials. ECs that were harvested from vein segments by scraping the luminal surface were directly seeded on polymeric implants [22]. Since then, it has been shown that up to 95% of seeded cells are lost in the first 24 hours after-implantation due to the pulsatile flow [23]. A currently favored method for creating endothelial lining of grafts is the "two-stage" strategy, whereby the extracted ECs undergo ex-vitro cell expansion before dense luminal seeding, and sometimes further bioreactor graft–EC culture before implantation. Using this approach, Teebken and colleagues seeded ECs and myofibroblasts from human saphenous veins on decellularized porcine aortas, resulting in vessel grafts with stable biomechanical properties [24]. Similarly encouraging results were obtained by others by seeding human umbilical vein ECs and adult human vascular SMCs onto decellularized porcine aortas [25, 26]. Quint and coworkers used a completely tissue-engineered vessel that was decellularized and seeded with endothelial progenitor cells (EPCs) isolated from peripheral blood [27]. When implanted in the pig carotid model, the EPC- and EC-seeded decellularized tissue-engineered vessel outperformed the vein graft by demonstrating a higher patency rate (100% vs. 38%), with a trend toward a lower neointimal response [27].

34.2.4.1 Native decellularized scaffolds of animal and human origin

A decellularized, non-vascular scaffold that has been extensively studied for more than two decades is the porcine-derived small-intestinal submucosa (SIS) [21]. This matrix is prepared by mechanically removing the mucosa and muscle from the small intestine, followed by a decellularization step. In a variety of soft-tissue applications, flat-sheet decellularized SIS is a successfully used clinical biomaterial. Unsurprisingly, SIS tubular grafts have been extensively studied as a vascular conduit material in animal models [28, 29]. In dog models, high patency rates have been reported in the aorta, in the carotid artery, and in the superior vena cava [28]. However, despite encouraging results from animal studies, early thrombosis (within 48 hours of implantation), low wall stability with subsequent aneurysm formation, the lack of elastic elements, and the probability of rupture hindered the SIS scaffolds' success as a small-diameter vessel graft [30, 31].

Because of their similarity in size to small-diameter human vessels, arteries and veins of human cadavers (allografts) and ureters of porcine origin (xenografts) have become commonly used vascular decellularized scaffolds. Xenograft heart valves of porcine origin treated with glutaraldehyde and mounted in a rigid stent are the most widely used cardiac bioprostheses. The xenografts' success as heart valves motivated the investigation of decellularized porcine matrices as scaffolds for small-diameter vascular grafts. The mechanical properties (tensile strength, compliance, and burst pressures) of decellularized porcine ureter scaffolds (<6 mm diameter) were examined and found to be comparable to those of fresh human saphenous vein samples [32]. Although the decellularization procedure does not affect the biomechanical properties of the xenograft scaffolds, the significant glycosaminoglycan content loss after decellularization ($\approx$60% loss of glycosaminoglycans, including heparan suflate proteoglycans) creates a thrombogenic surface, which is of special significance in small-diameter vessels. In addition the decellularization procedure exposes collagen, which is one of the most thrombogenic components of the sub-endothelial matrix responsible for the initiation of platelet adhesion [33]. This explains the observations in which EC-seeded porcine decellularized xenografts (ureters and iliac vessels) remained patent for 6 months, whereas non-seeded decellularized xenografts became occluded within a week [24, 34, 35]. Hence, endothelialization of decellularized xenografts is a crucial factor for blood vessel patency. This trend is also prevalent in heart valve applications, where decellularized allogeneic valve prostheses covered with autologous endothelial cells have already been implanted in humans [36].

Although decellularized porcine scaffolds support EC proliferation into a confluent monolayer, it has also been shown that cell migration into these scaffolds is inadequate, probably due to the very tight matrix organization specific to the aortic structure [35, 37]. To enhance the cellular infiltration into the xeonografts, Simionescu and co-workers prepared pure elastin scaffolds and pure collagen scaffolds by selectively removing the collagen or elastin component, to create more porous scaffolds for cell infiltration [38]. However, the seeded SMCs adhered and proliferated, forming multiple layers on scaffold surfaces, but rarely infiltrated the scaffolds [38]. These results showed that scaffold composition and architecture are cell-friendly, but additional signals are required in order to drive the cells inside the scaffolds.

An additional hurdle to the use of xenografts in vascular applications is the early-to-mid-term failure with porcine and bovine decellularized valve conduits related to immune response to the xenogenic materials. The SynerGraft (CryoLife) vascular graft is a conduit derived from porcine heart valve that is decellularized using a patented process. The authors of initial animal implantation studies of the SynerGraft porcine aortic valve xenografts reported finding little evidence of immunological rejection [39]. However, the implantation of SynerGraft porcine aortic valves in pediatric patients resulted in catastrophic failure associated with a strong inflammatory response suggestive of immune rejection [40].

The rationale for decellularization of xenogeneic scaffolds is that removal of the native cells from xenografts will remove antigenicity. Indeed, the histological analysis of the failed SynerGrafts revealed no histologically detectable residual cells or cell nuclei. These results suggest that decellularization disrupts the cells but does not adequately remove antigenic proteins from the xenografts. Thus, whilst the assessment of decellularization methods has relied primarily on histological cellularity, this type of analysis does not necessarily ensure removal of xenogeneic antigens from the tissue. To date, it is unclear to what extent a decellularization procedure needs to remove non-cellular integral components of the extracellular matrix. Of concern among known xenogeneic antigens is galactose-α-(1,3)-galactose (α-gal), which is widely accepted to be the first barrier to discordant xenotransplantation [41]. It has been estimated that as much as 1% of natural human IgG is directed against the α-gal moiety [41]. Glutaraldehyde treatment of xenografts can reduce immunogenicity by crosslinking the active moities, but glutaraldehyde has been demonstrated to induce its own set of drawbacks on the vasculature. It is a well-described phenomenon that glutaraldehyde release from cardiac implants delays endothelialization, and may cause toxic damage to the aortic wall, thus inducing scar formation [42].

Human cryopreserved allografts were introduced as hemodialysis access grafts and seem less prone (but not immune) to fibrosis, calcification, and degeneration than their xenograft counterparts. Particularly successful as hemodialysis access grafts (6 mm diameter) is CryoValve (CryoLife), a new generation of cryopreserved allografts that are decellularized and antigen-reduced [2].

Insofar as small-diameter vascular grafts are concerned, the development of allografts is currently limited to animal models. Decellularized human umbilical veins have shown potential for cellular integration and maintenance of the mechanical properties of native blood vessels [43]. When implanted into nude rats as abdominal aortic interposition grafts, decellularized human umbilical veins remained mechanically intact and patent for up to 8 weeks [44]. The implanted grafts were seeded with a confluent endothelial layer of human umbilical vein ECs (HUVECs) to tackle the thrombogenicity issue.

34.2.4.1 Tissue-engineered decellularized scaffolds

Another way of addressing the native decellularized scaffold's shortcomings is the new approach of using decellularized scaffolds of engineered origin. The advantage of this approach is that vascular grafts with the desired mechanical properties and dimensions can be created (Figure 34.6). One human donor provides a cell bank large enough to produce 74 small-diameter tissue-engineered vascular grafts [3]. Unlike native decellularized scaffolds (of animal or human origin),

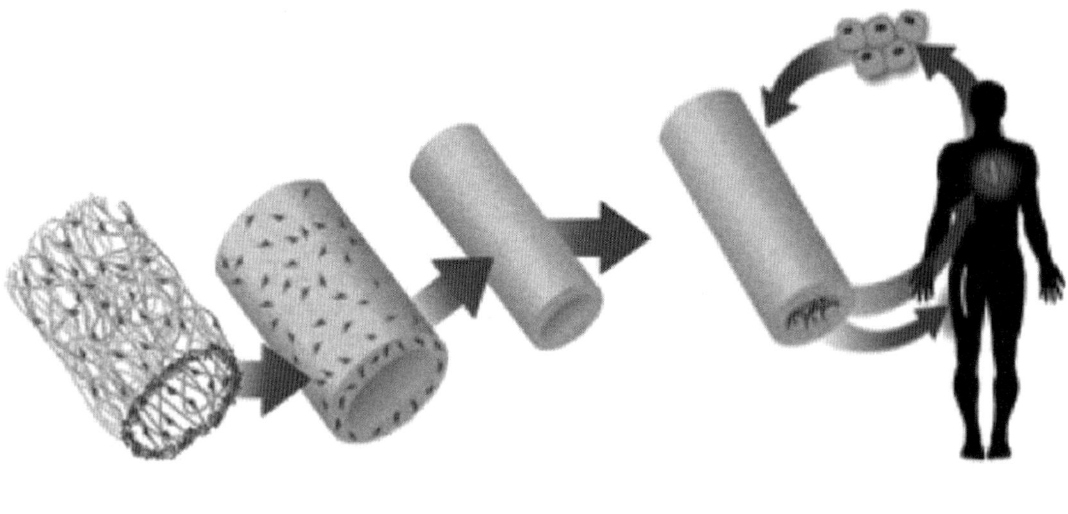

Figure 34.6 A schematic representation of the strategy for producing readily available TEVGs. Each graft is tissue-engineered by culturing human cells on a polymer scaffold that degrades as the cells produce extracellular matrix proteins to form a tubular tissue devoid of polymer. Cellular material is then removed via decellularization, leaving an extracellular matrix tube (the TEVG), which may be refrigerated until it is needed by the patient. TEVGs are then seeded with endothelial cells from the recipient. (Reproduced with permission from the authors [3].)

where branches must be ligated to create a continuous conduit, the engineered structures have no branches and are not tapered. Also, the diameter is a well-controlled parameter in engineered structures, allowing a complete match with the native bypassed artery. One group has described tissue-engineered vessels that were then decellularized using a series of detergents, creating an ECM tubular construct that is fully devoid of cells. Two types of decellularized grafts were created: large-diameter vessels (diameter 6 mm) that were implanted following decellularization in a baboon arteriovenous bypass model as-is; and small-diameter vessels (diameters 3 and 4 mm, derived from canine SMC) that were luminally seeded with ECs and implanted into canine recipients [3]. Both the large and the small decellularized TEVGs showed excellent function and patency rates, without graft infections or calcification.

In native vessel ECM provides resident cells with a complex combination of physical and molecular factors called the "cellular niche" dictating cell fate. The natural ECM "cellular niche" environment achieves this in part through cell-adhesion molecules and growth factors of the surrounding matrix. However, as discussed previously, the decellularization procedure of native and tissue-engineered scaffolds imparts a significant loss of glycosaminoglycan content, altering the ideal "cellular niche" environment. To restore the fine-balanced interplay between lacking environmental factors and reseeded cells the cell culture is commonly supplemented with growth factors, amino acids, and vitamins. The particular growth-medium "cocktail" used is tailored to cell type, and will be discussed in Section 34.3.

34.3 Cell sources for human blood vessel engineering

34.3.1 General cellular considerations for vascular engineering

The most challenging component to engineer is the TEVG's mechanical properties. Burst strength similar to that of saphenous veins (i.e. >1700 mm Hg) must be maintained after implantation (i.e. stable diameter after weeks to months of pulsatile loading in vivo). Mechanically robust TEVGs are classically obtained by inducing SMCs to deposit large amounts of collagen and/or elastin [43]. Collagen offers high tensile strength, while elastin contributes to the vessel compliance by acting as a recoil protein [43, 44]. To achieve a mechanically robust TEVG, adult cell sources (terminally differentiated cells) and progenitor cell sources of SMCs have been investigated. The adult cell source approach involves isolation of the desired cells, expansion to the desired cell number, and then a cell-seeding step for building the TEVG. The progenitor cell source approach adds a cell differentiation step before the initial cell expansion. Although historically adult stem cell sources were the preferred choice for tissue-engineering applications, progenitor cell sources offer new possibilities.

34.3.1.1 Adult cells from tissues (terminally differentiated)

34.3.1.1.1 Smooth muscle cells

Autologous SMCs isolated from patients themselves are the first cell choice for vessel engineering due to their non-immunogenic advantage. Both autologous and allogeneic SMCs have been utilized in different TEVG approaches.

One successful approach using SMCs for culturing a TEVG [4] utilized bovine SMCs that were seeded on a degradable polymer and cultured under mechanical stimulation for 8 weeks. This work demonstrated that, in a 3D environment, collagen synthesis by SMCs and crosslink formation could be supported by supplementing the cells with ascorbic acid, copper ions, amino acids, and growth factors [4, 45]. This work also demonstrated that pulsatile strain promotes a homogeneous cell distribution in the construct wall.

However, adult human SMCs can be limited by their early senescence, which can occur after 10–30 population doublings [46]. The building of a mechanically robust vessel requires as many as 40–60 population doublings for deposition of sufficient ECM protein [46]. In addition, the patient group most in need of autologous engineered grafts is elderly donors with vascular diseases. Older vascular cells deposit less

ECM than do younger cells, due to down-regulation of matrix production [43]. Therefore, the combined limited lifespan and low matrix production of elderly SMCs result in TEVGs with inferior mechanical properties. To address this issue, Dahl and co-workers applied an alternative approach. Using SMCs isolated from tissues from healthy adult human donors (aged 17–49 years), they produced tubular vascular constructs composed of secreted matrix proteins that were decellularized, thereby removing all antigenic cellular components. This allowed the production of non-immunogenic TEVGs from banked allogeneic cells.

Genetic manipulation approaches to overcoming human SMCs' early senescence have also been investigated. The limited replicative lifespan of elderly human SMCs is in part due to the progressive age-dependent shortening of the telomeres. The telomere is a region of repeating DNA sequences at the end of the chromosomes that shortens with each cell division. Introduction of ectopic telomerase through retroviral gene therapy can lengthen telomeres and can overcome senescence in some cell types [47–49]. As shown by Poh and co-workers, genetically manipulating SMCs' telomerase expression resulted in proliferation far beyond the cells' normal life span, generating mechanically superior vessels [47]. However, the ECM deposition in TEVGs still decreased as a function of donor age, despite lifespan extension using telomerase. In light of the cellular lifespan and limitations in ECM production, various investigators have also set out to identify alternative cell sources.

34.3.1.1.2 Fibroblast cells

While SMC-based vascular grafts recapitulate the medial layer of an artery, the adventitial layer is composed of fibroblasts and collagen. One of the earliest TEVG successes was based on a fibroblast/SMC co-culture. L'Heureux and colleagues cultured human autologous fibroblasts and SMCs from skin and vein biopsies under conditions with an elevated concentration of ascorbic acid to produce cells sheets, which were then fused into TEVGs [18]. However, this autologous approach required a 6–9-month culture period, in part due (perhaps) to the advanced age of many of the cell donors used in their studies.

Others have entrapped autologous fibroblasts from small skin biopsies in a fibrin gel [16]. In this method, a bioreactor imparted both cyclic distension and transmural flow, producing grafts with circumferentially aligned ECM and collagen after only 7–9 weeks of culture. The burst strength was $\approx$1400 mm Hg for the 4-mm vascular grafts, which was comparable to the native ovine femoral artery burst pressure (2297 $\pm$ 207 mm Hg). The suture retention force of the 4-mm grafts with entrapped PLA cuffs was 1.32 N, equal to the suture retention strength of human internal mammary artery (1.35 N) [50]. Others have obtained tubular constructs using ovine vascular myofibroblasts after only 28 days of dynamic culture [51, 52]. Although this underlines the general feasibility of obtaining human fibroblast-based TEVGs in relatively short time periods, the burst strength of the grafts when cultured under pulsatile flow for 28 days was $\approx$326.3 mm Hg, still much lower than the native artery burst pressure ($\approx$2297 mm Hg). The low mechanical strength of these short-time-cultured grafts limits their clinical applicability. Although SMC-based TEVGs exhibit contractile functionality, and express contractile proteins such as α-SMA, calponin-1, caldesmon-1, and smooth muscle myosin heavy chain (MHC), fibroblast-based TEVGs offer the advantage of easy harvesting from dermal biopsies.

34.3.1.1.3 Endothelial cells

Endothelial cells are sometimes used as a luminal vessel lining for TEVGs, in an attempt to reduce thrombosis, inflammation, and hyperplasia [3, 4, 9]. In native vessels, the endothelial cell layer prevents the adhesion of platelets and other blood components by acting as a physical barrier and by producing antithrombogenic factors such as NO, thrombomodulin, tissue-type plasminogen activator (tPA), and prostaglandin I_2 (PGI_2) [13, 24]. However, under static culture conditions the important antithrombogenic molecules are down-regulated, whereas undesirable pro-coagulant and pro-inflammatory molecules such as VCAM-1 and ICAM-1 are expressed [26, 27]. Despite this, even partial luminal EC coverage is correlated with a reduction of TEVG thrombosis and failure. This may be due to the presence of ECs at the time of implantation, which subsequently aid in recruitment of recipient ECs to the TEVG [3]. In addition, ECs secrete factors such as NO and prostacyclin that inhibit platelet activation, even if the EC layer is subconfluent [18]. Depending on the species under study, HUVECs have been utilized, though bovine, canine, and porcine ECs have also been used [4, 5, 48, 53].

34.3.1.2 Adult progenitor cells

Stem cells are defined by two main characteristics: the ability for self-renewal and the potential for differentiating into mature cell types. The various stem cell types are classified in general by their age and potency. Totipotent cells (e.g. embryonic stem cells) can give rise to almost every mature cell type, but are in a very early developmental stage. Although not discussed in this chapter, there are several excellent reviews of applications of pluripotent cells to vascular regeneration [54, 55]. Adult stem cells are typically restricted to differentiating into only a few mature cell types, but their application in vascular regeneration offers exciting opportunities. The main types used in TEVG building are mesenchymal stem cells, adipose-derived stem cells, and blood-derived EPCs.

34.3.1.2.1 Mesenchymal stem cells

Because of their ability to expand thousands-fold in culture, into multiple tissue lineages, mesenchymal stem cells (MSCs) have been actively studied in vascular engineering. It has even been postulated that MSCs can modulate immune responses by suppressing both B and T cell functions, thereby enhancing the acceptance of MSC by allogeneic recipients [56]. Thus, it may be feasible to use MSCs to construct autologous or allogeneic (off-the-shelf) TEVGs.

Cohnheim first described MSCs in 1867 [57]. They are easily accessible from the heterogeneous mononuclear cell fraction of the bone marrow, but can also be found in non-marrow tissues. The definition of MSCs is both inclusive and exclusive in nature, since these cells do not possess a unique marker that can be reliably used for isolation. The presence of cell surface markers, such as CD13, CD29, CD44, CD73, CD90, CD105, and CD166 suggests an MSC phenotype. MSCs must also lack CD14, CD31, CD34, CD45, and HLA-DR markers, which are found on various hematopoietic cell populations. These cells differentiate into a variety of cell lineages, including osteoblasts, adipocytes, chondrocytes, and myoblasts, using factors that are well defined and have been described extensively [58].

Being of particular interest to vascular tissue engineering, differentiation of human MSCs toward a smooth muscle cell lineage has been studied since its proof-of-concept demonstration in 1993 by Galmiche and colleagues [59]. Several cytokines, such as transforming growth factor β (TGF-β_1), basic fibroblast growth factor (bFGF), vascular endothelial growth factor (VEGF), and retinoic acid, are known to play a significant role in MSC differentiation to calponin-positive SMCs [60]. In addition, the environment of cell culture (i.e. cell–cell contact and ECM substrate), plays a key role in SMC differentiation [61]. Also, mimicking the dynamic environment of the circulatory system via mechanical conditioning, such as uniaxial cyclic strain, drives MSC progenitor cells to express SMC markers (α-SMA, h1-Calponin) and enhances ECM remodeling and synthesis [62, 63].

In efforts to circumvent the early senescence of terminally differentiated SMC, there is a recent trend of using MSC to produce TEVGs. Human bone-marrow-derived MSCs have been used to build TEVGs [64]. In a biomimetic culture system of mechanical cyclic strain and enriched Dubbecco's Modified Eagle's Medium the authors induced proliferation and differentiation phases to promote hMSC proliferation and SMC differentiation, respectively. After 8 weeks of culture the vessel grafts exhibited insufficiently good mechanical properties, with a burst pressure of 7–8 psi and a collagen production of 22.1 ± 7.8% of dry weight, which is approximately half of the collagen content of native vessels. However, the TEVGs stained positive for smooth muscle actin and calponin, confirming that SMC differentiation had been achieved in a 3D bioreactor environment. The MSCs were differentiated into calponin-expressing SMCs using TGF-β_1, PDGF-BB, and bFGF, cyclic mechanical strain, and fibronectin ECM protein stimulation. As summarized in Table 34.1, TEVGs have also been built

Table 34.1 Cell-based TEVGs summarized by approach and cell type

General approach	Specific approach	Time-course from culture to clinical implantation			Results	Disadvantages	Reference
		In-vitro culturing	Bioreactor	In-vivo clinical application			
Degradable polymeric scaffolds	Allogenic SMC cultured on degradable PGA scaffold	Expansion of SMCs	Culture of SMCs on PGA scaffolds for 8–10 weeks under pulsatile pressure	Clinical trials on baboon animal models	Mechanical properties comparable to those of native vessels (burst pressure of 2150 mm Hg)	Long lead-time (<2 months) for the production of a graft	[4]
	Mononuclear fraction of bone marrow seeded on degradable copolymer scaffold	None, the graft is implanted in patients immediately	None	Clinical trials in pediatric patients for low-pressure vessels	First clinical trial for TEVGs, with 32 months' patency without aneurysm formation or calcification	Low mechanical strength limiting applicability to low-pressure veins	[73]
	Differentiation of MSCs into SMCs, prior to seeding on degradable PGA scaffold	Select SMC-differentiated MSCs by selecting calponin^{+} cells	MSCs differentiated into SMCs on PGA scaffolds for 8 weeks of culture under pulsatile pressure	None	The tubular structures stained positive for smooth muscle actin and calponin, confirming SMC differentiation in a 3D bioreactor environment	Low mechanical strength, with a burst pressure of 8 psi	[64]
	Differentiation of ASCs into SMCs, prior to seeding on degradable PGA scaffold	Culture of ASCs with TGF-β_1 and BMP-4, and expansion of differentiated SMCs	ASCs differentiated into SMCs on PGA scaffolds with 8 weeks of culture under pulsatile pressure	None	The tubular structures stained positive for smooth muscle actin and calponin, confirming SMC differentiation in a 3D bioreactor environment	Low mechanical strength, with an elastic modulus of $\approx$10.5 MPa	[70]

Extracellular matrix- and protein-based scaffolds	Injection of cell and collagen into a tubular mold followed by solidification of the collagen scaffold	ECs, SMCs, and fibroblasts are expanded; the cells are then seeded solidified in a collagen tubular scaffold	None	None	Low mechanical strength (burst pressure of 40 mm Hg)	Irrespective of strengthening approach used, resulting grafts have low mechanical strength	[9]
	Neonatal dermal fibroblasts entrapped in fibrin gel	Expansion of neonatal dermal fibroblasts	Culture for 7–9 weeks in fibrin gel entrapment bioreactor under pulsed flow and stretch	None	A new type of pulsed flow–stretch bioreactor formed tubular structures	Burst strength 1400 mm Hg	[16]
	MSCs and HUVECs entrapped in collagen–fibronectin gel	Expansion of MSCs and HUVECs and seeding in a 3D gel construct	None	Implanted in immuno-compromised mice	The vessels remained functional for 130 days in mouse animal model	By themselves hMSCs could not form conduit for blood flow	[67]
Cell sheet	Flat sheets grown from fibroblasts are wrapped in tubular structures	Cell expansion for 6 months leading to production of cell sheets	Cell sheet tubular construct culture on porous mandrel, followed by seeding of luminal ECs and further bioreactor culture	Clinical trials in human (3 years)	Clinical trials have proved initial safety and good mechanical properties	Long lead-time (<6 months) for the production of a graft	[18]

from animal (ovine) bone-marrow-derived smooth muscle progenitor cells. These grafts exhibited a confluent endothelial monolayer, circumferentially aligned SMCs, and collagen levels similar to those in native veins 5 weeks after implantation [65].

Several promising approaches avoiding significant culture periods draw on the idea of directly implanting isolated undifferentiated MSCs or even bone marrow fractions in vivo to aid vascular regeneration. In fact, the first reported tissue-engineered blood vessel clinical trials in 2001 used an autologous mononuclear fraction of bone marrow seeded on a polycaprolactone–polylactic acid copolymer scaffold [38]. In later studies performed by the same group MSCs isolated from the bone marrow were directly seeded in the operating room on tubular grafts, and demonstrated at least 32 months' patency without aneurysm formation or calcification [6].

Hashi and co-workers used an approach whereby MSCs were seeded on PLLA nanofibrous aligned electrospun conduits. The nanofiber alignment mimicked native collagen fibrils, guiding cell organization in the grafts. The MSC-seeded conduits were implanted in rat carotid arteries, where long-term patency with well-formed endothelial and smooth muscle layers was observed. The long-term patency of the grafts was attributed to the antithrombogenic property of MSCs [56]. Although some researchers have demonstrated the ability to differentiate MSCs into ECs expressing typical ECs markers such as Flk-1, Tie-1, Tie-2, and vWF, others have reported their inability to differentiate MSCs into ECs in vitro [66, 67]. Thus, the capacity of MSCs to differentiate into ECs remains an unresolved, controversial issue.

34.3.1.2.2 Adipose-derived stem cells

Adipose-derived stem cells (ASCs) are mesenchymal cells that share many properties in common with the bone-marrow-derived MSCs. The surface immunophenotype of ASCs is broadly similar to that of bone-marrow-derived MSCs, but they lack CD106 expression, among other markers, suggesting that they are a distinct population of cells of mesenchymal origin. Just like MSCs, ASCs are capable of differentiating into multiple cell lineages, such as osteoblasts, chondroblasts, and adipocytes. Of interest to vascular regeneration is that processed human lipoaspirate-derived ASC have been differentiated into functional contractile SMCs [68]. In addition to their ease of harvest by minimally invasive liposuction, the key potential advantage of ASCs in vascular regeneration is their much greater numerical availability for harvest from adipose tissue, possibly rendering culture expansion unnecessary. Indeed, the authors of most clinical animal trials assessing ASCs used autologous preparations of cell pellets rich in ASCs from adipose tissue, without any subsequent culture steps. Another potential advantage is the isolation consistency of ASCs, which is unaffected by patient age, obesity, renal failure, and vascular disease [69]. As an example of this approach, Wang and co-workers successfully built small-diameter vessels utilizing human ASCs obtained from the stromal fraction of lipoaspirates [70]. The isolated ASCs were differentiated into functional SMCs, seeded on a PGA polymer scaffold and grown for 8 weeks in a pulsatile bioreactor system. The vessels grown under dynamic conditions had an elastic modulus of $\approx$10.5 MPa, suture retention strength of $\approx$1.23 N, and collagen deposition of about 50 mg/g of wet weight, which are all fractions of native arteries' values.

34.3.1.2.3 Blood-derived endothelial progenitor cells

Endothelial progenitor cells (EPCs) are defined as pre-differentiated adult stem cells that have the potential to proliferate and differentiate into mature endothelial cells. EPCs are pre-differentiated in the bone marrow and then mobilized into peripheral blood. They possess a strong proliferation capacity, and play an essential role in post-natal angiogenesis. Similarly to the identification of MSCs, the definition of EPCs is also exclusive in nature, in that isolated EPCs must lack hematopoietic cell population markers, while simultaneously presenting EPC surface markers, such as CD34, Flk-1 (VEGF-receptor-2, KDR), CD133, and VE-cadherin [70]. Of relevance to TEVG, it has been suggested that injured endothelium recovers in vivo by the adhesion of circulating EPCs to the exposed ECM and their subsequent differentiation and migration within the remaining endothelium [71]. Indeed,

$CD34^+$, VEGF-R-2^+, $CD133^+$ cells have been found lining the sites of neointima formation in vascular implants [70].

Inspired by this finding, synthetic PET grafts have been seeded with $CD34^+$ purified cells isolated from bone marrow, and implanted in a canine animal model. In addition to the high percentage of retained cells (cell coverage of 92% at explantation) the authors found histological evidence of increased microvessel formation [72]. There have also been some early attempts to seed a more purified population of EPCs on polycaprolactone electrospun scaffolds. Zhang and co-workers characterized isolated EPCs by selecting for $CD31^-$ but $CD34^+$ and $CD105^+$ cells from porcine peripheral blood. The authors also showed functional characteristics of the EPCs by measuring the uptake of acetylated low-density lipid (LDL). It was observed that the EPCs grow into a confluent layer within 24 hours of static culture time on electrospun scaffolds [71]. Quint and co-workers selected cells from porcine peripheral blood that express $CD31^+$, $CD144^+$, and von Willebrand factor in the absence of the hematopoietic marker CD45. The functional characteristics of the EPCs were shown by detecting the uptake of acetylated low-density lipid (LDL) and the formation of capillary-like tubes when they were cultured on Matrigel. The isolated EPCs and differentiated ECs were additionally exposed to laminar shear stress. Both types of cell showed an increase in production of endothelial nitric oxide synthase (eNOS). The production of NO is expected for functional ECs. Hence, the measured characteristics of porcine peripheral blood-derived EPCs closely resembled those of differentiated porcine ECs. The isolated EPCs were fluorescently labeled (GFP^+) and seeded on TEVGs, and their efficacy as a small-diameter arterial graft was assessed in a porcine animal model [53]. At the 30-day explant point an average of 35% luminal coverage of GFP^+ cells was found, proving that the seeded cells were retained, as opposed to the adhesion of EPCs from circulating peripherial blood. An additional encouraging observation was the high patency rate of 100% and a trend toward an attenuated neointimal response.

34.4 Conclusion

The development of TEVGs that are mechanically robust and biologically similar to native vessels is extremely challenging. From a clinical perspective, the time and cost requirements are imperative for the creation of implantable TEVGs for an age- and risk-appropriate patient population. To date, the most successful approaches have utilized differentiated vascular cells and still require long times for generation of TEVGs. Owing to their proliferative and differentiative capacity, stem cells open up new alternatives for obtaining autologous cells that may, in the long run, enable production of TEVGs in a more time-efficient manner.

REFERENCES

[1] Roger, V. L., Go, A. S., Lloyd-Jones, D. M. *et al.* 2011. Heart disease and stroke statistics – 2011 update: a report from the American Heart Association. *Circulation*, **123**, e18–209.

[2] Farber, A., Major, K., Wagner, W. H. *et al.* 2003. Cryopreserved saphenous vein allografts in infrainguinal revascularization: analysis of 240 grafts. *J. Vasc. Surg.*, **38**, 15–21.

[3] Dahl, S. L., Kypson, A. P., Lawson, J. H. *et al.* 2011. Readily available tissue-engineered vascular grafts. *Sci. Transl. Med.*, **3**, 68–9.

[4] Niklason, L. E., Gao, J., Abbott, W. M. *et al.* 1999. Functional arteries grown in vitro. *Science*, **284**, 489–93.

[5] Niklason, L. E., Abbott, W., Gao, J. *et al.* 2001. Morphologic and mechanical characteristics of engineered bovine arteries. *J. Vasc. Surg.*, **33**, 628–38.

[6] Mooney, D. J., Mazzoni, C. L., Breuer, C. *et al.* 1996. Stabilized polyglycolic acid fibre-based tubes for tissue engineering. *Biomaterials*, **17**, 115–24.

[7] Miller, D. C., Thapa, A., Haberstroh, K. M. and Webster, T. J. 2004. Endothelial and vascular smooth muscle cell function on poly(lactic-*co*-glycolic acid) with nano-structured surface features. *Biomaterials*, **25**, 53-61.

[8] Bilgen, B., Uygun, K., Bueno, E. M., Sucosky, P. and Barabino, G. A. 2009. Tissue growth modeling in a wavy-walled bioreactor. *Tissue Eng. Part A*, **15**, 761–71.

[9] Weinberg, C. B. and Bell, E. 1986. A blood vessel model constructed from collagen and cultured vascular cells. *Science*, **231**, 397–400.

[10] Peck, M., Gebhart, D., Dusserre, N., McAllister, T. N. and L'Heureux, N. 2012. The evolution of vascular tissue engineering and current state of the art. *Cells Tissues Organs*, **195**, 144–58.

[11] Orban, J. M., Wilson, L. B., Kofroth, J. A. *et al.* 2004. Crosslinking of collagen gels by transglutaminase. *J. Biomed. Mater. Res. A*, **68**, 756–62.

[12] Hirai, J. and Matsuda, T. 1996. Venous reconstruction using hybrid vascular tissue composed of vascular cells and collagen: tissue regeneration process. *Cell Transplant.*, **5**, 93–105.

[13] Haisch, A., Loch, A., David, J. *et al.* 2000. Preparation of a pure autologous biodegradable fibrin matrix for tissue engineering. *Med. Biol. Eng. Comput.*, **38**, 686–9.

[14] Grassl, E. D., Oegema, T. R. and Tranquillo, R. T. 2003. A fibrin-based arterial media equivalent. *J. Biomed. Mater. Res. A*, **66**, 550–61.

[15] Tschoeke, B., Flanagan, T. C., Koch, S. *et al.* 2009. Tissue-engineered small-caliber vascular graft based on a novel biodegradable composite fibrin–polylactide scaffold. *Tissue Eng. Part A*, **15**, 1909–18.

[16] Syedain, Z. H., Meier, L. A., Bjork, J. W., Lee, A. and Tranquillo, R. T. 2011. Implantable arterial grafts from human fibroblasts and fibrin using a multi-graft pulsed flow–stretch bioreactor with noninvasive strength monitoring. *Biomaterials*, **32**, 714–22.

[17] Berglund, J. D., Nerem, R. M. and Sambanis, A. 2004. Incorporation of intact elastin scaffolds in tissue-engineered collagen-based vascular grafts. *Tissue Eng.*, **10**, 1526–35.

[18] L'Heureux, N., Paquet, S., Labbe, R., Germain, L. and Auger, F. A. 1998. A completely biological tissue-engineered human blood vessel. *FASEB J.*, **12**, 47–56.

[19] McAllister, T. N., Maruszewski, M., Garrido, S. A. *et al.* 2009. Effectiveness of haemodialysis access with an autologous tissue-engineered vascular graft: a multicentre cohort study. *Lancet*, **373**, 1440–6.

[20] Hodde, J. P., Record, R. D., Tullius, R. S. and Badylak, S. F. 2002. Retention of endothelial cell adherence to porcine-derived extracellular matrix after disinfection and sterilization. *Tissue Eng.*, **8**, 225–34.

[21] Hiles, M. C., Badylak, S. F., Lantz, G. C. *et al.* 1995. Mechanical properties of xenogeneic small-intestinal submucosa when used as an aortic graft in the dog. *J. Biomed. Mater. Res.*, **29**, 883–91.

[22] Herring, M., Gardner, A. and Glover, J. 1978. A single-staged technique for seeding vascular grafts with autogenous endothelium. *Surgery*, **84**, 498–504.

[23] Rosenman, J. E., Kempczinski, R. F., Pearce, W. H. and Silberstein, E. B. 1985. Kinetics of endothelial cell seeding. *J. Vasc. Surg.*, **2**, 778–84.

[24] Teebken, O. E., Bader, A., Steinhoff, G. and Haverich, A. 2000. Tissue engineering of vascular grafts: human cell seeding of decellularised porcine matrix. *Eur. J. Vasc. Endovasc. Surg.*, **19**, 381–6.

[25] Amiel, G. E., Komura, M. and Shapira, O. *et al.* 2006. Engineering of blood vessels from acellular collagen matrices coated with human endothelial cells. *Tissue Eng.*, **12**, 2355–65.

[26] McFetridge, P. S., Daniel, J. W., Bodamyali, T., Horrocks, M. and Chaudhuri, J. B. 2004. Preparation of porcine carotid arteries for vascular tissue engineering applications. *J. Biomed. Mater. Res. A*, **70**, 224–34.

[27] Quint, C., Kondo, Y., Manson, R. J. *et al.* 2011. Decellularized tissue-engineered blood vessel as an arterial conduit. *Proc. Nat. Acad. Sci. USA*, **108**, 9214–9.

[28] Lantz, G. C., Badylak, S. F., Coffey, A. C., Geddes, L. A. and Blevins, W. E. 1990. Small intestinal submucosa as a small-diameter arterial graft in the dog. *J. Invest. Surg.*, **3**, 217–27.

[29] Sandusky, G. E. Jr., Badylak, S. F., Morff, R. J., Johnson, W. D. and Lantz, G. 1992. Histologic findings after in vivo placement of small intestine submucosal vascular grafts and saphenous vein grafts in the carotid artery in dogs. *Am. J. Pathol.*, **140**, 317–24.

[30] Badylak, S. F., Lantz, G. C., Coffey, A. and Geddes, L. A. 1989. Small intestinal submucosa as a large diameter vascular graft in the dog. *J. Surg. Res.*, **47**, 74–80.

[31] Teebken, O. E. and Haverich, A. 2002. Tissue engineering of small diameter vascular grafts. *Eur. J. Vasc. Endovasc. Surg.*, **23**, 475–85.

[32] Derham, C., Yow, H., Ingram, J. *et al.* 2008. Tissue engineering small-diameter vascular grafts: preparation of a biocompatible porcine ureteric scaffold. *Tissue Eng. Part A*, **14**, 1871–82.

[33] Stapleton, T. W., Ingram, J., Katta, J. *et al.* 2008. Development and characterization of an acellular porcine medial meniscus for use in tissue engineering. *Tissue Eng. Part A*, **14**, 505–18.

[34] Narita, Y., Kagami, H., Matsunuma, H. *et al.* 2008. Decellularized ureter for tissue-engineered small-caliber vascular graft. *J. Artif. Organs*, **11**, 91–9.

[35] Kaushal, S., Amiel, G. E., Guleserian, K. J. *et al.* 2001. Functional small-diameter neovessels created using endothelial progenitor cells expanded ex vivo. *Nature Med.*, **7**, 1035–40.

[36] Dohmen, P. M., Lembcke, A., Hotz, H., Kivelitz, D. and Konertz, W. F. 2002. Ross operation with a tissue-engineered heart valve. *Ann. Thorac. Surg.*, **74**, 1438–42.

[37] Walles, T., Puschmann, C., Haverich, A. and Mertsching, H. 2003. Acellular scaffold implantation – no alternative to tissue engineering. *Int. J. Artif. Organs*, **26**, 225–34.

[38] Simionescu, D. T., Lu, Q., Song, Y. *et al.* 2006. Biocompatibility and remodeling potential of pure arterial elastin and collagen scaffolds. *Biomaterials*, **27**, 702–13.

[39] Dohmen, P. M., Lembcke, A., Holinski, S. *et al.* 2007. Mid-term clinical results using a tissue-engineered pulmonary valve to reconstruct the right ventricular outflow tract during the Ross procedure. *Ann. Thorac. Surg.*, **84**, 729–36.

[40] Simon, P., Kasimir, M. T., Seebacher, G. *et al.* 2003. Early failure of the tissue engineered porcine heart valve SYNERGRAFT in pediatric patients. *Eur. J. Cardiothorac. Surg.*, **23**, 1002–6; discussion 6.

[41] Baumann, B. C., Forte, P., Hawley, R. J. *et al.* 2004. Lack of galactose-α-1,3-galactose expression on porcine endothelial cells prevents complement-induced lysis but not direct xenogeneic NK cytotoxicity. *J. Immunol.*, **172**, 6460–7.

[42] Ruffer, A., Purbojo, A., Cicha, I. *et al.* 2010. Early failure of xenogenous de-cellularised pulmonary valve conduits – a word of caution! *Eur. J. Cardiothorac. Surg.*, **38**, 78–85.

[43] Johnson, D. J., Robson, P., Hew, Y. and Keeley, F. W. 1995. Decreased elastin synthesis in normal development and in long-term aortic organ and cell cultures is related to rapid and selective destabilization of mRNA for elastin. *Circ. Res.*, **77**, 1107–13.

[44] McMahon, M. P., Faris, B., Wolfe, B. L. *et al.* 1985. Aging effects on the elastin composition in the extracellular matrix of cultured rat aortic smooth muscle cells. *In Vitro Cell Dev. Biol.*, **21**, 674–80.

[45] Davidson, J. M., LuValle, P. A., Zoia, O., Quaglino, D. Jr. and Giro, M. 1997. Ascorbate differentially regulates elastin and collagen biosynthesis in vascular smooth muscle cells and skin fibroblasts by pretranslational mechanisms. *J. Biol. Chem.*, **272**, 345–52.

[46] Sundaram, S. and Niklason, L. E. 2012. Smooth muscle and other cell sources for human blood vessel engineering. *Cells Tissues Organs*, **195**, 15–25.

[47] Poh, M., Boyer, M., Solan, A. *et al.* 2005. Blood vessels engineered from human cells. *Lancet*, **365**, 2122–4.

[48] McKee, J. A., Banik, S. S., Boyer, M. J. *et al.* 2003. Human arteries engineered in vitro. *EMBO Rep.*, **4**, 633–8.

[49] Bodnar, A. G., Ouellette, M., Frolkis, M. *et al.* 1998. Extension of life-span by introduction of telomerase into normal human cells. *Science*, **279**, 349–52.

[50] Syedain, Z. H., Weinberg, J. S. and Tranquillo, R. T. 2008. Cyclic distension of fibrin-based tissue constructs: evidence of adaptation during growth of engineered connective tissue. *Proc. Nat. Acad. Sci. USA*, **105**, 6537–42.

[51] Hoerstrup, S. P., Zund, G., Sodian, R. *et al.* 2001. Tissue engineering of small caliber vascular grafts. *Eur. J. Cardiothorac. Surg.*, **20**, 164–9.

[52] Braddon, L. G., Karoyli, D., Harrison, D. G. and Nerem, R. M. 2002. Maintenance of a functional endothelial cell monolayer on a fibroblast/polymer substrate under physiologically relevant shear stress conditions. *Tissue Eng.*, **8**, 695–708.

[53] Niklason, L. E. 1999. Techview: medical technology. Replacement arteries made to order. *Science*, **286**, 1493–4.

[54] Sundaram, S. and Niklason, L. E. 2012. Smooth muscle and other cell sources for human blood vessel engineering. *Cells Tissues Organs*, **195**(1–2), 15–25.

[55] Cheung, C. and Sinha, S. 2011. Human embryonic stem cell-derived vascular smooth muscle cells in therapeutic neovascularisation. *J. Molec. Cell Cardiol.*, **51**, 651–64.

[56] Hashi, C. K., Zhu, Y., Yang, G. Y. *et al.* 2007. Antithrombogenic property of bone marrow mesenchymal stem cells in nanofibrous vascular grafts. *Proc. Nat. Acad. Sci. USA*, **104**, 11915–20.

[57] Cohnheim, J. F. 1867. Über Entzündung und Eiterung. *Virchows Arch. Path. Anat. Physiol. Klin. Med.*, **40**, 1–79.

[58] Minguell, J. J., Erices, A. and Conget, P. 2001. Mesenchymal stem cells. *Exp. Biol. Med. (Maywood)*, **226**, 507–20.

[59] Galmiche, M. C., Koteliansky, V. E., Briere, J., Herve, P. and Charbord, P. 1993. Stromal cells from human long-term marrow cultures are mesenchymal cells that differentiate following a vascular smooth muscle differentiation pathway. *Blood*, **82**, 66–76.

[60] Gong, Z., Calkins, G., Cheng, E. C., Krause, D. and Niklason, L. E. 2009. Influence of culture medium on smooth muscle cell differentiation from human bone marrow-derived mesenchymal stem cells. *Tissue Eng. Part A*, **15**, 319–30.

[61] LeDuc, P., Ostuni, E., Whitesides, G. and Ingber, D. 2002. Use of micropatterned adhesive surfaces for control of cell behavior. *Methods Cell Biol.*, **69**, 385–401.

[62] Hamilton, D. W., Maul, T. M. and Vorp, D. A. 2004. Characterization of the response of bone marrow-derived progenitor cells to cyclic strain: implications for vascular tissue-engineering applications. *Tissue Eng.*, **10**, 361–9.

[63] Kurpinski, K., Chu, J., Hashi, C. and Li, S. 2006. Anisotropic mechanosensing by mesenchymal stem cells. *Proc. Nat. Acad. Sci. USA*, **103**, 16095–100.

[64] Gong, Z. and Niklason, L. E. 2008. Small-diameter human vessel wall engineered from bone marrow-derived mesenchymal stem cells (hMSCs). *FASEB J.*, **22**, 1635–48.

[65] Liu, J. Y., Swartz, D. D., Peng, H. F. *et al.* 2007. Functional tissue-engineered blood vessels from bone marrow progenitor cells. *Cardiovasc. Res.*, **75**, 618–28.

[66] Gang, E. J., Jeong, J. A., Han, S. *et al.* 2006. In vitro endothelial potential of human UC blood-derived mesenchymal stem cells. *Cytotherapy*, **8**, 215–27.

[67] Au, P., Tam, J., Fukumura, D. and Jain, R. K. 2008. Bone marrow-derived mesenchymal stem cells facilitate engineering of long-lasting functional vasculature. *Blood*, **111**, 4551–8.

[68] Rodriguez, L. V., Alfonso, Z., Zhang, R. *et al.* 2006. Clonogenic multipotent stem cells in human adipose tissue differentiate into functional smooth muscle cells. *Proc. Nat. Acad. Sci. USA*, **103**, 12167–72.

[69] DiMuzio, P. and Tulenko, T. 2007. Tissue engineering applications to vascular bypass graft development: the use of adipose-derived stem cells. *J. Vasc. Surg.*, **45**(Suppl. A), A99–103.

[70] Wang, C., Cen, L., Yin, S. *et al.* 2010. A small diameter elastic blood vessel wall prepared under pulsatile conditions from polyglycolic acid mesh and smooth muscle cells differentiated from adipose-derived stem cells. *Biomaterials*, **31**, 621–30.

[71] Zhang, X., Xu, Y., Thomas, V., Bellis, S. L. and Vohra, Y. K. 2011. Engineering an antiplatelet adhesion layer on an electrospun scaffold using porcine endothelial progenitor cells. *J. Biomed. Mater. Res. A*, **97**, 145–51.

[72] Cho, S.-W., Lim, S. H., Kim, I.-K. *et al.* 2005. Small-diameter blood vessels engineered with bone marrow-derived cells. *Ann. Surg.*, **241**, 506–15.

[73] Shinoka, T., Shum-Tim, D., Ma, P. X. *et al.* 1998. Creation of viable pulmonary artery autografts through tissue engineering. *J. Thorac. Cardiovasc. Surg.*, **115**, 536–45; discussion 545–6.

35

Stem cells for vascular engineering

Y. Eugene Chen, Changqing Xie and Bo Yang

35.1 Introduction

Normal blood vessels consist of three layers, including the tunica intima, the tunica media, and the tunica adventitia [1]. Each structural layer consists of distinct cell and matrix types. A monolayer of endothelial cells (ECs) lines the lumen of blood vessels to provide a continuous, selectively permeable, hemo-compatible blood-contacting surface. Meanwhile, ECs play a key role in various physiological and pathological processes including blood supply, metabolic homeostasis, immune cell trafficking, and inflammation [2]. Vascular smooth muscle cells (VSMCs) and pericytes cover the outside of the endothelium, protect the fragile channels from rupture, and contribute to the contraction and relaxation of the vessels [3]. The vascular wall extracellular matrix (ECM) is composed of structural proteins such as collagen and elastin and adhesion proteins such as fibronectin and laminin that determine mechanical strength, cell response, and ultimately hierarchical tissue organization [4]. An intact and functioning vasculature is crucial in order to maintain homeostasis and provides necessary nutrients and oxygen exchange to all parts of the body.

Diseases that affect the integrity of blood vessels lead to serious and often deadly outcomes. Vascular diseases are the major causes of morbidity around the world [5]. At present, approximately 12 million people in the USA are affected by peripheral vascular disease, but only approximately one in four of them has been diagnosed and is receiving treatment [6]. EC and SMC pathology has been implicated in various vascular diseases [7–10]. Current important therapeutic options for vascular disease incorporate the surgical implantation of stents or grafts and greatly reconstruct impaired vascular function to drain downstream tissues and organs. However, the implanted grafts may incompletely recover the functional integrity of the vasculature. In addition, these therapeutic methods neither provide long-lasting solutions nor prevent damage to downstream tissues and organs [11]. In this scenario, cell-based engineered vessel grafts may offer the opportunity to permanently and effectively treat many vascular diseases [11]. The regeneration of some or all of the vessel layers and their original properties may provide potentially functional vascular grafts. The use of autologous bypass grafts, including saphenous vein, internal mammary artery, and radial artery bypass grafts, remains an important therapeutic option for the treatment of coronary artery disease. However, many patients do not have a vessel suitable for use because of concomitant vascular disease, amputation, or previous harvest, and hence artificial grafts must also be used [12]. Therefore, vascular engineering has emerged as a promising approach to address the shortcomings of current options.

Vascular engineering is an interdisciplinary field that applies the principles of engineering and life sciences to the development of biological vessels in order to restore, maintain, or improve downstream vessel/tissue/organ functions [13]. Vascular engineering is involved in designing, controlling, and manipulating some of the signaling mechanisms driving vascular repair, and ultimately offers potential alternatives to the problem of suboptimal bypass conduits. Recent work has strongly demonstrated that

Table 35.1 Comparison of human ES cells, iPS cells, and adult stem cells

	ES cells	iPS cells	Adult stem cells
Origin	Blastocysts	Various cells	Various tissues
Culture conditions	Established	Established	Various and stringent
Differentiation potential	Pluripotent	Pluripotent	Multipotent/unipotent (some pluripotent, e.g. AFSCs)
Proliferation	Unlimited	Unlimited	Limited
Telomerase activity	High	High	Low
Scalability	Unlimited	Unlimited	Limited
Teratoma formation	Yes	Yes	No
Immunological rejection	High chance	Less chance	Less chance
Ethical issues	Yes	No	No

ES cells, embryonic stem cells; iPS cells, induced pluripotent cells; AFSCs, amniotic fluid stem cells.

tissue-engineered vascular grafts provide a possible readily available option for patients with vessel deficiency [14]. The reconstruction of a functional vessel needs the integration of ECs, VSMCs, and well-organized ECM. However, the use of autologous differentiated ECs to line the lumen and VSMCs to fasten the channel of a graft is hampered by the need to harvest a blood vessel from the patient and subsequently isolate and culture enough vascular cells to seed the conduit. Moreover, mature differentiated VSMCs have limited ability to proliferate and usually lose their contractile phenotype, followed by switching to a synthetic one during in-vitro expansion [15]. These limitations make it necessary to explore alternative and high-scale vascular cell sources for blood vessel engineering, since large numbers of functional vascular cells are usually required.

Stem cells offer unique advantages over isolated vascular cells due to their proliferative potential [16, 17]. Furthermore, available data have shown that the use of stem cells for vascular tissue engineering could potentially increase seeding efficiency, solve the cell sourcing difficulties, and reduce the time required in vitro [18]. Ultimately, the potential of stem cells to differentiate into different cell lines could be employed to construct vessels with different tissue layers from the same original cell source. The innovative use of stem cells for vascular tissue engineering has opened up new avenues for a fully engineered graft or blood vessel, although the characteristics differ among individual stem cell populations (Tables 35.1 and 35.2). In this review, we focus on different types of stem cells currently being investigated as potential sources for vascular engineering.

35.2 Pluripotent stem cells

Pluripotent stem cells have the capability to undergo unlimited self-renewal and differentiation into all somatic cell types [19]. There are several types of pluripotent stem cells, including embryonic carcinoma cells, embryonic stem (ES) cells, epiblast stem cells, embryonic germ cells, and induced pluripotent stem (iPS) cells [19].

35.2.1 Embryonic stem cells

ES cells are isolated from the inner cell mass (ICM) of blastocyst-stage embryos. ES cells have the capability of self-renewal and differentiation into all fetal and adult lineages. Under proper in-vitro culture conditions ES cells can be indefinitely propagated while retaining their differentiation potential.

35.2.1.1 Endothelial cell differentiation from ES cells

Embryoid body (EB) formation, with a three-dimensional (3D) structure, from ES cells is a

Table 35.2 Summary of characteristics of adult stem cells

Stem cells	Origin	Cell surface markers	Reference
MSCs	BM, umbilical cord blood, adipose, vessel wall, placenta	STRO-1$^+$, VCAM1$^+$, Sca-1$^+$, BMPR$^+$, c-kit$^+$, CD29$^+$, CD44$^+$, CD49$^+$, CD51$^+$, CD73$^+$, CD90$^+$, CD105$^+$, CD106$^+$, CD166$^+$, CD11b$^-$, CD14$^-$, CD34$^-$, CD45$^-$	[192]
EPCs	BM, peripheral blood, adipose, vessel wall, umbilical cord blood, spleen, liver, heart	CD34$^+$, AC133$^+$, Flk1$^+$, CD11b$^+$, CD62L$^+$, CD146$^+$, CD19$^-$, CD3$^-$, CD33$^-$	[193, 194]
ASCs	Adipose	CD10$^+$, CD13$^+$, CD29$^+$, CD34$^+$, CD44$^+$, ICAM1$^+$, CD71$^+$, CD90$^+$, CD105$^+$, VCAM1$^+$, c-kit$^+$, STRO-1$^+$, CD45$^-$, CD14$^-$, CD16$^-$, CD56$^-$, CD61$^-$	[154, 155]
NCSCs	Embryonic neural crest, dorsal root ganglia, gut, cornea, heart, BM skin	p75 Neurotrophin R$^+$, α4-integrin$^+$,	[166]
AFSCs	Amniotic fluid	c-kit$^+$, CD29$^+$, CD44$^+$, CD73$^+$, CD90$^+$, CD105$^+$, SSEA4 $^+$, CD45$^-$, CD34$^-$, AC133$^-$	[173]
HSCs	BM, fetal liver, placenta	CD34$^+$, c-kit$^+$, AC133$^+$, CD135$^+$, CD159$^+$, Sca-1$^+$, CD150$^+$, ABCG2$^+$, CXCR4$^+$, Lin$^-$, CD38$^-$, CD48$^-$, CD244$^-$	[195]
CSCs	Heart	c-kit$^+$, Sca-1$^+$, Islet1$^+$, Flk1$^+$, CD34$^-$, CD45$^-$, Lin$^-$	[196]

MSCs, mesenchymal stem cells; EPCs, endothelial progenitor cells; ASCs, adipose-derived stem cells; NCSCs, neural crest stem cells; AFSCs, amniotic fluid stem cells; HSCs, hemapoietic stem cells; CSCs, cardiac stem cells; BM, bone marrow; BMPR, bone morphogenetic protein receptor; VCAM, vascular cell adhesion molecule; ICAM, intercellular adhesion molecule; CXCR, chemokine (C–X–C motif) receptor; Flk, fetal liver kinase; ABCG, ATP-binding cassette, subfamily G; SSEA, stage-specific embryonic antigen.

well-characterized spontaneous differentiation that recapitulates early embryogenesis and involves various cell lineage progenitor cells. Human ES cells can spontaneously differentiate into hemangioblasts, forming blood islands that contain endothelial and hematopoietic progenitors [20], and organize within EBs into 3D vessel-like structures, in a pattern that resembles embryonic vascularization [20–23].

It was found that within EBs endothelial-cell-associated markers are expressed sequentially in a way that reflects in-vivo endothelial differentiation during embryonic development [24]. The expression of endothelial markers (CD31, VE-cadherin, CD34, and GATA2) increases during human EB differentiation, reaching a maximum during days 13–15 (GATA2 around day 18) [25], along with additional up-regulation of vasculogenic growth factors, including vascular endothelial growth factor (VEGF), angiopoietins 1 and 2, and platelet-derived growth factor-BB (PDGF-BB), endothelial markers (including VCAM1, Flt1, and 2), and transcription factors (including GATA1 and GATA3) [26]. In addition, several different vascular progenitor cell groups have been isolated from human EBs and further induced to differentiate to mature vascular cells. CD31$^+$, Flk1$^+$, VE-cadherin$^+$, CD45$^-$ cells isolated from 10-day-old human EBs constituted a population of primitive precursors that could be induced to mature into functional ECs in Medium-199 supplemented with 20% FBS, bovine pituitary extract, and VEGF for 7 days [27]. When cultured in media supplemented with VEGF, CD34$^+$ progenitor cells from 10 day-old EBs differentiate into ECs as characterized by immunohistochemistry and by functionality in in-vivo models where they are able to integrate into host vasculature [28]. Hematoangioblast cells from 3.5-day-old EBs expand in blast colony expansion media and further differentiate into hematopoietic cells, ECs, and SMCs, which are able to benefit vasculature reconstruction in a hindlimb ischemic model in mice [29].

Direct isolation of mature ECs from human EBs has also been explored through sorting either $CD31^+$ or von Willebrand factor (vWF) cells without isolating progenitor cells [25, 30]. Isolated ECs expressed CD34, Flk1, VE-cadherin, and vWF, and took up acetylated low-density lipid (LDL) [25], also forming capillary-like structures on Matrigel after several passages [30]. EBs cultured in media supplemented with VEGF for 14 days expressed higher levels of CD31, VE-cadherin, and vWF protein than did the control cells lacking VEGF [31]. EBs cultured in serum-free media, with the sequential addition of bone morphogenetic protein 4 (BMP-4), activin A, basic fibroblast growth factor (bFGF), VEGF-A, and transforming growth factor β (TGF-β)-inhibitory molecule SB-431542, yielded dramatically (10-fold) increased numbers of ECs (around 2% total yield) [32].

To circumvent EB formation, additional ECM or feeder cells have been investigated as a means to directly generate mature ECs from ES cells. Among those conditions, mouse bone-marrow-derived cell lines (S17, OP9, and MS-5) [33, 34], mouse yolk sac ECs (c166) [33], mouse embryonic fibroblasts (mEFs) [35], methylcellulose, and collagen have been shown to promote human ES cell differentiation toward early hematopoietic precursors with the subsequent potential to differentiate into ECs [36]. Human ES cells can differentiate to yield up to 20% of $CD34^+$ cells when co-cultured with OP9 cells and up to 10^7 $CD34^+$ cells with more than 95% purity can be isolated after 8–9 days of culture [34, 37]. Isolated $CD34^+$ cells display the phenotype of primitive hematopoietic progenitors as defined by co-expression of CD90, c-kit, and CD164, together with a lack of CD38 expression, and contain aldehyde dehydrogenase-positive cells as well as cells with verapamil-sensitive ability to efflux rhodamine 123 [34, 37]. Approximately 15% of the cells presented the $Flk1^+/TRA\text{-}1\text{-}60^-$ phenotype by day 8 after human ES cell colonies had been seeded on an OP9 layer [38]. $Flk1^+/TRA\text{-}1\text{-}60^-$ cells were then cultured on collagen-IV-coated dishes and treated with VEGF. As a result, $Flk1^+/TRA\text{-}1\text{-}60^-$ cells differentiated into cells with expression of EC markers, including CD34, VE-cadherin, CD31, and eNOS. In addition, when these cells were cultured in the absence of VEGF, all cells differentiated into SM α-$actin^+$, $calponin^+$ SMCs. When transplanted into a hindlimb ischemic mouse model, ECs in the early differentiation stage were incorporated into blood vessels and accelerated improvement of local blood flow [38]. Alternatively, human ES cells cultured on either S17 or M2–10B4 stromal cells derived from mouse bone marrow generated a large population of $CD34^+$ cells [39]. Culture on a human fibroblast (Hs27) feeder layer in the presence of BMP-4, VEGF, and bFGF and without serum was also shown to enrich a $CD34^+$ progenitor cell population to more than 10% that could differentiate into both ECs and SMCs upon further culture under cell-specific conditions, although functionality was not confirmed in vivo [40]. The authors of another study found that human ES cells seeded at high density on mEFs and grown in human ES cell differentiation media yielded 5%–10% $CD34^+$ cells by day 10 [35]. The $CD34^+$ population was then enriched via magnetic sorting and, when cultured in media containing VEGF and bFGF, developed the EC specific gene expression of CD31 and VE-cadherin. Importantly, when these cells were injected into SCID mice, they were incorporated into the vasculature within 2 days of implantation and persisted for 150 days [35]. During normal vascular development, ECM components, such as collagen, play an important role in guiding vascular cell differentiation. It has been shown that this role of ECM involves EC differentiation from ES cells. Undifferentiated human ES cells grown on collagen-IV-coated dishes for 6 days and strained through a 40-μm filter could further differentiate into ECs when cultured in VEGF [41]. $Flk1^+$ cells were isolated and re-cultured on collagen IV in VEGF in the presence or absence of 8-bromo-cAMP to induce arterial or venous ECs, respectively [41].

Although various methods of generating ECs from human ES cells have been tried, the recurring challenge is how to produce sufficient numbers of ECs for practical application, which will likely be resolved mostly by relying on insights into the signaling pathways that regulate commitment to the vascular lineage. BMP-4 was shown to accelerate commitment to the EC lineage via EB formation, as demonstrated by a shift in the peak of VE-cadherin$^+$, Flk1$^+$ cells from 12 to 7 days [42]. BMP-4 was also shown to promote human ES cell differentiation into CD34$^+$, CD31$^+$ cells at an early stage, when human ES cells were cultured on an Hs27 feeder layer for 10 days and then selected for expression of CD34 [40]. In addition, Wnt1-overexpressing M2–10B4 stromal cells as feeders in co-culture conditions generated four times more CD34$^+$ progenitor cells than did regular M2–10B4 stromal cells [39], although there were discrepancies regarding the effect of Wnt5 overexpression by the stromal cells in co-culture on the generation of CD34$^+$ progenitor cells [39, 43]. The TGF-β inhibitor SB-431542 could significantly increase the number of ECs generated from human ES and iPS cells. The cells were cultured as EBs in suspension in defined media for 4 days, followed by adherent culture for another 10 days. Cells isolated for CD31$^+$ expression, when subsequently expanded in the presence of SB-431542, yielded approximately six times more ECs than did the untreated controls [32].

35.2.1.2 Smooth muscle cell differentiation from ES cells

Common progenitor cells shared by EC and SMCs, either from EBs or from two-dimensional (2D) culture systems, have been discovered by studies on the differentiation of human ES cells [28, 38–40]. Isolated CD34$^+$ vascular progenitor cells from human EBs could also differentiate into SMC-like cells when treated with PDGF-BB. SMC-like cells expressed SM marker genes, including SM α-actin, SMMHC, SM22α, calponin, and caldesmon, and were able to contract in response to carbachol [28]. In addition, isolated CD34$^+$ cells from human ES cells cultured on either S17 or Wnt1-expressing M2–10B4 stromal cells differentiate to SMCs with further SMC culture conditions in media supplemented with PDGF-BB and TGF-β_1 [39]. Isolated CD34$^+$ progenitor cell population from human ES cells co-cultured with Hs27 feeder layer was also shown to differentiate into SMCs in basic medium MCDB131 with SMC supplements, which include insulin, transferrin, EGF, bFGF, PDGF-BB, ascorbic acid, heparin, hydrocortisone, sodium selenite, and monothioglycerol [40]. In addition, isolated Flk1$^+$, Tra-1-60$^-$ cells from human ES cells co-cultured with OP9 feeder layer could differentiate into SM α-actin$^+$, calponin$^+$ SMCs in the absence of VEGF [38].

Functional SMCs can be derived from human ES cells directly via culture on collagen IV in media supplemented with PDGF-BB [41, 44] and TGF-β_1 [44]. Furthermore, treatment with all-*trans* retinoic acid has been shown to induce SMCs directly from human ES cells with up to approximately 93% efficiency [45]. Alternatively, human EBs transferred to adherent culture on gelatin-coated dishes for 6 days and then transferred to smooth muscle growth media were shown to differentiate into functional SMCs with an efficiency of 55.26% for SMMHC and 96.81% for SM α-actin [46]. Recently, chemically defined protocols with sequential growth factor and signaling inhibitor cocktail have been employed to generate SMCs from human ES cells (>80% SMMHC$^+$ and SM α-actin$^+$). Derived SMCs exhibit contractile ability in response to vasoconstrictors and recapitulate the phenotypic switch upon the treatment of cytokines [47].

Collectively, the results summarized here suggest that ES cells are highly suited for vascular engineering since they renew themselves indefinitely and provide an inexhaustible source of vascular progenitor cells, although some challenges still remain to be solved before their widespread adoption can be considered.

35.2.2 Induced pluripotent stem cells

iPS cells are ES-like cells derived from various somatic cells, which are genetically reprogrammed to an ES cell state by forced expression of genes important for maintaining the pluripotency. It is not known whether iPS cells and ES cells differ in clinically significant ways [19]. iPS cells retain the advantages of human ES cells in that they can self-renew, and retain the potential to be differentiated into all cell types in the body [48, 49]. However, since they are derived from adult tissues, they bypass ethical controversies over relating to the use of embryos. Therefore, applying human iPS cells for future stem-cell-based therapy will be more acceptable than using human ES cells, given the lesser likelihood of there being ethical and political issues. The generation of patient-specific pluripotent cells presents more advantages than merely providing a source of cells for transplantation. Theoretically, there is a lower risk of allogeneic immune rejection since the transplanted iPS cells are derived from the patient who needs to be treated. Furthermore, using patient-derived iPS cells allows one to personalize the study and treatment of diseases, through the development of disease models and ultimately transfer of corrected genes to autologous progenitors. This is particularly important for diseases that lack corresponding in-vitro or animal models, such as disorders resulting from dysfunctions of the brain and heart. Such disease/mutation-specific cell lines also offer an opportunity to map out the developmental course of complex medical conditions, such as diabetes and Parkinson's disease, in a manner not possible through animal research alone or by observing patients. In fact, disease-specific iPS cell lines have already been created from patients suffering from amyotrophic lateral sclerosis [50], juvenile onset type 1 diabetes mellitus [51], Parkinson's disease [52], and spinal muscular atrophy [50, 51].

A new body of literature is emerging surrounding iPS cell differentiation into vascular cells [53–57]. Human iPS cells can generate $CD31^+$, $CD43^-$ ECs in co-culture with OP9 [28]. Although ECs derived from human iPS cells were capable of taking up acetylated LDL and forming capillary-vascular-like structures on Matrigel, these cells also underwent early cellular senescence (most of the ECs senesced after one passage) [42]. Human iPS cells cultured on an OP9 feeder layer differentiate to TRA-1-60^-, $Flk1^+$, VE-$cadherin^+$ or TRA-1-60^-, $Flk1^+$, VE-$cadherin^-$ cells. Furthermore, TRA-1-60^-, $Flk1^+$, VE-$cadherin^+$ can differentiate to $CD34^+$, $CD31^+$, $eNOS^+$ ECs with the treatment of VEGF when grown on collagen IV. Interestingly, sorted TRA1-60^-, $Flk1^+$, VE-$cadherin^-$ cells did not differentiate into ECs in the absence of VEGF, but differentiated into SM α-$actin^+$, $calponin^+$ cells with or without the presence of PDGF-BB [56], in a way that mirrors that described for ES cells above [38]. EC differentiation from human iPS cells was also achieved by administration of BMP-4 and VEGF. The derived ECs exhibited endothelial characteristics by forming capillary-like structures in Matrigel and incorporating acetylated LDL and improving blood perfusion and limb salvage in mouse ischemic hindlimb models [57].

iPS cells have been successfully differentiated into SMCs using an adherent monolayer culture differentiation system [58]. In the meantime, an iPS-derived EB differentiation approach is also applicable in terms of SMC differentiation [59]. In that study, iPS-derived EBs were alternatively seeded on gelatin-coated plates and maintained in SMC-specific medium for 10 days. Colonies with SMC-like morphology showed a characterisitic SMC-specific gene expression profile and acquired the SMC requisite functions, including augmented intracellular calcium influx in response to carbachol and KCl [59]. Furthermore, the effect of various scaffolds on iPS/SMC differentiation has been tested and the data suggest that iPS cell-derived SMCs can be an important cell source for personalized vascular tissue engineering applications [60].

Taken together, the accumulating insights into the vascular cell lineage differentiation potential of human ES and iPS cells highlight the promises of new tissue engineering approaches conducive to vascular differentiation with pluripotent stem cells.

35.3 Adult stem cells

Adult stem cells are relatively undifferentiated cells that reside in various tissues of the human body [61]. Adult stem cell therapies, such as bone marrow transplants to treat blood disorders, have been in place for decades [62]. A variety of adult stem cells has been identified by combination of negative and positive cell surface markers (Table 35.2) from different tissues or organs, including bone marrow [63–71], peripheral blood [63, 72], cord blood [73], heart [74], blood vessel wall [75], spleen [76], and adipose tissue [77, 78], and have been shown to have the capability to differentiate to vascular cells.

35.3.1 Mesenchymal stem cells

Mesenchymal stem cells (MSCs) were first identified in 1966 from bone marrow [79]. Since then, MSCs have recently been found in umbilical cord blood [80], adipose tissue [80], vessel walls [81, 82], hair follicles [83], and placenta [84]. Because of their ability to expand into multiple tissue lineages, MSCs from bone-marrow or non-marrow sources [85–94] have been shown to have enormous potential for engineering purposes. MSCs from these various sources had similar morphologies and immune properties, although they differ regarding the degree of difficulty of their isolation and their proliferation capacity in vitro [80].

Results from earlier studies have indirectly suggested that MSCs possess the ability to differentiate into ECs and SMCs in vivo [95, 96]. MSCs were able to differentiate to ECs in vitro in 2D culture with VEGF treatment as determined by the presence of vWF and the formation of characteristic capillary-like structures [97]. Furthermore, MSCs isolated from canine bone marrow and seeded on 3D tissue-engineered vascular grafts were shown to differentiate into ECs upon being subjected to shear stress [98]. In addition, these bone marrow cells were found to differentiate into ECs on biodegradable scaffolds after being fixed with fibrin glue and further maturated for only 4 hours, though their shear stress resistance after such short maturation has yet to be ascertained [99].

The differentiation of MSCs to VSMCs has been well documented and appears to be regulated not only by soluble factors but also by shear stress and cell–cell interactions. After confluent culture for 3–7 weeks, MSCs expressed SM α-actin^{+} microfilaments as well as other SMC-specific proteins such as metavinculin, caldesmon, SMMHC, and calponin [100]. MSCs have been shown to have a greater potential to differentiate into SMCs when exposed to TGF-β [83, 101, 102] or BMP-4 [83] or through over-expression of TGF-β_1 [103]. In the meantime, the importance of cell–cell interaction during MSC-to-SMC differentiation has been suggested in a study of co-cultured MSCs with ECs or fibroblasts, because the SM α-actin filament organization exhibited comprehensive disruption in the SMCs derived from MSCs if they were directly co-cultured with ECs [104]. Additionally, the significance of mechanical conditions has been shown during MSC-to-SMC differentiation. The use of cyclic strain promoted differentiation of bone marrow progenitor cells to SMCs, as evidenced by enhanced expression of SM α-actin and calponin and perpendicular alignment of cells relative to the direction of the applied strain [105].

Furthermore, different 3D culture systems also enhance SMC differentiation from MSCs. Adult human bone-marrow-derived MSCs exhibited the ability to differentiate into SMCs in a polyglycolic acid (PGA) mesh in a bioreactor system with multiple factors: PDGF, TGF-β, fibronectin, and cyclic strain. As a result, the cellularity and collagen production substantially improved the quality of the engineered vessel wall [106]. Differentiated SMCs and ECs from MSCs were seeded on decellularized arteries and subsequently implanted as carotid artery interposition grafts in the cell-donor dogs. The vascular grafts showed regeneration of endothelia, media, and adventitia within 8 weeks after implantation and were patent [107]. Histological observation showed the presence of endothelium, SMCs, elastin, and collagen after 2 months [108].

Additionally, MSCs are advantageous for regenerative medicine applications because they lack MHC class II molecules, which can elicit an immune response [109]. Thus, there is potential for allogeneic MSCs to be transplanted with limited risk for immune rejection, though it is uncertain whether the cells differentiated from MSCs are immunogenic. It will be important to resolve this uncertainty prior to their use in cell therapies, since blood vessels have direct contact with circulating immune cells.

35.3.2 Endothelial progenitor cells

Endothelial progenitor cells (EPCs) are a complex subject, and there remains intense debate regarding their definition and biology. In accord with their initial discovery, EPCs were defined as cells positive both for hematopoietic stem cell (HSC) markers such as CD34 and AC133 and for an endothelial marker protein such as Flk1 [110]. EPCs can be isolated from bone marrow [63], peripheral blood [63, 111], adipose tissue [112, 113], vessel walls [1, 2, 100, 114], umbilical cord blood [115] and possibly spleen [116, 117], liver [118, 119], and heart [120]. Increasing evidence indicates that they have the potential to differentiate into mature EC and contribute to the process of endothelium repair. The number of circulating EPCs increases in response to local ischemia [121], statins [122, 123], estrogen [117, 124, 125], erythropoietin [126] and VEGF [127]. Recent work indicates that EPCs play roles during the recovery processes including myocardial ischemia and infarction, limb ischemia, wound healing, and endogenous endothelial repair, as well as atherosclerosis and tumor vascularization [128]. Systemic administration of EPCs isolated from peripheral blood and expanded in vitro augmented naturally impaired neovascularization in an animal model of experimentally induced limb ischemia [129] and improved symptoms and collateral circulation of 45 patients with ischemic lower limb muscles [130].

Since EPCs can be endogenously triggered to differentiate into ECs [131], and $CD34^+$ EPCs from bone marrow contribute to the lining of grafts implanted in vivo [132, 133], EPCs have also been employed to create engineered vessel grafts [134–136]. $CD34^+$, $Flk1^+$ cells from human peripheral blood can differentiate into ECs when plated on fibronectin in vitro and home to sites of angiogenesis in hindlimb ischemia models in vivo, demonstrating their progenitor-like capabilities and their critical presence in the circulation [137]. $AC133^+$ cells from human peripheral blood differentiated more efficiently on fibronectin plates than they did when exposed to type I and IV collagens [138]. VEGF was shown to be critical for progenitor-to-EC transition [110, 139–141]. At the same time, the effect of shear stress on EC differentiation of EPCs has been established. On comparing EPCs cultured under static conditions with those exposed to laminar shear stress, the latter expressed higher levels of VE-cadherin, suggestive of a more differentiated phenotype [142]. This modulation in phenotype under natural conditions represents another important step toward a fully engineered vessel that can exhibit transferability from an in-vitro to an in-vivo environment.

On the other hand, engineered vessels have utilized biodegradable polymer 3D materials, including PGA–P4HB, poly-L-lactic acid (PLLA), and a PGA–PLLA combination, to demonstrate progenitor-to-EC differentiation on the scaffold [143–145]. For example, EPCs from peripheral blood can be seeded on the autologous fibrin segments in an in-vitro bioreactor culture system to generate fibrin tubes lined with an EC-like monolayer that has elasticity and burst strength [146]. Nevertheless, EPCs from umbilical cord can be seeded on a 3D porous polyurethane foam within a pulse-duplicator in-vitro system, which results in a favorable cell-to-polymer attachment, proliferation into the 3D tubular scaffolds, and further differentiation to ECs [147]. Isolated EPCs from the peripheral blood of sheep were expanded and seeded onto decellularized porcine iliac arteries and preconditioned by shear stress to simulate in-vivo arterial conditions. By pre-seeding endothelial progenitors onto the lumen of an engineered vessel, thrombosis is kept to a minimum, and the patency rate for grafts transferred from an in-vitro to an in-vivo environment can be augmented [148]. These results show that ECs grown on matrices have both the structural and the functional capabilities of blood vessels in vitro and in vivo.

The SMC differentiation potential of EPCs has been investigated too. The PDGF family has been shown to drive differentiation of EPCs to SMCs. PDGF-CC induced the differentiation of bone marrow cells into SMCs and stimulated their growth during vessel sprouting [149]. In the meantime, PDGF-BB not only enhances SMC differentiation from EPCs, but helps maintain the phenotype of synthetic-type SMC [150]. Furthermore, co-culture of $AC133^+$ EPCs with SMCs increases the expression of SMC-specific markers, including SM α-actin, SM22α and myocardin, and decreases the expression of the EC marker CD31 [151, 152]. Interestingly, $AC133^+$ EPCs could migrate into the intima and differentiate into SMC when co-incubated with human isolated pulmonary arteries [152]. Additionally, the potent TGF-β_1 inhibitor SB-431542 decreased SMC-stimulated EPC migration without affecting their functionality and adhesion capacity [151]. These results indicate that EPCs may differentiate into SMC-like cells under the control of TGF-β_1 signaling pathway [151, 152]. Thus EPCs may be an ideal source of cells for vessel engineering.

35.3.3 Adipose-derived stem cells

Human adipose tissue has been used to extract adipose-derived stem cells (ASCs) that are able to differentiate to osteoid, adipose, muscle, and cartilaginous cells [89, 153, 154]. ASCs can proliferate and express several common cell-surface antigens [155], namely, CD10, CD13, CD29, CD34, CD44, ICAM1, CD71, CD90, CD105, VCAM1, c-kit, and STRO-1. They are negative for the hematopoietic lineage markers CD45, CD14, CD16, CD56, CD61, E-selectin, and β_4 integrin, and for the EC markers CD31, VE-cadherin, and vWF [154, 156, 157].

Recent evidence suggests that ASCs have the ability to differentiate into vascular cells. ASCs could differentiate into ECs in response to local cues in vivo that contribute to angiogenesis and increased blood flow and capillary density, and be incorporated into mouse leg vasculature [112, 158]. In vitro, ASCs can spontaneously express the EC markers CD31 and vWF when cultured in methylcellulose [78]. When cultured in an EC-specific medium, namely EGM-2 containing 2% fetal bovine serum, supplemented with VEGF, bFGF, EGF, insulin-like growth factor 1 (IGF1), and ascorbic acid, Flk1$^+$ ASCs isolated from adipose tissue differentiate to ECs expressing VE-cadherin, vWF, and a lectin receptor, take up low-density lipoprotein and are incorporated into an EC tubular network [159]. A recent study showed that VEGF enhanced CD31$^-$, CD34$^-$, VCAM1$^-$, Flk1$^+$ ASCs differentiated in vitro into ECs [158]. In addition, CD34$^+$, CD31$^-$ ASCs can differentiate into ECs when cultured with EC growth medium supplemented with VEGF and IGF [112]. Furthermore, the so-derived EC-like cells promoted neovascularization in ischemic tissue and vessel-like structure formation in Matrigel plugs [78, 112].

The capacity of ASCs to differentiate into functional SMCs was also evaluated. To induce differentiation into SMCs, ASCs were cultured in smooth muscle inductive medium consisting of reduced serum-supplemented medium and heparin. ASCs were induced to differentiate into SMCs marked by the gene expression of SMC markers and their functional ability to contract and relax in direct response to pharmacological agents [160]. It was demonstrated that angiotensin II induces differentiation of ASCs into contractile SMC-like cells through ERK-dependent activation of the autocrine TGF-β_1 pathway [161]. A recent study has shown that a combined stimulation with TGF-β_1 and BMP-4 enhanced the expression of both early and mid-markers (SM α-actin, SM22α, calponin) as well as a late marker (SMMHC) of SMC differentiation, to levels similar to those in human umbilical artery SMCs [162]. More importantly, the so-differentiated SMC cells were functional in contracting a collagen matrix lattice when entrapped inside. The contractile function of SMCs differentiated from ASCs was further enhanced by direct exposure to KCl, which is consistent with what was described regarding human umbilical artery SMCs [162]. Also, sphingosylphosphorylcholine and TGF-β_1 promoted CD13$^+$, CD29$^+$, and CD90$^+$ ASCs from the peri-umbilical adipose tissue to differentiate to SMCs [163]. Furthermore, SMCs from ASCs showed a high level of collagen deposition, which was close to that of native vessels, when seeded on a 3D PGA unwoven mesh and further subjected to pulsatile stimulation in a bioreactor for 8 weeks [164]. In addition, and of relevance to vascular engineering, SMCs derived from ASCs exhibit contractile properties, adhere, and proliferate when seeded on the decellularized saphenous vein within a bioreactor [163].

35.3.4 Neural-crest-derived stem cells

Neural-crest-derived stem cells (NCSCs) are a transient, multipotent, migratory cell population unique to vertebrates that gives rise to diverse cell lineages including melanocytes, craniofacial cartilage and bone, smooth muscle, peripheral and enteric neurons, and glia [165]. Intriguingly, NCSCs exist not only in the embryonic neural crest, but also in different neural-crest-derived tissues in the fetal and adult organism [166]. When clonal GFP-labeled NCSCs were transplanted into the telencephalon of embryonic day-14 mice, 1.6% of NCSCs converted to cells that co-expressed endothelial phenotypes (that is, that bound to lectin and expressed VE cadherin) by embryonic day 16 [167]. In the presence of ECs, 6% of the NCSC population converted to cells with stable expression of multiple endothelial markers and the capacity to form capillary networks [167].

NCSCs are the progenitor cells of vascular SMCs distributed along the ascending and arch portions of the aorta, the ductus arteriosus, the innominate and right subclavian arteries, and the right and left common carotid arteries [168]. Various methods for differentiation of SMCs from NCSCs have been reported [169]. Skin-derived precursor cells (SKPs) derive from endogenous adult dermal precursors that exhibit properties similar to those of embryonic neural crest cells in terms of gene expression, differentiation potential in vitro and in vivo, and migration behavior in vivo [170]. Thus, biopsied skin samples may serve as alternative sources of vascular SMC for vascular engineering, as indicated by results from recent studies [171, 172]. Lineage analysis indicates that both hair and whisker follicle dermal papillae contain neural-crest-derived cells, and that SKPs from the whisker pad are of neural-crest origin [170]. Specifically, SKPs can be manipulated to differentiate into SMCs [172]. Adult SKPs derived from various species were differentiated in response to TGF signaling, which is known to direct NCSCs to a SMC lineage. Interestingly, under serum-free conditions, TGF-β-stimulated human SKPs can differentiate into SMCs with high efficiency. However, with respect to enhanced SMC differentiation, rat and human SKPs appear to have different responses to TGF signaling. That study showed that TGF-β not only enhances SMC marker expression in human SKPs, but also promotes SMC proliferation [172]. Therefore, SKPs may provide an additional source for large-scale SMC generation for vascular engineering.

35.3.5 Other adult stem cells

Amniotic fluid also contains a vast repository of progenitor cells that may be useful for bioengineering applications. Amniotic fluid stem cells (AFSCs) have been demonstrated to be pluripotent, with the capacity to give rise to multiple lineages, including representatives of all three embryonic germ layers [173]. Therefore, AFSCs hold great potential for a variety of therapeutic applications, including cell therapy for vascular diseases. AFSCs have been shown to express c-kit, CD29, CD44, CD73, CD90, CD105, and stage-specific embryonic antigen-4, but are negative for markers of the hematopoietic lineage (CD45) and of HSCs (CD34, AC133) [173]. It has been demonstrated that isolated AFSCs differentiate into EC-like cells when cultured in endothelial basal medium-2 supplemented either with bFGF in gelatin-coated dishes [174] or with VEGF, bFGF, EGF, IGF-1, heparin, ascorbic acid, and 10% FBS [175]. In these conditions, AFSCs differentiated and exhibited an EC-like morphology, formed cord-like structures, and took up acetylated LDL/lectin. Additionally, mRNA and protein levels of CD31 and vWF significantly increased in response to culture in EGM-2, with further up-regulation when stimulated by bFGF [174] or physiological levels of shear force [175].

HSCs from bone marrow can differentiate into multilineages that comprise the hematopoietic system in transplanted hosts for their entire lifespan. HSCs were the first progenitor cells reported to transdifferentiate into non-hematopoietic cells after bone marrow transplantation [64]. After local injection over the infarcted area, the bone-marrow-derived cells not only proliferated and generated de novo myocardium with various stages of maturation, but also differentiated into ECs in the mouse myocardial infarction model [67].

$CD34^+$, $Flt1^+$, $Flk1^+$ mononuclear cells isolated from human peripheral blood were shown to differentiate into SMCs when seeded onto a collagen type I matrix and exposed to PDGF-BB while differentiating into EC colonies when exposed to VEGF [176]. Recently, tissue-resident c-kit^+ stem cells that are capable of differentiating into the endothelial lineage have been isolated from the heart [74].

Thus, this group of adult stem cells may be additional sources for application in vascular engineering, although their potential has not yet been investigated.

35.4 Conclusion and prospects

Intensive research into vascular engineering is being performed in an effort to overcome the barriers to the construction of a fully engineered vessel for arterial replacement, a task that will certainly be facilitated by the impressive advances in our understanding of vascular differentiation from stem cells. Because of their proliferative capacity and growth potential, stem cells will be the next type of reliable cell source for vascular engineering in order to generate vascular grafts. As the prevalence of vascular disease continues to rise, investigation of this area will undoubtedly continue to grow and expand. However, more detailed studies including basic science and translation research must be performed before this new technology can serve in the clinical setting.

First, it is believed that there is remarkable heterogeneity of ECs in different organs [177], including general cell structure [178–181], cell surface markers, and protein and mRNA expression [182–184], which is mediated both by the microenvironment and by epigenetic modifications. Similarly, vascular SMCs exhibit comparably significant heterogeneity, with different embryonic origins in different vessels, or even within segments of the same vessel, different aspects of SMC function, and various SMC responses to environmental cues [169]. The other striking feature of vascular SMCs is that they are liable to undergo phenotypic switching between secretory and contractile phenotypes in response to environmental cues [9]. It remains a challenge to differentiate stem cells into a generic type of ECs and SMCs and further incorporate the heterogeneity of ECs and SMCs to generate clinically available engineered vascular grafts. Thus, future differentiation studies will require close examination of the signaling pathways that govern the EC- and vascular SMC-specific characteristics of a particular location.

Second, challenges remain in terms of better controlling and quantifying the kinetics of vascular differentiation, maturation, and final organization, since cell differentiation from stem cells and vasculogenesis during embryogenesis are complicated and poorly defined processes that are triggered by complex microenvironments, including growth factors, ECM, mechanical stress, cell–cell contact, cell–matrix interactions, and various molecular signal pathways [169, 185, 186]. Moreover, fundamental knowledge of the complex biological factors governing cell lineage destiny is not yet fully attainable, and protocols must be developed via refinement of stem cell differentiation to vascular cells before the potential translation of this technology to clinical use can be achieved. The beneficial effect of 3D culture systems in terms of generating engineered biocompatible grafts has been indicated. One of the potential future directions regarding generating engineering vessels in vitro may be the incorporation of ECMs with a biodegradable polymer material within a nanometer-scale scaffold that mimics in vivo nanometer-scale vascular environmental cues and would promote cell differentiation and maintain the mechanical needs for constructing biocompatible vessels [60, 187–189].

Third, although stem cells generated or isolated from individuals bearing genetic mutations, defects, and diseases could be very valuable for disease modeling [190] and toxicological studies, for the sake of personalized medicine, gene editing methods to correct genetic abnormalities for certain inherited diseases before application need to be established. Recently, highly efficient methods using zinc finger nuclease-mediated [52] or helper-dependent adenovirus-mediated [191] strategies have succeeded in modifying genes in iPS cells. Those technologies may be used to correct disease mutations prior to transplantation and to enable more precise cell models of human disease to be developed. The likelihood of engineering pluripotent stem cells to release therapeutic proteins, marker proteins, or suicide genes to facilitate human cell therapy with pluripotent stem cell lines should be studied further.

With better characterization of various stem cells in the future, the scientific community will be able to isolate and determine the most practical and feasible progenitors for vascular applications. It is hoped that better understanding of the biology of stem cells will provide strategies to additionally enhance neovascularization. In addition, the efforts to overcome some of the above-mentioned barriers that prevent successful translation of stem cell biology into clinical therapy should be helpful in terms of increasing our knowledge regarding vascular disease pathogenesis itself and therapeutics to prevent its onset and progression.

REFERENCES

[1] Humphrey, J. D. and Na, S. 2002. Elastodynamics and arterial wall stress. *Ann. Biomed. Eng.*, **30**(4), 509–23.

[2] Danese, S., Dejana, E. and Fiocchi, C. 2007. Immune regulation by microvascular endothelial cells: directing innate and adaptive immunity, coagulation, and inflammation. *J. Immunol.*, **178**(10), 6017–22.

[3] Jain, R. K. 2003. Molecular regulation of vessel maturation. *Nature Med.*, **9**(6), 685–93.

[4] Ruoslahti, E. and Engvall, E. 1997. Integrins and vascular extracellular matrix assembly. *J. Clin. Invest.*, **99**(6), 1149–52.

[5] Roger, V. L., Go, A. S., Lloyd-Jones, D. M. *et al.* 2011. Heart disease and stroke statistics – 2011 update: a report from the American Heart Association. *Circulation*, **123**(4), e18–209.

[6] Hirsch, A. T., Criqui, M. H., Treat-Jacobson, D. *et al.* 2001. Peripheral arterial disease detection, awareness, and treatment in primary care. *JAMA*, **286**(11), 1317–24.

[7] Cai, H. and Harrison, D. G. 2000. Endothelial dysfunction in cardiovascular diseases: the role of oxidant stress. *Circ. Res.*, **87**(10), 840–4.

[8] Celermajer, D. S., Sorensen, K. E., Gooch, V. M. *et al.* 1992. Non-invasive detection of endothelial dysfunction in children and adults at risk of atherosclerosis. *Lancet*, **340**(8828), 1111–15.

[9] Owens, G. K., Kumar, M. S. and Wamhoff, B. R. 2004. Molecular regulation of vascular smooth muscle cell differentiation in development and disease. *Physiol. Rev.*, **84**(3), 767–801.

[10] Ross, R. 1999. Atherosclerosis – an inflammatory disease. *N. Engl. J. Med.*, **340**(2), 115–26.

[11] Sun, G. and Gerecht, S. 2009. Vascular regeneration: engineering the stem cell microenvironment. *Regen. Med.*, **4**(3), 435–47.

[12] Arrigoni, C., Camozzi, D. and Remuzzi, A. 2006. Vascular tissue engineering. *Cell Transplant.*, **15**(Suppl. 1), S119–25.

[13] Langer, R. and Vacanti, J. P. 1993. Tissue engineering. *Science*, **260**(5110), 920–6.

[14] Dahl, S. L., Kypson, A. P., Lawson, J. H. *et al.* 2011. Readily available tissue-engineered vascular grafts. *Sci. Transl. Med.*, **3**(68), 68–9.

[15] Owens, G. K. 1995. Regulation of differentiation of vascular smooth muscle cells. *Physiol. Rev.*, **75**(3), 487–517.

[16] Kadner, A., Hoerstrup, S. P., Zund, G. *et al.* 2002. A new source for cardiovascular tissue engineering: human bone marrow stromal cells. *Eur. J. Cardiothorac. Surg.*, **21**(6), 1055–60.

[17] Lavik, E. and Langer, R. 2004. Tissue engineering: current state and perspectives. *Appl. Microbiol. Biotechnol.*, **65**(1), 1–8.

[18] Pankajakshan, D. and Agrawal, D. K. 2010. Scaffolds in tissue engineering of blood vessels. *Can. J. Physiol. Pharmacol.*, **88**(9), 855–73.

[19] 2011. Stem cell basics: what are the similarities and differences between embryonic and adult stem cells? In *Stem Cell Information*. Bethesda, MD: National Institutes of Health, US Department of Health and Human Services, http://stemcellsnihgov/info/basics/basics5.

[20] Risau, W., Sariola, H., Zerwes, H. G. *et al.* 1988. Vasculogenesis and angiogenesis in embryonic-stem-cell-derived embryoid bodies. *Development*, **102**(3), 471–8.

[21] Rafii, S. and Lyden, D. 2003. Therapeutic stem and progenitor cell transplantation for organ vascularization and regeneration. *Nature Med.*, **9**(6), 702–12.

[22] Choi, K., Kennedy, M., Kazarov, A., Papadimitriou, J. C. and Keller, G. 1998. A common precursor for hematopoietic and endothelial cells. *Development*, **125**(4), 725–32.

[23] Vittet, D., Prandini, M. H., Berthier, R. *et al.* 1996. Embryonic stem cells differentiate in vitro to endothelial cells through successive maturation steps. *Blood*, **88**(9), 3424–31.

[24] Choi, K., Chung, Y. S. and Zhang, W. J. 2005. Hematopoietic and endothelial development of mouse embryonic stem cells in culture. *Methods Molec. Med.*, **105**, 359–68.

[25] Levenberg, S., Golub, J. S., Amit, M., Itskovitz-Eldor, J. and Langer, R. 2002. Endothelial cells derived from human embryonic stem cells. *Proc. Nat. Acad. Sci. USA*, **99**(7), 4391–6.

[26] Gerecht-Nir, S., Dazard, J. E., Golan-Mashiach, M. *et al.* 2005. Vascular gene expression and phenotypic correlation during differentiation of human embryonic stem cells. *Dev. Dyn.*, **232**(2), 487–97.

[27] Wang, L., Li, L., Shojaei, F. *et al.* 2004. Endothelial and hematopoietic cell fate of human embryonic stem cells originates from primitive endothelium with hemangioblastic properties. *Immunity*, **21**(1), 31–41.

[28] Ferreira, L. S., Gerecht, S., Shieh, H. F. *et al.* 2007. Vascular progenitor cells isolated from human embryonic stem cells give rise to endothelial and smooth muscle like cells and form vascular networks in vivo. *Circ. Res.*, **101**(3), 286–94.

[29] Lu, S. J., Ivanova, Y., Feng, Q., Luo, C. and Lanza, R. 2009. Hemangioblasts from human embryonic stem cells generate multilayered blood vessels with functional smooth muscle cells. *Regen. Med.*, **4**(1), 37–47.

[30] Cho, S. W., Moon, S. H., Lee, S. H. *et al.* 2007. Improvement of postnatal neovascularization by human embryonic stem cell derived endothelial-like cell transplantation in a mouse model of hindlimb ischemia. *Circulation*, **116**(21), 2409–19.

[31] Nourse, M. B., Halpin, D. E., Scatena, M. *et al.* 2010. VEGF induces differentiation of functional endothelium from human embryonic stem cells: implications for tissue engineering. *Arterioscler. Thromb. Vasc. Biol.*, **30**(1), 80–9.

[32] James, D., Nam, H. S., Seandel, M. *et al.* 2010. Expansion and maintenance of human embryonic stem cell-derived endothelial cells by TGFβ inhibition is Id1 dependent. *Nature Biotechnol.*, **28**(2), 161–6.

[33] Kaufman, D. S., Hanson, E. T., Lewis, R. L., Auerbach, R. and Thomson, J. A. 2001. Hematopoietic colony-forming cells derived from human embryonic stem cells. *Proc. Nat. Acad. Sci. USA*, **98**(19), 10716–21.

[34] Vodyanik, M. A., Bork, J. A., Thomson, J. A. and Slukvin, I. I. 2005. Human embryonic stem cell-derived $CD34^+$ cells: efficient production in the coculture with OP9 stromal cells and analysis of lymphohematopoietic potential. *Blood*, **105**(2), 617–26.

[35] Wang, Z. Z., Au, P., Chen, T. *et al.* 2007. Endothelial cells derived from human embryonic stem cells form durable blood vessels in vivo. *Nature Biotechnol.*, **25**(3), 317–18.

[36] Zambidis, E. T., Peault, B., Park, T. S., Bunz, F. and Civin, C. I. 2005. Hematopoietic differentiation of human embryonic stem cells progresses through sequential hematoendothelial, primitive, and definitive stages resembling human yolk sac development. *Blood*, **106**(3), 860–70.

[37] Vodyanik, M. A. and Slukvin, I. I. 2007. Hematoendothelial differentiation of human embryonic stem cells. In *Current Protocols in Cell Biology*, Chapter 23, Unit 23.6.

[38] Sone, M., Itoh, H., Yamahara, K. *et al.* 2007. Pathway for differentiation of human embryonic stem cells to vascular cell components and their potential for vascular regeneration. *Arterioscler. Thromb. Vasc. Biol.*, **27**(10), 2127–34.

[39] Hill, K. L., Obrtlikova, P., Alvarez, D. F. *et al.* 2010. Human embryonic stem cell-derived vascular progenitor cells capable of endothelial and smooth muscle cell function. *Exp. Hematol.*, **38**(3), 246–57.

[40] Bai, H., Gao, Y., Arzigian, M. *et al.* 2010. BMP4 regulates vascular progenitor development in human embryonic stem cells through a Smad-dependent pathway. *J. Cell Biochem.*, **109**(2), 363–74.

[41] Gerecht-Nir, S., Ziskind, A., Cohen, S. and Itskovitz-Eldor, J. 2003. Human embryonic stem cells as an in vitro model for human vascular development and the induction of vascular differentiation. *Lab. Invest.*, **83**(12), 1811–20.

[42] Goldman, O., Feraud, O., Boyer-Di Ponio, J. *et al.* 2009. A boost of BMP4 accelerates the commitment of human embryonic stem cells to the endothelial lineage. *Stem Cells*, **27**(8), 1750–9.

[43] Woll, P. S., Morris, J. K., Painschab, M. S. *et al.* 2008. Wnt signaling promotes hematoendothelial cell development from human embryonic stem cells. *Blood*, **111**(1), 122–31.

[44] Vo, E., Hanjaya-Putra, D., Zha, Y., Kusuma, S. and Gerecht, S. 2010. Smooth-muscle-like cells derived from human embryonic stem cells support and augment cord-like structures in vitro. *Stem Cell Rev.*, **6**(2), 237–47.

[45] Huang, H., Zhao, X., Chen, L. *et al.* 2006. Differentiation of human embryonic stem cells into smooth muscle cells in adherent monolayer culture. *Biochem. Biophys. Res. Commun.*, **351**(2), 321–7.

[46] Xie, C. Q., Zhang, J., Villacorta, L. *et al.* 2007. A highly efficient method to differentiate smooth muscle cells from human embryonic stem cells. *Arterioscler. Thromb. Vasc. Biol.*, **27**(12), e311–12.

[47] Cheung, C., Bernardo, A. S., Trotter, M. W., Pedersen, R. A. and Sinha, S. 2012. Generation of human vascular smooth muscle subtypes provides insight into embryological origin-dependent disease susceptibility. *Nature Biotechnol.*, **30**(2), 165–73.

[48] Takahashi, K., Tanabe, K., Ohnuki, M. *et al.* 2007. Induction of pluripotent stem cells from adult human fibroblasts by defined factors. *Cell*, **131**(5), 861–72.

[49] Takahashi, K. and Yamanaka, S. 2006. Induction of pluripotent stem cells from mouse embryonic and adult fibroblast cultures by defined factors. *Cell*, **126**(4), 663–76.

[50] Dimos, J. T., Rodolfa, K. T., Niakan, K. K. *et al.* 2008. Induced pluripotent stem cells generated from patients with ALS can be differentiated into motor neurons. *Science*, **321**(5893), 1218–21.

[51] Park, I. H., Arora, N., Huo, H. *et al.* 2008. Disease-specific induced pluripotent stem cells. *Cell*, **134**(5), 877–86.

[52] Soldner, F., Laganiere, J., Cheng, A. W. *et al.* 2011. Generation of isogenic pluripotent stem cells differing

exclusively at two early onset Parkinson point mutations. *Cell*, **146**(2), 318–31.

[53] Choi, K. D., Yu, J., Smuga-Otto, K. *et al.* 2009. Hematopoietic and endothelial differentiation of human induced pluripotent stem cells. *Stem Cells*, **27**(3), 559–67.

[54] Feng, Q., Lu, S. J., Klimanskaya, I. *et al.* 2010. Hemangioblastic derivatives from human induced pluripotent stem cells exhibit limited expansion and early senescence. *Stem Cells*, **28**(4), 704–12.

[55] Homma, K., Sone, M., Taura, D. *et al.* 2010. Sirt1 plays an important role in mediating greater functionality of human ES/iPS-derived vascular endothelial cells. *Atherosclerosis*, **212**(1), 42–7.

[56] Taura, D., Sone, M., Homma, K. *et al.* 2009. Induction and isolation of vascular cells from human induced pluripotent stem cells – brief report. *Arterioscler. Thromb. Vasc. Biol.*, **29**(7), 1100–3.

[57] Rufaihah, A. J., Huang, N. F., Jame, S. *et al.* 2011. Endothelial cells derived from human iPSCs increase capillary density and improve perfusion in a mouse model of peripheral arterial disease. *Arterioscler. Thromb. Vasc. Biol.*, **31**(11), e72–9.

[58] Xie, C. Q., Huang, H., Wei, S. *et al.* 2009. A comparison of murine smooth muscle cells generated from embryonic versus induced pluripotent stem cells. *Stem Cells Dev.*, **18**(5), 741–8.

[59] Lee, T. H., Song, S. H., Kim, K. L. *et al.* 2010. Functional recapitulation of smooth muscle cells via induced pluripotent stem cells from human aortic smooth muscle cells. *Circ Res.*, **106**(1), 120–8.

[60] Xie, C., Hu, J., Ma, H. *et al.* 2011. Three-dimensional growth of iPS cell-derived smooth muscle cells on nanofibrous scaffolds. *Biomaterials*, **32**(19), 4369–75.

[61] Korbling, M. and Estrov, Z. 2003. Adult stem cells for tissue repair – a new therapeutic concept? *N. Engl. J. Med.*, **349**(6), 570–82.

[62] Bianco, P., Riminucci, M., Gronthos, S. and Robey, P. G. 2001. Bone marrow stromal stem cells: nature, biology, and potential applications. *Stem Cells*, **19**(3), 180–92.

[63] Asahara, T., Murohara, T., Sullivan, A. *et al.* 1997. Isolation of putative progenitor endothelial cells for angiogenesis. *Science*, **275**(5302), 964–7.

[64] Jackson, K. A., Majka, S. M., Wang, H. *et al.* 2001. Regeneration of ischemic cardiac muscle and vascular endothelium by adult stem cells. *J. Clin. Invest.*, **107**(11), 1395–402.

[65] Kamihata, H., Matsubara, H., Nishiue, T. *et al.* 2001. Implantation of bone marrow mononuclear cells into ischemic myocardium enhances collateral perfusion and regional function via side supply of angioblasts, angiogenic ligands, and cytokines. *Circulation*, **104**(9), 1046–52.

[66] Kocher, A. A., Schuster, M. D., Szabolcs, M. J. *et al.* 2001. Neovascularization of ischemic myocardium by human bone-marrow-derived angioblasts prevents cardiomyocyte apoptosis, reduces remodeling and improves cardiac function. *Nature Med.*, **7**(4), 430–6.

[67] Orlic, D., Kajstura, J., Chimenti, S. *et al.* 2001. Bone marrow cells regenerate infarcted myocardium. *Nature*, **410**(6829), 701–5.

[68] Orlic, D., Kajstura, J., Chimenti, S. *et al.* 2001. Mobilized bone marrow cells repair the infarcted heart, improving function and survival. *Proc. Nat. Acad. Sci. USA*, **98**(18), 10344–9.

[69] Reyes, M., Dudek, A., Jahagirdar, B. *et al.* 2002. Origin of endothelial progenitors in human postnatal bone marrow. *J. Clin. Invest.*, **109**(3), 337–46.

[70] Shintani, S., Murohara, T., Ikeda, H. *et al.* 2001. Augmentation of postnatal neovascularization with autologous bone marrow transplantation. *Circulation*, **103**(6), 897–903.

[71] Takahashi, T., Kalka, C., Masuda, H. *et al.* 1999. Ischemia- and cytokine-induced mobilization of bone marrow-derived endothelial progenitor cells for neovascularization. *Nature Med.*, **5**(4), 434–8.

[72] Iba, O., Matsubara, H., Nozawa, Y. *et al.* 2002. Angiogenesis by implantation of peripheral blood mononuclear cells and platelets into ischemic limbs. *Circulation*, **106**(15), 2019–25.

[73] Pesce, M., Orlandi, A., Iachininoto, M. G. *et al.* 2003. Myoendothelial differentiation of human umbilical cord blood-derived stem cells in ischemic limb tissues. *Circ. Res.*, **93**(5), e51–62.

[74] Beltrami, A. P., Barlucchi, L., Torella, D. *et al.* 2003. Adult cardiac stem cells are multipotent and support myocardial regeneration. *Cell*, **114**(6), 763–76.

[75] Campagnolo, P., Cesselli, D., Al Haj Zen, A. *et al.* 2010. Human adult vena saphena contains perivascular progenitor cells endowed with clonogenic and proangiogenic potential. *Circulation*, **121**(15), 1735–45.

[76] Werner, N., Junk, S., Laufs, U. *et al.* 2003. Intravenous transfusion of endothelial progenitor cells reduces neointima formation after vascular injury. *Circ. Res.*, **93**(2), e17–24.

[77] Lin, Y., Chen, X., Yan, Z. *et al.* 2006. Multilineage differentiation of adipose-derived stromal cells from GFP transgenic mice. *Molec. Cell Biochem.*, **285**(1–2), 69–78.

[78] Planat-Benard, V., Silvestre, J. S., Cousin, B. *et al.* 2004. Plasticity of human adipose lineage cells toward endothelial cells: physiological and therapeutic perspectives. *Circulation*, **109**(5), 656–63.
[79] Friedenstein, A. J., Piatetzky, S. II and Petrakova, K. V. 1966. Osteogenesis in transplants of bone marrow cells. *J. Embryol. Exp. Morphol.*, **16**(3), 381–90.
[80] Kern, S., Eichler, H., Stoeve, J., Kluter, H. and Bieback, K. 2006. Comparative analysis of mesenchymal stem cells from bone marrow, umbilical cord blood, or adipose tissue. *Stem Cells*, **24**(5), 1294–301.
[81] Pasquinelli, G., Pacilli, A., Alviano, F. *et al.* 2010. Multidistrict human mesenchymal vascular cells: pluripotency and stemness characteristics. *Cytotherapy*, **12**(3), 275–87.
[82] Pasquinelli, G., Tazzari, P. L., Vaselli, C. *et al.* 2007. Thoracic aortas from multiorgan donors are suitable for obtaining resident angiogenic mesenchymal stromal cells. *Stem Cells*, **25**(7), 1627–34.
[83] Liu, J. Y., Peng, H. F., Gopinath, S., Tian, J. and Andreadis, S. T. 2010. Derivation of functional smooth muscle cells from multipotent human hair follicle mesenchymal stem cells. *Tissue Eng. Part A*, **16**(8), 2553–64.
[84] Parolini, O., Alviano, F., Bagnara, G. P. *et al.* 2008. Concise review: isolation and characterization of cells from human term placenta: outcome of the First International Workshop on Placenta Derived Stem Cells. *Stem Cells*, **26**(2), 300–11.
[85] Erices, A., Conget, P. and Minguell, J. J. 2000. Mesenchymal progenitor cells in human umbilical cord blood. *Br. J. Haematol.*, **109**(1), 235–42.
[86] Goodwin, H. S., Bicknese, A. R., Chien, S. N. *et al.* 2001. Multilineage differentiation activity by cells isolated from umbilical cord blood: expression of bone, fat, and neural markers. *Biol. Blood Marrow Transplant.*, **7**(11), 581–8.
[87] Mareschi, K., Biasin, E., Piacibello, W. *et al.* 2001. Isolation of human mesenchymal stem cells: bone marrow versus umbilical cord blood. *Haematologica*, **86**(10), 1099–100.
[88] Lee, O. K., Kuo, T. K., Chen, W. M. *et al.* 2004. Isolation of multipotent mesenchymal stem cells from umbilical cord blood. *Blood*, **103**(5), 1669–75.
[89] Zuk, P. A., Zhu, M., Mizuno, H. *et al.* 2001. Multilineage cells from human adipose tissue: implications for cell-based therapies. *Tissue Eng.*, **7**(2), 211–28.
[90] Covas, D. T., Siufi, J. L., Silva, A. R. and Orellana, M. D. 2003. Isolation and culture of umbilical vein mesenchymal stem cells. *Braz. J. Med. Biol. Res.*, **36**(9), 1179–83.
[91] Romanov, Y. A., Svintsitskaya, V. A. and Smirnov, V. N. 2003. Searching for alternative sources of postnatal human mesenchymal stem cells: candidate MSC-like cells from umbilical cord. *Stem Cells*, **21**(1), 105–10.
[92] Fernandez, M., Simon, V., Herrera, G. *et al.* 1997. Detection of stromal cells in peripheral blood progenitor cell collections from breast cancer patients. *Bone Marrow Transplant.*, **20**(4), 265–71.
[93] Kuramochi, Y., Fukazawa, R., Migita, M. *et al.* 2003. Cardiomyocyte regeneration from circulating bone marrow cells in mice. *Pediatr. Res.*, **54**(3), 319–25.
[94] Zvaifler, N. J., Marinova-Mutafchieva, L., Adams, G. *et al.* 2000. Mesenchymal precursor cells in the blood of normal individuals. *Arthritis Res.*, **2**(6), 477–88.
[95] Davani, S., Marandin, A., Mersin, N. *et al.* 2003. Mesenchymal progenitor cells differentiate into an endothelial phenotype, enhance vascular density, and improve heart function in a rat cellular cardiomyoplasty model. *Circulation*, **108**(Suppl. 1), II253–8.
[96] Gojo, S., Gojo, N., Takeda, Y. *et al.* 2003. In vivo cardiovasculogenesis by direct injection of isolated adult mesenchymal stem cells. *Exp. Cell. Res.*, **288**(1), 51–9.
[97] Oswald, J., Boxberger, S., Jorgensen, B. *et al.* 2004. Mesenchymal stem cells can be differentiated into endothelial cells in vitro. *Stem Cells*, **22**(3), 377–84.
[98] Dong, J. D., Gu, Y. Q., Li, C. M. *et al.* 2009. Response of mesenchymal stem cells to shear stress in tissue-engineered vascular grafts. *Acta Pharmacol. Sin.*, **30**(5), 530–6.
[99] Shin'oka, T., Matsumura, G., Hibino, N. *et al.* 2005. Midterm clinical result of tissue-engineered vascular autografts seeded with autologous bone marrow cells. *J. Thorac. Cardiovasc. Surg.*, **129**(6), 1330–8.
[100] Galmiche, M. C., Koteliansky, V. E., Briere, J., Herve, P. and Charbord, P. 1993. Stromal cells from human long-term marrow cultures are mesenchymal cells that differentiate following a vascular smooth muscle differentiation pathway. *Blood*, **82**(1), 66–76.
[101] Seruya, M., Shah, A., Pedrotty, D. *et al.* 2004. Clonal population of adult stem cells: life span and differentiation potential. *Cell Transplant.*, **13**(2), 93–101.
[102] Kinner, B., Zaleskas, J. M. and Spector, M. 2002. Regulation of smooth muscle actin expression and contraction in adult human mesenchymal stem cells. *Exp. Cell Res.*, **278**(1), 72–83.
[103] Fierro, F. A., Kalomoiris, S., Sondergaard, C. S. and Nolta, J. A. 2011. Effects on proliferation and differentiation of multipotent bone marrow stromal cells

engineered to express growth factors for combined cell and gene therapy. *Stem Cells*, **29**(11), 1727–37.

[104] Ball, S. G., Shuttleworth, A. C. and Kielty, C. M. 2004. Direct cell contact influences bone marrow mesenchymal stem cell fate. *Int. J. Biochem. Cell Biol.*, **36**(4), 714–27.

[105] Hamilton, D. W., Maul, T. M. and Vorp, D. A. 2004. Characterization of the response of bone marrow-derived progenitor cells to cyclic strain: implications for vascular tissue-engineering applications. *Tissue Eng.*, **10**(3–4), 361–9.

[106] Gong, Z. and Niklason, L. E. 2008. Small-diameter human vessel wall engineered from bone marrow-derived mesenchymal stem cells (hMSCs). *FASEB J.*, **22**(6), 1635–48.

[107] Cho, S. W., Lim, S. H., Kim, I. K. *et al.* 2005. Small-diameter blood vessels engineered with bone marrow-derived cells. *Ann. Surg.*, **241**(3), 506–15.

[108] Zhao, Y., Zhang, S., Zhou, J. *et al.* 2010. The development of a tissue-engineered artery using decellularized scaffold and autologous ovine mesenchymal stem cells. *Biomaterials*, **31**(2), 296–307.

[109] Caplan, A. I. 2009. Why are MSCs therapeutic? New data: new insight. *J. Pathol.*, **217**(2), 318–24.

[110] Peichev, M., Naiyer, A. J., Pereira, D. *et al.* 2000. Expression of VEGFR-2 and AC133 by circulating human CD34(+) cells identifies a population of functional endothelial precursors. *Blood*, **95**(3), 952–8.

[111] Schmid, M. C. and Varner, J. A. 2009. Circulating endothelial progenitor cells. *Methods Molec. Biol.*, **467**, 139–55.

[112] Miranville, A., Heeschen, C., Sengenes, C. *et al.* 2004. Improvement of postnatal neovascularization by human adipose tissue-derived stem cells. *Circulation*, **110**(3), 349–55.

[113] Xue, S., Zhang, H. T., Zhang, P. *et al.* 2010. Functional endothelial progenitor cells derived from adipose tissue show beneficial effect on cell therapy of traumatic brain injury. *Neurosci. Lett.*, **473**(3), 186–91.

[114] Ingram, D. A., Mead, L. E., Moore, D. B. *et al.* 2005. Vessel wall-derived endothelial cells rapidly proliferate because they contain a complete hierarchy of endothelial progenitor cells. *Blood*, **105**(7), 2783–6.

[115] Murohara, T., Ikeda, H., Duan, J. *et al.* 2000. Transplanted cord blood-derived endothelial precursor cells augment postnatal neovascularization. *J. Clin. Invest.*, **105**(11), 1527–36.

[116] Heeschen, C., Aicher, A., Lehmann, R. *et al.* 2003. Erythropoietin is a potent physiologic stimulus for endothelial progenitor cell mobilization. *Blood*, **102**(4), 1340–6.

[117] Strehlow, K., Werner, N., Berweiler, J. *et al.* 2003. Estrogen increases bone marrow-derived endothelial progenitor cell production and diminishes neointima formation. *Circulation*, **107**(24), 3059–65.

[118] Cherqui, S., Kurian, S. M., Schussler, O. *et al.* 2006. Isolation and angiogenesis by endothelial progenitors in the fetal liver. *Stem Cells*, **24**(1), 44–54.

[119] Kordes, C., Sawitza, I., Muller-Marbach, A. *et al.* 2007. $CD133^+$ hepatic stellate cells are progenitor cells. *Biochem. Biophys. Res. Commun.*, **352**(2), 410–17.

[120] Messina, E., De Angelis, L., Frati, G. *et al.* 2004. Isolation and expansion of adult cardiac stem cells from human and murine heart. *Circ. Res.*, **95**(9), 911–21.

[121] Adams, V., Lenk, K., Linke, A. *et al.* 2004. Increase of circulating endothelial progenitor cells in patients with coronary artery disease after exercise-induced ischemia. *Arterioscler. Thromb. Vasc. Biol.*, **24**(4), 684–90.

[122] Vasa, M., Fichtlscherer, S., Adler, K. *et al.* 2001. Increase in circulating endothelial progenitor cells by statin therapy in patients with stable coronary artery disease. *Circulation*, **103**(24), 2885–90.

[123] Vasa, M., Fichtlscherer, S., Aicher, A. *et al.* 2001. Number and migratory activity of circulating endothelial progenitor cells inversely correlate with risk factors for coronary artery disease. *Circ. Res.*, **89**(1), E1–7.

[124] Al Attar, N., Carrion, C., Ghostine, S. *et al.* 2003. Long-term (1 year) functional and histological results of autologous skeletal muscle cells transplantation in rat. *Cardiovasc. Res.*, **58**(1), 142–8.

[125] Werner, N., Priller, J., Laufs, U. *et al.* 2002. Bone marrow-derived progenitor cells modulate vascular reendothelialization and neointimal formation: effect of 3-hydroxy-3-methylglutaryl coenzyme a reductase inhibition. *Arterioscler. Thromb. Vasc. Biol.*, **22**(10), 1567–72.

[126] Bahlmann, F. H., De Groot, K., Spandau, J. M. *et al.* 2004. Erythropoietin regulates endothelial progenitor cells. *Blood*, **103**(3), 921–6.

[127] Masuda, H. and Asahara, T. 2003. Post-natal endothelial progenitor cells for neovascularization in tissue regeneration. *Cardiovasc. Res.*, **58**(2), 390–8.

[128] Khakoo, A. Y. and Finkel, T. 2005. Endothelial progenitor cells. *Ann. Rev. Med.*, **56**, 79–101.

[129] Kalka, C., Masuda, H., Takahashi, T. *et al.* 2000. Transplantation of ex vivo expanded endothelial progenitor

cells for therapeutic neovascularization. *Proc. Nat. Acad. Sci. USA*, **97**(7), 3422–7.

[130] Tateishi-Yuyama, E., Matsubara, H., Murohara, T. *et al.* 2002. Therapeutic angiogenesis for patients with limb ischaemia by autologous transplantation of bone-marrow cells: a pilot study and a randomised controlled trial. *Lancet*, **360**(9331), 427–35.

[131] Asahara, T., Masuda, H., Takahashi, T. *et al.* 1999. Bone marrow origin of endothelial progenitor cells responsible for postnatal vasculogenesis in physiological and pathological neovascularization. *Circ. Res.*, **85**(3), 221–8.

[132] Bhattacharya, V., McSweeney, P. A., Shi, Q. *et al.* 2000. Enhanced endothelialization and microvessel formation in polyester grafts seeded with CD34(+) bone marrow cells. *Blood*, **95**(2), 581–5.

[133] Shi, Q., Rafii, S., Wu, M. H. *et al.* 1998. Evidence for circulating bone marrow-derived endothelial cells. *Blood*, **92**(2), 362–7.

[134] Barrilleaux, B., Phinney, D. G., Prockop, D. J. and O'Connor, K. C. 2006. Ex vivo engineering of living tissues with adult stem cells. *Tissue Eng.*, **12**(11), 3007–19.

[135] Isenberg, B. C., Williams, C. and Tranquillo, R. T. 2006. Small-diameter artificial arteries engineered in vitro. *Circ. Res.*, **98**(1), 25–35.

[136] Sales, K. M., Salacinski, H. J., Alobaid, N. *et al.* 2005. Advancing vascular tissue engineering: the role of stem cell technology. *Trends Biotechnol.*, **23**(9), 461–7.

[137] Wijelath, E. S., Rahman, S., Murray, J. *et al.* 2004. Fibronectin promotes VEGF-induced CD34 cell differentiation into endothelial cells. *J. Vasc. Surg.*, **39**(3), 655–60.

[138] Kanayasu-Toyoda, T., Yamaguchi, T., Oshizawa, T. and Hayakawa, T. 2003. CD31 (PECAM-1)-bright cells derived from AC133-positive cells in human peripheral blood as endothelial-precursor cells. *J. Cell Physiol.*, **195**(1), 119–29.

[139] Asahara, T., Takahashi, T., Masuda, H. *et al.* 1999. VEGF contributes to postnatal neovascularization by mobilizing bone marrow-derived endothelial progenitor cells. *EMBO J.*, **18**(14), 3964–72.

[140] Gehling, U. M., Ergun, S., Schumacher, U. *et al.* 2000. In vitro differentiation of endothelial cells from AC133-positive progenitor cells. *Blood*, **95**(10), 3106–12.

[141] Rehman, J., Li, J., Orschell, C. M. and March, K. L. 2003. Peripheral blood "endothelial progenitor cells" are derived from monocyte/macrophages and secrete angiogenic growth factors. *Circulation*, **107**(8), 1164–9.

[142] Yamamoto, K., Takahashi, T., Asahara, T. *et al.* 2003. Proliferation, differentiation, and tube formation by endothelial progenitor cells in response to shear stress. *J. Appl. Physiol.*, **95**(5), 2081–8.

[143] Dvorin, E. L., Wylie-Sears, J., Kaushal, S., Martin, D. P. and Bischoff, J. 2003. Quantitative evaluation of endothelial progenitors and cardiac valve endothelial cells: proliferation and differentiation on poly-glycolic acid/poly-4-hydroxybutyrate scaffold in response to vascular endothelial growth factor and transforming growth factor beta1. *Tissue Eng.*, **9**(3), 487–93.

[144] Matsumura, G., Miyagawa-Tomita, S., Shin'oka, T., Ikada, Y. and Kurosawa, H. 2003. First evidence that bone marrow cells contribute to the construction of tissue-engineered vascular autografts in vivo. *Circulation*, **108**(14), 1729–34.

[145] Wu, X., Rabkin-Aikawa, E., Guleserian, K. J. *et al.* 2004. Tissue-engineered microvessels on three-dimensional biodegradable scaffolds using human endothelial progenitor cells. *Am. J. Physiol. Heart Circ. Physiol.*, **287**(2), H480–7.

[146] Aper, T., Schmidt, A., Duchrow, M. and Bruch, H. P. 2007. Autologous blood vessels engineered from peripheral blood sample. *Eur. J. Vasc. Endovasc. Surg.*, **33**(1), 33–9.

[147] Schmidt, D., Breymann, C., Weber, A. *et al.* 2004. Umbilical cord blood derived endothelial progenitor cells for tissue engineering of vascular grafts. *Ann. Thorac. Surg.*, **78**(6), 2094–8.

[148] Kaushal, S., Amiel, G. E., Guleserian, K. J. *et al.* 2001. Functional small-diameter neovessels created using endothelial progenitor cells expanded ex vivo. *Nature Med.*, **7**(9), 1035–40.

[149] Li, X., Tjwa, M., Moons, L. *et al.* 2005. Revascularization of ischemic tissues by PDGF-CC via effects on endothelial cells and their progenitors. *J. Clin. Invest.*, **115**(1), 118–27.

[150] Miyata, T., Iizasa, H., Sai, Y. *et al.* 2005. Platelet-derived growth factor-BB (PDGF-BB) induces differentiation of bone marrow endothelial progenitor cell-derived cell line TR-BME2 into mural cells, and changes the phenotype. *J. Cell Physiol.*, **204**(3), 948–55.

[151] Diez, M., Musri, M. M., Ferrer, E., Barbera, J. A. and Peinado, V. I. 2010. Endothelial progenitor cells undergo an endothelial-to-mesenchymal transition-like process mediated by TGFβRI. *Cardiovasc. Res.*, **88**(3), 502–11.

[152] Diez, M., Barbera, J. A., Ferrer, E. *et al.* 2007. Plasticity of $CD133^{+}$ cells: role in pulmonary vascular remodeling. *Cardiovasc. Res.*, **76**(3), 517–27.

[153] Katz, A. J., Tholpady, A., Tholpady, S. S., Shang, H. and Ogle, R. C. 2005. Cell surface and transcriptional characterization of human adipose-derived adherent stromal (hADAS) cells. *Stem Cells*, **23**(3), 412–23.

[154] Zuk, P. A., Zhu, M., Ashjian, P. *et al.* 2000. Human adipose tissue is a source of multipotent stem cells. *Molec. Biol. Cell*, **13**(12), 4279–95.

[155] Gronthos, S., Franklin, D. M., Leddy, H. A. *et al.* 2001. Surface protein characterization of human adipose tissue-derived stromal cells. *J. Cell Physiol.*, **189**(1), 54–63.

[156] Musina, R. A., Bekchanova, E. S. and Sukhikh, G. T. 2005. Comparison of mesenchymal stem cells obtained from different human tissues. *Bull. Exp. Biol. Med.*, **139**(4), 504–9.

[157] Romanov, Y. A., Darevskaya, A. N., Merzlikina, N. V. and Buravkova, L. B. 2005. Mesenchymal stem cells from human bone marrow and adipose tissue: isolation, characterization, and differentiation potentialities. *Bull. Exp. Biol. Med.*, **140**(1), 138–43.

[158] Cao, Y., Sun, Z., Liao, L. *et al.* 2005. Human adipose tissue-derived stem cells differentiate into endothelial cells in vitro and improve postnatal neovascularization in vivo. *Biochem. Biophys. Res. Commun.*, **332**(2), 370–9.

[159] Martinez-Estrada, O. M., Munoz-Santos, Y., Julve, J., Reina, M. and Vilaro, S. 2005. Human adipose tissue as a source of Flk-1$^+$ cells: new method of differentiation and expansion. *Cardiovasc. Res.*, **65**(2), 328–33.

[160] Rodriguez, L. V., Alfonso, Z., Zhang, R. *et al.* 2006. Clonogenic multipotent stem cells in human adipose tissue differentiate into functional smooth muscle cells. *Proc. Nat. Acad. Sci. USA*, **103**(32), 12167–72.

[161] Kim, Y. M., Jeon, E. S., Kim, M. R. *et al.* 2008. Angiotensin II-induced differentiation of adipose tissue-derived mesenchymal stem cells to smooth muscle-like cells. *Int. J. Biochem. Cell Biol.*, **40**(11), 2482–91.

[162] Wang, C., Yin, S., Cen, L. *et al.* 2010. Differentiation of adipose-derived stem cells into contractile smooth muscle cells induced by transforming growth factor-β_1 and bone morphogenetic protein-4. *Tissue Eng. Part A*, **16**(4), 1201–13.

[163] Harris, L. J., Abdollahi, H., Zhang, P. *et al.* 2011. Differentiation of adult stem cells into smooth muscle for vascular tissue engineering. *J. Surg. Res.*, **168**(2), 306–14.

[164] Wang, C., Cen, L., Yin, S. *et al.* 2010. A small diameter elastic blood vessel wall prepared under pulsatile conditions from polyglycolic acid mesh and smooth muscle cells differentiated from adipose-derived stem cells. *Biomaterials*, **31**(4), 621–30.

[165] Huang, X. and Saint-Jeannet, J. P. 2004. Induction of the neural crest and the opportunities of life on the edge. *Dev. Biol.*, **275**(1), 1–11.

[166] Shakhova, O. and Sommer, L. 2010. Neural crest-derived stem cells. In The Stem Cell Research Community, editors. *StemBook*, doi/10.3824/stembook.1.51.1, http://www.stembook.org.

[167] Wurmser, A. E., Nakashima, K., Summers, R. G. *et al.* 2004. Cell fusion-independent differentiation of neural stem cells to the endothelial lineage. *Nature*, **430**(6997), 350–6.

[168] Majesky, M. W. 2007. Developmental basis of vascular smooth muscle diversity. *Arterioscler. Thromb. Vasc. Biol.*, **27**(6), 1248–58.

[169] Xie, C., Ritchie, R. P., Huang, H., Zhang, J. and Chen, Y. E. 2011. Smooth muscle cell differentiation in vitro: models and underlying molecular mechanisms. *Arterioscler. Thromb. Vasc. Biol.*, **31**(7), 1485–94.

[170] Fernandes, K. J., McKenzie, I. A., Mill, P. *et al.* 2004. A dermal niche for multipotent adult skin-derived precursor cells. *Nature Cell Biol.*, **6**(11), 1082–93.

[171] Fujiwara, H., Ferreira, M., Donati, G. *et al.* 2011. The basement membrane of hair follicle stem cells is a muscle cell niche. *Cell*, **144**(4), 577–89.

[172] Steinbach, S. K., El-Mounayri, O., DaCosta, R. S. *et al.* 2011. Directed differentiation of skin-derived precursors into functional vascular smooth muscle cells. *Arterioscler. Thromb. Vasc. Biol.*, **31**(12), 2938–48.

[173] De Coppi, P., Bartsch, G., Jr., Siddiqui, M. M. *et al.* 2007. Isolation of amniotic stem cell lines with potential for therapy. *Nature Biotechnol.*, **25**(1), 100–6.

[174] Perin, L., Sedrakyan, S., Da Sacco, S. and De Filippo, R. 2008. Characterization of human amniotic fluid stem cells and their pluripotential capability. *Methods Cell Biol.*, **86**, 85–99.

[175] Zhang, P., Baxter, J., Vinod, K., Tulenko, T. N. and Di Muzio, P. J. 2009. Endothelial differentiation of amniotic fluid-derived stem cells: synergism of biochemical and shear force stimuli. *Stem Cells Dev.*, **18**(9), 1299–308.

[176] Simper, D., Stalboerger, P. G., Panetta, C. J., Wang, S. and Caplice, N. M. 2002. Smooth muscle progenitor cells in human blood. *Circulation*, **106**(10), 1199–204.

[177] Aird, W. C. 2007. Phenotypic heterogeneity of the endothelium: II. Representative vascular beds. *Circ. Res.*, **100**(2), 174–90.

[178] Thorgeirsson, G. and Robertson, A. L., Jr. 1978. The vascular endothelium – pathobiologic significance. *Am. J. Pathol.*, **93**(3), 803–48.

[179] Nagy, Z., Peters, H. and Huttner, I. 1984. Fracture faces of cell junctions in cerebral endothelium during normal and hyperosmotic conditions. *Lab. Invest.*, **50**(3), 313–22.

[180] Wolburg, H., Neuhaus, J., Kniesel, U. *et al.* 1994. Modulation of tight junction structure in blood-brain barrier endothelial cells. Effects of tissue culture, second messengers and cocultured astrocytes. *J. Cell Sci.*, **107**(Part 5), 1347–57.

[181] Risau, W. 1995. Differentiation of endothelium. *FASEB J.*, **9**(10), 926–33.

[182] Aird, W. C. 2003. Endothelial cell heterogeneity. *Crit. Care Med.*, **31**(4 Suppl.), S221–30.

[183] Craig, L. E., Spelman, J. P., Strandberg, J. D. and Zink, M. C. 1998. Endothelial cells from diverse tissues exhibit differences in growth and morphology. *Microvasc. Res.*, **55**(1), 65–76.

[184] Garlanda, C. and Dejana, E. 1997. Heterogeneity of endothelial cells. Specific markers. *Arterioscler. Thromb. Vasc. Biol.*, **17**(7), 1193–202.

[185] Atkins, G. B., Jain, M. K. and Hamik, A. 2011. Endothelial differentiation: molecular mechanisms of specification and heterogeneity. *Arterioscler. Thromb. Vasc. Biol.*, **31**(7), 1476–84.

[186] Ferguson, J. E., 3rd, Kelley, R. W. and Patterson, C. 2005. Mechanisms of endothelial differentiation in embryonic vasculogenesis. *Arterioscler. Thromb. Vasc. Biol.*, **25**(11), 2246–54.

[187] Riha, G. M., Lin, P. H., Lumsden, A. B., Yao, Q. and Chen, C. 2005. Application of stem cells for vascular tissue engineering. *Tissue Eng.*, **11**(9–10), 1535–52.

[188] Hu, J., Sun, X., Ma, H. *et al.* 2010. Porous nanofibrous PLLA scaffolds for vascular tissue engineering. *Biomaterials*, **31**(31), 7971–7.

[189] Wei, G., Jin, Q., Giannobile, W. V. and Ma, P. X. 2007. The enhancement of osteogenesis by nano-fibrous scaffolds incorporating rhBMP-7 nanospheres. *Biomaterials*, **28**(12), 2087–96.

[190] Wu, S. M. and Hochedlinger, K. 2011. Harnessing the potential of induced pluripotent stem cells for regenerative medicine. *Nature Cell Biol.*, **13**(5), 497–505.

[191] Liu, G. H., Suzuki, K., Qu, J. *et al.* 2011. Targeted gene correction of laminopathy-associated LMNA mutations in patient-specific iPSCs. *Cell Stem Cell*, **8**(6), 688–94.

[192] Pontikoglou, C., Delorme, B. and Charbord, P. 2008. Human bone marrow native mesenchymal stem cells. *Regen. Med.*, **3**(5), 731–41.

[193] Miller-Kasprzak, E. and Jagodziński, P. P. 2007. Endothelial progenitor cells as a new agent contributing to vascular repair. *Arch. Immunol. Ther. Exp. (Warszawa)*, **55**(4), 247–59.

[194] Yoder, M. C. 2010. Is endothelium the origin of endothelial progenitor cells? *Arterioscler. Thromb. Vasc. Biol.*, **30**(6), 1094–103.

[195] Ratajczak, M. Z. 2008. Phenotypic and functional characterization of hematopoietic stem cells. *Curr. Opin. Hematol.*, **15**(4), 293–300.

[196] Di Nardo, P., Forte, G., Ahluwalia, A. and Minieri, M. 2010. Cardiac progenitor cells: potency and control. *J. Cell Physiol.*, **224**(3), 590–600.

36

Cardiac tissue regeneration in bioreactors

Loraine L. Y. Chiu, Boyang Zhang, Yun Xiao and Milica Radisic

36.1 Motivation for cardiac tissue regeneration in vitro

Myocardial infarction (MI) leads to the death of cardiomyocytes, and the infarct area becomes replaced by a fibroblastic scar tissue that has no contractile function. This reduces the pumping ability of the heart and the cardiac output. In addition, the scar tissue thins due to the lack of vasculature to provide oxygen and nutrients to the infarct site, thus leading to high wall stress and cardiac dilatation, which may ultimately lead to heart failure.

The adult heart has a limited regenerative capacity. The shortage of donor organs further suggests a need to develop new treatment strategies for cardiovascular diseases. Cardiac tissue regeneration can be achieved through several strategies, including (1) gene therapy, (2) cell transplantation, and (3) implantation or injection of biomaterials or engineered cardiac tissues. The goal of these cardiac tissue regeneration strategies is to repair the damaged myocardium through supporting vascularization and cell survival, in turn reducing wall thinning and preventing dilatation and heart failure. Gene therapy is not a specific topic of this chapter, in which the focus will be on bioreactors for cell expansion and engineering of cardiac tissues for cardiac tissue regeneration. Instead, we refer the reader to excellent reviews [1–3].

Since the damaged myocardium has limited capacity to regenerate, cell transplantation can replace the damaged and lost cells, thus attenuating pathological remodeling. However, cell transplantation is limited by the washout of cells from the injection site and the inability of injected cells to integrate with the native tissue. Solutions include delivering cells within a scaffold or hydrogel to support cell engraftment, and growing functional cardiac tissues that can be implanted and would integrate with the native tissue.

The classical approach to engineering cardiac tissues in vitro involves the incorporation of living cells and biomolecules into a scaffold, and the cultivation of the construct in a bioreactor. In-vitro cultivation within a bioreactor allows the cells to grow and form tissues, and ensures that the engineered cardiac tissues reach the desired level of functionality prior to use in vivo. More recently, novel approaches of cardiac tissue engineering have been developed in order to overcome the limitations of using conventional scaffolds. Cell sheet technology allows the engineering of cardiac constructs without scaffolds. Like conventional tissue engineering, it has benefits over cell injection since the tissues formed contain intact cell–cell junctions. It additionally avoids graft rejection due to inflammation, which is often caused by scaffold degradation upon implantation. Organ decellularization allows the engineering of whole hearts using decellularized cadaveric hearts as scaffolds. The decellularized heart is an ideal scaffold for cardiac tissue engineering because cultivated cells are exposed to the preserved cardiac architecture.

36.2 Approaches for cardiac tissue engineering

The goal of cardiac tissue engineering is to create new myocardium that can be electrically and mechanically integrated into the heart [4]. A functional cardiac patch for clinical applications should be mechanically stable (Young's modulus of 22–50 kPa [5]), of thickness comparable to the thickness of the human myocardium (~1 cm), and capable of electrical impulse propagation (27 cm/s for rat ventricle), and should have a high density of elongated and aligned cardiomyocytes (~10^8 cells/cm^3) with an intercapillary distance of ~20 μm. Cardiac tissue engineering requires (1) the isolation and expansion of cells, (2) tissue engineering scaffolds with biochemical and mechanical properties that are specifically suitable for the engineering of cardiac tissues, and (3) bioreactors that mimic the body environment.

36.2.1 Cells

Generally, cells for tissue engineering should be (1) expandable to achieve high numbers of cells, (2) compatible with the host without causing immune reactions, and (3) able to survive and maintain function in vitro and in vivo [6]. Cells for cardiac tissue engineering can be categorized into (1) primary cardiac cells, (2) embryonic stem cells, (3) induced pluripotent stem cells (iPSCs), (4) resident cardiac progenitor cells, and (5) adult progenitor cells from other native tissues.

36.2.1.1 Fetal and neonatal cardiac cells

Adult cardiac cells are the target cell source in cardiac regeneration since they are differentiated cardiomyocytes with developed contractile apparatus and can integrate with host cardiomyocytes through gap junctions and intercalated disks. However, they are present in low numbers and have little proliferative and developmental potential. The advantages of using fetal and neonatal cardiac cells include their greater proliferative and developmental potential than that of adult cardiac cells. These cells also showed efficacy in cardiac regeneration, since the injection of fetal or neonatal cardiomyocytes attenuated pathological ventricular remodeling by forming viable grafts, increasing the ventricle thickness, and improving left ventricular function [7, 8]. By contrast, injected adult cardiomyocytes were unable to survive both in acutely cryoinjured myocardium and in granulation tissue.

Contractile cardiac tissues have also been engineered using fetal or neonatal rat cardiomyocyte-enriched cell populations [9–12]. However, fetal or neonatal cardiac cells are not available in large numbers to provide the millions of cardiomyocytes required for cardiac tissue regeneration, thus motivating the search for alternative cell sources. Moreover, while fetal or neonatal cardiac cells from animals can readily be used, a direct translation to human studies will not be possible due to obvious ethical considerations involving the use of human cells.

36.2.1.2 Embryonic stem cells

Embryonic stem cells (ESCs) have been investigated intensively due to their ability to undergo indefinite propagation without losing the capacity to differentiate into all cell types. ESCs are commonly cultivated and differentiated in three-dimensional (3D) aggregates known as embryoid bodies (EBs). Quantification of "beating" EBs is commonly applied to assess cardiogenicity in ESCs. However, despite robust cardiomyogenicity in EBs, only 1%–5% of their total cell number consists of cardiomyocytes under standard culture conditions (i.e. plated on 0.1% gelatin-coated culture dishes and cultured in 80% knockout Dulbecco's Modified Eagle's Medium with 20% fetal bovine serum, 1 mM L-glutamine, 0.1 mM mercaptoethanol, and 1% non-essential amino acid stock [13]). The most efficient and reproducible protocols to date for differentiation of cardiomyocytes from pluripotent stem cells are those that have replicated the signaling pathways that regulate lineage commitment in the early embryo. With this approach, the earliest stages of cardiovascular development in ESC differentiation cultures were mapped, identifying a multipotent cardiovascular progenitor that displays the capacity to generate cardiac and vascular progeny [14, 15]. In mouse Flk1 and in humans KDR expression can be used to enrich for cardiac-specified mesoderm [16]. When isolated from the differentiated EBs and cultured as a monolayer, these progenitors generate contracting cardiomyocytes [14, 15]. As these progenitors differentiate, they progress through the developmental stages thought to be involved in the establishment of the cardiovascular lineages in vivo, for which specific cytokines are required. The combination of activin A and BMP4 on days 1–4 of EB differentiation induces a primitive-streak-like population and mesoderm development. Subsequent application of WNT inhibitor DKK1 and KDR ligand $VEGF_{165}$ significantly enhances the differentiation of KDR^{+} progenitors into cardiomyocytes [14, 15], while bFGF is added to support continued expansion of cardiovascular lineages.

Embryonic stem-cell-derived cardiomyocytes have been used to engineer cardiac tissues. Guo *et al.* [17] seeded mouse ESC-derived cardiomyocytes into circular molds with collagen type I and Matrigel to produce engineered heart tissues. Stevens *et al.* [18, 19] tricultured human ESC-derived cardiomyocytes with mouse embryonic fibroblasts and ESC-derived endothelial cells or human umbilical vein endothelial cells to generate scaffold-free cardiac patches.

36.2.1.3 Induced pluripotent stem cells

The recent advent of iPSCs has been considered as a solution for the ethical issues and immunological concerns associated with the usage of ESCs. Briefly, fully differentiated cells can be reprogrammed to have pluripotency like ESCs by introducing a set of transcription factors including Oct3/4, Sox2, c-Myc, and Klf4 [20]. Although the efficiency of current protocols for derivation of iPSCs is still low, iPSCs can serve as a novel cell source for cardiac tissue engineering.

Previously, Mauritz *et al.* [21] generated functional cardiomyocytes from mouse iPSCs. Importantly, human iPSCs, which were derived from reprogramming of adult fibroblasts, were differentiated into cardiomyocytes [22, 23]. The derivation of cardiomyocytes from iPSCs allows the generation of autologous human cardiomyocytes necessary for cardiac tissue regeneration [23]. Human embryonic stem cell and human iPSC-derived cardiomyocytes were previously cultured in collagen matrices using uniaxial mechanical stress conditioning and the addition of endothelial cells and stromal supporting cells [24]. The engineered human myocardium was transplanted onto hearts of athymic rats. The grafts resembled host myocardium and contained microvessels that were perfused by the host coronary circulation.

Fibroblasts, with their demonstrated ability to be transdifferentiated into skeletal muscle cells [25], have been considered as an attractive cell source for cardiac tissue engineering. Efe *et al.* [26] reprogrammed mouse embryonic fibroblasts (MEFs) directly into cardiomyocytes through over-expression of Oct4, Sox2, Klf4 and c-Myc. Reprogramming fibroblasts into cardiomyocytes is a very appealing approach since "on-site" therapy would be possible if the reprogramming could be done directly in the infarct area.

36.2.1.4 Cardiac progenitor cells

Recent studies have revealed evidence for DNA synthesis and an increase in the number of cardiomyocytes in diseased human hearts [27, 28]. Although it occurs at a very slow rate, the regeneration of cardiomyocytes in the heart seems to be an appealing solution for myocardial infarction. Endogenous regeneration of the myocardium may be due to (1) cardiomyocytes re-entering the cell cycle and dividing, or (2) the proliferation and differentiation of resident populations of cardiac progenitor cells (CPCs) [29]. Genetic manipulation or application of bioactive molecules can be used to alter the cell cycle control in adult cardiomyocytes in order to promote cell proliferation.

Urbanek *et al.* [30] reported that the increase in cardiac mass after human aortic stenosis is a result of combined myocyte hypertrophy and hyperplasia. The number of cells expressing stem cell markers and telomerase was increased in aortic stenosis. The cell clusters containing these stem cells made the transition to cardiogenic and myocyte precursors. There was also evidence of primitive myocytes turning into terminally differentiated myocytes. In a separate study, Urbanek *et al.* [31] found a cardiac stem cell pool in the human heart that is capable of promoting myocardial regeneration after infarction. The number of cardiac stem cells increased both in acute and in chronic infarcts. These cells were telomerase-competent dividing stem cells that were committed to the myocyte, smooth muscle, and endothelial cell lineages. This suggests the activation of cardiac stem cells in response to ischemic injury. However, chronic infarcts had fewer functionally competent cardiac stem cells in the viable myocardium than were present in acute cases, as indicated by the higher expression of markers of cellular senescence (i.e. p16 and p53), shorter telomeres, and greater apoptosis in cardiac stem cells of chronic infarcts. This underlies the progressive cardiac deterioration that leads to terminal cardiac failure in chronic infarcts. It was later reported that the myocardium has interstitial structures with stem cell niches that contain resident cardiac stem cells and lineage-committed cells [32]. These cells are connected through gap and adherens junctions to myocytes and fibroblasts, which act as supporting cells. The cardiac stem cells divide both symmetrically and asymmetrically, with a dominance of asymmetric division in which the cells give rise to one daughter cardiac stem cell and one daughter committed cell. This preserves primitive cells while generating myocyte progenitors, endothelial cells, and smooth muscle cells.

Laugwitz *et al.* [33] reported the identification of isl^+ cardiac progenitors in post-natal rat, mouse, and human myocardium. When co-cultured with neonatal myocytes, these $isl1^+$ cells underwent highly efficient conversion into the mature cardiac phenotype. Subsequent studies have identified CPCs in post-natal hearts with the expression of surface markers such as c-kit and Sca-1, and physiological properties such as the ability to efflux fluorescent dye and to form multicellular spheroids [34, 35]. However, these cell subpopulations are insufficient for cardiac repair without appropriate signaling. Bioactive molecules and biomaterials can be used to recruit these cells to the infarct region for *in situ* cardiac repair. In addition, these cells can be isolated and then expanded in vitro for further use in cardiac tissue regeneration.

Different resident stem cell populations have been used for cardiac repair. The injection of lin^-, $c\text{-}kit^+$ cells into the ischemic heart improved the regeneration of the myocardium [36]. In addition, cardiomyocytes were derived from the $isl1^+$ cardiac progenitor population [37]. These cells were then used to generate beating thin films [30]. Adult cardiac progenitors can also be isolated from explant cultures of human endomyocardial biopsies, and can be expanded as cardiospheres in vitro [38, 39]. These cardiosphere-derived cells improved cardiac regeneration in mice through direct differentiation and the secretion of angiogenic growth factor to improve cell survival [40]. However, it remains a challenge to generate high numbers of cardiac progenitor cells for cardiac tissue engineering.

36.2.1.5 Bone marrow cells

Bone-marrow-derived stem cells have elicited considerable interest in cardiac tissue engineering because there were reports of hematopoietic stem cells regenerating into cardiomyocytes [41]. Adult bone marrow cells have been used to regenerate and improve the functional properties of the myocardium [42–45]. Marrow-derived stromal cells, also referred to as mesenchymal stem cells (MSCs), have been applied in clinical trials, and this resulted in a significant improvement in ejection fraction [46]. However, subsequent studies showed that the improvement brought about by bone marrow cells was more likely due to their secretion of soluble factors and to their vasculogenic potential after transplantation rather than their differentiation into cardiomyocytes.

36.2.1.6 Adipose-derived cells

Besides bone marrow cells and cardiac progenitor cells, the adipose tissue is another source of autologous adult stem cells. A significantly higher density of MSCs is present in the adipose tissue than in the bone marrow (5% compared with 0.01%) [47]. Adipose-derived cells have been shown to improve cardiac tissue regeneration by direct differentiation and secretion of paracrine factors [48–50].

36.2.2 Scaffolds

The role of scaffolds in cardiac tissue engineering is to (1) support cell function, survival, proliferation, and differentiation; (2) allow infiltration of cells and blood vessels; and (3) provide mechanical support during tissue regeneration and degrade after the regenerated tissue has started to perform its proper function. Scaffolds should be biocompatible in terms of being non-toxic, causing a minimal immune response, and supporting cell attachment, survival, growth, proliferation, and differentiation. Biodegradability is also an important criterion for scaffolds used in cardiac tissue engineering. The scaffold should degrade while being replaced by the tissue formed by the seeded cells within the scaffold. In addition, the degradation products should be non-toxic, non-immunogenic, and readily removable from the body. Many natural biomaterials such as fibronectin and collagen are degraded in vitro and in vivo within days to weeks by cell-secreted enzymes [51]. Since these biomaterials are naturally occurring components of the extracellular matrix, seeded cells can also easily remodel their environment and lay down their own extracellular matrix components for tissue formation. Synthetic materials can be more easily modified to control biodegradation rate, but some may have toxic degradation products [51]. Scaffolds should also have appropriate tensile strength such that the engineered cardiac tissue can achieve simultaneous contraction with the native cardiac tissue. For example, the adult rat left-ventricular (LV) myocardium is anisotropic, with Young's modulus of ~160 kPa in the circumferential direction and ~85 kPa in the longitudinal direction [52]. Engelmayr *et al.* [52] previously designed an anisotropic scaffold based on poly(glycerol sebacate) to match the circumferential and longitudinal Young moduli of the adult rat right-ventricular (RV) myocardium (~55 kPa and ~20 kPa, respectively).

Many natural and synthetic biomaterials have been studied as scaffolds for cardiac tissue engineering. Natural biomaterials that have been used include collagen [53, 54], gelatin [11], alginate [9, 55], Matrigel [54], fibrin [56], and laminin [57]. Synthetic biomaterials include polyglycolic acid [58–62], poly-L-lactide [10], polyurethane [63], and poly(glycerol sebacate) [52].

Scaffolds can be tailored to any size or shape, and their mechanical properties can be controlled. McDevitt *et al.* [57] microcontact printed laminin onto a biodegradable polyurethane scaffold to control the spatial organization of cardiomyocytes. Zong *et al.* [10] seeded cardiomyocytes on finely textured matrices that had been fabricated by electrospinning of poly-L-lactide and polyglycolide. These matrices were mechanically stretched to attain oriented fibres. As a result, the seeded cells oriented and elongated along the fibre direction, in turn improving sarcomere development and contractile function. Zimmermann *et al.* [54] encapsulated neonatal rat cardiomyocytes in collagen type I/Matrigel into circular molds and applied unidirectional stretch to the tissue construct to engineer a heart tissue with functional and morphological properties of differentiated muscle. To decrease the immunogenicity of cultivation methods for eventual clinical application, these engineered heart tissues were cultivated under serum-free and Matrigel-free conditions [64].

Different scaffold structures have been created for cardiac tissue engineering. Engelmayr *et al.* [52] created an accordion-like poly(glycerol sebacate) scaffold to guide the orientation of CMs and achieve an anisotropic structure similar to that of the native myocardium. The honeycomb scaffold consisted of overlapping 200 μm × 200 μm squares at an angle of 45°. Cultivation of fibroblasts and cardiomyocytes in the scaffold led to aligned cells and contractile cardiac grafts with mechanical properties similar to those of the native rat right ventricle. To facilitate transport of oxygen and nutrients within the cardiac construct, porous collagen scaffolds have been used for the engineering of functional contractile cardiac patches [65]. Another strategy to improve mass transport was to mimic blood flow through a capillary structure by seeding cells in a scaffold with an array of channels, and cultivate the cardiac construct under perfusion with culture medium supplemented with perfluorocarbon, which is a synthetic oxygen carrier [66]. These cardiac constructs showed higher cell density and viability, mature cell morphology, and improved contractile properties.

Whole-heart decellularization provides an alternative method of generating a naturally derived scaffold with proper cardiac architecture. Ott *et al.* [67] decellularized cadaveric rat hearts by coronary perfusion with detergents, preserving the extracellular matrix, vascular structure, and chamber geometry. The decellularized heart acts as a scaffold for whole-heart engineering on reseeding it with cardiac cells and cultivating the construct in vitro. Whole-heart engineering is discussed further in Section 36.5.4. In a recent study, Godier-Furnémont *et al.* [68] seeded human mesenchymal progenitor cells (MPCs) in fibrin hydrogel onto decellularized sheets of human myocardium. The decellularization process preserved most elements of the extracellular matrix, as well as the underlying mechanical properties. The MPCs were conditioned with a low concentration of TGF-β to promote an arteriogenic profile of gene expression. After implantation of these constructs into the infarct bed in rats, significantly enhanced vascular network formation was observed. Echocardiography demonstrated the recovery of baseline levels of LV systolic dimensions and contractility.

Ruvinov *et al.* [29] recently described two bio-inspired materials for myocardial repair after MI. The first one is an alginate biomaterial with affinity-binding moieties, enabling the controlled binding of heparin-binding proteins. In this study, the biomaterial demonstrated the ability to increase scar thickness and prevent LV remodeling and dilatation. The second biomaterial, phosphatidylserine-presenting liposomes, was developed to mimic apoptotic cell bodies to bring activated macrophages into the anti-inflammatory state, in turn secreting high levels of anti-inflammatory cytokines such as TGF-β and interleukin-10. Treatment with the biomaterial resulted in angiogenesis, the preservation of small scars, and the prevention of ventricular dilatation and remodeling. *In situ*-forming biomaterials are beneficial for cardiac repair because of their ability to increase scar thickness and stabilize the infarct, thus reducing the wall stress and LV dilatation. In addition, the sustained presentation and delivery of biomolecules can further improve cardiac repair by eliciting appropriate cell activities such as cell survival, cell mobilization, growth factor release, and angiogenesis. Thus, cell-free bioactive biomaterials show great promise for *in situ* cardiac repair [29, 69].

Shimizu *et al.* [70] developed a novel alternative technology to engineer contractile cardiac grafts by layering monolayers of cell sheets without the use of matrix materials. Surfaces coated with a temperature-responsive polymer that is non-adhesive below 32 °C, poly-N-isopropylacrylamide, were used to culture neonatal cardiomyocytes. By lowering the temperature, cell sheets detached spontaneously, while preserving cell junctions and adhesive proteins, and could be stacked together [70, 71]. Cell sheet engineering is further discussed in Section 36.5.2. Another matrix-free self-organization approach involves spontaneous wrapping of confluent cardiomyocyte monolayers around a poly(glycolic acid) suture [72].

36.2.3 Bioreactors

Bioreactors are in-vitro culture systems that provide a monitored and controlled environment for cells to grow, expand, or assemble into an engineered tissue. The use of bioreactors for cardiac tissue regeneration can be divided into two main categories. First, bioreactors are necessary for the controlled growth and differentiation of cells prior to their use in cell transplantation or tissue engineering. These cells require controlled growth in vitro in order to expand to the large numbers necessary for cardiac tissue engineering. In addition, the differentiation of stem cells can be controlled through recapitulating the desired stem cell niche. Cell expansion and differentiation are influenced by the physiochemical (i.e. pH level, temperature, dissolved oxygen tension, hydrodynamic shear stress, osmolarity) and biochemical (i.e. nutrients, metabolic waste products, growth factors, cytokines) parameters in bioreactors [73]. Second, bioreactors are used to recreate the microenvironment that cells normally experience in the body, so as to provide biomimetic cues for aiding the formation of physiologically relevant cardiac tissues. Bioreactors for cardiac tissue engineering specifically focus on (1) improving mass transport of oxygen and nutrients to the cardiac tissue constructs in order to support the survival and growth of highly metabolically active cardiomyocytes, and (2) providing stimuli such as electrical pulses or mechanical loading to support the functional assembly of engineered myocardium through improvements in the ultrastructural differentiation of the tissue. Bioreactors are discussed in detail in Sections 36.3 and 36.4.

36.3 Bioreactors for cell expansion

Recent advances in pluripotent cell biology and biotechnology have shown promise for cell therapy to become available for many diseases. However, the robust production of pluripotent cells and their progeny necessary to provide the cell numbers required for clinical use remains challenging. To address this problem, several groups have designed different methods for scalable expansion of pluripotent cells. Among these methods, stirred-suspension bioreactors seem to be quite efficient and promising.

36.3.1 Anchorage-dependent cells

Undifferentiated pluripotent stem cells are anchorage-dependent and can be cultivated in large quantities in roller bottles [74]. Both MSCs and multipotent adult progenitor cells (MAPCs) are anchorage-dependent cells. Multiple-plate vessels are also used for cultivation of these cells since they have a large cultivation surface area to reduce the need for labor and the risk of contamination associated with the use of roller bottles. Simple stirred vessels such as spinner flasks and fermentors can also be used, in conjunction with monitoring and control of the environment. To use stirred vessels for anchorage-dependent cells, microcarriers are required in order to provide surfaces for attachment.

Microcarriers are either solid or macroporous. Solid microcarriers are made of crosslinked dextran, cellulose, or polystyrene. Cells grow on the external surface on these microcarriers. However, the exposure of cells to the bulk medium renders them susceptible to changes in the microenvironment due to mechanical agitation. Macroporous microcarriers have open pores in the interior for larger surface area, and are usually made of gelatin or collagen, to allow efficient diffusion of oxygen. Cells are grown in the internal pores, thus protecting them from mechanical forces arising from fluid flow. The high surface area in microcarrier culture systems also allows a higher cell density than in conventional static cultures.

Cardiospheres can be expanded as monolayers on fibronectin-coated surfaces [75]. Briefly, RV endomyocardial biopsies are cultured as explants on fibronectin-coated dishes. The cells surrounding the adherent explants are harvested by enzymatic digestion and these cardiosphere-forming cells are seeded on poly-D-lysine-coated dishes. The cells that adhere to the poly-D-lysine-coated dishes are discarded. The detached cardiospheres are then plated on fibronectin-coated flasks to be expanded as monolayers.

36.3.2 Pluripotent stem cells as aggregates

Aggregates such as EBs are often cultivated in suspension in mixed vessels such as stirred vessels or bubble columns [74]. However, since they are larger than single cells, they require more liquid pumping for suspension (i.e. large impellers, slow agitation rate). It is also necessary to control the agglomeration of these cell aggregates, since their large size can lead to limitations in oxygen transfer and subsequently to necrosis. Hence an agitation rate sufficiently high to break apart the colliding aggregates is required.

Gerecht-Nir *et al.* [76] were the first to describe the formation of differentiating human embryoid bodies (hEBs) in rotating bioreactors. The authors of this study compared hEB formation and differentiation in the high-aspect-ratio rotation vessel and slowly turning lateral vessel. Quantitative analyses of hEBs, DNA, and protein contents revealed a three-fold enhancement in hEB generation compared with conventional static culture.

Recent studies have focussed more on stirred bioreactors, since they are easier to work with. Subramanian *et al.* [77] cultured multipotent adult progenitor cells (MAPCs) as aggregates in stirred bioreactors, and this led to a 70-fold expansion in 6 days. Importantly, after this scalable expansion, MAPCs still kept their multipotent property of being able to differentiate into other progenitor cells.

Serra *et al.* [78] demonstrated the importance of controlled oxygen concentration at 30% air saturation to improve human embryonic stem cell (hESC) growth. Under this condition, the final yield of hESCs was improved 12-fold, and these cells were claimed to be of higher quality. This study demonstrated that stirred suspension bioreactors could be further optimized with better controlled conditions.

The formation of large EBs can also be prevented by using methylcellulose in the culture medium, using a small number of cells in hanging drops of medium, and by alginate encapsulation [74]. Encapsulation of cells in agarose controlled the agglomeration of mouse and hESCs during EB formation [79]. These encapsulated cells were then transferred to stirred cultures to produce 61-fold cell expansion, which was significantly higher than for non-encapsulated cells in stirred culture.

36.3.3 Stem cell differentiation

Stem cell cultivation requires both increasing cell number and retaining the self-regenerating and differentiation capabilities [74]. To derive purified cardiomyocytes, Zandstra *et al.* [80] first transfected ESCs with a fusion gene consisting of the α-cardiac myosin heavy chain promoter that drives the aminoglycoside phosphotransferase gene. The transfected cells were aggregated into EBs and cultured in a stirred suspension. After 9 days of differentiation, Geneticin (G418) and retinoic acid were added to select for cardiomyocytes. G418 kills non-cardiomyocytes and retinoic acid depletes undifferentiated ESCs to improve the cardiomyocyte yield. The cardiomyocytes derived had the contractile and structural characteristics of native cardiomyocytes.

Bauwens *et al.* [81] developed a perfusion fed bioreactor for the generation of ESC-derived cardiomyocytes. This system allows the manipulation of oxygen tension, which is an important culture parameter for improving the cardiomyocyte yield. In this study, ESCs were encapsulated in agarose hydrogel to control the size of the aggregates, and purified for cardiomyocytes by treatment with G418 and retinoic acid on day 9. Cultivation was performed in bioreactors with medium perfusion as well as monitoring and control of dissolved oxygen. The bioreactors were run at 4% and 20% oxygen tension to study the effect of hypoxic and normoxic conditions. The cardiomyocyte yield per input ESC was ~4 under the hypoxic condition, which is higher than had been found in previous studies.

To establish a more robust bioprocess for generating cardiomyocytes from hESCs, Niebruegge *et al.* [82] first generated large numbers of size-specified hESC aggregates by seeding hESCs on Matrigel patterns. It was found that control of aggregate size, stirred bioreactor culture, and hypoxia (4% oxygen tension) were all beneficial to cell growth and differentiation into cardiomyocytes.

Niebruegge *et al.* [83] reported the generation of pure cardiomyocytes from mouse EBs on a 2-l scale. The process parameters were further optimized in a 250-ml spinner flask to determine the duration of the differentiation phase, the timing of retinoic acid addition, and the rate of medium exchange for improving the cardiomyocyte yield. These conditions were applied to the 2-l automated perfusion-based bioreactor to produce 4.6×10^9 cardiomyocytes in a single run at day 16. The automated perfusion-based bioreactor produced five times the cardiomyocyte yield obtained with a manual fill-and-draw medium change. Medium consumption was also reduced by 40%. This study shows the potential in differentiation of ESCs on a large scale. To further improve the expansion and differentiation of stem cells, it will be essential to develop bioreactors equipped with online monitoring of the culture environment, as well as the cell properties (i.e. expression of cardiomyocyte markers, such as sarcomeric myosin, and markers for undifferentiated ESCs, such as Oct-4).

36.4 Bioreactors for engineered cardiac tissues

36.4.1 Design parameters for bioreactors for cardiac tissue engineering

An ideal bioreactor should be able to accomplish the following tasks: (1) establish spatially uniform cell seeding in scaffolds, (2) efficiently deliver oxygen and nutrients throughout the depth of the cultured tissue constructs, (3) minimize damaging shear stress on the tissue surface, and (4) provide stimulation cues that mimic the in-vivo environment [84–86]. In addition, bioreactors should have the capacity for automation, and should be equipped with control systems for engineering reproducible tissue constructs in a sterile environment. Within the last decade, many types of bioreactors have been developed, such as static flask reactors, spinner flask reactors, rotating-wall vessels, and direct perfusion bioreactors [84, 87–90]. Each type of reactor has its unique characteristics, and thus reactors should be selected on the basis of the needs of a specific application. When evaluating bioreactors, there are several key design parameters to consider.

36.4.1.1 Cell seeding in bioreactors

The length of time required for cell seeding and the uniformity of the seeding will directly affect the growth of the tissue construct. In a static flask reactor such as a culture dish or flask (Section 36.4.2.1), cells are seeded into the scaffolds by static loading. Although this is a widely used method due to its simplicity, low seeding efficiency and non-uniform cell distribution within the scaffolds are often reported [89]. In addition, the seeding process can take up to a day. A slightly more advanced reactor, the spinner flask reactor (Section 36.4.2.2), utilizes a stirring bar to circulate the medium around a tissue scaffold anchored inside the flask. Spinner flask reactors slightly improve the seeding efficiency by providing convection on the surface of the scaffold. However, surface convection cannot effectively deliver cells deep into the tissue construct, thus often resulting in a non-uniform cell distribution with a high cell density near the scaffold surface [89]. On the other hand, direct perfusion methods (Section 36.4.3.1) can effectively deliver cells into the tissue construct with a more uniform distribution [88]. Owing to the rapid delivery of cells into the scaffold, the decrease in cell viability during seeding with direct perfusion (at 0.5 or 1.5 ml/min for 1.5 or 4.5 hours) was significantly lower than with culture in orbitally mixed dishes (8.8 ± 0.8% and 56.3 ± 4.0%, respectively) [53].

36.4.1.2 Medium delivery

Efficient delivery of oxygen and nutrients into the cell-seeded scaffolds is critical for sustaining cell viability. Stem cells and progenitors also require soluble components such as dexamethasone, 5-azacytidine, oxytocin, or a combination of 5-azacytidine and TGF-β in the medium in order to differentiate [91]. Under static conditions, both the external and the internal mass transport between the tissue and the medium are governed by molecular diffusion, which is a slow process. By applying convective flow on the surface of the tissue construct in a spinner flask reactor, the external diffusion coefficient on the tissue surface can be improved. However, turbulent flow often induces a high level of shear stress that can potentially scar the tissue surface. For example, a 400-μm-thick fibrous capsule was formed near the tissue surface when the tissue construct was cultured in a spinner flask reactor, due to the turbulent eddies generated on the tissue surface [89]. In addition, it is difficult to model the turbulent flow and predict the exact shear on various locations of the tissue surface for studies. Rotating-wall vessels (Section 36.4.2.2) were introduced in order to provide predictable and gentler laminar flow on the surface of the tissue construct, which significantly minimizes tissue damage on the construct surface. However, both methods still rely on simple diffusion to feed medium into the interior of the tissue. This obstacle limits the thickness of the tissue construct to no more than 200 μm [89]. The direct perfusion method, on the other hand, drives the medium directly into the pores of the tissue engineering scaffold, and therefore significantly decreases the dependence on passive diffusion. The flow through the construct volume is laminar, and has velocities comparable to that of the blood flow in native tissue. Besides continuous perfusion, pulsatile injection can be implemented to mimic the paced flow of blood in the heart [88]. Cells cultured under direct perfusion were consistently shown to have much higher viability (81.6 ± 3.7%) than cells cultured under static conditions (47.4 ± 7.8%) [87, 88]. In addition, with direct perfusion, the molar ratio of the lactate produced to glucose consumed (L/G ratio) was close to 1, which indicates healthy aerobic cell metabolism in comparison with static culture conditions, under which the L/G ratio increased from 1 to 2, which signals transition to anaerobic metabolism due to lack of oxygen [87, 92].

Another solution to the mass-transfer problem is to engineer tissue constructs with vascular networks. We refer the reader to excellent reviews on vascularization of engineered cardiac tissues [93, 94].

36.4.1.3 Biomimetic cues

Growing a functional tissue amounts to more than just providing an adequate medium. Certain physiological cues (Section 36.4.3) must be applied to the cells in order to induce their maturation and proper assembly into a functional tissue [95, 96]. For cardiac tissue engineering, these external cues involve electrical stimulation mimicking the in-vivo environment, where the contractions of cardiomyocytes are synchronized and relayed through electrical wave propagation. To mimic the physical environment, external electrical pulses can be applied to the engineered cardiac tissue to induce many important aspects of tissue development, such as cell elongation and alignment in the direction of electrical propagation, positioning of mitochrondria between sarcomeres, and sarcomere development [97, 98]. Other forms of biomimetic cues include topographical cues and mechanical stimulation.

In addition to using biomimetic cues for cardiac tissue formation, cell differentiation can be induced in a similar manner. Although nowadays stem cells and progenitors are normally differentiated through co-culture with cardiac cells or pharmacological and genetic manipulation [91], low-frequency electromagnetic fields were previously used in differentiation of cardiospheres [99]. An increase in the expression of cardiac markers was observed in human cardiospheres and cardiosphere-derived cells after exposing them to extremely low-frequency electromagnetic fields tuned at the cyclotron energy resonance of the Ca^{2+} ion for 5 days.

36.4.2 Conventional bioreactors

36.4.2.1 Static bioreactors

The simplest class of bioreactor is the static bioreactor, such as multiwell plates, Petri dishes, and T-flasks. Static bioreactors are used by placing cells or a cell-seeded scaffold into the bioreactor, which contains a culture medium, and then subsequently putting the bioreactor into an incubator with temperature and gas controls. Oxygen and nutrients are made available to the cells within the construct through diffusion.

The advantages of static bioreactors are that they are easy to use, disposable, and inexpensive. A disadvantage is that the transport of oxygen, nutrients, and wastes depends on random diffusion, which is inefficient, especially for thick 3D constructs. Diffusion can support the viability only of a thin outer layer (100–200 μm) of the engineered tissue. Clinically relevant cardiac tissues should have a thickness of ~0.5 cm. Another drawback of static bioreactors is the non-uniform distribution of cells within the scaffold. Cells usually migrate to the bottom of the scaffolds due to gravity when cultivated in static bioreactors, and form a thin tissue there [100]. Static bioreactors can be placed on an orbital shaker to improve the cell distribution and gas or nutrient transport. The cell distribution can be further improved using rotary or perfusion systems (Sections 36.4.2.2 and 36.4.3.1).

36.4.2.2 Rotary bioreactors

The purpose of using rotational motion in bioreactors is to improve the cell seeding distribution as well as the transport and distribution of nutrients to the cell-seeded scaffold constructs. Rotary bioreactors include spinner flasks and rotating vessels.

Spinner flasks are flasks containing impellers that mix culture medium throughout the bioreactor volume. The cell-seeded scaffolds are stationary at the base of the bioreactor. The movement of the impeller provides a well-mixed environment for the constructs, in turn minimizing stagnant cell layers at the surface of the construct [85]. However, the disadvantage of such a bioreactor is the turbulent flow produced by the impeller's action, which results in high shear stresses that could damage the cells.

Rotating vessels involve the rotation of the entire bioreactor, thus providing a dynamic laminar flow environment for the tissue constructs. As a result, a microgravity environment is created, and one suspends the constructs in free-fall. There are two types of rotating vessels – slow lateral turning vessel (SLTV) and rotating-wall perfused vessel (RWPV) [85]. The SLTV consists of two concentric cylinders, with the outer cylinder rotating about the inner one and the tissue constructs suspended in the medium-filled annular space between the cylinders. In the RWPV, the outer and inner cylinders rotate in opposite directions. Moreover, medium inlets and outlets are placed at the ends of the cylinders and connected to a perfusion system. The disadvantage of rotating vessels is the non-uniform tissue growth and the collision of the constructs with the vessel wall.

In a study by Bursac *et al.* [101], scaffolds seeded with neonatal rat CMs were cultured in rotating bioreactors for 1 week. The resulting engineered cardiac tissues had superior molecular characteristics (i.e. higher levels of creatine kinase, myosin heavy chain and connexin-43) and electrophysiological properties (i.e. lower action potential duration) to those of cells cultured as monolayers.

36.4.3 Biomimetic bioreactors

36.4.3.1 Direct perfusion

Clinical applications require engineered heart tissues to have an area of 10–50 cm^2 and a thickness of several millimeters [51]. Perfusion bioreactors (Figure 36.1(A)) can improve mass transport of oxygen and nutrients to cardiac tissue constructs through convective flow [53, 55, 58, 65, 88, 102]. In a study by Carrier *et al.* [58], cell-seeded scaffolds were placed in a perfusion cartridge, with fluid flow through the construct. A peristaltic pump was used to provide perfusion. The enhanced mass transport maintains cell viability by reducing the time for which cells would be subjected to hypoxic conditions, further improving the spatial distribution of cells within the scaffold and allowing the cultivation of thicker tissue constructs [53, 58, 102].

In addition, Radisic *et al.* [65] designed a scaffold with a parallel array of cylindrical channels, which was then seeded with cardiac cells in Matrigel ($(0.5\text{–}1) \times 10^8$ cells/cm^3) and placed in the perfusion bioreactor. Mass transport occurred by axial convection and radial diffusion. The parallel channels mimicked the native capillaries. The culture medium was supplemented with perfluorocarbon, which acted as an oxygen carrier like hemoglobin [65]. The increased oxygen content in the group with oxygen-carrier-supplemented medium improved the cell density, cardiac protein expression and contractile properties of the tissue constructs compared with those of the unsupplemented controls [65].

Moreover, mechanical conditioning of cardiac tissue constructs to enhance tissue assembly can be achieved using perfusion bioreactors. Pulsatile flow conditions, which more closely resemble blood flow in the cardiovascular system than does continuous perfusion, have been used in perfusion bioreactors [88]. A pulsatile pump allows the control of pressures and flow waveforms. Pulsatile fluid flow was applied at physiologically relevant shear stresses and flow rates (1 Hz, 1.50 ml/min). Tissue constructs cultivated under pulsatile flow conditions had higher contractile amplitude than did constructs cultivated under static and non-pulsatile flow conditions. In a separate study, a multifunctional bioreactor was developed to provide flexibility in culturing different cardiac structures, including aortic valve and coronary artery, since it can simulate various physiological flow conditions [103].

36.4.3.2 Mechanical stimulation

Mechanical stimulation in the form of stretching has been applied to engineer functional cardiac tissues. In a study by Zimmermann *et al.* [54], a mixture of collagen type I, Matrigel, and neonatal rat cardiomyocytes was seeded into circular molds to form engineered heart tissues. After a week, these tissues were then transferred to a stretch device to expose the tissues to unidirectional cyclic stretch at 10% strain and 2 Hz for another week. Contracting ring-shaped engineered heart tissues resulted from the cultivation. Highly organized sarcomeres, adherens junctions, gap junctions, desmosomes, and a well-developed T-tubular system were shown in these engineered heart tissues, all of which are characteristic of native differentiated myocardium [54]. The rings were stacked to generate

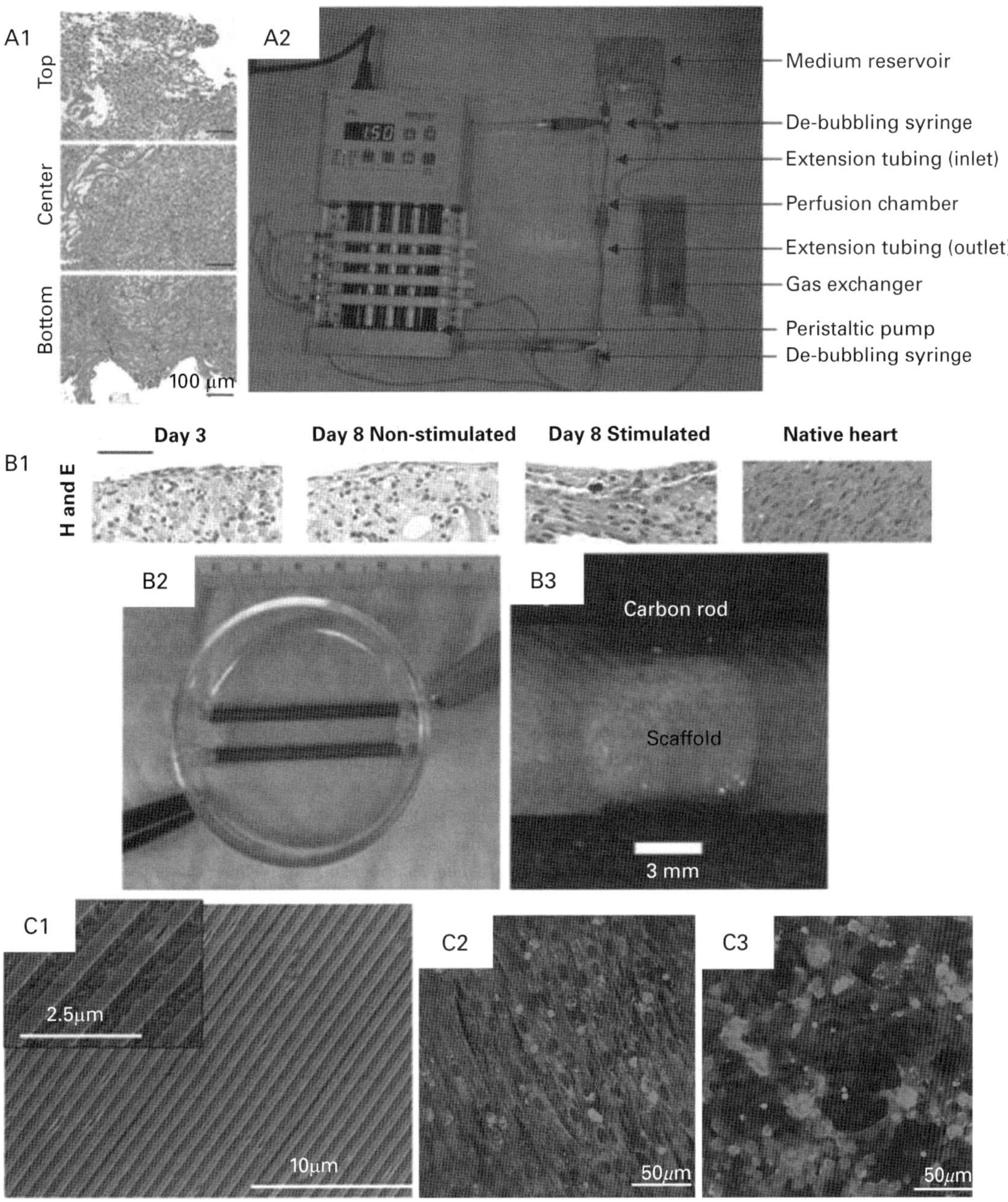

Figure 36.1 Various biomimetic bioreactors for cardiac tissue engineering. (A) A perfusion bioreactor. Reprinted by permission from Macmillan Publishers Ltd.: *Nature Protocols* [87], copyright (2008). (A1) A hematoxylin and eosin (H and E) stained cross-section of a collagen scaffold inoculated with C2C12 cells in Matrigel and seeded under direct perfusion for 4.5 hours. (A2) The setup of the perfusion system for cultivation of cardiac tissue constructs. (B) A bioreactor with electrical field stimulation [97, 98]. (B1) Representative sections with hematoxylin and eosin staining of cardiac tissue constructs at the end of preculture

multiloop engineered heart tissues, which were implanted in the rat MI model [104]. These large-force-generating engineered heart tissues showed electrical coupling to the native myocardium, prevented dilation, induced systolic wall thickening, and improved fractional area shortening of the infarcted hearts in comparison with sham treatment and implantation of non-contractile constructs [104]. Akhyari *et al.* [105] also showed that cyclical mechanical stretch (20% strain, 80 cycles/min for 14 days) increased cell proliferation, improved cell distribution, enhanced collagen matrix formation and organization, and yielded higher maximal tensile strength and resistance to stretch in cardiac grafts engineered from cardiac cells from children undergoing repair of tetralogy of Fallot.

36.4.3.3 Electrical stimulation

Cells within the engineered cardiac tissues can develop proper excitation–contraction coupling on being exposed to electrical pacing. Bioreactors that apply electrical field stimulation to cardiac tissue constructs have been shown to promote the assembly of functional engineered cardiac tissues (Figure 36.1(B)). These bioreactors involve placing cell-seeded scaffolds between two electrodes that are connected to an electrical stimulator. Electrical stimulation parameters such as voltage, frequency, and duration can be chosen to mimic the native myocardium conditions.

It had previously been shown that the use of electrical stimulation during the cultivation of neonatal cardiomyocytes led to the formation of mature beating tissues [97, 98, 106]. In a study by Radisic *et al.* [97], applying electrical stimulation at physiological pace (rectangular pulse, 2 ms, 5 V/cm, 1 Hz) markedly enhanced the contractile function of the tissue. After 8 days of cultivation under electrical stimulation, the engineered cardiac tissues had a decreased excitation threshold, which is the minimal voltage necessary to induce observable beating from the entire tissue construct. In addition, the tissues had an increased maximum capture rate, which is the maximum frequency at which synchronous construct contractions could be observed. Both are direct results of a much more robust ultrastructural differentiation of the tissue than with constructs cultured without electrical stimulation. The ultrastructural development involves cell elongation and alignment in the direction of the electrical signal followed by the development of well-aligned sarcomeres, which is the hallmark of mature cardiomyocytes. At the molecular level, electrical stimulation enhanced the expression of cardiac troponin I, sarcomeric α-actin, connexin-43, and α-myosin heavy chain.

The timing of the electrical stimulation was critical. Freshly isolated cardiac cells are usually first cultured for 3 days without stimulation to recover their surface channels and receptors prior to the application of electrical stimulation [97]. If electrical stimulation were applied too early, there would not be an adequate amount of connexin-43 gap junctions to induce contractile behaviour [97]. On the other hand, if electrical stimulation were applied too late, ultrastructural reorganization of the tissue would not result in effective whole-tissue contraction [97].

Electrical field stimulation with biphasic pulses was shown to improve the functionality of engineered cardiac tissues, as compared with no stimulation or stimulation with monophasic pulses, by enhancing 3D cell organization and increasing cell elongation, cell density, the density of cross-striations, and expression of connexin-43 [106]. It is thought that the first phase

Caption for Figure 36.1 (*cont.*) (day 3) and culture with or without electrical stimulation (day 8) [97] (copyright (2004) National Academy of Sciences, USA). The native ventricle is shown for comparison. (B2) A photograph of a typical electrical stimulation chamber. (Reprinted by permission from Macmillan Publishers Ltd.: *Nature Protocols* [98], copyright (2009).) (B3) An image of a scaffold positioned in between the electrodes. (Reprinted by permission from Macmillan Publishers Ltd.: *Nature Protocols* [98], copyright (2009).) (C) A combination of topographical cues and electrical field stimulation [109]. (Reproduced by permission of The Royal Society of Chemistry, http://dx.doi.org/10.1039/B810034A.) (C1) A microgrooved polystyrene surface (of period 1 μm, groove width 0.5 μm, and groove height 400 nm). (C2) Sarcomeric α-actinin staining of cardiomyocytes cultivated on the microgrooved surface. (C3) Smooth control.

of the biphasic pulse regime is the conditioning subthreshold prepulse and the second phase is the excitatory pulse, acting synergistically during stimulation [106].

Furthermore, the electrical stimulation parameters were optimized by systematically varying the electrode material and the amplitude and frequency of stimulation [107]. Carbon electrodes were found to have the highest charge-injection capacity, and were most suitable for engineering cardiac tissues, giving the best structural and functional properties [107]. The amplitude of 3 V/cm and frequency of 3 Hz were found to be the best parameters for engineering cardiac tissues with high tissue density, high concentrations of cardiac troponin-I and connexin-43, and improved contractile properties [107].

36.4.3.4 Multiple biomimetic cues

Even though electrical stimulation enhances the functional assembly of cardiomyocytes in scaffolds, medium diffusion through the interior of the scaffold still limits the thickness of the tissue (to 100–200 μm with passive diffusion). Electrical stimulation does not have any marked effect on construct cellularity or cell metabolism. To solve this issue, a direct perfusion method can be coupled with electrical stimulation to generate thick and functional cardiac tissues. Barash *et al.* [108] demonstrated that, with 4 days of medium perfusion (homogeneous fluid-flow regime) and electrical stimulation (74.4 mA/cm^2, 2 ms, bipolar, 1 Hz), cells elongated and striated in the direction of the electrical signal and expressed much higher levels of connexin-43. This study was coupled with computer modeling and simulation to reveal local stimulation conditions in static vessels. This enabled the transfer of the same current intensity to the perfusion cultivation system with a different geometry by changing the voltage amplitude.

Electrical stimulation and topographical cues were provided simultaneously in another setup (Figure 36.1(C)). The native myocardium is made of myocytes and myofibres aligned in parallel, with the orientation of the myofibres varying along the depth of the ventricular wall. The highest contraction force and impulse propagation velocity are found to occur along the long axis of the fibre. The structural organization on the nanoscale to macroscale is important for the pump function of the heart. Au *et al.* [109] created cell culture chips that had hot-embossed microgrooves between two gold electrodes electrodeposited at the two ends of the chip. The cardiomyocytes cultivated in this bioreactor system aligned in the direction of the microgrooves, with more elongation when microgrooves ran parallel to the electric field [109]. In addition, gap junctions were found at the cell–cell end junctions, whereas there was a punctate distribution of gap junctions in neonatal cells [109].

In a recent study, Kensah *et al.* [110] constructed a bioreactor with multiple features, including mechanical stimulation and direct real-time contraction force measurement, to culture and monitor engineered heart tissues at the same time. In this study, cardiomyocyte hypertrophy was induced by cyclic stretch, and a significantly higher systolic force was observed after β-adrenergic stimulation with noradrenalin. In addition, the results from this study showed the possibility of combining mechanical stimulation, real-time contraction force measurement, electrical stimulation, perfusion of the culture chamber, and microscope assessment during cultivation all within a single bioreactor system.

36.4.3.5 High-throughput bioreactors

The development of high-throughput bioreactors with arrays of cardiac microtissues is essential for producing highly controlled tissues with which to systematically study the parameters for cardiac tissue regeneration. For example, these microtissues could be used to study the effects of growth factors, perfusion, and electrical stimulation on the cultivation of cardiac patches for cardiac repair. They could also be used for testing the effects of cardiac drugs. Figallo *et al.* [111] developed a microbioreactor array for studying the effect of different flow configurations on the expression of cell differentiation markers by cultivated cardiomyocytes. Also, the microtissues created from bioreactor arrays could act as model systems and be injected with different stem and progenitor cells to evaluate the transplantation of these cells for cardiac tissue regeneration [112].

36.4.3.6 In-vivo bioreactors

The body can be utilized as a bioreactor. Neonatal rat cardiomyocytes were suspended in fibrin gel and seeded in silicone tubing that was then implanted around the femoral vessels in the groin region of rats [113]. After 3 weeks, there was a concentric ring of cardiac cells surrounding the femoral vessels, with tissue contractility and a significant amount of neovascularization. Morritt *et al.* [114] created an arteriovenous loop and placed it into a plastic chamber that was seeded with neonatal rat cardiomyocytes in Matrigel and implanted into the groin region of rats, which served as an in-vivo bioreactor. Spontaneously contracting constructs with extensive vascularization were found to have formed after 4 and 10 weeks of cultivation [114]. The maximum tissue thickness achieved was nearly 2 mm [114].

36.5 Examples and applications of cardiac tissue regeneration in bioreactors

36.5.1 Cell transplantation

Complex bioreactor technologies have allowed the 3D culture of primary and stem cells. Adult stem cells or MSCs have the capacity to form different tissues, including cardiac tissues, and thus play an important role in clinical research. Many groups have shown the efficacy of cell transplantation (of fetal ventricular cardiomyocytes, satellite cells from skeletal muscle, and neonatal skeletal myoblasts) in animal models (rat, canine, and rabbit) of heart failure [115–119].

There are several methods to deliver cells in cardiac regenerative therapy [120]. The first method is intravenous delivery, which involves cell infusion and the mobilization of the cells to the heart. Second, cells can be directly injected, either as a suspension of cells or as an injectable tissue, by surgical delivery. Third, cells can be delivered through a catheter as an intracoronary arterial infusion, intracoronary venous infusion, or direct myocardial injection. Finally, cells can be delivered surgically as an engineered patch or a cell sheet.

Menasché *et al.* [121] reported the first implantation of autologous myoblasts in a human patient with infarction. A muscle biopsy was extracted from the patient, and cells were cultivated in vitro [121]. The cells were then administered by intramyocardial injection into the peri-infarction region [121]. The treated patients had improved ejection fraction after ~11 months, but 40% of the patients required implantation of a defibrillator due to ventricular arrhythmia [122].

In a clinical investigation by Strauer *et al.* [123], patients with myocardial infarction were treated with intracoronary transplantation of autologous mononuclear bone marrow cells after a standard therapy. The infarct region had decreased significantly in the patients with cell therapy after 3 months, and was significantly smaller than that in patients treated with the standard therapy alone [123]. Cardiac function, as evaluated by the measurements of wall movement velocity, contractility, and LV end-systolic volume, was also improved [123]. Other clinical studies with transplantation of bone marrow cells have also revealed improvements in ejection fraction [124–126].

Human bone-marrow-derived MSCs have been transplanted for cardiac repair [46, 127]. In a clinical study by Hare *et al.* [127], allogeneic human bone-marrow-derived MSCs were administered intravenously. The treatment increased LV ejection fraction and reverse remodeling [127]. Treated patients were also less likely to experience arrhythmia [127]. A phase II clinical trial concerning using these cells for treatment after myocardial infarction has been approved [128].

Cardiac stem cells that had been isolated from the ventricle were delivered intravascularly in rats after reperfusion to mimic clinically relevant conditions for myocardial repair [129]. These cells contributed to myocardial regeneration by decreasing the infarct size and improving LV function, independently of cell fusion [129]. A phase I trial, The Cardiac Stem Cell Infusion in Patients with Ischemic Cardiomyopathy (SCIPIO) [128], on testing the safety and feasibility of a treatment involving an infusion of autologous c-kit$^+$

cardiac stem cells has begun at the University of Louisville. The procedure involves performing coronary artery bypass surgery and the removal of a small piece of the patient's cardiac tissue. The patient's own cardiac stem cells are then isolated, expanded and infused through catheterization. The ejection fraction increases after the surgery. The clinical trial is now ongoing, and 20 patients will be treated and compared against 20 control subjects. Another clinical trial, Cardiosphere-Derived Autologous Stem Cells to Reverse Ventricular Dysfunction (CADUCEUS) [128], is being conducted at the Cedars-Sinai Heart Institute in Los Angeles using cardiosphere-derived cells.

Human clinical trials have demonstrated the safety and modest benefits of cell therapy for cardiac repair. Other ongoing clinical studies of cell delivery for heart failure treatment include the use of $CD133^+$ (NCT01033617 and NCT00462774) and $CD34^+$ (NCT00480961) cells delivered intramyocardially. However, the clinical trials to date lack uniformity in the cell types used, cell dose, time of administration, delivery method and duration of study (Table 36.1) [128]. In addition, we refer the reader to extensive reviews of stem cell delivery for cardiac repair [34, 128].

The evaluation of cardiac cell therapy in vivo requires a large number of animals, cells, and reagents. Moreover, the risk-benefit profile of cell therapy in the rodent, which is the most frequently used animal model, differs from that in large animals such as swine, dogs, sheep, and humans. Song *et al.* [112] demonstrated that the engineered heart tissue can be used as an in-vitro model of healthy and diseased myocardium, and allows the study of differentiation and integration of injected cells in the cardiac environment. The engineered heart tissue can be a useful model system for pre-clinical studies, especially with the availability of human stem-cell-derived cardiomyocytes to create a human engineered myocardium. Advancements in bioreactor design (Section 36.4.3.5) will allow the miniaturization of these engineered tissues used as a high-throughput method for in-vitro evaluation of cell therapies.

36.5.2 Cell sheet engineering

Researchers have created 3D cardiac tissues in vitro without the use of scaffolds, by layering cell sheets (Table 36.2) [138–140]. This involves the culture of ventricular myocytes on a poly(N-isopropylacrylamide) (PIPAAm) grafted dish [138]. The cell sheets were released from the temperature-responsive culture surfaces by lowering the temperature from 37 °C to 20 °C [138]. Several sheets were then transferred and attached onto initial sheets [138]. However, four- and five-layer constructs showed disordered vasculature and large areas of connective tissues 1 month after implantation subcutaneously, due to primary ischemia [71]. Instead, these cell sheets can be transplanted in vivo layer by layer in a series of operations, in order to allow sufficient vascularization of the cell sheet prior to the subsequent implantation [71]. Grafts of thickness 0.84 ± 0.16 mm were achieved using 10 episodes of polysurgery [71]. The cell sheets could also be engineered from an in-vitro co-culture of CMs with endothelial cells to improve neovascularization [139]. Another method to form prevascularized networks in vitro is to seed human umbilical vein endothelial cells between myoblast sheets [140]. The endothelial cells formed capillary-like structures in a five-layer construct, and the networks connected to the host vessels after transplantation subcutaneously [140]. This enhanced neovascularization is important for the survival of the implanted grafts [140]. Alternatively, endothelial cell sheets can be first cultured from the endothelial cells and then sandwiched between the objective cell sheets [141]. This has been achieved with the objective cell sheets made of human dermal fibroblasts [141], and can be applied to cardiac cell sheets as well. Recently, the same group developed a bioreactor to culture layered cell sheets on perfused microchannels that are made of collagen.

Besides using temperature-sensitive cell culture dishes as bioreactors, polymerized fibrin-coated dishes were also used to engineer myocardial cell sheets from neonatal rat cardiomyocytes [142]. The fibrin layer was degraded by proteases that were secreted from the cultivated cells over the 4-day culture, and thus the engineered cell sheets could be easily detached from the plates [142].

Table 36.1 Clinical trials of cell transplantation to the heart

Cell type	Total number of patients	Administration time (post-MI)	Delivery method	Duration (months)	Significant results
Bone marrow cells	60	<5 days	Intracoronary	6–18	Increased ejection fraction at 6 months [124], but not at 18 months, compared with control [130]
Bone marrow mononuclear cells	204	3–7 days	Intracoronary	4–12	Improved ejection fraction at 4 months, revascularization and reduced death rates at 12 months [125]
Circulating blood-derived and bone-marrow-derived progenitor cells	20	4 days	Intracoronary	4	Improved LV remodeling, contractile function of infarct zone [131]
Bone marrow cells	18	5 months to 8.5 years	Intracoronary	3	Reduction in infarct size, improvement in ejection fraction and regional infarct wall-motion velocity [126]
Autologous cardiac stem cells	40 (estimated)	4 months	Intracoronary	Ongoing	Ongoing [128]
Cardiosphere-derived stem cells	30 (estimated)	Unspecified	Intracoronary	6–12	Ongoing [128]
Adipose-derived stem cells	27	Unspecified	Transendocardial	6	Stabilized infarct size and improved maximal oxygen consumption [132]
Bone-marrow-derived mononuclear progenitor cells	121	>3 months	Intracoronary	19	Reduction of natriuretic peptide serum levels at 3 months, and lower mortality in long-term follow-up [133]
Autologous bone marrow mononuclear cells	30	>3 months	Transendocardial	3–6	Improved quality-of-life scores after 6 months [134]
Bone-marrow-derived MSCs	78	10 days	Intracoronary	6	Increased LV ejection fraction and wall-motion velocity [46]
Bone-marrow-derived MSCs	53	1–10 days	Intravenous	6	Safe treatment, fewer adverse events, improved LV ejection fraction and reverse remodeling [127]
Peripheral blood stem cells	82	<14 days and >14 days	Intracoronary	6	Improved LV systolic function and reduced infarct size, efficacy of treatment less definite when cells were injected >14 days after MI [135]
Bone marrow mononuclear cells	28	Unspecified	Intracoronary	6	Increased LV ejection fraction [136]
Autologous skeletal myoblasts	23	>1 month	Delivery to the endocardial surface	12	Safe treatment [137]

Table 36.2 Cell sheet engineering

Cell type	Bioreactor	Number of cells	Cultivation time	Implantation	Reference
Neonatal cardiomyocytes	Temperature-responsive culture dishes Polymerized fibrin-coated dishes	$(1–4.8) \times 10^6$ (with/without ECs, $(2–8) \times 10^5$) $2.8 \times 10^5/cm^2$	4 days	Rat subcutaneous tissue, Rat MI	Shimizu *et al.* [138], Shimizu *et al.* [71], Sekine *et al.* [139], Miyagawa *et al.* [154], Itabashi *et al.* [142]
Skeletal myoblasts	Temperature-responsive culture dishes	5×10^6 to 1×10^7	16 hours to 4 days	Rat acute MI, Rat chronic MI, RV diastolic dysfunction, Porcine MI	Memon *et al.* [144], Siltanen *et al.* [145], Hoashi *et al.* [146], Miyagawa *et al.* [147]
Adipose tissue-derived mesenchymal stem cells	Temperature-responsive culture dishes	5×10^5 to 1×10^6	2–3 days	Rat chronic heart failure	Miyahara *et al.* [149], Okura *et al.* [150]
Human embryonic stem-cell-derived cardiomyocytes	Teflon-coated dishes on a rotating orbital shaker	$(0.125–3) \times 10^6$ (with ECs and fibroblasts at various ratios)	8 days	Rat skeletal muscle, Rat MI	Stevens *et al.* [18]
Rat or human cardiosphere-forming progenitor cells combined with cardiac stromal cells	Plates coated with poly-L-lysine and collagen type IV	21 ± 0.5 spheres per 100,000 viable stromal cells	4 weeks	Rat MI	Zakharova *et al.* [151]

Transplantation of cell sheets can be an effective method of delivering cells (i.e. primary cardiomyocytes, cardiac progenitors, or stem- cell-derived cardiomyocytes) to the infarcted myocardium after MI, by supporting cell retention and survival. A key advantage of cell sheet transplantation over cell injection is the preservation of cell–cell communication and cellular matrix, which are lost due to treatment with trypsin during cell isolation [143]. Cell sheet implantation rather than cell injection can better improve global cardiac function [143].

Several cell sources have been used for cell sheet engineering. Cell sheets made of autologous skeletal myoblasts were shown to improve systolic and diastolic performance in acute MI in rats [144]. The sheets reduced fibrosis and recruited hematopoietic stem cells through the release of growth factors (i.e. stromal-derived factor 1), in turn preventing cardiac remodeling [144]. Siltanen *et al.* [145] demonstrated that Bcl-2-expressing myoblast sheets increased pro-angiogenic paracrine signaling, endothelial cell proliferation, vascular density, and the number of myocytes in the infarct region, and in turn improved LV ejection fraction, compared with the wild-type myoblast sheets. Myoblast sheet transplantation also improved RV diastolic dysfunction in rats after RV failure due to chronic pressure overload [146]. The improvement was achieved by suppressing ventricular fibrosis and increasing capillary density [146]. The implantation of a single skeletal muscle cell sheet in the porcine heart gave increased myocardial perfusion, viable tissue, and improved cardiac function [147]. Importantly, a clinical trial using autologous skeletal myoblasts in cell sheets has been initiated in Japan, with successful treatment of one patient with dilated cardiomyopathy [148].

MSCs from the adipose tissue are another candidate for engineering cell sheets for cardiac repair since they are multipotent cells that can differentiate both into cardiomyocytes and into vascular endothelial cells [149]. Miyahara *et al.* [149] transplanted cell sheets made of adipose-tissue-derived MSCs onto the damaged myocardium. The cell sheet formed a thick tissue, with blood vessel formation and some differentiation into cardiomyocytes [149]. This reduced wall thinning and improved cardiac function in the rat MI model, in comparison with the fibroblast cell sheet control [149]. Further, Okura *et al.* [150] induced differentiation of human adipose-tissue-derived MSCs into cardiomyoblast-like cells with dimethysulfoxide. Sheets made of these cells were transplanted onto the infarcted myocardium in nude rats, and showed differentiation into human cardiac troponin I-positive cardiomyocytes, long-term improvement of cardiac function, and a higher survival rate [150]. Although the patches made of non-committed stem cells showed short-term improvement of cardiac function, the cells did not differentiate into cardiomyocytes, and the transplantation did not demonstrate long-term improvement [150].

Cell sheets composed of rat or human cardiac progenitor cells and cardiac stromal cells were transplanted onto the rat infarcted myocardium, and reduced wall thinning and increased capillary density compared with the untreated case [151]. The progenitor cells within the transplanted cell sheet survived and differentiated into cardiomyocytes [151]. Cardiac function, as evaluated by increased ejection fraction and reduced LV end diastolic pressure, was improved compared with that of the untreated case [151].

Stevens *et al.* [18] created cell sheets from embryonic stem-cell-derived cardiomyocytes. The cardiomyocytes were placed as a suspension into Teflon-coated low-attachment tissue culture dishes on a rotating orbital shaker, and grown into disk-shaped sheets of thickness 300–600 μm [18]. There was increased purity and maturation of the cells with time, with cardiomyocytes comprising 80% of the total cell population within the patch after 11 days [18]. The patches transmitted synchronous intracellular calcium transients, thus indicating electromechanical coupling [18]. These cardiomyocytes were also co-cultured with endothelial cells and fibroblasts to create prevascularized sheets that effectively integrated with the host coronary circulation after implantation [19].

Transplantation of cardiac constructs made of several cell sheets has shown success in terms of both functionality and integration with the native tissue. Electrical coupling between layers is essential for cell sheet engineering to be clinically relevant, since the sheets need to integrate together and to properly integrate with the host tissue as well. It was shown that two overlaid cardiomyocyte sheets were electrically coupled by 46 min after layering, and connexin-43 was detected between the sheets within 30 min [152]. A multilayer myocardial tube was formed by sequentially wrapping six neonatal rat cardiomyocyte sheets around a resected rat thoracic aorta to replace the abdominal aorta [153]. These myocardial tubes were spontaneously pulsing 4 weeks after implantation due to host blood flow [153], thus showing the ability of cell sheets to integrate with one another and with the native tissue. The four-layer cardiomyocyte cell sheet construct created by Shimizu *et al.* [70, 138] was implanted subcutaneously to show that it could achieve beating and survival for 1 year. The implantation of neonatal cardiomyocyte sheets into the infarcted myocardium showed attachment and integration of the sheet with the host myocardium, as indicated by connexin-43 expression and QRS complex with a single peak [154].

36.5.3 Cardiac patches

Cardiac patches engineered from cultivating cell-seeded scaffold matrices in bioreactors have been implanted in different MI models to show improvements in cardiac function. The use of cell-seeded scaffolds helps to provide mechanical support, while the transplanted cells engraft and repair the damaged tissue. This can greatly prevent recurrent dilatation. However, the cell types and scaffolds used varied greatly between studies. Table 36.3 summarizes the cell types, scaffolds, and bioreactors used in

Table 36.3 Examples of tissue-engineered cardiac patches that were implanted in animal or human models

Cell type	Scaffold	Bioreactor	Implantation
Fetal rat cardiomyocytes	Alginate porous scaffolds [9], gelatin mesh [11]	Static	Rat MI [9, 11] Rat subcutaneous tissue [11]
Neonatal rat cardiomyocytes	A mixture of collagen type I, Matrigel, and culture medium [155]	Circular molds then transferred to bioreactor with mechanical stretching [54, 104, 155]	Rat MI [54, 104, 155]
Human MSCs	Rat tail collagen type I	Tissue culture plates	Rat MI [156]
Rat vascular smooth muscle cells	Sponge polymer of ε-caprolactone-*co*-L-lactide reinforced with knitted poly-L-lactide fabric, polyurethane	Cell culture dishes	Rat MI [166]
Rat bone marrow cells	Polyglycolic acid cloth with collagen type I containing basic fibroblast growth factor	No cultivation prior to transplantation	Rat MI [158]
Human dermal fibroblasts	Knitted Vicryl mesh (90:10 poly (glycolide:lactide))	Multicavity bags	Mouse MI [157]
Human bone marrow cells	Collagen type I matrix	No cultivation prior to transplantation	Human MI [165]
Rat skeletal myoblasts	Polyurethane scaffolds coated with laminin	Silicone-coated dishes	Rat MI [167]

engineering some of the cardiac patches that were then implanted into animal MI models.

As an example, Leor *et al.* [9] cultured fetal rat cardiac cells within porous alginate scaffolds for 4 days to create cardiac constructs that were then implanted in rats with MI. The implanted grafts stimulated neovascularization, integrated into the host, attenuated LV dilatation, and prevented deterioration in LV contractility [9]. Similarly, Li *et al.* seeded fetal rat cardiac cells into a gelatin mesh to form a graft after 7 days of culture, and implanted the graft onto myocardial scar tissue to induce vessel infiltration and formation of junctions between implanted and recipient cardiac cells [11]. Zimmermann *et al.* [54] created engineered heart tissues by mixing neonatal cardiomyocytes with collagen type I, Matrigel and culture medium and casting the mixture in circular molds. On day 7, the tissues were transferred to a stretch device to be subjected to unidirectional cyclic stretch at 10% strain and a frequency of 2 Hz for seven more days [54]. The engineered tissues were vascularized and maintained an organized heart muscle structure and contractile function after being implanted to fit around the circumference of rat hearts for 14 days [155]. The implantation of large, 1–4-mm-thick engineered heart tissues onto myocardial infarcts in rats gave electrical coupling to the native myocardium after 28 days, and prevented dilatation, induced systolic wall thickening, and improved fractional area shortening compared with sham operation and implantation of non-contractile tissues [104].

Human MSCs were seeded in a collagen type I matrix to form a cardiac patch, which was then applied to the epicardial surface of the infarct area in the rat MI model [156]. The patch increased anterior wall thickness and fractional shortening and reduced systolic LV interior diameter [156]. Although the cells were engrafted after 1 week, there was no detection of human mesenchymal stem cells after 4 weeks, showing that long-term cell engraftment is not necessary for repair [156]. Studies have also involved the implantation of angiogenic patches engineered by using cells that secrete angiogenic growth factors [157], or scaffolds that contain these cytokines [158]. These patches stimulate the revascularization of the damaged tissue, which in turn enhances cardiac repair.

Human heart cells from children undergoing repair of tetralogy of Fallot were seeded on gelatin scaffolds and cultured with cyclical mechanical stress at 80 cycles/min for 14 days [105]. Mechanical stretch was found to increase cell proliferation, improve cell distribution, and increase mechanical strength of the graft by stimulating the formation of organized collagen matrix [105]. For more examples of different cell types and scaffolds used for engineering of cardiac patches that have been evaluated in vitro but not yet tested in vivo, we refer the reader to excellent reviews [159, 160]. Moreover, cell-free biomaterials have been implanted to enhance angiogenesis and create cardiac tissue by recruiting resident cells (as reviewed in [159]). For example, cell- free alginate hydrogel that was validated in extensive pre-clinical studies [161] successfully completed phase I clinical trials and is now moving to phase II studies as a medical device for treatment of MI and heart failure.

The drawback of engineered cardiac patches is the difficulty involved in translation of the technique to large-animal or human models. Most of the engineered patches cannot survive in vivo without immunosuppression due to the use of Matrigel and serum [159]. Scaffolds such as poly-L-lactide [162], elastomeric polyurethane [163], and collagen type I [164] have been used to reduce immunogenicity.

In a clinical trial by Chachques *et al.* [165], 20 patients with LV post-ischemic myocardial scars were subjected to implantation of bone marrow cells, with the last 10 patients having an additional collagen matrix seeded with bone marrow cells placed onto the scar. No death was reported, suggesting that the treatment using cell-seeded scaffolds was feasible [165]. Both bone marrow cell implantation alone and cell implantation in combination with implantation of cell-seeded scaffold led to improvements in scar area and thickness and ejection fraction compared with before treatment [165]. The cell-seeded grafts further improved cardiac function by reducing adverse LV remodeling and wall thinning, as indicated by the thicker infarcted wall with viable tissue in the cell-seeded matrix group than in the cell-therapy-alone group, thus minimizing the increase in cardiac wall stress and improving diastolic function [165]. The scaffold was shown to play an important role in allowing cell retention at the scar region and supporting cell survival [165].

36.5.4 Whole-heart engineering

Ott *et al.* [67] engineered a bio-artificial heart by first decellularizing cadaveric rat hearts by coronary perfusion, and then reseeding the decellularized heart by intramural injection of isolated neonatal cardiac cells and perfusion of endothelial cells into the vascular conduits. Heterotopic transplantation of a decellularized heart demonstrated the reperfusion of the organ when the aorta of the host was unclamped [67]. The recellularized heart was contracting after 8 days of cultivation in a working-heart bioreactor [67]. In the working-heart bioreactor, oxygenated medium with serum and antibiotics enters the left atrium and exits through the aortic valve [67]. There is pulsatile distention of the left ventricle and a compliance loop that is attached to the ascending aorta for coronary perfusion and afterload [67]. The effluent exits through the right atrium [67]. The heart was also exposed to electrical stimulation at 5–20 V [67]. Porcine [168, 169] hearts have also been decellularized to produce 3D scaffolds with intact chamber geometry and vascular architecture, preserved organ-specific extracellular matrix, and maintained mechanical integrity. The goal of whole-heart engineering is to generate autologous off-the-shelf bio-artificial hearts for transplantation through the use of stem or progenitor cells for recellularization [170].

36.6 Challenges and future studies

The main challenge in bioreactor design for cardiac tissue regeneration is the transition from laboratory-scale to industrial scale, which requires the generation of highly specialized bioreactors that perform standardized implementation of defined bioprocesses [89].

In a review, Martin *et al.* [89] described a vision for a closed-system bioreactor that can be used for automated production of tissue-engineered grafts. The closed-system bioreactor would store all the required reagents, such as culture medium, supplements, and scaffolds, at the appropriate temperature and humidity. To operate the bioreactor, a biopsy from the patient would be extracted by a surgeon and put into an on-site bioreactor at the hospital. This bioreactor should be able to automatically proceed with (1) cell isolation from the biopsy; (2) cell expansion; (3) cell seeding onto scaffolds; (4) culture of the tissue constructs until a desired graft has been generated, with the control of culture parameters based on inputs of data derived from clinical records of the patient, as well as monitoring of environmental culture parameters and tissue development; and (5) data analysis to provide the surgeons with a report on the tissue development, allowing them to plan for a timely implantation [89]. This system has been achieved for skin tissue engineering, with the manufacture of Dermagraft by Advanced Tissue Sciences [171]. However, it produced many defective batches due to limited control of the bioreactor system. Millenium Biologix has also used aspects of the OSTEO bioreactor system in the design of the on-site hospital-based Autologous Clinical Tissue Engineering System (ACTES) [89]. It would be ideal to achieve such a bioreactor system for cardiac tissue engineering so that engineered cardiac tissues can be grown with great control and uniformity.

There are many benefits to a single closed and automated system for cardiac tissue engineering. First, the ability to carry out autologous tissue engineering for the patients at the hospital eliminates the need to transfer specimens [89]. Second, it also eliminates the need for costly tissue engineering facilities and personnel, in turn reducing the cost of tissue-engineered products [89].

While the described bioreactor system can be used with resident stem cells, cardiac tissue engineering in the future will likely use ESCs or iPSCs. In this case, the bioreactor system will need to incorporate the following steps: (1) automatic directed differentiation, (2) selection of cardiomyocytes, (3) seeding of cells into scaffolds, (4) tissue culture with control of culture conditions and monitoring of tissue development, and (5) implantation of the engineered tissue. Alternatively, scaffolds and culture parameters could be designed such that stem cells can directly differentiate into cardiomyocytes on the scaffolds.

In the future, bioreactors both for cell expansion and for cardiac tissue engineering, whether they be conventional laboratory bioreactors or closed-system bioreactors, should be equipped with integrated systems to monitor and control (1) environmental factors, such as temperature, pH, and oxygen level; and (2) parameters indicating the developmental progress of engineered tissues, such as cell number, phenotype, and metabolism, as well as structural and functional properties of the tissue. Monitoring systems could include video microscopy, magnetic resonance imaging, and microcomputerized tomography for tissue properties [89]. The culture parameters should then be controlled on the basis of the data collected. Modeling will be essential in order to integrate the physicochemical data acquired in such a way as to predict the development of the tissue with time. Such analysis systems are currently available, including Stat Profile Critical Care Xpress and BioProfile 400 (Nova Biomedical) [89].

36.7 Summary

We have described here the important roles of cells, scaffolds, and bioreactors in cardiac tissue engineering. In particular, the expansion and differentiation of embryonic stem cells, induced pluripotent stem cells, and cardiac progenitor cells are essential for producing large numbers of cardiomyocytes to be used for cell transplantation, cell sheet engineering, and the engineering of cardiac patches or the whole heart. We discussed in detail the use of bioreactors for cell expansion and differentiation, and for engineering of cardiac tissues. The application of biomimetic cues in bioreactors, such as perfusion, electrical stimulation, and mechanical stimulation, has been shown to improve tissue morphology and contractility. In the future, the development of various high-throughput bioreactors will allow the engineering of cardiac microtissues for drug testing, evaluation of cell transplantation, and optimization of cardiac tissue culture conditions. Finally, we described many clinical applications of cardiac tissue engineering to demonstrate the promise that this field holds and to indicate the challenges which need to be overcome.

REFERENCES

[1] Holladay, C. A., O'Brien, T. and Pandit, A. 2010. Non-viral gene therapy for myocardial engineering. *Wiley Interdiscip. Rev. Nanomed. Nanobiotechnol.*, **2**(3), 232–48.

[2] Nabel, E. G. 1995. Gene therapy for cardiovascular disease. *Circulation*, **91**(2), 541–8.

[3] Vinge, L. E., Raake, P. W. and Koch, W. J. 2008. Gene therapy in heart failure. *Circ. Res.*, **102**(12), 1458–70.

[4] Laflamme, M. A. and Murry, C. E. 2011. Heart regeneration. *Nature*, **473**(7347), 326–35.

[5] Bhana, B., Iyer, R. K., Chen, W. L. *et al.* 2010. Influence of substrate stiffness on the phenotype of heart cells. *Biotechnol. Bioeng.*, **105**(6), 1148–60.

[6] Nerem, R. M. and Sambanis, A. 1995. Tissue engineering: from biology to biological substitutes. *Tissue Eng.*, **1**(1), 3–13.

[7] Müller-Ehmsen, J., Peterson, K. L., Kedes, L. *et al.* 2002. Rebuilding a damaged heart: long-term survival of transplanted neonatal rat cardiomyocytes after myocardial infarction and effect on cardiac function. *Circulation*, **105**(14), 1720–6.

[8] Reinecke, H., Zhang, M., Bartosek, T. and Murry, C. E. 1999. Survival, integration, and differentiation of cardiomyocyte grafts: a study in normal and injured rat hearts. *Circulation*, **100**(2), 193–202.

[9] Leor, J., Aboulafia-Etzion, S., Dar, A. *et al.* 2000. Bioengineered cardiac grafts: a new approach to repair the infarcted myocardium? *Circulation*, **102**(19, Suppl. 3), III56–61.

[10] Zong, X., Bien, H., Chung, C. Y. *et al.* 2005. Electrospun fine-textured scaffolds for heart tissue constructs. *Biomaterials*, **26**(26), 5330–8.

[11] Li, R. K., Jia, Z. Q., Weisel, R. D. *et al.* 1999. Survival and function of bioengineered cardiac grafts. *Circulation*, **100**(19, Suppl. 2), II63–9.

[12] Kofidis, T., Akhyari, P., Wachsmann, B. *et al.* 2003. Clinically established hemostatic scaffold (tissue fleece) as biomatrix in tissue- and organ-engineering research. *Tissue Eng.*, **9**(3), 517–23.

[13] Kehat, I., Kenyagin-Karsenti, D., Snir, M. *et al.* 2001. Human embryonic stem cells can differentiate into myocytes with structural and functional properties of cardiomyocytes. *J. Clin. Invest.*, **108**(3), 407–14.

[14] Kattman, S. J., Huber, T. L. and Keller, G. M. 2006. Multipotent flk-1+ cardiovascular progenitor cells give rise to the cardiomyocyte, endothelial, and vascular smooth muscle lineages. *Dev. Cell*, **11**(5), 723–32.

[15] Yang, L., Soonpaa, M. H., Adler, E. D. *et al.* 2008. Human cardiovascular progenitor cells develop from a KDR+ embryonic-stem-cell-derived population. *Nature*, **453**(7194), 524–8.

[16] Kouskoff, V., Lacaud, G., Schwantz, S., Fehling, H. J. and Keller, G. 2005. Sequential development of hematopoietic and cardiac mesoderm during embryonic stem cell differentiation. *Proc. Nat. Acad. Sci. USA*, **102**(37), 13170–5.

[17] Guo, X. M., Zhao, Y. S., Chang, H. X. *et al.* 2006. Creation of engineered cardiac tissue in vitro from mouse embryonic stem cells. *Circulation*, **113**(18), 2229–37.

[18] Stevens, K. R., Kreutziger, K. L., Dupras, S. K. *et al.* 2009. Scaffold-free human cardiac tissue patch created from embryonic stem cells. *Tissue Eng. Part A*, **15**(6), 1211–22.

[19] Stevens, K. R., Kreutziger, K. L., Dupras, S. K. *et al.* 2009. Physiological function and transplantation of scaffold-free and vascularized human cardiac muscle tissue. *Proc. Nat. Acad. Sci. USA*, **106**(39), 16568–73.

[20] Takahashi, K. and Yamanaka, S. 2006. Induction of pluripotent stem cells from mouse embryonic and adult fibroblast cultures by defined factors. *Cell*, **126**(4), 663–76.

[21] Mauritz, C., Schwanke, K., Reppel, M. *et al.* 2008. Generation of functional murine cardiac myocytes from induced pluripotent stem cells. *Circulation*, **118**(5), 507–17.

[22] Zwi, L., Caspi, O., Arbel, G. *et al.* 2009. Cardiomyocyte differentiation of human induced pluripotent stem cells. *Circulation*, **120**(15), 1513–23.

[23] Zhang, J., Wilson, G. F., Soerens, A. G. *et al.* 2009. Functional cardiomyocytes derived from human induced pluripotent stem cells. *Circ. Res.*, **104**(4), e30–41.

[24] Tulloch, N. L., Muskheli, V., Razumova, M. V. *et al.* 2011. Growth of engineered human myocardium with mechanical loading and vascular coculture. *Circ. Res.*, **109**(1), 47–59.

[25] Murry, C. E., Kay, M. A., Bartosek, T., Hauschka, S. D. and Schwartz, S. M. 1996. Muscle differentiation during

repair of myocardial necrosis in rats via gene transfer with MyoD. *J. Clin. Invest.*, **98**(10), 2209–17.

[26] Efe, J. A., Hilcove, S., Kim, J. *et al.* 2011. Conversion of mouse fibroblasts into cardiomyocytes using a direct reprogramming strategy. *Nature Cell Biol.*, **13**(3), 215–22.

[27] Bergmann, O., Bhardwaj, R. D., Bernard, S. *et al.* 2009. Evidence for cardiomyocyte renewal in humans. *Science*, **324**(5923), 98–102.

[28] Kajstura, J., Urbanek, K., Perl, S. *et al.* 2010. Cardiomyogenesis in the adult human heart. *Circ. Res.*, **107**(2), 305–15.

[29] Ruvinov, E., Harel-Adar, T. and Cohen, S. 2011. Bioengineering the infarcted heart by applying bio-inspired materials. *J. Cardiovasc. Transl. Res.*, **4**(5), 559–74.

[30] Urbanek, K., Quaini, F., Tasca, G. *et al.* 2003. Intense myocyte formation from cardiac stem cells in human cardiac hypertrophy. *Proc. Nat. Acad. Sci. USA*, **100**(18), 10440–5.

[31] Urbanek, K., Torella, D., Sheikh, F. *et al.* 2005. Myocardial regeneration by activation of multipotent cardiac stem cells in ischemic heart failure. *Proc. Nat. Acad. Sci. USA*, **102**(24), 8692–7.

[32] Urbanek, K., Cesselli, D., Rota, M. *et al.* 2006. Stem cell niches in the adult mouse heart. *Proc. Nat. Acad. Sci. USA*, **103**(24), 9226–31.

[33] Laugwitz, K. L., Moretti, A., Lam, J. *et al.* 2005. Postnatal isl1^{+} cardioblasts enter fully differentiated cardiomyocyte lineages. *Nature*, **433**(7026), 647–53.

[34] Segers, V. F. and Lee, R. T. 2008. Stem-cell therapy for cardiac disease. *Nature*, **451**(7181), 937–42.

[35] Passier, R., van Laake, L. W. and Mummery, C. L. 2008. Stem-cell-based therapy and lessons from the heart. *Nature*, **453**(7193), 322–9.

[36] Beltrami, A. P., Barlucchi, L., Torella, D. *et al.* 2003. Adult cardiac stem cells are multipotent and support myocardial regeneration. *Cell*, **114**(6), 763–76.

[37] Domian, I. J., Chiravuri, M., van der Meer, P. *et al.* 2009. Generation of functional ventricular heart muscle from mouse ventricular progenitor cells. *Science*, **326**(5951), 426–9.

[38] Messina, E., De Angelis, L., Frati, G. *et al.* 2004. Isolation and expansion of adult cardiac stem cells from human and murine heart. *Circ. Res.*, **95**(9), 911–21.

[39] Johnston, P. V., Sasano, T., Mills, K. *et al.* 2009. Engraftment, differentiation, and functional benefits of autologous cardiosphere-derived cells in porcine ischemic cardiomyopathy. *Circulation*, **120**(12), 1075–83, 7 pp. following 1083.

[40] Chimenti, I., Smith, R. R., Li, T. S. *et al.* 2010. Relative roles of direct regeneration versus paracrine effects of human cardiosphere-derived cells transplanted into infarcted mice. *Circ. Res.*, **106**(5), 971–80.

[41] Orlic, D., Kajstura, J., Chimenti, S. *et al.* 2001. Bone marrow cells regenerate infarcted myocardium. *Nature*, **410**(6829), 701–5.

[42] Jackson, K. A., Majka, S. M., Wang, H. *et al.* 2001. Regeneration of ischemic cardiac muscle and vascular endothelium by adult stem cells. *J. Clin. Invest.*, **107**(11), 1395–402.

[43] Deb, A., Wang, S., Skelding, K. A. *et al.* 2003. Bone marrow-derived cardiomyocytes are present in adult human heart: a study of gender-mismatched bone marrow transplantation patients. *Circulation*, **107**(9), 1247–9.

[44] Orlic, D., Kajstura, J., Chimenti, S. *et al.* 2003. Bone marrow stem cells regenerate infarcted myocardium. *Pediatr. Transplant.*, **7**(Suppl. 3), 86–8.

[45] Orlic, D., Kajstura, J., Chimenti, S. *et al.* 2001. Mobilized bone marrow cells repair the infarcted heart, improving function and survival. *Proc. Nat. Acad. Sci. USA*, **98**(18), 10344–9.

[46] Chen, S. L., Fang, W. W., Ye, F. *et al.* 2004. Effect on left ventricular function of intracoronary transplantation of autologous bone marrow mesenchymal stem cell in patients with acute myocardial infarction. *Am. J. Cardiol.*, **94**(1), 92–5.

[47] Fraser, J. K., Wulur, I., Alfonso, Z. *et al.* 2006. Fat tissue: an underappreciated source of stem cells for biotechnology. *Trends Biotechnol.*, **24**(4), 150–4.

[48] Bai, X. and Alt, E. 2010. Myocardial regeneration potential of adipose tissue-derived stem cells. *Biochem. Biophys. Res. Commun.*, **401**(3), 321–6.

[49] Bai, X., Yan, Y., Song, Y. H. *et al.* 2010. Both cultured and freshly isolated adipose tissue-derived stem cells enhance cardiac function after acute myocardial infarction. *Eur. Heart J.*, **31**(4), 489–501.

[50] Gaebel, R., Furlani, D., Sorg, H. *et al.* 2011. Cell origin of human mesenchymal stem cells determines a different healing performance in cardiac regeneration. *PLoS One*, **6**(2), e15652.

[51] Vunjak-Novakovic, G., Tandon, N., Godier, A. *et al.* 2010. Challenges in cardiac tissue engineering. *Tissue Eng. Part B Rev.*, **16**(2), 169–87.

[52] Engelmayr, G. C. Jr., Cheng, M., Bettinger, C. J. *et al.* 2008. Accordion-like honeycombs for tissue engineering of cardiac anisotropy. *Nature Mater.*, **7**(12), 1003–10.

[53] Radisic, M., Euloth, M., Yang, L. *et al.* 2003. High-density seeding of myocyte cells for cardiac tissue engineering. *Biotechnol. Bioeng.*, **82**(4), 403–14.

[54] Zimmermann, W. H., Didie, M., Wasmeier, G. H. *et al.* 2002. Tissue engineering of a differentiated cardiac muscle construct. *Circ. Res.*, **90**(2), 223–30.

[55] Dvir, T., Benishti, N., Shachar, M. and Cohen, S. *et al.* 2006. A novel perfusion bioreactor providing a homogenous milieu for tissue regeneration. *Tissue Eng.*, **12**(10), 2843–52.

[56] Kofidis, T., Lenz, A., Boublik, J. *et al.* 2003. Pulsatile perfusion and cardiomyocyte viability in a solid three-dimensional matrix. *Biomaterials*, **24**(27), 5009–14.

[57] McDevitt, T. C., Angello, J. C., Whitney, M. L. *et al.* 2002. In vitro generation of differentiated cardiac myofibers on micropatterned laminin surfaces. *J. Biomed. Mater. Res.*, **60**(3), 472–9.

[58] Carrier, R. L., Rupnick, M., Langer, R. *et al.* 2002. Perfusion improves tissue architecture of engineered cardiac muscle. *Tissue Eng.*, **8**(2), 175–88.

[59] Bursac, N., Papadaki, M., Cohen, R. J. *et al.* 1999. Cardiac muscle tissue engineering: toward an in vitro model for electrophysiological studies. *Am. J. Physiol.*, **277**(2, Part 2), H433–44.

[60] Carrier, R. L., Papadaki, M., Rupnick, M. *et al.* 1999. Cardiac tissue engineering: cell seeding, cultivation parameters, and tissue construct characterization. *Biotechnol. Bioeng.*, **64**(5), 580–9.

[61] Carrier, R. L., Rupnick, M., Langer, R. *et al.* 2002. Effects of oxygen on engineered cardiac muscle. *Biotechnol. Bioeng.*, **78**(6), 617–25.

[62] Papadaki, M., Bursac, N., Langer, R. *et al.* 2001. Tissue engineering of functional cardiac muscle: molecular, structural, and electrophysiological studies. *Am. J. Physiol. Heart Circ. Physiol.*, **280**(1), H168–78.

[63] Rockwood, D. N., Akins, R. E. Jr., Parrag, I. C., Woodhouse, K. A. and Rabolt, J. F. 2008. Culture on electrospun polyurethane scaffolds decreases atrial natriuretic peptide expression by cardiomyocytes in vitro. *Biomaterials*, **29**(36), 4783–91.

[64] Naito, H., Melnychenko, I., Didie, M. *et al.* 2006. Optimizing engineered heart tissue for therapeutic applications as surrogate heart muscle. *Circulation*, **114**(1 Suppl.), I72–8.

[65] Radisic, M., Park, H., Chen, F. *et al.* 2006. Biomimetic approach to cardiac tissue engineering: oxygen carriers and channeled scaffolds. *Tissue Eng.*, **12**(8), 2077–91.

[66] Radisic, M., Deen, W., Langer, R. and Vunjak-Novakovic, G. 2005. Mathematical model of oxygen distribution in engineered cardiac tissue with parallel channel array perfused with culture medium containing oxygen carriers. *Am. J. Physiol. Heart Circ. Physiol.*, **288**(3), H1278–89.

[67] Ott, H. C., Matthiesen, T. S., Goh, S. K. *et al.* 2008. Perfusion-decellularized matrix: using nature's platform to engineer a bioartificial heart. *Nature Med.*, **14**(2), 213–21.

[68] Godier-Furnémont, A. F., Martens, T. P., Koeckert, M. S. *et al.* 2011. Composite scaffold provides a cell delivery platform for cardiovascular repair. *Proc. Nat. Acad. Sci. USA*, **108**(19), 7974–9.

[69] Miyagi, Y., Chiu, L. L., Cimini, M. *et al.* 2011. Biodegradable collagen patch with covalently immobilized VEGF for myocardial repair. *Biomaterials*, **32**(5), 1280–90.

[70] Shimizu, T., Yamato, M., Isoi, Y. *et al.* 2002. Fabrication of pulsatile cardiac tissue grafts using a novel 3-dimensional cell sheet manipulation technique and temperature-responsive cell culture surfaces. *Circ. Res.*, **90**(3), e40.

[71] Shimizu, T., Sekine, H., Yang, J. *et al.* 2006. Polysurgery of cell sheet grafts overcomes diffusion limits to produce thick, vascularized myocardial tissues. *FASEB J.*, **20**(6), 708–10.

[72] Baar, K., Birla, R., Bolyut, M. O. *et al.* 2005. Self-organization of rat cardiac cells into contractile 3-D cardiac tissue. *FASEB J.*, **19**(2), 275–7.

[73] Rodrigues, C. A., Fernandes, T. G., Diogo, M. M., da Silva, C. L. and Cabral, J. M. 2011. Stem cell cultivation in bioreactors. *Biotechnol. Adv.*, **29**(6), 815–29.

[74] Ulloa-Montoya, F., Verfaillie, C. M. and Hu, W. S. 2005. Culture systems for pluripotent stem cells. *J. Biosci. Bioeng.*, **100**(1), 12–27.

[75] Smith, R. R., Barile, L., Cho, H. C. *et al.* 2007. Regenerative potential of cardiosphere-derived cells expanded from percutaneous endomyocardial biopsy specimens. *Circulation*, **115**(7), 896–908.

[76] Gerecht-Nir, S., Cohen, S. and Itskovitz-Eldor, J. 2004. Bioreactor cultivation enhances the efficiency of human embryoid body (hEB) formation and differentiation. *Biotechnol. Bioeng.*, **86**(5), 493–502.

[77] Subramanian, K., Park, Y., Verfaille, C. M. and Hu, W. S. 2011. Scalable expansion of multipotent adult progenitor cells as three-dimensional cell aggregates. *Biotechnol. Bioeng.*, **108**(2), 364–75.

[78] Serra, M., Brito, C., Sousa, M. F. *et al.* 2010. Improving expansion of pluripotent human embryonic stem cells in perfused bioreactors through oxygen control. *J. Biotechnol.*, **148**(4), 208–15.

[79] Dang, S. M., Gerecht-Nir, S., Chen, J., Itskovitz-Eldor, J. and Zandstra, P. W. 2004. Controlled, scalable embryonic stem cell differentiation culture. *Stem Cells*, **22**(3), 275–82.

[80] Zandstra, P. W., Bauwens, C., Yin, T. *et al.* 2003. Scalable production of embryonic stem cell-derived cardiomyocytes. *Tissue Eng.*, **9**(4), 767–78.

[81] Bauwens, C., Yin, T., Dang, S., Peerani, R. and Zandstra, P. W. 2005. Development of a perfusion fed bioreactor for embryonic stem cell-derived cardiomyocyte generation: oxygen-mediated enhancement of cardiomyocyte output. *Biotechnol. Bioeng.*, **90**(4), 452–61.

[82] Niebruegge, S., Bauwens, C. L., Peerani, R. *et al.* 2009. Generation of human embryonic stem cell-derived mesoderm and cardiac cells using size-specified aggregates in an oxygen-controlled bioreactor. *Biotechnol. Bioeng.*, **102**(2), 493–507.

[83] Niebruegge, S., Nehring, A., Bär, H. *et al.* 2008. Cardiomyocyte production in mass suspension culture: embryonic stem cells as a source for great amounts of functional cardiomyocytes. *Tissue Eng. Part A*, **14**(10), 1591–601.

[84] Barron, V., Lyons, E., Stevenson-Cox, C., McHugh, P. E. and Pandit, A. 2003. Bioreactors for cardiovascular cell and tissue growth: a review. *Ann. Biomed. Eng.*, **31**(9), 1017–30.

[85] Chen, H. C. and Hu, Y. C. 2006. Bioreactors for tissue engineering. *Biotechnol. Lett.*, **28**(18), 1415–23.

[86] Eschenhagen, T. and Zimmermann, W. H. 2005. Engineering myocardial tissue. *Circ. Res.*, **97**(12), 1220–31.

[87] Radisic, M., Marsano, A., Maidhof, R. *et al.* 2008. Cardiac tissue engineering using perfusion bioreactor systems. *Nature Protoc.*, **3**(4), 719–38.

[88] Brown, M. A., Iyer, R. K. and Radisic, M. 2008. Pulsatile perfusion bioreactor for cardiac tissue engineering. *Biotechnol. Prog.*, **24**(4), 907–20.

[89] Martin, I., Wendt, D. and Heberer, M. 2004. The role of bioreactors in tissue engineering. *Trends Biotechnol.*, **22**(2), 80–6.

[90] Pörtner, R., Nagel-Heyer, S., Goepfert, C., Adamietz, P. and Meenen, N. M. 2005. Bioreactor design for tissue engineering. *J. Biosci. Bioeng.*, **100**(3), 235–45.

[91] Chamuleau, S. A., van Belle, E. and Doevendans, P. A. 2009. Enhancing cardiac stem cell differentiation into cardiomyocytes. *Cardiovasc. Res.*, **82**(3), 385–7.

[92] Maidhof, R., Marsano, A., Lee, A. J. and Vunjak-Novakovic, G. 2010. Perfusion seeding of channeled elastomeric scaffolds with myocytes and endothelial cells for cardiac tissue engineering. *Biotechnol. Prog.*, **26**(2), 565–72.

[93] Iyer, R. K., Chiu, L. L., Reis, L. A. and Radisic, M. 2011. Engineered cardiac tissues. *Curr. Opin. Biotechnol.*, **22**(5), 706–14.

[94] Chiu, L. L., Radisic, M. and Vunjak-Novakovic, G. 2010. Bioactive scaffolds for engineering vascularized cardiac tissues. *Macromolec. Biosci*, **10**(11), 1286–301.

[95] Grayson, W. L., Martens, T. P., Eng, G. M., Radisic, M. and Vunjak-Novakovic, G. 2009. Biomimetic approach to tissue engineering. *Semin. Cell Dev. Biol.*, **20**(6), 665–73.

[96] Hecker, L. and Birla, R. K. 2007. Engineering the heart piece by piece: state of the art in cardiac tissue engineering. *Regen. Med.*, **2**(2), 125–44.

[97] Radisic, M., Park, H., Shing, H. *et al.* 2004. Functional assembly of engineered myocardium by electrical stimulation of cardiac myocytes cultured on scaffolds. *Proc. Nat. Acad. Sci. USA*, **101**(52), 18129–34.

[98] Tandon, N., Cannizzaro, C., Chao, P. H. *et al.* 2009. Electrical stimulation systems for cardiac tissue engineering. *Nature Protoc.*, **4**(2), 155–73.

[99] Gaetani, R., Ledda, M., Barile, L. *et al.* 2009. Differentiation of human adult cardiac stem cells exposed to extremely low-frequency electromagnetic fields. *Cardiovasc. Res.*, **82**(3), 411–20.

[100] Freed, L. E., Guilak, F., Guo, X. E. *et al.* 2006. Advanced tools for tissue engineering: scaffolds, bioreactors, and signaling. *Tissue Eng.*, **12**(12), 3285–305.

[101] Bursac, N., Papadaki, M., White, J. A. *et al.* 2003. Cultivation in rotating bioreactors promotes maintenance of cardiac myocyte electrophysiology and molecular properties. *Tissue Eng.*, **9**(6), 1243–53.

[102] Radisic, M., Papadaki, M., White, J. A. *et al.* 2004. Medium perfusion enables engineering of compact and contractile cardiac tissue. *Am. J. Physiol. Heart Circ. Physiol.*, **286**(2), H507–16.

[103] Morsi, Y. S., Yang, W. W., Owida, A. and Wong, C. S. 2007. Development of a novel pulsatile bioreactor for tissue culture. *J. Artif. Organs*, **10**(2), 109–14.

[104] Zimmermann, W. H., Melnychenko, I., Wasmeier, G. *et al.* 2006. Engineered heart tissue grafts improve systolic and diastolic function in infarcted rat hearts. *Nature Med.*, **12**(4), 452–8.

[105] Akhyari, P., Fedak, P. W., Weisel, R. D. *et al.* 2002. Mechanical stretch regimen enhances the formation of bioengineered autologous cardiac muscle grafts. *Circulation*, **106**(12, Suppl. 1), I137–42.

[106] Chiu, L. L., Iyer, R. K., King, J. P. and Radisic, M. 2011. Biphasic electrical field stimulation AIDS in tissue engineering of multicell-type cardiac organoids. *Tissue Eng. Part A*, **17**(11–12), 1465–77.

[107] Tandon, N., Marsano, A., Maidhof, R. *et al.* 2011. Optimization of electrical stimulation parameters for cardiac tissue engineering. *J. Tissue Eng. Regen. Med.*, **5**(6), e115–25.

[108] Barash, Y., Dvir, T., Tandeitnik, P. *et al.* 2010. Electric field stimulation integrated into perfusion bioreactor for cardiac tissue engineering. *Tissue Eng. Part C Methods*, **16**(6), 1417–26.

[109] Au, H. T., Cui, B., Chu, Z. E., Veres, T. and Radisic, M. 2009. Cell culture chips for simultaneous application of topographical and electrical cues enhance phenotype of cardiomyocytes. *Lab Chip*, **9**(4), 564–75.

[110] Kensah, G., Gruh, I., Viering, J. *et al.* 2011. A novel miniaturized multimodal bioreactor for continuous in situ assessment of bioartificial cardiac tissue during stimulation and maturation. *Tissue Eng. Part C Methods*, **17**(4), 463–73.

[111] Figallo, E., Cannizzaro, C., Gerecht, S. *et al.* 2007. Micro-bioreactor array for controlling cellular microenvironments. *Lab Chip*, **7**(6), 710–19.

[112] Song, H., Yoon, C., Kattman, S. J. *et al.* 2010. Interrogating functional integration between injected pluripotent stem cell-derived cells and surrogate cardiac tissue. *Proc. Nat. Acad. Sci. USA*, **107**(8), 3329–34.

[113] Birla, R. K., Dhawan, V., Dow, D. *et al.* 2009. Cardiac cells implanted into a cylindrical, vascularized chamber in vivo: pressure generation and morphology. *Biotechnol. Lett.*, **31**(2), 191–201.

[114] Morritt, A. N., Bortolotto, S. K., Dilley, R. J. *et al.* 2007. Cardiac tissue engineering in an in vivo vascularized chamber. *Circulation*, **115**(3), 353–60.

[115] Sakai, T., Li, R. K., Weisel, R. D. *et al.* 1999. Fetal cell transplantation: a comparison of three cell types. *J. Thorac. Cardiovasc. Surg.*, **118**(4), 715–24.

[116] Chiu, R. C., Zibaitis, A. and Kao, R. L. 1995. Cellular cardiomyoplasty: myocardial regeneration with satellite cell implantation. *Ann. Thorac. Surg.*, **60**(1), 12–18.

[117] Murry, C. E., Wiseman, R. W., Schwartz, S. M. and Hauschka, S. D. 1996. Skeletal myoblast transplantation for repair of myocardial necrosis. *J. Clin. Invest.*, **98**(11), 2512–23.

[118] Taylor, D. A., Atkins, B. Z., Hungspreugs, P. *et al.* 1998. Regenerating functional myocardium: improved performance after skeletal myoblast transplantation. *Nature Med.*, **4**(8), 929–33.

[119] Scorsin, M., Hagège, A., Vilquin, J. T. *et al.* 2000. Comparison of the effects of fetal cardiomyocyte and skeletal myoblast transplantation on postinfarction left ventricular function. *J. Thorac. Cardiovasc. Surg.*, **119**(6), 1169–75.

[120] Wu, K. H., Han, Z. C., Mo, X. M. and Zhou, B. 2011. Cell delivery in cardiac regenerative therapy. *Ageing Res. Rev.*, **11**(1), 32–40.

[121] Menasché, P., Hagège, A. A., Scorsin, M. *et al.* 2001. Myoblast transplantation for heart failure. *Lancet*, **357** (9252), 279–80.

[122] Menasché, P., Hagège, A. A., Vilquin, J. T. *et al.* 2003. Autologous skeletal myoblast transplantation for severe postinfarction left ventricular dysfunction. *J. Am. Coll. Cardiol.*, **41**(7), 1078–83.

[123] Strauer, B. E., Brehm, M., Zeus, T. *et al.* 2002. Repair of infarcted myocardium by autologous intracoronary mononuclear bone marrow cell transplantation in humans. *Circulation*, **106**(15), 1913–18.

[124] Wollert, K. C., Meyer, G. P., Lotz, J. *et al.* 2004. Intracoronary autologous bone-marrow cell transfer after myocardial infarction: the BOOST randomised controlled clinical trial. *Lancet*, **364**(9429), 141–8.

[125] Schächinger, V., Erbs, S., Elsässer, A. *et al.* 2006. Intracoronary bone marrow-derived progenitor cells in acute myocardial infarction. *N. Engl. J. Med.*, **355**(12), 1210–21.

[126] Strauer, B. E., Brehm, M., Zeus, T. *et al.* 2005. Regeneration of human infarcted heart muscle by intracoronary autologous bone marrow cell transplantation in chronic coronary artery disease: the IACT Study. *J. Am. Coll. Cardiol.*, **46**(9), 1651–8.

[127] Hare, J. M., Traverse, J. H., Henry, T. D. *et al.* 2009. A randomized, double-blind, placebo-controlled, dose-escalation study of intravenous adult human mesenchymal stem cells (prochymal) after acute myocardial infarction. *J. Am. Coll. Cardiol.*, **54**(24), 2277–86.

[128] Flynn, A. and O'Brien, T. 2011. Stem cell therapy for cardiac disease. *Expert Opin. Biol. Ther.*, **11**(2), 177–87.

[129] Dawn, B., Stein, A. B., Urbanek, K. *et al.* 2005. Cardiac stem cells delivered intravascularly traverse the vessel barrier, regenerate infarcted myocardium, and improve cardiac function. *Proc. Nat. Acad. Sci. USA*, **102**(10), 3766–71.

[130] Meyer, G. P., Wollert, K. C., Lotz, J. *et al.* 2006. Intracoronary bone marrow cell transfer after myocardial infarction: eighteen months' follow-up data from the randomized, controlled BOOST (BOne marrOw transfer to enhance ST-elevation infarct regeneration) trial. *Circulation*, **113**(10), 1287–94.

[131] Assmus, B., Schächinger, V., Teupe, C. *et al.* 2002. Transplantation of progenitor cells and regeneration

enhancement in acute myocardial infarction (TOPCARE-AMI). *Circulation*, **106**(24), 3009–17.

[132] Perin, E. C. and Willerson, J. T. 2011. $CD34^+$ autologous human stem cells in treating refractory angina. *Circ. Res.*, **109**(4), 351–2.

[133] Assmus, B., Fischer-Rasokat, U., Honold, J. *et al.* 2007. Transcoronary transplantation of functionally competent BMCs is associated with a decrease in natriuretic peptide serum levels and improved survival of patients with chronic postinfarction heart failure: results of the TOPCARE-CHD Registry. *Circ. Res.*, **100**(8), 1234–41.

[134] Perin, E. C., Silva, G. V., Henry, T. D. *et al.* 2011. A randomized study of transendocardial injection of autologous bone marrow mononuclear cells and cell function analysis in ischemic heart failure (FOCUS-HF). *Am. Heart J.*, **161**(6), 1078–87.

[135] Kang, H. J., Lee, H. Y., Na, S. H. *et al.* 2006. Differential effect of intracoronary infusion of mobilized peripheral blood stem cells by granulocyte colony-stimulating factor on left ventricular function and remodeling in patients with acute myocardial infarction versus old myocardial infarction: the MAGIC Cell-3-DES randomized, controlled trial. *Circulation*, **114**(1 Suppl.), I145–51.

[136] Tse, H. F., Thambar, S., Kwong, Y. L. *et al.* 2007. Prospective randomized trial of direct endomyocardial implantation of bone marrow cells for treatment of severe coronary artery diseases (PROTECT-CAD trial). *Eur. Heart J.*, **28**(24), 2998–3005.

[137] Dib, N., Dinsmore, J., Labadibi, Z. *et al.* 2009. One-year follow-up of feasibility and safety of the first U.S., randomized, controlled study using 3-dimensional guided catheter-based delivery of autologous skeletal myoblasts for ischemic cardiomyopathy (CAuSMIC study). *JACC Cardiovasc. Interv.*, **2**(1), 9–16.

[138] Shimizu, T., Sekine, H., Isoi, Y. *et al.* 2006. Long-term survival and growth of pulsatile myocardial tissue grafts engineered by the layering of cardiomyocyte sheets. *Tissue Eng.*, **12**(3), 499–507.

[139] Sekine, H., Shimizu, T., Hobo, K. *et al.* 2008. Endothelial cell coculture within tissue-engineered cardiomyocyte sheets enhances neovascularization and improves cardiac function of ischemic hearts. *Circulation*, **118**(14 Suppl.), S145–52.

[140] Sasagawa, T., Shimizu, T., Sekiya, S. *et al.* 2010. Design of prevascularized three-dimensional cell-dense tissues using a cell sheet stacking manipulation technology. *Biomaterials*, **31**(7), 1646–54.

[141] Asakawa, N., Shimizu, T., Tsuda, Y. *et al.* 2010. Prevascularization of in vitro three-dimensional tissues created by cell sheet engineering. *Biomaterials*, **31**(14), 3903–9.

[142] Itabashi, Y., Miyoshi, S., Kawaguchi, H. *et al.* 2005. A new method for manufacturing cardiac cell sheets using fibrin-coated dishes and its electrophysiological studies by optical mapping. *Artif. Organs*, **29**(2), 95–103.

[143] Villet, O. M., Siltanen, A., Pätilä, T. *et al.* 2011. Advances in cell transplantation therapy for diseased myocardium. *Stem Cells Int.*, 679171.

[144] Memon, I. A., Sawa, Y., Fukushima, N. *et al.* 2005. Repair of impaired myocardium by means of implantation of engineered autologous myoblast sheets. *J. Thorac. Cardiovasc. Surg.*, **130**(5), 1333–41.

[145] Siltanen, A., Kitabayashi, K., Pätilä, T. *et al.* 2011. Bcl-2 improves myoblast sheet therapy in rat chronic heart failure. *Tissue Eng. Part A*, **17**(1–2), 115–25.

[146] Hoashi, T., Matsumiya, G., Miyagawa, S. *et al.* 2009. Skeletal myoblast sheet transplantation improves the diastolic function of a pressure-overloaded right heart. *J. Thorac. Cardiovasc. Surg.*, **138**(2), 460–7.

[147] Miyagawa, S., Saito, A., Sakaguchi, T. *et al.* 2010. Impaired myocardium regeneration with skeletal cell sheets–a preclinical trial for tissue-engineered regeneration therapy. *Transplantation*, **90**(4), 364–72.

[148] Sawa, Y. 2010. Myocardial regeneration for heart failure [in Japanese]. *Nippon Rinsho*, **68**(4), 719–25.

[149] Miyahara, Y., Nagaya, N., Kataoka, M. *et al.* 2006. Monolayered mesenchymal stem cells repair scarred myocardium after myocardial infarction. *Nature Med.*, **12**(4), 459–65.

[150] Okura, H., Matsuyama, A., Lee, C. M. *et al.* 2010. Cardiomyoblast-like cells differentiated from human adipose tissue-derived mesenchymal stem cells improve left ventricular dysfunction and survival in a rat myocardial infarction model. *Tissue Eng. Part C Methods*, **16**(3), 417–25.

[151] Zakharova, L., Mastroeni, D., Mutlu, N. *et al.* 2010. Transplantation of cardiac progenitor cell sheet onto infarcted heart promotes cardiogenesis and improves function. *Cardiovasc. Res.*, **87**(1), 40–9.

[152] Haraguchi, Y., Shimizu, T., Yamato, M. *et al.* 2006. Electrical coupling of cardiomyocyte sheets occurs rapidly via functional gap junction formation. *Biomaterials*, **27**(27), 4765–74.

[153] Sekine, H., Shimizu, T., Yang, J., Kobayashi, E. and Okano, T. 2006. Pulsatile myocardial tubes fabricated

with cell sheet engineering. *Circulation*, **114**(1 Suppl.), I87–93.

[154] Miyagawa, S., Sawa, Y., Sakakida, S. *et al.* 2005. Tissue cardiomyoplasty using bioengineered contractile cardiomyocyte sheets to repair damaged myocardium: their integration with recipient myocardium. *Transplantation*, **80**(11), 1586–95.

[155] Zimmermann, W. H., Didié, M., Wasmeier, G. H. *et al.* 2002. Cardiac grafting of engineered heart tissue in syngenic rats. *Circulation*, **106**(12, Suppl. 1), I151–7.

[156] Simpson, D., Liu, H., Fan, T. H., Nerem, R. and Dudley, S. C. Jr. 2007. A tissue engineering approach to progenitor cell delivery results in significant cell engraftment and improved myocardial remodeling. *Stem Cells*, **25**(9), 2350–7.

[157] Kellar, R. S., Landeen, L. K., Shepherd, B. R. *et al.* 2001. Scaffold-based three-dimensional human fibroblast culture provides a structural matrix that supports angiogenesis in infarcted heart tissue. *Circulation*, **104**(17), 2063–8.

[158] Fukuhara, S., Tomita, S., Nakatani, T. *et al.* 2005. Bone marrow cell-seeded biodegradable polymeric scaffold enhances angiogenesis and improves function of the infarcted heart. *Circ. J.*, **69**(7), 850–7.

[159] Miyagawa, S., Roth, M., Saito, A., Sawa, Y. and Kostin, S. 2011. Tissue-engineered cardiac constructs for cardiac repair. *Ann. Thorac. Surg.*, **91**(1), 320–9.

[160] Jawad, H., Ali, N. N., Lyon, A. R., *et al.* 2008. Myocardial tissue engineering. *Br. Med. Bull.*, **87**, 31–47.

[161] Leor, J., Tuvia, S., Guetta, V. *et al.* 2009. Intracoronary injection of *in situ* forming alginate hydrogel reverses left ventricular remodeling after myocardial infarction in swine. *J. Am. Coll. Cardiol.*, **54**(11), 1014–23.

[162] Ozawa, T., Mickle, D. A., Weisel, R. D. *et al.* 2002. Optimal biomaterial for creation of autologous cardiac grafts. *Circulation*, **106**(12, Suppl. 1), I176–82.

[163] McDevitt, T. C., Woodhouse, K. A., Hauschka, S. D., Murry, C. E. and Stayton, P. S. 2003. Spatially organized layers of cardiomyocytes on biodegradable polyurethane films for myocardial repair. *J. Biomed. Mater. Res. A*, **66**(3), 586–95.

[164] Kofidis, T., Akhyari, P., Boublik, J. *et al.* 2002. In vitro engineering of heart muscle: artificial myocardial tissue. *J. Thorac. Cardiovasc. Surg.*, **124**(1), 63–9.

[165] Chachques, J. C., Trainini, J. C., Lago, N. *et al.* 2008. Myocardial assistance by grafting a new bioartificial upgraded myocardium (MAGNUM trial): clinical feasibility study. *Ann. Thorac. Surg.*, **85**(3), 901–8.

[166] Matsubayashi, K., Fedak, P. W., Mickle, D. A. *et al.* 2003. Improved left ventricular aneurysm repair with bioengineered vascular smooth muscle grafts. *Circulation*, **108**(Suppl. 1), II219–25.

[167] Siepe, M., Giraud, M. N., Pavlovic, M. *et al.* 2006. Myoblast-seeded biodegradable scaffolds to prevent post-myocardial infarction evolution toward heart failure. *J. Thorac. Cardiovasc. Surg.*, **132**(1), 124–31.

[168] Weymann, A., Loganathan, S., Takahashi, H. *et al.* 2011. Development and evaluation of a perfusion decellularization porcine heart model – generation of 3-dimensional myocardial neoscaffolds. *Circ. J.*, **75**(4), 852–60.

[169] Wainwright, J. M., Czajka, C. A., Patel, U. B. *et al.* 2010. Preparation of cardiac extracellular matrix from an intact porcine heart. *Tissue Eng. Part C Methods*, **16**(3), 525–32.

[170] Taylor, D. A. 2009. From stem cells and cadaveric matrix to engineered organs. *Curr. Opin. Biotechnol.*, **20**(5), 598–605.

[171] Naughton, G. K. 2002. From lab bench to market: critical issues in tissue engineering. *Ann. NY Acad. Sci.*, **961**, 372–85.

37

Bladder regeneration

Yuanyuan Zhang and Anthony Atala

37.1 Introduction

Bladder tissue engineering technology has provided an alternative treatment for patients with congenital bladder conditions (e.g. bladder exstrophy) and conditions such as radiation damage, infection, interstitial cystitis, neuropathic small bladder disease, and bladder cancer. To treat these end-stage bladder diseases, a partial or total cystectomy is often performed, followed by the creation of a neobladder or a continent urinary reservoir using intestinal segments to restore bladder capacity. However, using bowel tissue for this purpose may cause many side effects, although a recent study showed that all children with neurogenic bladder disease are at increased risk of bladder cancer regardless of exposure to intestinal tissue in the urinary tract [1]. Therefore, new clinical and surgical techniques are needed in order to allow these patients to live healthier and more normal lives. The authors of a clinical study recently reported that it is possible to engineer neobladder tissue using autologous cells seeded on biodegradable scaffolds [2] and that this engineered tissue can be used to enlarge the bladder volume and improve function for patients with neuropathic diseases. Additionally, increasing evidence indicates that the use of patients' own stem cells provides a promising alternative for patients with end-stage bladder diseases in cases in which healthy autologous bladder cells might not be available.

It has been known for a number of years that the bladder is able to regenerate generously over cell-free scaffolds in models in which 40% or less of the bladder is replaced with a biomaterial, because urothelium has a high reparative capacity [3]. However, bladder muscle tissue is less likely to regenerate in the same fashion as urothelium, which often leads to contraction or resorption of the graft. In addition, the inflammatory response toward the materials used to form the graft matrix may contribute to the resorption of cell-free grafts as well. The authors of an important dog study demonstrated that there was a major difference between matrices used with autologous cells (tissue-engineered matrices) and those used without cells [4]. The matrices seeded with cells prior to use in bladder augmentation retained most of their implanted diameter, whereas graft contraction and shrinkage occurred in matrices implanted without cells. As in previous studies, the histomorphology revealed a lack of muscle cells and a more aggressive inflammatory reaction in the unseeded matrices. Thus, for the replacement of bladder tissue, a biodegradable scaffold seeded with cells is preferred [2, 5–8]. Concomitant development of a healthy cell source and an optimal three-dimensional (3D) nanofibrous polymer scaffold are promising developments for use in patients with end-stage bladder diseases or bladder cancer who require cystoplasty. In this chapter, we will focus on the use of autologous bladder cells or stem cells, biodegradable scaffolds, and cell-seeding technology for regeneration and/or repair of the urinary bladder.

37.2 Cell sources

Autologous cell sources currently used for bladder regeneration are divided into two main categories: urological tissue (such as bladder, ureter and urine [9–13]) and non-urological tissues (bone marrow [14–19] and fat tissues [20, 21]). These cells can be fully differentiated, functional smooth muscle cells and urothelial cells or mesenchymal stem cells that are capable of differentiation into bladder cell types. When implanted mesenchymal stem cells are placed on an appropriate biodegradable scaffold, it seems that they can act as anti-fibrotic, angiogenic, anti-apoptotic, and mitotic agents [22] and that they can promote the development of a larger-sized bladder with less scarring.

37.2.1 Cells derived from bladder or ureter

Throughout the urinary tract, there are fully differentiated cells and stem/progenitor cells as well. Fully functional smooth muscle cells (SMCs), urothelial cells, and bladder stem cells are often mixed in cultures derived from tissue biopsies. Adult human bladder stem/progenitor cells have recently been described and characterized [9, 23]. It has been shown experimentally that the bladder neck and trigone area have a higher density of urothelial progenitor cells [24], and that these cells are localized in the basal region [25]. In the past, it was possible to grow urothelial cells in the laboratory setting, but only with limited success, because it was believed that urothelial cells had a natural senescence that was hard to overcome. However, several protocols that have improved urothelial growth and expansion by enhancing culture conditions to support proliferation and differentiation of urothelial progenitor cells have been developed over the last two decades [26–29]. It is now possible to expand a urothelial strain from a single surgical specimen that initially covers a surface area of 1 cm^2 to one covering a surface area of 4202 m^2 within 8 weeks [26]. Now, normal human bladder epithelial and muscle cells can be efficiently harvested from surgical material, then extensively expanded in culture, and their differentiation characteristics, growth requirements, and other biological properties can be studied [12, 26, 28–38]. In addition, human urothelial and muscle cells can be expanded in vitro, seeded onto polymer scaffolds, and allowed to attach and form sheets of cells.

Subsequently, these cell–polymer scaffold constructs have been implanted in animals after subtotal cystectomy. The bladders augmented with seeded matrices exhibited a 100% increase in capacity compared with bladders augmented with cell-free matrices, which generated only a 30% increase in capacity [4]. Histological analysis indicates that the non-seeded scaffolds resulted in a structure composed of normal urothelial cells with a thickened fibrotic submucosa and a thin layer of muscle fibers. Within the cell–polymer construct, viable cells appear able to self-assemble back into their respective tissue types, and they retain their native phenotype [39]. Normal cellular organization, consisting of a trilayer of urothelium, submucosa, and muscle, is also observed. Immunocytochemical analyses confirmed the muscle and urothelial phenotypes, and indicated the presence of neural structures [40]. These experiments, which were performed with polyglycolic acid-based scaffolds, have been repeated by other investigators, who found similar long-term results in large numbers of animals [41, 42]. Results of subsequent studies indicated that biodegradable scaffolds seeded with cells can be used without generating local or systemic toxicity [43].

After these successful large-animal experiments, bladder tissue engineered using autologous cells has been used clinically. A small clinical study was conducted starting in 1998. Seven patients were treated using a collagen–polyglycolic acid (PGA) scaffold seeded with their own cells, which had been taken from biopsies of bladder tissue several weeks before. These constructs were implanted either with or without omental coverage. The bladders reconstructed with the engineered bladder tissue created with the PGA–collagen cell-seeded scaffolds with omental coverage had greater compliance, lower end filling pressures, greater capacities and longer dry periods over time [44]. It is clear from this small study that the engineered bladders continued to improve with time, suggesting continued development in vivo. Although the experience is promising, it is just a start, and the technology is not yet ready for wide dissemination. Further experimental and clinical studies are being conducted.

37.2.2 Bone-marrow-derived stem cells

Adult stem cells are defined as clonogenic, self-renewing progenitor cells that reside in adult tissues and can generate one or more specialized types of cells required for the function of that tissue. The majority of adult tissues contain their own stem/progenitor cells that are capable of maintaining, generating, and replacing terminally differentiated cells within the tissue in response to physiological cell turnover or tissue damage resulting from injury. Stem cell populations in the bone marrow and the gastrointestinal tract were the first adult stem cell populations to be described, but in recent years adult stem populations have been demonstrated in most organs, tissues, and body fluids. Tissues that have especially large stem cell populations include adipose tissue [45], skeletal muscle [46], cord blood [47], amniotic fluid [48], and urine [9, 11, 13, 49–51]. These stem cells remain an area of intense study, since their potential for therapy may be applicable to a myriad of bladder diseases and other degenerative disorders. These cells are a particularly attractive option for bladder tissue engineering applications because they can be used in autologous cell therapies, thus avoiding any complications associated with immune rejection.

Currently, the best characterized types of multipotent stem cells are from bone marrow. Bone marrow stem cells (BMSCs) have been shown to differentiate into specialized cells, mainly mesodermal derivatives such as bone, cartilage, cardiac muscles, skeletal muscle, and fat. It has been suggested that, if BMSCs are placed on a proper biodegradable scaffold and implanted, they can act as anti-fibrotic, angiogenic, anti-apoptotic, and mitotic agents. Recently, BMSCs were evaluated as an alternative cell type for use in replacement of bladder SMCs. The potential of BMSCs to differentiate into cells with the characteristics of bladder SMCs was assessed in vitro [15] and in different animal models [5, 16–18, 52, 53]. Kanematsu *et al.* [53] showed that, in vitro, supernatants either from cultured rat bladder cells (conditioned media) or from media containing TGF-β and VEGF induced bone marrow cells to adopt an SMC phenotype. In a large-animal study [5], canine BMSCs proliferated at the same rate as primary cultured bladder SMCs in vitro, and they had a histological appearance and contractile phenotype similar to those of primary cultured bladder SMCs. Canine BMSCs had a significant contractile response to a calcium ionophore in vitro, and this response was similar to that seen in bladder SMCs but markedly different from fibroblasts. Immunohistochemical staining and Western blotting indicated that non-induced BMSCs expressed α-smooth muscle actin, but did not express desmin or myosin in vitro. More recently, we have investigated the impacts of soluble growth factors, bladder extracellular matrix (ECM), and 3D dynamic culture on cell proliferation and differentiation of human BMSCs into SMCs [15]. Myogenic growth factors (PDGF-BB and TGF-β_1) alone, or combined either with bladder ECM or with dynamic cultures, induced BMSCs to express smooth-muscle-specific genes and proteins. Either ECM or the dynamic culture alone promoted cell proliferation but did not induce myogenic differentiation of human BMSCs.

It is notoriously difficult to induce mesenchymal stem cells to differentiate into cell types of the endodermal lineage, such as urothelial cells. Additionally, there is no specific soluble growth factor that has been shown to enhance this differentiation. Using conditioned medium from urothelial cell cultures, we have shown that BMSCs can be induced to express the RNA transcript of uroplakin (Up)-Ia, but that co-culture with urothelial cells induces weaker expression of Up-Ia gene and protein in BMSCs. Although urothelial markers were expressed in BMSCs following urothelial induction, only about half of the BMSCs changed from a spindle shape to a polygonal shape after 14 days of differentiation [14].

In order to test this in vivo, bone marrow cells expressing green fluorescent protein (GFP) were transplanted into lethally irradiated rats. Eight weeks following transplantation, bladder domes were replaced with acellular matrix grafts. Two weeks after the graft procedure, GFP expression in the matrices indicated that the transplanted marrow cells had repopulated the graft. After 12 weeks, these cells had reconstituted the smooth muscle layer, with native SMCs also infiltrating the graft. In another rat study

[52], rapid regeneration of bladder SMCs and urothelium occurred on BMSC-seeded collagen matrices, whereas fibrotic changes were observed in the non-seeded matrix group 3 months after bladder augmentation. In a canine bladder cystoplasty model [5], small-intestinal submucosa (SIS) grafts seeded with BMSCs developed solid smooth-muscle bundle formations throughout the grafts, as did bladder-cell-seeded SIS grafts. However, bladder tissue regeneration did not occur in animals that received cell-free scaffolding. These results indicate that BMSCs may provide an alternative cell source for bladder tissue engineering. This is relevant for patients with bladder malignancies who require bladder augmentation or replacement but who do not have enough normal, non-malignant bladder cells for use in tissue engineering applications.

37.2.3 Adipose-derived stem cells

Other stem cell types, such as adipose stem cells [54–62] have been investigated as potential candidates for cell-based tissue engineering in bladder reconstruction. The advantages to using adipose stem cells are that they can be obtained in larger quantities, under local anesthesia, and with minimal discomfort. However, the major limitation is that adipose stem cells differentiate into only SMCs, not urothelial cells.

37.2.4 Urine-derived stem cells

We recently demonstrated that it is possible to isolate and expand cells from human urine [9]. Cells from human urine specimens could be consistently cultured on a long-term basis. However, the phenotype of the cultured human urine-derived cells was not that of primary urothelial cells. The primary cultures from urine did not show expression of the cytokeratins (CK7, CK13, and CK19/20), which are characteristic of epithelial cells; nor did the cells express the urothelial-specific protein uroplakin. After growth in medium containing higher levels of epidermal growth factor, the cells began to express the cytokeratin proteins and uroplakin [9]. However, after growth in myogenic differentiation medium, the cultured cells expressed markers consistent with smooth muscle, including α-smooth muscle actin (α-SM actin), desmin, calponin, and myosin [9]. This led us to conclude that the urine-derived cells were progenitors (initially designated urine-derived progenitor cells) capable of giving rise to both urothelium and bladder smooth muscle. Furthermore, we found that the cells displayed a surface marker phenotype consistent with mesenchymal stem cells and pericytes. Specifically, they expressed CD44, CD73, CD90, CD105, CD146, NG2, and PDGF-rβ, and they were negative both for hematopoietic markers and for endothelial markers including CD45, CD34, and CD31. The cells also display telomerase activity and grow for up to 20 passages in culture. We concluded that these cells were at least bipotential progenitors for the major bladder cell types. This result was surprising, because it was generally believed that muscle and epithelial cells in the bladder represented separate cell lineages derived from the mesoderm and endoderm, respectively. Most recently, we have observed that the urine-derived cells expressing mesenchymal stem cell markers can differentiate to yield the characteristic cell lineages obtained from mesenchymal stem cells, namely osteocytes, adipocytes, and chondrocytes [62], suggesting that they may represent a new type of stem cell that we term urine-derived stem cells (USCs).

The quality of cells obtained from the differentiation of USCs is similar to that of the biopsy-derived cells described above. When differentiated, USCs express all proteins characteristic of the various bladder cell lineages. Karyotype analysis has demonstrated that these cells are genetically stable. Importantly, there is a major cost advantage to using USCs – it costs about $50 to obtain cells from urine, versus about $5000 to isolate cells from a biopsy procedure [9]. About 1.4×10^9 urothelial cells and SMCs are required for bladder tissue regeneration [2]. One finds an average of about seven USCs per 100 ml of urine (in the range 5–10 cells/100 ml urine). The average population doubling was 31.3 (i.e. $2^{31.3} = 2.2 \times 10^9$). We estimate that one or two urine samples (about 15 cells/200 ml urine) expanded for 6–7 weeks would yield a sufficient quantity of healthy, low-passage cells (about 3×10^{10} cells) for clinical tissue engineering applications. This time frame is comparable to that required for expansion from a tissue biopsy (7–8 weeks) [63]. The USCs and the cells obtained through urological tissue biopsies come from the same urinary tract systems and have similar biological features. Therefore, collecting cells from urine could be an attractive alternative to the standard urological tissue biopsies currently used in cell therapy and tissue engineering.

There are many potential advantages to using USCs as a cell source for bladder tissue engineering. First, cells can be easily harvested by a non-invasive method and grown in culture without an isolation procedure using enzyme digestion. USCs do not require culture on a layer of feeder cells to support cell growth. Second, since invasive surgical biopsy procedures are not necessary to harvest cells from urine, patient morbidity and potential complications, such as urethral or bladder trauma and urinary tract infections, are avoided. Since USCs are autologous somatic cells, no ethical issues are involved in their use for tissue reconstruction, and no immune reaction to engineered implants should occur.

37.3 Biodegradable scaffolds

There are two tissue engineering technologies, i.e. cell-seeded and non-seeded, which have been used in bladder tissue engineering and regeneration studies. In cell-seeded tissue engineering, fully functional bladder cells or stem cells are used as a cell source seeded on biodegradable biomaterials for a large-size bladder tissue replacement. In non-seeded tissue engineering, a cell-free scaffold is implanted and recruits the host's own stem/progenitor cells, which then differentiate into the proper cell type required. This type of tissue engineering strategy, as described previously, can be used only for relatively small-sized bladder tissue repairs. The selection of a biodegradable scaffold is another critical factor for bladder tissue engineering. An ideal scaffold for bladder or other hollow organ tissue engineering must possess the proper mechanical/physical assets together with a highly porous structure. A scaffold with the appropriate biomechanical properties can maintain the correct shape of the bladder and its hollow structure during tissue regeneration. The porosity of the biomaterial aids cell infiltration into the matrix in vitro and promotes vascularization of cell-scaffold constructs at early stages of implantation. Currently, two types of scaffolds are commonly used in experimental and clinical applications for bladder tissue engineering: natural collagen acellular matrices, such as SIS derived from pigs [5, 11, 64–69], bladder submucosa (BSM) [4, 70], and bladder acellular matrix graft [20, 71, 72]; and synthetic polymers, such as PGA plus poly(lactic-*co*-glycolic acid) (PLGA) [48, 63] and a highly porous poly-L-lactic acid (PLLA) scaffold [14, 15].

Natural collagen acellular matrixes are produced by removing all cellular components from a piece of tissue to obtain a biological scaffold. This material contains numerous growth factors that promote tissue regeneration. In animal studies of partial cystoplasty, this type of biologically derived material alone (without seeded cells) facilitated tissue regeneration with infiltration of SMCs, vascularization, and innervation. However, the use of natural collagen matrices for bladder regeneration is limited by the size of the bladder defect to be replaced. In partial (30%–40%) cystoplasty, SIS alone (without seeded cells) can also facilitate tissue regeneration. Infiltration of SMCs, vascularization, and innervation can be observed at early stages, and muscle bundle formation is observed later after surgery in the dog model [73, 74]. However, a recent study showed that extensive bladder augmentation with either cell-seeded or cell-free natural collagen matrix did not improve bladder regeneration [75]. One reason for this finding is that the collagen matrix is too soft to maintain the shape of the organ during tissue remodeling, and as a result the scaffold collapses after implantation. Other concerns about the use of natural collagen matrices center on the possibility of residual porcine cellular and DNA content, which could still cause immunological reactions in vivo after implantation [76]. For replacement of large amounts of tissue, a PGA–PLGA cell-seeded scaffold is preferred. PGA–PLGA can provide a 3D structure to allow loading of more cells during the in-vitro phase, and this can lead to the formation of complete tissues in vivo. Importantly, a PGA–PLGA scaffold provides adequate physical properties to hold the shape of the implant and prevent collapse during tissue healing processes. Additionally, this material is highly porous, which facilitates gas and nutrition exchange, and promotes cell metabolism within the cell–scaffold composite. PGA–PLGA is also FDA-approved as a scaffold material, and has been used for many other types of clinical applications.

Biodegradable PLLA polymeric scaffolds are a new generation of synthetic polymer scaffold that possesses better biomechanical/physical features, with highly enhanced porosity. PLLA has been used successfully as a nanofibrous scaffold in the tissue engineering of several organs, e.g. bone, cartilage, and liver, both in vitro and in vivo [14, 15, 77, 78]. This nanostructured PLLA scaffold mimics natural ECM and provides macropores and micropores, and fibers with diameters that facilitate gas and nutrition exchange together with a better cell–matrix infiltration, thereby promoting cell metabolism. As a 3D, nanofibrous, porous polymer scaffold, PLLA possesses suitable macroporosity and interconnected microporosity to facilitate cell ingrowth and differentiation, and also has sufficient mechanical strength to prevent collapse of grafts after implantation [14, 15, 77, 78]. The PLLA scaffold maintains the physiological strength of the replaced tissue in vivo. This biodegradable scaffold can be maintained in the body for 3–6 months without any cytotoxic effects or immunological reactions [14, 15, 77, 78]. In our recent study, the growth-factor-induced BMSCs were grown on PLLA scaffold and the cells displayed abundant cell–matrix infiltration and SMC differentiation in vitro. The nanofibrous PLLA scaffolds enhance cell infiltration, muscle contractile phenotype expression, bladder tissue regeneration, vascularization, and tissue remodeling in vivo when seeded with human BMSCs induced with myogenic growth factors [14, 15]. The cell-seeded nanofibrous PLLA scaffold induced smooth muscle tissue regeneration with abundant formation of capillaries, superior to those induced by cell-seeded natural collagen matrix. The main advantage of using PLLA as a substrate is that its porous structure provides cellular interactions with the polymer, prompting cell migration, proliferation, and tissue formation in a 3D construct. This nanofibrous 3D PLLA polymer scaffold with a porous structure provides an optimal microenvironment for facilitating cell–matrix penetration and retention of myogenically differentiated BMSCs, thereby promoting tissue remolding with rich capillary formation in vivo. Therefore, fully functional bladder cells or differentiated stem cells seeded on this nanofibrous PLLA scaffold could potentially be used in cell-based tissue engineering in patients.

37.4 Cell seeding techniques and dynamic culture

Two main cell types, i.e. SMCs and urothelial cells, are used in bladder tissue engineering. To mimic in-vivo conditions, layered or sandwich co-culture techniques [28] are commonly used for cell seeding. For biomaterials with porous structures on both sides, such as PGA–PLGA and PLLA, the sandwich co-culture method might be preferable, since SMCs and urothelial cells can be adherent and penetrate on the lumen and serosa or lamina propria sides. For biomaterials that are porous only on one side, such as SIS and BSM, layered co-culture techniques appear to better induce organized cell sorting, formation of a well-defined pseudostratified urothelium, and the presence of multilayered smooth muscle cells with enhanced matrix penetration on the lamina serosa or propria side [11, 69, 70].

Dynamic culture with a bioreactor, i.e. culture that includes perfusion or rotation, has commonly been used for seeded scaffolds. Dynamic culturing mimics physiological environments and promotes cell adhesion, proliferation, infiltration, and differentiation [79, 80]. Several advantages are associated with dynamic culture conditions, namely (i) the even distribution of nutrition and oxygen supply leads to uniform growth of cells on the matrix; (ii) increased synthesis of endogenous ECM; and (iii) physiologically relevant mechanical forces (i.e. shear stress, pressure, and hydrodynamic compression) on the cultured cells. In this study, we used a simple bioreactor to provide a 3D culture setting that enhances the efficiency, yield, and homogeneity of bladder cell differentiation and also promotes cell–matrix infiltration. This culture system utilizes simple, efficient, and low-cost equipment for improving the culture environment. Unlike a perfusion bioreactor that requires a large set of equipment, a 3D dynamic culture bioreactor is easier to handle and carries less risk of contamination.

A dynamic culture is suitable both for sandwich and for layered co-culture techniques, as demonstrated in our study [11, 14, 70]. The cell–matrix infiltration is important in cell-seeded tissue engineering since it enhances cell differentiation and protects against cell loss during transplantation of the cell-seeded scaffold into the host. Several elements enhance cell–matrix infiltration: (i) a 3D porous scaffold with large pore size; (ii) a 3D dynamic culture bioreactor; (iii) interaction of epithelial and stromal cells in the co-culture system; and (iv) gradual seeding of cells on the matrix. Dynamic culture is beneficial for cells seeded both on natural collagen matrices and on synthetic polymer biomaterials. In BSM [70] and in SIS [11], the cells proliferated and adhered tightly on the surface of the serosa or lamina propria with good cell–matrix penetration in a sandwich co-culture via dynamic culture. Cells penetrated more deeply into the matrix while using the layered co-culture method. We did not observe significant loss of cells seeded on the bottom of the membrane due to gravity using the sandwich co-culture technique. Moreover, the bladder cells were seeded gradually over three days, which also resulted in better cell ingrowth than did a single seeding of all cells at once as described previously [69]. Use of the above methods in combination facilitates the formation of well-organized tubule-like structures in vivo with urothelial cells layered on the luminal side and SMCs infiltrated into collagen matrix, which might provide an alternative approach for reconstruction of anatomically correct urological macrotubular tissues. Our data demonstrated that significant enhancement of SMC penetration of the SIS or BSM membrane and multilayer urothelium formation had been achieved in dynamic culture. The same outcomes were observed for cell-seeded PLLA in dynamic culture. We have observed that adding growth factors to a dynamic culture system improves the efficiency of myogenically differentiated BMSCs in expressing SMC-specific transcripts and protein markers in vitro. Induced BMSC proliferated and underwent differentiation more rapidly in a 3D dynamic culture than they did in a static culture. Overall, our study showed that, using bladder ECM, SIS, or PLLA scaffolds, a dynamic culture could significantly promote cell proliferation, differentiation, and tissue formation in vitro.

37.5 Conclusions

Two types of tissue engineering technologies have been employed to build bladder tissue, cell-seeded and non-seeded. Cell-seeded technology uses scaffolds that are seeded in vitro with primary cultured cells obtained from a bladder biopsy. This composite graft is then implanted back in the host for carry-over of the regenerative process [2, 4, 5, 52, 63, 75]. The non-seeded technology uses cell-free biodegradable scaffolds to allow the natural process of regeneration to occur in vivo, and was successfully applied experimentally in partial (30%–40% tissue replacement) cystoplasty models [73, 74]. One may wonder which approach is to be preferred for large-scale bladder tissue replacement, since numerous investigations involving both technologies have been conducted over the years. Increasing evidence indicates that cells are necessary to achieve improved bladder tissue function when a large amount of bladder tissue is in demand. Further validation of the cell-seeded technology was demonstrated in a clinical trial involving bladder augmentation in myelomeningocele patients [5].

When implanted cells are placed on a proper biodegradable scaffold, they appear to behave as antifibrotic, angiogenic, anti-apoptotic, and mitotic agents [22], and they could promote the development of a larger-sized bladder with less scarring. However, several issues still need further investigation. First, it is uncertain whether the seeded cells proliferate and populate the scaffold themselves, or whether they act in a "feeder-cell-like" manner by recruiting and activating the resident progenitor cells to participate in the regeneration of bladder tissue. Alternatively, the seeded cells could perform both functions. Second, a method to efficiently promote angiogenesis in the early stages of implantation must be developed. Finally, it is necessary to improve nerve development in the implant so that the new organ will have the proper innervation to function as a normal bladder. More research is needed in these areas.

REFERENCES

[1] Higuchi, T. T., Granberg, C. F., Fox, J. A. and Husmann, D. A. 2010. Augmentation cystoplasty and risk of neoplasia: fact, fiction and controversy. *J. Urol.*, **184**(6), 2492–6.

[2] Atala, A., Bauer, S. B., Soker, S., Yoo, J. J. and Retik, A. B. 2006. Tissue-engineered autologous bladders for patients needing cystoplasty. *Lancet*, **367**(9518), 1241–6.

[3] de Boer, W. I., Schuller, A. G., Vermey, M. and van der Kwast, T. H. 1994. Expression of growth factors and receptors during specific phases in regenerating urothelium after acute injury in vivo. *Am. J. Pathol.*, **145**(5), 1199–207.

[4] Yoo, J. J., Meng, J., Oberpenning, F. and Atala, A. 1998. Bladder augmentation using allogenic bladder submucosa seeded with cells. *Urology*, **51**(2), 221–5.

[5] Zhang, Y., Lin, H. K., Frimberger, D., Epstein, R. B. and Kropp, B. P. 2005. Growth of bone marrow stromal cells on small intestinal submucosa: an alternative cell source for tissue engineered bladder. *BJU Int.*, **96**(7), 1120–5.

[6] Atala, A. 2006. Recent developments in tissue engineering and regenerative medicine. *Curr. Opin. Pediatr.*, **18**(2), 167–71.

[7] Atala, A. 2008. Bioengineered tissues for urogenital repair in children. *Pediatr. Res.*, **63**(5), 569–75.

[8] Zhang, Y. 2008. Bladder reconstruction by tissue engineering – with or without cells? *J. Urol.*, **180**(1), 10–11.

[9] Zhang, Y., McNeill, E., Tian, H. *et al.* 2008. Urine derived cells are a potential source for urological tissue reconstruction. *J. Urol.*, **180**(5), 2226–33.

[10] Zhang, Y. 2008. Autologous cell sources for urological applications. In Atala, A. and Denstedt, J., editors. *Biomaterials and Tissue Engineering in Urology*. Cambridge: Woodhead Publishing Limited.

[11] Wu, S., Liu, Y., Bharadwaj, S., Atala, A. and Zhang, Y. 2011. Human urine-derived stem cells seeded in a modified 3D porous small intestinal submucosa scaffold for urethral tissue engineering. *Biomaterials*, **32**(5), 1317–26.

[12] Tobin, M. S., Freeman, M. R. and Atala, A. 1994. Maturational response of normal human urothelial cells in culture is dependent on extracellular matrix and serum additives. *Surg. Forum*, **45**, 786.

[13] Bodin, A., Bharadwaj, S., Wu, S. *et al.* 2010. Tissue-engineered conduit using urine-derived stem cells seeded bacterial cellulose polymer in urinary reconstruction and diversion. *Biomaterials*, **31**(34), 8889–901.

[14] Tian, H., Bharadwaj, S., Liu, Y. *et al.* 2010. Differentiation of human bone marrow mesenchymal stem cells into bladder cells: potential for urological tissue engineering. *Tissue Eng. Part A*, **16**(5), 1769–79.

[15] Tian, H., Bharadwaj, S., Liu, Y. *et al.* 2010. Myogenic differentiation of human bone marrow mesenchymal stem cells on a 3D nano fibrous scaffold for bladder tissue engineering. *Biomaterials*, **31**(5), 870–7.

[16] Sharma, A. K., Hota, P. V., Matoka, D. J. *et al.* 2010. Urinary bladder smooth muscle regeneration utilizing bone marrow derived mesenchymal stem cell seeded elastomeric poly(1,8-octanediol-*co*-citrate) based thin films. *Biomaterials*, **31**(24), 6207–17.

[17] Sharma, A. K., Fuller, N. J., Sullivan, R. R. *et al.* 2009. Defined populations of bone marrow derived mesenchymal stem and endothelial progenitor cells for bladder regeneration. *J. Urol.*, **182**(4 Suppl.), 1898–905.

[18] Sharma, A. K., Bury, M. I., Marks, A. J. *et al.* 2011. A non-human primate model for urinary bladder regeneration using autologous sources of bone marrow-derived mesenchymal stem cells. *Stem Cells*, **29**(2), 241–50.

[19] De Coppi, P., Callegari, A., Chiavegato, A. *et al.* 2007. Amniotic fluid and bone marrow derived mesenchymal stem cells can be converted to smooth muscle cells in the cryo-injured rat bladder and prevent compensatory hypertrophy of surviving smooth muscle cells. *J. Urol.*, **177**(1), 369–76.

[20] Zhu, W. D., Xu, Y. M., Feng, C. *et al.* 2010. Bladder reconstruction with adipose-derived stem cell-seeded bladder acellular matrix grafts improve morphology composition. *World J. Urol.*, **28**(4), 493–8.

[21] Jack, G. S., Almeida, F. G., Zhang, R. *et al.* 2005. Processed lipoaspirate cells for tissue engineering of the lower urinary tract: implications for the treatment of stress urinary incontinence and bladder reconstruction. *J. Urol.*, **174**(5), 2041–5.

[22] Caplan, A. I. 2007. Adult mesenchymal stem cells for tissue engineering versus regenerative medicine. *J. Cell Physiol.*, **213**(2), 341–7.

[23] Oottamasathien, S., Williams, K., Franco, O. E. *et al.* 2007. Urothelial inhibition of transforming growth factor-β in a bladder tissue recombination model. *J. Urol.*, **178**(4, Part 2), 1643–9.

[24] Nguyen, M. M., Lieu, D. K., deGraffenried, L. A., Isseroff, R. R. and Kurzrock, E. A. 2007. Urothelial progenitor

cells: regional differences in the rat bladder. *Cell Proliferation*, **40**(2), 157–65.

[25] Kurzrock, E. A., Lieu, D. K., Degraffenried, L. A., Chan, C. W. and Isseroff, R. R. 2008. Label-retaining cells of the bladder: candidate urothelial stem cells. *Am. J. Physiol. – Renal Physiol.*, **294**(6), F1415–21.

[26] Cilento, B. G., Freeman, M. R., Schneck, F. X., Retik, A. B. and Atala, A. 1994. Phenotypic and cytogenetic characterization of human bladder urothelia expanded in vitro. *J. Urol.*, **152**(2, Part 2), 665–70.

[27] Scriven, S. D., Booth, C., Thomas, D. F., Trejdosiewicz, L. K. and Southgate, J. 1997. Reconstitution of human urothelium from monolayer cultures. *J. Urol.*, **158**(3, Part 2), 1147–52.

[28] Liebert, M., Hubbel, A., Chung, M. *et al.* 1997. Expression of mal is associated with urothelial differentiation in vitro: identification by differential display reverse-transcriptase polymerase chain reaction. *Differentiation*, **61**(3), 177–85.

[29] Puthenveettil, J. A., Burger, M. S. and Reznikoff, C. A. 1999. Replicative senescence in human uroepithelial cells. *Adv. Exp. Med. Biol.*, **462**, 83–91.

[30] Liebert, M., Wedemeyer, G., Abruzzo, L. V. *et al.* 1991. Stimulated urothelial cells produce cytokines and express an activated cell surface antigenic phenotype. *Seminars Urol.*, **9**(2), 124–30.

[31] Harriss, D. R. 1995. Smooth muscle cell culture: a new approach to the study of human detrusor physiology and pathophysiology. *Brit. J. Urol.*, **75**(Suppl. 1), 18–26.

[32] Freeman, M. R., Yoo, J. J., Raab, G. *et al.* 1997. Heparin-binding EGF-like growth factor is an autocrine growth factor for human urothelial cells and is synthesized by epithelial and smooth muscle cells in the human bladder. *J. Clin. Invest.*, **99**(5), 1028–36.

[33] Fauza, D. O., Fishman, S. J., Mehegan, K. and Atala, A. 1998. Videofetoscopically assisted fetal tissue engineering: skin replacement. *J. Pediatr. Surg.*, **33**(2), 357–61.

[34] Fauza, D. O., Fishman, S. J., Mehegan, K. and Atala, A. 1998. Videofetoscopically assisted fetal tissue engineering: bladder augmentation. *J. Pediatr. Surg.*, **33**(1), 7–12.

[35] Solomon, L. Z., Jennings, A. M., Sharpe, P., Cooper, A. J. and Malone, P. S. 1998. Effects of short-chain fatty acids on primary urothelial cells in culture: implications for intravesical use in enterocystoplasties. *J. Lab. Clin. Med.*, **132**(4), 279–83.

[36] Lobban, E. D., Smith, B. A., Hall, G. D. *et al.* 1998. Uroplakin gene expression by normal and neoplastic human urothelium. *Am. J. Pathol.*, **153**(6), 1957–67.

[37] Nguyen, H. T., Park, J. M., Peters, C. A. *et al.* 1999. Cell-specific activation of the HB-EGF and ErbB1 genes by stretch in primary human bladder cells. *In Vitro Cell. Developmental Biol. Animal*, **35**(7), 371–5.

[38] Rackley, R. R., Bandyopadhyay, S. K., Fazeli-Matin, S., Shin, M. S. and Appell, R. 1996. Immunoregulatory potential of urothelium: characterization of NF-kappaB signal transduction. *J. Urol.*, **162**(5), 1812–16.

[39] Oberpenning, F., Meng, J., Yoo, J. J. and Atala, A. 1999. De novo reconstitution of a functional mammalian urinary bladder by tissue engineering. *Nature Biotechnol.*, **17**(2), 149–55.

[40] Atala, A., Freeman, M. R., Vacanti, J. P., Shepard, J. and Retik, A. B. 1993. Implantation in vivo and retrieval of artificial structures consisting of rabbit and human urothelium and human bladder muscle. *J. Urol.*, **150**(2, Part 2), 608–12.

[41] Jayo, M. J., Jain, D., Ludlow, J. W. *et al.* 2008. Long-term durability, tissue regeneration and neo-organ growth during skeletal maturation with a neo-bladder augmentation construct. *Regen. Med.*, **3**(5), 671–82.

[42] Jayo, M. J., Jain, D., Wagner, B. J. and Bertram, T. A. 2008. Early cellular and stromal responses in regeneration versus repair of a mammalian bladder using autologous cell and biodegradable scaffold technologies. *J. Urol.*, **180**(1), 392–7.

[43] Kwon, T. G., Yoo, J. J. and Atala, A. 2008. Local and systemic effects of a tissue engineered neobladder in a canine cystoplasty model. *J. Urol.*, **179**(5), 2035–41.

[44] Atala, A., Bauer, S. B., Soker, S., Yoo, J. J. and Retik, A. B. 2006. Tissue-engineered autologous bladders for patients needing cystoplasty. *Lancet*, **367**(9518), 1241–6.

[45] Hanada, K., Dennis, J. E. and Caplan, A. I. 1997. Stimulatory effects of basic fibroblast growth factor and bone morphogenetic protein-2 on osteogenic differentiation of rat bone marrow-derived mesenchymal stem cells. *J. Bone Miner. Res.*, **12**(10), 1606–14.

[46] Saito, T., Dennis, J. E., Lennon, D. P., Young, R. G. and Caplan, A. I. 1995. Myogenic expression of mesenchymal stem cells within myotubes of mdx mice in vitro and in vivo. *Tissue Eng.*, **1**(4), 327–43.

[47] Caplan, A. I. 1995. Osteogenesis imperfecta, rehabilitation medicine, fundamental research and mesenchymal stem cells. *Connect Tissue Res.*, **31**(4), S9–14.

[48] da Silva Meirelles, L., Sand, T. T., Harman, R. J., Lennon, D. P. and Caplan, A. I. 2009. MSC frequency correlates with blood vessel density in equine adipose tissue. *Tissue Eng. Part A*, **15**(2), 221–9.

[49] Bharadwaj, S., Liu, G., Shi, Y. *et al.* 2011. Characterization of urine-derived stem cells obtained from upper urinary tract for use in cell-based urological tissue engineering. *Tissue Eng. Part A*, **17**(15–16), 2123–32.

[50] Bharadwaj, S., Wu, S., Hodges, S., Atala, A. and Zhang, Y. 2011. Skeletal muscle differentiation of human urine-derived stem cells for injection therapy in the treatment of stress urinary incontinence. *J. Urol.*, **184**(4), E681.

[51] Wu, S., Liu, Y., Bharadwaj, S. *et al.* 2011. Implantation of autologous urine-derived stem cells expressing vascular endothelial growth factor for potential use in genito-urinary reconstruction. *J. Urol.*, **186**(2), 640–7.

[52] Chung, S. Y., Krivorov, N. P., Rausei, V. *et al.* 2005. Bladder reconstitution with bone marrow derived stem cells seeded on small intestinal submucosa improves morphological and molecular composition. *J. Urol.*, **174**(1), 353–9.

[53] Kanematsu, A., Yamamoto, S., Iwai-Kanai, E. *et al.* 2005. Induction of smooth muscle cell-like phenotype in marrow-derived cells among regenerating urinary bladder smooth muscle cells. *Am. J. Pathol.*, **166**(2), 565–73.

[54] Sakuma, T., Matsumoto, T., Kano, K. *et al.* 2009. Mature, adipocyte derived, dedifferentiated fat cells can differentiate into smooth muscle-like cells and contribute to bladder tissue regeneration. *J. Urol.*, **182**(1), 355–65.

[55] Smaldone, M. C., Chen, M. L. and Chancellor, M. B. 2009. Stem cell therapy for urethral sphincter regeneration. *Minerva Urol. Nefrol.*, **61**(1), 27–40.

[56] Montzka, K. and Heidenreich, A. 2010. Application of mesenchymal stromal cells in urological diseases. *BJU Int.*, **105**(3), 309–12.

[57] Liu, J., Huang, J., Lin, T., Zhang, C. and Yin, X. 2009. Cell-to-cell contact induces human adipose tissue-derived stromal cells to differentiate into urothelium-like cells in vitro. *Biochem. Biophys. Res. Commun.*, **390**(3), 931–6.

[58] Lin, G., Wang, G., Banie, L. *et al.* 2010. Treatment of stress urinary incontinence with adipose tissue-derived stem cells. *Cytotherapy*, **12**(1), 88–95.

[59] Lin, G., Banie, L., Ning, H. *et al.* 2009. Potential of adipose-derived stem cells for treatment of erectile dysfunction. *J. Sex Med.*, **6**(Suppl. 3), 320–7.

[60] Jack, G. S., Zhang, R., Lee, M. *et al.* 2009. Urinary bladder smooth muscle engineered from adipose stem cells and a three dimensional synthetic composite. *Biomaterials*, **30**(19), 3259–70.

[61] Cavarretta, I. T., Altanerova, V., Matuskova, M. *et al.* 2010. Adipose tissue-derived mesenchymal stem cells expressing prodrug-converting enzyme inhibit human prostate tumor growth. *Molec. Ther.*, **18**(1), 223–31.

[62] Bharadwaj, S., Liu, G., Shi, Y. *et al.* 2013. Multipotential differentiation of human urine-derived stem cells: potential for therapeutic applications in urology. *Stem Cells*, **31**(9), 1840–56.

[63] Oberpenning, F., Meng, J., Yoo, J. J. and Atala A. 1999. De novo reconstitution of a functional mammalian urinary bladder by tissue engineering. *Nature Biotechnol.*, **17**(2), 149–55.

[64] Kropp, B. P. and Cheng, E. Y. 2000. Bioengineering organs using small intestinal submucosa scaffolds: in vivo tissue-engineering technology. *J. Endourol.*, **14**(1), 59–62.

[65] Kropp, B. P., Cheng, E. Y., Lin, H. K. and Zhang, Y. 2004. Reliable and reproducible bladder regeneration using unseeded distal small intestinal submucosa. *J. Urol.*, **172**(4, Part 2), 1710–13.

[66] Kropp, B. P., Rippy, M. K., Badylak, S. F. *et al.* 1996. Regenerative urinary bladder augmentation using small intestinal submucosa: urodynamic and histopathologic assessment in long-term canine bladder augmentations. *J. Urol.*, **155**(6), 2098–104.

[67] Kropp, B. P., Sawyer, B. D., Shannon, H. E. *et al.* 1996. Characterization of small intestinal submucosa regenerated canine detrusor: assessment of reinnervation, in vitro compliance and contractility. *J. Urol.*, **156**(2, Part 2), 599–607.

[68] Zhang, Y., Kropp, B. P., Lin, H. K., Cowan, R. and Cheng, E. Y. 2004. Bladder regeneration with cell-seeded small intestinal submucosa. *Tissue Eng.*, **10**(1–2), 181–7.

[69] Zhang, Y., Kropp, B. P., Moore, P. *et al.* 2000. Coculture of bladder urothelial and smooth muscle cells on small intestinal submucosa: potential applications for tissue engineering technology. *J. Urol.*, **164**(3, Part 2), 928–34; discussion 34–5.

[70] Liu, Y., Bharadwaj, S., Lee, S. J., Atala, A. and Zhang, Y. 2009. Optimization of a natural collagen scaffold to aid cell-matrix penetration for urologic tissue engineering. *Biomaterials*, **30**(23–24), 3865–73.

[71] Chen, B. S., Zhang, S. L., Geng, H., Pan, J. and Chen, F. 2009. Ex vivo functional evaluation of isolated strips in BAMG tissue-engineered bladders. *Int. J. Artif. Organs*, **32**(3), 159–65.

[72] Kikuno, N., Kawamoto, K., Hirata, H. *et al.* 2009. Nerve growth factor combined with vascular endothelial growth factor enhances regeneration of bladder acellular matrix graft in spinal cord injury-induced neurogenic rat bladder. *BJU Int.*, **103**(10), 1424–8.

[73] Badylak, S. F., Kropp, B., McPherson, T., Liang, H. and Snyder, P. W. 1998. Small intestional submucosa: a

rapidly resorbed bioscaffold for augmentation cystoplasty in a dog model. *Tissue Eng.*, **4**(4), 379–87.

[74] Kropp, B. P., Rippy, M. K., Badylak, S. F. *et al.* 1996. Regenerative urinary bladder augmentation using small intestinal submucosa: urodynamic and histopathologic assessment in long-term canine bladder augmentations. *J. Urol.*, **155**(6), 2098–104.

[75] Zhang, Y., Frimberger, D., Cheng, E. Y., Lin, H. K. and Kropp, B. P. 2006. Challenges in a larger bladder replacement with cell-seeded and unseeded small intestinal submucosa grafts in a subtotal cystectomy model. *BJU Int.*, **98**(5), 1100–5.

[76] Feil, G., Christ-Adler, M., Maurer, S. *et al.* 2006. Investigations of urothelial cells seeded on commercially available small intestine submucosa. *Eur. Urol.*, **50**(6), 1330–7.

[77] Ma, Z., Gao, C., Gong, Y. and Shen, J. 2005. Cartilage tissue engineering PLLA scaffold with surface immobilized collagen and basic fibroblast growth factor. *Biomaterials*, **26**(11), 1253–9.

[78] Ma, Z., Mao, Z. and Gao, C. 2007. Surface modification and property analysis of biomedical polymers used for tissue engineering. *Colloids Surf. B Biointerfaces*, **60**(2), 137–57.

[79] Sikavitsas, V. I., Bancroft, G. N., Holtorf, H. L., Jansen, J. A. and Mikos, A. G. 2003. Mineralized matrix deposition by marrow stromal osteoblasts in 3D perfusion culture increases with increasing fluid shear forces. *Proc. Nat. Acad. Sci. USA*, **100**(25), 14683–8.

[80] Bancroft, G. N., Sikavitsas, V. I., van den Dolder, J. *et al.* 2002. Fluid flow increases mineralized matrix deposition in 3D perfusion culture of marrow stromal osteoblasts in a dose-dependent manner. *Proc. Nat. Acad. Sci. USA*, **99**(20), 12600–5.

Index

Figures and tables are denoted in bold typeface